Tutorials in Clinical Chemistry

Tutorials in Clinical Chemistry

Ibrahim A. Hashim
University of Texas Southwestern Medical Center,
Dallas, TX, United States

ELSEVIER

Elsevier
Radarweg 29, PO Box 211, 1000 AE Amsterdam, Netherlands
The Boulevard, Langford Lane, Kidlington, Oxford OX5 1GB, United Kingdom
50 Hampshire Street, 5th Floor, Cambridge, MA 02139, United States

Notices
Knowledge and best practice in this field are constantly changing. As new research and experience broaden our understanding, changes in research methods, professional practices, or medical treatment may become necessary.

Practitioners and researchers must always rely on their own experience and knowledge in evaluating and using any information, methods, compounds, or experiments described herein. In using such information or methods they should be mindful of their own safety and the safety of others, including parties for whom they have a professional responsibility.

To the fullest extent of the law, neither the Publisher nor the authors, contributors, or editors, assume any liability for any injury and/or damage to persons or property as a matter of products liability, negligence or otherwise, or from any use or operation of any methods, products, instructions, or ideas contained in the material herein.

ISBN: 978-0-12-822949-1

For information on all Elsevier publications
visit our website at https://www.elsevier.com/books-and-journals

Publisher: Stacy Masucci
Acquisitions Editor: Patricia M. Osborn
Editorial Project Manager: Andrea R. Dulberger
Production Project Manager: Omer Mukthar
Cover Designer: Christian J. Bilbow

Typeset by STRAIVE, India

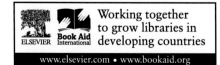

Working together
to grow libraries in
developing countries

www.elsevier.com • www.bookaid.org

Dedication

This book is dedicated to my late mother, Nemat,
and to my father, Abdelmoniem.
Without their sacrifice, endless support, and encouragement,
I would not have been able to pursue a rewarding career in
Clinical Biochemistry.

Ibrahim A. Hashim
Dallas, TX, United States

Contents

13. Biomarkers of malignancy

14. Therapeutic drugs and toxicology testing

Preface

Training in clinical chemistry (also known as clinical biochemistry, chemical pathology, or sometimes medical biochemistry) is acquired via different avenues that include didactic lectures on the pathophysiology of disease and on methodologies and practical aspects of testing, as well as through attendance of "sign-out" sessions, seminars, tutorials, and operational meetings.

This book provides tutorial sessions in all major topics in clinical chemistry with emphasis on practical applications to clinical practice.

The book is designed for those at or beyond postgraduate level. It is aimed at trainee clinical chemists, pathology residents, and medical students, and for those preparing for board and postgraduate examinations. The book is also helpful for those in practice, as well as serves as a teaching aid for teachers, instructors, mentors, and directors.

For ease of reference, laboratory values are presented in both conventional and SI units, when possible. Reference ranges are those used by the author's various laboratories and should only be used as a guide.

Ibrahim A. Hashim

Acknowledgments

My gratitude and thanks go to my wife Nahid and my children Huda, Yasir, Nada, and Hatim for their love, support, and encouragement and for putting up with my long work hours and frequent absence.

My deep affection and appreciation go to Huda for her outstanding graphic design and support for most of the figures in this book. Her talent is evident throughout.

I am grateful to my mentors, colleagues, and students for their support and encouragement and for the stimulating debates. I am indebted to my mentors and teachers—Drs. Michael Norman and Joan Butler (Kings College London); Professors Alan Shenkin and Bill Fraser (Royal Liverpool); and to Professors Erol Friedberg, Frank Wians, and James Malter—for providing me with the opportunity to fulfill my academic desire and facilitating my growth at such an esteemed academic institution as the University of Texas Southwestern Medical Center.

Abbreviations

ALK	alkaline phosphatase
CHF	congestive heart failure
CRH	corticotropin-releasing hormone
ED	emergency department
GH	growth hormone
GHRH	growth hormone-releasing hormone
GHRIH	growth hormone-release inhibiting hormone
Glu	glucose
GnRH	gonadotropin-releasing hormone
IP	inpatient
NTI	nonthyroidal illness
sCr	creatinine (serum)
STAT	*statim* immediate/urgent laboratory analysis request
TRH	thyrotropin-releasing hormone
uCr	creatinine (urine)

Reference intervals

Reference intervals used throughout this book are from the author's laboratories. Both conventional and SI units are reported for ease of reading. Conversion factors applied are shown below.

To convert conventional mass unit to SI units, multiply by:

Analyte	Units change	Multiplication factor
Acetaminophen	μg/mL to μmol/L	6.62
Bilirubin	mg/dL to μmol/L	17.1
Calcium	mg/dL to mmo/L	0.25
Carbamazepine	μg/mL to μmol/L	4.23
Cholesterol	mg/dL to mmo/L	0.0259
Cortisol	μg/dL to nmol/L	27.6
Creatinine	mg/dL to μmol/L	88.4
Digoxin	ng/ml to nmol/L	1.28
Ethanol (alcohol)	mg/dL to mmo/L	0.217
Gentamicin	μg/mL to μmol/L	2.09
Glucose	mg/dL to mmo/L	0.0555
Lactate	mg/dL to mmo/L	0.111
Magnesium	mg/dL to mmo/L	0.4114
Phenobarbital	μg/mL to μmol/L	4.31
Phenytoin	μg/mL to μmol/L	3.96
Phosphate	mg/dL to mmo/L	0.323
PTH (parathyroid hormone)	pg/mL to pmol/L	0.1061
Salicylate	μg/mL to mmol/L	0.00727
Testosterone	ng/ml to nmol/L	0.0347
Theophylline	μg/mL to μmol/L	5.55
Thyroxine, free (FT4)	ng/dL to pmol/L	12.9
Triiodothyronine, free (FT3)	pg/mL to pmol/L	0.0154
Valproate	μg/mL to μmol/L	6.93
Vancomycin	μg/mL to μmol/L	0.69

Chapter 1

Endocrine system disorders

Introduction

The clinical chemistry laboratory is central to the investigation and management of endocrine disorders. This chapter is divided into four sections and describes the thyroid, parathyroid, pituitary, and adrenal glands, as well as the gonads pathophysiology and their respective laboratory investigations. Of particular emphasis are hormones measurement and factors affecting their determination and interpretation.

The thyroid gland

Structure

The thyroid gland is located anteriorly in the neck attached to the trachea and the larynx. It weighs about 15–25 g in adults. It comprises right and left lateral lobes with each lobe being 4 cm in length, 2 cm in width, and 2–3 cm in thickness. The gland is highly vascular with blood supplied from two pairs of arteries and receives double the volume of blood reaching the kidney, at 5 mL per minute per gram of tissue. The cellular composition includes follicular cells (thyrocytes), parafollicular cells, and Kupffer cells (Fig. 1).

Embryologically, the thyroid is derived from the floor of the pharyngeal cavities and migrates to its final position in the neck. Defective embryological travel of thyroid tissue may be realized by an absent thyroid tissue, and that the tissue may be in different location anatomically, commonly as a lingual thyroid, with 70% of such patients exhibiting no thyroid tissue in the neck. This is relevant, as biochemical evidence for circulating parathyroid hormone (PTH) and for calcium homoeostasis are surrogate markers of a posteriorly imbedded parathyroid glands. PTH measurement is often sought for confirmation of a functional ectopic thyroid before removal of the glandular tissue mistaken for a cyst.

Function

The thyroid gland synthesizes and releases thyroid hormones as well as thyroglobulin. Thyroid hormones are essential for normal growth, development, and for general metabolism. They stimulate protein synthesis, lipids, and glucose metabolism, as well as bone turnover where for instance, increased bone resorption due to increased thyroid hormones leads to the hypercalcemia seen in hyperthyroidism.

Iodine is an essential constituent of thyroid hormones (three iodine moieties in triiodothyronine and four iodine moieties in thyroxin), and that iodine deficiency results in goiter, thyroid nodules, and hypothyroidism. Global fortification programs (salt iodination) although helped reduced the global incidence of goiter, iodine deficiency remains a problem probably due to limited salt intake or to consumption of processed food with high content of non-iodized salt.

Iodide deficiency is present in Africa and Asia as well as among pregnant women in developed countries and that differences in iodine status affect the prevalence of hypothyroidism where a shift from severe to mild iodine deficiency decreases the prevalence of hypothyroidism. Cretinism (impaired mental and physical development during both in utero and childhood) occurs in states of severe iodine deficiency and is secondary to the deficiency in thyroid hormones during fetal and early infancy development.

Thyroid hormones and metabolism

Iodine is absorbed in the stomach and small intestine and is transported bound to pendrin (an 85 kDa carrier protein for iodide and chloride) to the thyroid gland. Iodine is taken up to against a concentration gradient by the sodium-iodide transporter protein present in thyrocytes basal membrane. It is stored in the follicular cells and oxidized by thyroid peroxidase in the presence of hydrogen peroxide and iodinate tyrosine residues.

Thyroxine (T4) and triiodothyronine (T3) are formed following mono- (position 3) and di-iodination (positions 3 and 5) of tyrosine amino acids of the thyroglobulin protein. Iodination is catalyzed by thyroid peroxidase (TPO) in the presence of hydrogen peroxide, producing both mono- and diiodotyrosine residues respectively. This differential iodination gives rise to both T4 and T3 where combination of two diiodotyrosine produces thyroxine (T4), whereas a combination of a mono- and a diiodotyrosine produces triiodothyronine (T3) (Fig. 2). Thyroid hormones are then released into circulation following proteolysis of thyroglobulin.

Thyroxine (T4) is the major hormone produced within the thyroid tissue with a T4 to T3 ratio of about 10 to 1. Daily synthesis being about 80 μg (100 nmol) for T4 and 6 μg (8 nmol) for T3.

Tutorials in Clinical Chemistry. https://doi.org/10.1016/B978-0-12-822949-1.00011-5

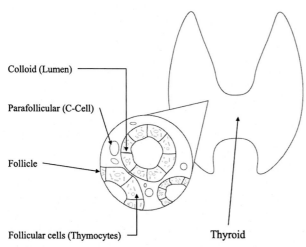

FIG. 1 Thyroid structure diagram illustrating the two lobes, follicular and parafollicular cells.

Thyroid hormones exert their actions within the nucleus (Fig. 2) and at the transcription action following binding of the biologically active T3 to its nuclear receptor. The nuclear receptors are encoded for by an α- and β-genes encoding alpha 1, and beta 1, 2, and 3. Several nuclear regulator proteins and transcription factors mediate the transcription activity. Mutations in the receptors (β form) lead to thyroid hormone resistance. Such mutations are also associated with thyroid cancer, pituitary tumors, growth and mental retardation, and metabolic abnormalities.

Additionally, thyroid hormone action is also via transmembrane binding, at the mitochondria, and in the cytoplasm. Such actions are termed nongenomic. At cell membrane, thyroid hormones activate ERK1/2 leading to sodium/hydrogen exchange, and T3 activates phosphatidylinositol 3-kinase and modulates the Na-K ATPase activity. Primarily, T3 acts on the mitochondria stimulating

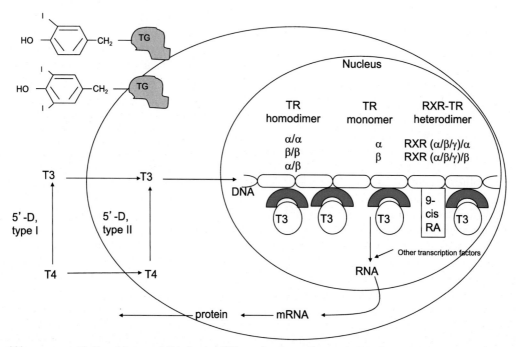

FIG. 2 Thyroid hormones metabolism: Mono- and di-iodination (5′D type I and type II respectively) of tyrosyl residues in thyroglobulin (TG) results in mono- and diiodotyrosine which are cleaved from the thyroglobulin molecule. A mono- and a diiodotyrosine combine to form T3, whereas two diiodotyrosine combines to form T4. Peripheral and cytoplasmic deiodinase isoenzymes I and II respectively convert T4 to T3 which binds to DNA nuclear thyroid hormone receptors leading to upregulation of metabolism. Daily production in normal thyroid tissue is about 86 μg and 6.6 μg of T4 and T3 respectively with a respective synthesis ratio of 13:1. *9-Cis RA*, 9-Cis retinoic acid binds to and activates RXR; *RXR*, retinoid X receptors (forms heterodimer with TR) and similar to the TRs play important role in transcription; *TR*, T3 receptor. *(Modified from several sources; Brent GA. Mechanisms of thyroid hormone action. J Clin Invest. 2012;122(9):3035–3043. https://doi.org/10.1172/JCI60047. Epub 2012 Sep 4. PMID: 22945636; PMCID: PMC3433956. Mondal S, Raja K, Schweizer U, Mugesh G. Chemistry and biology in the biosynthesis and action of thyroid hormones. Angew Chem Int Ed Engl. 2016;55(27):7606–7630. https://doi.org/10.1002/anie.201601116. Epub 2016 May 25. PMID: 27226395. Bassett JH, Harvey CB, Williams GR. Mechanisms of thyroid hormone receptor-specific nuclear and extra nuclear actions. Mol Cell Endocrinol. 2003;213(1):1–11. https://doi.org/10.1016/j.mce.2003.10.033. PMID: 15062569. Darras VM, Houbrechts AM, Van Herck SL. Intracellular thyroid hormone metabolism as a local regulator of nuclear thyroid hormone receptor-mediated impact on vertebrate development. Biochim Biophys Acta. 2015;1849(2):130–141. https://doi.org/10.1016/j.bbagrm.2014.05.004. Epub 2014 May 17. PMID: 24844179. Sinha R, Yen PM. Cellular action of thyroid hormone. In: Feingold KR, Anawalt B, Blackman MR, et al., eds. Endotext [Internet]. South Dartmouth, MA: MDText.com, Inc.; 2018:2000. PMID: 25905423.)*

proton leak which leads to heat production also secondary to increased cellular oxygen consumption. Thyroid hormones also act on the mitochondrial genome via imported isoforms of nuclear T3 receptors (TRs) to affect several mitochondrial transcription factors.

Synthesis and release of thyroid hormones by the thyroid gland are stimulated by thyrotropin-stimulating hormone (TSH) which is secreted by the anterior pituitary and is under feedback inhibition by circulating thyroid hormones. Furthermore, the synthesis and release of TSH are stimulated by hypothalamic thyrotropin-releasing hormone (TRH). TRH production is also under negative feedback control by thyroid hormones which modulate the release of TSH in response to TRH. Low thyroid hormone levels lead to increased TSH and TRH secretion (Fig. 3).

Released thyroid hormones are transported tightly bound to proteins. The main binding proteins are albumin, prealbumin, and thyroxine-binding globulin (TBG). Although 99.97% of T4 is protein bound, the relative proportional binding is varied being 60%–75% to TBG, 5%–30% to prealbumin, and 10% bound to albumin. Binding to albumin and prealbumin is with reduced affinity compared to that with TBG making bound thyroid hormones easily available to tissues constituting what is termed bioavailable forms.

As for T3, 99.7% is bound; however, T3 binding to TBG is 10-fold weaker than that for T4.

While there are relatively higher albumin and prealbumin levels compared to TBG, binding affinities are higher to TBG. This extensive protein binding dictates that only 0.05% T4 and 0.5% T3 are available as "free hormones" for entry into cells and that this free fraction correlates better than total hormone levels with clinical thyroid status.

Although, in molar terms free T4 is 50-fold more than free T3, differences in protein binding and in respective half-life, T4 and T3 being 5–7 days, and 1–2 days respectively, lead to overall relative circulating concentrations ratio of 3 to 1. Although 20% of circulating T3 is secreted by the thyroid tissue, the majority (>80%) is derived from mono-deiodination of T4 in peripheral tissues.

Deiodinase isoenzymes

Selenocysteine-containing deiodinase isoenzymes (DIO) are responsible for the synthesis of the different thyroid hormones. DIO1 and DIO2 convert T4 to the relatively much more active T3 and is inhibited in nonthyroidal illness. DIO3 and DIO1 convert T4 to the relatively inactive rT3 whereas they convert T3 to 3,3'-T2 (3,3'-diiodothyronine). It is the relative activity as well as tissue distribution of the different isoforms that imparts the specific pathway, independent of the hypothalamic pituitary regulation of thyroid hormones.

As stated above, conversion of T4 to T3 is catalyzed by iodotyrosine deiodinase isoforms types 1, 2, and 3. Isoform type 1 is predominant in the liver, kidney, thyroid, and pituitary, whereas isoform 2 is predominant in the thyroid, breast and central nervous system, whereas isoform 3 is predominant in brain and skin, fetal liver, and in the placenta during pregnancy. Considered an oncofetal protein, type 3 is overexpressed in hemangiomas leading to increase in rT3 production, and low T3 and T4 and to concomitant increase in TSH levels.

This peripheral tissue conversion is inhibited or switched to the biologically inactive isomer, 3, 3', 5' triiodothyronine (reverse T3 (rT3)) catalyzed by deiodinase isoforms 1 and 3, in patients with acute illness and in generalized nonthyroidal illness, as well as by certain iodine-containing pharmacological agents (Fig. 4).

Reverse triiodothyronine (rT3)

Whereas T3 is the most active thyroid hormone, rT3 is the third most abundant. It is produced following deiodination of the inner ring of T4 (Fig. 4) by the membrane-bound selenocysteine containing deiodinase enzyme. The inner deiodination results in rT3 which has several 100-fold lower affinity (association constant) for the nuclear thyroid

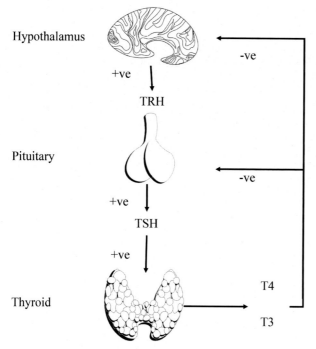

FIG. 3 Hypothalamic-pituitary-thyroid axis. Hypothalamic TRH stimulates pituitary TSH synthesis and release. TSH stimulates the thyroid gland synthesis of thyroid hormones. The production of TRH and TSH is under feedback inhibition by thyroid hormones. *(Modified from Stathatos N. Thyroid physiology. Med Clin North Am. 2012;96(2):165–173. https://doi.org/10.1016/j.mcna.2012.01.007. Epub 2012 Feb 1. PMID: 22443969.)*

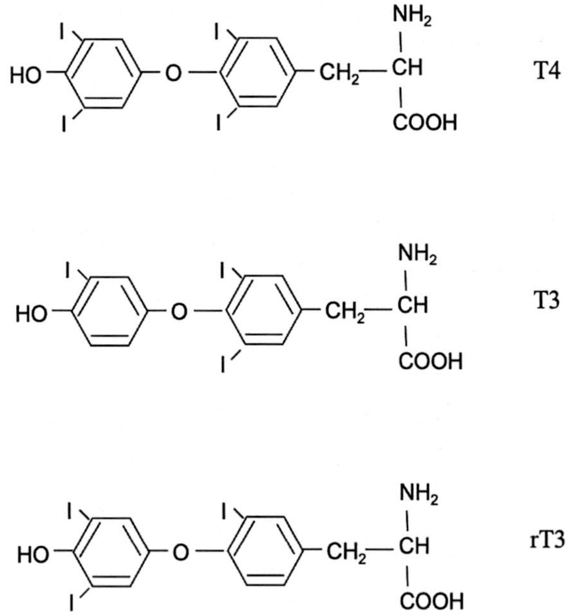

FIG. 4 Chemical structure of T4, T3, and rT3 showing respective positions of the iodide molecule. T3 and rT3 carry three iodide molecules, and T4 has four iodide molecules.

hormone receptors (TR-α and β) compared to T3. Therefore, it is likely to represent a conversion to the inactive thyroid hormones. However, it binds to the extra-nuclear thyroid hormone receptors (recently identified) and that the biological significance is unclear.

During acute nonthyroidal illness and starvation, physiological response includes increased conversion of T4 to rT3. Deiodinase enzyme is expressed in the placenta and is thought to protect the fetus from maternal T3. This causes higher circulating rT3 in the mother.

rT3 is >99% protein bound to TBG, transthyretin, and albumin with higher affinities than T3 but lower than T4. Relative binding of rT3 compared to that of T4 is 38% for TBG, 3.2% for prealbumin (transthyretin), and 50% to albumin compared to 9%, 1.4%, and 5% for T3 as compared to T4 percentage binding respectively.

Serum concentration of rT3 is about 17 ng/mL, tenth that of T3 concentration of about 140 ng/mL. In addition to immunoassays, it is measured using liquid chromatography mass spectrophotometry (LCMSMS) methods. The increase of rT3 in nonthyroidal illness is secondary to inhibition of deiodinase 1 reducing the conversion of T4 to T3 and deiodination of rT3. T4 is reduced by a separate mechanism of hypothalamic response to nonthyroidal illness (NTI) and starvation by reducing both circadian rhythm and concentration of TSH. This results in reduced T4 levels.

Amiodarone inhibits 5′deiodination of T4 (which normally leads to T3 production) resulting in high T4 and rT3 at the expense of the biologically active T3. Deiodinase 3 which converts T4 to rT3 is predominantly present in brain

and skin. rT3 is rapidly cleared by further deiodination by deiodinase 1 expressed in the liver and kidney to 3,3 T2.

Nonnuclear receptors recently identified include those in the nontranscriptional truncated forms of TR-α (p30 TR-α-1) and plasma membrane integrin-β-3. rT3 positively correlates with all-cause mortality most likely due to adverse effects of nonthyroidal illness. There is currently no evidence to support the routine measurement of rT3 in the management of thyroid replacement therapy. Although it remains controversial, however some advocate for rT3 measurement in optimizing thyroid hormone replacement therapy.

Thyroid hormones enter the tissue via a number of transport mechanism that are enzymes dependent and tissue specific. Mutations in receptor monocarboxylate transporter 8 (MCT8) gene lead to severe psychomotor retardation with elevated T3 levels.

In summary, thyroid hormones' mode of action is different from that of other hormones where they bind to DNA receptors stimulating transcription and protein synthesis. T3 is metabolically more potent than T4, considered to be prohormone, on a molar basis and is probably the physiologically active hormone. Mutations in the T4 and T3 binding to the DNA receptors have been reported and known to result in thyroid resistance syndromes. T3 binds to nuclear thyroid hormone receptors and that mutations in the receptor genes lead to decreased affinity for T3 binding expressed as T3 resistance syndrome.

Thyroid hormones binding proteins

The concentration of thyroid hormones binding proteins may change due to a variety of physiological, pathological, or pharmacological reasons. For instance, TBG rises during pregnancy where a new steady state is reached, so that free hormone concentrations remain relatively constant. Steroids increase TBG levels and thus measured total thyroid hormones. Increased proteins (TBG, albumin, and prealbumin) loss is seen in renal dysfunction and in protein losing enteropathies or to reduced synthesis in liver dysfunction. Additionally, albumin and prealbumin are negative phase reactants and their concentration decline during inflammatory conditions. Decreased levels are seen in protein energy malnutrition and in hypervolemic (volume overload) states.

TBG, a serine protease inhibitor produced by the liver. Approximately 27 different mutations have been identified contributing to the variable inherited TBG levels ranging from partial to complete deficiency. The most common is partial deficiency with a prevalence of 1:4000, and complete deficiency has an incidence of 1 in 15,000 in male newborns. Normal TBG levels range from 1.1 to 2.1 mg/dL and in complete TBG deficiency level are below 0.5 mg/dL.

Decreased TBG levels are seen in terminal illness, with possible role for interleukin-6 (IL-6), and due to increased rate of metabolism in hyperthyroidism. Androgens cause decrease in TBG levels, whereas estrogens elevation, as in pregnancy, cause elevation in TBG levels.

TBG deficiency although does not lead to adverse metabolic affects, due to presence of normal active free thyroid hormones; however, it can result in confusing thyroid testing results (low values) when measuring total thyroid hormones. These factors must be considered when interpreting thyroid function tests to avoid misinterpretation and inappropriate interventions.

Thyroid hormone resistance

Mutations in the T3 nuclear receptors TR-α and β have been described. In patient with the autosomal dominant mutations in the TR-β, the pituitary has a higher set point for thyroid hormone suppression of TSH and a biochemical finding of a relatively high TSH in the presence of high thyroid hormones. The biochemical findings are more subtle in TR-α mutations with borderline T4, a slightly high T3 and TSH. rT3 is low in this group compared with elevated levels in the TR-β mutations.

Thyroid function tests (TFTs)

Thyroid disorders are common with 3%–5% prevalence. Thyroid function testing strategy varies between laboratories and has been a subject of much debate. Most laboratories offer a first-line assessment using TSH alone and or via a reflex protocol where either total or free T4 is performed if TSH values were abnormal with follow up tests (e.g., T3) according to initial results and clinical symptoms.

Tests that examine the cause of thyroid dysfunction include thyroidal antibodies, in autoimmune thyroiditis, and thyroglobulin in patients with carcinoma of the thyroid.

Thyroid stimulating hormone (TSH)

There is linear-logarithmic relationship between TSH and thyroxine. A doubling of T4 results in 100-fold decrease in TSH. This relationship supports the use of TSH as primary test of thyroid function and in monitoring response to therapy. Although TSH levels are very sensitive to changes in thyroid hormones levels (due to the logarithmic-linear relationship) measuring TSH alone without T4 level risks missing secondary hypothyroidism where T4 will be low. Therefore, the finding of a low FT4 suggests either primary hypothyroidism where TSH is high or secondary hypothyroidism where TSH is inappropriately low.

TSH, a 26 kDa, consists of an alpha and beta subunit. The alpha subunit is common to LH and FSH, whereas the beta unit confers TSH biological specificity. It is produced by the anterior pituitary in response to hypothalamic TRH and stimulates T4 and T3 synthesis and release by the thyroid gland. Similar to TRH, TSH is under negative feedback inhibition by circulating T4 and T3 hormones (Fig. 3).

In most laboratories, TSH is measured by sensitive immunoassays (third or fourth generation) with lower limit of detection being 0.01 and 0.001 mIU/L respectively, therefore it can reliably distinguish between normal and suppressed TSH levels. Liquid chromatography-mass spectrometry (LCMSMS) methods are increasing being used for the measurement of TSH and of thyroid hormones.

In primary hyperthyroidism, TSH levels are usually <0.02 mIU/L, whereas in nonthyroidal illness, it is often between 0.1 and 0.01 mIL/L. TSH being the most reliable predictor of thyroid status in the majority of cases, as it examines the status of the feedback loop. TSH is raised in overt primary hypothyroidism and is useful as a predictor of incipient hypothyroidism in patients on long-term follow-up after treatment for thyrotoxicosis.

However, in secondary hypothyroidism, due to pituitary insufficiency, TSH levels may be normal or low. TSH may be low in euthyroid sick patients or those with multinodular goiter, ophthalmic Graves' disease or a single autonomous nodule. For these reasons, it is advisable to include thyroxine measurement in the first-line test repertoire.

Thyroid hormones (T4 and T3)

Thyroid hormones, namely T4 and T3, may be measured as either total form (free and protein bound forms) or as free hormone (FT4, FT3). Measuring free hormones is more challenging due to the relatively lower concentrations (ng/dL/pmol/L) compared to the total hormones (μg/dL/nmol/L) with various applications utilized described as one or two step assays, and either labeled hormone, labeled analog or labeled antibody methodologies (Fig. 5).

Requirement for the free hormone assays is that the assay conditions, such as incubation period, ionic strength, and pH, and that binding to the antibody does not affect the equilibrium between bound and free hormone.

The number of free hormones in equilibrium is a function of binding affinity and concentration of the binding protein. Therefore, if the binding protein affinity and or concentration decrease, the circulating-free hormones increase. Although albumin is more predominant, changes in TBG binding are more significant than those due to prealbumin and albumin.

In circulation, the total hormone level is influenced by the concentration of their binding proteins as well as respective affinities. There are also congenital abnormalities such as those for TBG as well the presence of hormone autoantibodies interfering with the measurement assay.

The total hormone assay reagents incorporate 8-anilino-i-naphthalene-sulphonic acid or salicylate to release hormones from their binding proteins.

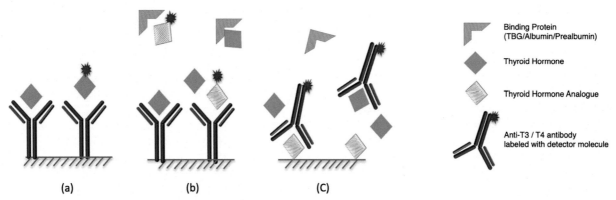

FIG. 5 Thyroid hormone assays configurations. (A) Solid phase antibody sequesters a small fraction of free hormone. After washing, labeled hormone is then added. Measure labeled hormone bound to solid phase. (B) Free hormone in serum competes with labeled hormone analog for solid phase antibody binding sites. Measure labeled analog. Hormone analog must bind antibody but not interact with binding proteins. (C) Free hormone in serum competes with solid phase analog hormone for binding labeled antibody. Coupling of analog hormone to solid phase further reduces interactions with binding proteins. In the labeled antibody format, labeled antibodies compete with sample free hormone with solid phase bound hormone. Coupling of the hormone to the solid phase reduces interaction with binding proteins (Fig. 5).

Measurement methodologies and their accuracy for free hormones have been debated. The assays for free hormone are either indirect assays which require two measurements, that of the total hormone and an uptake test, or use of direct assays. Less frequently performed, is to calculate free hormone index.

The direct assays include a two-step labeled hormone method where initial incubation with patient sample, followed by washing, then by addition of labeled analog, requires the use of high avidity antibodies and a short second incubation period. In the one-step direct method, with the advantage of shorter testing time, and in the labeled antigen format, sample in addition to a labeled analog are added together, there is no separation step in this assay format, and thus it is important that the labeled chemically modified analog does not bind to thyroid hormone binding proteins (Fig. 5).

Equilibrium dialysis methods

Considered to be the reference method where measurement is uninfluenced by changes in binding proteins. So much so that some manufactures will adjust the assay reagent protein content to ameliorate results to those obtained by equilibrium dialysis methods.

Physical separation of free from bound by equilibrium dialysis and ultra-filtration, often following an overnight incubation, followed by measuring the free hormones by a sensitive assay, more often by liquid chromatography-mass spectrometry (LCMSMS). The prolonged assay incubation time and need for a sensitive assay limits its routine availability and often the often few samples with discordant thyroid results are sent to a reference laboratory for analysis.

Total thyroxine (T4)

Minor interference is seen in rare instances when T4 autoantibodies are present. Measured total thyroxine level varies with concentration of binding proteins, low binding protein

concentrations causes a low total measurement; however, this is often obvious and unlikely to cause problems when interpreted in conjunction with TSH levels.

Free thyroxine

The measurement of free hormones may pose technical problems because binding of the free hormone in an immunoassay disturbs the equilibrium between circulating natural free and bound hormone. Ideally, a free T4 assay should be independent of binding protein concentrations and should give constant results after sample dilution (secondary to addition of assay reagents). This is usually not the case and free hormone assay must be interpreted with caution. However, it is very useful as a second-line test when alterations in TBG are suspected, or in borderline cases with normal binding proteins.

A low FT4 in the presence of high TSH confirms clinical suspicion for primary hypothyroidism, whereas the finding of low TSH suggests secondary hypothyroidism.

In patients treated for hyperthyroidism, circulating TSH levels will be suppressed for a while, and the FT4 measurement provides assessment of thyroid status.

Total triiodothyronine (T3)

Total T3 is measurement is most useful as a second-line test in suspected hyperthyroidism and in patients with T3 thyrotoxicosis (i.e., in the presence of normal FT4).

In patients with hypothyroidism, total and free T3 is often within normal levels and are thus unhelpful. Total T3 levels decline slightly throughout life.

Thyroglobulin

Circulating thyroglobulin levels roughly mirror the size of the thyroid gland (0.5–1.0 ng/mL thyroglobulin per gram of thyroid tissue).

Several immunoassays are available for the measurement of thyroglobulin; however, they are subject to interference by circulating antithyroglobulin antibodies. The prevalence of the antibodies being 10% in the general population and up to 25% in patients with differentiated thyroid cancer.

Due to the marked variability between assays, the same assay should be used for serial measurements of thyroglobulin. Furthermore, antithyroglobulin antibodies should always be measured. The presence of antithyroglobulin antibodies limits the measurement of thyroglobulin, and it is recommended that thyroglobulin is not reported in those cases.

Successful treatment is evident by thyroglobulin levels <0.2 ng/mL (using a highly sensitive assay with functional sensitivity of 0.1 ng/mL or less is required). The sensitivity for determining residual disease or early detection of recurrence is improved following stimulation using recombinant TSH. Stimulated thyroglobulin levels <0.5 to 1.0 ng/mL in the absence of interfering antithyroglobulin antibodies has a 98%–99.5% sensitivity for identifying cancer-free patients following therapeutic interventions.

Its measurement has been suggested to be helpful when assessing patient compliance in the setting of a high FT4 and high TSH levels.

Reference intervals

There are significant age, and slight gender and ethnicity-related reference intervals for TSH and for thyroid hormones. However, there continue to be a debate on the upper normal limit for TSH. Most clinical laboratories report 4.5 mIU/L defined by the National Health and Nutrition Examination Survey III data. Recalculation of the reference intervals using a subset who were nonpregnant, had undetectable thyroid autoantibodies, and not on medication likely to affect thyroid function, the upper limit was found to be 4.12 mIU/L. Some professional societies and investigators recommend the use of 2.5 mIU/L as the upper normal limit. It is certainly worthwhile considering the lower limit for young adults. The NHNES II showed lower upper limit at 3.24 mIU/L in African American between the ages of 30 and 39 years suggesting an impact of age and ethnicity on TSH reference intervals.

High TSH values are observed at birth (up to 40 mIU/L) and decline to normal adult values within a month following birth (Table 1). Use of age-related reference intervals in neonates is important to avoid unnecessary investigations and therapy interventions. TSH to FT4 ratio is high at term; up to 4.5, decreasing to 3.8 at 3 days, 2 at 10 weeks, 1.2 at 14 months and to 1 at greater than 14 years. TSH and free T4 reference intervals in use by the author's laboratory are shown in Table 1 below. The data is for full term neonates. Values for premature neonates may differ.

Furthermore, in pregnancy, maternal TSH levels change with gestational age as well as with number of fetuses.

TABLE 1 TSH and free T4 reference intervals in use by the author's laboratory.

Age	TSH (mIU/L)	FT4 (ng/dL)
0–24 h	4.1–40.2	1.17–3.4
24–48 h	3.2–29.6	1.13–4.1
0–72 h	2.6–17.3	1.27–3.5
0–4 days	2.2–14.7	1.37–3.0
97–120 h	1.8–14.2	1.07–2.5
5–6 days	1.4–12.7	1.0–2.5
6–7 days	1.0–8.3	1.07–2.4
3–30 days	0.65–6.5	0.8–1.8
>30 days	0.45–4.5	0.8–1.8

TSH values are significantly higher at birth and decline quickly. The data is for full term neonates. Values for premature neonates may differ.

Circulating TSH levels decline during the first trimester with nadir at 10 weeks of gestation, possibly due to increased hCGβ, and returning to baseline at 16–18 weeks. Additionally, gestational TSH levels are lower in twin pregnancy compared to singleton.

Limitations with free home assays

Interferences

Interference in measurement is either analyte specific (such as molecular heterogeneity, binding to proteins) and or assays specific such as presence of interfering antibodies. Thyroid testing is based on immunoassays. There are a number of pitfalls and interferences that can affect their performance and must be assessed.

Free thyroid hormones assays are subject to variability in binding proteins concentration and to their binding affinities.

Circulating thyroid hormones are displaced from binding proteins by drugs such as salicylate, heparin, and free fatty acids. Additionally, autoantibodies interfere with binding, free hormone equilibrium, and assay reaction. The assays are also subject to interference by heterophile antibodies and HAMA (see later and Chapter 17 on analytical methods). There is significant assay-to-assay variability with limitations in standardization between different manufacturers.

Binding proteins

Changes in thyroid hormones due to changes in binding proteins is often more that those due to actual thyroid function alterations. In otherwords, changes in the proteins are more common than those related to thyroid function. The principal binding proteins are thyroid binding globulin (TBG), albumin, and prealbumin to a small extent.

Abnormalities in thyroid binding globulin (TBG)

The majority of thyroid hormones is bound to TBG and thus changes in its circulating concentrations influence thyroid hormone measurements. The total thyroid (bound plus free) is most affected. Although there are congenital abnormalities in TBG production leading to deficiency or excess levels, physiological changes due to pregnancy are more common. Elevated estrogens increase TBG synthesis by about 2.5-fold and thus leads to falsely elevated (1.5-fold) total thyroid hormones levels. Free thyroid hormones levels are not elevated and depending on the assay format slight decline in levels may be observed.

Thyroxine binding globulin is measured directly by immunoassay and is a useful confirmatory test when congenital or pharmacological changes in TBG are suspected.

Abnormalities in albumin levels and in binding

Significant changes in circulating albumin concentration may cause assay bias and some manufacturers supplement their reagents formulations with albumin to reduced effect of serum binding in the one step assays. This ameliorates bias seen in patients with low circulating albumin levels. It is of note that possible differences in binding properties of albumin between reagent batches and lot numbers may be present. The addition of albumin to the reagents also ameliorates the often very high nonesterified fatty acids (often high in patients with hypoalbuminemia). It also limits positive bias in patients with nonthyroidal illness.

Familial dysalbuminemia

In patients with familial dysalbuminemia, structural changes in albumin and prealbumin due to genetic mutation cause increased binding affinity to thyroid hormones. Enhanced binding affinity causes bias in the free thyroid hormones causing falsely low levels. A condition termed familial dysalbuminemic hypothyroxinemia.

Similar to that observed for TBG, changes in albumin concentrations seen in late pregnancy (due to volume distribution) and those in pathological losses (nephrotic syndrome), vascular leakage and redistribution (sepsis), and those due to decreased synthesis (chronic liver disease). Measurement of total thyroid hormones are discrepant. Free homes levels are mildly affected as the degree of change is assay dependent. Impact of free hormone measurements becomes more apparent at extremes of alterations in levels of binding proteins. Measurement by equilibrium dialysis methods often resolves the discrepancy.

Limitation with TSH measurements

A common consultative query is as to why the TSH remains elevated despite claims of compliance with thyroxine replacement therapy. The assumption often being laboratory error, or the presence of interference in TSH measurement. There are a number of isolated reports of human antimouse antibodies (HAMA) and heterophile antibody interferences. In the authors experience, this is often a case of noncompliance with testing protocol where FT4 is often within the reference intervals having been taken recently, and the fact that TSH takes about 6–8 weeks to normalize. The presence of elevated thyroglobulin levels supports the suspicion for poor compliance with dietary limitations, or the intake of interfering drugs, or issues related to absorption.

Monitoring TSH as a marker for adequate replacement therapy cannot be used in patients with central hypothyroidism where in those patients, thyroxine (T4) measurements are used to assess both compliance and adequacy. TSH is measured 4–12 weeks following initiation of therapy, then every 6 months, and then annually once stable. In some patients, FT3 may be low despite normalized TSH and for that reason its measurement is unhelpful.

Human antianimal antibodies, e.g., HAMA antibodies interfere with TSH measurement by immunoassays and in FT4 assay by equilibrium dialysis. Biotin interferes with biotin-based immunoassays (mimicking hyperthyroidism with a falsely low TSH and falsely high FT4). Drugs that interfere with protein bindings such as heparin will displace T4 and lead to a false elevated FT4. Changes in binding proteins (albumin, TBG) seen in protein losing conditions, acute illness, and pregnancy affect measurement of thyroid hormones (free and total). Equilibrium dialysis and LCMSMS methodologies are less influenced by changes in protein concentrations.

Autoantibodies

Antibodies directed toward thyroid tissue, receptors and hormones, although play a role in the pathogenesis and have diagnostic utility as discussed, they cause interference in a number of thyroid function assays.

Antiperoxidase antibodies

Circulating polyclonal antibodies, also termed antimicrosomal antibodies, directed toward thyroid peroxidase enzyme required for the iodination and synthesis of thyroid hormones. The antibodies have both diagnostic and prognostic values, where they are elevated in most patients with autoimmune thyroiditis. It is also elevated in about 20% of patients with no biochemical abnormalities (TSH, thyroid hormones). Among those patients, 50% will develop overt hypothyroidism.

Anti-TSH receptor antibodies

Two distinct anti-TSH receptor antibodies are encountered leading to either hypothyroidism or to hyperthyroidism. The stimulating antibodies also known as thyroid stimulating immunoglobulin (TSI) elevated in Graves' disease.

The other antibodies type are competitive inhibitors of TSH binding. The antibodies cross the placenta and are responsible for the transient neonatal hypothyroidism seen in pregnancy and Graves' disease. Switching between the respective stimulatory and inhibitory functions of the TSI and TSH receptor blocking antibodies is seen in hypothyroid patients on thyroxine replacement and in hyperthyroid patients on antithyroid drugs. The antibody detection assays are complex and utilize thyroid tissue competing for binding with labeled TSH or indirectly by measuring cAMP levels stimulated by the action of the antibodies on the receptor.

Heparin effect

Heparin causes in vivo induction of lipoprotein lipase leading to increase in nonesterified fatty acids with resultant increase in FT4 and FT3 results as the fatty acids compete for free hormone protein binding. Similarly, in vitro, lipase in a time- and temperature-dependent manner will also cause an elevation in nonesterified free fatty acids and thus elevated free T3 and T4 levels.

Interfering antibodies

Two groups of antibodies may interfere with hormones measurements. They are heterophile antibodies and human antimouse antibodies (HAMA). The prevalence of the antibodies in circulation is unknown, but could as high as 20% in patient with autoimmune disorders and those with occupational exposure to animals such as animal house workers.

The antibodies interfere by participating in the assay antibody antigen reaction by either effecting binding between capture and detection antibody in the absence of the thyroid hormone antigen (Fig. 6). The interference is assay dependent with those employing mouse monoclonal antibodies being more susceptible. Furthermore, the interference can either be positive or negative in nature. The presence of HAMA antibodies can be measured directly or removed following sample pretreatment using proprietary material.

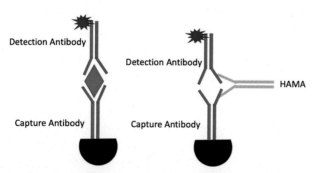

FIG. 6 Possible configurations for HAMA / heterophile antibodies interference. (*Modified from Heterophilic Blocking Reagent (HBR), Scan-Brief, 1 (1), Scantibodies Laboratory, Inc., Santee, CA, USA.*)

The antibodies are adsorbed following incubation with adsorbent material possibly containing mouse serum. Patient samples are reanalyzed for hormonal content following treatment with blocking and adsorption tubes.

Biotin interference

Circulating biotin following ingestion of high dosage either via over-the-counter vitamin supplements intake or via prescription therapy in patients with nutritional deficiency, those with inborn errors of metabolism, and in patients with multiple sclerosis.

Avidin-biotin binding characteristics are widely utilized in the development of immunoassays. Antibodies and antigens can be easily biotinylated. Detector reagents such as peroxidase enzymes (horseradish peroxidase, alkaline phosphatase), or separator molecules (such as magnetic beads) are linked to avidin. The strong avidin-biotin binding facilitates formation of required antibody antigen complex, their separation and development of the detection system following separation and washings. Additionally, several biotin molecules can be attached and thus improving assay sensitivity. The presence of high levels of biotin binds to assay avidin reagents and thus interfere in the assay's reaction. Depending on the assay formulation, this can cause falsely elevated levels (such as in competitive FT4 assays) and falsely low sandwich assays (as in TSH). Therefore, in patients with high levels of biotin levels, a biochemical finding of falsely low TSH and falsely high FT4 is suggestive of false impression of hyperthyroidism.

Drugs interreference

Medication interfere with thyroid hormone metabolism in three ways, interference with absorption of exogenous (therapeutic T4) by calcium, iron supplements, interference with synthesis and secretion such as by lithium and amiodarone, and tyrosine kinase inhibitors, and at the hypothalamic-pituitary-thyroid axis by dopamine, bexarotene, octreotide, and ipilimumab, or due to increased clearance (enhanced metabolism) by phenytoin, carbamazepine, and interference with peripheral conversion and metabolism by glucocorticoids and beta blockers such as propranolol inhibits conversion of T4 to T3 and decreases clearance of rT3. Amiodarone inhibits the mono-deiodination of (5'-deiodinase activity) of T4 that is reduced conversion of T4 to T3.

Antigen-excess "hook-effect"

Some manufacturers add excess antibodies to improve assays sensitivity (favored in some situations) for example improved sensitivities in third and fourth generational TSH assays. The addition of excess antibodies helps overcome the presence of large concentration of the analyte e.g., TSH and tumor markers thyroglobulin and calcitonin where

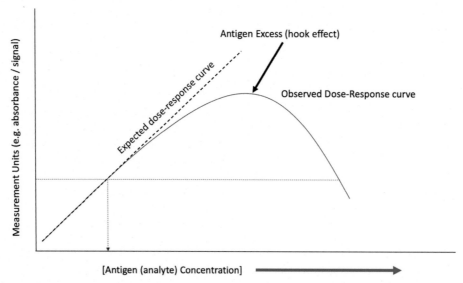

FIG. 7 Expected dose-response curve (-----). However, the observed dose-response curve (___) initially increases as expected before reaching a plateau and a decline due to antigen excess (hook-effect). In situations with antigen excess, antibodies of the assay (sandwich or complimentary) each occupied by an antigen molecule, due to the antigen excess, and a sandwich complex is not formed. Washing, nonreacting components washes away antigen-antibody complex and thus exhibits a drop in the signal (or absorbance measurement units) giving a falsely low result.

elevated levels may exceed the antibody sandwich binding capacity and results in falsely low values, a phenomenon termed antigen excess (hook effect) (Fig. 7).

Thyroid disorders

Thyroid gland disorders are common, affecting about 20 per 1000 of the population with prevalence in females 5–6 times that in males. Thyroid autoimmune disorders being the most common leading to either hypothyroidism (Hashimoto's thyroiditis) or to hyperthyroidism (Graves' disease). Although geographical differences in incidence of autoimmune thyroid disorders exist, the increased risk for females than males is uniform.

The prevalence of hypothyroidism among women ranges from 19 to 27 per thousand females and 1.6 to 2.3 thousand males. The prevalence of overt hypothyroidism is 14–19 per 1000 females and compares with less than 1 per 1000 males.[1]

Thyroid disorders are characterized by the presence of various autoantibodies to thyroid peroxidase, to thyroglobulin, and to TSH receptor. In patients with Hashimoto's thyroiditis, patients will have antibodies to peroxidase and to thyroglobulin leading to thyroid tissue destruction and fibrosis.

Circulating antiperoxidase antibodies (TPO), antithyroglobulin antibodies, anti-TSH receptor antibodies (either blocking TSH receptor or stimulating thyroid antibodies (TSI)) are diagnostic and are often present. There is however no correlation between anti-TPO titer and disease activity. Less than 15% of patients with Hashimoto's will exhibit negative antibody findings. In patients with

Graves' disease anti-TSH receptor antibodies are stimulating in nature, although a smaller percentage of blocking are present with the relative proportion suggestive of disease severity. A number of autoantibodies influence thyroid function assessment, for instance, antibodies directed against TSH receptors results in prolonged TSH suppression (Table 2).

Loss of immune tolerance to thyroid antigens leads to autoantibodies formation. Thyroid peroxidase (TPO), thyroglobulin (Tg), and TSH receptor are target antigens in autoimmune thyroid disorders. Antigen presenting cells such as microphages, dendritic cells accumulate within the thyroid gland and present antigens to B and T lymphocytes. T-helper (CD4+) and cytotoxic CD8+ T-cell destroying thyroid parenchyma and exposing the antigens followed by antibodies production by B-lymphocytes.

A number of drugs affect TSH and thyroid hormones synthesis and release. For instance, cardiac drugs, such as amiodarone inhibits peripheral T4 to T3 conversion, with a biochemical pattern of elevated T4, reduced T3 and elevated TSH since T3 is the biologically active hormone. Some drugs interfere with TSH assays.

Thyroid function tests being the most commonly requested endocrine laboratory investigation, although there is no clear evidence supporting screening for thyroid disorders, its measurement during annual physical examination and during presentations at general practice suggest that screening is already taking place. Clinical presentation is varied and this often triggers thyroid function testing, for example, in patients with dyslipidemia, infertility, fatigue, tiredness, myopathy, cold and heat intolerance, among other common symptoms.

TABLE 2 Autoantibodies involved in the etiology of thyroid dysfunction and their diagnostic utility.

Antibodies	Hypothyroidism	Hyperthyroidism	Comment
Anti-TPO	>80% in Graves' disease and Hashimoto's thyroiditis		Antigen: Intracellular thyroid peroxidase enzymes. Present in 2%–5% subclinical and euthyroid women following thyrocytes destruction. Crosses placental barrier
Anti-TSHR		90% in Graves' disease 10% in Hashimoto's thyroiditis	Antigen: Extracellular Crosses placental barrier Fetal risk for neonatal hyperthyroidism Stimulating antibodies more common than receptor blocking
Anti-TG	>50% in Hashimoto's thyroiditis	>50% in Graves' disease	Antigen: Intrafollicular Thyroglobulin assay interference

TG, thyroglobulin; *TPO*, thyroid peroxidase (previously known as thyroid microsomal antibodies); *TSHR*, thyroid stimulating hormone receptor. *(Modified from Fröhlich E, Wahl R. Thyroid autoimmunity: role of anti-thyroid antibodies in thyroid and extra-thyroidal diseases. Front Immunol. 2017;8:521. https://doi.org/10.3389/fimmu.2017.00521. PMID: 28536577; PMCID: PMC5422478.)*

Thyroid disease, related to under or over production of thyroid hormones, may be insidious in onset and present with a wide variety of symptoms. Thyroid swelling or goiter may be present. There is often a strong family history of thyroid disease. Carcinoma of the thyroid is rare representing <1% of human malignancies.

Hyperthyroidism

The incidence of hyperthyroidism is 0.5–1.4/1000/year in women with 6:1 ratio compared to men.

Clinical features of excessive secretion of thyroid hormones may include tiredness, weight loss, heat intolerance, sweating, tremor, palpitations, and diarrhea. There is marked individual variation in the dominant symptoms.

The commonest cause is Graves' disease, an autoimmune disorder of unknown etiology (thyroid stimulation IgG antibodies against the TSH receptor of the thyroid follicular cell are present), other causes of hyperthyroidism include toxic multinodular goiter, solitary toxic nodule and excess administration of thyroid hormones. Graves' disease patients may have diffuse thyroid enlargement with bruit, ophthalmopathy or pretibial myxedema. Untreated Graves' disease has a natural history of remission and relapse. Treatment of hyperthyroidism varies according to the age of the patient and severity of the disease. Treatment modalities include: antithyroid or β blocking drugs, subtotal thyroidectomy, or radiotherapy using ^{131}I. Almost all cases of hypothyroidism have suppressed TSH level. Total T4 is usually elevated but may be normal in the early stages of the disease, with elevated total T3 in T3 thyrotoxicosis,

Long-term follow-up after treatment is essential. Patients may relapse, particularly after drug treatment, and up to 45% may become hypothyroid following ^{131}I therapy or surgery.

Thyroid failure occurs within 6 months of destructive therapy but is usually transient.

Biochemical follow-up includes measurement of TSH and thyroid hormones as measurement of TSH alone may be misleading due to prolonged suppression.

Determining the ratio of FT4 to FT3 is helpful in determining the cause of thyrotoxicosis. Total T3 to total T4 less than 20 is indicative of Graves' disease (autoimmune destructive disease) rather than subacute thyroiditis induced thyrotoxicosis. However, total hormone measurement is limited by changes in protein binding levels as discussed earlier. Free T3 to Free T4 ratio more than 4.4 (10^{-2} pg/ng) is indicative of Graves' disease.

T3 thyrotoxicosis

Hyperthyroidism due to T3 thyrotoxicosis is characterized by suppressed TSH levels <0.01 mIU/L and FT4 levels within the normal range. Causes of T3 thyrotoxicosis are iodine deficiency or during the early stages of thyrotoxicosis caused by an autonomous thyroid nodule, multinodular goiter, or Graves' disease. The prevalence of T3 thyrotoxicosis is 1%–5%, with some populations being as high as 16%.

Toxic multinodular goiter

Toxic multinodular goiter is the most common thyroid disease worldwide with more than 300 million cases. It is secondary to abnormal thyroid follicular cell growth due to continued hyperstimulation by TSH. Hyperplasia progressing to nodular degeneration of the thyroid tissues. The incidence of toxic multinodular goiter correlates with iodine intake being higher in geographical areas low in iodine.

Diffused (nonnodular) goiter in Graves' disease (autoimmune) thyroiditis is the most common cause of hyperthyroidism in pregnancy. However, toxic multinodular goiter is also a common cause.

Thyroid storm

Thyrotoxicosis crisis is also known as thyroid storm. Although relatively rare, mortality remains high approaching 10%–20% and represents the end stage of a severe thyrotoxicosis accompanied by compromised organ function.

Autoimmune Graves' disease is the most common form of thyrotoxicosis associated with circulating TSH receptor stimulating antibodies. The pathophysiology of thyroid storm is not fully understood; however, it is related to ensued hypermetabolic state and consequent increase in oxygen consumption as well as to increase in sympathetic nervous system activity. Exposure of increased numbers of beta-1 adrenergic receptors to the stress induced high catecholamine levels may contribute to the storm. The transition to thyroid storm usually is associated with existing comorbidities such as infection, myocardial infarction, diabetic ketoacidosis, pregnancy, surgery, and trauma.

Although rapid laboratory assessment of thyroid status by measuring TSH and thyroid hormones is helpful, waiting for the results in cases with high clinical suspicion may cause critical delay in the initiation of effective life-saving therapies.[2]

TSH adenomas

TSH secreting adenoma (TSH-omas) are very infrequent and account for about 0.5%–2% of all pituitary adenomas. The prevalence in the population being about 1–2 in a million. The majority (75%) of patients will have symptoms of hyperthyroidism in the setting of elevated TSH and the presence of a pituitary mass. The mass may lead to visual field defects in about 25% of cases. However, this is less common due to early detection because of the frequent routine measurement of thyroid function tests (TSH and free T4). TSH levels are detectable and often range from 3.2 to 7.4 mIU/L in the presence of high free thyroxin ranging from 26.2 to 56.8 pmol/L (2.0 to 4.4 ng/dL).

The above biochemical profile is similar to that encountered in the syndromes of thyroid hormone resistance. Thus, correct diagnosis is essential for appropriate treatment as well as to prevention of neurological and endocrinological complications associated with TSH-omas.

TSH-omas are part of the multiple endocrine neoplasia type I syndrome (MEN-1). Although 70% will secrete only TSH, the remaining 30% often secrete other pituitary hormones in addition to TSH. Most commonly GH and prolactin and patients may exhibit clinical symptoms of acromegaly and or amenorrhea.

For the biochemical findings described above, exclusion of methodological interference is often considered.

Presence of anti-T4 and anti-T3 antibodies, abnormal albumin and prealbumin as in familial dysalbuminemic hyperthyroxinemia (see below) may lead to false FT4 and FT3 results. Use of direct free hormone assays and equilibrium dialysis method will rule out such interference as a cause of the elevated free thyroid hormones. Falsely elevated TSH may be due the presence of interfering heterophile antibodies. Those are screened for using human antimouse antibodies (HAMA) detection assays or by treating patient sample with blocking material prior to repeat analysis.

Patients with TSH-oma have high circulating alpha subunit and thus a high alpha subunit to TSH ratio is seen in contrast to patients with resistant thyroid syndrome, where the ratio is normal or low.

The use of the dynamic T3 suppression test has been used in the diagnosis of TSH-oma. T3 supplement (80–100 µg/day is taken for 8–10 days), where lack of TSH suppression supports the diagnosis of TSH-oma. The test is contraindicated in the elderly and those with coronary heart disease. Another dynamic test, TRH stimulation (200 µg given intravenously) does not result in increase in either TSH nor in alpha subunit levels in 85% of TSH-oma cases.

Hypothyroidism

The incidence of hypothyroidism is 2.8–5.0/1000/year in women and much lower in men 0.3–1.2/1000. About 5% remain undiagnosed, at least in Europe. The incidence is higher in patients with autoimmune disorders (e.g., diabetes). The probability of hypothyroidism increases with age in contrast to no age relationship for hyperthyroidism. Biochemically, it is characterized by high TSH and low thyroid hormones levels.

Chronic autoimmune thyroiditis (Hashimoto's) is the most common cause of hypothyroidism in iodine-sufficient regions. Thyroid peroxidase and antithyroglobulin antibodies are present in most cases and confirm the diagnosis. Thyroid peroxidase antibodies are elevated in 11% of the general population; however, the presence of the antibodies predicts progression to overt hypothyroidism in patients with biochemical subclinical hypothyroidism. Genetic and environmental associations with hypothyroidism include vitamin D and selenium deficiency as well as genetic variants for thyroid peroxidase antibodies showing association with higher TSH concentration and overt hypothyroidism.

Fourteen percent of patients treated with amiodarone (iodine-containing drugs restricting thyroid hormone production) develop hypothyroidism due to iodine overload blocking thyroid hormone synthesis (Wolff-Chaikoff effect). Similarly, lithium interferes with thyroid hormone synthesis and release where 8% of patients on lithium therapy required T4 replacement 18 months later. Hypothyroidism is also observed in patients on tyrosine kinase inhibitors (more in those on sunitinib compared with sorafenib). Hypothyroidism is common (80%) after radiotherapy for the hyperthyroid and require replacement therapy.

Clinical features are varied and include a spectrum of no symptoms to tiredness, weight gain, cold intolerance, bradycardia, dry skin and hair and hoarseness. In children, the dominant features are reduction in growth velocity and arrest of pubertal development. The definition of hypothyroidism is based on biochemical markers, and this remains a matter of debate where some patients on T4 replacement with biochemical markers within the reference intervals remain symptomatic. Subclinical hypothyroidism (biochemical abnormalities), thyroid hormones within reference intervals and a TSH slightly outside the reference intervals, improve clinically when given thyroxine.

Hypothyroidism may be primary due to destruction of the thyroid tissue (autoimmune), or secondary due to central deficiency in pituitary TSH or tertiary deficiency in hypothalamic TRH. Peripheral hypothyroidism (<1%) is rare and is due to consumptive hypothyroidism or reduced sensitivity to thyroid hormones.

The commonest causes of hypothyroidism are failure of the gland due to autoimmune atrophy (TSH receptor blocking antibodies), Hashimoto's thyroiditis, postradio iodine or surgical treatment of hyperthyroidism, and drugs (e.g., lithium).

Secondary hypothyroidism due to a pituitary insufficiency is less common and hypothalamic hypothyroidism is rare.

A raised TSH with low thyroxine is indicative of primary hypothyroidism. Total T3 is a poor indicator of thyroidal production and is not useful in the diagnosis of hypothyroidism.

Treatment is by oral administration of T4, and ideally, the dose given should maintain TSH within the reference range. Total T4 levels are typically high normal or moderately raised (100–190 nmol/L, 7.8–14.7 µg/dL) when the patient is clinically euthyroid.

Individual set point for each patient is narrower than the interindividual variability. Therefore, the adequacy of T4 replacement as determined by TSH seems to be specific to the individual rather than the general statistical reference intervals. This is supported by the findings of persistent symptoms in 5%–10% of patients with biochemical evidence of adequacy.

Few patients with rare polymorphism (Thr92Ala) in the DIO2 gene coding for the deiodinase 2 enzyme converting T4 to T3 are thought to benefit from combination of T3 and T4 replacement therapy.

Congenital hypothyroidism

Congenital hypothyroidism can be due to dysfunction of the hypothalamic pituitary thyroid axis at birth, or to abnormal development of either the thyroid, the pituitary, or the hypothalamus, or to impaired thyroid hormones action. The incidence of congenital hypothyroidism ranges from 1 in 16,000 to 1 in 20,000. It can either be transient or persistent and increasing among patients with eutopic (normally located) thyroid gland, whereas those with thyroid dysgenesis did not significantly change. About a third (28%–38%) of eutopic thyroid patients have transient congenital form, and about half (38%–51%) had persistent hypothyroidism.

The observed increase in incidence over time was attributed in part to changes in TSH cut off values (from 20–25 mIU/L to 6–10 mIU/L) leading to doubling in the incidence. Other reasons include increasing survival of preterm infants and shifting in demographics with the largest increase in those mildly affected. Most importantly, the active newborn screening has significantly reduced incidence of mental retardation secondary to congenital hypothyroidism.

It is thus relevant that clinical laboratories report TSH values accompanied with appropriate neonatal reference intervals.

Congenital dysfunction is associated with either mutations in thyroperoxidases, dual oxidase system (generates hydrogen peroxide required in iodine incorporation), and in the anoctamin-1 iodine transporter.

Mutations in the thyroperoxidase (DUOX2 and DUOX2A) result a spectrum from congenital hypothyroid to euthyroid goiter in adults. The mutations in DUOX2 occurs in 65% of permanent cases and 35% in transient cases.

Neonatal screening by measuring TSH and in some programs also total T4 for detection of congenital hypothyroidism takes place at birth and at 10–14 days of age for low weight, premature, and sick neonates. An abnormal neonatal screen should be followed by measuring neonatal serum TSH and FT4.

Nonthyroidal illness

Patients with acute or chronic illnesses may have abnormal thyroid function tests due to a variety of factors, e.g., reduced peripheral conversion of T4 to T3, changes in binding protein concentrations, and alterations in hypothalamic-pituitary-thyroid axis. Typically, total T3 is usually decreased, total T4 and free T4 may be decreased and that TSH is often normal or slightly decreased. Unless there are clear clinical signs to suggest a thyroid disorder, thyroid function tests are best delayed until other illness is resolved.

This biochemical picture is encountered in patient in critical care setting (intensive care units). It occurs during the initial acute phase illness, which is thought to have a beneficial effect of directing metabolism to the acute response, however, in long-term illness, suppression of TRH synthesis and release results in reduced TSH synthesis and thus low thyroid hormones. Infusion of TRH induces TSH and thyroid hormones synthesis and a beneficial anabolic metabolic state.

Mild hypothyroidism/mild hyperthyroidism

The term subclinical hypothyroidism or subclinical hyperthyroidism are terms often used when the thyroid hormones are within the normal range, but the TSH is either above the normal range >4.5 mIU/L or below the normal range ≤0.4 mIU/L receptively.

Subclinical hypothyroidism

In subclinical hypothyroidism, when the patients were put on thyroxine replacement therapy, they felt much better.

Patients with subclinical hypothyroidism are at increased risk for cardiovascular disease, hypertension, and dyslipidemia.

In addition to feeling better, when placed on thyroxin replacement it reduces risk for cardiovascular disease (risk based on age and extent of TSH elevation).

Subclinical hyperthyroidism

In subclinical hyperthyroidism, patients are classified as mild when TSH is between 0.4 and 0.1 mIU/L, where 65%–75% of patients and severe when TSH is below 0.1 mIU/L.

Progression to overt hyperthyroidism is likely when TSH is <0.1 mIU/L. Patients with severe subclinical hyperthyroidism are at risk of atrial fibrillation, heart failure, coronary heart disease, osteoporosis, bone fracture, and dementia.

Thyroid resistance syndrome

Mutations in the T3 nuclear receptors TR-α and β have been described. In patient with the autosomal dominant mutations in the TR-β, the pituitary will have a higher set point for thyroid hormone suppression of TSH and a biochemical finding of a relatively high TSH in the presence of high thyroid hormones. The biochemical findings are more subtle in TR-α mutations with borderline T4, slightly high T3 and TSH. rT3 is low in this group compared with elevated levels in the TR-β mutations.

This is the most common form of syndromes of resistance to thyroid hormones. It exhibits an autosomal dominant mode of inheritance. The prevalence is variable from1 in 19,000 to 1: 40,000 in two different neonatal screening studies that employed both TSH and free T4.

Several mutations located in the functional areas of the T3 binding domain and adjacent hinge region. This results in reduced T3 binding to tissues. A new variant of thyroid hormone resistance of the alpha (α) subunit has recently been described (RTH-α). Biochemically, the syndrome is characterized by elevated thyroid hormones levels (FT4 and FT3), principally T4 in the presence of normal or slightly elevated TSH.[3]

The elevated TSH is a reflection of the impaired sensitivity of the hypothalamic-pituitary access to thyroid hormones. Clinically, the patient is able to maintain or to attain euthyroid status because of the compensation.

In the beta form, the phenotypic presentation depends on the degree of destruction and distribution of thyroid homoreceptors where there is variable coexistence of hypothyroid or thyrotoxic manifestations. However, in the alpha receptor mutations, the phenotype is that of hypothyroidism with normal TSH and a borderline low FT4.

Organs influenced by thyroid function

Certain organs and their functions are affected by thyroid hormones. Acting on the liver, thyroid hormones stimulate proteins synthesis and lipid metabolism where a fall in cholesterol levels reflects degradation exceeding synthesis. Increased muscle metabolism evident by increased creatine kinase and increased bone resorption in excess of mineralization evident by increased alkaline phosphate and osteocalcin levels, and on the gonadal hormones activity secondary to changes in sex-hormone binding globulin (SHBG) levels.

Thyroid malignancy

The incidence of thyroid cancer has been increasing from 5 in 100,000 in the 1990 to 15 in 100,000 in 2017, at a faster rate than any other cancer, and this has been attributed to overdiagnosis. Low-risk tumors are incidentally detected from a large subclinical reservoir of disease. The American Thyroid Association guidelines issued in 2015 recommended a risk basis approach to histological fine needle aspiration biopsies where nodules <1 cm in size should in general not be biopsied. Differentiated thyroid cancer is the most common type.

Thyroglobulin

Thyroglobulin (TG) a 66 kDa protein containing many tyrosyl residues synthesized by thyroid follicular cell. Carbohydrates and iodine constitute 8%–10% of its molecular weight. It is stored within the colloid of the follicular lumen and is released under the control of TSH. Circulating levels reflects thyroid tissue mass. $T_{1/2}$ 65 h. Posttotal thyroidectomy TG levels takes about a month to clear form the body. Incidence of antibodies is double that of the general population. Higher in women but gender-related reference ranges are not necessary. The values are geographically sensitive (that is influenced by iodide status). Assays interference by antithyroglobulin antibodies is common. Twenty percent of patients have antithyroglobulin antibodies.

Thyroglobulin measurement is helpful in the management of patient with differentiated thyroid carcinoma (DTC). Its levels decline posttreatment, and knowing the decay time is helpful in determining the persistence detection (remnant tissue or metastases).

Thyroglobulin assays

Thyroglobulin immunoassays are amenable to significant interference from circulating antithyroglobulin antibodies. Earlier first-generation thyroglobulin assays suffered from poor sensitivity, imprecision, and wide bias between methods.

Competitive assays measure free and antibody bound thyroglobulin, whereas immunometric assays measure free thyroglobulin (nonantibody bound). There is discordance between competitive and immunometric assays mostly secondary to the presence of antibody interference.

It is widely preferred not to report negative values (undetectable levels) for thyroglobulin in samples with positive antibodies in patients who have documented disease. Twenty percent of patients will exhibit circulating antithyroglobulin antibodies. Alternatively, serial measurements of the antibodies titers (levels) are useful and have prognostic value. The antibody levels decline following successful surgical resection of the tumor and that cured patient will become negative. Patients with detectable antibodies suggests recurrence of the disease.

There are two types of thyroglobulin assays (Class 1 and 2). In class 1 assays, normal individuals have no detectable antibodies. Whereas class 2 assays report a normal antibody range. Although both assays are standardized against the same MRC reference preparation, reportable values are different between the two assays and thus cannot be used interchangeably.

Recently, liquid chromatography mass spectrophotometry based assays for thyroglobulin are becoming available. They are free from antibody interference.

Thyroglobulin decay following surgical and/or radioactive treatment of differentiated thyroid carcinoma (DTC) is helpful in predicting recurrence early.

Calcitonin

Produced by the neuroendocrine parafollicular "C" cells of the thyroid gland and its function remains to be elucidated. A low-molecular-weight 32 amino acid peptide following cleavage from procalcitonin. It is metabolized by the kidney with circulatory half-life of 5 min. It is secreted in response to hypercalcemia where it has a calcium reducing action by inhibiting osteoclastic bone activity, and thus reduces bone resorption. It also inhibits kidney reabsorption of calcium and phosphate by the kidney. Secretion of calcitonin is also stimulated by gastrin, secretin, glucagon, and cholecystokinin.

The performance of several immunoassays has improved overtime with increased sensitivity and lack of interference from procalcitonin. The latter elevated in patients with sepsis and inflammation. The majority of normal individuals (56%–88%) will exhibit low calcitonin levels (below the functional sensitivity of the assay) with about 10% having levels >10 pg/mL. Due to the larger mass of the C-cells in men, they exhibit higher calcitonin levels compared to females.

Similar to thyroglobulin, lack of standardization among available immunoassays dictates that serial measurements be performed by the same assay or that a new baseline established if the assay platforms to change.

Calcitonin excess as in medullary carcinoma of the thyroid and deficiency as in postsurgical resection does not lead to bone demineralization, nor to hypercalcemia. Thus, its measurement has no value in investigation of calcium homeostasis per se, however, its measurement in patients suspected of medullary thyroid carcinoma, similarly postresection of medullary thyroid carcinoma is helpful. Basal levels correlate with medullary carcinoma tumor burden. The test sensitivity can be enhanced following intravenous administration of calcium when detecting possible residual MTC tissue (3–6 months postsurgical intervention). Levels below detection limit of the assay correlates with improved survival and a 5% recurrence rate. Levels are monitored every 6 months for the first year and then annually afterward to detect recurrence.

Undetectable calcitonin levels indicate successful resection, whereas increasing calcitonin levels indicates recurrence. Additionally, calcitonin level below 150 pg/mL is suggested to indicate localized tumor and distant metastasis for levels greater than 150 pg/mL and often greater than 1000 pg/mL.

Calcitonin is small molecule cleared by the kidney and thus renal impairment leads to falsely elevated levels. High levels are seen in patients with autoimmune thyroiditis, hyperparathyroidism, malignancy of the prostate, gastrointestinal, and neuroendocrine tumors as well as in patients with large-cell lung cancers.

Possible surrogate biomarker is carcinoembryonic antigen (CEA) produced by medullary thyroid carcinoma. Combined elevation of calcitonin and CEA suggestive of disease progression. Increasing CEA in the presence of stable or decreasing calcitonin levels suggest poorly differentiated medullary carcinoma of the thyroid.

Serial measurement every 6 months and a doubling of the levels in less than 6 months correlates with 5 and 10 years survival rates of 23% and 15% respectively.[4] If doubling time is >24 months the 5 and 10 years survival rates are high at 100%.

The molecular exhibits molecular heterogeneity which may be reflected by the different response in different immunoassays. Therefore, serial measurements using different assays are best to be avoided. This is further emphasized by the assay-dependent reported levels among normal subjects ranging from nondetectable to above 10 pg/mL. Higher levels are seen among normal men compared to women a reflection of gland size.

TRH test

Measurement of TSH following intravenous administration of TRH (200 µg) allows assessment of the hypothalamic-pituitary-thyroid axis particularly in secondary hypothyroidism; however, its use is in decline due to the improved sensitivity of TSH assays and is mainly restricted to diagnosis of thyroid hormones resistance and suspected TSH secreting pituitary adenoma investigations. A normal response (baseline <4 mIU/L and an increase in TSH >2 mIU/L at

20 min following TRH administration) indicates a euthyroid state. An absent or impaired response is seen in primary hyperthyroidism or secondary hypothyroidism.[5]

Parathyroid glands disorders

Normally, there are two pairs of oval shaped glands localized behind the thyroid gland. Each weighing 30–60 mg with 0.3–0.5 cm in diameter.

The glands synthesize and secrete parathyroid hormone (PTH) responsible for the maintenance of calcium homeostasis.

Parathyroid hormone (PTH) secreted by the chief cells of the parathyroid glands as needed (with few secretory granules for storage).

PTH plays important physiological role in calcium and phosphate homeostasis. Its secretion is regulated by ionized calcium via a calcium sensing receptor (CaSR). However, the relationship is not linear, and for any given ionized calcium concentration, PTH concentration is lower when the ionized calcium is rising than when it is falling suggesting that it is not the only control mechanism. Lithium stimulates parathyroid hormone secretion and thus increase renal calcium reabsorption.

In addition to calcium, phosphate, and magnesium, PTH secretion is regulated by Klotho and fibroblast growth factor 1 (FGF23). They are expressed in many tissues including the kidney, bone, and the parathyroid. Via binding to its complex Klotho-FGF receptor 1-c splicing form (FGFR1c), FGF23 acts on the parathyroid gland to decrease PTH mRNA and thus circulating PTH levels. It also acts on the kidney proximal tubules to suppress phosphate reabsorption and on renal 1,25-$(OH)_2$ vitamin D synthesis.

In patients with chronic kidney disease, both PTH and FGF23 levels are increased. This may be a reflection of decreased renal clearance, secondary to hyperphosphatemia. The presence of parathyroid resistance to FGF23 is supported by finding of decreased Klotho-EGFR1c complex in parathyroid glands in patients with end-stage kidney disease.

Calcium and phosphate homeostasis are interlinked. It includes magnesium, and endocrine functioning of the parathyroid gland. Calcium and phosphates metabolism are discussed in detail in Chapter 2 on electrolytes.

The hormone exhibits diurnal variation with 50% nadir at 9 a.m. and a 50% peak at 2 a.m. This is helpful diagnostically, where measurement at 10 a.m. improves the test performance for hyperparathyroidism (unexpectedly high PTH levels otherwise would be nadir in normal).

It is made up of 115 aa pre-pro-PTH and undergoes both hepatic and renal metabolism. Several PTH molecular forms are identified. They include 1–84 amino acid intact molecule, smaller fragments with longer half-life 1–34 N with biological activity, and a less biologically active 7–84 mid molecule fragment (see Fig. 8) which accumulates in patients with impaired renal function (reduced GFR).

PTH measurement

Intact (1–84 amino acid) PTH form measurement is preferred and is helpful in the investigation of calcium abnormalities (hyper- and hypocalcemia). Its measurement is helpful investigation of secondary hyperparathyroidism seen in patients with chronic kidney disease, in patients with hypocalcemia, hyperphosphatemia, vitamin D deficiency and in patients following bariatric surgery. Intact PTH is measured intraoperatively and postparathyroid surgery as aid in surgical resection and management of parathyroid adenoma (see later).

PTH is measured using antibody based immunoassays. Several generational assays have since been developed with sequential improvement in both specificity and sensitivity.

In the first generation assays, although using single polyclonal antibody that detects the 84 PTH molecule, it also cross-reacts against the C-terminal nonbioactive fragments that accumulate in patients with reduced renal clearance. The cleaved PTH molecule was found in 50% of uremic patients and up to 20% of normal individuals.

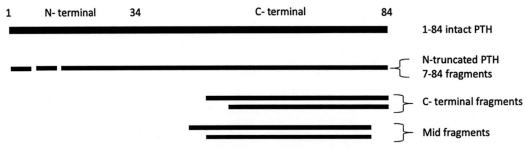

FIG. 8 PTH molecular heterogeneity influencing its biological activity and half-life in the circulation. Intact PTH 1–84 amino acids, the most biological active, with short half-life (2–4 min) and circulating concentration of about 1–5 pmol/L. In contrast, the fragments are of lower relatively lower biological activity and marked circulating levels that are 5–20 time that of the intact PTH. *(Modified from Henrich LM, Rogol AD, D'Amour P, Levine MA, Hanks JB, Bruns DE. Persistent hypercalcemia after parathyroidectomy in an adolescent and effect of treatment with cinacalcet HCl. Clin Chem. 2006;52(12):2286–2293. https://doi.org/10.1373/clinchem.2006.070219. Epub 2006 Nov 14. PMID: 17105782.)*

The second generation assays, developed in collaboration with the Nichol's institute, and hence sometimes referred to as the Nichol's assays, employ two monoclonal antibodies, a capture antibody directed against the C-terminal half of the molecule 39–84 and a detection antibody directed against the first amino terminal half 1–34. The second-generation assays recognize both intact PTH as well as inactive fragments.

The finding of elevated second-generation PTH assay in some patients with renal dysfunction and are discordant with bone status suggested the presence of additional interference. The discovery of a nearly intact PTH variant with 4–7 amino acids missing but remained detectable in the second generation assays lead to the development of a third-generation assays where the capture C-terminal antibody is the same, but the N-terminal detection antibody is specifically directed against the 1–4 amino acids. This facilitated the detection of only what is termed the biologically active 1–84 PTH, the nicked molecule is not biologically active. However, there are difference in performance between the third- and second-generational assays in patients with normal renal function.

The third generation assay is the most widely used assay in current practice with formulations in automated analyzers providing results within 20 min some offer reduced incubation time (9–11 min) and thus facilitating intraoperative assessment of PTH levels (see later).

There is, however, lack of standardization among the various immunoassays, and thus considerable assay variability. However, in most cases it is used in trending, the extent of increase (several folds) above the upper limit of normal. The lack of standardization, in the investigation of primary hyperparathyroidism, does not impair its utility as precise concentration and is irrelevant. Whereas, in patients with secondary hyperparathyroidism (due to renal cause) with 2–9-fold increase in PTH levels, PTH third generational assay better reflects therapy success compared to that by the second generational assay due to interference by accumulating fragments in impaired renal function.

The relative amount of C-terminal fragment to that of the intact 1–84 molecule is variable. The ratio is high in patients with impaired renal function. Interestingly, calcium concentration influences the relative ratio with low ratios seen in hypocalcemia in contrast to the high ratios observed in hypercalcemia.

Most of the biological activity is exhibited by the 1–34 fragment and that the C-terminal fragments do not bind PTH1R.

Posttranslational modification (in the 12–18 amino acid region) is seen in patients with carcinoma and such molecular transformation although detectable by the third generation PTH assays, the immunoreactivity is lower when compared with the older less specific second generation assays. A ratio >1 is suggestive of parathyroid carcinoma.

Similarly, posttranslational modifications of the PTH molecule in either healthy subjects, or in those with primary hyperparathyroidism and or chronic kidney disease may lead to misleading PTH values and misinterpretation. This is further complicated by the lack of standardization among the various commercially available PTH assays.

The performance of PTH assays is important for normocalcemic hyperparathyroidism, in distinguishing between parathyroid carcinoma and benign disease. Posttranslational modification (12–18 aa region) seen in carcinoma is detected by third generation assays which give lower value compared to second generation assays. A ratio >1 suggestive of parathyroid carcinoma. In general, the utility of the assays is hindered by lack of assay standardization, posttranslational modification present in healthy and in patients with primary hyperparathyroidism or chronic kidney disease. Use of the same sassy in serial measures help reduced variations due to those limitations.

In addition to the above discussed immunoassays, several liquid chromatography mass spectrophotometric methods (LCMSMS) are in use. The methods offer enhanced specificity and sensitivity, however, they are influenced by the enrichment method (antibody used often directed at the C-Terminal), requires tryptic cleavage (arginine or lysine), i.e., 1–13 aa fragment denotes iPTH, 7–84 fragment are not detected by LCMSMS.

There are slight differences between corresponding plasma and serum PTH values. Circulating PTH biological variabiliy is about 20% in normal subjects and 30% in patients with chronic kidney disease, thus the PTH relative change value (also termed critical difference) is 54% and 72% respectively.

There appears to be race-related stratification in circulating PTH levels; it is higher in African American. Additionally, PTH levels are associated with BMI, and increase with age. It is 20% lower in patients with vitamin D sufficiency.

PTH assays are subject to interference by heterophile antibodies and by human antimouse antibodies (HAMA). Elevated immunoglobulins in patients with autoimmune disorders and high autoantibodies such as rheumatoid factors are known as heterophile antibodies. Circulating anti mouse antibodies (often seen in patients being treated by OKT3, an immunosuppressant drug used to treat acute transplant rejection). Use of HAMA blocking agents or the use of alternative assays that employs antibodies raised in other species such as rabbit and goat polyclonal antibodies avoid the observed interference.

Pathophysiology

Dysfunction in parathyroid glands is characterized either by hyper or hyposecretion of PTH.

The dysfunction is suspected in patients with hypercalcemia or hypocalcemia in the presence of inappropriately high-normal, or decreased PTH levels respectively.

The finding of hypercalcemia should be repeated in two different occasions within a period of 3 months. Mild increase in calcium over a very long period of time could be suggestive of primary hyperparathyroidism, whereas an acute rise in calcium levels over a short period of time is suggestive of malignancy as the cause. Therefore, clinical assessment guides the subsequent investigations for the hypercalcemia.

The finding of elevated PTH or unsuppressed PTH in the presence of hypercalcemia is indicative of primary hypothyroidism and the finding of hypophosphatemia supports the diagnosis. Finding of suppressed PTH in the presence of hypercalcemia indicates malignancy which is confirmed by the presence of elevated parathyroid hormone related peptide (protein) (PTHrp).

Increased levels of one alpha hydroxy vitamin D (1,25-$(OH)_2$ vitamin D) in the presence of hypercalcemia, suppressed PTH and/or PTHrp levels suggest the presence of granulomatous disease. The latter is due to increased one alpha hydroxylase activity which converts 25-(OH) vitamin D to the active 1,25-$(OH)_2$ vitamin D.

Hyperparathyroidism

Primary hyperparathyroidism has an estimated prevalence of 1–7 cases per 1000 adults. It is the most common cause of hypercalcemia among the ambulatory population, with malignancy being the most common among hospitalized patients. The incidence of hyperparathyroidism is poorly defined showing a wide range from 0.41 to 21.6 cases per 100,000 annually. Single adenoma is most common, double adenomas represent 15% of cases, and multiglandular adenomas represent 10%–15%.

In primary hyperparathyroidism, 80%–85% is due parathyroid adenoma, 15% due to primary parathyroid hyperplasia, and <5% to parathyroid carcinoma. The incidence of parathyroid adenomas peaks in the fifth and sixth decade of life being more common in females with 2:1 female to male ratio. Occurring more frequently in lower lobe, it can weigh from 300 mg to several grams with size ranging from few millimeters to more than 10 cm. Parathyroid adenoma is found in both multiple endocrine neoplasia syndrome types 1 and 2 with type 1 being more common.

Secondary hyperparathyroidism in patients with chronic kidney disease is characterized by elevated PTH levels in the presence of hypocalcemia, hyperphosphatemia, as well as low 1,25-$(OH)_2$ vitamin D levels, and high FGF23. Elevated PTH levels suggest renal osteodystrophy is often seen in patients with renal impairment.

Hyperphosphatemia, hypocalcemia of renal disease as well as reduced 1,25-$(OH)_2$ vitamin D leads to increased PTH synthesis and release by the parathyroid. Additionally, impaired renal function leads to downregulation of the PTH, vitamin D, and calcium sensing receptors. Parathyroid hyperplasia and bone disorders are the most clinical complication as well as cardiovascular disease.

Prolonged secondary hyperthyroidism leads to tertiary hyperparathyroidism evident in the significant proportion of patients with chronic kidney disease who maintain increased levels of PTH following kidney transplant.

PTH measurement is helpful in patients who undergone bariatric surgery. In such patients, calcium and vitamin D absorption are decreased leading to secondary hyperparathyroidism. The prevalence 5 years postsurgery of secondary hyperparathyroidism is about 63%. It is suggested that monitoring PTH levels postoperatively and that levels >65 pg/mL indicates calcium or vitamin D deficiency.

Clinical symptoms vary from mild to severe. Nonspecific symptoms of fatigue, mild depression, or cognitive impairment. Progressive and long-standing hypercalcemia leads to renal impairment, nephrolithiasis, gastrointestinal disturbances, peptic ulcer, pancreatitis, bone pain, secondary bone fractures, and psychosis.

Parathyroidectomy is performed in symptomatic patients with or without osteoporosis, in patients with impaired renal function (GFR <60 mL/min/1.73 m^2), patients with recurrent kidney stones, and patients with hypercalciuria, in patients <50 years old with calcium levels increased by 1 mg/dL above upper limit of normal. It is worth noting that PTH levels are not included in the decision criteria. However, its measurement is required in the discrimination between primary hyperparathyroidism and other causes of hypercalcemia. The use of intact PTH assay is preferred in the setting of renal impairment due to accumulation of c-mid molecule fragments which interferes in some of the older PTH assays.

The laboratory plays an important role in the diagnosis and management of hyperparathyroidism. The finding of elevated—inappropriate detectable PTH levels in the setting of hypercalcemia confirms the diagnosis.

Additionally, the laboratory plays a major role during surgical resection of the parathyroid adenoma.

Peripheral PTH levels are measured perioperatively and that a circulating PTH levels of ≥50% in circulating PTH levels 10 min following resection indicates successful resection of parathyroid adenoma.[6]

PTH third generation assay performs better, it detects more rapid decline in PTH compared to the second generation assays as the latter detects C-terminal fragments (which have longer half-life) more pronounced in patients with chronic kidney disease.

Additionally, in patients with secondary hyperparathyroidism, it takes longer for circulating PTH levels to decline by ≥50% at 10 min when using the third generation assays, and longer at 15 min when using the second generation assay. It is preferable that the same PTH generational assays be used for perioperative and postsurgical studies.

Patients' calcium levels must be closely monitored at postsurgical removal of parathyroid adenoma. However, PTH levels >15 pg/mL at 20 min postsurgery eliminated the need for close monitoring of calcium levels for possible postsurgical hypoparathyroidism.

With the availability and use of intraoperative PTH the decision to conclude the parathyroid surgery following removal of one or more enlarged glands avoids subjectively and affords an objective assessment of removal of the offending gland rather than reliance on visual appearance.

Patients with hypercalcemia following parathyroid surgery indicates the presence of adenoma tissue and possible failure of surgery. Such patients undergo selective parathyroid sampling and exploration. Samples are collected from various anatomical blood drainage sites and sent to the laboratory for PTH measurement. Samples with highest PTH gradient levels are identified by their anatomical sources creating a "hot" biochemical spot. The patient then undergoes another surgical procedure guided by the biochemical profile established (Fig. 9).

Hypoparathyroidism

Hypoparathyroidism is rare in contrast to hyperparathyroidism. It is characterized by hypocalcemia (total calcium adjusted for albumin or ionized calcium) and inappropriately low PTH levels in the presence of hyperphosphatemia, often the findings confirmed at least twice over a 6-month period confirms hypoparathyroidism.

There is often associated low $1,25$-$(OH)_2$ vitamin D levels (due to reduced activation of 1-alpha hydroxylase secondary to the reduced or absent PTH), and the presence of relatively high urinary calcium levels inappropriate for the hypocalcemia.

The incidence of hypoparathyroidism varies among different countries and populations and ranges from 5.3 to 27 per 100,000. It is thus a relatively rare disorder of calcium homeostasis.

The most common causes of hypoparathyroidism are neck surgery (accounting for 75% of cases), genetic causes (<10% of cases) include commonly (60% of children) in DiGeorge syndrome associated with microdeletion in chromosome 22q11.2 where it lacks the T box protein 1 required for parathyroid and thymus development, familial hypoparathyroidism (mutation in the pre-proPTH gene), auto-immune polyendocrine syndrome type1 (APS-1) due to autosomal recessive mutations in the autoimmune regulatory gene (AIRE). The mutation results in lack of self-immunotolerance and thus destruction of parathyroid gland. The diagnosis is made when two of the triad hypoparathyroidism, adrenal insufficiency, and or mucocutaneous candidiasis are present.

Autosomal dominant hypocalcemia (ADH) is a gain of function mutation of the calcium sensing receptor 1 (CaSR1) (type 1) or the G11-alpha (type 2) proteins. The hypocalcemia is not always accompanied by low PTH, the levels are inappropriately low for the calcium levels. There is hypercalciuria with renal calcification as a complication more prominent in type 1.

There are a number of rare genetic mutations associated with low PTH levels; they include syndromes associated with deafness and renal dysfunction, bone dysplastic syndrome (Kenny-Caffey syndrome), abnormalities of parathyroid-specific transcription factors (GCM2) or SOX_3, and disorders of intracellular PTH processing.

Other causes of hypoparathyroidism include hypomagnesemia (magnesium is required for PTH biological activity), parathyroid gland destruction due to deposition of iron (hemochromatosis), copper (Wilson's) disease, and by metastatic infiltration by tumors.

Long-term complication of hypoparathyroidism include neuromuscular irritability the extent of which depends on the rate of change in circulating calcium levels, prolonged hypocalcemia leads to cataracts formation, dry scaly skin, brittle nails, coarse and thin hair, renal stones (due to prolonged hypercalciuria, the risk for stone formation is fivefold greater than in normal subjects), renal impairment (partly due to calcification), cardiovascular manifestation (prolonged Q2 interval, polymorphic ventricular arrhythmia (torsade De pointes)) are consequences of the persistent hypocalcemia in hypoparathyroidism, reduced bone remodeling (due to lack of PTH which stimulates replacement of mature bone with younger bone thus causing increased bone density evident by dual X-ray absorptiometry studies), acute neurological dysfunction secondary to hypocalcemia and chronic neurological manifestations associated with basal ganglia calcification where the ensued hyperphosphatemia is thought to play a role.

Summary

Thyroid

- Thyroid hormones (T4 and T3) are produced in the thyroid following mono- and di-iodination of tyrosyl amino acid on the thyroglobulin molecule.
- Synthesis is regulated by feedback of TSH and TRH from the anterior pituitary and hypothalamus respectively.
- The majority of T4 and T4 is bound TBG ($\sim$70%), prealbumin ($\sim$20%), and albumin ($\sim$10%). Albumin and prealbumin bound fractions are described as "bioavailable" due to weaker binding compared to TBG and delivery to tissues.
- About 0.05% of T4 is free compared with 0.5% of T3.
- Most of T3 (70%) is produced in peripheral tissue following deiodination of T4.
- Hypothyroidism more prevalent in women, an autoimmune disorder, often anti-TPO is detected. Thyroid hormones are low in the presence of elevated TSH levels.
- Hyperthyroidism an autoimmune disorder with elevated TPO, anti-TSH receptor, and thyroid stimulating immunoglobulins. Thyroid hormones are elevated in the presence of suppressed TSH.

Sample	Anatomic Site	Time	[PTH] pg/mL	Fold increase in PTH from lowest PTH value= 79.8 pg/mL
1a	RT. Atrium	10:20	79.8	0.00
1b	Azygous			
1	SVC	10:21	171.8	115.29
2	R. Innominate Vein	10:28	152.2	90.73
3	L Brachiocephalic Vein Proximal	10:24	158.7	98.87
4	L. Brachiocephalic Vein Distal	10:26	217.8	172.93
5	Mediastinal Vein #1			
6	L. Subclavian Vein	10:33	95.5	19.67
7	R. Subclavian Vein	10:38	91.0	14.04
8	Proximal R. Internal Jugular Vein	10:39	273.5	242.73
9	Proximal L. Internal Jugular Vein	10:56	118.5	48.50
10	Mid L. Internal Jugular Vein	11:02	109.4	37.09
11	Distal L. Internal Jugular Vein	11:06	103.9	30.20
12	L.Inferior Thyroid Vein	11:36	101.6	27.32
13	L. Mid Thyroid Vein	11:32	103.4	29.57
14	L. Superior Thyroid Vein	11:28	110.9	38.97
15	L. External Jugular Vein Proximal	11:40	102.3	28.20
16	L. External Jugular Vein Mid	11:47	102.5	28.45
17	L. External Jugular Vein Distal	11:45	100.2	25.56
18	L. Prox. Vertebral Vein	11:39	100.8	26.32
19	L. Mid Vertebral Vein	-	-	-
20	L. Distal Vertebral Vein	11:45	98.2	23.06
21	R. Proximal (2nd) Int. Jugular Vein	11:57	316.4	296.49
22	R. Mid Internal Jugular Vein	11:56	238.4	198.75
23	R. Distal Internal Jugular Vein	11:54	102.3	28.20
24	R. Superior Thyroid Vein	12:09	82.4	3.26
25	R. Mid Thyroid Vein	12:22	94.8	18.80
26	R. Inferior Thyroid Vein	12:21	456.6	472.18
27	R. Proximal Exterior Jugular Vein	11:53	100.2	25.56
28	R. Mid Exterior Jugular Vein	11:52	97.8	22.56
29	R. Distal External Jugular Vein	11:51	88.2	10.53
30	R. Inferior Vertebral Vein	-	-	-
31	R. Mid Vertebral Vein	-	-	-
32	R. Distal Vertebral Vein	11:50	90.8	13.78
33	L. Cephalic Vein	-	-	-
34	L. Brachial / Basilic Vein	-	-	-
35	L. Antecubital Vein	-	-	-
24	R. Superior Thyroid Vein	12:09	82.4	3.26
25	R. Mid Thyroid Vein	12:22	94.8	18.80
26	R. Inferior Thyroid Vein	12:21	456.6	472.18

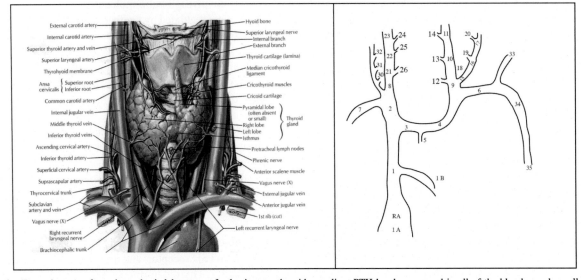

FIG. 9 Example report from the author's laboratory of selective parathyroid sampling. PTH levels measured in all of the blood samples collections from the respective anatomical sites. The PTH levels are represented as gradients of fold increase from the lowest PTH value. Samples with high PTH gradients region(s) are indicated as regional on the anatomical depiction of the patient's gland. This biochemical "hot spot" guides the surgeon during the second attempt to resect the remaining adenomatous tissue. This is helpful as scar tissue and damage from the initial operation limits visual inspection of the remaining parathyroid glands.

- Biochemical abnormalities in patients with nonthyroidal illness exhibit suppressed TSH in the presence of normal thyroid hormone levels.
- Mutations in the thyroid hormone receptor beta (TRβ) gene leads to thyroid resistance syndrome evident by the presence of elevated TSH and elevated thyroid hormone levels.
- Disorders leading to changes in proteins levels such as liver disease, protein losing enteropathies, renal dysfunction, as well as genetic abnormalities leads to erroneous total thyroid hormone levels.
- In addition to influencing total thyroid hormone levels, extreme changes in binding protein levels and in their binding affinities, may also impact free thyroid hormone measurements. Isotope-dilution liquid chromatography mass spectrometry (ID-LCMSMS), a reference method for the measurement of free thyroid hormones, is often utilized when there is discrepancy in free thyroid hormone determinations.
- The log-linear relationship between TSH and thyroid hormones as well as the availability of high sensitivity TSH assays (third and fourth generations) has favored TSH as a reliable predictor of thyroid function and in the monitoring of adequacy of thyroid hormone replacement therapy.
- There is age-related TSH reference ranges. TSH is elevated in neonates during the first week of life. TSH is suppressed during the first trimester of gestation. Use of age-related and gestational age-specific reference intervals for TSH is recommended.
- Assays employing the biotin-avidin system may be interfered with by the presence of circulating biotin following intake of high doses of biotin. Interference often exhibits a reduced TSH and elevated free thyroid hormones representing biochemical finding of hyperthyroidism erroneously.
- Drugs may interfere with free thyroid hormone measurements such as salicylate that causes displacement of thyroid hormones from the binding proteins.

Parathyroid glands

- Individual has two pairs of parathyroid glands located posteriorly in each thyroid lope.
- Parathyroid glands secrete PTH which plays significant role in calcium homeostasis.
- PTH acts in concert with 1,25-(OH)$_2$ vitamin D to absorb both calcium and phosphate in the intestine.
- Magnesium is essential for PTH secretion and action.
- Measurement of intact PTH 1–84 is preferred. Older assays are influenced by PTH fragments and midmolecule that accumulate in patients with impaired renal function.
- Most of the biological activity is exhibited by the 1–34 amino acid segment of PTH.

- Hyperparathyroidism has prevalence of about 7 cases per 1000. It is the most common cause of hypercalcemia among ambulatory population, whereas malignancy is the most common cause among hospitalized patients.
- The majority (about 85%) of hyperparathyroidism is due to parathyroid adenoma.
- Decline of PTH levels (intraoperatively) by 50% or more confirms successful resection of the parathyroid adenoma.
- Hypoparathyroidism is rare compared to hyperparathyroidism. It is often secondary to neck surgery, or more rarely to genetic causes. It is characterized by hypocalcemia and hyperphosphatemia.

The pituitary

The pituitary gland

The pituitary gland located in the pituitary fossa (Sella turcica). It weighs about 0.5–1.0 g. The pituitary gland itself is divided into the anterior and posterior parts, and these are embryologically, anatomically and functionally discrete. The anterior pituitary receives blood supply via the portal vessels, whereas the posterior pituitary has direct arterial blood supply and is not influenced by portal circulation (Fig. 10). Interference in this blood flow causes pituitary dysfunction (see later). Specific hypothalamic hormones reaching the pituitary stimulates their respective anterior pituitary hormones secretion, whereas those reaching the posterior pituitary are stored and released as needed. The synthesis and release of most hypothalamic and pituitary hormones are under feedback inhibition by their target hormones (Fig. 10). Furthermore, hypothalamic peptides are pharmacology available and can be used, although rarely, in dynamic investigation of pituitary function (see later).

Anterior pituitary

Hormones and their control

Anterior pituitary hormones, their controlling hypothalamic peptides, and their effects or target are shown in Table 3. Each hormone is individually discussed in details (see later).

Adrenocorticotrophic hormone (ACTH) (corticotrophin)[7]

ACTH a 39 amino acid peptide with the 1–24 amino acid peptide being the biologically active N-terminal portion. Preopiomelanocortin (POMC) a 246 amino acid peptide is the precursor of ACTH. It is cleaved by proteinases (proconvertases 1–3) to produce ACTH, melanocyte stimulating hormone (α- and β-MSH), β-lipotropin, and β-endorphin (Fig. 11). Additionally, POMC is synthesized by several peripheral tissues, with proteinases present in the heart,

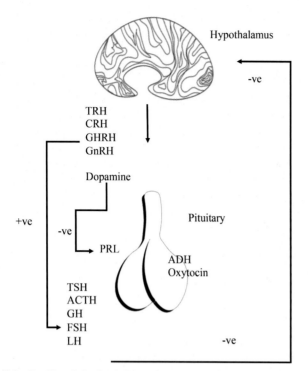

FIG. 10 Hypothalamic-pituitary axis; hypothalamic hormones/peptides stimulate synthesis of pituitary thyrotropin (TSH), adrenocorticotrophic hormone (ACTH), growth hormone (GH), follicle stimulating hormone (FSH), and luteinizing hormone (LH) which in turn inhibits the synthesis and release of their respective stimulating hypothalamic hormones. In contrast, prolactin produced by the anterior pituitary is under tonic inhibition by hypothalamic dopamine. Antidiuretic hormone (ADH) and oxytocin are produced in the hypothalamus and stored in the posterior pituitary.

TABLE 3 Hypothalamic and pituitary hormones and their respective target organs and subsequent endocrine hormonal release.

Hypothalamic hormones	Pituitary hormones	Target organ (feedback inhibiting hormone (s))
CRH	ACTH	Adrenal (cortisol)
GnRH	FSH/LH	Gonads (testosterone, estradiol, progesterone)
GHRH/GHRIH	GH	Liver, muscle (IGFs)
TRH	TSH	Thyroid (thyroxine, triiodothyronine)
Dopamine (PIH)	Prolactin	Mammary glands (milk secretion)

ACTH, adrenocorticotropic hormone; *CRH*, corticotrophin releasing hormone; *FSH*, follicle stimulating hormone; *GH*, growth hormone; *GHRH*, growth hormone releasing hormone; *GHRIH*, growth hormone release inhibiting hormone; *GnRH*, gonadotropic releasing hormone; *IGFs*, insulin like growth factor-1; *LH*, luteinizing hormone; *TRH*, thyrotropin releasing hormone; *TSH*, thyrotropin stimulating hormone.

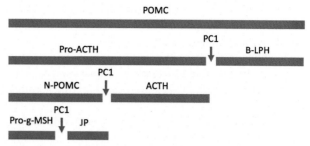

FIG. 11 ACTH structure and processing in the anterior pituitary mediated via prohormone convertase 1 (PC1) and via prohormone convertase 2 (PC2), carboxypeptidase E (CPE), and peptidyl amidating monooxygenase (PMA) in the hypothalamus and skin, leading to biologically active and immune-based assays activity of practical interest. *(Modified from Stevens A, White A. ACTH: cellular peptide hormone synthesis and secretory pathways. Results Probl Cell Differ. 2010;50:63–84. https://doi.org/10.1007/400_2009_30. PMID: 19888563.)*

placenta, lung, thyroid, and adrenal gland. ACTH synthesis and release is stimulated by hypothalamic CRH, arginine, vasopressin (ADH—antidiuretic hormone), Interleukins 1 and 6 (and therefore in inflammatory conditions). Adrenal cortisol inhibits ACTH release via a negative feedback inhibition (Fig. 10).

Earlier difficulties with ACTH measurement supported measuring cortisol as a surrogate marker. It is labile and is easily oxidized. It is degraded by proteases and by repeat freeze thawing. Additionally, it exhibits significant binding to glass and thus collection and storage in glass tubes as well as repeated freeze thawing should be avoided. Some laboratories recommend the use of protease inhibitors such as Trasylol to inhibit proteolytic cleavage as well as adding mercaptoethanol (antioxidant) to stabilize ACTH. Degraded fragments are not detected by most immunoassays. Reports of macroforms of ACTH, presumably a result of defective cleavage of precursor protein interferes in some commercially available immunoassay. Such molecular heterogeneity leads to discordance among ACTH immunoassays. ACTH has a marked diurnal rhythm, the nadir being at midnight. Levels start to rise at 2:00 a.m., reaching a peak around 6:00–8:00 a.m. then fall thought the rest of the day. Samples have, therefore, to be taken at a set time, usually between 9:00 a.m. and 10:00 a.m. Stress elevates ACTH levels.

Gonadotrophins

The gonadotrophins follicle-stimulating hormone (FSH) and luteinizing hormone (LH) are dimeric made of alpha and beta subunits. They share the alpha subunit with TSH and hCG, whereas the beta subunits confer their respective specificity. Their synthesis and release is stimulated by hypothalamic decapeptide gonadotropic-releasing hormone (GnRH). Its release is modified by circulating estrogens, androgens, progesterone as well as inhibins. LH and FSH stimulates gonadal synthesis and secretion of estradiol and testosterone respectively which control both GnRH and FSH and LH in a negative feedback inhibition at the hypothalamus and anterior pituitary respectively (Fig. 10). FSH and LH are secreted in a pulsatile fashion with a periodicity of 1–2 h, although this pulsatile release is essential for physiological response, it does not interfere with their interpretation in routine practice, but frequent sampling may be necessary for academic purposes. The pulsatile fashion is mimicked during therapeutic protocols in hypogonadism to effect fertility. Subnormal levels are found with weight loss. They are routinely measured using automated immunoassays in the assessment of infertility with little assays limitations.

Growth hormone (GH)

This is a 20–22 kDa protein synthesized by the anterior pituitary (somatotrophs) in response to hypothalamic 44 amino acid growth hormone releasing hormone (GHRH). GH exhibits molecular heterogeneity with 20 and 22 kDa circulating variants. The 22 kDa is considered to be a glycosylated form of the hormone. In circulation, 50% of growth hormone is bound to a 191 amino acid growth hormone binding proteins (GHBP).

It is anabolic hormone stimulating hepatic gluconeogenesis, protein synthesis, and lipolysis. It is produced in a pulsatile fashion lasting 1–2 h at midnight, following onset of sleep, and in response to stress. Small irregular spikes of secretion may occur during the day but become very marked during sleep or orthodox sleep (non-rapid eye movement sleep). This gives a sort of diurnal rhythm. The physiological action of GH is mediated via insulin-like growth factors (IGFs) produced by hepatocytes in response to GH.

IGF-1 is bound to several (1–5) binding proteins (IGF-1BPs). The one most relevant when assessing GH status is binding protein-3 (IGFBP3).

Control of GH and GHRH is via negative feedback inhibition by somatostatin (14 amino acid peptide). Growth hormone release inhibitory hormone (Ghrelin) a 28 amino acid peptide produced by epithelial cells lining the fundus of the stomach, stimulates GH release in concert with GHRH controlling both time and amplitudes of its release.

Estrogen levels increase the sensitivity of GH responses to a variety of stimuli. Starvation (as opposed to overnight fasting), stress, and exercise elevate GH levels. Glucose ingestion suppresses GH levels, but oral protein hydrolysates or amino-acid infusions stimulate GH secretion. GH status is assessed in patients with acromegaly, gigantism, or short stature. Dynamic testing suppression (in suspected excess production) and stimulation (in suspected deficiency) is often required to confirm diagnosis.

Thyrotropin (thyroid stimulating hormone) TSH

A 26.6 kDa molecular-weight glycoprotein made up of two subunits alpha and beta unit with the latter required for thyroid receptor binding and thus affords specificity. Both units are significantly glycosylated (up to 31% of its molecular weight) and together are required for biological activity. Changes in carbohydrate structure give rise to isoforms that may have different biological and immunological activities; however in clinical practice, most assays in routine use do not detect changes in carbohydrate structure. The alpha subunit is common with gonadotropins and chorionic gonadotrophin. The long half-life at 50 min for TSH allows a single measurement as sufficient to reflect circulating levels. TSH release is very sensitive to changes in free hormone levels with a logarithmic-linear relationship where a 2-fold change in T4 reflects 100-fold change in TSH. The hormone exhibits both pulsatile and circadian rhythm synthesis and release where increased levels are seen between midnight and 4 a.m. This is however not reflected in thyroidal (T4, T3) hormones levels. Notably, most statistical reference intervals are often based on morning values.

Thyroid hormones exert negative feedback inhibition on both TRH and TSH and thus control the hypothalamic-pituitary-thyroidal axis (Fig. 10). The widely reported reference range for TSH in adult is 0.45–4.5 mIUL/L, however in 95% of individuals, free of thyroid disease, will have TSH values 0.3–2.5 mIU/L. Individual variability within a TSH set-point is about 0.75 mIU/L.

There are age-related changes in TSH, and levels are elevated in neonates in the presence of elevated and normal thyroid hormone. Levels approach those of adults 4–8 weeks of age.

Secretion of TSH is inhibited by elevated dopamine and glucocorticoids, inflammatory cytokines (IL-1 and TNF-α) often seen in patients with nonthyroidal illness. Similarly, catecholamines and leptin stimulates TRH release which in turn stimulates TSH synthesis and release.

Assays for TSH measurements are mainly sandwich immunoassays employing a capture and detector antibodies. Few reports suggest interference due to heterophile antibodies. Generational classification of TSH immunoassays assays are related to their functional sensitivity with 0.1 being second generation and 0.01 a third generational assay. Most current assays in routine use are either third or fourth generation making it more reliable to detect TSH levels far below lower reference 0.45 mIU/L. The reference intervals for TSH remain debated with upper limit of normal ranging from 2.5 mIUl/L to 4.5 mIU/L. Although higher lower level often around 0.45 mIU/L are reported, patients on thyroid therapy experience improved symptoms when TSH levels are about 2.5 mIU/L. There are method-related differences and until methods traceability are established by in vitro diagnostics, the universal use of reference intervals is not feasible.

Prolactin (PRL)

Prolactin, a 23–25 kDa polypeptide made of 198 amino acids, is secreted by lactotrophs in a pulsatile fashion with peaks every 1–5 min. The hormone exhibits molecular heterogeneity with significant proportion >60% glycosylated. PRL is under positive inhibition by hypothalamic dopamine. Interruption in portal blood supply by mass occupying lesion causing stalk compression leads to hyperprolactinemia due to lack of dopamine. Drugs interfering with dopamine production, such as antipsychotic, antiemetics, and tranquilizers, lead to hyperprolactinemia due to removal of the dopamine prolactin inhibitory action.

There is a two- to threefold rise in plasma levels during deep sleep and even daytime naps elevate PRL. The effect of estrogens is shown by men having lower levels than postmenopausal women who, in turn, have a lower PRL than premenopausal women. Levels are extremely high during pregnancy but fall by the 6th day postpartum. PRL secretion and lactation are thereafter maintained by the suckling reflex. PRL is another "stress" hormone with elevated levels in stress. Prolactin-producing adenoma is the most common pituitary adenoma. The adenoma is defined by its radiological size, a microadenoma <1 cm, and a macroadenoma >1 cm.

About 10%–20% of patients with hyperlactinemia will exhibit macroprolactin. It is circulating prolactin complexed with immunoglobulin and/or prolactin aggregates that exhibits immunoreactivity in some immunoassays. This causes false hyperprolactinemia as it is often devoid of biological activity. The high molecular weight complex is precipitated using polyethylene glycol, and that less than 40% of the prolactin recovered suggests the presence of macroprolactin as a cause of the false hyperprolactinemia.

Pituitary disorders and their investigation

Assessment include measurement in basal states, measurement following dynamic stimulation when hypofunction is suspected and dynamic suppression when hyperpituitarism is suspected. Basal state measurements are often not helpful except for prolactin disorders, however, measurement of the respective hormone following a dynamic procedure will improve test sensitivity, alleviate effect of stress, assess reserve capacity, and elucidate the presence of ectopic hormonal production (see separate sections below).

Anterior hyperpituitarism

Adrenocorticotrophic hormone (ACTH)

Hypersecretion of ACTH leads to hypercortisolism and to Cushing's disease. It is synthesized and released either from the anterior pituitary or form ectopic extra-pituitary sources such as carcinoma of the lung, carcinoid, or pheochromocytoma.

A state of hypercortisolism need to be confirmed in a patient with clinical signs and symptoms suggestive of Cushing's, such as catabolic wasting, purple striae secondary to increased capillary fragility, moon face, buffalo hump.

The differential diagnosis of Cushing's syndrome depends on proper laboratory evaluation. Biochemical investigations involve initial diagnostic test followed by confirmatory test if necessary.

ACTH and thus cortisol production exhibits diurnal rhythm elevated in the morning with a nadir in the evening. The loss and disturbance in the diurnal rhythm is often an early sign of dysfunction but requires several timed samples and thus impractical.

Cortisol is produced by the adrenal glands in response to ACTH released from the anterior pituitary. The findings of elevated cortisol in the presence of elevated ACTH indicates an ACTH dependent Cushing's disease, whereas the findings of an elevated cortisol in the presence of a suppressed ACTH suggest an adrenal or exogenous source for the cortisol. In the ACTH-dependent Cushing's, the source of ACTH needs to be confirmed. It could originate from the anterior pituitary or from an extra-pituitary ectopic source.

In the presence of elevated cortisol, normal or elevated ACTH levels (50–100 pg/mL) is diagnostic of ACTH dependent Cushing's. The initial screening for Cushing's syndrome (confirm state of hypercortisolism) is via measurement of 24 h urinary free cortisol levels or by measuring 8 a.m. serum cortisol levels following an overnight 1 mg dexamethasone suppression. Late-night salivary cortisol measurement is increasingly being used. Salivary cortisol being a surrogate marker for serum cortisol and has the advantage of being collected at home in a low stress environment.

Furthermore, markedly elevated ACTH >100–200 pg/mL is suggestive of ectopic ACTH. Falsely low ACTH may be seen and is often due to big form of ACTH that is missed by some immunoassays. Additionally, the diagnosis is confirmed following a high dose dexamethasone suppression test. Adequate suppression of >80% suppression of urine free cortisol suggests hypothalamic-pituitary disorder, whereas failure of suppression; cortisol >15 µg/dL and ACTH >15 pg/mL indicates the presence of ACTH-producing tumor.

ACTH-dependent Cushing's (Cushing's disease)

The source of ACTH (pituitary versus ectopic source) is investigated following its measurement in samples obtained by invasive inferior petrosal sinus sampling (IPSS) procedures. Blood samples are collected at −15, −5, 0, 1, 3, 5, 10, 15, and 30 min following administration of CRH (1 µg/kg body weight). ACTH levels are measured at all time points and cortisol at −15, 5, and 15 min.

The procedure is performed by intervention radiology and assisted by clinical chemistry in preparation of protocol, in paired sample tubes, and in interpretation of laboratory findings. Correct sample tube type and additives are essential, ACTH binds to glass, and thus those are avoided at all stages of sample collection and processing, additionally ACTH is labile and thus storage of blood tubes on crushed ice, prompt plasma separation in refrigerated centrifugation, and aliquots stored frozen until analysis are all essential steps to preserve sample quality.

CRH injection is often used at the beginning of the procedure to improve test sensitivity. It helps eliminate alterations in ACTH and cortisol due the stress of the procedure and a reliable baseline is thus obtained. For a patient weighing less than 200 pounds (90.9 kg), the dose is 1 µg CRH/kg body weight. For a patient equal to or more than 200 pounds (≥90.9 kg), the entire vial of CRH (100 µg) is used.

Interventional radiologist establishes two inferior petrosal catheters (labeled as Left and Right). Remembering that the catheters will cross overlap at the optic chiasm. Correct labeling is thus important as it is used to interpret lateralization and assists with subsequent surgical intervention.

Peripheral blood samples for cortisol measurements are collected from peripheral vein at −15, +5, and +15 min following administration of CRH. Blood samples are collected from the inferior petrosal sinus using the two IPSS catheters and at −15, −5, 0, 1, 2, 3, 5, 10, 15, and 30 min following CRH injection. Similarly, peripheral venous samples are collected for ACTH measurement. ACTH levels are measured for all peripheral and IPSS samples. Cortisol levels are measured in peripheral samples collected at −15, −5, and +15 min.

The presence of IPSS ACTH ≥ three folds of peripheral ACTH suggests pituitary source with petrosal ACTH values 40% more to one side suggests tumor lateralization to that side (Table 4). This is helpful in guiding surgical intervention. Lateralize is not always accurate with about 7%–15% failure rate in experienced centers. The addition of prolactin measurement to the IPSS procedure has been suggested to improve the discrimination between pituitary and ectopic ACTH source in borderline cases. False negative results may occur caused by inadequate cannulation due to anatomical anomalies. ACTH values corrected for prolactin levels are suggested to improve the test utility in selected cases and may eliminate unnecessary search for an ectopic ACTH-producing neoplasm. Several formulas and cutoff points have been suggested (Table 4).

A report is generated (see case examples below) includes all ACTH and cortisol measurement and interpretation. Pituitary as a source for ACTH is indicated when a gradient of 3 or greater for IPSS and peripheral ACTH levels is obtained for at least two samples in one of the IPSS catheters. Additionally, a 40% increase in ACTH on one side of the IPSS catheter suggests lateralization and that the pituitary tumor is located on the side of the higher ACTH. When the ACTH gradient between IPSS and peripheral venous blood is low, this indicates ectopic source for the ACTH (often lung lesion, e.g., carcinoma). Intermediate gradients in the

TABLE 4 Interpretive criteria for inferior petrosal sinus sampling (IPSS).

Ratio/gradient	Magnitude of ratio	Interpretation
(R or L) IPSS/PV	≥3.0	Pituitary ACTH-producing adenoma
RIPSS/LIPSS	>1.4	Pituitary adenoma located on the same side as the elevated ACTH levels
(R&L) IPSS/PV	<2.0	Primary adrenal tumor or ectopic ACTH syndrome
(R&L) IPSS/PV	≥2.0 but <3.0	Abnormal pituitary ACTH secretion

Ratio of IFPS ACTH to peripheral level >3.0 suggests pituitary sources for ACTH ratio >1.7 cutoff (without CRH stimulation), with possible lateralization to either the right or left side respectively (if >40%). Ratios less than 2 suggests extra pituitary sources of ACTH, i.e., ectopic (commonly lung), or to primary cortisol producing adrenal tumor. *IPSS*, inferior petrosal sinus specimen; *LIPSS*, left IPSS; *PV*, peripheral vein; *RIPSS*, right IPSS. (Criteria as described in England et al.[8])

greater than 2 but less than 3 indicates abnormal pituitary ACTH secretion.

The below IPSS study (Fig. 12) shows ACTH and cortisol values obtained during the study at the specified time points. Ratio of IPSS to peripheral vein ACTH was greater than 3 in both the left and the right IPS in at least 2 samples. Suggesting pituitary source for the ACTH. Furthermore, the ratio of ACTH in the left IPS to the right catheter samples was predominantly greater than 1.4 compared with less than 1.4 for most samples in the right catheter. This suggests lateralization to the left. In conclusion, the study indicates a pituitary source for ACTH and a left lateralization of the gland. The latter is helpful during surgical intervention.

The below IPSS study (Fig. 13) shows ACTH and cortisol values obtained during the study at the specified time points. Ratio of IPSS to peripheral vein ACTH was less than 3 (actually were less than twofold) in both the left and the right IPS in at least 2 samples (actually in all study samples). Suggesting nonpituitary source for the ACTH. Furthermore, the ratio of ACTH in the left IPS to the right catheter samples and vice versa was as expectedly less than 1.4. In conclusion, the study indicates a nonpituitary ectopic source for ACTH.

Postoperative assessment for remission and recurrence is important since remission rate for Cushing's disease is 59%–95% with 20% recurrence. Annual or semiannual assessment of cortisol status is performed. CRH stimulation test exhibits sensitivity and specificity of 93% and 71% for relapse respectively. Additionally, immediately postoperative ACTH and corresponding cortisol levels predict patients

Specimen Time	[Cortisol], ug/dL	[ACTH], pg/mL			ACTH Gradients							
			Left	Right	Left-Side/PV Ratio		Right-Side/PV Ratio		Left-to-Right Side Ratio		Right-Left Side Ratio	
Time, min	NRR: 7.0-25.0	PV	LIFPS	RIFPS	LIFPS/PV	Ratio	RIFPS/PV	Ratio	LIFPS/RIFPS	Ratio	RIFPS/LIFPS	Ratio
-15	3.4	26	56	42	2.15	Between 2 and 3	1.62	less than 2	1.33	less than 1.4	0.75	less than 1.4
-5		32	86	88	2.69	Between 2 and 3	2.75	Between 2 and 3	0.98	less than 1.4	1.02	less than 1.4
0		34	460	64	13.53	greater than 3	1.88	less than 2	7.19	greater than 1.4	0.14	less than 1.4
1		35	431	77	12.31	greater than 3	2.20	Between 2 and 3	5.60	greater than 1.4	0.18	less than 1.4
3		33	789	76	23.91	greater than 3	2.30	Between 2 and 3	10.38	greater than 1.4	0.10	less than 1.4
5	5.8	32	1470	106	45.94	greater than 3	3.31	greater than 3	13.87	greater than 1.4	0.07	less than 1.4
10		46	125	63	2.72	Between 2 and 3	1.37	less than 2	1.98	greater than 1.4	0.50	less than 1.4
15	9.6	43	56	201	1.30	less than 2	4.67	greater than 3	0.28	less than 1.4	3.59	greater than 1.4
30		52	60	71	1.15	less than 2	1.37	less than 2	0.85	less than 1.4	1.18	less than 1.4

FIG. 12   ACTH levels in peripheral blood and in left and right inferior petrosal sinus samples. ACTH in IPSS was ≥3 times that in peripheral circulation and >3 times on the left compared to the right IPSS suggesting pituitary source of ACTH that is lateralized to the left.

Specimen Time	[Cortisol], ug/dL	PV	Left	Right	Left-Side/PV Ratio		Right-Side/PV Ratio	
Time, min	NRR: 7.0-25.0	PV	LIFPS	RIFPS	LIFPS/PV	Ratio	RIFPS/PV	Ratio
-15	101.7	234	270	289	1.15	less than 2	1.24	less than 2
-5		233	275	295	1.18	less than 2	1.27	less than 2
0		231	268	297	1.16	less than 2	1.29	less than 2
1		219	256	283	1.17	less than 2	1.29	less than 2
3		241	283	281	1.17	less than 2	1.17	less than 2
5	102.6	225	270	295	1.20	less than 2	1.31	less than 2
10		232	261	266	1.13	less than 2	1.15	less than 2
15	100.7	219	251	278	1.15	less than 2	1.27	less than 2
30		197	265	257	1.35	less than 2	1.30	less than 2

FIG. 13   ACTH levels in peripheral blood and in left and right inferior petrosal sinus samples. ACTH in peripheral samples is ≥ three folds higher that in IPSS samples (both left and right). Suggesting ectopic sources pituitary of ACTH. It is worth noting that IPSS ACTH is suppressed compared with peripheral levels. This is due to suppression by the high circulating cortisol levels and that the pituitary feedback inhibition response is intact.

likely to show recurrence. The use of CRH alone or in combination with desmopressin remains controversial. The addition of desmopressin to CRH does not appear to be of value.

Investigating adrenal sources of cortisol is discussed in the section on adrenal glands.

Follicle stimulating hormone (FSH) and luteinizing hormone (LH)

Pituitary tumors which secrete gonadotrophins are rare and have been described infrequently, while some so called "functionless" tumors have been found to secrete FSH and LH when grown in vitro. Gonadotroph pituitary neuroendocrine tumors express FSH and LH evident by immunohistochemistry studies but are not secreted and thus elevated levels are not detected in the circulation.

Growth hormone (GH)

Hypersecretion of growth hormone causes gigantism before epiphyseal fusion, i.e., before puberty and causes acromegaly in adults (following epiphyseal fusion). As already mentioned, stress, exercise, and starvation elevate GH levels and so single estimates are of little value in the diagnosis of acromegaly. Normally, 75 g of oral glucose suppresses GH to undetectable levels, whereas in acromegaly no GH suppression occurs and in 20% of patients, GH levels rise even higher, known as the paradoxical rise. It is also worth considering blood glucose results because acromegalics can have impaired glucose tolerance or frank diabetes. High calcium levels may indicate hyperparathyroidism as part of the multiple endocrine adenoma syndrome. An elevated serum IGF-1 is a useful confirmatory test for acromegaly and also serves as a baseline to monitor the results of therapy. However, the main assessment of treatment depends on periodic GH measurements throughout the day.

Basal GH measurements are thus helpful to rule out GH as a cause of acromegaly and of gigantism.

IGF-1 varies with age and an age-specific reference interval must be applied when interpreting their values.

The 75 g glucoses tolerance test (GTT) is used to suppress GH levels. Limitations of the test, however, include lack of suppression supports the presence of GH secreting pituitary adenoma. However, the test fails in patients with liver disease, chronic kidney disease, malnutrition, and in GH resistance (Laron syndrome due to GH binding proteins abnormalities). Additionally, the use of GTT in patient with diabetes is inappropriate.

GH respond to TRH or to LHRH in acromegalic patients showing a rise in GH level. This is helpful when other tests are equivocal. In contrast, dopamine infusion causes a decline in GH in acromegaly. Those tests, however, are not routinely performed.

Rarely ectopic GHRH (usually by pancreatic endocrine tumor) causes increased GH levels. The syndrome is diagnosed by measuring GHRH levels.

GH levels >1 µg/L and a nadir of ≥0.4 µg/L following GTT and elevated IGF-1 indicates active disease. Whereas GH levels >2.0 µg/L suggest deterioration. Controlled disease is achieved when random GH levels are <1 µg/L or a nadir of <0.4 µg/L following GTT and that IGF-1 levels are within normal limits.

TSH

Pituitary tumors secreting TSH are rare (0.5%–2%) with less than 1% of all pituitary adenomas cause of thyrotoxicosis characterized by markedly elevated thyroid hormones in the presence of a measurable TSH levels. A similar biochemical profile is that of thyroid hormone resistance syndromes. About 30% of TSH secreting adenoma are mixed cosecreting mostly prolactin, or growth hormone, or gonadotropins to a lesser extent.

Prolactin (PRL)

Hyperprolactinemia leads to oligo and amenorrhea, galactorrhea and infertility, breast enlargement (in male) gynecomastia, and impotence. The presence of large tumors (space occupying lesion) may also lead to visual field defects. The main limitation in the investigation of hyperprolactinemia is that there is no dynamic test to distinguish the raised PRL due to stress from that of other causes. If the level is very high, it is unlikely to be due to stress, but if only moderately elevated the test should be repeated to ascertain if hyperprolactinemia is sustained.

Sustained hyperprolactinemia in women inhibits gonadotrophin pulsatility, inhibits the positive feedback of estrogen, and inhibits the effect of gonadotrophin on the ovary. Patients thus present with infertility, amenorrhea, and less frequently with galactorrhea. In men, it causes hypogonadism resulting in loss of libido.

Prolactin release is under inhibition by dopamine and therefore hyperprolactinemia can result from inhibition of dopamine activity or stalk compression due to space occupying lesion interrupting portal circulation and thus delivery of dopamine.

Inhibition of dopamine activity by drugs (particularly those interfering with dopamine release, antipsychotic, antiemetic, and tranquilizers) other drugs include contraceptives.

Hyperprolactinemia is seen in patients with prolactin secreting (lactotrophs) tumors. The tumors may produce solely prolactin, or be mixed with GH secretion and rarely with ACTH evident by immunochemical staining.

Prolactin levels >5000 mIU/L (>235 ng/mL) are suggestive of prolactinoma. Levels <5000 mIU/L (<235 ng/mL) may be seen in microadenoma or in stalk compression.

In primary hypothyroidism (possibly due to increased hypothalamic TRH levels), prolactin is in the range of 1000–2000 mIU/L (47–94 ng/mL). Similar levels are seen in patients with chronic kidney disease possible to stress or to reduced metabolism and clearance. Assessment of thyroid and kidney function elucidates the secondary causes of hyperprolactinemia.

Pregnancy and lactation as well as stress are the most common causes of hyperprolactinemia. Measurement of hCGβ confirms pregnancy as the cause. TRH dynamic test offers little value in determining the cause of hyperprolactinemia.

Macroprolactin

Circulating macroprolactin causes hyperprolactinemia where there are variabilities in susceptible to interferences in among the different immunoassays. Polyethylene glycol precipitation is used to investigate its presence (see Chapter 17).

Antigen excess (hook effect)

prolactin levels can be extremely high >100,000 mIU/L (>4700 ng/mL) which is beyond the assay analytical measuring range of the assay. This may cause a falsely low prolactin level (due to hook effect). Repeat samples analysis following sample dilution resolves the issue; however, most assays in routine clinical practice offer a large analytical measurement range, and this is rarely encountered in current practice, despite it being cited in older textbooks and often considered by obstetrician and endocrinologist as a more common cause of false low prolactin levels (see Chapter 17).

Anterior hypopituitarism

Anterior hypopituitarism may result from direct damage to the pituitary through compression by tumors, vascular disorders, surgery, radiotherapy, and inflammatory lesions or, indirectly, due to hypothalamic tumors which remove the controlling peptide hormone activity. It is often difficult to distinguish between hypothalamic and pituitary disease on biochemical grounds alone. These disorders produce varying degrees of hypopituitarism from unitrophic deficiency (usually GH) to panhypopituitarism. In addition, there are a group of disorders in which there is an isolated trophic hormone deficiency (e.g., GH, gonadotrophin) without any anatomical lesion, and these are ascribed to lack of the appropriate hypothalamic releasing hormone. The symptoms and signs can be deduced from considering the hormones involved (lack of ACTH; pale skin, torpor crisis, lack of GH; dwarfism in children, lack of FSH/LH; amenorrhea, male hypogonadism, lack of TSH; dry skin/hair, torpor and lack of prolactin; failure of lactation). Detailed biochemical investigation and findings are described separately below.

Patients with a suspicion of hypothalamic-pituitary disease require pituitary function testing to determine the need for replacement therapy. Causes of hypofunction include nonfunctioning pituitary tumor, craniopharyngioma, meningioma, inflammatory condition, and sarcoidosis.

Adrenocorticotrophin hormone (ACTH)

Isolated ACTH deficiency is rare and is often due to pan hypopituitarism where other hormones are also low. A number of ACTH stimulation tests are used, Tthey include measurement of ACTH following injection of 250 μg CRH and measuring ACTH at times 0, 30, and 60 min following injection. Other dynamic test includes metyrapone test, where metyrapone blocks cortisol synthesis, the reduction in cortisol stimulates the production of ACTH under normal conditions, lack of adequate ACTH repose to the developing hypocortisolemia indicates ACTH deficiency.

Another test not widely used and is to assess ACTH status to stress induced by hypoglycemia with intravenous insulin in a dose of 0.15 U/kg. To insure the test has been sufficiently provocative, blood glucoses are collected, and the nadir should be <2.2 mmol/L (<40 mg/dL). The test may be dangerous due to the induced hypoglycemia and is contraindicated in a number of conditions.

Follicle stimulating hormone (FSH) and luteinizing hormone (LH)

FSH and LH and are produced in response to the pulsatile secretion of hypothalamic gonadotropin releasing hormone (GnRH).

Isolated LH deficiency is rare (0.1%). Deficiency can be congenial or acquired and can be due to hypothalamic, pituitary, or gonadal dysfunction. Low levels are observed secondary to exogenous testosterone administration. The incidence of hypogonadotropic hypogonadism is 1 in 10,000 to 1 in 86,000, and that nearly 60% are associated with Kallmann syndrome (see below).

Investigation of low FSH and LH involves measurement of testosterone and estradiol as well as dynamic testing. In the latter, GnRH is administered intravenously in a dose of 100 μg that will stimulate LH release in a normal individual, and in 40% there will also be a rise in FSH. Lack of FSH release is not significant. In children the converse is true, where FSH but not LH exhibits a rise.

Genetical mutations leading to failure in GnRH release and delivery to the pituitary. Mutations in the KISS1 gen that encodes hypothalamic kisspeptin hormone regulate GnRH and hence gonadotropins secretion. The causes of Kallmann syndrome are characterized by reduced steroids hormones, absence of puberty, and secondary sexual characteristics.

Additionally, mutations in the LH-β subunit or its receptor result in nonfunctional unit and thus clinical presentation of hypogonadism. However, LH levels may be elevated or within the normal limit despite low testosterone and gonadal steroids.

Prolonged physical exercise and extreme weight loss causes elevated corticotrophin releasing hormone (CRH) levels. Elevated CRH inhibits the pulsatile release of GnRH and thus leads to LH and FSH deficiency. Additionally, elevated CRH stimulates pituitary synthesis and release of ACTH which in turn stimulates adrenal synthesis and release of cortisol. Excessive circulating cortisol levels inhibits pituitary synthesis and secretion of LH, and thus ovarian estrogens and progesterone. Administration of exogenous glucocorticoids will exert the same inhibitory effect on LH synthesis and release.

Hyperprolactinemia of any cause (prolactinoma, Sheehan's syndrome, etc.) will inhibit LH and FSH synthesis and secretion from the pituitary. Sheehan's syndrome caused by infarct and hemorrhage of the anterior pituitary in pregnancy and during delivery (the increase in the size of the pituitary tissue during pregnancy exceeds the blood supply), the anterior pituitary hormones are either absent (panhypopituitarism) or decreased leading to low or undetectable LH and FSH levels and the associated clinical personation of hypogonadotropic hypogonadism.

Growth hormone (GH)

GH deficiency, a rare cause of short stature in childhood, could be isolated, idiopathic, or in combination with other pituitary disorders leading to short stature and poor growth in children. Other causes include hypothyroidism (high TSH, low thyroid hormones), chronic kidney disease (elevated urea and creatinine), malnutrition, and gastrointestinal disorders (fat malabsorption and presence of antigliadin antibodies).

The finding that testosterone in boys and estradiol in girls augment endogenous growth hormone secretion and thus IGF-1 circulating levels, and that prepubertal or patients with constitutional pubertal delay will often results in suboptimal growth hormone response following provocation, although not widely practiced, 50% of endocrinologists prefer to prime prepubertal children (testosterone in boys, 100 mg intramuscular injection for 7–10 days or oral 10–20 μg of ethinyloestradiol for 48–72 h in girls), some investigators use ethinyloestradiol for boys to avoid the intramuscular injections.

In the rare Laron dwarfism due to deficient GH receptor or to mutations in the receptor, patients' GH level is elevated in the presence of low IGF-1 level.

Dynamic tests are required to investigate GH disorders. The diagnosis of GH deficiency requires two positive GH provocative tests (due to likelihood for a false positive test). Low IGF-1 and IGFBP-3 levels support the diagnosis of GH deficiency.

Inulin-like growth factor 1 (IGF-1) mainly produced by the liver stimulated by GH In the circulation, it is bound to a number of binding proteins (IGF-1 BPs) with IGFBP-3 being the major carrier. Measurement of IGF-1 and its associated binding protein IGFBP-3 are preferred over GH as they are comparatively more stable and do not require provocative testing.

However, normal values vary with age and pubertal Tanner stage and thus appropriate reference intervals need be applied. Furthermore, chronic renal disease, diabetes, hypothyroidism, and nutritional deficiency cause low IGF-1 concentrations.

IGF-1 has a high specificity >90% but relatively low sensitivity (50%–70%) particularly in children less than 5 year old. The high specificity for IGF-1 suggests that low values are highly predictive of GH deficiency, but a normal level does not exclude deficiency.

A number of pharmacological stimulation tests are available; they include clonidine, arginine, glucagon, and GHRH administration, including nonpharmacological moderate to intense 20 min exercise, and measurement at the onset of deep sleep. A GH levels ≥ 7 ng/mL following any of the above dynamic test is considered as normal response and rules out GH deficiency.

More than one dynamic test is required as only 80% of normal children will respond to any single test. However, when using two stimulation tests 95% of normal children responded adequately. Commonly applied investigations of GH deficiency are summarized in Table 5.

TABLE 5 Summary of biochemical investigations of suspected GH deficiency.

Biomarker	Test	Comment
Grow hormone	Random	Unreliable affected by stress,
	Stimulated: Provocation tests Normal response Basal <10 mIU/L (<3.33 ng/mL) increases >20 mIU/L (>9.9 ng/mL)	Clonidine, arginine, exercise, hypoglycemia (insulin induced-not widely used)
IGF-1 and IGFBP-3	Random	Levels influenced by chronic kidney disease, nutritional status
Genetics tests	Idiopathic growth hormone deficiency	Several genes (including those associated with combined pituitary hormones deficiency)

IGF-1, insulin-like growth factor 1; *BP-3*, IGF-1 binding protien-3.

Genetic testing

Although not routinely available, testing for genes associated with growth hormone deficiency include genes that are part of the MPHD (POU1F1, PROP1, LHX3, LHX4, HESX1, OTYX2, SOX2, SOX3, GLI2, GLI3, FGFR1, FGES, and PROKR2). Patients with idiopathic growth hormone deficiency more commonly exhibit mutations in the GH1, GHRHR, and RNPC3 genes.

Genetic studies are warranted in children with idiopathic growth hormone deficiency with early severe (>3SD below the mean) growth failure, positive family history and consanguinity, and extremely low peak hGH and IGF-1/IGFBP-3 levels.

Thyrotropin-stimulating hormone (TSH)

Congenital hypothyroidism is a collection of disorders affecting the hypothalamic pituitary thyroid axis. Untreated patients develop cretinism and severe mental and growth retardation.

The majority (85%) of cases are due to thyroid dysfunction and the remaining 15% due to central (hypothalamic pituitary cause). The latter includes either isolated TSH deficiency which accounts for 40% of central causes, or part of a combined pituitary hormones deficiencies. Since hypothalamic TRH stimulates both TSH and prolactin, isolated central deficiency affects both TSH and prolactin.

Thyroid dysfunction as a cause of congenital hypothyroidism is an autosomal recessive disorder. The disorder is attributed to a s mingle base substitution in the codon for the 29th amino acid of the TSH β subunit gene.

Mutations in one of the five genes (IGSF1, IRS4, TBL1X1, TRHR, and TSHB) have been described.

The level of TSH before and after 200 µg intravenous TRH injection is used to assess the extent of TSH release.

One of the considerations is that, particularly in hypothalamic disease, TSH may be elevated but biologically inactive or with reduced activity.

Prolactin

Low basal prolactin levels are indicative of prolactin deficiency. This is often clinically obvious as in reduced lactation postpartum due to pituitary infarction (pituitary hypertrophy and reduced blood supply) as seen in Sheehan's syndrome. Although dynamic stimulation tests may be used, and prolactin release can be judged following TRH stimulation or by the insulin stress test. The latter is rarely used and not recommended. This is discussed in detail in Chapter 8.

Posterior pituitary hormones

Microscopically, the tissue of the posterior pituitary is neuronal in origin and represent an extension of the neurological hypothalamus. Hormones synthesized in the hypothalamus and stored in the posterior pituitary, this is in contrast to the anterior pituitary made up of specialized cells where respective homes are synthesized. The hormones stored in the posterior pituitary include arginine vasopressin (AVP) also termed antidiuretic hormone (ADH) and the hormone oxytocin.

Antidiuretic hormone (ADH) hypersecretion

Synthesized by the hypothalamus and stimulated by an increase in blood osmolality detected by the osmoreceptors, similarly a fall in extracellular fluid volume is detected by hypothalamic baroreceptors. ADH plays an important part in water metabolism. When fluid is withheld, the osmotic pressure of the blood increases and the osmoreceptors in the hypothalamus are activated and AVP secretion is increased. This causes an increase in permeability of the collecting tubules and an antidiuresis develops in an attempt to restore the plasma oncotic pressure to normal. Conversely, when fluid is given the oncotic pressure falls, AVP secretion is suppressed, and a diuresis occurs.

There are conditions where ADH secretion is inappropriately raised, e.g., cortisol deficiency, but the important hypersecretory state arises from ectopic production of AVP by nonendocrine tumors, particularly small cell bronchial carcinoma. This gives rise to a dilutional hyponatremia and a high urine osmolality. ADH increases water permeability of distal tubules of the collecting duct facilitating water reabsorption.

Decreased ADH activity

Main clinical interest is centered on decreased ADH activity which gives rise to the syndrome of diabetes insipidus (DI). There are two types: (1) cranial (sometimes called neurogenic or central) and (2) nephrogenic.

Cranial DI results from destruction of the ADH-producing nuclei in the hypothalamus (damage to the posterior pituitary alone does not produce DI) and it is, therefore, relatively infrequent compared with anterior hypopituitarism. Nephrogenic DI on the other hand results from the failure of ADH action on the kidney. This may be due to a rare sex-linked recessive disorder or certain drugs may be responsible.

Although the symptoms of polyuria and polydipsia are quite characteristic of DI, they are mimicked by patients with primary polydipsia (compulsive water drinking). Tests are, therefore, necessary to make the distinction. The simplest of these is the 8-h water deprivation tests. Since it is dangerous for patients to lose more than 5% body weight during the procedure, patients have to be weighed before and during the test. Samples are taken throughout for plasma and urine osmolality. A random urine osmolality >300 mOsmol/L rules out diabetes insipidus, often serum osmolality being <300 mOsmol/L and urine osmolality >600 mOsmol/L. High serum osmolality 300 mOsmol/L in the presence of inappropriately low <300 mOsmol/L urine osmolality is indicative of diabetes insipidus.

Having diagnosed DI the distinction between cranial and nephrogenic types can be made by assessing the response of urine osmolality to desmopressin (DDAVP) administration. When the water deprivation test is repeated after DDAVP, a greater than 150% rise in osmolality indicates cranial DI and a less than 50% rise points to the nephrogenic cause. DDAVP may be administered at the end of the water deprivation test without the need to repeat the entire test (Fig. 14).

The water deprivation test can be refined by including plasma copeptin measurements as well as osmolality. Some centers prefer to measure the plasma AVP response to infusion of 5% saline. However, copeptin assays are technically difficult and only performed in a few centers.

Diabetes insipidus characterized by the inability of the kidney to concentrate the urine and thus maintain an appropriate plasma osmolality as well as normovolemia. It is due to deficiency of ADH (hypothalamic-cranial DI), nephrogenic DI (inability of the collecting duct to response to ADH), or to primary polydipsia (excessive and inappropriate drinking of water) in psychogenic polydipsia.

Nephrogenic DI (impaired renal response to ADH) is a sex-linked recessive. ADH activity is also impaired in hyperglycosuria (diabetes mellitus), in hypercalcemia and in hypokalemia. It is also influenced by drugs such as lithium.

Investigation of patients suspected of diabetes insipidus (e.g., with polyuria (>3 L/24 h)), water deprivation test (used to stimulate ADH secretion) is perfomed. Urine and serum osmolality are measured following a prolonged water deprivation. Adequate ADH release and action at the distal tubule and the ability of the kidney to concentration the urine is exhibited by an elevated urine osmolality.

In patients with plasma sodium >147 mmol/L, copeptin levels ≥21.4 pmol/L is suggestive of nephrogenic diabetes insipidus and values ≤4.9 pmol/L are suggestive of central diabetes insipidus.

In patients with normal sodium and copeptin levels in the indeterminant, it can be measured following arginine stimulated. Levels ≤3.8 pmol/L suggests central diabetes insipidus and >3.8 pmol/L suggests primary polydipsia. In borderline cases, copeptin is measured following hypertonic stimulated release where levels ≤4.9 pmol/L suggests central diabetes insipidus and levels >4.9 pmol/L suggestive of primary polydipsia.

Patients with plasma sodium <135 mmol/L is suggestive of polydipsia as a cause of hypotonic polyuria and polydipsia. Copeptin is the C-terminal fragment of arginine vasopressin (AVP). It is stable compared to AVP that has short half-life in circulation and poor stability. Copeptin is stable for up to 7 days at room temperature and that several commercial assays are available. As the C-terminal of AVP, it correlates with AVP levels and thus considered a stable surrogate marker of AVP. Elevated basal (unstimulated) levels are indicative of

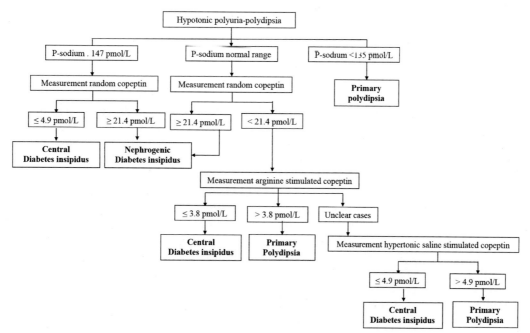

FIG. 14 Copeptin-based investigation of patients suspected of diabetes insipidus. *(Modified from Refardt J. Diagnosis and differential diagnosis of diabetes insipidus: update. Best Pract Res Clin Endocrinol Metab. 2020;34(5):101398. https://doi.org/10.1016/j.beem.2020.101398. Epub 2020 Feb 28. PMID: 32387127.)*

nephrogenic diabetes insipidus. Using either arginine or hypertonic solution, stimulated copeptin levels discriminate between central and primary polydipsia. Elevated levels post-stimulation suggest primary polydipsia whereas suppressed levels indicate central diabetes insipidus. An algorithm for the utility of copeptin in the diagnosis and differential of causes of diabetes insipidus is outlined in Fig. 14.

Oxytocin

A pleotropic peptide hormone, nine peptides long (Cys-Tyr-Ile-Gln-Asn-Cys-Pro-Leu-Gly-NH$_2$), is best known for its roles in partition and lactation. It is produced in the hypothalamus and stored in the posterior pituitary. Extra pituitary sources of oxytocin include uterus, placenta, corpus luteal, heart, and testis. It is structurally similar to vasopressin (differ by two amino acids) located on the same chromosome 20. A precursor preprohormone is made up of the signal peptide, oxytocin, and neurophysin.

It is released from the posterior pituitary in response to stimuli such as suckling, parturition, and stress.

Its functions range from a role in reproduction, general health, growth, immunity, antiinflammatory, antioxidant, and also implicated in social behavior and adaptation.

The original function of oxytocin is stimulation of contraction of the smooth uterine muscle during labor, milk ejection during lactation.

The oxytocin receptor is a member of the class I G protein-coupled receptor coupled to phospholipase C. The receptor is high affinity and requires magnesium (Mg^{2+}) and cholesterol for binding.

Hormonal measurement considerations

Most hormones including all those from the pituitary are typically analyzed by immunoassay methods, although chromatographic method (LCMSMS) are increasingly being used.

This means that immunological/structural activity rather than biological activity is measured and although this does not appear to mater in most clinical situations, it is possible to obtain a high level of immunoreactivity hormone which is biologically inactive, an example being TSH in hypothalamic disease and macroprolactin in false hyperprolactinemia. Assays specificity remains problematic for some analytes such as the small and structurally similar steroids. Another point of importance is that particularly with pituitary and adrenocortical disease, only limited diagnostic information is given by single tests and usually dynamic function studies involving gland suppression and stimulation need to be carried out. Additionally, hormone responses can be influenced by systemic disease and the activity of other endocrine organs, examples being the impairment of growth hormone (GH) release by high cortisol or low gonadal steroid levels.

Summary

- The human pituitary consists of anterior and posterior structures.
- ACTH, GH, LH, FSH, and PRL are secreted and released by the anterior pituitary.

- ADH, oxytocin are synthesized in the hypothalamus and stored in the posterior pituitary before being released into the circulation.
- Excessive ACTH secretion results in ACTH dependant hypercortisolism and is associated with either Cushing's disease (pituitary sources) or ectopic ACTH production (commonly the lung).
- ACTH deficiency leads to adrenal insufficiency and a state of hypocortisolism.
- Growth hormone excess due to a GH secreting tumors results in acromegaly (prior to epiphyseal bone fusion) and to gigantism postfusion.
- GH stimulates hepatic synthesis and release of IGF-1 which circulates mainly bound to IGFBP-3. The latter are better indicators for GH excess.
- GH suppression and provocation tests are essential for diagnosis of GH deficiency and excess as the latter is influenced by physiological factors such as stress. Suppression of suspected excess is achieved following glucose tolerance test (75–100 g glucose). Provocation tests include clonidine, arginine, and exercise.
- Hyperprolactinemia is caused by either pituitary adenoma (of the lactotrophs), or by interference with dopamine release as in stalk compression or use of dopamine antagonist.
- Prolactin exhibits molecular heterogeneity and up to 20% of patients may exhibit macroprolactin (high molecular weight complex of prolactin bound to antiprolactin antibody or aggregates of prolactin) which causes interference in some immunoassays. The prevalence thus depends on assays susceptibility.
- Isolated LH of FSH deficiency is rare. Often occur combined as part of panhypopituitarism syndrome. Genetic mutations leading to dysfunction LH β submits and or its receptor have been reported and lead to hypogonadism and Kallmann syndrome.
- Growth hormone deficiency can be isolated or combined with other pituitary hormones.

- Isolated TSH deficiency is a rare cause of congenital hypothyroidism.
- Prolactin deficiency (often secondary to postpartum Sheehan syndrome) is clinically suspected when there is postpartum lactation failure. Prolactin levels are low among other pituitary hormones.
- Antidiuretic hormone deficiency or reduced activity leads to diabetes insipidus. It can either be due to hypothalamic deficiency (cranial diabetes mellitus) or to impaired renal responsiveness to ADH (nephrogenic diabetes insipidus). Measurement of ADH (vasopressin) is not widely available, and that water deprivation test is often performed to investigate patients suspected of diabetes insipidus.
- Oxytocin, a pleotropic peptide hormone best known for its roles in partition and lactation. It is produced in the hypothalamus and stored in the posterior pituitary.

The adrenal gland

Introduction

This section describes the pathophysiology and laboratory investigation of common adrenal gland dysfunction.

Structure/function

The adrenal gland is pyramidal in shape; 2–3 cm wide, 4 cm long, and 1 cm thick. Two glands each sitting on the epic od each kidney. Blood supply is from the adrenal artery (from the vena cava) venous drainage with the right vein being shorter than the left adrenal vein. The right adrenal vein enters directly into the vena cava, whereas the left adrenal vein enters the left renal vein.

The adrenal gland is divided into two parts, the outer cortex (made up of glomerulosa, reticularis, and fasciculate) which produces mineralocorticoids, glucocorticoids, and androgens respectively, and an inner medulla which produces catecholamine (Fig. 15).

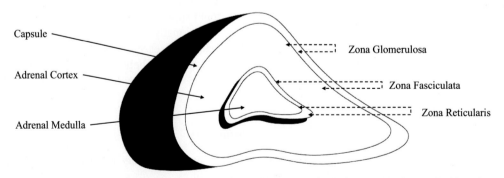

FIG. 15 Adrenal gland structure showing the capsule, the cortex, and medulla. Microscopically the areas are characterized into the zona glomerulosa, zona fasciculata, and zona reticularis. *(Modified from Hahner S, Ross RJ, Arlt W, et al. Adrenal insufficiency. Nat Rev Dis Primers. 2021;7(1):19. https://doi.org/10.1038/s41572-021-00252-7. PMID: 33707469.)*

The adrenal cortex

The adrenal cortex itself is divided into the inner reticularis and fasciculate zones, and the outer glomerulosa (Fig. 15). The inner zones produce glucocorticoids (principally cortisol) and androgens (DHEA), while the glomerulosa secretes mineralocorticoids (aldosterone).

Glucocorticoids (cortisol)

All the adrenal steroids including cortisol are formed from cholesterol in a series of enzymatic steps (Fig. 20), the initial one being under the control of ACTH. ACTH also causes adrenocortical hyperplasia. ACTH has a marked diurnal rhythm which is reflected in the early morning rise in plasma cortisol with the nadir during the night. This diurnal variation is overridden in stress when ACTH and hence cortisol levels are elevated.

Most of the plasma cortisol is bound to cortisol binding globulin (CBG) or transcortin and it is only the free form that is biologically active. Like other binding proteins, CBG is increased by pregnancy and oral contraceptive (OC) use. Cortisol has several physiological effects, the main ones being to take part in the maintenance of blood glucose levels and protein waste activity. Cortisol has a mineralocorticoid activity.

Measured by immunoassays where a rapid result required for immediate management can be obtained and reported as in patients suspected of adrenal crisis/insufficiency. Furthermore, in patients undergoing adrenal venous sampling (AVS) cortisol results are markedly elevated and exceed the immunoassay analytical measurement range. From a practical point, samples must be analyzed with and without dilution (minimum 1:5) so that cortisol result can be obtained during the initial assays run, as results are often awaited by interventional radiology to assure adequate cannulation prior to patient discharge.

Androgens (dehydroepiandrosterone (DHEA))

Quantitatively, although the most important adrenal androgen is DHEA, its activity is extremely weak. Conversion to androstenedione (itself weak) and testosterone, both in the gland and in periphery, accounts for the main androgen activity. As with cortisol, control is via ACTH, but there is no feedback mechanism.

Mineralocorticoids (aldosterone)

Aldosterone produced by the zona glomerulosa and is the main mineralocorticoid steroid. Its synthesis is induced by angiotensin II and is a constituent of the renin-angiotensin aldosterone system (RAAS). Renin is an aspartic protease enzyme produced and secreted by the proximal glomerular epithelioid cells of the afferent arterioles at the juxtaglomerular apparatus. It is released in response to low serum sodium, decreased extraocular fluid and blood volume, to decreased arterial pressure and to increased sympathetic activity. Renin cleaves 10 peptides representing angiotensin I from angiotensinogen. The latter is an alpha-2 globulin produced be hepatocytes, the kidney and other tissue, released angiotensin I is further cleaved by angiotensin converting enzyme (ACE) present in pulmonary capillaries, endothelial cells, and also in renal epithelial cells. Angiotensin II is the active form which stimulates aldosterone production. Angiotensin III is produced following removal of position one aspartic acid, but its activity is modest compared to angiotensin II.

A number of factors such as painful stimuli, upright posture, and decreased renal perfusion pressure stimulate renin production while recumbency and increased perfusion pressure are suppressive. Aldosterone itself has a negative feedback effect on renin secretion. In effect Angiotensin II is the main effector substance of RAAS.

Aldosterone is the main hormone responsible for sodium retention, potassium excretion, and blood fluid and volume regulation. As sodium is reabsorbed, water follows along the ensued concertation gradient.

Aldosterone can be measured by both immunoassays and by LCMSMS. Prior sample extraction may be required to improve assays specificity and sensitivity.

Similar to and complimentary to aldosterone, renin measurement is important in the assessment of hypertension. Renin can either be measured directly by immunoassays (mass units) or by its activity. In the activity assay, renin converts angiotensinogen to angiotensin 1. The latter is measured and reflects renin activity. The reaction is allowed to proceed for a specified period of time, and the angiotensin 1 produced is measured in terms of activity per unit time.

ACTH plays a minor role in mineralocorticoid control, the main mechanism being via the renin-angiotensin system.

The adrenal medulla

Catecholamine synthesis and metabolism

The secretory products of the adrenal medulla are the catecholamines, dopamine, noradrenaline, and adrenaline. Epinephrine release is controlled by sympathetic nervous system. They constitute a class of neurotransmitter hormones playing a role in the development of neurological, endocrine, and cardiovascular disorders. Most metabolism of catecholamines take place in the same cells where they are produced. Under normal status, the rate of catecholamines leakage is counterbalanced by sequestration. The rate of leakage exceeds that of baseline release, the contribution of catecholamines leakage to circulating levels predominates. Monoamine transporter sequesters 90% of leaked catecholamines back into the storage vesicles with

10% escaping sequestration and is metabolized in circulation. Thus, under resting states, much more catecholamines are metabolized secondary to leakage from vesicles than is metabolized after active exocytotic release.

They are formed from tyrosine in a number of enzymatic steps. Phenylalanine is metabolized to tyrosine as the first committed step in the reaction. Series of hydroxylases, decarboxylases, and methyl transferases play a role in the formation of catecholamines (Fig. 16).

Sympathetic nerves contain monoamine oxidase (MAO) but not catechol-*O*-methyltransferase (COMT). Thus, metabolism of norepinephrine leads to production of DHPG but not normetanephrine in intraneuronal metabolism and consequently metanephrine and normetanephrine are exclusively derived from nonneuronal chromaffin cell of the adrenal medulla.

The most interesting of these is the methylation process whereby noradrenaline is converted to adrenaline. The enzyme concerned is phenyl ethanolamine-*N*-methyl transferase, and it appears to be induced by the high levels of cortisol coming from the adrenal cortex. It is for this reason that only the medulla produces adrenaline while sympathetic nerve endings, and most of the brain, can only synthesize noradrenaline. This is why it was stated at the beginning there was a slight exception to functional separation of cortex and medulla.

In the cells, catecholamines are stored in granules where they are protected from degradation. There is also a releasable pool which responds to sympathetic nerve stimulation. Following release of catecholamines, they may be re-taken up by the cells, stored, and made available for re-secretion. On the other hand, they may be metabolized in the peripheral tissues by MAO or COMT to form normetadrenaline, metadrenaline and vanillylmandelic acid (VMA) (Fig. 17). These together with catecholamines are excreted in urine. Similarly, the excretion product of dopamine is homovanillic acid (HVA).

Function

It is very difficult to determine the physiological function of the adrenal medulla because it is a minor source of catecholamines. Consequently, hypofunction of the adrenal medulla, e.g., after bilateral adrenalectomy, has no clinical implications. On the other hand, tumors which excessively secrete catecholamines are important, the most prominent being the pheochromocytoma.

Adrenal disorders

Common adrenal disorders involving the clinical biochemistry laboratory are those of hyperfunction (Cushing syndrome, Conn's syndrome (hyperaldosteronism), catecholamines

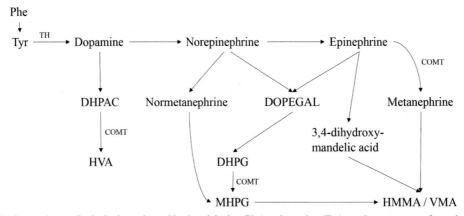

FIG. 16 Catecholamines pathways. In the brain, amino acids phenylalanine (Phe) and tyrosine (Tyr) are the precursors of catecholamines production. Catecholamine-*o*-methyl transferase (COMT), tyrosine hydroxylase (TH), dihydroxyphenyl glycolaldehyde (DOPEGAL), methoxyhydroxyphenylglycol (MHPG), dihydroxyphenyl glycol (DHPG), dihydroxyphenyl acetic acid (DHPAC), homovanillic acid (HVA), and 4-hydroxy-3-methoxy-mandelic acid (HMMA). (*Modified from Eisenhofer G, Kopin IJ, Goldstein DS. Catecholamine metabolism: a contemporary view with implications for physiology and medicine. Pharmacol Rev. 2004;56(3):331–349. https://doi.org/10.1124/pr.56.3.1. PMID: 15317907.*)

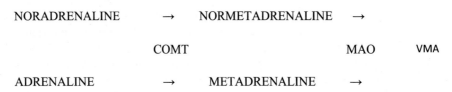

FIG. 17 Noradrenaline and adrenaline are methylated by catecholamine methyl transferase (MAO) and catechol-*o*-methyl transferase (COMT) to normetadrenaline and metadrenaline which are metabolized to vanillylmandelic acid (VMA) by monoamine oxidase.

(pheochromocytoma and neuroblastoma), and hypofunction (Addison disease). The disorders can either be primary of the adrenal or secondary. However, there is an important third category with a mixture of hyper- and hyposecretion of steroid, namely congenital adrenal hyperplasia, represents a group of metabolic disorders due to deficiency in one of the enzymes in the steroid pathways.

Cushing's syndrome

Patients with Cushing's syndrome are characterized by high circulating cortisol levels and often present with truncal obesity, striae, hypertension, myopathy, signs of virilization in women, etc. The clinical features are caused by excessive secretion of cortisol together with varying amounts of androgen.

It has several causes: (a) pituitary-dependent adrenal hyperplasia due to excessive ACTH, also called Cushing's disease, (b) adrenocortical tumors (adenoma and carcinoma) where ACTH is suppressed in the presence of markedly elevated cortisol, and (c) ectopic ACTH syndrome (extra-pituitary secretion of ACTH) as in small cell lung carcinoma.

The vast majority of patients with a provisional diagnosis of Cushing's syndrome have simple obesity with or without striae, perhaps with some hirsute and menstrual irregularity. It is, therefore, important to have a screening test to separate those with a probable adrenal problem for further study. The schedule of investigation of a suspected case would therefore be a screening test, if positive, confirmatory tests and then only if these are positive proceed to investigate the cause.

The often used screening test, a 9:00–10:00 a.m. plasma cortisol level, is often unhelpful. The level could be high because of stress or due to oral contraceptive use, while in a proportion of patient's morning plasma cortisol levels can be normal, the syndrome being due to inappropriately high levels during the afternoon and night. Most investigators would, therefore, recommend the overnight dexamethasone suppression test. Dexamethasone is given in a dose of 1–2 mg last thing at night. In a normal person, this suppresses ACTH secretion by the negative feed-back mechanism and the plasma cortisol next morning is suppressed to <150 nmol/L (<5.4 μg/dL). In Cushing's disease the pituitary is resistant to suppression while in the other two conditions, adrenal steroid and ACTH secretion are autonomous. The test is not infallible; depressed patients frequently fail to suppress, hence the need for confirmatory tests.

Tests which can be used to confirm the diagnosis of Cushing's syndrome are: (a) 24 h urine free cortisol test, which has the highest sensitivity and has been recommended as the first line of investigation, however, accurate 24 h urine collection could be difficult, (b) short and long, high and low dose dexamethasone suppression tests , and (c) diurnal rhythm studies.

The diagnosis is confirmed by finding a high urinary cortisol levels, failure of suppression with dexamethasone, and lack of diurnal rhythm

If the index of suspicion is very high but the investigations are negative, then the tests should be repeated at intervals because of the possibility of cyclical Cushing's disease (Table 6).

Having decided a patient has Cushing's syndrome, then the following tests can be used to determine the cause: (1) serum electrolytes (hypokalemic alkalosis suggests ectopic ACTH syndrome), (2) plasma ACTH (suppressed in adrenal tumors, if very high suggests ectopic ACTH syndrome), (3) prolonged high dose dexamethasone suppression test (suppression of plasma cortisol after dexamethasone 8 mg daily for 3 days strongly favors pituitary dependent disease, (4) CRH and metyrapone tests (excessive response of cortisol to CRH or 11-deoxycortisol to metyrapone favors pituitary dependent disease), (5) plasma androgens (a disproportionate elevation compared with plasma cortisol favors adrenal carcinoma), and (6) venous sampling (a search for ACTH gradients will help distinguish ectopic and pituitary ACTH dependence). ACTH levels >100 ng/L are often seen in patients with ectopic sources (e.g., small cell carcinoma of the lung). Investigation of ACTH-dependent Cushing's (Cushing's disease) is discussed in detail in "The pituitary" section.

Loss of cortisol circadian rhythm in Cushing syndrome results in high overnight serum cortisol levels.

Use of saliva as a sample type for cortisol measurement in the investigation of Cushing syndrome is increasingly being used. Saliva is an ultrafiltrate, and thus, assays detecting low free cortisol values are required. Salivary cortisol correlated with serum free cortisol levels and thus a midnight (late night 23 h) home collected saliva is used is a simple initial screen in patients suspected of hypercortisolism. There are no clear established cut values when using saliva sample and variabilities among assays limit its routine use.

It is worth noting that the majority (80%) of patients with ectopic ACTH exhibit hypokalemic alkalosis which is only observed in about 10% of patients with pituitary source of ACTH.

Conn's syndrome (primary hyperaldosteronism)

Primary aldosteronism is characterized by autonomous secretion of aldosterone from a single or bilateral glands. The prevalence is estimated to be 5%–20% among patients with hypertension.

One of the most common causes of secondary hypertension is primary aldosteronism. There are several causes of primary hyperaldosteronism, but the commonest is an aldosterone secreting adenoma or Conn's syndrome. The main features of the disorder are spontaneous hypokalemia and alkalosis in a hypertensive patient.

TABLE 6 Biochemical investigation of adrenal Cushing's.

	Biochemical tests	Comments
Initial investigation	24 h UFC (Sensitivity: 71%, Specificity: 73%)	Urine collection subject to errors. Increased levels due to stress or in obesity
	LDDST (1 mg overnight) Dose taken at bedtime about 23 h, and a blood sample collected at 9 h a.m.	Cortisol suppressed in normal (<50 nmol/L (<1.8 µg/dL) or undetectable). (Sensitivity: 54%, Specificity: 41%)
	LNSC (Sensitivity: 93%, Specificity: 96%)	Blood collection at night (hospital stay/phlebotomy visit required). Elevated levels due to stress
Secondary investigation	ACTH and cortisol measurement	ACTH suppressed in adrenal cause, elevated in pituitary source (Cushing's disease-ACTH dependent)
ACTH source	IPSS	Source of ACTH (elevated IPSS ACTH indicate pituitary source), Low IPSS suggests ectopic ACTH source
	HDDST (2 mg)	2 mg orally every 6 h for 48 h. normal response is >50% suppression of cortisol levels from basal at 24 and 48 h (80% of patients with pituitary dependent ACTH suppress, and 10% of ectopic ACTH suppress).
	CRH stimulation test	CRH (CRF-41) 100 µg intravenously. 25% increase in ACTH from basal in 80% of pituitary dependent ACTH. Extremely rare response to CRH in ectopic ACTH.

Once a state of hypercortisolism (Cushing's syndrome) is established, secondary investigations are targeted toward identifying the cause (that is pituitary vs adrenal source). *UFC*, Urine free cortisol; *LNSC*, late night serum cortisol; *HDDST*, high dose dexamethasone suppression test; *LDDST*, low dose dexamethasone suppression test; *IPSS*, inferior petrosal sinus sampling.
Modified from Raff H, Carroll T. Cushing's syndrome: from physiological principles to diagnosis and clinical care. J Physiol. *2015;593(3):493–506. https://doi.org/10.1113/jphysiol.2014.282871. Epub 2015 Jan 5. PMID: 25480800; PMCID: PMC4324701.*

The most common cause of primary aldosteronism is bilateral hyperplasia of the zona glomerulosa of the adrenal gland with aldosterone-producing adenoma being the second most common. The latter is cured following unilateral surgical excision of the adenoma containing adrenal gland.

Establishing the diagnosis of primary aldosteronism is a multistep process. Initial biochemical assessment is determining the aldosterone renin ratio (ARR). A range of ARR threshold have been suggested to account for the variability and lack of standardization with a positive screen ranging from >20 ng/dL per ng/mL/h up to >50 ng/dL per ng/mL/h.

The diagnosis is made by finding a raised plasma aldosterone in the presence of suppressed renin activity. However, certain conditions have to be fulfilled. Diuretics have to be stopped at least 4 weeks and hypotensive agents 1 week before the test. Unrestricted sodium intake is encouraged for a week, and the patient is admitted and sodium loaded. The following day plasma for aldosterone and renin assays are withdrawn at 8:00 a.m. (supine) and noon (4 h upright). As well as a high aldosterone and low renin in the "supine" sample, the "upright" specimen usually shows a paradoxical fall in plasma aldosterone in Conn's syndrome (Table 7).

The main biochemical difficulty can be differentiating primary from secondary hyperaldosteronism. In the latter, there is an elevated plasma aldosterone in response to ascites, renal artery stenosis, etc. However, in these conditions the hyperaldosteronism is renin mediated so in contrast to Conn's syndrome, renin activity is high rather than low. If doubt exists a captopril test will be helpful. The drug is without effect in Conn's syndrome but, being an ACE inhibitor, lowers plasma aldosterone in the secondary form.

Adrenal venous sampling

Adrenal venous sampling is widely used in the investigation of primary hyperaldosteronism (Table 7). The procedure performed by interventional radiology usually when imaging studies were inconclusive.

When investigating hyperaldosteronism, posture studies have an accuracy of 84%, adrenal CT 73%–90% accuracy, adrenal scintigraphy 72%–90% accuracy compared with 95% accuracy for adrenal venous sampling. Retrospective review of imaging studies and histopathology of tissue suspected of aldosterone adenoma often reveals high percentages of discordance.[9]

Therefore, adrenal venous sampling is performed with continuous cosyntropin infusion. This reduces fluctuations in cortisol levels secondary to stress.

The clinical chemistry laboratory plays an important role in the appropriate measurements of cortisol and aldosterone. Localized cortisol and aldosterone values are usually extremely high 10 to several 100-folds higher than peripheral levels and thus often beyond the analytical measurement range of the assay. High and serial dilutions are

TABLE 7 Screening and confirmatory modalities for primary hyperaldosteronism.

Procedure	Test	Normal response	Comment
Screening	Aldosterone renin ratio (ARR)	20–30 (55–83 pmol/L)	Lower if measured by LCMSMS
Confirmation	Fludrocortisone suppression	Suppressed aldosterone	
	Oral saline load	Urine sodium excretion >200 mmol/day	Urine sample collected at 3 days
	Intravenous saline load	Aldosterone <6 ng/dL (171 pmol/L) by LCMSMS <8 ng/dL (222 pmol/L) by immunoassay	Aldosterone level remains high in primary aldosteronism
	Captopril challenge test (furosemide upright test)	Plasma aldosterone is decreased by >30%, and plasma renin is increased, and ARR is reduced. A postcaptopril plasma aldosterone ≤11 ng/dL (≤305 pmol/L)	Captopril blocks angiotensin II production causing aldosterone suppression
	Adrenal venous sampling (AVS)	Unstimulated: ≥2 or ≥5 following ACTH. Lateralization ≥2 (unstimulated) or ≥4 after ACTH (1–24)	Endocrine Society (2016) and European Society of Hypertension (2020) recommendation
		≥10 while continuous ACTNH infusion. Lateralization ≥3	American Society of Endocrinology (2009)
		ACTH stimulated ≥5. Lateralization ≥2.6 (or aldosterone concentration > 1400 ng/dL on one side)	Japan Society of Endocrinology (2009)
		Selectivity ≥2 and lateralization ≥4	French Society of Endocrinology (2016)

Different but similar guidelines are in use by different endocrinologists. Aldosterone levels are measured either without ACTH stimulation or following a bolus injection of ACTH 1–24 or during a continuous infusion of ACTH with cutoff values ≥2, and ≥4 or 5, or 10 for diagnosis of aldosteronism and ≥4 for lateralization.
Modified from Reincke M, Bancos I, Mulatero P, Scholl UI, Stowasser M, Williams TA. Diagnosis and treatment of primary aldosteronism. Lancet Diabetes Endocrinol. *2021;9(12):876–892.*

required. Cortisol levels are urgently required as they are used to assess success of cannulation prior to removal of stents and discharge of patient from recovery suite. When cortisol values are indicative of unsuccessful cannulation, a repeat collection is often attempted. The clinical chemistry laboratory needs to have the assay ready and uninterrupted and that samples are processed both neat and at appropriate dilutions to facilitate obtaining a value immediately and avoid unnecessary delay due to requirement for sample dilutions. Successful cannulation is when adrenal veins cortisol is at least threefold higher than inferior vena cava levels. In some studies, a gradient of at least 5 to 1 is required.

Success of the procedure is operator dependent. It is difficult to catheterize the short (5–8 mm) right adrenal vein (RAV) and to close proximity to the posterior surface of the inferior vena cava (IVC). Procedure failure ranging from 10% to 38%. Cortisol measurement is helpful in assessing degree of dilution of adrenal venous blood. Calculating the aldosterone cortisol (A/C) ratio corrects for varying degree of dilution due to adrenal venous effluent with blood from the inferior phrenic vein (*left side*) or IVC (*right side*). Continuous infusion of ACTH removes possibility of ACTH surges due to stress affecting aldosterone levels.

Aldosterone levels are corrected for cortisol levels and are compared to both right and left sampling sources. A dominant side is identified and a ratio of dominant (aldosterone cortisol ratio) to nondominant ratio suggest lateralization to that side. The ratio must exceed 4 to indicate laterality. Furthermore, ratio less than 2 suggests bilateral adrenal hyperplasia (Figs. 18 and 19).

Adrenal samples require extensive sample dilution prior to analysis to facilitate timely results.

The above case is a representative laboratory findings and analysis in a patient with left aldosterone producing adenoma. The AVS cannulation was successful since adrenal veins cortisol levels were at least 3–5-fold higher than the inferior vena cava cortisol (in this above case is more than 23-fold). When correcting aldosterone levels for cortisol, the left adrenal vein aldosterone is the dominant at 4.94 versus 0.27. For lateralization, a contralateral ratio of greater than 4 for cortisol adjusted aldosterone levels for both right and left adrenal vein samples. This was found to be at 18.37 for the above case suggesting a left lateralization of an aldosterone-producing adenoma.

A representative laboratory findings and analysis in a patient with bilateral hyperaldosteronism is secondary to

Specimen Source	During ACTH Infusion		A/C Ratio $(x10^{-3})$	$C_{RAV\ and\ LAV}$ $\geq 3C_{IVC}$	Adrenal Vein A/C Ratio				$(A/C)_{Dominant}$ $(A/C)_{Nondominant}$
	[Aldo] ng/dL	[Cortisol] ug/dL			Dominant (D)	D/IVC	Nondominant (ND)	ND/IVC	
RAV	187.0	695.6	0.27	Yes	4.94	2.60	0.27	0.14	18.37
LAV	2840.0	575.2	4.94	Yes					
IVC (SRV)	46.0	24.2	1.90	*Yes*	◄ Overall AVS successful?				
PV	46.0	24.2	1.90	*Yes*	◄ $C_{PV} \geq 20$ ug/dL?				

FIG. 18 Biochemical findings in a patient being investigated for aldosterone producing adenoma. Aldosterone cortisol ratio indicate left aldosterone producing adenoma (example from the author's laboratory).

Specimen Source	During ACTH Infusion		A/C Ratio $(x10^{-3})$	$C_{RAV\ and\ LAV}$ $\geq 3C_{IVC}$	Adrenal Vein A/C Ratio				$(A/C)_{Dominant}$ $(A/C)_{Nondominant}$
	[Aldo] ng/dL	[Cortisol] ug/dL			Dominant (D)	D/IVC	Nondominant (ND)	ND/IVC	
RAV	3000.0	1287.2	2.33	Yes	2.33	1.72	2.33	1.72	1.00
LAV	2800.0	1200.8	2.33	Yes					
IVC (SRV)	61.0	45.1	1.35	*Yes*	◄ Overall AVS successful?				
PV	25.0	35.2	0.71	*Yes*	◄ $C_{PV} \geq 20$ ug/dL?				

FIG. 19 Biochemical findings in a patient being investigated for aldosterone-producing adenoma. Aldosterone cortisol ratio is similar and both less than 4 indicating bilateral adrenal hyperplasia without indication of aldosterone producing adenoma (example from the author's laboratory).

adrenal hyperplasia. The AVS cannulation was successful since adrenal veins cortisol levels were at least 3–5-fold higher than the inferior vena cava cortisol (in this above case is more than 26-fold). When correcting aldosterone levels for cortisol, both left and right adrenal veins aldosterone ratios were similar (less than twofold differences), very similar in this case indicating lack of dominance.

Which is further confirmed by a ratio of 1 when the left adrenal vein aldosterone is the dominant at 4.94 versus 0.27. For lateralization a contralateral ratio of greater than 4 for cortisol adjusted aldosterone levels ratios for both right and left adrenal vein samples is required. Lack of dominance in this case was further confirmed by a ratio of 1. This was found to be at 18.37 for the above case suggesting lack of lateralization and the presence of bilateral hyperaldosteronism production.

Congenital adrenal hyperplasia (CAH)

In CAH, there is a spectrum of disease depending on the severity of the condition. In the most severe expression, neonates present with salt loss and may die in Addisonian crisis. In addition, females have virilization of their external genitalia leading to sexual ambiguity. No such clue is, of course, present in boys. Those that survive into childhood develop increasing virilization which mimics puberty in boys (precocious pseudo-puberty). Initially, growth is rapid but epiphyses fuse prematurely and dwarfism is the end result. Affected girls may present with primary amenorrhea.

CAH results from an inherited deficiency of one of these enzymes (Fig. 20). This may cause subnormal production of cortisol, or aldosterone, or both. Although six defects have been described only the commonest, which is 21-hydroxylase deficiency, will be discussed. Since this enzyme is involved in both cortisol and aldosterone synthesis, its deficiency will result in reduced secretion of both steroids which results in the Addisonian-like clinical picture. As in Addison's disease the negative feedback will be activated inducing ACTH hypersecretion which causes adrenocortical hyperplasia and stimulates adrenal steroidogenesis up to the enzyme block. This excessive production of cortisol precursors serves as substrates for the alternative pathway, notable androstenedione and testosterone. Enhanced secretion of these accounts for the virilization.

In the case of 21-hydroxylase deficiency, diagnosis is made by finding a raised level of plasma 17α-hydroxyprogesterone, the metabolite immediately proximal to the block. Samples have to be taken at least 48h after birth to avoid delivery stress and interference from placental steroids. Patients are treated with a glucocorticoid, and if there is salt loss, they need a mineralocorticoid in the form of fludro-hydrocortisone as well. The glucocorticoid not only replaces the cortisol deficiency but suppresses ACTH leading to a fall in adrenal androgen production. Biochemically, the effectiveness of therapy is judged by monitoring plasma 17-OH-progesterone and testosterone levels while pediatricians also take growth patterns into consideration. A recent advance has been the introduction of 17-OH-progesterone assays on blood spots on filter paper so that patients can collect timed samples at home throughout the day.

Adrenal size increase (hyperplasia) under the sustained stimulation by ACTH due to the lack of feedback inhibition by cortisol. Genetic mutations leading to the deficiency on one or more of the enzymes (Fig. 20) with 21-hydroxylase being the most common. Diagnosis is made by finding of elevated enzymes precursor 17-OH progesterone in the case of 21 hydroxylase deficiency. Adrenal androgens are also

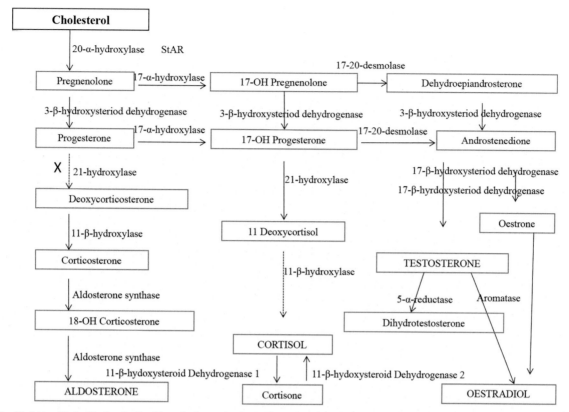

FIG. 20 Cholesterol is the biochemical backbone in the synthesis of aldosterone, cortisol, testosterone, and estradiol. Deficiencies in the enzymes, most commonly, 21-hydroxylasde and 11-beta hydroxylase cause accumulation of 17-OH-propgesterone in the first and 11-deoxycortisol in the second enzyme with concomitant increased production of androgens leading to the observed virilization.

In congenital adrenal hyperplasia, deficiency in the enzymes in the adrenal steroid synthesis pathway diverts accumulating precursors to androgen synthesis pathways. Nonclassical congenital adrenal hyperplasia is what is relevant here occurring at the prepubertal period with 21 hydroxylase deficiency being the most common exhibiting an elevated 17-OH progesterone. *(Modified from Rege J, Turcu AF, Else T, Auchs RJ, Rainey WE. Steroid biomarkers in human adrenal disease. J Steroid Biochem Mol Biol. 2019;190:273–280).*

raised (androstenedione), testosterone, dehydroepiandrosterone sulfate (DHEAS) causing the mentioned virilization. However, in 17 α-hydroxylase deficiency, androgen and cortisol levels are low, thus leading to female phenotype in the genetic male patient. Increased mineralocorticoids lead to salt retention and thus to hypertension.

17-OH progesterone is measured to determine the adequacy of steroid glucocorticoids replacement treatment.

Addison disease

Adrenal insufficiency following autoimmune destruction of the whole adrenals is the most common cause in developed countries, whereas infection (tuberculosis) in the leading cause in developing countries. Elevated ACTH due to lack of cortisol feedback inhibition leads to hyperpigmentation (ACTH has melanocyte stimulating activity), hyponatremia and hyperkalemia (lack of aldosterone). Samples for cortisol are collected prior to steroid replacement preferred, however, since dexamethasone is often used, the assay does not cross react with dexamethasone and some assays cross react with prednisolone although to variable degree.

Dynamic stimulation tests

Synacthen stimulation test (synthetic ACTH, the first 24 amino acids) is injected intramuscularly or intravenous (250 μg), cortisol levels >20 μg/dL (>500 nmol/L indicates a normal response and adequate adrenal function and reserve). Cortisol is measured in samples 0, 30, and 60 min following injection. Although an increment of 7 μg/dL (18 nmol/L) from basal is considered normal, stress may affect the results and prove a false low response therefore peak cortisol is more reliable.

Catecholamines disorders

Disorders of catecholamine are either inherited deficiency of enzymes involved in the steroid synthesis pathway leading to pheochromocytoma or to malignancy as in neuroblastoma.

Pheochromocytoma

Tumors of the adrenal medulla are classified as pheochromocytomas (Pheo "brown-back," Chromo "color" cytoma "mass of cells" as in Greek terminology). Brown-black color of the tissue due to oxidation of catecholamines when dichromate fixative is applied. They are rare tumors with incidence of 0.005%–01% of the general population and from 0.1% to 0.2% of the adult hypertensive population and may represent up to 60% of all adrenal incidentalomas with the majority being benign and 25% being malignant. The majority are clinically silent and about 50% are diagnosed at autopsy.[10] Recurrence of pheochromocytoma after resection occurs in about 6.5%–16.5% of cases where tumor size greater than 5 cm is a predictor of recurrence periodic testing for plasma or urine metanephrines is warranted for prompt diagnosis. Surveillance is recommended at 1, 6, and 12 months following treatment and imaging studies at 1 year. Annual laboratory values are recommended.

Clinical presentation is common to over 30 disorders. That is triad episodes of hypertension, anxiety and palpitation, and profuse sweating during an attack. Overall, they account for 0.2–0.6 of both systolic and diastolic hypertensions. Hereditary cases are usually benign whereas 10% are malignant.

Catecholamine hypersecretion produces a variety of clinical features such as hypertension, paroxysmal blanching, palpitations, sweating, psychic changes, impaired glucose tolerance, weight loss, etc. Pheochromocytoma thus mimics a variety of other diseases including diabetes mellitus and thyrotoxicosis. Depending on the storage, release, and metabolism of the catecholamines, symptoms may or may not be prominent. If the former, tumors are discovered early when they are small, while in the latter tumors grow large. This difference may be reflected in the results of tests.

The diagnosis is established by finding an elevated plasma fractionated metanephrines or elevated 24 h urinary fractionated metanephrines. Plasma metanephrines are considered superior to that of urine with less false positives.

Values indicative of positive findings include plasma metanephrines levels that are >4 times upper limit of normal and have a 100% probability of presence of tumor.

A result was considered to be normal if following clonidine stimulation, normetanephrine was less than 4 times the upper limit of normal and was reduced to below the age-adjusted upper limit of normal 3 h after clonidine administration or decreased at least 40% compared with baseline with a 100% sensitivity and 96% specificity.

As for dopamine, methoxytyramine, a metabolite of dopamine formed following methylation of dopamine by catechol-o-methyl transferase, is indicative of dopamine excess.

Small tumors less than 1 cm do not release much catecholamines and thus difficult to be detected whereas some tumors release only dopamine. The fractionated metanephrines are norepinephrine, epinephrine. Norepinephrine is the predominantly synthesized by the sympathetic ganglia and that epinephrine is synthesized in the adrenal medulla following norepinephrine N-methylation by phenylethanolamine N-methyltransferase (Figs. 16 and 17) which is localized to the adrenal medulla and stimulated by adrenal cortex cortisol.

Free normetanephrine and metanephrine circulating at low concentration have short half-life and are conjugated to sulfate by sulfotransferase isoenzyme, thus the sulfated metabolites have longer half-life, present 20–40-fold higher concentrations, and excreted into the urine.

The diagnostic tests vary from center to center, but urine studies are usually favored compared with blood. It is preferable to measure adrenaline and noradrenaline, metadrenaline and normetadrenaline, and vanillylmandelic acid (VMA). This has the advantage of estimating the initially released catecholamines and the later appearance of metabolites, so a longer period after an attack is covered. Up to three collections may be necessary to detect abnormally high levels when the symptoms are paroxysmal and it is best to ask the patient to collect during an "attack." If the ratio of VMA to catecholamines is high (reflecting rapid inaction), the tumors are likely to be large. If adrenaline and metadrenaline are increased, the tumor will probably be found in the adrenal gland. However, if necessary the site can be determined with venous sampling and plasma catecholamine assays. It is important to remember a variety of food-stuffs and drugs interfere with the tests.

If tests prove positive, then dopamine and homovanillic acid (HVA) levels may give additional information since these tend to be secreted by malignant pheochromocytomas and primitive neuroblastomas.

Finally, a positive finding will lead to consideration of the pheochromocytoma being a part of multiple endocrine neoplasia. There are a number of pheochromocytoma-associated clinical syndromes.

Normal metanephrines do not exclude pheochromocytoma. Effective tumor localization is improved by functional imaging with [123]I- metaiodobenzylguanidine (MIBG) scintigraphy of ^{68}Ga-DOTATATE-PET-CT.

Inheritance is autosomal dominant for pheochromocytoma-predisposing germline mutations. That is offspring of a carrier has 50% chance of inheriting the parent's mutation.

Unilateral or bilateral pheochromocytoma develops in 50% of patients with those associated syndromes. RET mutation carriers will likely have medullary thyroid carcinoma (calcitonin measurement). Patients with pheochromocytoma who are also of the MEN-2A, 20% of patients will have hyperparathyroidism.

Patients with mutations SDHx, TMEM127, MAX mutations will generally only exhibit pheochromocytoma and paragangliomas. Minority of patients with SDHx mutation will have gastrointestinal stromal tumors, renal-cell carcinomas, or pituitary adenomas (the 3P's syndrome: pheochromocytoma, paraganglioma, and pituitary adenoma).

Catecholamines measurement

Catecholamines are measured by chromatographic-based techniques where all metabolites are identified and quantified. Earlier methods used HPLC linked to electrochemical detector with recent development of LCMSMS methods. Although chemical screening methods are available for rapid analysis, they lack specificity. The diagnostic performance of the different catecholamine metabolites is shown in Table 8.

Following an overnight fast, blood ideally collected at a supine position after 15–20 min of intravenous catheters insertion. This is not practical for ambulatory population and clinics. Caffeinated beverages, strenuous physical exercise, smoking should be avoided 8–12 h prior to blood collections. Acetaminophen is reported to interfere with some normetanephrine assays, and cessation 5 days prior to testing has been recommended.

Measurement of catecholamines is subject to interferences by many compounds (Table 9). The following can influence catecholamines results as follows;

Dopamine, epinephrine, and norepinephrine cause negative interference in enzymatic creatinine assays, whereas the alkaline picrate Jaffe method is not affected.

Neuroblastoma

Elevated homovanillic acid (HVA), dopamine (DA), and vanillylmandelic acid (VMA) are diagnostic in neuroblastoma. The relative ratios have been associated with tumor staging. The sensitivity of combined analytes is 81.5% in stage one neuroblastoma.

TABLE 8 Diagnostic performance of catecholamines fractions.

	Sensitivity (%)	Specificity (%)
Plasma metanephrines	89.5–100	79.4–97.6
Urine metanephrines	85.7–97.1	68.6–95.1
Plasma (free metadrenalines)	99	89
Urine (fractionated metanephrines)	97	64
Plasma (catecholamines)	81	81
Urine (catecholamines)	85	86
Urine (total metanephrines spectrophotometry)	74	93
Urine vanillylmandelic acid (VMA)	62	93

Modified from Farrugia FA, Charalampopoulos A. Pheochromocytoma. Endocr Regul. 2019;53(3):191–212.

TABLE 9 Drugs and metabolites interfering in the determination of catecholamines when using different sample and different methods.

Drug	Effect
Tricyclic antidepressants	Increases catecholamines/metanephrines (Urine/Plasma)
Monoamine oxidase inhibitors	Increases metadrenalines (Urine/Plasma)
Calcium channel blockers	Increases cats (Urine/Plasma)
Nicotine	Increased cats (Urine/Plasma)
Caffeine	Increases cats (Urine/Plasma) HPLC interference
Methyldopa	HPLC interference
Labetalol	HPL interference
Levodopa	HPLC interference. Increases cats and metadrenalines (Urine/Plasma)

Modified from Grouzmann E, Lamine, F. Determination of catecholamines in plasma and urine. Best Pract Res Clin Endocrinol Metab. 2013;27:713–723.

Approximately 90% of neuroblastoma exhibit high levels of urinary HVA and VMA. Although screening increased the incidence of neuroblastoma, data on mortality reduction were inconsistent and on balance screening did not reduce mortality, and at least in some instances lead to harm (surgical complications). Currently, screening for neuroblastoma is not recommended. This may be influenced by the nature of the tumors where some regress spontaneously without intervention and that those that are aggressive often detected clinically prior to screening and results availability. They have the ability for spontaneous regression suggesting a wait and see strategy in some cases.

Summary

- The adrenal gland structure constitutes the cortex and the medulla. The adrenal cortex is made up of zona glomerulosa (secretes mineralocorticoids—aldosterone) and an inner zona fasciculata (secretes glucocorticoids (cortisol)) and androgens (DHEA).
- States of hypercortisolism is either due to cortisol production in response to excessive unabated ACTH production by an anterior pituitary tumor (Cushing's disease), or by an ectopic ACTH producing tumor (lung cancer) or to primary adrenal production.
- Aldosterone is the main hormone responsible for sodium retention, potassium excretion, and blood fluid and volume regulation.
- Aldosterone and renin levels are measured in the assessment of patients with hypertension.

- Primary aldosteronism is characterized by autonomous of secretion of aldosterone from a single or bilateral glands.
- The clinical features of Cushing syndrome are caused by excessive secretion of cortisol together with varying amounts of androgen.
- Cushing's disease describes pituitary dependent adrenal hyperplasia due to excessive ACTH.
- Urinary free cortisol has the highest diagnostic efficiency for Cushing syndrome. Other test modalities include lack of AM cortisol suppression following either low dose or high dosage dexamethasone suppression test.
- CAH results from an inherited deficiency different steroid pathway enzymes leading to subnormal production of cortisol, or aldosterone, or both and to adrenal hyperplasia secondary to the sustained ACTH stimulation.
- Diagnosis is made by finding of elevated enzymes precursor 17-OH progesterone in the case of 21 hydroxylase.
- Adrenal insufficiency following autoimmune destruction of the whole adrenals is the most common cause in developed countries.
- Catecholamine hypersecretion produces a variety of clinical features such as hypertension, paroxysmal blanching, palpitations, sweating, psychic changes, impaired glucose tolerance, weight loss.
- The diagnosis is established by finding an elevated plasma fractionated metanephrines or elevated 24 h urinary fractionated metanephrines. Plasma metanephrines are considered superior to that of urine with less false positives.
- Catecholamines are measured by chromatographic-based techniques where all metabolites are identified and quantified (using HPLC linked to electrochemical detector or by LCMSMS methods).
- Elevated homovanillic acid (HVA), dopamine (DA), and vanillylmandelic acid (VMA) are diagnostic in neuroblastoma.

The gonads

Introduction

This section describes the gonads (testis and ovaries) their structure and function and biochemical investigations of their dysfunction.

The testis and ovaries are the steroid secreting glands of the hypothalamic-pituitary-gonadal axis. Secreting testosterone and estradiol and progesterone in the male and female respectively; those hormones play a fundamental role in fertility and in the phenotypical primary and secondary sexual characteristics.

Similar to other endocrine pathology, disorders of the gonads are manifested by either an underproduction or overproduction of their hormones with resultant clinical features and symptoms. In states of gonadal dysfunction (hypo or hyperfunction), patients for investigation present with infertility, hirsutism, among other symptoms.

Dysfunction at the prepubertal stage leads to absent puberty and primary amenorrhea in female. Postpubertal onset results in impotence and infertility in male and infertility, secondary amenorrhea, and premature menopause.

Biochemical tests in the assessment of gonadal function include measurement of testosterone (total and free forms), estradiol, progesterone, anti-Mullerian hormone, inhibin, as well as pituitary hormones (FSH and LH).

The testis

Structure/function

In the male, there are two oval-shaped glands termed testicles. They are the site of spermatogenesis. Anatomically they are contained in the scrotum and hangs outside the body. Each testicle is connected to an epididymis leading to the vas deference.

The testes play a dual role as secretor of the androgen, testosterone, and as producer of spermatozoa.

Spermatogenesis takes place in the seminiferous tubules and under the influence of testosterone (produced by the Leydig cells) and the Sertoli cells producing inhibin, activin, and anti-Mullerian hormone (AMH), where LH stimulates testosterone secretion. FSH regulates Sertoli cell functions.

Depending on whether the ovum is fertilized by an X or a Y spermatozoon will determine the gender of the fetus. The primitive gonad of the fetus remains undifferentiated for about 6 weeks. The Y chromosome contains a testis-determining factor (TDF) and with differentiation of the primitive gonad to a testis comes secretion of testosterone and Mullerian inhibiting factor (anti-Mullerian hormone).

This fetal testosterone is responsible for development of the Wolffian ducts, vas deferens, epididymis, and seminal vesicles. If there is no Y chromosome then no TDF, hence absence of Mullerian inhibiting factor with development of Mullerian duct, uterus, fallopian tubes, and upper vagina.

The testis remains quiescent from the neonatal period until the onset of puberty when, under the influence of gonadotrophin releasing hormone (GnRH) from the hypothalamus, the pituitary increases the output of gonadotrophins FSH and LH which in turn lead to maturation of the seminiferous tubules, testicular enlargement, and stimulation of the Leydig cells to increase testosterone secretion. This initial stimulation of the testis occurs during sleep, eventually, as adulthood approaches, extending into daytime. This stimulation of LH in particular appears to be pulsatile in nature, occurring approximately every 90 min.

GnRH effect on LH is more marked than that on FSH. Causes release of LH in a pulsatile fashion, FSH pulsatility is less marked when compared to LH. Amplitude and frequency are important for adequate testosterone production.

LH is under negative feedback inhibition by testosterone. FSH secretion is inhibited by inhibin and stimulated by activin both produced by the Sertoli cells.

Inhibin is a dimer with alpha and beta subunits of 20 and 15 kDa molecular weights respectively. There are two forms of the beta subunits giving rise to inhibin A and B forms. In males, inhibin B is the more important form and is different from inhibin A measured in maternal serum for fetal risk assessment for aneuploidy. Both FSH and testosterone are necessary for inhibin production. Activin is a dimer of inhibin B subunit, and it stimulates FSH release.

Basal FSH and estradiol levels are used to assess ovarian reserve before initiating fertility treatment. Day 3 FSH levels >20–25 IU/L are suggestive of poor reproductive outcome. Basal estradiol >75–80 pg/mL are associated with poor stimulation and pregnancy outcome. Inhibin B produced by the developing follicles in addition to FSH and estradiol is used to assess ovarian function. Day 3 inhibin B <45 pg/mL has a pregnancy rate of 7% and spontaneous abortion of 33% compared with 26% and 3% when inhibin B is >45 pg/mL respectively.

At 7 weeks of gestation, anti-Mullerian hormone (AMH) is produced by the testicular Sertoli cells. It leads to regression of the Mullerian ducts initiating male phenotype development. Lack of AMH during embryogenesis causes development of the Mullerian ducts to internal female organs, uterus, fallopian tubes, and upper two-thirds of the vagina.

Testosterone

Testicular androgens promote secondary sexual characteristics which include development of pubic hair, enlargement of the penis in length and girth, pigmentation of the scrotum, growth of axillary, and other body hair such as the beard. Deepening of the voice, enlargement of the larynx, onset of libido, potency and male aggression are also secondary sexual characteristics brought about by increased secretion of testosterone.

Testosterone circulates in both a protein-bound and free unbound forms. It is generally accepted that the biologically active form of the hormone is the free form. About 1%–2% of circulating testosterone is in the unbound form; the rest is bound to a saturable sex-hormone binding globulin (SHBG), 60% strongly bound, and to the nearly unsaturable albumin fraction, 38% weakly bound. Albumin binds testosterone much less avidly than does SHBG which displays a much higher affinity constant with testosterone. It is argued that testosterone bound to SHBG is therefore biologically unavailable. Alterations in the circulating levels of binding protein may therefore dictate the fraction of the biologically active hormone that is available to the target organ known as bioavailable testosterone.

SHBG levels, and hence total testosterone, are affected by several factors. SHBG is increased in pregnancy, hyperthyroidism, cirrhosis, estrogen, and anticonvulsant use. Furthermore, it is decreased in hypothyroidism, glucocorticoids and androgens use, obesity, in poly cystic ovary syndrome, and in nephrotic syndrome.

Normal levels of circulating total testosterone in the adult male are unequivocally distinct from those of the adult female. In the male, the levels of testosterone vary between 10 and 35 nmol/L (288 and 1000 ng/dL) and in the female between 1 and 3 nmol/L (29 and 87 ng/dL).

In the adult male, a testosterone level greater than the upper limit of normal is of questionable significance. In the prepubertal male an increase in serum testosterone is of considerable significance and may be a sign of precocious puberty, resulting in pubertal changes before the appropriate age and height are reached.

Testosterone is converted to the more biologically active 5-α dihydroxytestosterone by the enzyme 5-α reductase. Additionally, testosterone is converted to estrogen by aromatase activity.

Of greater importance is a finding of a serum testosterone below normal in the male indicating the possibility of primary gonadal failure (associated with raised gonadotrophins) or hypopituitarism (hypo gonadotrophic hypogonadism). Other causes of hypogonadism (manifested by low testosterone) may be hyperprolactinemia, isolated gonadotrophin deficiency (Kallmann syndrome) or some of the intersex states such as Klinefelter's syndrome (47XXY). Although Klinefelter's may show either low or normal testosterone, the gonadotrophins, in particular FSH, are generally elevated.

The finding of low serum testosterone levels (at least two morning levels) less than 9–12 nmol/L (250–350 ng/dL) and elevated FSH and LH levels suggests primary hypogonadism. The finding of inappropriately low/normal LH and FSH levels suggests secondary hypogonadism.

Testosterone measurement

Testosterone is a C-19 steroid bound to SHBG (80%: men, 60%: women), and to albumin and cortisol binding globulin. Free testosterone is about 2% in men and 1% in women.

Production in men by testis is 24 μmol/Day and 0.04 μmol/Day by adrenal cortex. In women, production by ovary and adrenal cortex is 0.02 μmol/Day. 50% from peripheral conversion from androstenedione. Testosterone is converted to 5-α-hydroxy testosterone and is excreted as 17 oxosteroids, 1% excreted as testosterone glucuronide. Peripheral synthesis not significant in men. However, in women, 50% of testosterone is derived from peripheral conversion.

Testosterone is predominantly and tightly bound to SHBG, however, there is wide variation in SHBG due to diet, BMI, insulin concentration, age, and to pathological causes. This leads to changes in circulating free testosterone levels. Free testosterone is measured directly using highly sensitive immunoassays or by LCMSMS following equilibrium dialysis.

Bioavailable Testosterone (readily available, that is non-SHBG bound testosterone level is obtained following ammonium sulfate precipitation and is calculated as follows: Free testosterone $(\%) = 6.11 - 2.38 \text{Log SHBG} \times 10^{-9}$ or free testosterone $(\%) = 2.28 - 1.38 \log \text{SHBG} \times 10^{-8}$.

Assessment of testosterone status involves measurement of total testosterone (bound and free), free testosterone, bioavailable testosterone (fraction bound to albumin and prealbumin), and calculated free testosterone index with several formulas for its calculation. The formulas do not take into account changes in the binding proteins SHBG, albumin and prealbumin and their binding affinities. However, the calculations appear to perform well in males compared to females where the free androgens index performs better. In the latter, it corrects for changes in SHBG but not in albumin levels.

Use of formulas in the elderly and in patients with low albumin is problematic.

Investigation of suspected hypogonadism requires measurement of circulating FSH, LH, testosterone, SHBG, and prolactin. Hyperprolactinemia can be associated with primary hypothyroidism (TRH stimulates prolactin secretion). Increased SHBG can be the result of T4 stimulated hepatic synthesis.

In addition to the measurement of baseline tests mentioned above, the following dynamic challenge tests may be helpful; (1) clomiphene stimulation test—assesses gonadotrophin reserve by competing for hypothalamic receptors which results in increased gonadotrophin secretion is a normal response, (2) hCG stimulation test—for assessment of primary testicular failure. Intramuscular injection of hCG on 3 consecutive days should result in an increase of testosterone into the normal adult range if adequate testicular reserve is present, (3) GnRH—targets the pituitary as the site of hormone deficiency. Administration of the releasing hormone should result in increased release of gonadotrophins within 120 min, in particular LH in the adult and FSH in the prepubertal.

Testicular dysfunction

Testicular and ovarian dysfunction is characterized by; (1) delayed puberty: FSH and LH >20 U/L, FSH elevated (selective impairment of tubular function), low testosterone. Repeat analysis is required to confirm pattern. In a boy, testosterone levels near normal adult lower limit suggest spontaneous pubertal development, (2) hypogonadism: Male with low testosterone. Female with low estradiol/progesterone, (3) gynecomastia: in androgen deficiency and or estrogen excess.

Testicular hypogonadism in men is characterized by inability to maintain normal levels of testosterone, normal sperm (count and function) or both. Gonadotrophins (LH and FSH) are both elevated due to the lack of negative feedback from testosterone.

Primary and secondary dysfunction

Primary testicular failure is either due to congenital and inherited disorders such as in Klinefelter syndrome, chromosomal abnormalities or to acquired causes as in iatrogenic drugs chemotherapy and radiation. Mechanical and trauma damage (bilateral testicular torsion), systemic disease, and sickle cell disease.

In patients with primary testicular dysfunction, biochemical findings include low testosterone, elevated LH and FSH levels in addition to morphologically impaired spermatogenesis.

Similarly, secondary causes of testicular dysfunction are either congenital as in GnRH mutations (deficiency in GnRH) (see "The pituitary" section), or acquired due to hyperprolactinemia, critical illness, nutritional (obesity and eating disorders leading to severe weight loss). Pituitary damage (infiltrative disease, sarcoidosis, hemochromatosis), infection, and pituitary damage; apoplexy, trauma, and infarct (causes of panhypopituitarism).

Semen analysis

Cornerstone to the assessment of male fertility is semen analysis. Normal sperm parameters (count, motility, structure) rule out male infertility as a cause for lack of conception. Sperm parameters in essence reflects testicular function. Normal semen volume is about 1.5 mL.

As for sperm numbers (count), lack of standardization makes it difficult to define absolute values, however, sperm counts blew 20 million are associated with higher percentage of infertile men compared with their fertile counterpart. The lower reference limit is considered to be $\geq 15 \times 10^6/\text{mL}$ ejaculate.

Sperm motility (quality of motion) a marker of vitality where total motility (progressive and nonprogressive) of $\geq 40\%$ is considerd normal, similarly, a progressive motility at $\geq 32\%$ is considered normal.

Shape (structure): Sperm morphology (structure) is subjective and difficult to asssess, however 4%–10% of sperms appear normal ($\geq 4\%$ is required for in vitro fertilization procedures). Live and high vitality of at least 58% of sperms are considered normal.

A number of DNA-based assays have been developed. They evaluate the extent of DNA damage and the impact of DNA damage on reproductive outcomes. An example method is the sperm chromatin structure assays that uses flow cytometry to assess the intensity of acridine orange fluorescence that binds to native and fragments DNA. The percentage of DNA fragmentation termed DNA fragmentation index is determined. DNA fragmentation index (DFI) of ≤15% is considered normal, >15% to 25% considered fair, and ≥25% to 50% considered poor with DFI ≥50% considered extermely poor.

Experience suggests that most males presenting with impotence have a normal plasma testosterone and a psychological cause (rather than endocrine) should be sought.

The ovaries

Structure/function

The ovaries are two oval-shaped glands located in the pelvic and constitute the female reproductive organ. Anatomically located on both sides of the uterus and adjacent to the fallopian tubes. At birth, the ovaries contain about 1–2 million ovum and that about 300 will eventually mature and are released for the purpose of fertilization.

At maturity, the ovaries produce estrogen, progesterone, inhibin, and androgens. Estrogens are responsible for the development of the female secondary sexual characteristics such as body habitus, breast development, and endometrial changes. Progesterone supports the fertilized ovum and prepares the uterus for pregnancy and for implantation of the embryo. In combination with estrogen, it drives the menstrual cycle changes.

In the female, 50% of circulating testosterone is produced by the ovaries, and the rest is secondary to conversion of DHEA and androstenedione to testosterone.

Unlike the male, the female gonads act in a cyclical fashion in both the frequency of the hormonal production and in the resultant physical events. For convenience, the menstrual cycle can be assumed to last 28 days with ovulation occurring midway between each menstrual period. Starting from day 1 of the menstrual blood flow, the sequence of hormonal events is as illustrated in Fig. 21.

Upon maturity of oocyte (ovum), the ovulatory phase (rupture of follicle and release of oocyte) is marked by increase in LH initiating the ovulatory phase. The corpus luteum (a temporary endocrine structure in the ovaries) secrets progesterone preparing the uterus for possible implantation of a fertilized ovum (embryo) characterized by the luteal phase.

Estradiol exerts both a negative and a positive feedback to the hypothalamus/pituitary, the positive feedback stimulating LH secretion from the pituitary at midcycle, and then a negative feedback, facilitated through the hypothalamus.

Like the testis, the ovaries remain dormant until puberty and then, like the male, gonadotrophin is released in a pulsatile fashion initially during sleep, FSH being the predominant gonadotrophin prepuberty. Postpuberty, the amplitude of the LH pulses is greater than that of FSH.

Superimposed on this pulsatile release of gonadotrophins is the normal changes in the menstrual cycle.

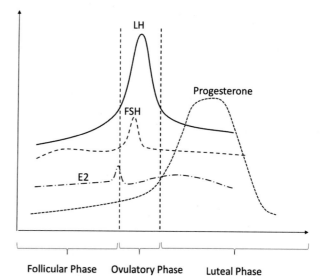

FIG. 21 Hormonal profile during the menstrual cycle. Increasing circulating levels of FSH and LH hormones reach peak levels at the midcycle (ovulatory phase). Progesterone reaches peak during the luteal phase and used to assess the adequacy of the luteal phase. *(Modified from Baker FC, Driver HS. Circadian rhythms, sleep, and the menstrual cycle. Sleep Med. 2007;8(6):613–622. https://doi.org/10.1016/j.sleep.2006.09.011. Epub 2007 Mar 26. PMID: 17383933.)*

Unlike the male gonad, the female eventually runs out of ova and the menopause ensues, characterized biochemically by a decline in the level of circulating estradiol and a concomitant increase in gonadotrophin secretion. Cessation of menses with a rise in gonadotrophin, especially FSH, with levels in excess of 20 IU/L, in women over the age of 40 (but sometimes earlier) is an indication of 1° ovarian failure.

The commonest cause of amenorrhea, however, is pregnancy characterized by a very high level of serum chorionic gonadotrophin levels and detected in the urine in the form of positive urine pregnancy test.

Amenorrhea is usually the presenting symptom in ovarian dysfunction. It is conveniently divided into primary and secondary amenorrhea. Primary amenorrhea is when there has never been menstruation and secondary when menstruation has ceased.

Anti-Mullerian hormone (AMH)

AMH, dimeric glycoprotein produced by the granulosa cells of the developing ovarian follicle and is used to assess ovarian reserve, which is a measure of oocyte quantity and quality. AMH levels decline with age and become undetectable at menopause. At 7 weeks of gestation, it is produced by the testicular Sertoli cells. It leads to regression of the Mullerian ducts initiating male phenotype development. Lack of AMH during embryogenesis causes development of the Mullerian ducts to internal female organs, uterus, fallopian tubes, and upper two-thirds of the vagina.

A number of immunoassays on automated analyzers are now available with improved precision and agreement between the different assay platforms. However, sensitivity remains a limitation for some of the assays.

It causes regression of the Mullerian ducts and embryologically in its absence and absence of testosterone, the ducts differentiate into female internal genitalia as its initially describes in 1947. Several biological function and importance was later identified.

Ovarian dysfunction

Ovarian dysfunction is characterized by infertility, amenorrhea, and hirsutism among others.

Biochemically characterized by low estradiol and progesterone levels. Laboratory investigations involve measuring various gonadal steroids and pituitary hormones and are often repeated to confirm the pattern.

Ovarian failure can arise as a result of hypogonadism or hypergonadism; both are discussed separately below.

Primary ovarian failure (hyper gonadotrophic hypergonadism)

Primary ovarian failure characterized by markedly elevated LH and FSH levels can be due to autoimmune disease, radiation damage or surgical removal, congenital hypoplasia, Turner's syndrome (45 XO), and to pure gonadal dysgenesis (46XX or 46XY).

Hypogonadotropic hypogonadism

Hypogonadotropic hypogonadism syndrome occurs in both men and women. It is caused by dysfunction at any point of the hypothalamic-pituitary-gonadal axis. It is classified as either primary indicating a dysfunction of the gonads (testis in men and ovaries in women). Or secondary due to dysfunction in either the pituitary or the hypothalamus.

The disorders are seen in patients with obesity, psychogenic disorders (e.g., anorexia nervosa), Kallmann syndrome, hyperprolactinemia, neoplastic or infiltrative disease, e.g., pituitary adenoma, vascular, traumatic insult, superagonist administration, and in athlete's hypogonadism.

Feedback suppression

Feedback suppression of androgens is seen in; congenital adrenal hyperplasia, virilizing tumors (adrenal or ovarian), and following androgen administration, e.g., anabolic steroid, whereas feedback suppression of estrogens is seen in estrogen producing tumors.

Secondary ovarian failure

Causes of secondary amenorrhea include pregnancy (the most common cause), in primary ovarian failure, menopause—physiological, premature ovarian failure (as for primary amenorrhea), in hypo gonadotrophic hypogonadism (as for primary amenorrhea), vascular (Sheehan's Syndrome), pituitary surgery, in excess sex steroid production, polycystic ovarian disease, congenital adrenal hyperplasia, virilizing tumors, androgen administration, e.g., anabolic steroids, and estrogen producing tumors.

Biochemical investigation of polycystic ovary syndrome (PCOS)

Polycystic ovary syndrome (PCOS) is the most common endocrine dysfunction during reproductive age affecting about 8%–13% of women. The pathogenesis is complex and includes genetic and environmental components. The system is characterized by a state of hyperandrogenism (infertility, hirsutism, acne, and alopecia).

There is chronic anovulation in the presence of elevated LH. Testosterone levels are 50%–150% increased among 90% of patients. In addition, patients have elevated androstenedione and Prolactin. Other biochemical abnormalities include insulin resistance (exacerbated by the hyperandrogenism stimulated adipose tissue accumulation), dyslipidemia, and impaired glucose tolerance. There is correlation between the prevalence of PCOS and obesity with prevalence being 4.3% and 14% in women with BMI $<25\,kg/m^2$ and $>30\,kg/m^2$ respectively.

It is postulated that the presence of high anti-Mullerian hormone (AMH) levels promotes hypothalamic GnRH and thus LH and FSH increased production.

There is no specific diagnostic test for PCOS; however, the syndrome is characterized by the presence of androgens excess (testosterone, DHEA), radiological evidence of polycystic ovaries, and anovulation. The presence of two of the three prior criteria satisfies the Rotterdam criteria (Table 10) for the diagnosis of PCOS.

Thyroid dysfunction (TSH and free thyroxin measurement), hyperprolactinemia (prolactin measurement), and late onset congenital adrenal hyperplasia, Cushing's

TABLE 10 Rotterdam criteria for phenotypes of PCOS (A–D).

Phenotype	Androgens excess	Ovulatory dysfunction	Ultrasound evidence for PCO
A	X	X	X
B	X	X	
C	X		X
D		X	X

Modified from Hoeger KM, Dokras A, Piltonen T. Update on PCOS: consequences, challenges, and guiding treatment. J Clin Endocrinol Metab. 2021;106(3):e1071–e1083.

disease, androgens producing tumors must be excluded as a cause of anovulation, hirsutism, amenorrhea, and androgens excess prior to making a diagnosis of PCOS.

Hyperandrogenism in the form of elevated testosterone is characteristic of PCOS. In females, 50% of testosterone is produced by the adrenal cortex, the rest is produced by interstitial cells of the ovaries and from peripheral conversion. The majority (99%) is protein bound mainly to SHBG and albumin, and only 1% is free and considered to be the active form as it diffuses reaching its DNA receptors.

Technical limitations include the fact that in normal women, circulating testosterone levels are much lower (0.2–2.86 nmol/L (0.06–0.82 ng/mL)) when compared to men (9.0–27.8 nmol/L (2.84–8.0 ng/mL)) respectively. Additionally, the presence of high circulating levels of estrogens requires careful consideration for possible interference and overestimation. For instance, measurements following extraction as well as the application of LCMSMS-based methods have significantly improved the accuracy and reproducibility of female testosterone measurements.

Combined measurement of SHBG and total testosterone facilitates calculation of the free androgen (testosterone) index. With the availability of reliable free testosterone measurement this is not frequently used. Slightly elevated testosterone (3–4 nmol/L (0.86–1.5 ng/mL)) in the presence of elevated free testosterone or its calculated index as well as an elevated androstenedione supports the diagnosis of PCOS. Whereas an extracted testosterone level less than 5.0 nmol/L (<1.5 ng/mL) makes the diagnosis unlikely. Normal DHEAS level distinguishes ovarian from adrenal sources (where it is elevated) when both testosterone and androstenedione are elevated.

The biologically active free testosterone may be calculated (estimated) as the free testosterone index $\%FT = 6.11 - 2.38 \log SHBG \times 10^{-9}$ or $\%FT = 2.28 - 1.38 \log SHBG \times 10^{-8}$ expressed as a percentage or measured. The concentration of free testosterone (upper limit of normal is 1.06 ng/dL) much lower than that of total testosterone (upper limit of normal 6 ng/dL) and thus requires a highly sensitive method.

Solvent extraction is preferred when measuring testosterone in female sera. Extraction is also recommended when estradiol is <82 pg/mL (<300 pmol/L). Androstenedione or DHEAS should be measured if testosterone is normal, and there is high index of suspicion for hyperandrogenism.

Antimullerian hormone (AMH) considered a surrogate marker of number of follicles per ovary (often determined by ultrasound); however, there is lack of assays standardization and thus marked variability among the different studies. In patients with PCOS, median AMH levels ranged from 20 to 81.6 pmol/L compared with normal subjects levels of 16.7–33.5 pmol/L. Levels are two to three folds higher in PCOS compared with normal women, but often overlap between patients and normal women and is more apparent in the adolescence stage.

Comorbidities of PCOS include metabolic syndrome, cardiovascular risk, diabetes, dyslipidemia, hypertension, psychological and emotional disorders. A1c should be measured every 3 years and assessed for type 2 DM using an oral glucose tolerance test initially performed during the first trimester and repeated in the second trimester.

Hirsutism

Hirsutism is a state of excessive hair growth in a female but of a male pattern. Hypertrichosis is excessive hair in a normal female distribution of nonsexual distribution. Hirsutism with a prevalence of 5%–15% reflects a state of hyperandrogenism.

Hirsutism is seen in a number of disorders including; polycystic ovary syndrome (PCOS) (71% of cases), idiopathic hyperandrogenism (15% of cases), idiopathic hirsutism (10% of cases), late onset congenital adrenal hyperplasia (3% of cases), androgens secreting tumors (e.g., ovarian and adrenal tumors (0.3% of cases)), iatrogenic causes (androgens treatment, anabolic steroids use, valproate intake), pituitary and adrenal disorders (acromegaly, prolactinoma), Cushing's syndrome, and thyroid disorders, and stress (the latter are rare causes and the relative prevalence is undefined).

Late onset (nonclassical) CAH commonly due to 21-hydroxylse deficiency leading to elevated levels of the precursor 17-hydroxyprogesterone.

Onset of hirsutism as well as clinical presentation provide clues to the cause. A rapid onset within few months in contrast to several months up to a year is often related to androgens producing tumors, compared to other causes in the latter.

Biochemical measurements include morning testosterone, thyroid function tests (TSH/FT4), prolactin, dehydroepiandrosterone (DHEA) and dehydroepiandrosterone sulfate (DHEAS), and 17-hydroxyprogesterone.

Adrenal androgens secreting tumors are associated with markedly elevated cortisol, DHEA and DHEAS levels.

Diagnostic sensitivity of 17-OH progesterone measurement is improved post-ACTH stimulation where elevated levels but are ≤1000 ng/dL suggest the patient is heterozygous carrier of 21-hydroxlase deficiency, and that levels >1000 ng/dL indicate the presence of late onset (nonclassical) CAH.

Mildly elevated testosterone suggests PCOS, whereas elevated testosterone in the presence of normal ovulation, and that ovarian and adrenal dysfunction is ruled out, the patient likely has idiopathic hyperandrogenism.

Idiopathic hirsutism is by elimination of all other causes that is when biochemical investigations were all unremarkable.

Iatrogenic causes of hirsutism are due to intake of drugs such as valproate, cyclosporine (Sandimmune), danazol, diazoxide, glucocorticoids, and testosterone, as well as use of anabolic steroids.

There is no correlation between the extent of hirsutism and testosterone levels. Free testosterone is the biologically active form, and its measurement is preferred. However, it is often difficult to measure reliably, the preferred methodology being equilibrium dialysis-mass spectrometry. Steroid assays suffer from limitations due to interference from similar steroids and changes in protein binding. For instance, the changes in sex hormone binding globulin (SHBG) seen during pregnancy, in patients with hepatic and renal dysfunction interferes with steroid-antibody binding.

Puberty

This is a process of physiological and psychological maturation. The onset of which is determined by familial, genetic, and neuroendocrine factors. Those factors are modulated by environmental, psychological, nutritional, and physical exercise confounders.

Activation of neuroendocrine network by kisspeptin leads to pulsatile release of GnRH. The secretion of kisspeptin by the hypothalamus is in itself pulsatile in nature. The result is pulsatile production of LH, the amplitude and frequency of which is central to the development of puberty.

Delayed puberty

Delayed puberty describes the absence of thelarche at the age of 13 years in girls (lack of breast development) and 14 years in boys (lack of testicular enlargement). It is defined as the absence of physical signs of puberty by 2–2.5 standard deviation above the mean age. It affects approximately 2% of adolescents.

Patients with delayed puberty exhibit low basal FSH and LH levels and also low levels following GnRH stimulation test.

Precautious puberty

Precautious puberty denotes the onset of puberty, development, and appearance of secondary sex characteristics before the age of 8 years in girls and before age of 9 years in boys.

It is 8 times more common in girls than boys. Premature breast development, pubic hair, and growth acceleration raise concerns often among patients and their parents.

Patients with high clinical suspicion for central precautious puberty are diagnosed following a GnRH stimulation test. A peak LH >5–7 mIU/mL at 30 min is diagnostic.

Administration of therapeutic GnRH is the mainstay. It suppresses the required pulsatile LH production and thus declines progression in pubertal characteristics within 3–6 months.

Gynecomastia

Gynecomastia is the enlargement of male breast, frequently seen in newborns, adolescents, and the elderly. In 25% of cases, it often resolves spontaneously and is termed a physiological form.

It is often due to imbalance between estradiol and testosterone ratio. Increased estradiol to testosterone ratio (that is in all forms of male hypogonadism) contributes to gynecomastia.

Gynecomastia is present in about 70% of patients with Klinefelter syndrome, the most common chromosomal anomaly associated with hypogonadism.

Estrogen excess is seen in feminizing adrenal tumors due to increased adrenal estrogens. Other causes of estrogens excess, in addition to exogenous administration, is secondary to reduced clearance and to increased aromatization. Increased production of hCG leads to gynecomastia, where hCG increases aromatase activity in Leydig cells resulting in excess estradiol levels compared to reduced testosterone levels.

Hyperthyroidism results in increased testosterone, SHBG, and estradiol. The increased SHBG binds testosterone and thus reduces the biologically active free testosterone in relation to the increased estradiol and thus leads to gynecomastia. Similarly, hypothyroidism results in reduced testosterone production and thus impaired ratio to estradiol and thus also leads to gynecomastia. Hypothyroidism among other causes of hyperprolactinemia results in secondary hypogonadism and hence associated with gynecomastia.

Adipose tissue converts testosterone to estradiol via aromatization and is the main source of estradiol in obesity. Aromatase activity increases with age and explains the gynecomastia seen among the elderly.

In addition to exogenous estrogen and growth hormone, a number of therapeutic drugs cause gynecomastia, they include: ketoconazole, spironolactone, and calcium channel blockers, methotrexate, cisplatin, vincristine, melphalan, amiodarone, amphetamines, digoxin, methadone, cannabinoids, among many others.

Summary

- The testis and ovaries are the steroid secreting glands of the hypothalamic-pituitary-gonadal axis.
- Biochemical tests in the assessment of gonadal function include testosterone (total and free forms), estradiol, progesterone, anti-Mullerian hormone, inhibin, as well as pituitary hormones (FSH and LH).
- Testicular androgens promote secondary sexual characteristics.
- Testosterone circulates in both a protein-bound and free unbound forms. It is generally accepted that the biologically active form of the hormone is the free form. About 1%–2% of circulating testosterone is in the unbound form.
- Testosterone is converted to dihydrotestosterone via 5-α hydroxylase enzyme.
- Primary testicular failure is either due to congenital and inherited disorders such as in Klinefelter syndrome, chromosomal abnormalities, or to acquired causes.

- During the menstrual cycle, increasing circulating levels of FSH and LH hormones reach peak levels at the midcycle (ovulatory phase). Progesterone reaches peak during the luteal phase and used to assess the adequacy of the luteal phase.
- Anti-Mullerian hormone (AMH) is produced by the granuloma cells of developing follicles and is used to assess ovarian reserve, which is a measure of oocyte quantity and quality.
- Primary ovarian failure characterized by markedly elevated LH and FSH levels.
- Polycystic ovary syndrome (PCOS) is the most common endocrine dysfunction during reproductive age affecting about 8%–13% of women. There is chronic anovulation in the presence of elevated LH. Testosterone levels are 50%–150% increased in 90% of patients.
- Hirsutism is a state of excessive hair growth in a female but of a male pattern.
- Patients with delayed puberty exhibit low basal FSH and LH levels and also low following GnRH stimulation test.
- In patients with high clinical suspicion for central precautious puberty is diagnosed following a GnRH stimulation test. A peak LH >5–7 mIU/mL at 30 min is diagnostic.
- Gynecomastia is often due to imbalance between estradiol and testosterone ratio.
- Gynecomastia is present in about 70% of patients with Klinefelter syndrome, the most common chromosomal anomaly associated with hypogonadism.

References

1. Tunbridge WM, Evered DC, Hall R, et al. The spectrum of thyroid disease in a community: the Whickham survey. *Clin Endocrinol (Oxf)*. 1977;7(6):481–493.
2. Carroll R, Matfin G. Endocrine and metabolic emergencies: thyroid storm. *Ther Adv Endocrinol Metab*. 2010;1(3):139–145.
3. Pappa T, Refetoff S. Resistance to thyroid hormone beta: a focused review. *Front Endocrinol (Lausanne)*. 2021;12:656551.
4. Laure Giraudet A, Al Ghulzan A, Auperin A, et al. Progression of medullary thyroid carcinoma: assessment with calcitonin and carcinoembryonic antigen doubling times. *Eur J Endocrinol*. 2008;158(2):239–246.
5. Esfandiari NH, Papaleontiou M. Biochemical testing in thyroid disorders. *Endocrinol Metab Clin North Am*. 2017;46(3):631–648.
6. Rodgers SF, Lew JI. The parathyroid hormone assay. *Endocr Pract*. 2011;17(Suppl. 1):2–6.
7. Stevens A, White A. ACTH: cellular peptide hormone synthesis and secretory pathways. *Results Probl Cell Differ*. 2010;50:63–84.
8. England RW, Geer EB, Deipolyi AR. Role of venous sampling in the diagnosis of endocrine disorders. *J Clin Med*. 2018;7(5):114. https://doi.org/10.3390/jcm7050114. PMID: 29757946; PMCID: PMC5977153.
9. Rehan M, Raizman JE, Cavalier E, Don-Wauchope AC, Holmes DT. Laboratory challenges in primary aldosteronism screening and diagnosis. *Clin Biochem*. 2015;48(6):377–387.
10. Farrugia FA, Charalampopoulos A. Pheochromocytoma. *Endocr Regul*. 2019;53(3):191–212.

Further reading

Wassner AJ, Brown RS. Congenital hypothyroidism: recent advances. *Curr Opin Endocrinol Diabetes Obes*. 2015;22(5):407–412.

Dashe JS, Casey BM, Wells CE, et al. Thyroid-stimulating hormone in singleton and twin pregnancy: importance of gestational age-specific reference ranges. *Obstet Gynecol*. 2005;106(4):753–757.

Chinoy A, Murray PG. Diagnosis of growth hormone deficiency in the paediatric and transitional age. *Best Pract Res Clin Endocrinol Metab*. 2016;30(6):737–747.

Hoeger KM, Dokras A, Piltonen T. Update on PCOS: consequences, challenges, and guiding treatment. *J Clin Endocrinol Metab*. 2021;106(3):e1071–e1083.

Bilezikian JP. Hypoparathyroidism. *J Clin Endocrinol Metab*. 2020;105:6.

Kola B, Grossman AB. Dynamic testing in Cushing's syndrome. *Pituitary*. 2008;11(2):155–162.

Halsall DJ, Oddy S. Clinical and laboratory aspects of 3,3′,5′-triiodothyronine (reverse T3). *Ann Clin Biochem*. 2021;58(1):29–37.

Matheson E, Bain J. Hirsutism in women. *Am Fam Physician*. 2019;100(3):168–175.

Sansone A, Romanelli F, Sansone M, Lenzi A, Di Luigi L. Gynecomastia and hormones. *Endocrine*. 2017;55(1):37–44.

Hung A, Ahmed S, Gupta A, et al. Performance of the aldosterone to renin ratio as a screening test for primary aldosteronism. *J Clin Endocrinol Metab*. 2021;106(8):2423–2435.

Reincke M, Bancos I, Mulatero P, Scholl UI, Stowasser M, Williams TA. Diagnosis and treatment of primary aldosteronism. *Lancet Diabetes Endocrinol*. 2021;9(12):876–892.

Dye AM, Nelson GB, Diaz-Thomas A. Delayed puberty. *Pediatr Ann*. 2018;47(1):e16–e22.

Chapter 2

Electrolytes and fluid balance

Introduction

Water and electrotype balance is essential for organ and body functions. Water and electrolyte imbalance is common among hospitalized patients and is also present among outpatients particularly those on long-term medications. The kidney, primarily as well as other organs including those of the endocrine system, maintains fluid homoeostasis. This chapter describes the pathophysiology of water and electrolytes disorders and their biochemical assessment.

Water and extracellular fluid homoeostasis

Total body water content represents 58%–60% of body weight in males and about 50%–55% in females and is distributed throughout the intra- and extracellular space with approximately two-thirds being intracellular, with intracellular fluid being double that in the extracellular space. Therefore, a 70 kg man will have 42 L with 28 L being intracellular and 14 L extracellular. The latter is distributed between the vascular space with 2.8–3.5 L (4%–5% of body weight) and the interstitial space with 10.5–11.2 L (15%–16% of body weight). Interstitial fluid returns to the venous systems vial the lymphatics. Blood volume is about 5 L made up of 2 L of red blood cells (RBCs) and 3 L of plasma water.

Water total body content is maintained by a number of homeostatic mechanisms (see later). Water intake is either orally (controlled by thirst) or intravenously (by medical therapeutic fluid management) and can be lost via the kidney, intestine, lungs, and skin. Losses can be either sensible (under physiological control) or insensible due for instance to environmental factors such as sweat and breathing rate (lungs). Water losses are about 800 mL daily to reduce body heat (higher amount in hot dry environment), 900 mL per day for minimal urinary function of excretion of urea and metabolic products.

Formulas for the calculation of body water depend on gender, weight, and height. They include the Watson formula: [$-2.097 + 0.2466 \times$ weight (kg) $+ 0.1069 \times$ height (cm)] for females, and [$+2.447 + 0.3362 \times$ weight (kg) $+ 0.1074 \times$ height (cm) $- 0.09156 \times$ age (years)] for males and the Hume formula:

[$-35.270121 + 0.183809 \times$ weight (kg) $+ 0.34454 \times$ height (cm)] for females, and [$-14.012934 + 0.296785 \times$ weight (kg) $+ 0.194786 \times$ height (cm)] for males.

Water diffuses freely through aquaporin membrane channels between various fluid compartments often down a concentration gradient to achieve osmotic balance.

Osmolarity defined as the concentration of osmotically active substances expressed as osmoles per liter of solution, whereas osmolality represents the concentration of osmotically active substances expressed as osmoles per solute per kilogram of solvent. It is directly proportional to the colligative properties of the solution, that is osmotic pressure, freezing point depression, vapor pressure lowering, and increase in boiling point. It is the freezing point depression and less common vapor pressure properties that are utilized in the measurement of samples osmolality (see later and Chapter 17 on analytical methods).

Factors contributing to fluid distribution

Water and electrolyte homeostasis are closely interlinked. Water follows sodium down a concentration gradient that is dependent on several factors including concentrations (osmolality) of significant solutes (see later), their relative size, charge, associated molecules and their extent and ability to dissociate, membranes permeability, colloidal oncotic pressure, presence of active and passive transport mechanisms, intact osmotic sensory organs, among others. Imbalances in electrolytes and water can be due to internal redistribution between the various body compartments and to external factors reflecting balance between input and output.

Sodium, potassium, and glucose are considered as effective osmolytes (osmotically active substances), whereas urea is considered ineffective due to its diffusible property.

To understand fluid balance and mechanism of maintenance of homeostasis, physiochemical principles as well as metabolism of contributing biomolecules are highlighted below:

Extracellular proteins

Albumin is the major circulating intravascular protein at 40 g/L. Since diffusion depends on the size of the molecules,

Tutorials in Clinical Chemistry. https://doi.org/10.1016/B978-0-12-822949-1.00015-2

proteins are not diffusible and thus provide oncotic pressure and therefore, albumin being the main driving force for colloidal oncotic pressure. This helps retain fluid within the intravascular space. In contrast, albumin concentration in interstitial space is about 10 g/L.

The overall content of albumin is however equal between the intravascular and interstitial fluid, that is 40 g/L for a total volume of 3 L (120 g) and 10 g/L for a volume of about 12 L (120 g), respectively.

One additional protein-associated factor contributing to water distribution between body fluid compartments is the contribution of the net charge on the predominant extracellular albumin. The negative charge on albumin coupled with its confinement within the extracellular fluid causes ion redistribution between extracellular and intracellular compartments, known as the Gibbs-Donnan effect.

Sodium is attracted by the negatively charged albumin, whereas chloride and bicarbonate are repelled out of the intravascular capillary space. This effect causes a change in ionic concentrations between intravascular and interstitial fluid. This difference, known as the anion gap, in ion concentation is small about 0.4 mmol/L but significant compared to the albumin concentration of 0.6 mmol/L (expressed in SI units) and that for every 1 g/L decrease in albumin level, anion gap will decrease by 0.25 mmol/L. Both albumin and associated ions contribute to the colloid osmotic pressure of about 24 mmHg (albumin contributes 13 mmHg and ions due to the Gibbs-Donnan effect contribute 11 mmHg).

Electrolytes

The majority of the osmotic cation sodium and its associated chloride and bicarbonate (HCO_3^-) anions are present extracellularly (Table 1). Their concentrations (osmolality) thus determine the extracellular volume as water is freely permeable between the extra- and intracellular fluid compartments and its movement follows osmolality gradient.

Metabolites and solutes

Major solutes contributing to osmolality are glucose and urea (blood urea nitrogen (BUN)). However, since those do not dissociate, one millimole equates one milliosmole compared with nearly fully dissociating sodium chloride and sodium bicarbonate (i.e., one millimole nearly equates to two milliosmole). Intracellular accumulation of metabolites and macromolecules such as organic phosphates and their associate cations increases intracellular osmolality and thus draws water into the cells.

Osmolality

Osmolality of body fluids is determined by the number of dissolved solutes such as electrolytes, glucose, and urea.

Some molecules dissociate fully and thus equally contribute to osmolality, whereas some for instance, sodium chloride dissociates into sodium and chloride although at not exactly at twofold but at 1.86. Distribution of these osmotically active particles depends on the permeability of the membrane and the size of the particles concerned. Proteins are examples of nondiffusible ions.

Urea and glucose contribute to osmolality, whereas urea diffuses into cells slowly, glucose is actively transported into cells and metabolized, however in diabetes, metabolism is impaired and glucose accumulates leading to increased intravascular osmolality and thus to cells dehydration.

Colligative properties (freezing point and vapor pressure) of a fluid change following addition of solutes to solvents. In clinical practice, fluid osmolality is widely measured by determination of the freezing point depression. The more osmotic the particles present the higher the osmolality and the lower the freezing point. The deviation (i.e., depression) from the point ((temperature (freezing or dew)) expected for a solvent (e.g., water) corresponds to the concentration of solutes. In practice, repeated measurement of osmolality (by freezing point depression) is dependent on sample application technique and on instrument proper calibration, variability in measurement is about 3 and 5 mOsmol/L for serum and urine samples, respectively.

Vapor pressure-based osmolality measurement is not widely used in clinical laboratories. The instrument does not in reality measure vapor pressure, in essence it measures decrease in dew point temperature of water caused by the decrease in vapor pressure of the serum/urine by the presence of solutes. It uses thermocouples (electrodes that measure temperate) where temperature differences are recorded as voltage difference. In addition to its poor imprecision when compared to freezing point depression methodology, it does not measure voltage (temperature) changes that is due to volatile substances. This technique is thus not suitable for alcohols (ethanol, methanol, isopropanol) which escape and increase the vapor pressure rather than lowering it therefore not useful in the determination of osmolar gap due to alcohols, often the clinical indication for osmolality testing.

Calculated osmolality

Osmolality can also be estimated by calculation using the predominant and most osmotically active circulating solutes. They are sodium, urea, and glucose. As indicated above sodium is present as sodium chloride and does not fully dissociate, and the presence of the associated chloride is accounted for by multiplication of the sodium by 1.86.

TABLE 1 Relative distribution of electrolytes, in a 70 kg man, in the different fluid compartments (extracellular (ECF) and intracellular fluid (ICF) compartments).

Electrolyte	Total body content	ECF			ICF
Sodium	3700 mmol 30% complexed in bone 70% freely exchangeable	Blood: 135–145 mmol/L	142 mmol/L	Gastric: 20–120 Small intestine: 120 Feces (diarrhea): 50 Rectal mucus: 100 Bile: 140 Pleural/peritoneal: 140	4–10 mmol/L 10–20 mmol/L
Potassium	3600 mmol 90% exchangeable	3.5–5.0 mmol/L	4.3 mmol/L	Gastric: 10–15 Small intestine: 10 Feces diarrhea: 30 Rectal mucus: 40 Bile: 5 Pleural peritoneal: 5	120–150 mmol/L
Chloride	85–115 g in adult (0.15% of body weigh)	113 mmol/L	104 mmol/L	Gastric: 110 Small intestine: 100 Feces (diarrhea): 50 Rectal mucus: 100 Bile: 100 Pleural/peritoneal: 100	5 mmol/L
Bicarbonate		26 mmol/L	24 mmol/L		10 mmol/L
Calcium (60 kg) 99% in bone	25,000 mmol (1 kg)	9 mmol/L	2.5 mmol/L		4.0 mmol/L
Phosphate	85% free inorganic phosphate ions HPO_4^{2-}, HPO_4^{1-}, PO_4^{3-} 10% bound to proteins 5% complexes with calcium, magnesium, or sodium At pH 7.4 HPO_4^{2-}, to $H_2PO_4^{1-}$, is 4:1	0.8–1.45 mmol/L (inorganic) Higher in children Diurnal rhythm (0.2 mmol/L)	2 mmol/L		130.0 mmol/L (organic)
Magnesium	21–28 g 60% in bone 20% skeletal muscle 19% in other cells 1% extracellular	0.65–1.05 mmol/L 20% bound to plasma protein 30% Complexed to various ligands 50% free ionized	1.1 mmol/L		34.0 mmol/L

Serum concentrations of electrolytes are not always representative of total body content, and that states of critical body sufficiency or excess may not be obvious when measured in plasma. The large amount of intracellular organic phosphate with its anion charge causes retention of the large intracellular K concentration cation to maintain ionic balance.

Modified from several sources including; Seifter JL. Body fluid compartments, cell membrane ion transport, electrolyte concentrations, and acid-base balance. *Semin Nephrol.* 2019;39(4):368–379. doi:https://doi.org/10.1016/j.semnephrol.2019.04.006. PMID: 31300092. Petraccia L, Liberati G, Masciullo SG, Grassi M, Fraioli A. Water, mineral waters and health. *Clin Nutr.* 2006;25(3):377–385. doi:https://doi.org/10.1016/j.clnu.2005.10.002. Epub 2005 Nov 28. PMID: 16314004. Shrimanker I, Bhattarai S. Electrolytes. [Updated 2022 Jul 25]. In: *StatPearls [Internet].* Treasure Island, FL: StatPearls Publishing; 2022. Available from: https://www.ncbi.nlm.nih.gov/books/NBK541123/. Sobotka, L, Allison S, Stanga Z. Basics in clinical nutrition: water and electrolytes in health and disease. *e-SPEN Eur e-J Clin Nutr Metab.* 2008:e259ee266. doi:https://doi.org/10.1016/j.eclnm.2008.06.004. Physiology of adult *Homo sapiens*—Urinary apparatus. https://www.ufrgs.br/imunovet/molecular_immunology/kidney.html. Accessed 3 March 2023. Hill LL. Body composition, normal electrolyte concentrations, and the maintenance of normal volume, tonicity, and acid-base metabolism. *Pediatr Clin North Am.* 1990;37(2):241–256. doi:https://doi.org/10.1016/s0031-3955(16)36865-1. PMID: 2184394.

Osmolality may be calculated using a number of formulas. The most widely used is the osmolality $= 1.86 \times [Na^+] + urea/2.8 + glucose/18$. When measuring urea and glucose in conventional units (mg/dL). Division by 2.8 and 18 is not required for urea and glucose respectively when measured in SI units. Normal osmolality values are between 280 and 290 mOsmol/L.

Urea is included in the equation although it is not considered an effective solute due to its ability to diffuse between ECF and ICF. Potassium is mostly intracellular, and its extracellular concentration is relatively small and thus not included in the calculation.

Homeostasis

Precise regulation of the ECF composition occurs by controlling the volume of water and the amount of sodium. Other sensors are concerned with volume regulation. A decrease in blood volume or flow is sensed by specialized juxtaglomerular cells in the kidney resulting in renin production which results in angiotensin I release and subsequent aldosterone production by the adrenal glands which causes the kidney to retain sodium and associated water (see Chapter 1 on endocrine testing).

Changes in the osmolality are detected by specialized cells in the hypothalamus which regulate the amount of antidiuretic hormone (ADH or arginine vasopressin) release. Increased osmolality increases ADH production. ADH acts on the distal renal tubule to cause water retention. Thirst center is stimulated when osmolality exceeds 295 mOsmol/L.

The sensitivity of ADH secretion to osmolality is higher than in response to circulating volume. One to two percent change in osmolality is required to induce ADH section, compared with a change in >10% of circulating volume to trigger ADH secretion.

Osmolality measurements help mainly in the interpretation of low serum sodium concentration, assessing renal function, compulsive water drinking states, and in cases of poisoning. Where a discrepancy exists between measured osmolality and calculated osmolality, this indicates the presence of an exogenous or abnormal levels of osmotically active particle.

Rapid exchanges of extracellular solute concentrations cause cell dehydration with slower changes having less effect. When urea and glucose concentration increase in abnormal states, e.g., renal failure and diabetic ketoacidosis (DKA) respectively, these solutes contribute significantly to the osmolality. Urea diffuses into cells slowly, but glucose can be actively transported into cells (and metabolized). In diabetic ketoacidosis however, metabolism of glucose is impaired, and persistent hyperglycemia can lead to cellular dehydration.

Abnormalities in water distribution and extracellular fluid osmolality

Water homeostasis is interlinked with both sodium alone and other osmotically active substances. Increased absorption of sodium as in states of hyperaldosteronism (Conn's syndrome) and/or increased losses as in hypoaldosteronism in adrenal insufficiency, in both conditions, water as described accompanies sodium movement along a concentration gradient leading to both hyper- and hyponatremia, respectively.

In pathological conditions, rapid changes of extracellular solute concentrations affect cell hydration; slower changes have less effect. Speed of change is more important than absolute levels in controlling fluid shifts. It is very important when correcting osmotic imbalance not to be "overzealous" in attempting to restore normality as cerebral hydration may be altered dramatically causing damage.

The effective osmolality of a solution is sometimes referred to as tonicity. Isotonic solutions have the same osmolality as body fluids, usually close to 285 mOsmol/L. Adequacy of fluid replacement is assessed and monitored via measurement of serum electrolytes, urine serum osmolality and by clinical assessment.

Fluid replacement therapy options are 5% dextrose which contributes to both ECF and ICF volume. It restores total body water. Isotonic sodium chloride (0.9% NaCl) distributes throughout the ECF mainly both plasma and interstitial space. Replacement therapy is to make up for losses that have occurred and to keep up with anticipated losses over the following 24 h.

Daily water intake is estimated at about 2300 mL with contribution from facultative intake (1000 mL), water in food (800 mL), and drinks (500 mL). Water from body metabolism includes contributions from carbohydrates oxidation (200 mL), lipids and protein oxidation (100 mL). Metabolism of 100 calories from fat, carbohydrates, or protein yields 14 mL of water. Daily water insensible losses are variable (500–700 mL) and influenced by environmental factors such as ambient temperature (150–200 mL per day for every degree (°C) increase above 37°C).

Sweat accounts for about 100 mL, evaporation in breathing (350–400 mL) losses increase to 650 mL in hyperventilation and in cold environment where P_{H2O} air is about 0. Obligatory renal losses, required to dispose of about 600 mOsmol/day of dissolved metabolic waste, are about 500 mL. Exercise and hyperthermia, infection, renal dysfunction, and metabolic disorders significantly alter insensible body water losses and must be closely monitored and regularly assessed.

Sodium pathophysiology

A 70 kg man has a total body sodium of 3700 mmol. Seventy percent is freely exchangeable with the remaining

30% complexed in bone. The majority of sodium is extracellular, the ECF concentration is 135–145 mmol/L and ICF concentration is only 4–10 mmol/L (Table 1).

Sodium is freely filtered at the glomerulus, and the vast majority (99.6%) of this filtered load is reabsorbed. Most is reabsorbed in the proximal tubule (65%) with the loop on Henle (25%) and the distal tubule (10%) accounting for a smaller proportion of reabsorption. Urinary sodium excretion is controlled by aldosterone and atrial natriuretic peptide.

Obligatory sodium normal daily losses are 5 mmol in sweat and 5 mmol in feces. In pathological conditions, however, the intestinal tract may be a major route of sodium loss for example in infantile diarrhea.

Daily body requirement for sodium is 1–2 mmol representing about 1% of a normal dietary intake of 130–26 mmol.

Adaptation to variations in sodium intake are not as prompt as adaptation to water intake and it can take several days to decrease urinary sodium loss to less than 5 mmol/day when a sodium free diet is consumed (amount of reabsorbed compared to filtered load represents about 5%–10%). Therefore, urinary sodium levels vary considerably (40–220 mmol/day) with dietary intake. There is large diurnal variation in urinary sodium with low levels during the night representing 20% of those excreted during daylight, changes in blood pressure being the main contributing factor.

Clinical disorders

Sodium and water homeostasis are intimately related, and when assessing sodium metabolism, it is essential to understand the factors controlling fluid balance. While hypernatremia is not as common in clinical practice but is usually a sign of relative water deficit and patients despite being water depleted and hypernatremia may not experience thirst, hyponatremia in hospital practice usually means water retention.

Hyponatremia

Understanding causes of hyponatremia, defined as serum sodium levels less than 130 mmol/L, is important as it is; (1) the most common electrolyte disorder in laboratory and clinical practice, (2) associated with increased morbidity and all-cause mortality, (3) difficult to correctly diagnose and manage and requires understanding of its pathophysiology, and (4) possibly a result of measurement errors, e.g., in pseudohyponatremia where sodium correction is not required.

Hyponatremia, generally defined as blood sodium concentration below the lower limit of normal (about 135–130 mmol/L) is a laboratory finding and of different etiology. Blood sodium levels less than 120 mmol/L are considered life threatening and requires immediate notification and medical attention.

Sodium levels less than 120 mmol/L are associated with nausea, generalized weakness, and mental confusion, whereas ocular palsy occurs at 110 mmol/L and severe mental impairment at 90–105 mmol/L. Blood sodium concentration <135 mmol/L will be used to represent hyponatremia for the purpose of this chapter.

The etiology of hyponatremia directs its medical intervention. Acute hyponatremia (occurring in less than 48 h) results in increased intracranial pressure with possible brain herniation and is a medical emergency, whereas chronic hyponatremia (occurring >48 h) requires slow correction to prevent osmotic demyelination. Rapid swelling and shrinkage of brain cells is a serious consequence of the rapid alteration in sodium concentration. In addition to actual sodium level, the rate of change is important where clinical symptoms may present at higher than stated sodium levels in situations of acute changes.

Hyponatremia is the most prevalent (up to 30%) electrolyte abnormality among hospitalized patients. The prevalence is, however, variable depending on the disorder and medication and is highest among tertiary care and high-risk patients. Among ambulatory patients, several studies showed wide prevalence from 1.7% in the NHANES study to 6.9% in the Dallas Heart Study and about 5% in a Rotterdam study. However, regardless of the patient type and location, there is positive association between hyponatremia, morbidity, and all-cause mortality. Mortality doubles among the 10% of hospitalized patients with severe hyponatremia (<120 mmol/L) with a U-shaped association between baseline sodium levels and subsequent cardiovascular disease mortality.

In additional to laboratory findings and clinical correlation, assessment for volume status is essential when investigating hyponatremia. Assessment of orthostatic hypotension, pulse rate, and skin turgor is essential and should always guide diagnosis and therapeutic intervention. Lack of such information often makes it difficult for clinical laboratories to investigate a finding of hyponatremia.

Sodium and water homeostasis are interlinked and observed abnormalities in sodium cannot be assessed without consideration of the body's volemic status. Hyponatremia is a state of relative water excess in comparison to sodium concentration, although water excess is not always the sole cause of hyponatremia. Sodium is predominantly extracellular at 140 mmol/L compared with about 4 mmol/L intracellular. In condition to sodium loss, water freely diffuses down a concentration gradient into the cells leading to expansion.

Hyponatremia could be due to poor sample collection. Contamination with intravenous fluid leads to spurious hyponatremia when fluid sodium content is less than half that of serum such as in dextrose infusion. This is seen in busy emergency and hospital units. A simple call and repeat collection often resolve the issue. Furthermore, iatrogenic or hospital acquired hyponatremia account for 40%–75% of patients.

Laboratory investigations of hyponatremia include measurement of serum and urine osmolality, urine sodium levels, and possibly serum aldosterone and cortisol levels. Although urine measurements are often considered helpful when investigating hyponatremia, urine osmolality measurement is superfluous and urine sodium is helpful only when its deficit is not due to renal impairment.

Central to the investigation of hyponatremia is serum osmolality. Sodium is the predominant extracellular solute and major contributor to osmolality. Other constituents include glucose and urea. Normal osmolality being 280–295 mOsmol/L and is maintained by arginine vasopressin (AVP) with osmo-receptor regulating its secretion.

Calculated osmolality is helpful in identifying solutes via osmolar gap and for laboratories that do not have access to an osmometer. Several formulas are in use with the following being more widely used (osmolality = 2 [Sodium] + Glucose/18 + Urea/2.8). However, calculation is not helpful in patients with pseudohyponatremia and in those with other unmeasurable solutes on board such as mannitol and glycine. A rule of thumb, compensation of 1.6–2.4 mmol of sodium is applied to every 100 mg/dL glucose that is above 100 mg/dL.

A difference >10 mOsmol/L between measured and calculated osmolality is to consider a gap and suggests the presence of an osmotically active substance. Measurement of osmolarity is thus helpful to identify nonhypotonic hyponatremia.

Approximately 93% of serum is water. Since sodium is diluted in the aqueous phase. For a mean concentration of 154 mmol/L, this represents (154 × 0.93 = 142 mmol/L). The presence of large amount of triglycerides and/or proteins occupies more of the water sample and thus falsely presents a state of hyponatremia. Osmolality will be normal as lipids and proteins do not contribute to its measurement. For each 1 mg/dL of lipids, sodium will decrease by 0.002 mmol/L, and for every 8 g/dL of protein, it decreases by 0.25 mmol/L. When using indirect measurement ISE (which dilutes sample prior to measurement exaggerates the water content of serum following multiplication by the dilution factor leading to the observed pseudohyponatremia). In otherwords, sample dilution exaggerates the reported sodium value (falsely low). Direct measurement (no premeasurement sample dilution occurs) as in point-of-care devices, blood gas instruments with ISE modules, dray chemistry analyzers, have lower influence on measured sodium.

For instance in patients receiving large dose immunoglobulins infusion (25/kg over 2–5 days), an approximate 3 mmol/L decrease in reported sodium levels is observed. Elevated immunoglobulins in multiple myeloma cause hyponatremia by an additional ionic mechanism where the negatively charged globulins displace sodium interacting with chloride cause a hyperchloremic hyponatremic states. This is in contrast to glucose, mannitol, sucrose, sorbitol, glycerol, maltose, glycine, and radiological contrast media drawing water from intracellular compartments to intravascular. One hundred milligrams per deciliter increase in glucose indicates a 2.4 mmol/L decrease in sodium.

Of note that elevated osmolality due to high urea has little effect on sodium movement as urea is diffusible and has no tonicity (ability to exert osmotic gradient between compartments).

Sodium is measured using ion selective electrode. Historically, there are two approaches, one involves diluting the sample prior to measurement (indirect method) and the other uses neat undiluted sample (direct methodology). The earlier method historically needed to acquire the necessary large volume of sample for the older methodologies. Although newer technologies require small sample volume, the tradition of diluting the sample continues. A large number of laboratories (83%) continue to measure sodium levels using an indirect methodology.

Hyponatremia in patients with normal osmolality (isotonic) suggests the presence of pseudohyponatremia. This is confirmed by the presence of elevated lipids and/or proteins.

Plasma water represents 93% of total plasma volume with the remainder accounted for by lipids and proteins. Most biochemistry analytes are measured in the plasma water fraction but are reported in reference to total plasma volume. It is assumed that little change in plasma volume takes place and thus the difference is ignored, however, for the predominant extracellular analyte sodium, changes in lipids and in protein concentration influence available plasma water causing what is termed exclusion effect.

This is not apparent in methodologies that measure sodium directly in plasma water, and it reflects actual concentration in the available plasma water. However, when applying a dilution step prior to sample analysis (in-direct). When diluting a fixed volume of sample, when using in-direct methods, only 93% of that volume is plasma water containing sodium, that fraction becomes lower in situations of elevated proteins and/or lipids. Thus, when results are calculated back it only considers the total applied volume and thus exaggerates the dilution and the exclusion effect and a falsely low sodium result is reported.

When using direct methods, results are however converted to plasma volume concentration by introducing a correction factor of 0.93 termed the flame mode (flame photometry is indirect methodology). This is recommended by clinical and laboratory standards institute (CLSI) and supported by the fact that the majority of clinical laboratories (83%) use indirect methods. The relationship between changes in protein/lipids concentrations and their exclusion effect on electrolytes concentration is nonlinear and thus it is not possible to apply a predictive and corrective factor. Laboratories without access to direct ISE methodologies (such as point-of-care testing and blood gas instruments) may wish in extreme cases consider measuring sodium following removal of lipemia by ultracentrifugation.

Measuring sodium levels using a direct methodology that does not include dilution helps identify the presence of pseudohyponatremia. Additionally, measurement of glucose, triglycerides, and proteins may help identify the cause of pseudohyponatremia.

Hyperglycemia causes dilutional apparent hyponatremia. High glucose results in movement of water from intracellular to extracellular space thus diluting sodium concentration. Additionally, hyperglycemia may result in osmotic diuresis leading to high osmolality. Sodium levels can be corrected for the glucose concentration by adding 1.6–2.4 mmol for every 100 mg/dL glucose above 100 mg/dL. In the absence of hyperglycemia, the presence of osmolar gap suggests the presence of other solutes such as mannitol.

Hyponatremia associated with low osmolality (hypotonicity) is seen in patients with heart failure, liver cirrhosis and in those exhibiting the syndrome of inappropriate antidiuretic hormone (SIADH) secretion. Conditions where relative water excess or loss of sodium or both exist. In SIADH, excess extracellular fluid, decreased water excretion due to excess AVP or (due to renal impairment inability to excrete excess body water), water accumulates in the extracellular space resulting in hyponatremia. There is no reliable relationship between AVP and etiology of hyponatremia; hence, its measurement is not helpful in most cases. Its measurement is, however, helpful in assessing normal osmoregulation following therapeutic intervention.

In addition to release by the hypothalamic pituitary axis in response to osmotic stimulation, ectopic production of AVP unrelated to sodium concentration is seen in patients with squamous cell carcinoma of the bronchus. This leads to excess water retention and hyponatremia.

SIADH is suspected when there is hypoosmolality, urine osmolality is inappropriately (high and/or higher than serum) concentrated (>100 mOsmol/L). Urinary sodium is often >30 mmol/L, there is normal renal, adrenal, thyroid, cardiac and liver functions, the patient is not on diuretics, and that water restriction reverses sodium wasting and corrects the ensuing hyponatremia. Drugs leading to SIADH include; chlorpropamide, carbamazepine, cyclophosphamide, and selective serotonin reuptake inhibitors.

Hyponatremia in patients with heart failure is a result of increased production of B-type natriuretic peptide (BNP). The latter is produced in response to stretched atrial ventricular tissue and causes urinal sodium loss. Heart failure leads to reduction in GFR and thus water excretion. Additionally,

there is none osmotic release of AVP all results in reabsorption of sodium and water and hyponatremia. Measurement of urinary sodium in the absence of renal impairment supports the hypothesis. Furthermore, volume overload due to heart failure could be inferred by the finding of elevated BNP.

The ensued hyponatremia activates renin angiotensin aldosterone system leading to increased sodium absorption and accompanied water absorption. Urinary sodium will be low <20 mmol/L. Urine sodium measurement is helpful only if the deficit is not due to renal impairment.

In patients with liver cirrhosis, portal hypertension and thus atrial vasodilatation causes activation of the renin angiotensin aldosterone system as well as AVP with sodium and water retention leading to hyponatremia. This explains the reason for a low spot urine sodium concentration. There is also water accumulation secondary to reduction in GFR; however, the major mechanism for hyponatremia appears to be nonosmotic release of AVP.

Patients with reduction in renal impairment and glomerular filtration rate will exhibit hyponatremia and water overload. Water intake in excess of limited urine output results in hyponatremia. AVP release is suppressed due to volume overload. In patients with nephrotic syndrome, if serum albumin falls below 2 g/dL, intravascular hypovolemia may cause non osmotic stimulation of AVP leading to hyponatremia.

In patient where the extracellular fluid is normal, a relative water excess causes a normal or low urea, low uric acid and a urinary sodium ≥20–30 mmol/L. Fluid accumulation secondary to AVP causes the above observation. An elevated urine osmolality >100 mOsmol/L is consistent with SIADH where serum osmolality is often <275 mOsmol/L.

Endocrine causes of hyponatremia include primary and secondary glucocorticoid deficiency. Isolated cortisol deficiency causes elevated AVP. Aldosterone remains intact. Hypothyroidism causing hyponatremia thought to be due to reduced GFR due to secondary reduction in cardiac output and peripheral vascular resistance. Increasing blood osmolality stimulates AVP release which in turn increases distal tubules permeability and facilitates reabsorption of water and thus reducing serum osmolality but in turn increasing that of urine. Expansion of extracellular volume inhibits renin-angiotensin-aldosterone system with resultant loss of sodium in urine. Sodium urinary excretion levels typically >30 mmol/24 h. SIADH is characterized by the above findings, and that hypouricemia is a common finding.

Disorders associated with SIADH include malignancy, small cell carcinoma of the lung being the most common, CNS disorders, pulmonary disease, drugs, among others such as ACTH deficiency. Adrenal insufficiency either primary or secondary leads to hyponatremia via loss of sodium in the urine.

Patients with hypovolemia (extracellular fluid loss) due to gastrointestinal disorders, diuretic therapy, exercise associated, and cerebral salt losing (following subarachnoid hemorrhage, head injury, or neurological procedures) increased natriuretic peptide has been suggested as a mechanism this is however, euvolemic rather than hypovolemic state associated with SIADH. Loss of sodium leads to hypovolemia and in turns stimulates AVP secretion (baroreceptor mediated AVP prelease). All exhibit hyponatremia although the mechanism may be different. Laboratory findings are those of elevated urea, elevated creatinine and urea/creatinine ratio, elevated uric acid and a reduced urinary sodium <20–30 mmol/L.

Hyponatremia among athletes is attributed to excessive water intake in the presence of extrarenal loss of sodium. There is also increased AVP production in response to the hypovolemia further exacerbating the hyponatremia.

Drugs used in the management of renal and endocrine disorders may lead to hyponatremia. They include, amiodarone, angiotensin II receptor blockers, angiotensin converting enzyme inhibitors, bromocriptine, as well as diuretics. Furthermore, the development of hyponatremia depends on the duration of use, for instance, frusemide causes hyponatremia within the first 3 months of therapy, whereas thiazide diuretics induces hyponatremia within 2 weeks of therapy.

Management of hyponatremia is costly with an estimated annual cost ranging from $1.6 to $3.6 billion. It occurs in 1% of hospitalized patients is invariably asymptomatic. Severe hyponatremia with sodium less than 125 mmol/L occurs in about 0.2% of hospitalized patients and if occurring rapidly can result in clinical symptoms. Identifying the cause of hyponatremia requires a methodical approach with history, examination, and laboratory tests required to make the correct diagnosis.

Dietary free sodium may only reduce urinary sodium to less than 5 mmol/day after several days compared with more immediate changes following water restriction and changes. Water and sodium homeostasis are interlinked and assessment of both is required for interpreting sodium abnormalities. For instance, a common asymptomatic mild hyponatremia (130 mmol/L) occurs in (1%) among inpatients and symptomatic severe hyponatremia (<125 mmol/L) in 0.2% are often due water excess rather than sodium depletion.

Similarly, conditions of hypernatremia are often associated with relative water deficit rather than sodium excess. Therefore, plasma sodium is not an accurate representation of body sodium content, and it is important to note that in life-threatening sodium excess or depletion, a normal plasma sodium levels may be obtained. The measurement of plasma sodium is influenced by excess lipid and protein levels. Those displace water from a blood sample resulting in lower measured sodium per liter of plasma than per liter of plasma water (pseudohyponatremia).

Pseudohyponatremia

In patients with severe hyperlipidemia or hyperproteinemia, the measured serum sodium concentration may be low caused by the way sodium is measured. The presence of lipids and/or proteins displace water from a blood sample resulting in a measured concentration of sodium lower per liter of plasma than the concentration per liter of plasma water (see above and Fig. 1).

Potentiometric measurement using ion-selective electrodes. Prior to measurement, the sample may be diluted using manufacturer recommended diluent (often high ranging from 1:16 to 1:34) to reduce sample viscosity (matrix effect) and speed up the electrode—sample interaction and thus obtaining results.

Measurement of undiluted sample is termed "direct" measurement. Those are often in use in point-of-care testing instruments including those included in blood gas analyzers.

In the presence of hyperlipidemia and/or hyperproteinemia, prior sample dilution exaggerates the displacement and falsely reported hyponatremia is reported. This is not encountered when using direct measurements. Clinical chemistry laboratories will often be asked to perform direct potentiometric measurements when pseudohyponatremia is suspected on results obtained from automated main analyzers.

In the absence of direct potentiometry, the impact of lipids (triglycerides) on indirect sodium measurement can be estimated as follows; first, percentage plasma water is estimated using the formula, plasma water $(\%) = 99.1 - (1.1 \times 10^{-5} \times$ (triglycerides in mmol/L)) $- (0.07 \times$ protein concentration in g/L). The measured indirect sodium is then multiplied by 0.93 and the product divided by calculated serum water (%). Triglyceride is used as its impact is higher than cholesterol by about 2.5 folds as triglyceride has a larger molecular weight (885.4 g/mol) than cholesterol (386.7 g/mol).

Potassium pathophysiology

The total body potassium of the average 70 kg man is 3600 mmol. Ninety percent is exchangeable, and the majority of the potassium is in the intracellular fluid (ICF). A very small fraction of the potassium is in the extracellular fluid (ECF) distributed uniformly between plasma and interstitial compartments (3.5–5.0 mmol/L). Intake of potassium is variable 30–100 mmol/day. Potassium loss is equally variable and mainly controlled by the kidney.

Total body potassium is 3600 mmol in a 70 kg man. Ninety percent of which is exchangeable and the majority being in intracellular fluid. Very small amount 3.5–5.0 mmol/L is present extracellularly and distributed between plasma and interstitial compartments. Potassium intake and loss is variable. Loss is mainly controlled by the kidney.

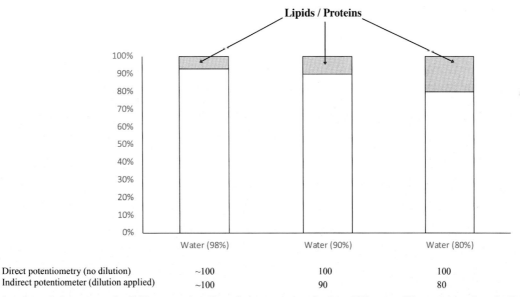

FIG. 1 Displacement of plasma water by lipids or proteins. Normal plasma contents is about 92% water, 8% nonaqueous (proteins/lipids, with no sodium content), as the amount of lipids and proteins contents by percentage increase (no sodium/electrolytes content), reported concentration depends on the method applied. If direct potentiometry (no sample dilution) relative accurate electrolytes (sodium content is reported) when sample dilution occurs prior to measurement, the extent of displacement by nonaqueous components is exaggerated (often dilution is 1 in 10) and thus exaggerated. Direct Potentiometer, e.g. (ion selective electrodes on blood gases instruments—no sample dilution occurs). Indirect potentiometry is ion selective electrode on automated chemistry analyzers, flame photometric methods (that dilutes samples prior to analysis to reduce serum viscosity effect). *(Modified from Seguna D, Imbroll M, Gruppetta M. Pseudohyponatraemia—a literature review. Malta Medical School Gazette. 2019;03(01):8–12.)*

Potassium is essential in maintaining cellular function. In association with sodium and the Na^+-K^+-ATPase pump which pumps sodium out of the cells and potassium into the cell maintaining a potassium gradient across cell membrane with intracellular potassium larger than that outside the cell. This established potential difference across cell membrane is essential for cellular function, particular in muscle and nerve cells (excitable cells). Hyperkalemia decreases membrane potential, whereas hypokalemia causes hyperpolarization and membranes nonresponsiveness.

Additionally, intracellular potassium is essential for maintenance of acid base status via exchange with hydrogen ions.

Ninety percent of filtered K is passively reabsorbed in the proximal tubule. Small amount passively released in the distal tubules. Factors favoring increased K loss is due to increased Na reabsorption, increased intracellular K, and decreased hydrogen ion secretion. Daily potassium intake is about 100 mmol with balance maintained via renal and gastrointestinal (stool) loss of about 90 and 10 mmol/day respectively.

Disturbances in K metabolism present the most critical electrolytes emergencies. Hyperkalemia usually due to redistribution between intracellular and extracellular compartments. Whereas hypokalemia may result from redistribution of K between intracellular fluids and extracellular fluids but more usually reflects potassium depletion. Both hyper- and hypokalemia present with weakness, cardiac arrhythmias, renal tubular damage, and polyuria in hypokalemia. Hyperkalemia as well as hypokalemia impairs myocardium electrical conduction leading to cardiac dysfunction, arrhythmia, and sudden death. Hypokalemia potentiates effects of digoxin and causes ECG changes and muscle tetany.

Similar to Na^+ a patient may have marked total body K loss and yet present with hyperkalemia as in diabetic ketoacidosis. Causes of hyperkalemia include acidosis, acute renal failure, aldosterone antagonists administration, Addison's disease, and artifactual (e.g., hemolysis), Hypokalemia is caused by diarrhea, diuresis, drugs, e.g., diuretics, distribution, decreased intake, diabetes mellitus, and distal tubular disorders.

Hyperkalemia may be acutely lowered by infusion of insulin and glucose, and stabilization of the endocardium by 10% calcium gluconate. Correction of acidosis if present can treat hypokalemia. Long-term treatment can be accomplished by restriction of intake and use of K binding resins.

Hypokalemia is corrected by correcting the cause (one of the above). K supplements may be prescribed or acute infusion of K although the later should be done carefully.

Circulating potassium is normally 3.5–4.5 mmol/L. However, disturbances in potassium metabolism often require immediate identification and management. They usually occur as a result of redistribution of potassium between the intracellular and extracellular compartments and reflects potassium excess and/or tissue depletion even in the presence of hyperkalemia.

Hyperkalemia

Defined as circulating potassium levels above 4.5 mmol/L and levels above 6.0 mmol/L are often considered critical requiring immediately intervention. Clinical manifestations include weakness and irritable "twitchy muscles," fearfulness and paresthesia, cardiac arrhythmias, myocardial infarction, and cardiac arrest.

Causes of hyperkalemia include acute renal failure, acidosis, hypoaldosteronism, drugs therapy (aldosterone antagonists), Addison's disease, as well as artifactual hemolysis.

With potassium being predominantly intracellular, slight leakage causes a significant rise in plasma potassium levels. Termed in vitro sample hemolysis, is the most common cause of hyperkalemia and is secondary to leakage of intracellular components into plasma. This is associated with suboptimal sample collection practices leading to RBC rupture and leakage of contents.

In some pathology, the RBC may be fragile and thus more susceptible to rupture such as states of hypo- and hypervolemia, hyperglycemia and hyperlipidemia, use of chemotherapy, disorders of RBCs and presence of immature RBCs. Hemolysis is routinely detected by determining serum indices (HIL). This is a spectrophotometric measurement of hemoglobin (H), icterus (I), and lipemia (L) by recoding absorbances at (320–450 and 540–580 nm), (400–540 nm), and at (300–700 nm) respectively and that the amount of free hemoglobin correlates with the extent of hemolysis. Significant impact for analytes such as potassium, phosphates, enzymes (AST and LDH) present in relatively high intracellular concentration compared to plasma will cause significant increase even in slight degree of hemolysis. The presence of hyperlipidemia detected by lipemic index affects RBC membrane fragility and thus susceptibility to leakage and rupture.

Reduced renal clearance is a common cause of hyperkalemia in patients with renal insufficiency and high levels are often encountered >7.0 mmol/L and often an indication for dialysis. Aldosterone reabsorbs filtered sodium and secretes potassium. Patients with adrenal insufficiency (hypoaldosteronism) exhibit hyponatremia and hyperkalemia. Acidosis (metabolic) causes hyperkalemia and often seen in lactic and ketoacidosis. It is secondary to insulin deficiency and to hyperosmolality rather than to the degree of acidemia. It is associated with type-4 renal tubular acidosis. Intracellular acidosis (high H^+) causes potassium to shift out of cells (a rise of 0.6 (range 0.2–1.7) mmol/L for every 0.1 unit reduction in pH) to maintain intracellular neutrality. Although this is more pronounced in metabolic acidosis, mild hyperkalemia is seen in patients with respiratory component acidosis, but the mechanism is unclear.

Treatment for hyperkalemia includes; infusion of insulin and glucose and stabilization of the myocardium can be accomplished by giving intravenous calcium gluconate. Correction of an acidosis if present can treat the hyperkalemia.

Hypokalemia

Defined as serum potassium less than 3.5 mmol/L the lower limit of reference intervals with levels <2.5 mmol/L considered critical and needs immediate attention. It is a common electrolyte disturbance among hospitalized patients. Clinical manifestations include severe weakness, tetany, cardiac arrhythmias, ECG changes, polyuria and renal dysfunction, and increased sensitivity to digoxin medication.

Causes leading to hypokalemia include gastrointestinal losses (diarrhea), renal losses (hyperaldosteronism—Conn's syndrome), distal tubular disorders, drugs (diuretics), and diabetes mellitus (total body potassium is low despite diabetic ketoacidosis hyperkalemia), and to a lesser extent secondary to reduced potassium intake (feeding disorders).

In contrast to the hyperkalemia seen and described in metabolic acidosis above, the reverse is true, where metabolic alkalosis results in intracellular shift of potassium leading to hypokalemia.

Treatment includes correcting the cause. Prescription of supplements (patients with hypokalemia very often have total body potassium deficits in excess of 500 mmol).

Chloride pathophysiology

Chloride, the principal anion in the body. Often not discussed due to its association with sodium and that its role, except for few important pathophysiology, remains not clear. A molecular weight of 35.5 Da, it is the predominant extracellular anion. Concentrations being about 110 mmol/L in circulation, 50–110 mmol/L in various other extracellular fluid, and 5 mmol/L intracellularly (Table 1).

It plays a role in maintaining electrical neutrality and that hyperchloremia accompany hypernatremia (maintaining neutrality) during active sodium reabsorption. It also helps in osmotic pressure maintenance. Circulating chloride levels are influenced by gastrointestinal loss of bicarbonate, in renal tubular acidosis, in compensated respiratory alkalosis, in mineralocorticoid deficiency and excess, salt losing pyelonephritis, and in gastrointestinal excessive chloride loss. Its measurement is helpful in the interpretation of complex acid base status where high levels are often seen in primary or compensated acidosis, in contrast low levels are indicative of either primary or compensated alkalosis.

Source being mainly dietary salt absorbed in the small intestine (7.9–11.8 g/day, and 5.8–7.8 g/day) in adult men and women, respectively.

A number of chloride channel abnormalities are described. They include mutations in the cystic fibrosis transmembrane conductance regulator (CFTR) gene leading to inhibition of the chloride channels. Congenial bilateral aplasia of the vas deference causes a chloride channel dysfunction, Barter's disease causing decreased renal tubular chloride transport leading to reduced renal reabsorption of both sodium and chloride.

Chloride shift

Hemoglobin inside red blood cells also provide a buffer system for H^+ where it binds to negatively charged Hb^- (Fig. 2). HCO_3^- is exchanged for chloride (known as the chloride shift, Bohr effect).

Hyperchloremia

High plasma chloride levels are seen associated with hypernatremia. It is also seen secondary to bicarbonate loss, such as in diarrhea (gastrointestinal loss), renal tubular acidosis, mineralocorticoid deficiency, and in compensated respiratory alkalosis.

Hyperchloremic acidosis is a complication of renal tubular acidosis caused by a defect in chloride excretion.

Hypochloremia

Low chloride levels defined as blood chloride level <95 mmol/L. It is encountered following loss in vomiting (loss of gastric HCL) and following nasogastric suction. In excess use of loop diuretics, and in mineralocorticoid excess associated metabolic alkalosis by increasing reabsorption of bicarbonate and reduced secretion in the renal distal tubule. In patients with urine chloride <10 mmol/L, the hypochloremia is due to chloride responsive alkalosis. Urinary chloride levels >40 mmol/L in patients with hypochloremia are indicative of volume overload. Hypochloremia and associated metabolic alkalosis are seen in patients with Bartter syndrome, a heterogeneous group of inherited tubular disorders.

Diabetes insipidus

It was mentioned that assessing water dysregulation is interlined and abnormalities in water metabolism must be investigated in relation with electrolytes such as Na and K (this is discussed in the respective sodium and potassium pathophysiology sections).

Specific to water is the mechanism of water reabsorption in the distal convoluted tubules and collecting ducts of the nephron (see Chapter 3 on renal function).

ADH increases permeability of renal tubules and allow water diffusion into interstitial fluid compartment and thus to intravascular blood stream compartment restoring both osmolality and hypovolemia. The primary driving force being intravascular blood osmolality where increased osmolality causes release of ADH from the posterior pituitary (see Chapter 1 on endocrine testing). Failure in ADH production and/or resistance to its action at the distal tubules causes cranial and nephrogenic diabetes insipidus, respectively.

In patients with cranial (central) diabetes insipidus clinical symptoms become apparent when at least 80% of ADH activity is lost. Nephrogenic diabetes insipidus is characterized by adequate ADH levels but lack of distal tubules response to ADH.

Osmolality measurements are performed when investigating ADH is rarely measured in the investigation of diabetes insipidus where serum and urine osmolality measurements are routinely and usually performed. The finding of inappropriately low urinary osmolality compared to serum suggests DI. Random urine osmolality >750 mOsmol/L excludes diabetes insipidus.

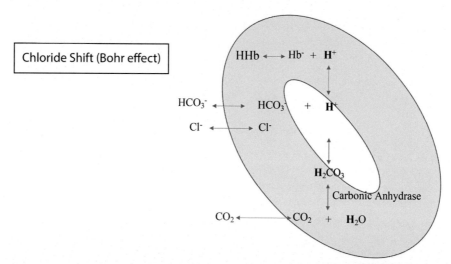

FIG. 2   Red blood cell hemoglobin as a buffer system buffering hydrogen and regenerating bicarbonate. Neutrality is maintained by exchange for chloride ions a process known as the Bohr effect. *(Modified from Jensen FB. Red blood cell pH, the Bohr effect, and other oxygenation-linked phenomena in blood O2 and CO2 transport. Acta Physiol Scand. 2004;182(3):215–227. doi:https://doi.org/10.1111/j.1365-201X.2004.01361.x. PMID: 15491402.)*

Patients being investigated for DI are subjected to water deprivation test. Water intake is restricted for up to 8 h during which serum and urine osmolality are measured on serial samples. The test is terminated if body weight loss is >3% or serum sodium >145 mmol/L. A normal patient concentrates the urine in response to water deprivation, and DI is excluded if urine to serum osmolality ratio is ≥2. Patients failing to concentrate the urine suggest lack of ADH activity and an increase in urine osmolality by >50% following ADH administration suggests cranial DI and a ≪10% rise in osmolality suggest resistance to ADH. Ten to fifteen percent increase in urine osmolality suggests partial deficiency.

Syndrome of inappropriate ADH secretion (SIADH)[1]

This characterized by euvolemic hyponatremia. It represents a state of water overload and is diagnosed according to the following findings: dilutional hyponatremia supported by appropriately low plasma osmolality, urinary osmolality is higher than plasma osmolality, persistent renal sodium excretion >30 mmol/24 h, absence of hypotension, hypovolemia, and edema forming states, normal cardiac, renal, hepatic, thyroid, and adrenal functions, and commonly encountered hypouricemia.

Characterized by a plasma sodium less than 135 mmol/L, osmolality usually less than 270–280 mOsmol/L, and a urine osmolality >100 mOsmol/L (typically in the range of 250–1400 mOsmol/L).

ADH secretion is inhibited when plasma osmolality is below 275 mOsmol/L (plasma sodium <135 mmol/L). Urine osmolality low about 50–100 mOsmol/L in the absence of ADH.

Clinical disorders associated with SIADH include neoplasm (small cell bronchial carcinoma), central nervous system disorders, nonneoplastic pulmonary disease, use of certain drugs (e.g., chlorpromazine, carbamazepine, etc.). SIADH is also seen in patients with porphyria, ACTH deficiency, and patients undergoing in vitro fertilization treatments and exhibiting hyperstimulation syndrome.

Hypernatremia

Hypernatremia defined as blood sodium levels >145 mmol/L. It is often secondary to water loss and dehydration. Endocrine causes of hypernatremia are hyperaldosteronism and Cushing's syndrome. Elevated aldosterone corticosteroids (with mineralocorticoid activity) respectively lead to excessive sodium reabsorption. Causes and biochemical findings in hypernatremia are summarized in Table 2.

TABLE 2 Clinical and biochemical findings in various volemic states in patients with hypernatremia.

Volume status	Clinical findings	Blood sodium (mmol/L)	Urine sodium (mmol/L)
Hypovolemia (low total body water and sodium)	Renal loss (acute/chronic)	>145	>20–30
	Drugs diuretics		<20–30
	Osmotic diuresis		<20–30
	Extrarenal loss (gastrointestinal, sweat, fistula, burn)		<20–30
Euvolemia	SIADH	~135–145	>20–30
Total body water may be slightly low, total body sodium may be slightly increased	Renal loss (DI)		<20–30 to >20–30
	Nonrenal fever, hyperventilation		
Hypervolemia	Iatrogenic intake (e.g., Intravenous solutions)	>145	>20–30
Total body water and sodium (high)	Hyperaldosteronism (Conn's syndrome)		<20–30
	Cushing's syndrome		

Modified from Muhsin SA, Mount DB. Diagnosis and treatment of hypernatremia. *Best Pract Res Clin Endocrinol Metab.* 2016;30(2):189–203. doi:https://doi.org/10.1016/j.beem.2016.02.014. Epub 2016 Mar 4. PMID: 27156758. Liamis G, Filippatos TD, Elisaf MS. Evaluation and treatment of hypernatremia: a practical guide for physicians. *Postgrad Med.* 2016;128(3):299–306. doi:https://doi.org/10.1080/00325481.2016.1147322. Epub 2016 Feb 23. PMID: 26813151. Pfennig CL, Slovis CM. Sodium disorders in the emergency department: a review of hyponatremia and hypernatremia. *Emerg Med Pract.* 2012;14(10):1–26. Epub 2012 Sep 20. PMID: 23114652.

Hyperaldosteronism

Hyperaldosteronism causes hypernatremia and associated hypokalcmia duc to aldostcronc action on the renal tubules of sodium reabsorption in exchange for potassium. The prevalence of hyperaldosteronism is 0.05% with Conn's syndrome representing 80% of cases, followed by bilateral adrenal hyperplasia (15%–20%), adrenocortical carcinoma (<5%), and a rare form <1% of glucocorticoid suppressible hyperaldosteronism. Patients present with hypertension and mild hypernatremia, hypokalemic alkalosis, and urinary potassium daily excretion in excess of 30 mmol. Secondary causes of hyperaldosteronism include liver cirrhosis, renal nephrotic syndrome, Bartter's syndrome, renal tubular acidosis, excessive renin production (renovascular, hypertension, renin-secreting tumors), and in response to extra renal sodium loss (vomiting, diarrhea, hemorrhage) (see Chapter 1 for the renin-angiotensin-aldosterone action).

Investigation of hyponatremia

Clinical and biochemical assessment of blood and urinary sodium and osmolality often reveals the underlaying cause.

In hypovolemic state (serum osmolality is high), the reduced blood volume stimulates the juxtaglomerular to release Rennin, which converts liber angiotensinogen to angiotensin-I, the latter is converted to angiotensin II by ACE in the lung. Angiotensin-II acts on the adrenal glands to release aldosterone which causes reabsorption of filtered sodium and accompanied water which restores the blood volume. Similarly, the increased osmolality stimulate ADH release which inhibit water loss and this help restores volume, hypervolemia is more important that osmolality and thus predominates evident by the low urinal sodium levels. Lack of the regulatory process is evident by high urinary sodium levels due to the causes shown in Table 3 (see Chapter 1 on adrenal for more on the renin-angiotensin-aldosterone system).

TABLE 3 Clinical assessment of hyponatremia can be based on volume status, i.e., hypervolemic, euvolemic and hypovolemic states.

Volume status	Clinical findings	Blood sodium (mmol/L)	Urine sodium (mmol/L)
Hypervolemia (high total body water and sodium)	Cardiac (failure)	>145	<20–30
	Liver (cirrhosis)		<20–30
	Nephrotic syndrome		<20–30
	Renal (ARF, CRF)		>20–30
Euvolemia	SIADH	~135–145	>20–30 (normal salt intake)
Total body water may be slightly high, total body sodium may be slightly increased	Pituitary/adrenal hypocortisolism		
	Hypothyroidism		
	Drugs (carbamazepine)		
Hypovolemia	Sweat	<135	<10 (nonrenal)
Total body water and sodium (low)	Gastrointestinal loss (vomiting, diarrhea)		
	This space loss (burns, peritoneal, pancreatic)		
	Renal (nephritis)/RTA-II		>20–30 (renal)
	Adrenal failure (Addison's, (Hypoaldosteronism))		
	Osmotic diuresis (DKA)		
	Diuretics		

Clinical, biochemical, and possible causes are listed. *ARF*, acute renal failure; *CRF*, chronic renal failure; *DKA*, diabetic ketoacidosis; *RTA*, renal tubular acidosis; *SIADH*, syndrome of inappropriate ADH.
Modified from several sources; Ball SG, Iqbal Z. Diagnosis and treatment of hyponatraemia. *Best Pract Res Clin Endocrinol Metab*. 2016;30(2):161–173. doi:https://doi.org/10.1016/j.beem.2015.12.001. Epub 2015 Dec 30. PMID: 27156756. Pfennig CL, Slovis CM. Sodium disorders in the emergency department: a review of hyponatremia and hypernatremia. *Emerg Med Pract*. 2012;14(10):1–26. Epub 2012 Sep 20. PMID: 23114652. Ball S, Barth J, Levy M, Society for Endocrinology Clinical Committee. SOCIETY FOR ENDOCRINOLOGY ENDOCRINE EMERGENCY GUIDANCE: emergency management of severe symptomatic hyponatraemia in adult patients. *Endocr Connect*. 2016;5(5):G4–G6. doi:https://doi.org/10.1530/EC-16-0058. PMID: 27935814; PMCID: PMC5314809.

In hypervolemic, both extracellular sodium and body water are elevated, states, aldosterone is inhibited causing loss of sodium into the urine (>20 mmol/L), the exception being in patient with cardiac failure where reduction in juxtaglomerular apparatus and GFR stimulates the rennin-angiotensin-aldosterone pathway cause reabsorption of sodium and exacerbation of the hypervolemia. Urinary sodium will be low (<10 mmol/L).

In euvolemic state, extracellular sodium is within normal range extra cellular body water may be slightly high, urinary sodium is often >20 mmol/L. In hypovolemic state, both blood and extracellular sodium are low with increased urinary sodium loss >20 mmol/L. In cases of extra renal and nongastrointestinal losses, sweat and skin loss is usually the case, in the latter urinary sodium is low <10 mmol/L.

In the presence of hyponatremia, hyper osmolality (hypertonic hyponatremia) suggests the presence of an osmotically active substances (glucose, mannitol ethylene glucose, etc.), whereas in the presence of normal osmolality suggests pseudohyponatremia as described above (high triglycerides proteins, paraproteins).

Biochemical investigation of hyperkalemia

Hyperkalemia defined as blood potassium levels above the upper limit of normal of 5.0 mmol/L. Pseudohyperkalemia can be due to sample hemolysis (leaking from red blood cells) due to incorrect phlebotomy, sample handing and transportation. Some patients are higher risk for hemolysis incudes those with fragile RBC membrane due to drugs, lipidemia blood viscosity, and visemic status. Additional patient with leukocytosis (>790,000/cm^3) and thrombocytosis (>100,000/cm^3) causes an elevated in potassium when collecting serum samples. Clotting (destruction of platelets) releases potassium and cause an elevation of about 3 mmol/L in absence leukocytosis and in normocythemia. Higher potassium levels are seen in patient with polycythemia and leukocytosis.

Increase potassium intake (therapeutic potassium supplementation when using potassium losing diuretics), as well as intravenous lines contamination leads to spurious hyperkalemia. On the other hand, true hyperkalemia can be due to reduced potassium clearance (i.e., reduced glomerular filtration rate in renal failure), use of potassium losing diuretics, renal tubular acidosis (type IV) (hyporeninemic hypoaldosteronism), adrenal failure hypoaldosteronism (Addison's disease), and isolated hypoaldosteronism. Other causes of hyperkalemia include, increased potassium release from cells due to in vivo hemolysis, trauma, rhabdomyolysis, tumor lysis syndrome, secondary causes include acidosis, insulin deficiency, hyperosmolality, and drugs as immunosuppressants, beta blockers causing increased potassium movement form intracellular to extracellular space.

It is important to note that circulating levels may not reflect tissue content. Potassium is predominantly intracellular and thus the duration of pathology (actue versus) influences the observed change in postassium levels.

Interference with its exchange mechanisms in the renal tubules. In renal tubular acidosis hydrogen ions competes with potassium for exchange in the distal tubules. Reduced potassium excretion at the proximal tubules in hyporeninemic hypoaldosteronism state. In patients with Addison's disease, lack of cortisol which has moderate mineralocorticoid activity simulates what is observed for hypoaldosteronism (also secondary to adrenal tissue damage). Drugs are also major cause for hyperkalemia. Antihypertensive medications and diuretics inhibiting the renin-angiotensin-aldosterone system (angiotensin converting enzyme (ACE) inhibitors, angiotensin II inhibitors, potassium sparing diuretics (spironolactone (aldosterone receptor antagonist), amiloride, and triamterene)).

Biochemical investigation of hypokalemia

Hypokalemia defined as blood levels below lower limit of normal <3.5 mmol/L. Hypokalemia can be due to either increased loss, transcellular compartments shift and to decreased intake (Fig. 3).

Gastrointestinal losses in diarrhea, laxative abuse, Zollinger-Ellison syndrome (increased gut motility), malabsorption and due to either adenoma of the colon, blood loss or to chemotherapy. Loss due to excess sweat is also seen. Transcellular shift leading to hypokalemia is often seen in patients with alkalosis, where H ions competes for K transport, thyrotoxicosis, beta-adrenergic drugs, insulin over dosage, as well as in hypokalemic periodic paralysis. Due to the extrarenal losses and transcellular shifts discussed urinal potassium levels are often less than 15 mmol/L. Renal loses are seen in patients with primary hyperaldosteronism, Cushing's syndrome (cortisol having mineralocorticoid activity) as well as several genetic disorders such as Liddle's syndrome, CAH due to 11-β hydroxysteroid dehydrogenase deficiency, Barter's syndrome, and Gitleman's syndrome. This patient will exhibit marked alkalosis. Whereas in patients with renal tubular acidosis types I and II the hypokalemia is accompanied with metabolic acidosis. A number of drugs cause urinal loss of potassium include potassium losing diuretics, nephrotoxic drugs, cisplatin. Iatrogenic hypokalemia is observed following dialysis.

Measuring urinary potassium level is helpful in the investigation of hypokalemia. Levels <15 mmol/24 h (or <1.5 mmol/mol for potassium creatinine ratio) suggest nonrenal losses such as gastrointestinal (vomiting, diarrhea) or rare genetic autosomal dominant mutations in the CACNA1S gene (HOKP type I) encoding the alpha-1-subunit of L-type calcium channels, or to mutations in the SCN4A (HOKP type II) encoding the Na$^+$ channel

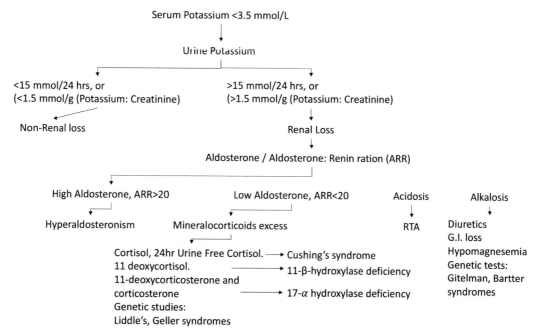

FIG. 3 Biochemical investigation of hypokalemia. The main component when investigating hypokalemia is to determine the route of loss (renal versus extrarenal). In the renal loss category, assessment for drugs intake, endocrine disorders, and of rare genetic mutations affecting renal handling of potassium. The nonrenal losses are those via gastrointestinal and transcellular shift. Assessment of potassium intake and of the patient acid-base status are required. *ARR*, aldosterone renin ratio; *RTA*, renal tubular acidosis. *(Modified from Kardalas E, Paschou SA, Panagiotis A, Muscogiuri G, Siasos G, Vryonidou A. Hypokalemia: a clinical update. Endocr Connect. 2018;7:135–146.)*

causing muscle periodic paralysis due to the hypokalemia (hypokalemic periodic paralysis). Although the Na and Ca channels are the primary defect, this leads to cation leak and to hypokalemic periodic paralysis and that the latter is potentiated by insulin.

In patients with urinary potassium >15 mmol/24 h (> 1.5 mmol/mol random urine potassium to creatinine ratio) indicates renal loss. Among hypertensive patients, elevated aldosterone (aldosterone renin ratio) suggests hyperaldosteronism as the cause of hypokalemia, if aldosterone (aldosterone renin ratio) is inappropriately low, assessment for metabolic disorders (mineralocorticoids excess, Cushing's syndrome, 11-β hydroxylase deficiency, 17-α-hydroxylase deficiency, Liddle's syndrome (mutation leading to increased distal sodium reabsorption and thus hypokalemia)), Geller's syndrome (familial activating mutation of the mineralocorticoid receptor exacerbated by pregnancy due to progesterone and leads to hypokalemia). In normotensive and hypotensive patients, acidosis (low bicarbonate) suggests renal tubular acidosis, and use of diuretics, magnesium deficiency, Bartter syndrome (secondary hyperaldosteronism to defective sodium reabsorption leading to hypokalemia), or Gitelman syndrome (familial hypokalemia and hypomagnesemia). Mutations in the sodium chloride and magnesium transporters in the distal nephron, secondary hyperaldosteronism leading to hypokalemia are suspected in the presence of alkalosis (high bicarbonate levels).

Genetic testing for the various rare and familial mutations may be required in the investigation of the rare causes of hypokalemia.

Calcium pathophysiology

Calcium is the most abundant cation in the human body. In an average 60 kg man, there will be 25,000 mmol (1 kg) of calcium. Ninety nine percent of calcium is bound with phosphate in the crystalline structure of bone. The extracellular fluid (ECF) contains 22.5 mmol of calcium with 9 mmol in the plasma (Table 1). Normal circulating calcium levels often range from 2.15 mmol/L (8.6 mg/dL) to 2.6 mmol/L (10.4 mg/dL).

Within the ECF calcium is present as free ionized calcium and protein bound calcium. It is the ionized calcium which is physiologically important, but most clinical chemistry laboratories will measure total calcium. The major calcium binding protein present in plasma is albumin, and changes in albumin concentration will affect total calcium levels independently of the ionized calcium. A formula can be used to adjust the calcium measured for changes in albumin concentration. Binding of calcium to proteins is dependent upon pH. As the number of negative charges on proteins varies with hydrogen ion concentration, acidosis increases and alkalosis reduces circulating ionized calcium.

About 45% of circulating calcium is bound to predominantly plasma proteins, mainly albumin. The reminder is free ionized calcium (45%) with minor component (10%) complexed with anions such as phosphate and citrates.

Total calcium is widely and easily measured in automated chemistry analyzers and is component of both the basic and metabolic panel profiles. Total calcium reacts with o-cresolphthalein complexone in alkaline condition giving a violet-colored complex, the intensity of which is proportional to the total calcium levels. Although the ionized form is the diffusible active form, it is analytically less convenient to measure requiring special sample precautions. Changes in blood pH alter the equilibrium constant of the albumin-ionized calcium fraction. Hydrogen ions displace ionized calcium from protein binding, and thus, the sample acid-based status must be maintained to reflect circulating levels. Samples for ionized calcium are handled as for a blood gas specimen. A whole blood sample in the presence of heparin as anticoagulant, filling the tube to avoiding trapped air bubbles, and avoid delay in analysis by prompt transportation to the laboratory and analysis. Thus, measurement of ionized calcium is recommended when there are major changes in blood pH.

Changes in circulating protein levels influence total calcium levels, whereas ionized calcium is not affected. Therefore, in patients with marked changes in protein concentration, hypoalbuminemia, hyperglobulinemia, in patients with hepatic and renal dysfunction.

Measured total calcium levels can be adjusted for changes in albumin concentration. The formula most widely used being total calcium plus 0.02 (40 − albumin level) when calcium is reported in mmol/L and plus 0.8 (4.0 − albumin level) when reported in mg/dL units. Ionized calcium is measured using ion-selective electrode (ISE) and requires maintenance of the sample acid base status and rapid analysis.

Calcium homeostasis

Calcium homeostasis is maintained by the gut, kidneys, and bones. The fluxes of calcium are under the control of parathyroid hormone and vitamin D.

Parathyroid hormone (PTH) is important for rapid control of calcium concentration. An increase in PTH results in release of calcium from bone (bone resorption), increased calcium reabsorption and phosphate excretion at the kidney, and stimulation of renal 1-alpha hydroxylation of 25-hydroxyvitamin D (25-OH vitamin D) to its active 1,25 dihydroxy vitamin D ($1,25\text{-}(OH)_2$ vitamin D).

In concert with PTH, $1,25\text{-}(OH)_2$ vitamin D absorbs calcium and phosphate from the intestine, renal calcium reabsorption, and calcium release from bone. All lead to calcium influx and maintenance of normal calcium levels.

Hypercalcemia

Hypercalcemia is defined as serum calcium two standard deviations above the normal mean calcium levels in at least

two samples at least 1 week part over a period of three months.[2] Normal circulating calcium levels usually range from 2.15 to 2.6 mmol/L (8.6 to 10.4 mg/dL).

Hypercalcemia defined as serum calcium >10.4 mg/dL (2.60 mmol/L) is a common finding, the setting of ambulatory primary care (about 1%) and inpatient hospital population (about 1%–4%).

The prevalence is variable and depends on the cause of the hypercalcemia. Hypercalcemia secondary to hyperparathyroidism, most common among adults greater than 65 years old, has a prevalence of 1–7 cases per 1000 adults and an annual incidence ranging from 0.41 to 21.6 cases per 100,000. Primary hyperparathyroidism being the predominant cause in the general population with malignancy being the predominant cause among hospital population.

Primary hyperparathyroidism and malignancy accounting for 90% of all cases of hypercalcemia. This as well as the causes of the remaining 10% require careful investigation.

The diagnosis of hypercalcemia is made when the albumin-corrected calcium concentration is two standard deviations above the mean normal value in at least two samples that are at least 1 week apart over a period of 3 months. Symptomatic patients present with nausea, vomiting, mental disturbance, depression, polyuria, abdominal pain (peptic ulcer, renal colic), constipation, bone pain.

When investigating causes of hypercalcemia, it helps to define the cause as either PTH related or non-PTH hypercalcemia. The finding of an elevated PTH level or PTH level that is not appropriately suppressed in the presence of hypercalcemia indicates possible hyperparathyroidism. Additionally, mildly elevated calcium is often seen in patients with hyperparathyroidism this is in contrast to the markedly elevated calcium in patients with hypercalcemia of malignancy (non-PTH).

Non-PTH-related hypercalcemia includes vitamin D toxicity, thyrotoxicosis (thyroid hormones stimulate RANK-ligand-mediated bone resorption), adrenal insufficiency, pheochromocytoma (part of the multiple endocrine neoplasia type II, some secrete PTH-related peptide, and/ or directly stimulating bone resorption), certain drugs such as thiazide diuretics (in about 8% of patients, increased renal reabsorption of calcium resulting in hypercalciuria), and lithium (stimulating PTH secretion and thus increased renal calcium reabsorption), supplementation with calcium and vitamin D in patients with renal failure, and therapeutic recombinant PTH. A familiar form characterized by hypocalciuric hypercalcemia due to genetic abnormalities in calcium sensing and thus continued PTH action at the kidney with continued reabsorption of filtered calcium. Other causes of mild hypercalcemia include prolonged immobilization (prominent when there is high bone turnover such as in young persons) (Table 4).

Humeral hypercalcemia in malignancy is due to either production of PTH-related peptide (PTHrp) by the tumor,

TABLE 4 Classification, causes of hypercalcemia, and associated biochemical measurements.

Hypercalcemia causes	Disorders	Biochemical findings
PTH-related		
Hyperparathyroidism	• Adenoma, hyperplasia, carcinoma, secondary and tertiary hyperparathyroidism • Familial hypocalciuric hypercalcemia • Ectopic PTH	• Elevated PTH (includes mildly elevated and within normal limits in the presence of hypercalcemia), i.e., inappropriate PTH levels for the calcium levels. • Low urinary calcium in the presence of hypercalcemia • Malignancy-rare
Non-PTH related		
Malignancy		
	• Humoral hypercalcemia of malignancy. • Osteolysis (bone metastatic involvement)	• PTHrp (PTH-related peptide) (lung, esophagus, skin, cervix, breast, kidney)
Endocrine causes	• Thyrotoxicosis • Adrenal insufficiency • Pheochromocytoma • Vasoactive intestinal Peptide (VIPoma)	• Elevated thyroid hormones with suppressed TSH • Elevated metanephrines • Elevated VIP
Vitamin D related	• Vitamin D intoxication • Granulomatous disease (sarcoidosis, tuberculosis, histoplasmosis, etc.)	• 25-OH vitamin D levels are markedly elevated • 1,25-$(OH)_2$ vitamin D levels elevated or within normal limits in the presence of suppressed PTH and PTHrp/ (Increased 1-alpha-hydroxylation of 25-OH Vit D) [lymphoproliferative and granulomatous]
Drugs		
	• Lithium, thiazide diuretics, recombinant PTH, calcium, and antiacids	• Lithium • PTH
Other causes		
	• Immobilization • Renal dysfunction	• Creatinine/BUN

Modified from Minisola S, Pepe J, Piemonte S, Cipriani C. The diagnosis and management of hypercalcaemia. *BMJ*. 2015;350:h2723.

typically squamous carcinoma's, or infiltration by the tumors and local osteolysis, mostly seen in hematological malignancy. Additionally, malignant cells and granulomas overexpress 1-alpha-hydroxylase which increases the conversion of 25-OH vitamin D to the active form 1,25-$(OH)_2$ vitamin D (calcitriol) leading to increased intestinal absorption of calcium and the presence of hypercalcemia and hypercalciuria (due to renal overflow).

Hypercalcemia secondary to pheochromocytoma is thought to be either related to production of PTHrp activity or to direct bone resorption.

Hypercalcemia of malignancy is observed in 2.7% of patients with cancer in adults and much lower 0.5%–1% in children.

Other causes of hypercalcemia include vitamin D excess (toxicity), thyrotoxicosis, adrenal insufficiency, drugs such as thiazide diuretics and lithium. Lithium stimulates parathyroid hormone secretion and thus increases renal calcium reabsorption. Thiazide diuretics increase renal reabsorption of calcium with 8% of people developing hypercalcemia while on thiazides.

In patients with familial hypocalciuric hypercalcemia, there is increased production of PTH and reabsorption of calcium from the kidney in the presence of hypercalcemia. There is alteration in calcium sensing receptor decreasing its sensitivity to hypercalcemia (see later).

Investigations of hypercalcemia

A stepwise diagnostic approach in the investigation of hypercalcemia is recommended (Fig. 4). In outpatient settings, the finding of hypercalcemia should be repeated in

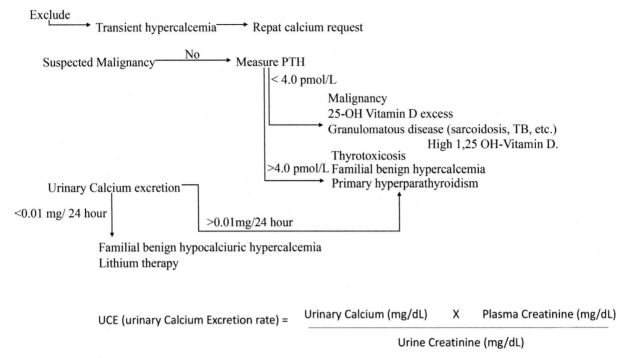

Exclude
→ Transient hypercalcemia → Repat calcium request

Suspected Malignancy —— No —→ Measure PTH

< 4.0 pmol/L

Malignancy
25-OH Vitamin D excess
Granulomatous disease (sarcoidosis, TB, etc.)
High 1,25 OH-Vitamin D.
Thyrotoxicosis
>4.0 pmol/L Familial benign hypercalcemia
→ Primary hyperparathyroidism

Urinary Calcium excretion

<0.01 mg/ 24 hour

>0.01mg/24 hour

Familial benign hypocalciuric hypercalcemia
Lithium therapy

$$UCE \text{ (urinary Calcium Excretion rate)} = \frac{\text{Urinary Calcium (mg/dL)} \quad X \quad \text{Plasma Creatinine (mg/dL)}}{\text{Urine Creatinine (mg/dL)}}$$

FIG. 4   Algorithm for the biochemical investigation of hypercalcemia. Initial finding of hypercalcemia is confirmed by repeat measurement at a separate instance to rule out transient hypercalcemia (immobilization, etc.). This is followed by PTH measurement where the finding of suppressed levels <4.0 pmol/L suggests either malignancy, granulomatous disease, or vitamin D toxicity, or familial hypercalcemia, or hyperthyroidism. The latter is investigated by measuring TSH and thyroid hormones. Elevated PTH suggest hyperparathyroidism and is associated with elevated urinary calcium. The finding of low urinary calcium suggests the presence of familial hypocalciuric hypercalcemia, or drug therapy (interfere with renal calcium handling such as lithium). (*Modified from Tonon CR, Silva TAAL, Pereira FWL, et al. A review of current clinical concepts in the pathophysiology, etiology, diagnosis, and management of hypercalcemia. Med Sci Monit. 2022;28:e935821. doi:10.12659/MSM.935821. PMID: 35217631; PMCID: PMC8889795.*)

two different occasions within a period of 3 months. Mild and gradual increase in calcium levels over a very longtime period could be suggestive of primary hyperparathyroidism, whereas a rapid and acute rise in calcium levels over a short period of time is suggestive of malignancy as the cause of hypercalcemia. Therefore, clinical assessment guides the subsequent investigations for the hypercalcemia.

As discussed earlier, total calcium levels are influenced by albumin levels where patients with significantly low albumin exhibit a false normal or low calcium levels. Calcium levels are preferably corrected for albumin levels (described above) or that ionized is measured if available.

The finding of elevated PTH or unsuppressed PTH in the presence of hypercalcemia is indicative of primary hypothyroidism the finding of hypophosphatemia supports the diagnosis.

Finding of suppressed PTH in the presence of hypercalcemia indicates malignancy which is confirmed by the presence of elevated PTHrp. The characteristics and thus performance of PTH assays is important when investigating patients with calcium disorders. Third generational assays are commercially available with antibodies directed at different epitopes of the PTH molecule and thus either measuring the intact 1–84 amino acid PTH molecule, fragments of the PTH molecule (mid molecule c-fragments),

and/or N-terminal fragments. The intact 1–84 PTH assays is considered as the gold standard, as it supposedly free for interference by PTH fragments circulating in renal dysfunction. The second and third generation assays offer improved specificity and sensitivity and are thus preferred (see Chapter 1 on endocrine testing). The finding of elevated or near normal PTH levels in the presence of hypercalcemia suggests primary hyperparathyroidism is the most likely diagnosis. Renal function should also be evaluated.

It helps differentiate between parathyroid carcinoma and benign disease. Posttranslational modification (12–18 aa region) seen in carcinoma is detected by third generation assays that gives lower value compared to second generation assays where ratio > 1 suggestive of parathyroid carcinoma.

Increased 1-alpha-hydroxy vitamin D in the presence of hypercalcemia suppressed PTH and PTHrp indicates the presence of granulomatous disease.

The finding of a mildly elevated or an inappropriately suppressed PTH requires ruling out of benign familial hypocalciuric hypercalcemia by measuring urinary calcium levels. Familial hypocalciuric hypercalcemia is a rare autosomal dominant disorder. It results from mutations in the calcium sensing receptor gene (CASR) leading to reduced receptor activity.

Either a 24-h urinary calcium levels or more commonly a random urine sample corrected for calcium measurements corrected for creatinine is used.

Vitamin D 25 level is determined. The finding of low levels of vitamin D impairs calcium urinary reabsorption and thus complicates the diagnosis of familial hypocalciuric hypercalcemia, and it is recommended that patient vitamin D status is restored before assessment of urinary calcium levels.

Reduced renal calcium clearance (calcium to creatinine ratio clearance value is less than 0.01) is strongly suggestive of familial hypocalciuric hypercalcemia. Serum magnesium level in familial hypocalciuric hypercalcemia is typically in the high range of normal or moderately increased.

Other causes of hypercalcemia include dehydration which can be considered as false hypercalcemia due to the increase in albumin levels and that concentration of ionized calcium is within normal range.

Prolonged immobilization leads to hypercalcemia secondary to increased bone resorption. It is more evident in young growing adults. Patients with acute renal failure secondary to rhabdomyolysis exhibit hypercalcemia in the presence of hyperphosphatemia.

Management of hypercalcemia includes establishing the cause, rehydrating with 0.9% sodium chloride, use of calcitonin (inhibits bone resorption and decreases renal tubular reabsorption). It has a short-lived action with onset within 2 h and drug tolerance reached within 2 days,

phosphate, and glucocorticoids as well as bisphosphonates (inhibit osteoclast activity) are frequently used. Denosumab, a fully humanized monoclonal antibody binds to RANK-like ligands and inhibits the maturation, activation, and function of osteoclasts. Prednisolone inhibits 1-alpha-hydroxylase and activates 24-hydroxylase thus directing vitamin D hydroxylation to the inactive 24,25 vitamin D form.

Hypocalcemia

Hypocalcemia defined as serum calcium levels <7.2 mg/dL (1.80 mmol/L). Causes of hypocalcemia include, hypoparathyroidism, pseudohypoparathyroidism, vitamin D deficiency, hypomagnesemia, renal impairment, drugs, tumor lysis syndrome, acute pancreatitis, and rhabdomyolysis (Fig. 5).

Symptoms of hypocalcemia include paresthesia, numbness, tingling, behavioral disturbance, tetany, convulsion, and cataracts in patients with chronic hypocalcemia.

About 5%–8% of hospitalized patients exhibit hypocalcemia mostly due to the presence low albumin. Adjusting measured calcium levels for albumin levels using the formula described above often resolves the apparent hypocalcemia among immobilized patients.

Causes of hypocalcemia may best categorized as PTH-mediated (hypoparathyroidism) and non-PTH causes (e.g., vitamin D deficiency).

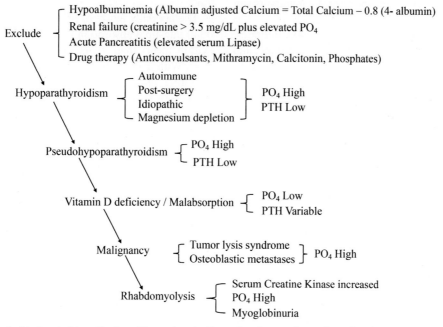

FIG. 5 Algorithm for the biochemical investigation of hypocalcemia. Hypocalcemia secondary to hypoalbuminemia, renal dysfunction, pancreatitis, and to drug therapy are easily exclude, inappropriately low PTH indicates hypoparathyroidism. Vitamin D levels are assessed. Hypocalcemia is encountered in tumor lysis syndrome and in patients with rhabdomyolysis. (*Modified from various sources including Pepe J, Colangelo L, Biamonte F, et al. Diagnosis and management of hypocalcemia. Endocrine. 2020;69(3):485–495. doi:https://doi.org/10.1007/s12020-020-02324-2. Epub 2020 May 4. PMID: 32367335.*)

Stepwise approach to the investigation of hypocalcemia is preferred. Hypocalcemia is confirmed by correcting for albumin (as discussed above) or by measuring ionized calcium if available. The latter is preferred in the presence of acid base disorders. Hypoalbuminemia is often encountered in critically ill and immobilized hospitalized patients.

Once hypocalcemia is confirmed (albumin correction and repeat measurement), biochemical investigation includes measurement of PTH, phosphate, as well as assessment of renal function (glomerular filtration rate). Assessment of GFR is required to rule out renal impairment as a primary cause of hyperphosphatemia. The presence of hyperphosphatemia in renal failure may also be due to either primary hypoparathyroidism or more commonly to secondary hyperparathyroidism. PTH levels are elevated in chronic kidney disease secondary to the hyperphosphatemia, hypocalcemia (leading to secondary hypoparathyroidism). Patients with renal impairment will exhibit low $1,25\text{-}(OH)_2$ Vitamin D due to reduced 1-α-hydroxylase activity (converting 25-OH vitamin D to the active $1,25\text{-}(OH)_2$ vitamin D) and high FGF23. Patients will exhibit renal osteodystrophy.

Magnesium levels are measured since magnesium is required for both PTH secretion and action. Hypomagnesemia may cause a misinterpretation of the possible hypoparathyroidism (low PTH). Attempts to correct the hypocalcemia without correcting hypomagnesemia will not improve and reverse the hypocalcemia (ineffective PTH). Causes of hypomagnesaemia are discussed below. Similarly, the presence of hypermagnesemia in patients with renal impairment may inhibit PTH activity.

Drugs may cause hypocalcemia (e.g., loop diuretics, anticonvulsants, phosphate, EDTA, magnesium sulfate, and bisphosphonates).

Hypocalcemia and low PTH may be associated with the autoimmune polyendocrine syndrome type 1 (APD1) supported by the presence of at least two of either Addison's disease, hypoparathyroidism, and mucocutaneous candidiasis.

Genetic disorders to be considered include the rare deletions of 22q11.2 which is characterized by hypoparathyroidism, autoimmune disorders, cognitive disorders, gastrointestinal and renal dysfunction in the young. Resistance to PTH action characterized by hypocalcemia, hyperphosphatasemia, and elevated PTH levels. Clinically, the patient is of short stature, brachydactyly, obese, and exhibits cognitive impairment.

Patients with hypophosphatemia. Elevated alkaline phosphatase and severe 25-OH vitamin D deficiency and hypocalcemia support the diagnosis of osteomalacia or rickets. The presence of normal vitamin D levels and elevated PTH in the presence of hypocalcemia and hypophosphatemia suggest the presence of vitamin D-dependent rickets (VDDR) or resistant rickets (hypocalcemia vitamin D-resistant rickets (HVDRR)).

Hypocalcemia in patients with pancreatitis and rhabdomyolysis is due to sequestration of calcium. Serum amylase and creatine kinase levels are measured retrospectively.

Phosphate pathophysiology

Phosphorus is a major constituent of all tissues and plays important roles in structure and in metabolism. It is incorporated into phospholipids of cell membranes and nucleic acids. Inorganic phosphate is a major constituent of hydroxyapatite of the bone serving as a body store for phosphate. It is present in phosphoproteins involved in metabolism in high energy metabolism. Examples being ATP, creatine phosphate, and in phosphoproteins involved in high energy metabolism such as muscle contraction, neurological functions, and electrolytes transport.

It is involved in many biochemical reactions and in cell signaling and metabolism examples being phosphate containing (ADP, NAD, cyclic-AMP, cyclic-GMP). It is involved in glucose phosphorylation by glucose-6-phosphate in glycolysis, in delivery of oxygen to tissue, in erythrocytes 2,3-diphopsphglycerate. Additionally, phosphate has an important role as a urinary buffer in its HPO_4^{2-} form.

Phosphate homeostasis

A healthy adult will contain 630 g (22 mol) of phosphate, 85% of which is present in the bone as hydroxyapatite, 10%–15% in skeletal muscle, and <1% in the extracellular fluid.

Dietary daily intake of phosphate is about 50 mmol with small intestinal absorption being higher in its soluble form (within meat) than in its insoluble form (within vegetables). With average absorption being 60%–70% of intake. Therefore, plasma inorganic phosphate varies with diet, exercise, age and demonstrates a marked circadian rhythm. Large changes in phosphate can be due to redistribution from the ECF to the ICF and vice versa.

Changes in phosphate may accompany calcium deposition or resorption of the bone. Direct control of plasma phosphate is achieved mainly by the kidney where tubular resorption is reduced by PTH with 80%–90% of phosphate filtered through the glomerulus is reabsorbed in the renal proximal tubules.

The amount of phosphate absorbed exceeds the daily requirement and that serum phosphate level is maintained via homeostatic control of intestinal absorption and renal handling of phosphate excretion and reabsorption. Absorption of phosphate in the intestine is attained by either passive transport of phosphate across tight junctions between cells and that the rate of absorption is directly proportional to the dietary phosphate contents. An active vitamin D-dependent absorption takes place via a sodium-phosphate transporter expressed in the brush border of enterocytes. The active absorption component becomes important when dietary phosphate content is low. Intestinal absorption of phosphate is reduced in the presence of aluminum hydroxide containing antiacid, glucocorticoids, high magnesium, and in hypothyroidism.

Homeostatic regulation of circulating phosphate levels is influenced by phosphate movement between extra-intracellular compartments. This transcellular movement is enhanced by respiratory alkalosis and by insulin.

Hormonal control of phosphate homeostasis is shown in Fig. 6. PTH has a phosphaturic effect by reducing the number of phosphate transporters in the proximal renal tubules. It stimulates the internalization and degradation of the sodium phosphate transporters (Fig. 6).

The active form of vitamin D (1,25-OH vitamin D) enhances intestinal absorption of phosphate by upregulating the sodium phosphate transporter. It's role in renal tubules remains unclear but shown to increase renal proximal transporters and thus reabsorption of phosphate.

Fibroblast growth factor 23 (FGF23) produced primarily by osteocytes and by osteoblast to a smaller extent is central to phosphate and calcium metabolism. Its expression is normally suppressed by phosphate regulating gene present on chromosome X. It has a net hypophosphatemic effect where it inhibits renal tubular reabsorption of phosphate by suppressing the expression of the sodium phosphate transporters in the proximal renal tubules. Although

1,25-$(OH)_2$ vitamin D stimulates FGF23 synthesis, the latter enhances breakdown of 1,25-$(OH)_2$ vitamin D by stimulating CYP 24. It is worth noting that FGF23 also inhibits PTH synthesis.

Total phosphate concentration in plasma is 3.9 mmol/L of which only 0.8–1.3 mmol/L is an inorganic phosphate. Ninety percent of the inorganic phosphate is present in a free form, 6% is complexed with calcium magnesium, whereas 10% is protein bound. Under normal acid base status, the majority of the free and organic phosphate is in the HPO_4^{2-} form compared to $H_2PO_4^-$ in a 4:1 ratio. The ratio decreases under acidic states and increases in alkaline states.

Hyperphosphatemia

The incidence of hyperphosphatemia among hospitalized patients without end-stage renal disease is reported to be about 12%. Among patients with renal disease who are on dialysis the incidence of hyperphosphatemia is 50%–74%.[3]

Acute severe hyperphosphatemia when associated with symptomatic hypercalcemia can be life-threatening. Phosphate levels bind to calcium causing precipitation and deposition of calcium phosphate in soft tissues leading to calcification this may occur in any organ including the myocardium, lungs, liver, skin, cornea, and conjunctiva. Vascular calcification can produce a syndrome of systemic calciphylaxis.

Causes of hyperphosphatemia falls into the following categories: transcellular shift, decreased renal excretion, acute phosphate load, and artifactual hyperphosphatemia due to preanalytical and analytical factors. Hypoparathyroidism decreased PTH levels (Fig. 7).

Preanalytical factors contributing to false hyperphosphatemia include hemolysis due to either poor sample collection or delayed sample processing due to intracellular phosphate leakage from erythrocytes (hemolysis).

The presence of excess immunoglobulins is seen in patients with multiple myeloma, Waldenström's macroglobulinemia interfere with the phosphate phosphomolybdate complex formation, or possibly by phosphate binding to the negatively charged paraproteins. This is however not seen in all patients with multiple myeloma.

The most common cause of hyperphosphatemia is renal impairment. However, in early renal impairment, phosphate concentrations are often within normal levels by initial elevation of FGF23 which decreases proximal tubular reabsorption. Significant hyperphosphatemia is observed once the GFR is below 20%–30% of normal or below 30 mL/min. Reduced GFR leads to decreased secretion and increased retention of phosphate. Impaired renal synthesis of 1,25-$(OH)_2$ vitamin D leads to secondary hyperparathyroidism seen in patients with kidney disease which results in increased osteoclastic bone resorption and the release of calcium and phosphate. Acidosis

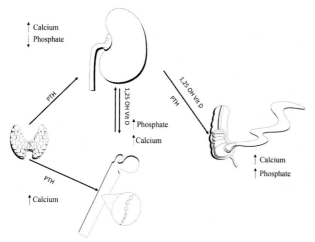

FIG. 6 Phosphate metabolism. Regulation of serum phosphate by PTH, 1,25 vitamin D, and fibroblast factor 23 (FGF23). PTH acts on the kidney be stimulating exertion of phosphate and reabsorption of calcium. It also stimulates 1,25 hydroxylase enzyme which converts 25-OH vitamin D to the active 1,25-OH Vitamin D. The latter reabsorbs calcium and excrete phosphate into the urine. 1,25-OH vitamin D and PTH acts on the gastrointestinal tract to reabsorb both phosphate and calcium. PTH causes calcium resorption from the bone and is inhibited by FGF23. The latter is stimulated by 1,25-OH vitamin D. *(Modified from Leung J, Crook M. Disorders of phosphate metabolism. J Clin Pathol. 2019;72(11):741–747. doi:https://doi.org/10.1136/jclinpath-2018-205130. Epub 2019 Aug 29. PMID: 31467040.)*

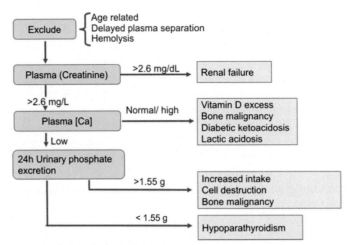

FIG. 7 Algorithm for the investigation of hyperphosphatemia. The most common cause of hyperphosphatemia is increased phosphate reabsorption and reduce glomerular filtration rate. Other causes include artifacts due to hemolysis and delayed sample processing and serum/plasma separation from cells, hypoparathyroidism, pseudohypoparathyroidism, acromegaly, excessive phosphate intake, tissue damage, tumor lysis syndrome, malignancy and in neonates (physiological high levels). *(Modified from Leung J, Crook M. Disorders of phosphate metabolism. J Clin Pathol. 2019;72(11):741–747. doi:https://doi.org/10.1136/jclinpath-2018-205130. Epub 2019 Aug 29. PMID: 31467040. García Martín A, Varsavsky M, Cortés Berdonces M, et al. Phosphate disorders and clinical management of hypophosphatemia and hyperphosphatemia. Endocrinol Diabetes Nutr (Engl Ed). 2020;67(3):205–215. [in English, Spanish]. doi:https://doi.org/10.1016/j.endinu.2019.06.004. Epub 2019 Sep 26. PMID: 31501071.)*

seen in patients with renal failure causes transcellular shift of phosphates from cells further contributing to hyperphosphatemia down an electronegativity gradient. This is also observed in patients with diabetic and lactic acidosis.

Excessive phosphate load due to either exogenous or indigenous sources leads to hyperphosphatemia particularly when there is impaired or excessive phosphate excretion. Endogenous increase loads of phosphates is seen in patients with cumulative syndrome due to breakage of cells and leakage of phosphate into the circulation, in patients with rhabdomyolysis due to the high content of phosphate in muscles, patient was hematological malignancies lymphoblast a particularly high in phosphorus. Exogenous sources of phosphates include ectopic skin applications or enemas widely used to treat constipation in both children and adults.

Tumor lysis syndrome is characterized by hyperphosphatemia and also hyperkalemia. In patients with impaired renal function, the hyperphosphatemia may be present before chemotherapy due to spontaneous cell death. Hyperphosphatemia is also seen in patients with vitamin D toxicity due to the increased intestinal absorption. Increased intake in milk (milk alkali syndrome).

PTH has phosphaturic affect and thus hyperphosphatemia is seen in patients with hypoparathyroidism. Growth hormone and IGF-I increases renal phosphate reabsorption and thus elevated levels seen in patients with acromegaly exhibit mild hyperphosphatemia.

Elevated thyroid hormones in thyrotoxicosis leads to hyperphosphatemia caused by increased tissue catabolism, bone resorption, and renal phosphate reabsorption. Reduced PTH secondary to the ensued hypercalcemia contributes to the hyperphosphatasemia.

A rare loss of function mutation affecting FGF23 causes either a reduction in circulating phosphate levels or end organ resistance in hypophosphatemic familial tumoral calcinosis.

Hypophosphatemia

Defined as serum phosphate less than 0.8 mmol/L with levels <0.3 mmol/L considered critically severe hypophosphatemia and requires immediate attention. Incidence of hypophosphatemia among hospitalized patients is 2.2%–3.1%. The incidence is, however, much higher (29%–34%) among patients in the intensive care, and 30% among patients with chronic alcoholism.

Patients with hypophosphatemia exhibit muscle weakness, respiratory and cardiac insufficiency. Hypophosphatemia leads to reduction in 2,3-diphosphoglycerate (2,3-DPG) increasing its affinity of hemoglobin for oxygen, reducing oxygen release into tissue. In patients with severe hypophosphatemia (<0.3 mmol/L), a range of clinical features are from proximal myopathy, tremors, seizures, confusion, cardiomyopathy, congestive heart failure, and respiratory failure.

Among many factors (Fig. 8), hypophosphatemia is mainly due to either decreased intake, or to increased renal excretion, transcellular redistribution, increased cellular uptake associated with high carbohydrate diet, insulin therapy, and hungry-bone-syndrome.

Most common causes in intensive care patients are decreased intestinal absorption, increased renal, and/or gastrointestinal losses.

Diuretic therapy, magnesium deficiency, vitamin D deficiency, hyperparathyroidism, enteral/parenteral nutrition

Hypophosphatemia

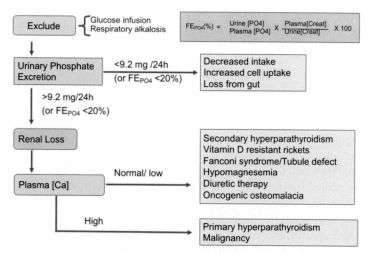

FIG. 8 Algorithm for the investigation of hypophosphatemia (serum/plasma <0.81 mmol/L (<2.5 mg/dL)). *(Modified from García Martín A, Varsavsky M, Cortés Berdonces M, et al. Phosphate disorders and clinical management of hypophosphatemia and hyperphosphatemia. Endocrinol Diabetes Nutr (Engl Ed). 2020;67(3):205–215. [in English, Spanish]. doi:https://doi.org/10.1016/j.endinu.2019.06.004. Epub 2019 Sep 26. PMID: 31501071.)*

in malnourished or alcoholic patients, secondary to transcellular shift due to ketoacidosis and to lactic acidosis in diabetic ketoacidosis, ingestion of nonabsorbable antacids (magnesium/aluminum salts). Congenital syndromes associated with hypophosphatemia include Fanconi syndrome, Wilson's disease, and X-linked hypophosphatemia crickets also known as vitamin D is resistant rickets. Multiple myeloma and heavy-metal intoxication leads to phosphate wastage by the affected renal tubules.

Increased intracellular pH seen in respiratory alkalosis stimulates phosphofructokinase with increased glycolysis and utilization of phosphate into the intermediate this leads to shift in phosphate from extracellular to intracellular and to hypophosphatemia.

Urinary phosphate levels ≪3.3 mmol/day (100 mg) indicates nonrenal loss as a cause of hypophosphatemia. Other causes for phosphate loss are gastrointestinal loss (diarrhea, vomiting).

False hypophosphatemia is observed in the presence of bilirubin levels and in presence of mannitol which binds the phosphate assay reagent molybdate.

Hyperventilation and respiratory alkalosis causes hypophosphatemia with values as low as 0.3 mmol/L. It is seen in a patient with septicemia, liver disease, salicylate intoxication, head injury, heat stroke, acute gout, and in mechanically ventilated patients.

Administration of insulin and glucose causes a shift of phosphate from the extracellular space to the intracellular causing a significant decrease in plasma phosphate concentration. Severe hypophosphatemia is seen in patients with nutritional deficiencies following refeeding and may precipitate cardiac failure and death.

Renal disease causes hyperphosphatemia however no phosphate levels are seen in up to 90% of patients in post renal transplant and about 6%–27% of patients have persistent low serum phosphate levels months or years later.

Primary hyperparathyroidism causes a reduction in the tubular maximum reabsorption of phosphate this leads to an initial increase in phosphate excretion and as a decrease in circulating phosphate levels however a steady state is reached, and significant phosphate depletion is not seen. This explains the moderately low phosphate level seen in the presence of hypercalcemia secondary to hyperparathyroidism. Hyperparathyroidism secondary to vitamin D deficiency results in significant hypophosphatemia due to reduce intestinal absorption and to renal phosphate wasting by PTH.

Symptoms and signs of hypophosphatemia vary and are dependent on the severity and the chronicity of phosphate depletion. Moderate and mild hypophosphatemia usually has few clinical manifestation clinical changes such as rickets or osteomalacia often the only consistent abnormality found.

Biochemical investigation of hypophosphatemia is shown in Fig. 8.

Magnesium homoeostasis

Magnesium is the most abundant divalent cation intracellularly followed by calcium. The body content of magnesium is 21–28 g (~1 mol) with 65% in bone bound to the surface of hydroxyapatite increasing the solubility of phosphorus and calcium, 34% intracellular compartment (soft tissue, muscle, myocardium, liver), and 1% is extracellular.

Normal circulating magnesium levels range from 0.7 to 1.1 mmol/L. It is present in several forma, free ionized form, bound to protein, or complexed with phosphates, citrates, bicarbonate, and sulfate. Under normal physiological conditions 23%–31% is bound to protein, 5%–11% is complexed with an ounce, and 59%–72% is present in the free form. Magnesium exhibits seasonal variation as well as ethnic variation where African Americans have lower magnesium levels.

Ionized magnesium is the biologically active form. When measuring total magnesium, significant changes in total proteins alters the proportion of free ionized magnesium and therefore measuring total magnesium may not represent magnesium status in nephrotic and protein losing enteropathies. Accurate measurement of ionized magnesium is performed by ion selective electrodes (ISE) and is dependent on using an ionophore specific for magnesium.

Magnesium is central to many biological functions. It is an essential cofactor for many (>300) enzymes such as alkaline phosphatase. It plays an important role in carbohydrate metabolism, insulin secretion, proteins, and nucleic acid synthesis. For instance, it is strongly bound to ATP forming a complex that is required for many rate limiting kinases.

Magnesium competes with ionized calcium for cellular membrane binding sites and inhibits calcium activity. Similar to calcium, its binding is pH dependent. It influences potassium balance between intra and extracellular compartment by inhibiting potassium chloride "transporters."

Magnesium is central to calcitonin stimulation, parathyroid hormone secretion an action, osteoblast adhesion, and thus to bone formation.

The main site for magnesium absorption is the small intestine, renal reabsorption and negative feedback maintains magnesium homeostasis. Similar to calcium, PTH absorbs magnesium at the kidney and in concert with vitamin D absorbs magnesium at the intestine. High fat, protein, calcium, and phosphate dietary content as well as alcohol, decrease the availability of magnesium in diet and reduces its absorption. Magnesium excretion is mostly vis the kidney and to smaller extent via the skin in sweat. Recommend daily intake is 10–15 mmol (300–400 mg/day).

When using heparin as anticoagulant, it should be at low concentration as it interferes with ionized magnesium measurement, similarly silicon used in vacutainer coating causes falsely elevated ionized magnesium due to a surfactant effect which changes the selectivity of magnesium selective electrode.

Although assays for the measurement of ionized magnesium are commercially available, total magnesium measurement remains the mainstay in clinical laboratories. The need to maintain the acid-base status of the specimen, free ionized magnesium concentration is PH dependent and magnesium binding to protein is increased at increased pH, thus requirement for rapid measurements of ionized magnesium. Lack of standardization among commercial commercially available assays has made measuring ionized a magnesium less favorable.

The high magnesium concentration inside red blood cell means that falsely elevated magnesium levels are seen in hemolyzed samples.

Plasma levels are not reliable indicator of body stores. However, persistent hypomagnesemia may indicate magnesium deficiency.

Magnesium disorders

Magnesium abnormality among 5%–10% of hospitalized patients. Magnesium disorders are those leading to either hypermagnesemia or hypomagnesemia. Causes and biochemical investigation are described below.

Hypermagnesemia

It is defined by a serum magnesium level >1.2 mmol/L (2.5 mg/dL). The prevalence among outpatients ranges from 3% to 10%. Hypermagnesemia is rare in patients with normal renal function, and it is mostly seen in patients with impaired renal function.

Although reduced renal reabsorption leads to hypomagnesemia (described below), this is overridden by the progressive reduction in glomerular filtration and thus magnesium excretion.

Although only 15% of patients with chronic kidney disease exhibit hypermagnesemia, the majority have normal magnesium and levels and few even hypomagnesemia. This is thought to be a reflection of reduced dietary intake (often top also reduce potassium). Other factors among renal patients include vitamin D deficiency, use of diuretics, and the low magnesium content in dialysate fluid and that the often present hypoalbuminemia in patients undergoing dialysis facilitates the removal of ionized and nonprotein bound fractions contributing to the negative balance.

False hypermagnesemia is commonly seen in poorly collected and handled blood samples. Delayed sample processing and separation from cells cause leakage of magnesium from red blood cells. Samples with slight hemolysis, often not apparent to the naked eye, results in hypermagnesemia, spectrophotometric assessment of hemolysis index provides a more sensitive indication for false hypermagnesemia.

Patients with in vivo hemolysis seen in coagulopathies will also exhibits hypermagnesemia. The extent may not be significant in the presence of intact renal function.

Magnesium levels >1.7–2.1 mmol/L are associated with neurological and cognitive dysfunction, confusion, absent deep tendon reflexes, gait disturbances, nausea and vomiting. Levels >3 mmol/L is associated with cardiovascular symptoms and dysrhythmia.

Hypermagnesemia is seen in patients taking oral antiacid, intravenous therapy. High dose magnesium sulfate is given in the management of preeclampsia to prevent seizures and treatment of severe hypertension. Therapeutic serum levels are in the range from 1.8 to 3.0 mmol/L often following a loading dose of 2.5–5 g and a maintenance dose of 1–2 g/h for 6–12 h.

Hypomagnesemia

Hypomagnesemia is common among hospitalized patients (up to 11%) with high incidence (50%–65%) among patients in intensive care units, defined as serum magnesium levels <0.75 mmol/L (1.8 mg/dL).

Causes of hypomagnesemia may be classified as either as renal or nonrenal causes. Nonrenal causes include gastrointestinal losses secondary to inflammatory bowel disease, diarrhea, vomiting, gastrointestinal malignancy, decreased intake (malnutrition, alcoholism), reduced absorption due to decreased surface area (bariatric surgery, intestinal resection), reduced absorption secondary to vitamin D deficiency.

Renal causes include impaired reabsorption, tubular damage (acute tubular necrosis), syndrome of inappropriate ADH, osmotic diuresis, polyuria, and proteinuria. There are a number of inherited disorders affecting renal reabsorption of magnesium, they include, hypercalciuric hypomagnesemia due to mutations in CLDN.16, 19, KB, and CASR genes, in Gitelman-like hypomagnesaemia, Kearns-Sayre syndrome mitochondrial hypomagnesemia.

Other causes are sepsis, refeeding syndrome and hungry bone syndrome, citrate chelation following blood transfusion (citrate as anticoagulant in blood bags).

Drugs inhibiting magnesium reabsorption include diuretics, anti-EGFR inhibitors, antibiotics (aminoglycosides, cyclosporine, tacrolimus), and insulin therapy (shift magnesium into cells).

There is increased requirement for magnesium during pregnancy due to fetal demand, tissue distribution, and to increased renal output. If not corrected, the ensued hypomagnesemia may lead to premature labor, preeclampsia (patients at risk for developing preeclampsia exhibited lower magnesium levels compared with normal counterpart), and to fetal growth retardation. However, currently there is no consensus on the benefit of magnesium supplementation.

False hypomagnesemia is encountered when blood tubes collections were contaminated with anticoagulants (such as EDTA or citrate) during multiple tubes collections and that are out of sequence.

Hypomagnesemia leads to hypocalcemia where PTH action on the bone is impaired in the presence of low magnesium. Low magnesium levels also inhibit PTH secretion by parathyroid glands. Additionally, magnesium is essential for the metabolism of vitamin D. It is a cofactor for its synthesis, transport and conversion to the active 1,25-(OH)$_2$ Vitamin D for, thus magnesium, deficiency leads to vitamin D resistance and must be assessed during supplementation of vitamin D deficiency.

An algorithm for the investigation of hypomagnesaemia is shown in Fig. 9. Loss (urinary levels >2.43 mg/day renal loss) whereas urinary levels <2.43 mg/day indicates nonrenal in the presence of hypomagnesemia. A 24 h urine magnesium sample is preferred over random urine as magnesium excretion varies with dietary intake, diurnal rhythm, and the added advantage of assessing daily urine volume for renal function.

Fractional excretion of magnesium is calculated as follows; FE_{Mg} = Serum Creatinine × Urine Magnesium/0.7 × Serum Magnesium × Urine Creatinine.

Where serum magnesium is multiplied by 0.7 to account for the nonalbumin bound fraction. Fractional excretion of ≥4% indicates renal loss of magnesium similarly for a daily magnesium urinary excretion of >1 mmol/day (2.43 mg/day).

Diuretics

Diuretics are widely used to increase urine flow and thus reduce body fluid volume. Most diuretics inhibit sodium reabsorption, reducing cellular, and tubular osmotic gradient (high osmotic pressure on the lumen side), thus results in reduced water reabsorption and net water loss. The receptors for the diuretics, with the exception of spironolactone, are on the luminal surface. The diuretics diffuse across tubular cells reaching their receptors.

Diuretics action is mainly on one of four classes and thus acts at four different sites at the nephron (Fig. 10). Loop diuretic (act at the thick ascending tubule, site II), thiazide diuretics (act at the distal convoluted tubule, site III), potassium sparing (act at the aldosterone sensitive distal collecting duct, site IV), carbonic anhydrase inhibitors, osmotic mannitol (proximal tubules).

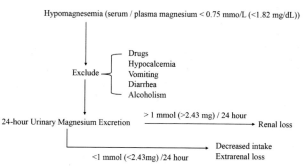

FIG. 9 Biochemical investigation of hypomagnesemia. Hypomagnesemia is due to either renal or nonrenal causes. Renal losses are conformed by measuring urinary magnesium levels (24 h urine collection or in an early morning random urine with values corrected for creatinine concentration). Nonrenal causes are those of gastrointestinal nature and are assessed clinically. *(Modified from Tucker BM, Pirkle JL Jr, Raghavan R. Urinary magnesium in the evaluation of hypomagnesemia. JAMA. 2020;324(22):2320–2321. doi:https://doi.org/10.1001/jama.2020.18400. Erratum in: JAMA. 2021;326(20):2081. PMID: 33125046.)*

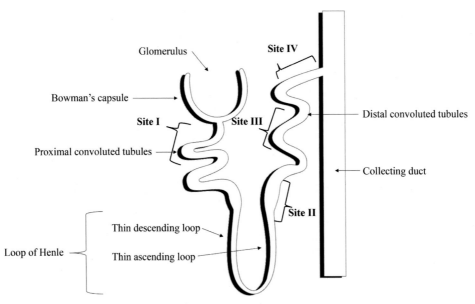

FIG. 10 Nephron sites of action of the different classes of diuretics described above. *(Modified from Lant A. Diuretics. Clinical pharmacology and therapeutic use (Part I). Drugs. 1985;29(1):57–87. doi:https://doi.org/10.2165/00003495-198529010-00003. PMID: 3882391.)*

TABLE 5 Mechanisms and sites of action of common diuretics.

Diuretic class	Target channels	Nephron region	Comments
Thiazides	Na$^+$ Cl$^-$ symport	III (cortical ascending loop and distal convoluted tubule)	Binds competitively to the chloride binding site. Inhibit 3%–5% of filtered Na$^+$
Loop diuretics (e.g., furosemide)	Na$^+$ K$^+$-2Cl$^-$ symport	Site II (thick ascending tubule)	Electroneutral transports and is activated once all sites are occupied. When blocked ~25% of filtered sodium would not be reabsorbed. Some sodium is reabsorbed at the expense of potassium via aldosterone at the collecting duct.
K-sparing diuretics	ENaCs, ROMK, AQP2	Site IV (distal collecting duct).	Weak diuretics (maximum 1%–2% of Na lost). Inhibits aldosterone action
Carbonic anhydrase inhibitors	Biochemical reaction: $(H_2O + CO_2 \rightleftarrows H_2CO_3 \rightleftarrows H^+ + HCO_3^-)$	Site I (proximal convoluted tubule)	Inhibits carbonic anhydrate and thus limit available H$^+$ for Na/H$^+$ exchange

AQP2, aquaporin channel 2 (water channel); *ENaCs*: epithelial sodium channels; *ROMK*, renal outer medullary potassium channel.
Modified from Wile D. Diuretics: a review. *Ann Clin Biochem*. 2012;49(Pt 5):419–431.

The different groups have different targets on the nephron and different mechanism of action. Channels of respective communication and actions are shown in Table 5.

Thiazides and thiazide-like diuretics

Chlorothiazide derived from addition of two sulfomoyl groups to sulfonamide. The original compounds were benzothiadiazide derivatives, this class of diuretics are named "thiazide" diuretics. The thiazide-like group are not true benzothiazides but are heterocyclic variants having the same pharmacological action.

Thiazide diuretics act on at the cortical portion of the ascending loop if Henle zone III (Fig. 10). They inhibit sodium-chloride channel (symport). There are not as effective as the loop diuretics as they can only inhibit up to a maximum of 3%–5% of the flittered sodium present in the tubular fluid.

The sodium chloride symporter derives its energy from Na-K-ATPase antiport in the basolateral membrane. The latter maintains a low sodium concentration in the tubular cell facilitating an electrochemical gradient that favors sodium reabsorption.

The binding of sodium to its site ion the symporter facilitates K binding, and both leads to confirmational change those transfers both Na and Cl across the luminal membrane. Thiazide diuretics act by competitively inhibiting Cl binding, and thus, the symporter and conformational change is dysfunctional and Na is not transported across the tubular membrane.

Thiazides also increase K and H exchange for Na at the distal convoluted tubule, and that mutations in the Na-Cl symporter lead to Gitelman's syndrome of hypokalemic alkalosis.

Thiazides also cause reabsorption of calcium at the distal convoluted tubule and have been used to reduce urinal calcium levels in patients at risk of developing kidney stones.

Loop-diuretics

This category includes furosemide, bumetanide, and torsemide. They all inhibit Na^+/K^+-$2CL^-$ channel. The channel is located in region II of the nephron (hence the designation of the diuretics "loop diuretics" (Fig. 10) and activated when it's all four sites are occupied. The four are transported from the tubular lumen into the tubular cells, entered Na^+ is further transferred into the circulation by the Na^+ K^+-ATPase pump.

This second transporter facilitate additional Na transfer at the first step of uptake from the tube lumen.

Two other receptors play a role here, the renal outer medullary potassium channel (ROMK) and a basolateral chloride channel (CLCN). The addition of Na facilitates movement of CL. Additionally, K taken up by the Na K ATPase channel is recycled back into the lumen by an ATP-dependent ROMK channel. The product is net uptake of Na and secretion of Cl and K.

Blocking this Na K Cl channel prevents reabsorption of about 25% of filtered Na and aldosterone will reabsorb some of the blocked Na but at the expense of K (hence K losing diuretic).

Mutations in the Na K Cl gene (NKCC) causes hypokalemia, hypercalciuria, and metabolic alkalosis named Bartter's syndrome and thus resembling patients on loop diuretics.

Potassium sparing diuretics

This group includes amiloride, triamterene. At the distal tubule and collecting ducts, a sodium transporter mechanism termed epithelial sodium channels located in the principal cells in the luminal membrane. Those channels are aldosterone sensitive and are inhibited by amiloride (used to be named amiloride-inhibitable sodium channel), and triamterene. Also, it is indirectly inhibited by spironolactone and eplerenone.

The diuretics act at site IV (Fig. 10) to decrease the number of open epithelial NA channels.

Spironolactone is synthetic steroid aldosterone competitive antagonist.

Aldosterone induced protein (expressed following aldosterone binding to the hormone -sensitive elements). The aldosterone induced proteins activate silent epithelial sodium channels. This the spironolactone are aldosterone antagonist and thus indirectly impacts the epithelial sodium channels.

This category are weak diuretics capable of maximum excretion of 1%–2% of the filtered sodium. Thus, their main use is in conjunction with thiazide and loop diuretics to minimize potassium loss.

Epithelial Na channels are made up of three subunits α, β, and γ. Alpha transports Na, β, and γ enhances Na^+ transport by α. Mutations β and γ subunits render it more functional leading to sodium retention and hypertension in an autosomal dominant fashion (Liddle's syndrome).

Carbonic anhydrase inhibitors

This category includes acetazolamide acts at the proximal tubules site I of the nephron (Fig. 10).

The enzyme carbonic anhydrase catalyzes the CO_2 and water reaction by several thousand folds.

The diuretic works be decreasing availability of H to the Na-H exchanger, thus reducing Na and chloride reabsorption and inability to neutralize luminal HCO_3^-. This results in alkaline urine and bicarbonate loss, and to hyperchloremic metabolic acidosis (normal anion gap due to the high Cl).

Other diuretics include those causing osmotic diuresis such as mannitol, urea, isosorbide, and glycerin. Mannitol is the only one remaining in use in this group, a polyalcohol, filtered at the glomerulus but not reabsorbed by the tubule increasing tubular fluid osmolality and reducing water reabsorption. Thus, this diuretic causes water diuresis and not like the other diuretics that lead to natriuresis (sodium loss and thus its accompanied water). The action could be located at the AQP water channels present at the proximal tubules and the thin descending limb of Henle. Theophylline and caffeine (1,3,7-trimethylzanthine) are methylxanthine they increase GFR by relaxing smooth muscles of the afferent arterial bed often glomerulus, by directly inhibiting salt reabsorption at the proximal tubules.

Urinary electrolytes[4]

The measurement of urinary electrolytes (sodium, potassium, and chloride) although helpful in the investigation of electrolytes disorders, it is not routinely performed, limitations being the very wide reference intervals which renders their interpretation difficult, the interplay between the many pathophysiological factors, and in addition to the difficulty in obtaining a urine sample in an outpatient setting. However, the wide ranges seen in urine is a reflection of the physiological tight control and maintenance of blood electrolytes.

Urine electrolytes abnormalities of clinical significance are usually of value when assessing inpatient in critical care. They are of value when the patient acid base status and/or blood electrolytes are abnormal, in hypovolemic states, and in kidney injury. The value of spot urine sodium is in the differentiation between hypovolemia and euvolemic states (often difficult to diagnose clinically) as described above. A spot urine sodium concentration greater than 20 mmol/L in euvolemic states is suggestive of SIADH as the cause for hyponatremia.

Methods of electrolytes measurement

The electrolytes sodium (Na^+), potassium (K^+), chloride (Cl^-), magnesium (ionized) (Mg^{2+}), and calcium (ionized) (Ca^{2+}) are measured using electrodes selective to the ionized electrolyte. Spectrophotometric methods utilizing a chemical enzymatic as well as inductively coupled plasma or atomic absorption spectrophotometry are available (see Chapter 17 on analytical methods for detailed description).

Ion-selective electrodes (ISEs)

Ion selective electrodes measure potential difference (potentiometry) between a reference electrode and an ion-specific elector in the presence of that particular ion (e.g., sodium, potassium, chloride, calcium, or magnesium). The potential difference generated is proportional to the logarithmic concentration of the ion being measured (the Nernst equation ($E = E_0 + S \log kc$) where E, electrode potential; E_0, a constant dependent on the electrode system; S, slope of the electrode (i.e., change in mV produced for a given change in activity of an ion); k, activity coefficient of an ion (=1 for an ion in an infinitely dilute solution); c, concentration of the ion).

The ISEs are available in automated clinical chemistry laboratory-based analyzers, point-of-care devices , and in blood gases instruments.

The essential component of the electrode system is the selectivity of the membrane to the ions to be measured. Selectivity, and thus specificity, is achieved by the use of membranes. The membranes are made up of either porous glass, crystalize or polymeric material. Although glass membranes are frequently used for pH measurement, polymeric membranes are widely used for measurement of sodium, potassium, chloride, ionized calcium, and magnesium (see Chapter 17 on analytical methods for more details).

When measuring ions, the difference between concentration and molality is expressed by formula Na (concentration) = Sodium molality × mass concentration of water in kg/L. Normally the mass concentration of water in normal blood is 0.93 kg/L. thus when measuring ionic concentration it is corrected for a 0.93 volume, however, in the presence of water displacing molecules such as proteins and lipids, the mass concentration of water in kg/L of blood becomes less at about 0.8 kg/L. Thus, the difference between concentration and molality becomes greater (up to 20%). Direct methodologies are a reflection of molality (less affected by proteins and lipids), whereas methodologies requiring dilution (indirect ISEs) are affected by the presence of proteins and lipids. The water phase is diluted giving results lower than that obtained by molality.

Acceptable performance variability for sodium is ± 4 mmol/L, whereas for potassium is ± 0.5 mmol/L. There is a difference between whole blood sodium and potassium as determined by point of care devices (such as blood gas instruments) and in plasma by laboratory based clinical chemistry analyzers. Although the differences do not pose clinical limitations in most cases where in cases of rapidly changing electrolytes levels it may be relevant. Whole blood point of care often exhibits slight negative bias. Of note is the lack of serum indices particularly for hemolysis when using whole blood point of care instruments. Hemolysis due to either poor sample collection and handling or to intravascular in vivo hemolysis will not be detected and falsely elevated potassium levels may be reported.

The methods are classified as either direct or indirect. Indirect measurement involves dilution of the sample prior to measurement. This is widely used in large, automated chemistry analyzers to reduce sample viscosity, to reduce measurement time, and to extend electrode working life. In the direct approach, the sample is measured directly without prior dilution. The latter is used in blood gases analyzers where whole blood samples are applied onto the instrument without any prior processing/dilution to preserve sample integrity for blood gases measurement.

The electrodes used (known as membranes) are highly selective (e.g., Ca^{2+} electrode has a Ca:Mg selectivity ratio of 300:1, i.e., negligible interference of Mg in the measurement of Ca).

Potassium ion selective electrode

The potassium ion selective electrode is unique in that it incorporates the antibiotic valinomycin. Dimensions of the cavity inside the ring structure of valinomycin closely match the radius of K^+. When electrode with a valinomycin-containing electrode comes in contact with serum, K^+ enters the membrane, leaving behind the counter ion, Cl^-, on the other side of the membrane. At equilibrium, this charge separation creates a membrane potential that is proportional to the activity of K^+.

Spectrometric methods

Total calcium, total magnesium, and bicarbonate concentrations are measured spectrophotometrically. Calcium reacts with cresolphthalein complexone in alkaline/acidic condition forming a colored complex, the intensity of the color is proportional to the calcium concentration.

Total magnesium is measured enzymatically with three different reaction methodologies available. They are either based on hexokinases, isocitrate dehydrogenase, or glycerol kinase. The rate of the conversion of NADP to NADPH in the first two systems is monitored and correlated to the total magnesium concentration. In the glucokinase, hexokinase, or glucose-6-phophayte dehydrogenase, glucose and Mg-ATP (in the presence of enzyme) is converted to glucose-6-phosphate (G-6-P) and Mg-ADP. G-6-P plus NADP (in the presence of glucose-6-phosphate dehydrogenase) is converted to NADPH. Similarly, for isocitrate dehydrogenase, Potassium isocitrate plus NADP (in the presence of magnesium and isocitrate dehydrogenase) produces 2-oxoglutarate and NADPH and CO_2. The rate of change in NADP or NADPH is monitored spectrophotometrically and is proportional to the respective analyte conecntration.

The glycerol kinase method utilizes glycerol and hydrogen peroxide where the development of a colored product is proportional to the concentration of magnesium.

Bicarbonate reacts with phosphoenolpyruvate in the presence of phosphoenolpyruvate carboxylase (PEPC). The phosphoenolpyruvate accepts bicarbonate and is converted to oxaloacetate. The latter is converted to malate in the presence of malate dehydrogenase and NADH. The latter is converted to NAD analog. The rate of NADH disappearance is monitored at 415 nm and is directly proportional to the concentration of bicarbonate in the specimen.

Bicarbonate concentration may be derived mathematically using the Henderson-Hasselbalch equation $[H_2CO_3] = 0.03 \times pCO_2$, often applied when using whole blood sample on a blood gas analyzer.

Other methodologies of historical interest include flame emission spectroscopy (FES), and gravimetric methods (where the ion is bound in an ion exchanger column and selectively eluted, converted to a weighable precipitate of its salt (e.g., sodium sulfate in the case of sodium)). Other methods include inductively coupled plasma-atomic emission spectroscopy (ICP-AES). Atomic absorption spectroscopy (AAS) methodologies can be used for the measurement of sodium and potassium often in tissues (for research purposes) with graphite furnace atomic absorption spectroscopy (GFAAS) being more sensitive than AAS. The methodology is not applicable to chloride, fluoride, and iodine. Those methods are not used in routine practice.

Summary

- Water and electrotypes balance is closely interlinked and are essential for organ and body functions. Water follows sodium down a concentration gradient that is dependent on several factors.
- Water content represents 60% of body weight and is distributed throughout the intra- and extracellular space with approximately two-thirds being intracellular.
- Albumin being the main driving force for colloidal oncotic pressure.
- Osmolality of body fluids is determined by the number of dissolved solutes such as electrolytes, glucose, and urea.
- Osmolality is measured using freezing point depression. Vapor pressure-based instruments are not suitable when volatile alcohols are present.
- Osmolality may be calculated using a number of formulas. The most widely used is (Osmolality = $1.86 \times [Na^+] + $ urea/2.8 + glucose/18). When urea and glucose are measured in conventional units (mg/dL).
- A difference >10 mOsmol/L between measured and calculated osmolality is consider a gap and suggest the presence of an osmotically active substance.
- A reduction in blood volume is sensed by the juxtaglomerular cells and renin angiotensin aldosterone is released, the latter stimulating sodium absorption and associated water.
- Changes in osmolality are detected by hypothalamic cells, and causes release of antidiuretic hormone (ADH) in response.
- Hyponatremia (sodium <130 mmol/L) is the most encountered electrolyte disorder in clinical biochemistry laboratory.
- Pseudohyponatremia is secondary to the presence of large amounts of triglycerides, proteins and/or glucose.
- Hyperkalemia describes potassium >4.5 mmol/L. Causes include in vitro and in vivo hemolysis, renal impairment, acidosis, adrenal insufficiency, and secondary to drugs therapy.
- Hypokalemia defined as serum potassium less than 3.5 mmol/L the lower limit of reference intervals with levels <2.5 mmol/L considered critical and needs immediate attention.
- Causes leading to hypokalemia include gastrointestinal losses and renal losses.
- Calcium is the most abundant cation in the human body.
- About 45% of circulating calcium is bound to predominant plasma proteins, mainly albumin. The reminder is free ionized calcium (45%) with minor component (10%) complexed with anions such as phosphate and citrate.
- PTH and 1,25-$(OH)_2$ vitamin D maintain normal calcium levels.
- Primary hyperparathyroidism being the predominant cause of hypercalcemia in the general population with malignancy being the predominant cause among hospital population.
- Hypercalcemia in malignancy is due to either production of PTH-related peptide (PTHrp) by the tumor, bone resorption, or to various factors.

- Magnesium abnormality is present in 5%–10% of hospitalized patients. Hypermagnesemia mostly associated with reduced renal clearance.
- Causes of hypomagnesemia may be classified as either as renal or nonrenal causes.
- There are four classes of diuretics: Loop diuretic (act at the thick ascending tubule, site II), thiazide diuretics (act at the distal convoluted tubule, site III), potassium sparing (act at the aldosterone sensitive distal collecting duct, site IV), and carbonic anhydrase inhibitors, osmotic mannitol (proximal tubules).

References

1. Decaux G, Musch W. Clinical laboratory evaluation of the syndrome of inappropriate secretion of antidiuretic hormone. *Clin J Am Soc Nephrol.* 2008;3(4):1175–1184.
2. Minisola S, Pepe J, Piemonte S, Cipriani C. The diagnosis and management of hypercalcaemia. *BMJ.* 2015;350:h2723.
3. Leung J, Crook M. Disorders of phosphate metabolism. *J Clin Pathol.* 2019;72(11):741–747.
4. Umbrello M, Formenti P, Chiumello D. Urine electrolytes in the intensive care unit: from pathophysiology to clinical practice. *Anesth Analg.* 2020;131(5):1456–1470.

Further reading

Pepe J, Colangelo L, Biamonte F, et al. Diagnosis and management of hypocalcemia. *Endocrine.* 2020;69(3):485–495.

Nadar R, Shaw N. Investigation and management of hypocalcaemia. *Arch Dis Child.* 2020;105(4):399–405.

Berend K, van Hulsteijn LH, Gans RO. Chloride: the queen of electrolytes? *Eur J Intern Med.* 2012;23(3):203–211.

Wile D. Diuretics: a review. *Ann Clin Biochem.* 2012;49(Pt 5):419–431.

Van Laecke S. Hypomagnesemia and hypermagnesemia. *Acta Clin Belg.* 2019;74(1):41–47.

Chapter 3

Renal function

Introduction

The kidney plays essential role in excretion of nitrogenous waste, drugs, and metabolites, in maintaining water and electrolytes balance, in acid-base homeostasis, and as an endocrine organ playing a role in calcium metabolism and in erythropoiesis.

This chapter describes the pathophysiology of the kidney and the utility of biomarkers in the diagnosis and management of renal dysfunction.

Kidney structure and function

Most individuals will have two kidneys with each kidney weighing about 150 g, although solitary kidney occurs in 1:2400 individuals.

The Nephron is the functional unit of the kidney (Fig. 1) with each kidney containing about one million nephrons (0.4–1.2 million).

The nephron may be short or long depending on the location of the glomerulus within the cortex. The different functional segments of the nephron are the Bowman's campus which house the glomerulus, the proximal and distal convoluted renal tubules, the descending and ascending loop of Henle, and the collecting duct (Fig. 1). Detailed description of each area is discussed below. The different segments of the nephron differ in their function and metabolic activity and are influenced by their surrounding environment as well as hydrostatic pressure and blood supply and are discussed in detail below.

Both kidneys receive 20%–25% of the resting cardiac output via renal arteries. There is mostly one renal artery per kidney, although multiple arteries may exist. They originate from the aorta and exit the kidney via renal veins draining into the vena cava. Most (90%) of the blood reaching the kidney supplies the rich and highly active proximal tubular tissue located in the renal cortex.

The glomerulus

The glomerulus (renal capsule) comprises a capillary network enclosed within the Bowman's capsule (Fig. 2) and are supported by the glomerulus basement membrane. The capillary endothelial cells are in contact but circular fenestrations between them allow for filtration.

The narrowing of the blood vessels and formation of capillaries results in a perfusion pressure of at least 50–60 mmHg required to overcome the hydrostatic and oncotic pressures opposing filtration. Cont rol of this pressure is maintained intrinsically and irrespective of systemic pressure in the range of 80–200 mmHg. Less than 80 mmHg causes a rapid decline in glomerular filtration rate (GFR).

Epithelial cells lining the urinary side of the glomerular basement membrane (podocytes) are relatively impermeable to proteins with molecular weight greater than 66 kDa. Furthermore, the basement membrane is rich in negatively charged polyanionic glycoproteins such as heparin sulfate which provide the main barrier to the passage of polyanions such as albumin.

The glomerular filtration rate (GFR) is considered the best indicator of kidney function in health and in disease. A reduction in GFR will result in accumulation of nitrogenous waste and metabolites, impair drug clearance, and could be an indication of reduced kidney mass and thus impaired endocrine functions as well. The reduction in GFR is a reflection of the reduction in the number of functioning unit, the nephron (see later).

Cells of the macula densa (small portion of the of the distal tubule located beside the glomerulus), lining the afferent and efferent arteriole coupled by the anatomical return of the collecting duct and the ascending loop of Henle to the capsule compose a tubule-glomerular feedback (TGF) mechanism. Those are collectively known as the juxtaglomerular apparatus area indicated in Fig. 3. This area is responsible for renin secretion, sensing of the sodium in the macular densa, and thus the ability to influence fluid balance via sodium reabsorption and adjustment glomerular filtration flow rate. Renin-producing cells of the afferent and efferent arterioles are in close contact with cells of the macula densa.

Therefore, anatomically, several types of cells including, vascular smooth muscle cells, endothelial cells, mesangial cells, macula densa cells, and renin secreting granular cells constitute the juxtaglomerular apparatus. With the exception of the macula densa cells, the above cells are tightly coupled by gap junctions with calcium (Ca^{2+}) flux

Tutorials in Clinical Chemistry. https://doi.org/10.1016/B978-0-12-822949-1.00009-7

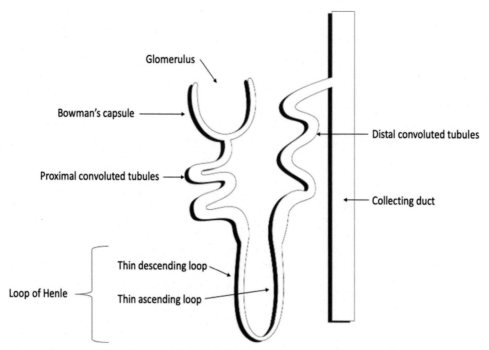

FIG. 1 The nephron. The functional unit of the kidney. It comprises, the glomerulus constituting Bowman's capsule, proximal and distal convoluted tubules, lope of Henle, and collecting duct. *(Modified from McMahon AP. Development of the mammalian kidney. Curr Top Dev Biol. 2016;117:31–64. doi:https://doi.org/10.1016/bs.ctdb.2015.10.010. Epub 2016 Jan 23. PMID: 26969971; PMCID: PMC5007134.)*

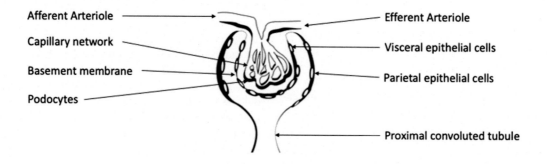

Bowman's capsule

FIG. 2 Bowman's capsule showing glomerular blood vessels (afferent and efferent arterioles), the capillary network and the narrow diameter of the efferent arterioles leads to development in hydrostatic pressure within the capsule facilitating ultrafiltration. The ultrafiltrate enters the proximal convoluted tubules where most are reabsorbed (see later). *(Modified from McMahon AP. Development of the mammalian kidney. Curr Top Dev Biol. 2016;117:31–64. doi:https://doi.org/10.1016/bs.ctdb.2015.10.010. Epub 2016 Jan 23. PMID: 26969971; PMCID: PMC5007134.)*

mediating intracellular communication and thus any required physiological response (Fig. 3).

In summary, the juxtaglomerular apparatus controls the release of renin and that of the glomerular hemofiltration dynamics.

Proximal tubules

A tightly coiled, proximal convoluted tubule, beginning from the Bowman's capsule and progressing toward the renal medulla. It is about 14mm in length with cylindrical

cells lining the tubule. The tubule can be divided into three segments based on metabolic activity, for instance the first and second segment have rapid reabsorption activity compared to the third segment, the amount of cellular mitochondria content (reflecting energy requirement), and type of brush border. Susceptibility to toxins is also varied for example segment three is more susceptible to mercury toxicity.

Reclamation of most of the glomerular filtrate, 75% of water and electrolytes (Na and Cl) and 100% of glucose, nearly all of the amino acids, micronutrients, and variable

Juxtaglomerular Apparatus

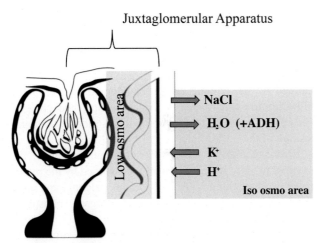

FIG. 3 Illustration showing areas of the juxtaglomerular apparatus (JGA). It comprises afferent and efferent arterioles, their epithelia cells, the macula densa cells, and the ascending loop of Henle, the distal convoluted tubules and the collecting ducts of the nephron in close proximity to the Bowman's campus. The areas of the macula densa are considered hypotonic compared to the area that surrounds the collecting duct (see Fig. 4). *(Modified from McMahon AP. Development of the mammalian kidney. Curr Top Dev Biol. 2016;117:31–64. doi:https://doi.org/10.1016/bs.ctdb.2015.10.010. Epub 2016 Jan 23. PMID: 26969971; PMCID: PMC5007134.)*

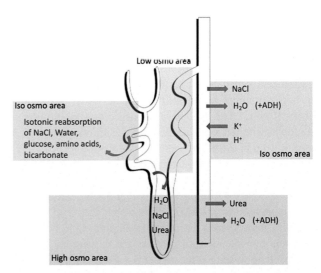

FIG. 4 Reabsorption, excretion, and development of countercurrent multiplication. Areas of variable degree of osmolality facilitates passive diffusion of water in the presence of ADH. *(Modified from Sands JM, Layton HE. The physiology of urinary concentration: an update. Semin Nephrol. 2009;29(3):178–195. doi:https://doi.org/10.1016/j.semnephrol.2009.03.008. PMID: 19523568; PMCID: PMC2709207.)*

amounts of bicarbonate, calcium, magnesium, and urate takes place at the proximal convoluted tubule. Reabsorption is energy dependent for most with some passive reabsorption down an osmotic concentration gradient.

The active reabsorption establishes an osmotic and electrical gradient between the lumen and surrounding renal tissue facilitating passive diffusion of water and chloride respectively. It is important to note that the active reabsorptive process is saturable, for instance excessive filtered glucose (as in diabetes) may exceed the re-absorptive capacity and thus exceeds renal threshold appearing in the urine (diabetes mellitus (sweet urine)).

In addition to the main and extensive re-absorptive activity, there is secretory activity associated with tubular metabolism and secondary to the active re-absorptive process, hydrogen ions as an example (Figs. 4 and 5).

Loop of Henle

The loop of Henle comprises the thin descending and ascending limbs and the thick ascending limb. The main role of the loop of Henle is to generate concentrated urine that is hypertonic with respect to plasma. Although the thin limbs are structurally similar they have different absorptive capacity and permeability to water.

The thick ascending limb lined with cuboidal cells similar to those of the proximal tubules, at its tip it is closely associated with the glomerulus and the efferent arterioles. This association forms the juxtaglomerular apparatus.

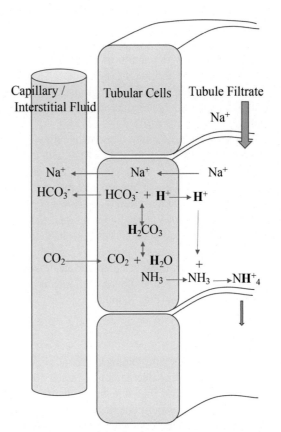

FIG. 5 Renal tubular handling of electrolytes and acid-base balance. *(Modified from Wagner CA, Imenez Silva PH, Bourgeois S. Molecular pathophysiology of acid-base disorders. Semin Nephrol. 2019;39(4):340–352. https://doi.org/10.1016/j.semnephrol.2019.04.004. PMID: 31300090.)*

The arteriolar cells contain renin and is innervated with sympathetic nerve fibers. Renin is released in response to decreased efferent arteriolar pressure and decreased intraluminal sodium. Renin, with its proteolytic activity converts plasma angiotensinogen to angiotensin I which is converted by lung angiotensin converting enzyme (ACE) to angiotensin II which is a potent vasoconstrictor and stimulator of aldosterone release. This results in both restoring blood pressure and in increased sodium reabsorption respectively. The active reabsorption of sodium and associated chloride maintains and increases the surrounding medullary tissue hyperosmolality. Of importance is that the ascending limb is impermeable to water and thus water does not accompany the reabsorbed sodium and the luminal fluid becomes relatively hypoosmolal. In contrast, the descending limb is permeable to water and thus water passively diffuses across down the osmotic gradient established by the high osmolality of the surrounding interstitial tissue. This process of water handling and development of an osmotic gradient is termed counter current multiplication.

Distal convoluted tubules

The distal convoluted tubules link the ascending limb of the loop of Henle and the collecting duct. The distal tubule is relatively shorter compared to the proximal tubule. Little adjustment of electrolytes (Na and Cl) takes place at this site. It is regulated by the action of both aldosterone and arginine vasopressin (antidiuretic hormone (ADH)). The anatomical association with the juxtaglomerular apparatus helps facilitate the intricate regulation of blood volume and osmolality.

ADH released in response to blood osmolality and when volume decreases by more than 5%–10% with decreases >10%, even in the presence of hypoosmolality, volume restoration prevails regardless of blood osmolality. Aldosterone is released in response to a reduced blood flow or pressure in the afferent renal arterioles and to hyponatremia. Aldosterone stimulates sodium reabsorption and its associated water and thus restores blood volume and pressure. Potassium and hydrogen ions are excreted in exchange for the absorbed sodium (Figs. 4 and 5). The excretion of hydrogen ions is central to bicarbonate reabsorption (Figs. 4 and 5).

Collecting duct

The combined drainage and joining of about six distal tubule's form the collecting duct which ultimately drain into the renal calyx. Last and fine adjustment of urine electrolytes (Na, Cl, K) and water content and thus urinary concentration occurs via the combined action of aldosterone and ADH. The collecting duct is permeable to urea and thus some urea diffuses out of the collecting duct into the interstitial tissue of the medulla (Fig. 4).

Functions of the kidney

The glomerulus of the nephron facilitates ultrafiltration of blood. The barrier to filtration of blood cells and proteins is primarily mechanical, furthermore anion proteins are retarded by the anionic charge on glomerular membrane (ultrafiltration thus depends on size, shape, and charge), whereas the nephron tubular components modify the composition of the ultrafiltrate.

Each day, 200 L of passive plasma ultrafiltrate enters the nephron, most of which is actively reabsorbed by the proximal convoluted tubules (70% of sodium, calcium, and magnesium, 100% of the potassium and inorganic phosphate reabsorption).

Handling and maintenance of water, electrolytes, and acid-base balance is interlinked (Fig. 4). For instance, water reabsorption is associated with sodium and phosphate reabsorption. Sodium and hydrogen ion exchange facilitates bicarbonate reabsorption. In addition to the above countercurrent and energy-dependent process, there is also active reabsorption of glucose, uric acid, and amino acids, and low molecular weight proteins such as β-2-microglobulins occur via analyte specific receptors (proteins by endocytosis in tubular epithelial cells via megalin and cubilin receptors). Mutations in those receptors lead to tubular proteinuria.

The process of reabsorption is either passive down a concentration gradient, or an energy requiring active process such as aldosterone reabsorption of sodium and its associated analytes and water, or via countercurrent osmotic multiplication gradient. Reabsorption of water in the proximal tubules is isosmotic compared with process at the distal tubule where the countercurrent multiplication causes passive diffusion down a concentration gradient through tubular membrane. Permeability of the membrane is regulated by vasopressin (antidiuretic hormone (ADH)) acting on the intercalated and principal cells lining the distal tubule. ADH secretion is influenced by osmolality and to some extent by volume as discussed earlier.

Maintaining a hypertonic interstitial area (i.e., of high osmolality) is essential to the functioning of the kidney. This is achieved via anatomical differences in permeability to water and to urea and via active absorption of solutes (Fig. 4).

Metabolic functions of the kidney

The kidney's metabolic functions are (a) excretion of nonvolatile metabolites such as urea, creatinine, uric acid, phosphates, sulfates, as well as toxins, drugs, and their metabolites, (b) maintain homeostasis of body fluid volume and electrolytes levels, (c) maintain acid-base homeostasis, (d) an endocrine role in renin and 1,25 dihydroxy vitamin D synthesis, and for PTH-regulated calcium and phosphate levels, and for erythropoietin synthesis.

In addition to re-absorption of filtered material, the kidney maintains a stable urine plasma osmolality ratio. The ability of the kidney to concentrate urine is the tubular function most frequently affected by disease. In normal individuals, the urine to plasma osmolality ratio varies between 1.1 and 3.0. Fluid restriction in a normal subject will result in a urine plasma osmolality ratio exceeding 4.5. Determination of this ratio is useful for distinguishing prerenal failure (where the ratio >1.5).

The above functions depend on presence of normal blood supply, intact glomeruli, and tubular cells, and on normal secretion and feedback control of hormones acting on the kidney.

Excretory function: Assessment of the glomerular filtration rate (GFR)

As stated, the kidney excretes nitrogenous waste and regulates body fluids. The excretory function depends on the glomerular filtration and on the tubular excretion and reabsorption.

The glomerular filtration rate (GFR) is routinely assessed by measuring clearance of endogenous circulating creatinine. Theoretically, GFR is the volume of plasma from which a substance is completely cleared. The GFR is considered the best overall index of kidney function.

At the glomerulus level, passive ultrafiltration of the plasma (200 L) entering the tubules every day depends on blood flow, normal glomeruli, the difference between hydrostatic pressure and plasma oncotic pressure (low albumin leads to low oncotic pressure and to fluid accumulation), the ultrafiltrate contains the same concentrations as in plasma. Furthermore, the very large volume of filtrate facilitates adequate elimination of waste such as urea and metabolites. Changes in filtration rate alters the total amount of water and solute but not the composition of the filtrate.

At the tubular level, active reabsorption (transport) requires energy (ATP) and thus function is impaired by enzyme poisons, hypoxia, and cell death. From the 200 L filtered, only 2 L of urine is formed (1%) with composition far different from that of plasma. The active transport of charged ions (isosmotic transport at the proximal tubules and ion exchange at the distal tubules) produces the electrochemical gradient.

Excretory function of the kidney is assessed by measurement of the glomerular filtration rate (GFR), see later. As described above, the plasma ultrafiltrate constituents is similar to that of plasma, however, the urine constituents are different where metabolites and toxic end products predominate. Urea and creatinine are product of ammonia and creatine respectively. Ammonia, an intermediary metabolite of proteins and amino acids is converted to urea in hepatocytes and the rate of production varies with dietary protein intake and extent of deamidation. Similarly, muscle phosphocreatine is metabolized to creatinine, the amount produced proportional to muscle mass with daily output of about 10 mmol (0.1 g).

Determining the glomerular filtration rate (GFR)

Glomerular filtration rate is measured as the clearance of a biomarkers from the circulation. GFR is measured either using an endogenous biomarker such as creatinine or cystatin C or in a dynamic study following administration of an exogenous substance such as iohexol and determining its clearance rate.

Determining the GFR is important to assess and monitor kidney function and is essential in therapeutic dosing of certain medications. The incidence of kidney disease in the United States is increasing for instance from the 10% in 1994 to 15% in 2021. This requires frequent monitoring to aid early intervention. Furthermore, the determination of GFR is not only to assess kidney function, but is also a potent predictor of cardiovascular disease and early mortality.

Endogenous markers of GFR

Both creatinine and urea can be used as endogenous markers of the glomerular filtration rate; however, they are not ideal markers as not all of the urea is excreted where about 40%–60% is reabsorbed via passive diffusion in the tubules resulting in underestimation of the GFR. Additionally, the amount of urea produced is influenced by dietary protein content.

Whereas although not influenced by dietary proteins content, creatinine is actively secreted by the peritubular capillaries and thus overestimates GFR by about 10%–20%. Coincidently, one of the assays used to measure creatinine levels overestimates serum creatinine levels, and this is thought to compensate for the excreted creatinine overestimation.

Creatinine

Circulating creatinine, a 113 Da amino acid derivative, and as described above is a better marker than urea as the latter is influenced by dietary proteins and is diffusible down a concentration gradient which means diffuse back into the circulation.

Creatinine is a breakdown product of dietary meat and muscle creatine phosphate and that its production is related to muscle mass. In routine clinical practice, creatinine is measured using two main methodologies that have been standardized to the isotope dilution mass spectrometry reference methodology.

One of the commonly used method known as the Jaffe assay with the original format described over a century ago

TABLE 1 Example drugs and metabolites interference with the two commonly used creatinine assays.

Metabolite/ compound	Jaffe-based method	Creatinase enzyme-based method
Bilirubin	−ve	N/A
Ketones	+ve	N/A
Pyruvate	+ve	N/A
Ascorbic acid	+ve	−ve
Streptomycin	+ve	
Aminoglycosides	+ve (at toxic levels)	
Cephalosporins	+ve (variable)	N/A
Dopamine	−ve	−ve
Catecholamines	N/A	−ve
Hemoglobin (sample hemolysis)	−ve	N/A

The interference is variable and can lead to either falsely elevated creatinine values (+ve interference) or to falsely decreased creatinine levels (−ve interference). N/A indicates lack of significant interference reported. Modified from Peake M, Whiting M. Measurement of serum creatinine—current status and future goals. *Clin Biochem Rev.* 2006;27:173–184.

in 1886, where creatinine reacts with picric acid under alkaline condition producing an orange colored complex with a maximum absorbance at 520 nm. The method is influenced by many drugs metabolites leading to either falsely high or low creatinine values (Table 1).

The second method is enzymatic, and is increasingly being used, employs the enzyme creatinase and the reaction is monitored by measuring production of quinine imine chromogen. The alkaline picrate chemical methodology is subject to interference by both bilirubin and ketones where high bilirubin causes falsely low creatinine value, and the presence of ketone bodies interferes causing a falsely high creatinine value. However, the enzymatic method, although exhibits no interference from the latter two metabolites, a number of drugs and their metabolites such as L-dopa and catecholamines interfere producing falsely low creatinine levels (Table 1).

Several point of care testing platforms for creatinine measurement are increasingly becoming available. The assays are primarily enzymatic but are amperometry-based methods where hydrogen peroxide produced in the reaction is oxidized at a platinum electrode and that the current produced is proportional to creatinine concentration. This assay format is not affected by catecholamines.

Measuring creatinine clearance requires timed collection of a urine sample. However, fewer 24-h timed urine collections are being performed and less so in an outpatient setting. This is due to difficulty and inconvenience of

collection as well as significant variability in urine volume and in collection practices. Even in the relatively controlled environment of in-patient collection, variability is more than 10% among serial collections. Therefore, allowing for both analytical and biological variability a critical difference of 33% must be exceeded for clinical significance.

Given the frequency of serum creatinine measurement, being a constituent of basic and complete metabolic panels, and thus more readily available, calculated GFR estimates are more widely utilized via use of several formulae using serum creatinine levels, age, race, gender, and body size. The original and still sparingly used is the MDRD formula derived from the Modification of Diet in Renal Disease (MDRD) study equation (Table 2). Major limitation of the MDRD formula is the imprecision and systematic underestimation at higher levels as it was developed in patients with chronic kidney disease (CKD), and thus, the formula does not allow reliable estimation for GFR beyond that of 60 mL/min/1.73 m^2, that is prior to CKD stage 3. Additionally, the formulae applies a correction factor for race which poses difficulty as the later is a social construct rather than a biological determinant and its use is discouraged. The inclusion of the non-GFR determinants of creatinine clearance include age, gender, and ethnicity with assumption that those are associated with muscle mass; however, the imprecision observed suggests those are not the only contributors.

The most widely used formulae being the CKD-EPI, and Cockcroft Gault and some laboratories may still offer the MDRD-IV formula.

CKD-EPI derived by the Chronic Kidney Disease Epidemiology Collaboration research group in 2009 and the equation (Table 2) was an improvement on the MDRD equation where estimated GFR is now reported for CKD stages 1 and 2. However, the equation led to reduced estimation of the stage 3 and 2 at the expense of increased prevalence of stage 1. Recently, following public outcry on race related discrepancy in healthcare and outcry on the accurate determination of race, a refit of the formulae was developed (Table 2) eliminating the race component. The emphasis being race is a social construct and thus not an exact determination.

The Cockcroft and Gault formulae (Table 2) includes body weight in the calculation and is frequently used by pharmacy to aid therapeutic regimens and dosing. Body weight is not typically available in laboratory information system and may not be interfaceable from hospital clinical databases or even electronically available, laboratories thus rely on available data such as creatinine levels, age and gender. Ethnicity is a variable that most laboratories used to account for both by providing both data for black and nonblack subjects.

Urea (blood urea nitrogen (BUN))

Urea is a 60 Da molecule and constitutes two nitrogen groups. Urea and BUN are often used interchangeably;

TABLE 2 Summary of formulas applied in the calculation (estimation) of the glomerular filtration rate (eGFR).

GFR estimation formulas	Equation	Comments
CKD-MDRD 4-V	eGFR = 175 × (Serum Creatinine)$^{-1.154}$ × (age)$^{-0.203}$ × 0.742 (if female) or × 1.212 (if black). eGFR is expressed in milliliters per minute per 1.73 m^2	Discontinued and should not be used. eGFR values are reported up to 60 mL/min/1.73 m^2. Higher values are reported as >60 mL/min/1.73 m^2. 1.73 m^2 is the correction for body surface area (standardized to a n adult mass of 63 kg and height of 1.7 m).
CKD-EPI	Male: eGFR = 141 × min(Scr/0.9, 1)$^{-0.411}$ × max(Scr/0.9, 1)$^{-1.209}$ × 0.9938^{Age} × 1.159 (if black) Female: eGFR = 144 × min(Scr/0.7, 1)$^{-0.329}$ × max(Scr/0.7, 1)$^{-1.209}$ × 0.9938^{Age} × 1.159 (if black)	Use not recommend and revised in 2021 (see below) a re-fit version without the race factor adjustment (see below).
CKD-EPI re-fit (2021)	eGFR = 142 × min(Scr/κ, 1)$^{\alpha}$ × max(Scr/κ, 1)$^{-1.200}$ × 0.9938^{Age} × 1.012 [if female] κ = 0.7 (females) or 0.9 (males) α = −0.241 (female) or −0.302 (male). min(Scr/κ, 1) is the minimum of Scr/κ or 1.0 max(Scr/κ, 1) is the maximum of Scr/κ or 1.0	Revised 2021. Reference to and race correction factor removed. Recommended for routine use.
CKD-EPI Cystatin C	eGFR = 133 × min(Scys/0.8, 1)$^{-0.499}$ × max(Scys/0.8, 1)$^{-1.328}$ × 0.996^{Age} × 0.932 [if female]	Revised year 2021
CKD-EPI Creatinine-Cystatin C	eGFRcr-cys = 135 × min(Scr/κ, 1)$^{\alpha}$ × max(Scr/κ, 1)$^{-0.544}$ × min(Scys/0.8, 1)$^{-0.323}$ × max(Scys/0.8, 1)$^{-0.778}$ × 0.9961^{Age} × 0.963 [if female] κ = 0.7 (females) or 0.9 (males) α = −0.219 (female) or −0.144 (male) min(Scr/κ, 1) is the minimum of Scr/κ or 1.0 max(Scr/κ, 1) is the maximum of Scr/κ or 1.0	Revised year 2021
Cockcroft-Gault	(140 − age) × body weight (kg)/(serum creatinine (μmol/L) × 72). For female multiply by 0.85	Drug dosage determination
Schwarz (pediatric)	K × (height in cm)/sCre K = 0.33 in premature infants K = 0.45 in term infants to 1 yr age	Applied to pediatric population

CKD, chronic renal disease; *CKD-EPI*, epidemiological collaboration; *MDRD*, Modification of Diet in Renal Disease; *4-V*, four variables that are creatinine, age, gender, and race.
Modified from Shahbaz H, Gupta M. Creatinine clearance. In: *StatPearls [Internet]*. Treasure Island, FL: StatPearls Publishing; 2022. PMID: 31334948.

however, the amounts are very different, the term urea represents the whole molecule (with two nitrogen) and BUN represents only the nitrogen contents of the molecule with 28 Da. Urea is (NH$_2$)$_2$CO. A molecular weight of 60 Da compared with the two nitrogen at 28 Da. Thus, urea is approximately twice (2.14 that of BUN).

Urea is measured using the enzyme reagent, urease. There are little or no known interferences. Although, creatinine is a better maker for GFR as urea is diffusible and levels may be affected by extra-renal factors, i.e., volume status, high protein load (diet and upper gastrointestinal bleeding), and GI bacterial action, however, its level is used to initiate therapy and to monitor dialysis efficacy hence the uremic status classification.

Circulating levels of urea and creatinine depend mainly on glomerular function and are inversely related to the glomerular filtration rate (GFR). Although urea and creatinine are insensitive; GFR, however, may fall by 50% before urea and creatinine are elevated above the reference ranges. The markers can be used to exclude the presence of severe renal disease and are used to monitor progress of disease. GFR depends upon the net pressure exerted across the glomerular membrane, the physical state of the membrane and its total surface area. GFR can be determined as the clearance from peripheral blood of any substance which is excreted solely by glomerular filtration. Creatinine clearance is used clinically for determining GFR. Creatinine production is relatively constant, so the serum level varies little over a 24 h period. Dietary restrictions are not required, and fluid intake need not be controlled during measurement. A 24 h urine collection and a blood sample taken during the collection (often at mid point) need to be analyzed simultaneously. In any clearance measurement, the biggest source of error is the timed urine collection.

For such a substance, let P = plasma concentration, U = urine concentration, V = urine flow in mL/min. At the steady state, the rate of filtration at the glomerulus = The rate of appearance in the urine. $GFR = \dfrac{U \times P}{V}$. The normal value for the GFR is around 125 mL/min. This corrected for a unique body surface area ($\times 1.73 \, m^2$). This generalized approach has been questioned and individualized calculation of body surface areas is recommended. There are two formulas for the calculation of body surface area (BSA).

The Schlich formula, for women $BSA = 0.000975482 \times W^{0.46} \times H^{1.08}$, and for men $BSA = 0.000579479 \times W^{0.38} \times H^{1.24}$. The Du Bois formula, $BSA = 0.007184 \times W^{0.425} \times H^{0.725}$, surface area reported as m^2.

Cystatin C

Cystatin C, a 13 kDa low-molecular-weight nonglycosylated protein present on the surface of all nucleated cells. There is no clear pathology associated with lack of or increased cystatin C levels and that it is considered a product of a house keeping gene.

It is a suitable endogenous marker and is superior to creatinine in that is it is freely filtered and not actively secreted and not influenced by body mass. There is no correlation between its level and lean body mass. This makes it suitable for assessment of kidney function in children and the elderly and those with conditions affecting muscle mass. In the original CKD-EPI formula, incorporation of cystatin C reduced the correction factor for black ethnicity from 1.159 to 1.08. Additionally, cystatin C exhibits a lower degree of intraindividual biological activity (25%) compared to creatinine at 93%. The upper limit of reference interval being 3–4 standard deviation from the mean for cystatin C compared with 13 for creatinine.

Its routine measurement was limited by the relatively expensive cost of test compared to creatinine, but it is becoming more affordable and increasingly being used in specific circumstances such as aid in decision making for those near or at cut-off limits or near decision limits of a more costly procedure.

Furthermore, cystatin C values have been incorporated into several of the eGFR formulas (Table 2) and that patients who had cystatin C added to the creatinine-based eGFR formular resulted in about 17% of them being reclassified into a higher eGFR value often $\geq 60 \, mL/min/1.73 \, m^2$.

Exogenous markers of GFR

A number of exogenous GFR markers are available, although not widely used. They include inulin, iothalamate, and iohexol. The latter is increasingly being used (see below).

Inulin

Inulin, a plant polysaccharide meets all of the required characteristics of a marker of filtration (nonmetabolized, freely filtered, not reabsorbed or actively excreted). Inulin is injected intravenously, and serial blood samples collected. It is considered the gold standard when measuring GFR. Three sets of 15 min apart successive serum, and urine samples are obtained during a 2 h clearance study (continuous infusion of 1% inulin). The clearance of inulin is reported as the average of the three sets of samples collections.

Prior to the procedure, the patient is well hydrated by drinking 500 mL of water orally 30 min prior to infusion. Additionally, 60 mL of water is given at 30, 60, and 90 min following the start of inulin infusion.

The inulin infusion rate is maintained at 300 mL/h for the first 30 min (loading dose) and reduced to 100 mL/min for the remaining 90 min of the test. Blood samples are collected at 45, 75, and 105 min after the start of inulin infusion, and the corresponding urine samples are collected at between 30 and 60 min, between 60 and 90 min and between 90 and 120 min. The patient having emptied the bladder at 30 min after start of infusion. Several modifications of the protocol minimizing sample collection to a single sample have been proposed.

Although commercial assays are available, the measurement is cumbersome mostly due to logistical issues with patient handling (fasting and well hydrated), requiring admission and clinical supervision of the procedure.

Iothalamate

Sodium iothalamate is used to measure GFR. Two combined approaches are in use. The first is following a bolus injection of iothalamate, and the second is a continuous rate infusion. Renal clearance is determined once a steady state is maintained.

In this test, patients are hydrated with 750 mL water orally over 45 min. A bolus iothalamate (456 mg) injection is given over 2–3 min. The patient hydration is maintained with 250 mL of water every hour throughout the study. Venous blood samples are collected prior to and 5, 10, 15, 30, 45, 60, 90, 120, 150, and 180 min following iothalamate dosage. The bolus approach is followed, 2 h later (washout period) with a continuous infusion study. A priming dose of 228 mg iothalamate followed by a 2.5 h constant rate infusion designed to establish a plasma concentration of about 20 mg/L. Blood samples are drawn prior to and 30, 60, 90, 120, 150, and 180 min following start of infusion. At the beginning of both approaches, the patient empties the bladder, and urine samples collected at 30 min intervals throughout the studies.

Iothalamate clearance calculated following measurement of plasma and urinary iothalamate levels. When using constant rate infusion, clearance is calculated using the formula ($Clp = k_{el} \cdot V_d$, where k_{el} is the elimination rate constant and V_d is the volume of distribution). Iothalamate plasma concentration in the bolus portion of the study is calculated as follows ($Ct = Ae^{-\alpha t} + Be^{-\beta t}$, where Ct is the concentration in plasma at time t, A and B are y-intercepts, and α and β are disposition rate constants). Complex statistical analysis and graphical analysis are required to obtain the GFR.

Iohexol

Iohexol, a radiology contrast media with ideal GFR characteristics. It is measured by LCMSMS and its rate of clearance (following administration) is calculated using serial timed blood samples. The analytes follow a two-compartment system. First compartment of distribution is influenced by the drug pharmacodynamics and the second compartment is that of clearance. Calculations involved either use of a single- or a two-compartment model. An example of both calculations for iohexol is shown in Fig. 6.

Plasma disappearance protocol for kidney donors (a GFR >80 mL/min indicate a good kidney to donate). Multiple samples collection may be extended up to collection at 24 h in patients with reduced GFR (Table 3).

TABLE 3 Actual iohexol study values obtained following injection of dosage collected at the specified time intervals.

Sample (S) number	Time (min)	Iohexol (µg/mL)
S0 (baseline)	0	0
S1	10	355.8
S2	20	178.1
S3	30	134.0
S4	50	106.1
S5	80	82.7
S6	120	52.4
S7	180	42.9
S8	240	28.3

Example data from the author's laboratory.

Estimated GFR (eGFR)

The glomerular filtration rate can be estimated via a number of mathematical formulas. Several formulas are historically in use (Table 2). The rational being estimation is easily obtained and can be used as a guide as to when to intervene or when an accurate measurement is needed. However, significant differences between estimated and measured GFR must be taken into account. Measurement of GFR (rather than estimation) is recommended in patients with rapidly changing renal function, those with metabolic muscle wasting diseases, and in those where accurate measurement of GFR is required (e.g., potential donor of kidney transplant).

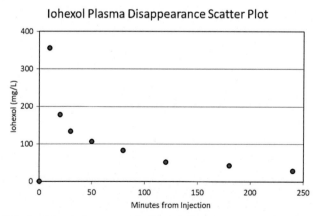
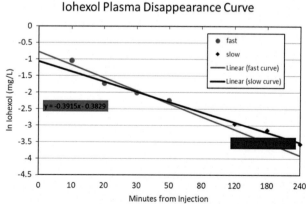

FIG. 6 Iohexol clearance study. Iohexol disappearance over time is plotted. The slow and fast clearance is shown. Iohexol clearance is 132 mL/min/1.73 m². The eGFR-CKD-EPI was estimated lower at 114.3 mL/min/1.73 m². *(Example data from the author's laboratory.)*

There are often significant differences between estimated and measured GFR and that they exceed ±15% about 43% to 57% of the time.

The Minimal Diet in Renal Disease (MDRD) formula

The MDRD equation was developed in 1999 using data from 1628 patients with chronic kidney disease. The equation was later in 2005 updated to reflect the use of a standardized and traceable creatinine assays which yields serum creatinine values that are 5% to 10% lower. The updated equation is $eGFR = 175 \times (Serum\ Creatinine)^{-1.154} \times (age)^{-0.203} \times 0.742$ (if female) or $\times 1.212$ (if black). eGFR is expressed in milliliters per minute per 1.73 m^2, and race is indicated as either black or not. The term for race thought to reflect a higher average serum creatinine level among black subjects partly owing to increased muscle mass and or to creatinine metabolism. When using the MDRD formula, eGFR values are only reported up to 60 mL/min/1.73 m^2 and any value above 60 mL/min is reported as ">60." In several studies, when using the MDRD formula, 91% of the eGFR values are within 30% of the measured GFR values. Furthermore, the mean difference between estimated and measured GFR ranges from −5.5 to 0.9 mL/min/1.73 m^2. In general, the MDRD formula is thought to underestimate GFR among women and young patients.

Chronic kidney disease-epidemiological studies (CKD-EPI) formula

CKD-EPI formula was developed in 2009 using 8254 subjects and is widely adopted and increasing being used. It has recent been revised with race correction (reference to African American or black ethnicity) removed. CKD-EPI formula was only about 4% in use (at least in the United States) at the time the modified CKD-EPI was published.

CKD-EPI will report actual values beyond 60 mL/min/1.73 m^2, and throughout the whole GFR range. It was developed from a population young and middle aged with GFR of about 70 mL/min/1.73 m^2. It gives a higher GFR values when comparted to the MDRD formula.

eGFR is used in diagnosis and in management of kidney disease (dialysis and evaluation for transplantation), medication dosage adjustment, use of radiology contrasts, media. It uses creatinine and/or cystatin C to calculate the GFR with creatinine being widely available and measured as part of biochemical and screening profiles. When calculating (estimating) the GFR several biological, factors are considered. There is age (body size and metabolism), gender (male/female muscle mass, and hormonal metabolism), body weight, and race. The latter although may contribute to creatinine metabolism and handing as well as genetic

variations, the race definition in itself is a social and not a biological construct. Inclusion of race in the eGFR equation overestimates GFR by about 20%. The explanation being that black race (African American) have a higher muscle mass and or variable clearance handling by the kidney.

Eliminating the race factor from the CKD-EPI equation results in reassignment of African American and black patients from stage 3a to 3b (a higher stage of kidney dysfunction). Given wide national concern over the impact of including an unreliable subjective and individually declared race to determine degree of kidney function lead to joint workforce by the National Kidney Foundation and American Society for Nephrology in 2021 recommended the use of a modified CKD-EPI (termed refit) where the original data were reanalyzed in the absence of race components.

When stratifying for race, 10.4% would miss CKD3 stage diagnosis, 0.7% would miss nephrology consult, and 0.1% would miss transplant (data from the author's laboratory). There is a race disparity with African American being three times more likely than non-Hispanic white to have kidney failure. The disparity exceeds that is due to prevalence. Thirty-six percent of African American are receiving dialysis, but the proportion receiving kidney transplant is lower than their non-Hispanic white counterpart patients.

Cockcroft-Gault formula

The Cockcroft and Gault formula was developed in the early 1970s from 249 men with creatinine clearance 30–130 mL/min. The formula includes age and weight in the calculation ($C_{Cr} = \{((140 - age) \times weight)/(72 \times S_{Cr})\} \times 0.85$ (if female)) and is widely used by pharmacy in drug dosage adjustment.

Its use is discouraged by some professional organizations due to the fact that it was not adjusted for body surface area and at the time of its development the creatinine assays used at the time were not standardized and not traceable to the ID-MSMS (see above). It is thought to overestimate GFR by about 20%. However, its utility in drugs with wide therapeutic range did not exhibit significant differences when using other formulas. Howevere, this is not the case for drugs with narrow therapeutic range where the formula is less reliable in assessing the risk for nephrotoxicity.

Homeostatic function: Fluid volume balance

Fluid balance is predominantly a tubular function. The function of the renal tubules is assessed by measuring the following; urine volume, urine osmolality (concentration), reabsorption of filtered electrolytes, glucose and amino acids, low molecular weight proteins (i.e., assessment of reabsorption of filtered β-2-microglobulin). The ability of the renal tubules to concentrate the urine as required to maintain blood volume and osmolality is assessed via a water deprivation test (see later) and the ability to acidify the urine assessed following an acid load test.

Only 10% of filtrate is excreted (2 L out of 200 L). Final urine composition is different from the filtrate. Active reabsorption requires energy (ATP) and is impaired by hypoxia, enzyme poisons, and by cell death. The active transport results in electrochemical gradient (isoosmotic at the proximal tubules) and ionic exchange at the distal tubules. >70% of filtered Na, Ca, Mg are reabsorbed and all of the K is re-absorbed. Phosphate reabsorption is incomplete. Bicarbonate is regenerated/recovered in exchange for Na and H ions (Loss of H in metabolic compensation and acid base balance). Glucose, urate, and amino acids have respective receptor-mediated active reabsorption processes.

Water reabsorption depends on isosmotic reabsorption from the proximal tubules via aldosterone action (isosmotic water accompanied sodium reabsorption). A high osmolality medulla (achieved through a counter current multiplication) and changes in collecting duct permeability via the action of ADH all facilitate water reabsorption.

The net filtration pressure at the glomerulus is 15 mmHg. This is calculated by subtracting the glomerular hydrostatic pressure in the glomerular capillaries (about 55 mmHg) from the colloid osmotic pressure due to the presence of proteins, mainly albumin, at about 30 mmHg, and the capsular hydrostatic pressure which is the back pressure that opposes filtration. The net filtration pressure at the glomerulus is then (55 mmHg − 15 mmHg − 30 mmHg). This is maintained irrespective of the systemic pressure for a systemic pressure of >200 and <80 mmHg. Reduction in the filtration area is reduced when glomerular damage occurs (due to various pathology).

Changes in efferent blood pressures stimulate the renin-angiotensin system. Renin is secreted by the myoepithelial juxtaglomerular cells in the walls of the afferent arterioles. The juxtaglomerular region is made of these cells, plus the adjacent epithelial cells (macula densa) of the distal convoluted tubules and the nearby Lacis cells (extraglomerular mesangial cells). All comprise the juxtaglomerular apparatus with results in production of renin in response to reduction in arteriolar pressure. Renin converts angiotensinogen to angiotensin I which is in turn converted to the active angiotensin II by the lung angiotensin converting enzyme (ACE).

Acid-base homeostasis/balance

The kidney is important in maintaining acid-base status. It excretes acidic metabolites, reabsorbs and generates bicarbonate (HCO_3^-), and excretes H ions and ammonia (Fig. 5). Therefore, helping in maintaining blood pH. The kidney is much slower than the lung when compensating to adjust blood pH. See Chapter 15 on blood gases and acid-base balance for detailed discussion.

Endocrine functions and laboratory investigation

The kidney plays an important endocrine role. It is responsible for the conversion of 25-OH vitamin D to its active form 1,25-(OH)$_2$ vitamin D via 1-alpha hydroxylation. Parathyroid hormone acts on the kidney stimulating calcium reabsorption and phosphate excretion. Renin synthesis by the juxtaglomerular apparatus leads to conversion of angiotensinogen to angiotensin. With ultimate endpoint of sodium reabsorption by aldosterone. The kidney produces erythropoietin which stimulates erythropoiesis. Endocrine disorders associated with water and electrolytes imbalance are diabetes insipidus and aldosterone abnormalities.

1,25 Hydroxy cholecalciferol (1,25-(OH)$_2$ vitamin D)

The kidney synthesizes the active form of vitamin D (1,25-(OH)$_2$ vitamin D) via hydroxylation of 25-OH vitamin D by the renal interstitial 1-α hydroxylase enzyme. The enzyme is activated by parathyroid hormone (see Chapters 1 and 2).

Renal osteodystrophy is associated with increased risk for fracture and is thought to be due to impaired mineralization due to combined abnormalities in calcium, phosphate, parathyroid hormone (PTH), and vitamin D metabolism. Levels of 1,25-(OH)$_2$ vitamin D decline with reduced GFR with the reductions seen earlier than those seen with PTH. Significant reduction in levels of 1,25-(OH)$_2$ vitamin D is not seen until the eGFR declines below 40 mL/min/1.73 m^2. Although deficiency is common among patients with chronic kidney disease, the primary cause for the decline in 1,25-(OH)$_2$ vitamin D is thought to be the increase in FGF23 levels (inhibiting 1-α hydroxylase activity and stimulating 24-hydroxylase) rather than the loss of functioning renal mass.

Renin aldosterone activity

Renin is produced by the epithelial cells lining the efferent and afferent arterioles as part of the juxtaglomerular apparatus response to changes in fluid balance.

Renin activates the release of angiotensinogen and its activation to angiotensin I. The latter is converted to active angiotensin II by ACE in the lung and acts on the adrenal glands to produce aldosterone, and the later acts on the renal tubules to reabsorb sodium and excrete potassium.

Diabetes insipidus

Diabetes insipidus (DI) characterized by the inability of the kidney to concentrate the urine and thus maintain an appropriate plasma osmolality as well as normovolemia. It is due to deficiency of ADH (hypothalamic-cranial DI), to nephrogenic DI (inability of the collecting duct to response to available ADH), or to primary polydipsia (excessive and inappropriate drinking of water) in psychogenic polydipsia.

Nephrogenic DI (impaired renal response to ADH) a sex-linked recessive disorder. Other causes leading to inability to reabsorb water include hyperglycosuria (diabetes), hypercalcemia, hypokalemia, and the presence of drugs, e.g., lithium. All interfere with ADH action.

Measurement of basal and stimulated urine and serum osmolality are central to the investigation of patients suspected of diabetes insipidus (see Chapter 1 on endocrine system disorders for more details). It is an assessment of the kidneys' ability to concentrate the urine.

For a patient with polyuria (>3 L/24 h), a water deprivation test is used to stimulate and assess ADH secretion. Urine and serum osmolality are measured. Adequate ADH release and action at the distal tubule and the ability of the kidney to concentration the urine exhibited by an elevated urine osmolality.

In patients with plasma sodium >147 mmol/L, copeptin levels ≥21.4 pmol/L is suggestive of nephrogenic diabetes insipidus, and copeptin values ≤4.9 pmol/L are suggestive of central diabetes insipidus.

In patients with normal sodium and copeptin levels in the indeterminant, it can be measured following arginine stimulation where copeptin levels ≤3.8 pmol/L indicate central diabetes insipidus and levels >3.8 pmol/L suggests primary polydipsia. In borderline cases, copeptin is measured following hypertonic-stimulation where copeptin ≤4.9 pmol/L suggests central diabetes insipidus levels and levels >4.9 pmol/L are suggestive of primary polydipsia.

Patients with plasma sodium <135 mmol/L are suggestive of polydipsia as a cause in the presence of hypotonic polyuria.

Erythropoietin

Erythropoietin (EPO) a glycoprotein peptide hormone of 30.4 kkDa molecular weight produced by the peritubular cells of the kidney in response to tissue hypoxia. The lower the tissue oxygen partial pressure (pO_2) the higher the production of EPO. A number of commercially available EPO stimulating agents (epoetin alpha, darbepoetin alpha, and methoxy polyethylene glycol-epoetin beta) are administered to patients with chronic kidney disease who are anemic and either receiving dialysis or are about to receive dialysis. A number of immunoassays are available for the measurement of circulating EPO levels.

Reduction in renal mass (peritubular cells) and thus EPO production results renal anemia. Both EPO and its stimulating pharmacological agents stimulate differentiation of erythroid progenitor cells. Mature CD34+ hematopoietic stem cells express EPO receptors on their cell surface. Risk factors EPO administration include increased thrombotic events and increased blood viscosity. The latter

in the presence of low oxygen is associated with vasodilation and thus increased risk for ischemic attack and myocardial infarction.

Kidney disorders and biomarkers

Given the excretory, homoeostatic, and endocrine functions of the kidney, assessment of those functions is routinely performed. The spectrum of abnormalities detected reflects the functions of the various anatomical areas of the kidney and often reflects either a glomerular or tubular component, mixed components are often present with biomarkers indicating predominance of as well as transition from one predominant form to another. There is a spectrum of conditions in which the proportions of tubular and glomerular dysfunction vary. The biochemical findings will depend on the relative contributions from these two components. Glomerular function is more commonly assessed than that of tubular function. Additionally, the dysfunction may be acute in nature, chronic, or acute on a chronic dysfunction. Blood and urine biomarkers of kidney function that are in routine use include urea (BUN), creatinine, electrolytes (Na, K, chloride, phosphate, and bicarbonate), 1,25-(OH)$_2$ vitamin D, erythropoietin, urinary proteins, urine, and plasm osmolality.

Kidney dysfunction

Causes of renal dysfunction are best described as prerenal, renal (intrinsic), and postrenal. Although the disorders and presentations are those of a spectrum. This classification helps with the discussion on the biochemical investigation.

With few exceptions, kidney biopsy remains the cornerstone for the evaluation of glomerular disease.

Prerenal causes of dysfunction

Prerenal causes of renal dysfunction are those affecting blood volume and thus glomerular filtration. It is characterized by reduced GFR and a normal (intact) renal tubular function. The reduction in GFR causes increased circulating urea (BUN) and creatinine levels. The reduced blood flow (filtration rate) stimulates aldosterone production which results in increased tubular sodium reabsorption in exchange for potassium and hydrogen ions.

The kidney receives about 25% of the cardiac output and reduction in volume and pressure is seen in circulatory failure, congestive heart failure, and myocardial injury.

The prevalence of prerenal (acute kidney injury) secondary to prerenal causes is about 9% among hospitalized patients and 50% among patients in critical care units.

Prerenal uremia progresses to tubular involvement (acute tubular necrosis) as the reduced GFR causes a reduction in nutrients and oxygen reaching the tubules now highly active in the reabsorption of sodium and water. This causes tissue ischemia and thus tubular necrosis.

It occurs in 3.2%–9.6% of hospital admission and in 2.1% and 22.1% among patients in intensive care. Acute kidney injury (AKI) leads to end stage renal disease (ESRD), early progression to chronic kidney disease (CKD) and associated with morbidity and mortality. Predisposing factors for AKI include reduced eGFR, proteinuria (albumin creatinine ratio (ACR) $\geq$ 30 mg/g), and CKD, advanced age, male gender, and African American (black) race.

The association between proteinuria and AKI has been attributed to chronic stress of proximal tubular membrane due to maximal albumin reabsorption causing tubular stress and injury.

Biomarkers indicating risk for AKI are eGFR and ACR and are more useful than stratification by age, gender, or by race.

ADH production is increased leading to increased water reabsorption to correct the hypovolemia and an apparent high urine osmolality (see later).

Aldosterone causes increased sodium (and associated water) and increased excretion of potassium and hydrogen ions in exchange. The increased sodium reabsorption leaves less tubular sodium available for exchange with H and potassium. This leads to acidosis (accumulation of H ions) and to hyperkalemia. There is also hyperuricemia and hyperphosphatemia, and that urine volume is reduced.

Urinalysis results are often within normal limits in patients with prerenal uremia but without tubular involvement, that is without acute tubular necrosis.

The patient is diagnosed with acute kidney injury if any of the following occurs, increased creatinine by more than 0.3 mg/dL (26 μmol/L) in 48 h or an increase in creatinine level by at least 1.5 times basal levels occurring over a week period.

In patients with acute tubular necrosis, the rate of rise in creatinine is higher at 0.3–0.5 mg/dL per day. BUN creatinine ratio is normally 10:1; however, it is much higher at 20:1 in prerenal uremia and is about 15:1 in patients with acute tubular necrosis.

The markedly increased BUN (urea) in prerenal uremia is due to the increased passive reabsorption at the proximal tubules in response to sodium and accompanied water reabsorption due to hyperaldosteronism seen in prerenal uremia and reduced GFR.

In the hypovolemic states, fractional excretion of sodium (FENa) is low secondary to hyperaldosteronism. Urinary sodium is less than 20 mmol/L with FENa being less than 1%. FENa is >2% in patients with acute tubular necrosis. Similarly, urea is exerted by the renal tubules and in patients with intact renal tubules but with prerenal uremia, and the fractional excretion rate of urea (FEU) is less than 35% compared with >50% in patients with acute tubular necrosis.

The reduced GFR and ensued kidney injury are associated with initial reduction in urine volume at a rate of $\leq$0.5 mL/kg/h.

In prerenal causes, the renal tubules are able to concentrate the urine. Urine osmolality is higher than 500 mOsmol/L compared to acute tubular necrosis where osmolality is less than 450 mOsmol/L.

Intrinsic renal dysfunction

Prerenal and postrenal dysfunction can both lead to intrinsic renal damage and to dysfunction if no urgent intervention was done to restore glomerular filtration.

Glomerular nephritis is often secondary to an immunological and inflammatory component, and that measurement of the respective antibodies indicates the immunological and/or infection nature.

However, intrinsic renal damage can also result from other systemic causes such as sepsis, autoimmune disorders, deposition of amyloids, proteins, light chains as well as blood cells, calcinosis secondary to prolonged hypercalcemia, administration of nephrotoxic drugs, chemotherapeutic agents as well as radiological contrast media.

Membranous nephropathy is a rare presentation of glomerular basement membrane disorder secondary to deposition of antiphospholipase A2 receptor causing glomerular damage and proteinuria. The immunological and physical insult leads to a reduction in GFR, to decreased membrane selectivity and to increased permeability leading to increased protein leakage.

In intrinsic renal dysfunction, creatinine and urea increase in tandem in contrast to that seen in prerenal uremia.

Thus, increased creatinine and urea and the presence of proteins and/or blood in the urine are the whole mark of glomerulonephritis.

The antibodies often measured are antiglomerular basement membrane antibody, antineutrophil cytoplasmic antibodies (ANCA) in vasculitis, antinuclear antibodies (ANA), and anti-dsDNA in systemic lupus erythematosus (SLE), antistreptolysin antibodies in poststreptococcal glomerulonephritis. Phospholipase A2 receptor antibodies are highly specific for the diagnosis of primary membranous nephropathy with 70%–75% of patients with primary membranous nephropathy. Its measurement helps defines the cause of nephrotic syndrome eliminating the need for biopsy. Values below 14 RU/mL are considered negative.

Reduced tubular function in the presence of normal glomerular function

Although progression to tubular dysfunction often follows glomerular dysfunction secondary to reduced GFR; however, tubular dysfunction in the presence of normal and intact glomerular function occurs. This is often due to selective tubular damage by autoimmune and or toxic agents.

Biochemical findings include polyuria, not encountered in glomerulonephritis, and is due to inability to reabsorb electrolytes and associated water. There are high urinary sodium levels in relation to patient hydration. There is hypokalemia, low plasma bicarbonate with metabolic acidosis, hypophosphatemia, and hypouricemia.

Postrenal dysfunction

Obstruction of urinary flow due to either kidney stones, ureter blockage, prostatic hypertrophy, bladder neoplasm, or inflammation. Both serum creatinine and urea will be elevated. The cause for obstruction, although often diagnosed using radiological procedures (ultrasound, contrast CT, etc.). Biochemical investigations are those of PSA measurement in prostate hyperplasia and cancer. Kidney stone analysis is obtained to assess cause and risk for recurrence.

Biochemical findings

Biochemical makers of kidney function discussed above are used to diagnose and assess the extent of prerenal, intrinsic, and postrenal dysfunction. Renal dysfunction may also present as acute, chronic uremic syndrome, or a combination of acute on chronic. Furthermore, biomarkers indicate either a glomerular component alone, a tubular component alone, or mixed glomerular and tubular dysfunction.

Urea (blood urea nitrogen) and creatinine

Elevated circulating urea and creatinine indicate reduced glomerular filtration rate. The extent as well as their respective elevation is helpful in assessing both cause and extent of GFR reduction. Concomitant increase indicates reduced GFR due to prerenal, intrinsic renal cause, such as glomerular nephritis, glomerular damage, or postrenal cause. Prerenal and postrenal obstruction causes of reduced GFR will ultimately lead to intrinsic renal damage.

Creatinine is constantly produced with relatively small normal variation. It has an inverse relationship with GFR (shown in Fig. 7). However, disproportionate increase in BUN to creatinine with a ratio exceeding 10:1 suggests prerenal cause leading to reduced renal blood flow. Causes include circulatory failure, blood loss, hypovolemia, and cardiac dysfunction. Urea diffuses from the lumen to interstitial fluid and into the circulation. It is a reflection of reduced blood flow (forces acting at the glomerulus being those of blood flow, hydrostatic pressure, and opposed by the colloidal osmotic pressure of the luminal fluid/ultrafiltrate).

The reduced hydrostatic pressure and associated hypovolemia stimulate renin angiotensin I production, and the resultant angiotensin II causes increased aldosterone

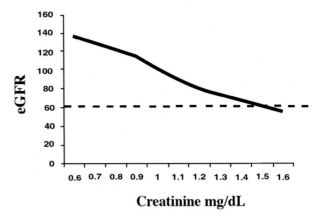

FIG. 7 Relationship between creatinine concentration and calculated eGFR. *(Data from the author's laboratory.)*

production (see above and Chapter 2 on electrolytes and fluid balance). Aldosterone stimulates reabsorption of sodium (with accompanied water) to restore normovolemia. This results in reduced urinary sodium and increased urinary osmolality. A urinary sodium less than 20 mmol/L and a urine/plasma osmolality of >1.5 is indicative of prerenal causes for the observed renal dysfunction. This obviously depends on an intact functioning tubules.

The reduced luminal sodium for exchange with hydrogen ions and thus loss of bicarbonate in the urine and accumulation of interstitial hydrogen results in acidosis with decreased plasma bicarbonate levels (Fig. 8).

Chronic and acute renal dysfunction

Patients with acute kidney failure may progress to chronic kidney disease if not managed appropriately. Additionally, patients with chronic kidney disease may develop an acute kidney failure episode. Biochemical changes are those of rapid and is exacerbated worsening in function. Examples include multiple myeloma patients with chronic kidney disease where reduced GFR and increasing disease burden (monoclonal proteins and/or free light chains) may deposit on the glomerulus and/or cause acute tubular injury.

Chronic kidney disease (CKD) describes a gradual decline in kidney function. It is defined as the persistence of kidney dysfunction for 3 months or more regardless of the cause. Interventions are required to halt decline and prevent progression to kidney failure. The clinical biochemistry laboratory plays a significant role in the detection, monitoring response to therapy and thus management of patients. GFR defines the five stages of chronic kidney disease and its progression (Table 4).

Renal tubular acidosis (acid-base status)

The kidneys play an important role in maintaining the acid-base status (see Chapter 15 on blood gases and acid base

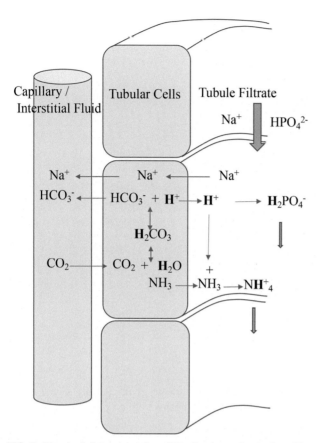

FIG. 8 Renal tubular regeneration of bicarbonate, and excretion of hydrogen in association with ammonia and phosphate. Urea creatinine ratio is 10–15:1 and rises in tandem in renal failure, urea, and creatine rise in tandem in renal failure. BUN:Creatinine ratio >20:1 imply prerenal failure. *(Modified from Wagner CA, Imenez Silva PH, Bourgeois S. Molecular pathophysiology of acid-base disorders. Semin Nephrol. 2019;39(4): 340–352. doi:https://doi.org/10.1016/j.semnephrol.2019.04.004. PMID: 31300090.)*

TABLE 4 Five stages of kidney disease in use by treatment guidelines by the National Kidney Foundation.

Stage	GFR (mL/min/m²)	Condition
1	>90	Damage with either normal or increased GFR
2	60–89	Damage with either normal or decreased GFR
3A	45–59	Moderate decline in GFR
3B	30–44	Moderate-to-severe decline in GFR
4	15–29	Severe decline in GFR
5	<15	Kidney failure

Stages 5D describes kidney failure patients undergoing chronic dialysis, 5T represents end-stage kidney failure patients who undergone kidney transplant.
Modified from https://kidneyfoundation.cachefly.net/professionals/KDOQI/ guidelines_ckd/p4_class_g1.htm. Accessed 18 February 2023.

balance). Urine pH is normally slightly acidic at 5.5–6.5. However, depending on the pathophysiology and dietary intake, it ranges from 4.5 to 8.0 and to some extent it reflects that of blood, except in renal tubular acidosis. High-protein diet produces an acidic urine where a high citrate content causes an alkaline urine.

An alkaline urine supports the finding of urinary tract infection; this is due to the presence of a urea-splitting microorganism and is found in patients with struvite and ammonium phosphate crystals (calculi). An acidic urine is often associated with uric acid crystals (calculi).

Renal tubular acidosis (RTA) is defined as the inability of the kidney to acidify the urine pH to below 5.5. There are three different types of RTA.

Type I RTA: This depicts the inability of the distal tubules to excrete hydrogen ions. Although hydrogen ions are excreted in isolation, it is accompanied with bicarbonate, ammonia, and phosphate with a net effect of hydrogen ion loss. Presentation is that of blood acidosis in the presence of an alkaline urine.

Type II RTA: This type describes the inability of the proximal tubules to reabsorb bicarbonate. With an initial alkaline urine that becomes acidic upon depletion of the filtered bicarbonate load.

Type III: It is a rare form with combined features of both distal and proximal RTAs. In type 4, hyperkalemic acidosis is present caused by abnormal acid and potassium excretion in the collecting duct.

The different RTA types, their defect, and biochemical findings are summarized below (Table 5).

Urinalysis investigation

Biochemical investigation of the urine provides clues on the etiology and course of the kidney disease. Midstream urine collection is preferred to minimize contamination and that analysis performed within 2h of collection yields appropriate results. Refrigeration and protection from light are recommended.

Urine volume

Urine volume is diagnostic and may indicate the nature of the kidney dysfunction. Normal urine volume is dependent on intake and on body hydration and is about 0.8–2.0L per day. Volumes in excess of 2.5L per day is considered polyureic. Causes of polyuria include drugs (use of diuretics, mannitol, anticholinergics (thirst stimulant), osmotic diuresis (secondary to hyperglycemia or hypercalcemia, urea), excessive fluid intake (psychogenic polydipsia), hypothalamic disorders (diabetes insipidus).

Oliguria, defined as a urine output less than 400mL/day. It is often a reflection of reduced glomerular filtration rate due to either prerenal, intrinsic renal damage or postrenal

TABLE 5 Summary of renal tubular acidosis classification and biochemical findings.

	Distal (type 1) RTA	Proximal (type 2) RTA	Hyperkalemic (type 4) RTA
Primary defect	Decreased distal acid excretion or increased H^+ membrane permeability	Decreased proximal reabsorption of HCO_3^-	Reduced excretion of acid and K^+ in the collecting duct
Urine pH	>5.3	<5.5	<5.5
Serum HCO_3^-	10–20 mmol/L	16–20 mmol/L	16–22 mmol/L
Serum K^+	Low (<3.5 mmol/L)	Low (<3.5 mmol/L)	High (5.5–6.5 mmol/L)
Dynamic diagnostic tests	Positive urinary anion gap after NH_4^+ loading test	Fractional excretion of HCO_3^- >15% or urine pH >7.5 after HCO_3^- loading test Glycosuria, hypophosphatemia, and hypouricemia indicates Fanconi syndrome	Urinary K^+ <40 mmol/L or fractional K^+ excretion <20%, abnormal serum aldosterone, with near-normal renal function

Initial anion gaps are normal in all of the three RTA types.
Modified from Palmer BF, Kelepouris E, Clegg DJ. Renal tubular acidosis and management strategies: a narrative review. *Adv Ther.* 2021;38(2):949–968.

obstruction. It often follows an episode of acute renal failure. In prerenal circulatory failure, fractional excretion of sodium $(FE_{Na} = ((Urine_{Na} \times Plasma_{Creatinine})/(Plasma_{Na} \times Urine_{creatinine})) \times 100)$ is <1 compared with >2 in patients with oliguria secondary to intrinsic acute renal failure.

An initial oliguria is often followed by polyuria during the recovery phase. Oliguria is observed in deteriorating kidney function and is followed by anuria (failure to pass any urine). Causes of oliguria include renal circulatory insufficiency secondary to circulatory shock, hemorrhage, dehydration, vomiting, and diarrhea. Intrinsic renal causes include glomerular nephritis, acute tubular necrosis, nephrotoxic damage, and polycystic kidney disease. Postrenal causes include obstructive uropathy secondary to renal calculi, prostatic hypertrophy, and to pelvic tumors.

Urine appearance

Urine color and appearance may provide a clue to some degree of pathophysiology. For example, suggest concentrated vs dilute urine, a dark urine color indicates a concentrated urine. A turbid appearance indicates either pyuria due to urinary tract infection or to stagnant urine (urea splitting bacteria) respectively, or due to precipitated phosphate crystals in alkaline urine, lipids, and high proteins. A red pinkish-colored urine indicates blood or myoglobin presence. The presence of conjugated bilirubin in urine contributes to the dark color of the urine observed in patient with cholestatic liver disease.

Odor of the urine may also give a clue to the pathophysiology. For instance, a pungent odor suggests urinary tract infection, diabetic ketoacidosis gives a fruity sweet odor, and maple syrup odor indicates maple syrup urine disease.

Urine concentration

The concentration of the urine sample is indicative of both intrinsic and extrinsic kidney dysfunction.

Diluted urine sample is seen in diabetes insipidus, use of diuretics, adrenal insufficiency, and impaired renal function. Concentrated urine sample is seen in patients with diabetes and glucosuria, syndrome of inappropriate antidiuretic hormone (SIADH), and hypovolemia. The degree of urine concentration is objectively assessed using either specific gravity or osmolality measurement.

Urine specific gravity

Specific gravity measurement detects ionic species only as indication for urine concentration. Normal specific gravity ranges from 1.003 to 1.030, and thus, patient hydration status with specific gravity <1.010 indicates adequate hydration, whereas a value >1.020 indicates relative dehydration and circulatory insufficiency as a cause for oliguria. Values <1.010 indicate intrinsic renal failure as a cause for oliguria. Specific gravity also provides insight into the urine concentrating ability of the kidney. Specific gravity often correlates with urine osmolality; however, it does not allow for contribution by glucose and other osmotic substances to the urine concentration. Patients with intrinsic renal disease-specific gravity resemble that of the glomerular filtrate at 1.010.

Osmolality

Urine osmolality can vary from 13 to 1400 mOsmol/L reflecting a dilute and a highly concentrated urine respectively. Urine volume can vary from 13% of filtered water to an obligatory minimal volume of 500 mL/24 h. Urine osmolality >500 mOsmol/L suggests prerenal cause of an oliguria, whereas levels <300 indicate acute renal failure as a cause of oliguria.

Urine volume (anuria, oliguria, and polyuria) is diagnostic. High and dilute volume indicating inability to concentrate the urine (diabetes insipidus), excessive hypotonic fluid intake (polydipsia), a high volume in the presence of high osmolality (diuresis) in glycosuria (diabetes mellitus), hypercalciuria (secondary to hypercalcemia (hyperparathyroidism and or malignancy)). This causes a higher urine flow rate due to both the osmotic substances present and to reduced reabsorption of sodium (increased concentration gradient against which the sodium is reabsorbed) resulting in reduced interstitial tonicity. Secondary causes are due to drugs (thiazides and lithium).

There are different formulas in use for the determination of osmolar gap (see later). Sources of errors when estimating osmolar gap include, the presence of; hyperproteinemia, hyperlipidemia, and hypomagnesaemia.

Conditions and subtances influencing osmolar gap include alcohol and or ethylene glycol ingestion, alcoholic or diabetic ketoacidosis, osmolar therapy (e.g., mannitol, glycerol administration), etc.

Osmolality is measured using freezing point depression (other method, such as vapor pressure measurement is also available but as not widely used. It is helpful when dealing with volatile substances, e.g., alcohols). The more osmotic particles present, the higher the osmolality and the lower the freezing point. Osmolality measurement is helpful in assessment of hyponatremia and in determining osmolar gap in suspected osmotic substance. Different formulas are in use for example; osmolality = $2 \times Na + [urea] + [Glucose]$ in mmol/L (normal 280–290 mOsmol/L). Others use 1.86 instead of 2 representing incomplete dissociation of Na Cl. The difference between measured and calculated osmolality is termed osmolal gap and indicates the presence of an osmotically active substance (s) unaccounted for by the different formulas.

Proteinuria

Measurement of urinary protein level is essential in the detection and assessment of kidney function. Normally little or no protein is detectable. Proteins with molecular weight less than 11 kDa are filtered through the glomerular, but most proteins are reabsorbed and/or metabolized by the proximal renal tubules, and thus, the detection of significant proteins in the urine suggests kidney damage.

Low-molecular-weight proteins are often associated with tubular damage compared with larger molecular weight proteins that are characteristic of glomerular dysfunction. Therefore, proteinuria is the hallmark of either glomerular or tubular dysfunction or both.

Furthermore, more than 99.9% of low-molecular-weight proteins are reabsorbed, and thus, the appearance in the urine of low-molecular-weight proteins reflects renal proximal tubular dysfunction.

The presence of Bence-Jones protein indicates monoclonal paraprotein mediated renal dysfunction.

Proteins detected in the urine include albumin and globulins and those secreted by the nephron. Levels exceeding 150 mg/day (or 10–20 mg/dL, influenced by urine concentration) are considered clinically significant and require detailed investigation. Proteinuria could be transient or persistent. In transient proteinuria, changes in glomerular function cause protein loss into the urine seen in congestive heart failure, dehydration, exercise, seizure, and fever.

Orthostatic proteinuria is seen following prolong standing, and it is confirmed by obtaining a negative sample after 8 h of being recumbent.

Persistent proteinuria is due to either glomerular or tubular dysfunction and or to overflow. Albumin, the predominant serum protein even in significant proteinuria where it often constitutes 60%–90%, and being of relatively high molecular weight, it appears in the urine when there is glomerular damage. The appearance of low-molecular-weight proteins reflects tubular dysfunction of either impaired reabsorption or decreased metabolism. In purely tubular dysfunction, low-molecular-weight proteins, often less than 2 g/day, exceed albumin levels. High circulating low-molecular-weight proteins overwhelm the absorptive capacity of the renal tubules. It is, however, often a continuum and mixed composition of proteins reflecting involvement of both glomerular and tubular components to variable degree is observed.

Normally very little proteins <150 mg/day appear in the urine with albumin being the most contributor. Levels are below detection by urine strip testing. Other proteins are of low molecular weight serum proteins, or those derived from the renal tubules and the lower urinary tract.

Due to the low concentration in urine, albumin is measured using immunoturbidimetry based assays. Either a 24 h urine (normal levels being <30 mg/day) or albumin creatinine ratio for a random urine collection (normal levels being <30 mg/g) are recommended measurements.

Urine volume as indicated above is variable and urine creatinine is used to correct for changes in urine volume. This is applied to both albumin (reported as albumin creatinine ration (ACR)) and to total protein measurements (reported as urine protein creatinine ratio (PCR)) and is used to measure albuminuria and assess the degree of renal impairment.

ACR measurement is preferred over protein creatinine ratio (PCR) for its higher sensitivity in patients with low levels of proteinuria.

A repeat analysis of ACR is preferred for initial samples with values between 30 and 700 mg/g using an early morning sample. This is not necessary for samples with initial ACR ≥700 mg/g. When ACR is 700 mg/g or more, protein creatinine ratio may be used to monitor disease progression and response to therapy.

ACR is measured in adults with DM (type I or II) in adults and children, in adults with eGFR <60 mL/min/1.73 m², in adults with eGFR of 60 mL/min/1.73 m² or more if there is strong suspicion of CKD.

Additionally, ACR >20 mg/g in patients with AKI is associated with better outcome than other forms of AKI, but this is not the case among critically ill patients.

ACR is used to guide diagnosis and management of CKD for instance; in patients with eGFR of 45–59 mL/min/1.73 m² sustained for 3 months directs the use of eGFR incorporating cystatin C help confirm or rule out CKD when ACR is <30 mg/g.

ACR guides the use of renin angiotensin inhibitors ACE inhibitors, angiotensin-II-receptor blockers offered to CKD patients without DM. Severity and risk of adverse outcomes, e.g., for diabetes and ACR ≥30 mg/g (category A2 or A3), hypertension and ACR ≥300 mg/g (ACR category A3), ACR ≥700 mg/g irrespective of hypertension or cardiovascular disease are shown below (Tables 6 and 7).

Urine ACR is vital for assessing risk for and monitoring progression of kidney disease and the impact of interventions but also is used to determine when a cystatin C-based eGFR estimation is indicated.

Laboratories are encouraged to offer a kidney profile that includes both eGFR and urine ACR to increase ordering of the latter when assessing kidney function. ACR screening is not performed in 35% of dietetic patients and in 4% hypertensive patients.

Most glomerular disease is associated with significant proteinuria. Albumin and creatinine or protein to creatinine ratio in a random urine spot is commonly used. Although there is poor agreement between those random urine results and 24 h urine protein measurements, the latter suffers from inaccuracy and difficulty with complete collections, storage, and handling particularly in children. Up to 50% of errors in 24 h GFR measurement is due to incomplete collections.

Persistent proteinuria is a risk factor for progressive loss of GFR, and its reduction is a goal for all glomerular diseases.

Qualitative urinary albumin dipstick results often reported as negative, 1+, 2+, or >2+ those results are often considered to represent albumin creatinine ratio (ACR) values of <10, 10–29, 30–299, and ≥300 mg/g, and that they may be categorized as normal (or mild albuminuria), moderate, or severe albuminuria respectively (Tables 6 and 7).

Similarly: Urine protein creatinine ratio: UPC ratio: A1 <150 mg/g (normal to low), 150–500 mg/g (moderate), >500 mg/g (severe).

ACR may be predicted from urine protein dipstick readings. The variables are gender, the presence diabetes, and of hypertension. Common classification of severity of albumin and proteinuria is shown in Table 6.

Glucosuria

Filtered glucose is reabsorbed by the proximal tubule and has a threshold of 180 mg/dL (10 mmol/L). This re-absorption threshold is overwhelmed in diabetes with glucosuria, and it decreases in pregnancy with glucose appearing in the urine at much lower glomerular filtrate levels (about 90 mg/dL (5 mmol/L)). Additionally, intrinsic tubule dysfunction as in Fanconi syndrome, glucose appears in the urine at lower glomerular filtrate levels.

Hematuria

The presence of hematuria and proteinuria is of pathological significance and suggests intrinsic glomerular kidney

TABLE 6 Excretion rates are timed collections.

	AER (mg/day)	PER (mg/day)	ACR (mg/g)	PCR (mg/g)	Protein dipstick
Normal to mildly increased	<30	<150	<30	<150	Negative/trace
Moderately increased	30–300	150–500	30–300	150–500	Trace–1+
Severely increased	>300	>500	>300	>500	>1+

Correction of random samples (untimed—preferred early morning concentrated samples) is preferred due to difficulties with obtaining accurate timed collections. *ACR*, albumin creatinine ratio; *AER*, albumin excretion rate; *PCR*, protein creatinine ratio; *PER*, protein excretion rate. Multiply by 0.113 to convert from mg/g to mg/mmol of creatinine. Urinary albumin creatinine ratio (ACR) and associated stage of chronic kidney disease. Urine albumin and protein daily excretion rates ≫2200 and 3500 are seen in nephrotic syndrome.
In use by the author's laboratory and modified from KIDGO. https://kidneyfoundation.cachefly.net/professionals/KDOQI/guidelines_ckd/p4_class_g1.htm. Accessed 18 February 2023.

TABLE 7 Risk of adverse outcomes in adults by GFR and ACR category.

	A1 ACR <3 mg/g Normal-mild increase	A2 ACR 3–300 mg/g Moderately increased	A3 ACR >300 mg/g Markedly increased
G1 (≥90 mL/min/1.73 m²) Normal or high GFR	Low risk	Moderate risk	High risk
G2 (60–89 mL/min/1.73 m²) Mild reduction in GFR	Low risk	Moderate risk	High risk
G3a (45–59 mL/min/1.73 m²) Mild-moderate reduction	Moderate risk	High risk	Very high risk
G3b (30–44 mL/min/1.73 m²) Moderate-severe reduction	High risk	Very high risk	Very high risk
G4 (15–29 mL/min/1.73 m²) Severe reduction	Very high risk	Very high risk	Very high risk
G5 (<15 mL/min/1.73 m²) Kidney failure	Very high risk	Very high risk	Very high risk

Modified from KIDGO. https://kidneyfoundation.cachefly.net/professionals/KDOQI/guidelines_ckd/p4_class_g1.htm. Accessed 18 February 2023.

dysfunction. Hematuria represents passage of red blood cells into the urine. It is observed in glomerular dysfunction, polycystic kidney disease, malignancy, nephrolithiasis, trauma and vascular injury, anticoagulant therapy, hematological disorders (sickle cell disease, thrombocytopenia), and strenuous exercise. Microscopic investigation of urine is required to identity the cause where the presence of white blood cells indicates infection, the presence of RBC sediments excludes hemoglobin in clear urine.

The presence of hyaline casts with or without epithelial cells in urine sediment indicates intrinsic interstitial kidney disease, similarly, in glomerular nephritis, the presence of red blood cells cast and hematuria. The presence of granulated cast suggests tubular dysfunction.

Hematuria is defined as presence of ≥3 red blood cells per high power field (hpf) microscopy in two or three urine samples, and this is to rule out benign exercise-associated hematuria witch is negative on repeat sample 48h later.

Frank hematuria occurs in glomerular, renal, and those of urological etiologies. In the glomerular form, accompanied by significant proteinuria, erythrocytes casts and dysmorphic red blood cells are the whole mark with 20% of patients present with hematuria alone. IgA nephropathy is the most common cause of glomerular hematuria.

Renal hematuria form is often secondary to tubular interstitial, renovascular, and/or metabolic disorders. Similar to that of glomerular hematuria, it is often associated with significant proteinuria; however, there are no associated dysmorphic red blood cells or erythrocytes casts.

The urological form of hematuria is often secondary to malignancy, calculi, and infections. In contrast to the two renal intrinsic forms, urological hematuria is often devoid of significant proteinuria despite the hematuria, and the microscopic dysmorphic red blood cells and erythrocytes casts. Among patients with urological hematuria, 20% will have urinary tract malignancy.

Red blood cells (RBCs)

RBCs in small amount are present in normal urine. Marked hematuria indicates significant pathology requiring further investigation and attention. Intact RBCs could be of tubular or ureteral origin, irregular RBCs indicates glomerular source and may indicate glomerulonephritis. There is a distinction between hematuria and hemoglobinuria, and all could indicate positive peroxidase including myoglobin. Hemoglobinuria may indicate in vivo hemolysis and coagulopathy, and myoglobinuria indicates rhabdomyolysis.

Hematuria whether macro- or microhematuria is always associated with glomerular disorder and that the identification of red cell cast identifies nephritic causes. Additionally, resolution of hematuria is associated with complete clinical remission and is important finding in assessing the activity of the IgA nephritis and antineutrophil cytoplasmic antibody vasculitis.

Urinary casts, crystals, and sediments

Casts observed in urinary sediments represent aggregation of Tamm-Horsfall large molecular weight glycoprotein secreted by renal tubular cells. Other serum proteins, fat bacteria, elements within the sediment will be trapped within

TABLE 8 Urinary cast characteristics and associated renal pathology.

Cast type	Constituents	Pathophysiology
Hyaline	Mucoproteins	Normal, pyelonephritis, chronic kidney disease
Erythrocyte	Red blood cells	Glomerulonephritis
Leukocyte	White blood cells	Pyelonephritis, glomerulonephritis, interstitial nephritis
Epithelial	Renal tubule cells	Acute tubular necrosis, interstitial nephritis, nephritic syndrome, allograft rejection, heavy metals toxicity
Granular	Variable cell types	Advanced renal disease
Waxy	Variable cell types	Advanced renal disease
Fatty	Lipid-laden renal tubule cell	Nephrotic syndrome
Broad	Variable cell types	End-stage renal disease

Modified from Simerville JA, Maxted WC, Pahira JJ. Urinalysis: a comprehensive review. *Am Fam Physician*. 2005;71(6):1153–1162.

the cast, which is molded by the tubules. This in effect provides a biopsy of the lumen of the nephron and represent the condition of the nephron at the time the cast was formed.

Cast formation is enhanced by the presence of proteins and acidic pH and thus casts are unlikely to be seen in dilute and alkaline urine (urine sample becomes alkaline due to storage may therefore give falsely negative casts results). Inclusions in the cast may comprise Tamm-Horsfall protein, RBCs, WBCs, epithelial cells, fat, and or bacteria, etc. (Table 8). The inclusions give the casts waxy and granular appearance and cylindrical appearance with rounded ends.

Hyaline casts are primarily made up of Tamm-Horsfall protein, and their presence suggests tubular injury. Other cast made up of proteins and contains cellular material of renal tissue origin. The casts indicate the site within the nephron as well as the pathophysiology associated with their formation (Table 8).

Crystals

Assessment of risk for calculi formation and investigation of causes of existing and past calculus is central to patient management. It often requires analysis of calculus composition for identification of cause and of precipitating factors (see below).

Urine dipstick (strip testing)

A reagent strip (chemical pads) often termed dipstick. A strip of reagent pads with specific reagents for the separate detection of albumin, glucose, ketones, blood, nitrates, bilirubin, pH, and leukocyte esterase (Table 9). It provides mostly a qualitative and for few a semiquantitative analysis.

Nephrolithiasis

The prevalence of nephrolithiasis (renal calculi) is increasing worldwide (doubled over a period of 6 years in the United States) with an annual incidence of 8 case per 1000 adults. The stones are formed in either the ureter, pelvis, or the bladder. The etiology varies from urinary tract infection in the developing world to dehydration, hot climate, and the presence of comorbidities (obesity, hypertension, gout, and fatty liver disease).

Stones form when the urinary constituent such as calcium, oxalate, urate, phosphate exceed their saturation concentration, often due to presence of concentrated urine. Exceeding their solubility and often the presence of a nucleation facilitates the formation of kidney stones. Those relative amounts of the components are dependent on the diet intake, and some have genetic cause in tubular handling such as cysteine (excess presence in urine). Development of stones are influenced by urine concentration, urine pH, urine stagnation, and presence of urinary tract infection.

Clinical presentation in the acute setting is of intermittent abdominal and flank pain often accompanied by nausea, vomiting, and malaise. About 90% of kidney stones pass spontaneously (small stones <6 mm) with only half of those >6 mm where medical intervention is required.

Biochemical assessments are used to assess the cause of as well as to assess risk for stone formation. The availability of extracorporeal shock wave lithotripsy in the management of nephrolithiasis, which leads to stones destruction and passing into the urine, little stone material is thus available for analysis to determine its constituents and thus cause. Measurement of urinary calcium, phosphate, oxalate, uric acid, citrate, magnesium, sodium, pH, nitrates, and culture

TABLE 9 Urinalysis dipstick test analytes, their respective methodologies, and special considerations.

Test	Method principle	Comment
pH	Uses protein error of indicators	pH ranges from 5.0 to 9.0
Glucose	Glucose oxidase	
Ketones	Sodium nitroprusside or nitro ferrocyanide and glycine	It detects acetone and acetoacetate but does not detect beta hydroxybutyrate which is often present early in diabetic ketoacidosis.
Albumin	Protein error of indicator	Detects 5–10 mg/dL (trace), 30 mg/dL (1+), 100 mg/dL (2+), 300 mg/dL (3+), and 1000 mg/dL (4+)
Nitrate	Based on diazotization reaction of nitrite with aromatic amine-producing diazonium salt.	Bacteria reduces nitrates to nitrites (many gram negative, some gram positive). A negative result does not rule out urinary tract infection (UTI) (not sensitive). Poor storage produces false positive strips.
Leukocyte esterase	Leukocyte esterase is produced by neutrophils	Pyuria associate with UTI.
Blood (hemoglobin/red blood cells)	Peroxidase activity	Detects hemoglobin, myoglobin, and red blood cells. The red blood cells can be seen as speckles on the pad whereas a homogeneous color indicates either hemoglobin or myoglobin. Additional testing is required to identify myoglobin.
Bilirubin (urobilinogen)	Bilirubin reacts with diazonium salt in acid medium forming azodye	Urobilinogen end product of direct bilirubin it indicates Biliary obstruction, hepatocellular disease, hemolysis.
Specific gravity	Change in pH and color of bromothymol blue from blue green to yellow green. Ionic solutes release protons and decrease pH.	Normal range from 1.003 to 1.030

Modified from Urine dipstick kit insert; One + Step®, Urine reagent strip, Exeter, United Kingdom.

is performed to determine cause as well as assess risk for stone formation. Fifty percent of patients with history of stone will have recurrence formation and therefore assessment of metabolic cause for stone formation is important.

This often performed on a time urine samples preferably in a 24 -h urine sample. However, urine pH and assessment for possible infection are assessed using an early morning urine sample.

Serum measurement of calcium and phosphate, uric acid, sodium, potassium, chloride, and bicarbonate are measured for the assessment of hyperparathyroidism, gout, renal dysfunction, and of renal tubular acidosis as a precipitating cause.

Analysis of the stone provides the best indication for the cause and identifies those rate stone of rare metabolic dysfunction xanthine and cysteine stones. With the advent use of extracorporeal shock wave lithotripsy, stones are fragmented and passed (often stones 0.5–2 cm diameter).

The majority of stones are calcium oxalate (70%–90%) which are calcium containing stones, followed by struvite stones (calcium ammonium phosphate) also known as infection stones, uric acid stones (10%), cysteine stone and more rarely those due to inherited xanthine disorders, cystinosis, and those triggered by renal tubular disorders (defect in basic amino acids reabsorption) cysteine, ornithine, arginine, and lysine (COAL).

The presence of calcium oxalate is due to increased urinary oxalate, whereas the presence of calcium phosphate stones is due to the presence of hypercalciuria. This is because the solubility of calcium oxalate is lower than that for calcium phosphate (saturation exceeded). Calcium oxalate stones are variable in size, and have a refractile square envelope shape.

Concentrated urine that is acidic favors production of uric acid stones, whereas alkaline urine favors production of struvite stones and calcium oxalate stones. Treatment thus is aimed at maintaining a urinary pH of about 6.5 and production of a dilute and large urinary volume which provides the best prevention modality. Uric acid crystals are yellow to orange brown in color. They are diamond or barrel shaped. Triple phosphate crystals are often associated with alkaline urine and urinary tract infection. They are colorless and have the coffin lid appearance. Cysteine crystals, a colorless (translucent, white), have a hexagonal shape, and they are present in acidic urine.

Citrate and magnesium have protective roles where the magnesium competes with calcium with oxalate and has a higher solubility and thus prevents calcium oxalate formation, similarly, citrate competes with oxalate for calcium and has a much higher solubility. Magnesium and citrate in addition to their therapeutic role, their measurement is used to assess risk for stone formation.

Stones formers that suggest genetic component (familial) or recurrent and is not due to those mentioned above require analysis for amino acids and for xanthine analysis.

Summary

- The nephron is the functional unit of the kidney.
- The nephron incudes; Bowman's campus which house the glomerulus, the proximal and distal convoluted renal tubules, the descending and ascending loop of Henle, and the collecting duct.
- The glomerulus (renal capsule) comprises a capillary network enclosed within the Bowman's capsule.
- The narrowing of the blood vessels and formation of capillaries results in a perfusion pressure of at least 50–60 mmHg is required to overcome the hydrostatic and oncotic pressures opposing filtration.
- The kidney's metabolic functions are (a) excretion of nonvolatile metabolites such as urea, creatinine, uric acid, phosphates, sulfates, as well as toxins, drugs, and their metabolites, (b) maintain homeostasis of body fluid volume and electrolytes levels, (c) maintain acid-base homeostasis, (d) providing an endocrine role for renin, 1,25-(OH)$_2$ vitamin D synthesis, and for PTH regulated calcium and phosphate levels, and for erythropoietin synthesis.
- Creatinine and urea as well as cystatin C are used as endogenous markers of the glomerular filtration rate.
- A number of exogenous GFR markers are available, although not widely used. They include inulin, iothalamate, and iohexol. The latter is increasingly being used.
- The glomerular filtration rate can be estimated via a number of mathematical formulas.
- CKD-EPI (2021) formula is widely adopted and increasing being used. It has recently been revised with race correction factor removed.
- Fluid balance is predominantly a tubular function.
- The kidney is important in maintaining acid-base status.
- Erythropoietin a glycoprotein peptide hormone with 30.4k kDa molecular weight produced by the peritubular cells of the kidney in response to tissue hypoxia.
- Urine osmolality can vary from 13 to 1400 mOsmol/L reflecting a dilute and a highly concentrated urine, respectively. In prerenal causes, the renal tubules are able to concentrate the urine. Urine osmolality is higher than 500 mOsmol/L compared in acute tubular necrosis where osmolality is less than 450 mOsmol/L.
- Prerenal and postrenal dysfunction can both lead to intrinsic renal damage and dysfunction.
- Glomerular nephritis, often secondary to an immunological and inflammatory component.
- Postrenal dysfunction is secondary to obstruction of urinary flow due to either kidney stones, ureter blockage, prostatic hypertrophy, bladder neoplasm, or inflammation.
- Biochemical investigation of the urine provides clues on the etiology and course of the kidney disease.
- Proteinuria is the hallmark of either glomerular or tubular dysfunction or both.
- Stones form when the urinary constituent such as calcium, oxalate, urate, phosphate exceed their saturation concentration, often due to presence of concentrated urine. Stone composition and urine analysis help indentify the cause.

Further reading

Simerville JA, Maxted WC, Pahira JJ. Urinalysis: a comprehensive review. *Am Fam Physician.* 2005;71(6):1153–1162.

Fontenelle LF, Sarti TD. Kidney stones: treatment and prevention. *Am Fam Physician.* 2019;99(8):490–496.

Schoener B, Borger J. Erythropoietin stimulating agents. In: *StatPearls.* Treasure Island, FL: StatPearls Publishing; 2022.

Manzoor H, Bhatt H. Prerenal kidney failure. In: *StatPearls.* Treasure Island, FL: StatPearls Publishing; 2022.

Horio M, Imai E, Yasuda Y, Hishida A, Matsuo S, Japanese Equation for Estimating GFR. Simple sampling strategy for measuring inulin renal clearance. *Clin Exp Nephrol.* 2009;13(1):50–54.

Taubert M, Ebert N, Martus P, van der Giet M, Fuhr U, Schaeffner E. Using a three-compartment model improves the estimation of iohexol clearance to assess glomerular filtration rate. *Sci Rep.* 2018;8(1):17723.

Hamm LL, Nakhoul N, Hering-Smith KS. Acid-base homeostasis. *Clin J Am Soc Nephrol.* 2015;10(12):2232–2242.

Stevens LA, Coresh J, Greene T, Levey AS. Assessing kidney function—measured and estimated glomerular filtration rate. *N Engl J Med.* 2006;354(23):2473–2483.

Ferguson TW, Komenda P, Tangri N. Cystatin C as a biomarker for estimating glomerular filtration rate. *Curr Opin Nephrol Hypertens.* 2015;24(3):295–300.

Kaminska J, Dymicka-Piekarska V, Tomaszewska J, Matowicka-Karna J, Koper-Lenkiewicz OM. Diagnostic utility of protein to creatinine ratio (P/C ratio) in spot urine sample within routine clinical practice. *Crit Rev Clin Lab Sci.* 2020;57(5):345–364.

Palmer BF, Kelepouris E, Clegg DJ. Renal tubular acidosis and management strategies: a narrative review. *Adv Ther.* 2021;38(2):949–968.

Chapter 4

Liver function

Introduction

This chapter describes hepatic functions and biomarkers used in the investigation of their disorders. That is markers of hepatic synthetic and detoxification functions, markers of hepatocytes injury and infection, and those of liver architecture such as cholestasis, fibrosis, and malignancy.

A generalized use of the term liver function tests should be avoided as the enzymes frequently measured as part of the "function" tests such as alanine aminotransferase (ALT), aspartate transaminase (AST), and alkaline phosphatase and gamma glutamyl transferase (γGT) are indicators of tissue integrity and not function compared to that of albumin where reduced albumin may reflect reduced liver function, increased bilirubin may reflect impaired bilirubin conjugation and or excretion, as well as impaired production of coagulation markers and detoxification and or elimination of toxic elements and metabolites (e.g., ammonia in urea synthesis) (see later). The functions and thus biochemical tests for their assessment depend on the presence of intact liver architecture.

Liver structure

The is liver located in the upper right quadrant of the abdomen. It weighs about 22 g/kg body weight. It thus varies with age being about 1.5 kg in a 70-year-old man.

The liver is made of two major lobes, a large right and a smaller left lobe (Fig. 1), and two further smaller lobes lying between the major right and left lobes, namely the quadrate and caudate lobes associated with venous drainage.

The functional unit of the liver, the acinus, is central to the role of the liver in homeostasis. The liver has a unique lobular structure where hepatocytes are arranged lining hepatic artery and portal vein and bile ducts. The structural integrity of the liver is important for both its important functions, ability to transport material from the blood into the bile, and to receive adequate blood supply.

The liver is unique among body organs in that it receives two blood supplies with over 200 L of blood daily passing through (30 mL/min/kg body weight representing about 100–130 mol/min/100 g liver). Hepatic artery (from heart—Aorta) is low in flow and high in oxygen content, portal vein (from the intestine) that is high in flow, low in oxygen, high in supply of nutrients, and in bacterial antigens. The portal blood delivers about 80% of the blood and 20% of the oxygen to the liver. The hepatic artery delivers the remaining 20% of blood volume and about 80% of the oxygen.

Blood flow is unidirectional from the portal vein to the hepatic artery. Hepatocytes spreading between portal and hepatic veins are divided into three zones based on their oxygen supply. Zone *one* is closest to the portal vein, and zone *three* is adjacent to the hepatic vein. Zone *two* is located in between. Overall although that anatomical boundaries between the three zones do not exist, differences in the composition of the blood which they receive dictate their function that level of oxygen and nutrients and metabolites as well as synthesized proteins develop them into diffuse but heterogeneous areas and thus a reflection of their ensued respective environment. For instance, zone one receives blood that is rich in oxygen thus exhibiting the highest the area performing the highest oxidative function that is those associated with respiratory chain, citric acid cycle and fatty acid oxidation, protein synthesis, gluconeogenesis, and formation of bile, whereas glycolysis, ammonia synthesis, and detoxification occurring predominantly in zone three. The bile duct drains bile from the liver to the intestine with storage in the gall bladder.

The liver structure/function relationship is three dimensional and is often difficult to visualized and is represented diagrammatically in Figs. 1 and 2. Parenchymal cells constitute the majority (80%) of the hepatocytes. Hepatocytes are arranged in single-cell sheets supported in place by collagenous material. Epithelial microvilli covering both sides of the sinusoid increase the surface area for exchange with blood enhancing both absorption and excretion. Kupffer cells are present in the sinusoidal space. Kupffer cells are phagocytic cells in sinusoids removing foreign antigens and antibody-antigen complexes. Understanding the functional microheterogeneity of hepatocytes dictated by the blood environment is important when assessing liver injury and dysfunction. Importantly, the liver has the ability to regenerate following injury, which is the rationale behind the long-term management of liver disease.

Hepatic function and assessment

As this chapter outlines, the liver is vital organ. It is central to essential homeostatic metabolism, and that liver failure is incompatible with life without a liver transplant.

Tutorials in Clinical Chemistry. https://doi.org/10.1016/B978-0-12-822949-1.00008-5

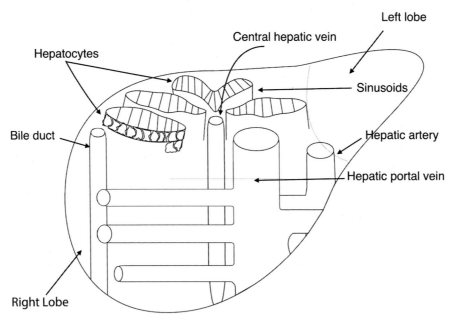

FIG. 1 Schematic diagram of the liver and associated vasculature and ducts. Liver is divided histologically into lobules. At the center of the lobule is the central vein. At the periphery of the lobule are portal triads. *(Modified from Abdel-Misih SR, Bloomston M. Liver anatomy. Surg Clin N Am. 2010;90(4):643–653. https://doi.org/10.1016/j.suc.2010.04.017. PMID: 20637938; PMCID: PMC4038911.)*

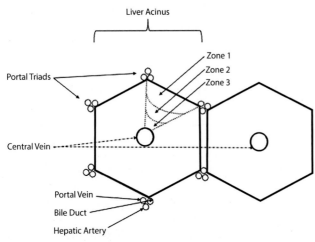

FIG. 2 Schematic illustration of the functional unit (acinus) showing vasculature (central vein and triad) and the zonal (1, 2, and 3) assignment of the acinus. *(Modified from Kietzmann T. Metabolic zonation of the liver: the oxygen gradient revisited. Redox Biol. 2017;11:622–630. https://doi. org/10.1016/j.redox.2017.01.012. Epub 2017 Jan 17. PMID: 28126520; PMCID: PMC5257182.)*

Synthetic function

The liver has large reserve capacity with functional deficiency apparent at a late stage in its dysfunction. Hepatocytes are the major functioning cells site of metabolism and synthetic function. In addition to its synthetic function of all proteins (except antibodies) including most clotting factors, glucose, lipids, and lipoproteins, it is the main site for detoxification of intermediary metabolites and toxins as in deamination conversion of ammonia (intermediary metabolite) to urea,

glucuronidation of toxins and their metabolites, synthesis of lipid soluble compounds for excretion into bile, and conversion into water soluble compounds for urinary excretion.

The liver has an endocrine role where it forms 25-OH vitamin D via hydroxylation of cholecalciferol from dietary and from in vivo synthetic sources, produces IGF-1 (insulin-like growth factor-1), and angiotensinogen. It is also responsible for the metabolism of hormones and those will be discussed separately.

Carbohydrates

The liver has a central role in the metabolism of carbohydrates maintaining the body's energy needs. Hepatocytes are the main metabolism site for glucose metabolism (carbohydrates metabolism discussed in detail in Chapter 6 on Diabetes). Maintenance of glucose and energy level is attained by hepatic glycolysis (breakdown of glucose to provide ATP), hepatic glycogenolysis (breakdown of glycogen to provide glucose for energy). In the presence of excess glucose, glucose is stored as glycogen (gluconeogenesis).

Maintaining adequate glucose levels requires both an acute immediate and a long-term regulation. Allosteric control by metabolic intermediates as well as posttranslational modifications provides the rapid acute control mechanism where gene expression of metabolizing enzymes facilitates the long-term control mechanism.

Glycolysis

Circulating glucose is taken up by glucose receptors (GLU) on sinusoidal membrane. Glucose is metabolized to pyruvate which in tissue rich in mitochondria is converted to acetyl-CoA by pyruvate dehydrogenase to provide energy in the form of ATP. In tissue lacking mitochondria or in ischemic environment, pyruvate is converted to lactate (Fig. 3).

The rate-limiting enzyme, glucokinase, converts glucose to glucose-6-phosphate. The enzyme acts as a glucose sensor and is activated in the presence of high glucose levels. Furthermore, it does not undergo allosteric inhibition by its product (glucose-6-phophate).

Gluconeogenesis

Glucose per se is obligatory for red blood cells and brain metabolism as energy source. At times of low availability of glucose, such as in between meals or during prolonged fasting, glucose is derived de novo from glycogen precursors. However, there is limited glycogen storage (about 75 g), and metabolism will then turn to inefficient gluconeogenesis from pyruvate and lactate. Pyruvate is converted to oxaloacetate by pyruvate carboxylase, and eventually converted to glucose (Fig. 3). Sources of pyruvate include amino acids or via lactate converted to pyruvate by lactate dehydrogenase.

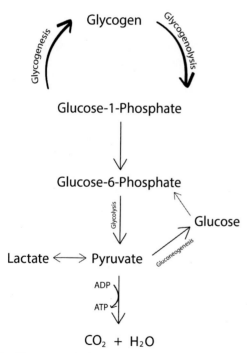

FIG. 3 Glucose metabolism showing glycolysis, gluconeogenesis, and glycogen metabolism. *(Modified from Rigoulet M, Bouchez CL, Paumard P, et al. Cell energy metabolism: an update. Biochim Biophys Acta Bioenerg. 2020;1861(11):148276. https://doi.org/10.1016/j.bbabio.2020.148276. Epub 2020 Jul 24. PMID: 32717222. Han HS, Kang G, Kim JS, Choi BH, Koo SH. Regulation of glucose metabolism from a liver-centric perspective. Exp Mol Med. 2016;48(3):e218. https://doi.org/10.1038/emm.2015.122. PMID: 26964834; PMCID: PMC4892876.)*

During prolonged periods of fasting or starvation, energy demand is met by ketones bodies.

Mitochondrial acetyl-CoA (derived from fatty acids oxidation) is a key allosteric activator of pyruvate carboxylase. It is also key substrate in the citric acid cycle combining with oxaloacetate to form citric acid (Fig. 4). The cycle produces three NADH, one $FADH_2$, one ATP, and one GTP (Table 1). NADH and $FADH_2$ are essential for the oxidative reduction reactions.

Impaired glucose synthesis and thus persistent hypoglycemia are encountered in acute hepatic failure (as in acetaminophen toxicity). Hyperglycemia is more common in patients with chronic liver disease secondary to the inability of the liver to store glycogen. Glucose metabolism is summarized in Fig. 3.

Proteins

The liver synthesis most blood proteins with the exception of immunoglobulins. Proteins synthesized by the liver include the predominantly circulating albumin, prealbumin, alpha-1-antitrypsin, alpha- and beta microglobulins, ceruloplasmin binding proteins, ferritin and haptoglobin, and IGF-1 and IGF binding proteins among many others.

Some of the proteins are termed acute phase proteins (Table 2) where levels either significantly increase as in alpha-1-antitrypsin, C-reactive protein termed positive acute phase proteins whereas others such as albumin, transferrin levels decline and are termed negative acute phase proteins.

In addition to protein synthesis, the liver is central to their degradation and metabolism in process of deamidation (see later under ammonia metabolism).

Albumin

Albumin is the major protein synthesized and secreted by the liver, accounting for about 50% of the total hepatic protein production and represent about 50%–60% of total serum proteins. Albumin has a biological half-life in plasma of about 21 days, and therefore, significant falls in albumin concentration in plasma are slow to occur in association with reduced synthesis. The finding of hypoalbuminemia is therefore a feature of advanced chronic liver disease, secondary to reduced liver mass and to inhibition of its synthesis by inflammatory cytokines (namely interleukim-6), albumin is thus a negative acute phase protein.

However, in chronic liver disease, reduced albumin concentration may also be associated with normal or occasionally above normal synthesis rates, and in these cases, other contributing important factors include abnormal distribution of the albumin pool and abnormal loss of albumin particularly into ascitic fluid. Low albumin levels may also be seen in patients presenting with severe and acute hepatic damage particularly when of several weeks duration.

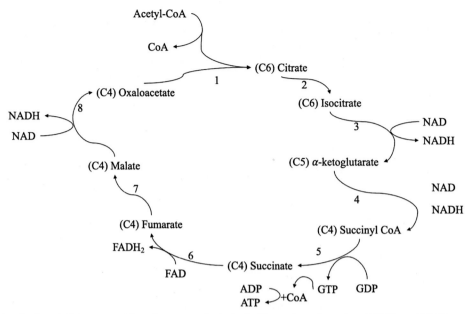

FIG. 4 Citric acid cycle. Acetyl-CoA an essential starting reactant in the cycle. The cycle produces three NADH, one $FADH_2$, one ATP, and one GTP. NADH and $FADH_2$ are essential for the oxidative reduction reactions. In the succinyl synthetase step, CoA is replaced by a phosphate group which is transferred to ADP to form ATP. 1: citrate synthase, 2: aconitase, 3: isocitrate dehydrogenase, 4: α-ketoglutarate dehydrogenase, 5: succinyl-Co-A synthetase, 6: succinate dehydrogenase, 7: fumarase, 8: malate dehydrogenase. *(Modified from Bender DA. Tricarboxylic acid cycle. In: Caballero B, ed. Encyclopedia of Food Sciences and Nutrition. 2nd ed. Academic Press; 2003:5851–5856. ISBN 9780122270550. https://doi.org/10.1016/B0-12-227055-X/01363-8. https://www.sciencedirect.com/science/article/pii/B012227055X013638. Rigoulet M, Bouchez CL, Paumard P, et al. Cell energy metabolism: an update. Biochim Biophys Acta Bioenerg. 2020;1861(11):148276. https://doi.org/10.1016/j.bbabio.2020.148276. Epub 2020 Jul 24. PMID: 32717222.)*

Additionally, circulating albumin level is reduced due to urinary loss in renal dysfunction (glomerular nephritis and nephrotic syndrome), and in protein losing enteropathies.

Normal circulating levels range from 3.5 to 4.0 g/dL. Albumin is measured either colorimetrically or nephelometrically and turbidimetrically. The colorimetric assays are used for serum albumin levels at the higher concentrations compared with that in urine and other body fluids (see Chapters 10 and 17) where nephelometric and turbidimetric methods provide the required sensitivity (the nephelometric/turbidimetric antibody-antigen reaction methods applicable for the 1000-fold difference—milligrams versus grams). As for the chemical method, the cationic albumin at acidic pH 4.1 binds to bromocresol green (BCG) anion and the albumin-BCG complex (blue green) is measured photometrically at 610 nm. The color intensity is directly proportional to the albumin concentration. There is no significant interference from either hemolysis, bilirubin, or lipidemia encountered in clinical practice; however, possible interference is reported in patients with macroglobulinemia.

In the nephelometric/immunoturbidimetric albumin methods, albumin assays employ antibodies directed against different epitopes on the albumin molecule. The generated albumin antibody complex causes turbidity in the reaction vessel, the level of which is directly proportional to the albumin concentration. The common analytical measurement range (AMR—see Chapter 17) for this type of assay is 0.03–0.4 g/L compared with the often AMR of 1–60 g/L in the colorimetric method.

Alpha-fetoprotein

Alpha-fetoprotein, a 70 kDa glycoprotein, is normally synthesized by liver during fetal life and is the predominantly circulating protein in fetal blood. The AFP gene is one of the four albumin gene family with the AFP gene expression regulated at the prescription level with upstream enhancers and silencer regions. The enhancers are blocked following fetal liver development and thus maintains albumin gene transcription. In hepatocellular carcinoma, there is overexpression of AFP, thought to be due to hypermethylation and to impaired silencing, in part.

In normal adults, AFP is present in plasma at low concentrations (<20 μg/L). Therefore, measurement of circulating AFP levels in adult in clinical practice is of great value in the diagnosis of hepatocellular carcinoma in which it is increased in 70%–90% of cases. Addition of AFP measurement to ultrasound significantly increases the sensitivity to 63% for early detection of hepatocellular carcinoma in patients with cirrhosis.

AFP may be transiently increased after acute liver injury with mildly elevated levels encountered in patients with cirrhosis. It is routinely measured using automated immunoassays analyzers. Markley elevated levels are encountered in patients with hepatocellular carcinoma, the levels of which

TABLE 1 Energy production by the different available pathways.

Pathway	Site	Energy input	FADH$_2$	NADH	Substrate level phosphorylation	ATP count
Glycolysis	Cytoplasm	2 ATP	None	2 NADH	4 ATP	2 ATP
Pyruvate to acetyl-CoA	Mitochondria	None	None	2 NADH	None	None
TCA	Mitochondria	None	2 FADH$_2$	6 NADH	2 ATP	2 ATP
ETC	Mitochondria		2 FADH$_2$			4 ATP
ETC	Mitochondria			10 NADH		28 ATP

ETC, electron transport chain; *TCA*, tricarboxylic acid cycle (citric acid cycle).
Modified from Dunn J, Grider MH. Physiology, adenosine triphosphate. [Updated 2022 Feb 17]. In: *StatPearls [Internet]*. Treasure Island, FL: StatPearls Publishing; 2022. Available from: https://www.ncbi.nlm.nih.gov/books/NBK553175/. Bonora M, Patergnani S, Rimessi A, et al. ATP synthesis and storage. *Purinergic Signal*. 2012;8(3):343–357. https://doi.org/10.1007/s11302-012-9305-8. Epub 2012 Apr 12. PMID: 22528680; PMCID: PMC3360099.

TABLE 2 Major proteins synthesized by the liver and changes in their circulating levels during the acute phase response.

Protein	Half-life	Function	Acute phase response
Albumin	21 days	Oncotic pressure, carrier protein	Negative
Alpha-1-antitrypsin	4–5 days	Exhibits antiprotease activity. High affinity for neutrophil elastase	Positive
Fibrinogen	3–5 days	Fibrin-based blood clot formation	Positive
Ceruloplasmin	4–5 days	Copper-carrying has ferroxidase activity (iron metabolism)	Positive
Haptoglobin	5 days (free form), few minutes (when bound to hemoglobin)	Binds free hemoglobin (during hemolysis)	Positive
Ferritin	12 h	Iron storage	Positive
Transferrin	8–10 days	Iron transporter in circulation	Negative
Prealbumin	2–3 days	Transport protein (thyroid hormones, retinol)	Negative
Thyroxine binding globulin (TBG)	5 days	T4 binding	Negative
C-reactive protein	19 h	Nonspecific acute phase protein. Binds Lys phosphatidylcholine expressed on dead/dying cells and on bacteria	Positive
Serum amyloid A	35 h	Nonspecific acute phase reactant. Binds to bacterial outer membrane protein—A.	Positive
Alpha-1-acid glycoprotein (orosomucoid)	2-3 days	Transporter protein (serotonin, histamine, platelet activating factor, melatonin).	Positive
IGF-1	10–15 min (free) 30–90 min (IGFBP)-bound	Growth-mediated GH action.	Negative

Modified from Gabay C, Kushner I. Acute-phase proteins and other systemic responses to inflammation. *N Engl J Med*. 1999;340(6):448–454. https://doi.org/10.1056/NEJM199902113400607. Erratum in: *N Engl J Med*. 1999;340(17):1376. PMID: 9971870.

may exceed the analytic measurement range of the assays and may also lead to antigen-excess effect resulting in falsely low AFP values. Serial dilutions of patient samples may be required to provide actual AFP value and to detect antigen-excess "hook effect" when using assays with limited analytical measurement range.

Total serum protein (the globulins pattern)

Albumin, discussed above, constitutes the major component of circulating proteins, the remainder are many proteins classified into defined electrophoretic mobility zones where the presence of a specific pattern (see later and Chapter 10) observed often indicates the presence of chronic liver disease. Chronic liver disease is characterized by a fall in serum albumin concentration and a rise in serum globulins which is related to the severity and duration of the disease.

The globulins are an extremely heterogeneous group of proteins several of which are synthesized in the liver (lipoproteins, haptoglobin, ceruloplasmin, iron-transport proteins, etc.).

When subjected to separation by protein electrophoresis, the presence of β-γ (beta-gamma) bridging (see Chapter 10) and an increased polyclonal gammopathy and hypoalbuminemia (leading to a globulin gap) is characteristic of cirrhosis and chronic liver disease. The β-γ (beta-gamma) bridging is thought to be due to elevated circulating

IgA levels. Although not used for diagnosis, the pattern may indicate additional testing if not expected due to the large hepatic reserve capacity.

Immunoglobulins

Although not synthesized by the liver, immunoglobulin levels are associated with certain hepatic disorders. They are increased in most patients with chronic liver disease. IgG increases in chronic active hepatitis, IgA increases in alcoholic cirrhosis, and IgM increases in primary biliary cirrhosis. However, these changes are of little diagnostic value.

Hormones

The liver is considered an endocrine organ that plays a role in hormone synthesis and metabolism and in the synthesis of binding proteins to which may hormones are predominantly bound.

The liver synthesizes 25-hydroxy vitamin D, insulin-like growth factor-I (IGF-1), angiotensinogen. The liver also synthesizes prealbumin, albumin, thyroid binding globulin (TBG, and sex hormone binding globulin (SHBG), and cortisol binding globulin (CBG)), which are predominant binding proteins for thyroid hormones, testosterone, estradiol sex hormones, and cortisol respectively.

The liver is the main site for the synthesis of hormones binding proteins. Steroid hormones include glucocorticoids, mineralocorticoids, and sex steroids which are lipophilic and are bound to proteins in circulation. The binding proteins are either specific to the hormones such as cortisol binding globulin ((CBG), sex hormones binding globulin (SHBG) and thyroxin binding globulin (TBG)) or afford nonspecific binding such as prealbumin and albumin.

The liver is the major site for the synthesis of the main storage form 25-hydroxy vitamin D (calcidiol) through the 25 hydroxylation of dietary and subcutaneously derived vitamin D. Hydroxylation is via hepatic multiple cytochrome P450 mixed-function oxidases located in the mitochondria, endoplasmic reticulum, and microsomes.

There is decreased vitamin D synthesis in chronic liver disease, cirrhosis, and cholestasis which are associated with osteomalacia, osteopenia, and osteoporosis. About 40% of chronic liver disease patients are at risk of developing osteoporotic fracture. The etiology is probably complex and in addition to low vitamin D levels include upregulation of inflammatory IL-6 which stimulates osteoclastic bone resorption.

In liver dysfunction such as in cirrhosis, there is estrogen-androgen imbalance with relatively higher estrogens compared to androgens, and the patients thus exhibit hypogonadism. In addition to variation in SHBG levels, high early in compensated liver cirrhosis to decreased levels in decompensated cirrhosis, there is increased peripheral conversion of androgens to estrogens in cirrhosis.

The liver deiodinase-1 converts T4 to the biologically active T3 at the tissue level. Changes in thyroid hormones levels in liver dysfunction are variable. However, alterations in liver disease are attributable to reduced synthesis of thyroid hormones binding proteins. Low TBG levels cause low total thyroxine (T4) and low total triiodothyronine (T3) levels. A pattern often seen in patients with nonthyroidal illness syndrome.

IGF-1 is a 70 amino acid polypeptide hormone. It is predominantly synthesized in the liver in response to pituitary growth hormone and thus considered an intermediary for the actions of growth hormone. In patients with liver cirrhosis, IGF-1 levels are low and is associated with diabetes due to hepatic, skeletal muscle, and adipose tissue insulin resistance. In addition to lipid abnormalities, the severity of liver steatosis correlates with a decrease in IGF-1 levels.

The liver is the main site for the synthesis of angiotensinogen. It is the substrate for renin which converts it to the active angiotensin-I. The atter is further acted upon by angiotensin converting enzyme in the lung to produce the potent vasoconstrictor angiotensin-II which stimulates aldosterone synthesis by the adrenal gland. The liver is able to produce near-normal angiotensinogen until the end stage of liver failure.

Several proteins predominantly produced by hepatocytes that regulate metabolic activities associated with insulin action, growth, and obesity have been identified. They are termed hepatokines and include fetuin-A (acts on skeletal muscle and adipose tissue decreasing insulin sensitivity), fibroblast growth factor-21 (acts on adipose tissue and brain to increase insulin sensitivity), activin E (acts on adipose tissue increases fatty acids oxidation), Tsukushi (acts on adipose tissue increasing thermogenesis), and glycoprotein nonmetastatic melanoma protein B (acting on adipose tissue increasing lipogenesis). Currently, none of the hepatokines has clinical diagnostic utility, but in research term support, the role of the liver has an important endocrine organ.

In summary, the liver plays several endocrine functions from direct role in the endocrine functions of the pituitary (IGF-1 synthesis), the thyroid (TBG synthesis and conversion of T4 to T3), adrenal (angiotensinogen, CBG), and the gonads (SHBG synthesis and sex hormones metabolism).

Coagulation factors

The liver is central to the synthesis and function of clotting factors and that patients with chronic liver disease are at increased risk of bleeding and coagulopathy. It is the site of synthesis of all clotting factors with the exception of von Willebrand factor.

Details are beyond the scope of this chapter, but decreased hepatic synthesis of clotting and inhibitory factors, accompanied with decreased clearance of activated factors, states of hyperfibrinolysis, and platelets dysfunction results in increased risk of morbidity and mortality.

Liver-associated coagulopathy leads to intravascular coagulation and fibrinolysis. Both bleeding and inappropriate clotting occur. Vitamin K, a fat-soluble vitamin, requires intact hepatobiliary system for its intestinal absorption. Thus, low levels are seen in cholestatic liver disease. It is a cofactor for many of the coagulation factors (factors I, II, V, VII, IX, X, XI, XIII and proteins C and S). It is required for γ-carboxylation of glutamic acid residues present in factors amino-terminal region. The increased fibrinolysis is thought to be due to reduced hepatic clearance of plasminogen activators (particularly tissue plasminogen activator). The impaired coagulation synthesis is reflected by prolonged PT and INR. However, activate partial thrombin time (aPTT) is not affected due to production of factor VII and von Willebrand factors by other body organs.

Since patients with cirrhosis are at risk of sepsis, this leads to hypocoagulation state and hyperfibrinolysis and thus to bleeding, particularly esophageal bleeding due to the ensued portal hypertension seen in patient with advanced liver disease. Consequently, the presence of both pro- and hypocoagulable states in patients with cirrhosis, PT, INR, and aPTT are not reliable markers of risk of bleeding in cirrhosis. Additionally, the ensued thrombocytopenia (due to sequestration in spleen), reduction of thrombopoietin level all collectively increase the risk of bleeding.

Bile formation and secretion

Bile is a complex mixture of cholesterol, cholesterol esters, bile salts (taurocholate and glycocholate), proteins, and bile pigments. Normal human bile contains about 25% of the monoglucuronide and almost 75% of the diglucuronide accompanied by traces of unconjugated bilirubin.

Bile is predominantly produced by hepatocytes and modified by cholangiocytes lining the bile ducts. It is actively secreted into bile ducts leaving the liver via hepatic bile duct and stored in that gallbladder.

Disturbance in the relative constituents of bile causes them to precipitate which leads to the formation of gallstones. Bile acids accumulate in cholestatic liver disease with elevated circulating levels. The clinical presentation of itching and biochemical markers suggestive of cholestatic liver disease requires additional investigation as bile acids salts are not routinely measured and thus require a high degree of clinical suspicion.

Upon entry of dietary fat and protein into the duodenum, cholecystokinin is released from the duodenal mucosa and at the gallbladder causes contraction of the gallbladder, in the fed state the gallbladder constricts to a variable degree (50%–90%) and the concentrated bile enters the duodenum. In the intestine, the bile acids enable the transport of fatty acids to the sites of absorption. They are reabsorbed at the terminal ileum and transported via the portal vein and extracted by the liver. Bile acids not extracted by the liver are shunted into the peripheral circulation and re-taken up by the liver with small fraction excreted into the urine.

Enterohepatic circulation

Bile acids synthesized in the liver (about 800–1000 mL per day) and excreted into the bile duct, enter the intestine they are absorbed and via the portal blood and to the liver for resecretion into the bile, a cycle constituting the enterohepatic circulation (Fig. 5). The majority of those in circulation are cholic acid, chenodeoxycholic acid, deoxycholic acid, and ursodeoxycholic acid often fractionated using liquid chromatography-mass spectrometry or measured as total bile acids and bile salts.

Metabolism and detoxification

The liver is central to the metabolism of many biomolecules and drugs. It is responsible for the conjugation of bilirubin, detoxification thru glucuronidation, conjugation, of drugs. This converts many of the otherwise fat-soluble material to that is water soluble to facilitate removal by the kidney. It contributes to digestion by producing bile and aids in hydrogen ion homeostasis. The liver reserves large capacity, and therefore, dysfunction is often realized at an advanced stage.

Additionally, 10–20 g of daily nitrogenous was in the form of ammonia from deamidation of surplus amino acids from protein degradation. Ammonia is neurotoxic and must be detoxified and excreted. Ammonia is converted to urea in the urea cycle and excreted into the urine (see later).

Bilirubin metabolism

Bilirubin is a yellow tetrapyrrole biomolecule derived from the metabolism of iron-containing protoporphyrin heme, mainly found in hemoglobin. Hemoglobin is metabolized to heme and globin within the mononuclear phagocytic system. Bilirubin reaches the liver bound to albumin where it is released, conjugated, and excreted into the bile (see later).

An adult normally produces about 450 μmol of bilirubin daily (about 250–350 mg), 80% of which arises from breakdown of red blood cells (RBCs) and thus hemoglobin. Bilirubin is insoluble in water and is transported in plasma almost totally bound to albumin. It is taken up by liver cells where it is conjugated with glucuronic acid by UDP-glucuronyl transferase enzyme (hepatic 1A1 isoform of uridine diphosphoglucose glucuronyl transferase) to mono- and di-glucosiduronates (glucuronides) water-soluble conjugates.

Normal circulating serum bilirubin level is <17 μmol/L (<1 mg/dL) with about 75% being unconjugated and thus albumin bound. Men tend to have higher bilirubin concentrations than women and in the population as a whole, the distribution is skewed to the right. Minor increases in bilirubin concentrations therefore need to be interpreted with caution.

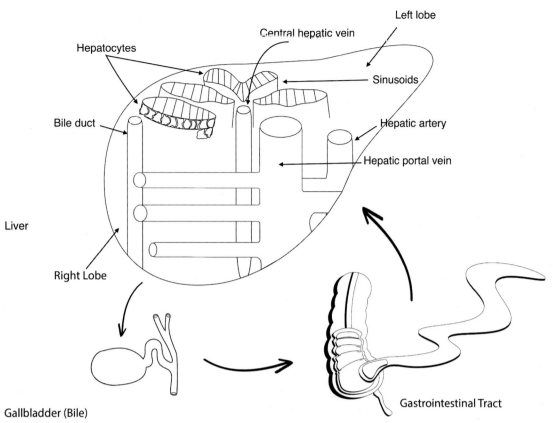

FIG. 5 Enterohepatic circulation: Circulation of bile acids (salt), bilirubin, and other metabolites from the liver to the bile, small intestine, absorbed by enterocytes, and retuned back to the liver. *(Modified from Di Ciaula A, Garruti G, Lunardi Baccetto R, et al. Bile acid physiology. Ann Hepatol. 2017;16(suppl 1: s3–105):s4–s14. https://doi.org/10.5604/01.3001.0010.5493. PMID: 29080336).*

Jaundice is a clinical sign and is not observed until the bilirubin concentration in plasma exceeds about 40 μmol/L (2.3 mg/dL). Literally, the patient appears yellow (obvious in the sclera, skin, and mucous membranes). The most common molecular cause of jaundice is a raised bilirubin concentration in tissues as well as in plasma.

Conjugated bilirubin is released into the bile canaliculi and gallbladder into the intestine. Conjugated bilirubin is not absorbed from the jejunum or upper ileum; however, in the terminal ileum and colon, the conjugates are attacked by bacteria to form a group of colorless tetrapyrroles known collectively as stercobilinogen, most of which are excreted in feces. Some of the stercobilin is absorbed into the circulation (portal vein), and most is excreted from the body by way of bile. Small amounts of these stercobilin tetrapyrroles are found in urine in which they are known collectively as urobilinogen.

Unconjugated hyperbilirubinemia may be due to excessive hemoglobin breakdown exceeding normal conjugation capacity of the liver such as in hemolysis, or to decreased or deficient UDP enzyme activity seen in patient with Gilbert's syndrome (see later).

Conjugated hyperbilirubinemia is often due to impaired excretion and thus suggests biliary obstruction, hepatitis (infective or toxic and ischemia), autoimmune cholestatic liver diseases, as well as secondary to drugs and total paracentral nutrition intake and in neonates receiving breast feeding.

Analysis of bilirubin fractions identifies the cause and possible etiology. Rarely, the increased bilirubin is purely unconjugated or conjugated, both reactions are often present, however, to variable degree.

Hyperbilirubinemia may be classified as predominantly unconjugated or predominantly conjugated. In predominantly unconjugated bilirubinemia, the causes include increased bilirubin production (e.g., hemolysis) exceeding hepatic conjugation capacity, primary failure of bilirubin uptake or conjugation, and mixed pathogenesis. Predominantly conjugated hyperbilirubinemia is encountered in biliary obstruction (intrahepatic or extrahepatic), primary failure of bilirubin transport, and in hepatocellular damage.

Unconjugated bilirubin, which is water insoluble and predominantly bound to albumin in the plasma, does not appear in urine even in the case of unconjugated hyperbilirubinemia. Unconjugated bilirubin increases by up to twofold with prolonged fasting and by up to 30% with strenuous exercise in men. It is 15%–30% lower in African Americans and by up to 50% with pregnancy, 15% with oral contraceptives, and artifactually decreased by up to 50% by light exposure.

The diazo method is commonly used for the measurement of bilirubin whereas conjugated bilirubin reacts directly and rapidly (hence the term direct bilirubin), and unconjugated bilirubin reacts relatively slowly and requires the addition of an accelerator such as caffeine, sodium benzoate, or methanol (hence termed indirect bilirubin).

The endpoint following addition of the reaction accelerator is total bilirubin; thus bilirubin measured early in the reaction is conjugated bilirubin, and the difference following addition of the accelerator is calculated as unconjugated bilirubin.

The diazo method is subject to interference by low levels of hemolysis as well as lipemia and in the presence of paraproteins (particularly IgM). However, paraprotein interference is variable being either positive or negative. Interference by hemolysis is particularly evident in samples from newborns and infants where obtaining a high-quality sample is challenging. Capillary samples for instance most likely represent interstitial fluid as well as capillary blood content and collection practices of repeated squeeze and warming contributes to the observed high hemolysis and thus sample rejection rates.

In the diazo method (based on the Jendrassik-Grof diazo method), acidified sodium nitrite produces nitrous acid that reacts with sulfanilic acid to form a diazonium salt. The latter reacts with bilirubin to form isomers of azobilirubins (red color recorded at 570 nm and at 660 nm secondary wavelength). Hemolysis greater than 20 mg/dL interferes with the direct bilirubin measurement leading to false negative results. The mechanism of hemolysis interference with direct bilirubin is not completely understood, and the measurement wavelength, albumin, reagents, all playing a role, falsely low bilirubin levels are observed.

Measuring direct bilirubin enzymatically utilizing vanadate and bilirubin oxidase is not influenced by the above interference. Bilirubin oxidase in the presence of vanadate (VO^{3-}) in acid medium (pH 3.0) catalyzes the conversion of bilirubin to biliverdin which is measured spectrophotometrically at 450 nm and 546 nm. Hemolysis up to 1000 mg/dL does not affect the direct bilirubin assay.

Some methods, that apply filters, allow the measurement of albumin bound conjugated bilirubin fraction termed (δ (delta)-bilirubin) as in the dry chemistry system Vitros (Ortho Clinical Diagnostics).

Direct bilirubin is more susceptible to interference by hemolysis than total bilirubin and that falsely low bilirubin results are observed. This is particularly relevant when collecting capillary samples from neonates with high degree of hemolysis. Inability to record direct and or total bilirubin impairs the ability to identify biliary atresia in neonates

with neonatal hyperbilirubinemia. The use of enzymatic Vanadate method overcomes this limitation.

Disorders of bilirubin metabolism

Disorders of bilirubin metabolism include those (a) affecting the conjugation process where unconjugated bilirubin exceeds the conjugation capacity of the liver (e.g., hemolysis) and (b) disorders affecting excretion of conjugated bilirubin (e.g., cholestasis and obstruction).

Bilirubin levels >40 μmol/L (2.3 mg/dL) are considered abnormal and present as jaundice. It may not be obvious in patients with darker skin; however, the sclera yellow discoloration is easy to notice.

Total bilirubin as well as conjugated and unconjugated fractions are often measured in clinical practice. Although there is rarely totally unconjugated bilirubin and totally conjugated bilirubin, there is often a relative distribution of both that are characteristic of the ensued hepatic disorder (see later).

Predominantly unconjugated bilirubin

Isolated increase in unconjugated bilirubin is secondary to excessive bilirubin production exceeding the liver conjugation ability as with hemolysis. It is also secondary to impaired bilirubin uptake and or conjugation. The most common cause of unconjugated hyperbilirubinemia is neonatal jaundice and inherited Gilbert syndrome (see later).

Predominantly conjugated bilirubin

Conjugated hyperbilirubinemia is a characteristic of cholestatic biliary disease where conjugated bilirubin accumulates due to biliary obstruction or to impaired excretion (Dubin-Johnson syndrome see later).

Neonatal jaundice

During fetal life, the infant accumulates higher levels of hemoglobin compared to maternal circulation to aid extract required oxygen from maternal blood, at birth the newborn does not require that additional hemoglobin and the developing liver has an excess load (given that neonatal red blood cells have a reduced lifespan) to convert to bilirubin.

Up to 50% of neonates will develop physiological jaundice by 48 h of life. Bilirubin level rarely exceeds 200 μmol/L (11.7 mg/dL) with mostly being unconjugated (indirect bilirubin) with direct conjugated fraction not exceeding 20%, and all return to normal levels within the 7–10 days of life.

A direct (conjugated bilirubin) that represents >15% of total bilirubin in patients with prolonged jaundice is considered abnormal.

In physiological jaundice, direct (conjugated) bilirubin constitutes less than 10 μmol/L (<0.6 mg/dL). Physiological jaundice is usually harmless and is often associated with breast feeding.

Neonates with trauma may have sustained hyperbilirubinemia, secondary to any associated bleeding, where each gram of hemoglobin yields 600 μmol (35 mg) of bilirubin.

Causes of neonatal hyperbilirubinemia therefore include hypovolemia, hemolysis, polycythemia, rhesus incompatibility, infection, breastfeeding, hypoglycemia, hypothyroidism, and hepatic prematurity, biliary atresia, inborn error of metabolism (glyucose-6-phphatse dehydrogenase deficiency, where 20%–30% of patients develop hemolysis).

Critical to determination of bilirubin levels is avoidance of risk of kernicterus due to severe unconjugated hyperbilirubinemia of >500 μmol/L (>30 mg/dL) in the presence of physiological hypoalbuminemia. Phototherapy and or exchange transfusion if often instituted.

A laboratory limitation is interference of sample hemolysis (common among neonatal samples), use of chemical assays with high degree of tolerance to hemolysis (e.g., Vanadate method) is thus recommended.

Prolonged jaundice, exceeding 10 days of birth requires detailed investigation to include bilirubin fractions. Bilirubin fractions are unconjugated bilirubin (also known as alpha (α) bilirubin), mono-conjugated (monoglucuronide (termed beta (β) fraction)), di-conjugated (diglucuronide (termed gamma (γ) fraction)), and an albumin bound conjugated fraction (termed delta (δ) fraction).

Delta (δ) bilirubin is different from unconjugated α-bilirubin. The latter although insoluble and is present bound to albumin and to plasma proteins, delta bilirubin is conjugated and esterified bilirubin that is covalently bound to albumin and to other serum proteins. Determined as total bilirubin minus the sum of direct and indirect bilirubin. Formed by spontaneous transesterification of bilirubin glucuronide esters to exposed carboxyl groups on serum proteins, predominantly albumin. Delta bilirubin coccus when conjugated bilirubin is in excess thus it is only observed in patients with cholestasis.

Transcutaneous measurement of bilirubin is increasingly being used in neonatal settings. In healthy infants before discharge and they are used to assess the need for laboratory-based bilirubin measurement.

Biliary atresia

Biliary atresia is a serious condition in neonatal period due to bile duct obstruction with about 1:12–18,000 worldwide newborn has biliary atresia.

The patient has favorable outcomes if the disorder is detected and treated within the first 30–45 days of life and early identification is important as it defines surgical intervention versus medical management. The prolonged jaundice is predominantly conjugated direct bilirubin, elevated bile acids, and presence of pale stool.

Measurement of different bilirubin forms (direct, indirect) helps in early identification of the disorder. The limitation being lack of laboratory derived age-specific reference interval for the various fractionated bilirubin fragments and interference by hemolysis (discussed earlier).

Delta bilirubin (delta bilirubin = total bilirubin − direct bilirubin − indirect bilirubin) a covalently albumin bound bilirubin increase in proportion to that of the conjugated direct bilirubin in patients with biliary atresia and a strong indicator of cholestasis similar to that of direct conjugated bilirubin, however, its measurement is widely available.

Inherited disorders of bilirubin metabolism

Inherited disorders of bilirubin metabolism include those (a) affecting the conjugation process (Crigler-Najjar and Gilbert syndromes) and (b) those affecting excretion of conjugated bilirubin (Dubin-Johnson and Rotor syndromes).

Crigler-Najjar syndrome

Crigler-Najjar syndrome is a rare autosomal recessive genetic disorder characterized by inability to conjugate bilirubin. It affects 0.6–1 million newborns worldwide. Presenting as congenital nonhemolytic jaundice. It is due to the absence in Crigler-Najjar type I or significantly decreased activity in Crigler-Najjar type II of the conjugating enzyme UDP-glucuronosyl transferase.

In Crigler-Najjar type I, the patient exhibit severe unconjugated hyperbilirubinemia with values often >340 μmol/L (>19.8 mg/dL) in the first few days of life.

In Crigler-Najjar type II, a milder form with serum bilirubin often below 340 μmol/L (<19.8 mg/dL), the enzyme activity is reduced and not completely deficient compared to type I.

Gilbert syndrome

Gilbert syndrome is a milder heterozygous form of Crigler-Najjar syndrome without manifestation of liver dysfunction. The disorder is present in about 2%–7% of the population. It is common among 5% of males and rare in females. The disorder is characterized by an intermittent unconjugated hyperbilirubinemia in the absence of hemolysis. Total serum bilirubin is usually about 20–50 μmol/L (1.2–2.9 mg/dL) and rarely exceeding 85 μmol/L (4.9 mg/dL). The conjugating enzymes are reduced at about 30% activity.

Hyperbilirubinemia is exaggerated by fasting, surgery, infection, physical exertion, and alcohol ingestion. Bilirubin is 3–4 times upper limit of normal bilirubin levels and liver enzymes remain within the normal range. Urine bilirubin and urobilinogen are negative or not detected.

Diagnosis is established by finding intermittent unconjugated hyperbilirubinemia in the absence of hemolysis and normal complete blood count, Coombs test, haptoglobin, and lactate dehydrogenase levels.

Dubin-Johnson and Rotor syndromes

Dubin-Johnson is a rare disorder characterized by conjugated hyperbilirubinemia. Bilirubin is typically in the 2–5 mg/dL (34–85 μmol/L) rarely rising to 20–25 mg/dL (340–428 μmol/L). The extent of jaundice is enhanced by fasting and stress.

It is a benign disorder with normal life expectancy, and patients do not to cirrhosis or fibrosis. The diagnosis is required so to as rule out other hepatobiliary disorders that require management. Livre enzymes are often within normal limits.

In the Dubin-Johnson syndrome, there is adequate conjugation activity, but the liver is unable to excrete conjugated bilirubin, there is liver lipofuscin pigmentation in contrast to Rotor syndrome that does not have pigmentation. The finding of elevated conjugated bilirubin is indicative of cholestasis. A protein bound form (delta (δ) bilirubin) accumulates with obstruction and falls slowly during recovery with half-life of 20 days.

Other inborn errors of metabolism affecting the liver

Hepatic heme-related disorders include porphyria (see Chapter 12 on metabolic disorders).

Deamination of ammonia

Ammonia is the intermediary metabolite following breakdown and metabolism of proteins. It is produced in the small and large intestine from bacterial proteases, ureases, amino oxidases with the main contributor being the hydrolysis of glutamine. It is absorbed and the portal hepatic vein contains ammonia levels 5–10 times those found in venous blood. Other sources of glutamine are direct synthesis by muscles, lymphocytes, and the kidney.

Ammonia reaching the liver is converted to urea in the in the urea cycle (Krebs-Henseleit) (Fig. 6) in the periportal hepatocytes as it transverse the hepatocytes to the central hepatic vein. It is also cleared by the kidney where it plays a buffering role (in the excretion of H ions and thus maintenance of the acid base homeostasis).

Elevated ammonia levels are observed when there is imbalance between increased production and decreased clearance. Increased production is that due to increased gastrointestinal protein load such as high protein diet or in gastrointestinal bleed. Decreased clearance is seen in advanced liver disease with decreased liver mass as in cirrhosis, acute and chronic liver failure, and portal systemic shunting of blood. Inborn errors of metabolism (urea cycle defect) lead to markedly elevated ammonia levels (often exceeding 1000 μmol/L). Inborn errors of dibasic amino acids (lysine, ornithine) and errors in the metabolism of organic acids (propionic, methylmalonic and isovaleric acids) (see "Inborn errors of metabolism" section in Chapter 12).

Artifactual hyperammonemia is seen in delayed blood cell separation, environment contamination (processing and handling in urine analysis area, use of ammonia containing bench and equipment cleaning reagents). Historically, smoking by both patient and phlebotomy staff thought to cause artifactual environmental contamination.

In the kidney's tubular cells, glutamine is metabolized to glutamate and alpha-ketoglutarate with production of ammonia. Ammonia diffuses into the tubular lumen where it combines with H ions facilitates excretion of H (Fig. 7). Therefore, ammonia accumulates in patients with renal failure.

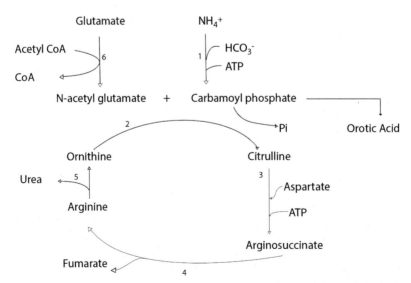

FIG. 6 Urea cycle (deamidation of ammonia). Enzymatic steps (1–6) that have been identified as possible deficiencies in the metabolism of ammonia and synthesis of urea. 1: carbamoyl phosphate synthetase, 2: ornithine carbamoyl transferase, 3: argininosuccinate synthetase, 4: arginosuccinate lyase, 5: arginase, 6: *N*-acetylglutamate synthetase. *(Modified from Summar ML, Mew NA. Inborn errors of metabolism with hyperammonemia: urea cycle defects and related disorders. Pediatr Clin N Am. 2018;65(2):231–246. https://doi.org/10.1016/j.pcl.2017.11.004. Epub 2018 Feb 2. PMID: 29502911.)*

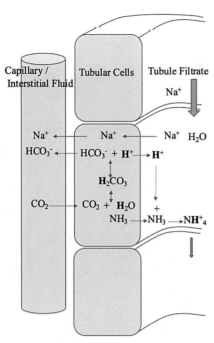

FIG. 7 Renal excretion of ammonia. *(Modified from Wagner CA, Imenez Silva PH, Bourgeois S. Molecular pathophysiology of acid-base disorders. Semin Nephrol. 2019;39(4):340–352. https://doi.org/10.1016/j.sem-nephrol.2019.04.004. PMID: 31300090.)*

Ammonia is toxic, it enters the central nervous system (CNS) by passive diffusing down a concentration gradient, and the rate of entry depends on plasma concentration and on pH ($NH_4^+ + H_2O$) at very low pH, and the predominant species ($NH_3 + H_3O^+$) when pH is moderately low/high.

Mitochondrial metabolism of ammonia produces reactive oxygen substances leading to oxidative stress, impaired mitochondrial permeability, and impaired ATP synthesis.

Therefore, the biochemical investigations of hyperammonemia will often require all or some of the following assessments: sample integrity, liver tests (bilirubin, AST, ALT), renal function tests, toxicology (Acetaminophen), serum and urine amino acids and or organic acids.

Measurement of ammonia

Measurement of ammonia is essential in the investigation of hepatic dysfunction. Since the liver has high reserve capacity, hyperammonemia is encountered in advanced liver disease.

The measurement of ammonia utilized the reaction below,

$$NH_4^+ + 2\text{-Oxoglutarate} + NADPH \xrightarrow[340\,nm]{GLDH}$$

$$L\text{-Glutamate} + NADP^+ + H_2O$$

Plasma with EDTA as the preservative is preferred. Heparin preservative is not recommended as it interferes in some of the assays producing significantly low ammonia results. The mechanism of interference is not clear and appears to be method dependent, possibly by interfering with assay reagent buffer system and reagent salt content.

Hemolyzed samples are not suitable and samples preferably kept on ice during transportation and plasma immediately separated by centrifugation. The sample is analyzed immediately and within 30 min (<2 h on ice). The assay has a linearity limit of linearity up to 600 μmol/L thus dilution is required for those with inborn errors of metabolism where ammonia is often above 600 μmol/L. There are significant interferences as mentioned previously with environmental contamination by ammonia, high protein diet, drugs (e.g., anticonvulsants). Prolonged venostasis during phlebotomy should be avoided.

Lymphocytes have high glutaminase activity that increases following stimulation in immunological challenge. The reaction products being glutamate, aspartate, and ammonia (30%).

The graph (Fig. 8) shows the rate of in vitro ammonia production when whole blood samples are left unseparated at room temperature.

Drugs detoxification

The liver is central to detoxification and metabolism of many drugs (e.g., acetaminophen). Detoxification takes place at hepatocytes surrounding hepatic vein. It involves oxidation, reduction, hydrolysis, followed by conjugation with glucuronic acid, sulfate, or glutathione.

The perivenular cells have higher cytochrome P450 activity and high glucuronic acid, whereas sulfate conjugation by sulfotransferase occurs predominantly in the periportal hepatocytes.

Superoxide dismutase, catalase, and glutathione peroxidase are present in high concentration in in the periportal hepatocytes. Perivenular hepatocytes have relatively lower concentration of these protective enzymes which may explain in part their susceptibility to oxidative damage.

Many drugs cause mild elevation in aminotransferase (with ALT being more predominant compared to AST). This may indicate mild hepatic inflammation and injury. Some dugs induce a cholestatic enzymes pattern they include antibiotics (Augmentin), macrolides, ceftriaxone, anticonvulsants, herbal supplements, statins, and antituberculosis medication.

Acetaminophen toxicity

The clinical laboratory often receives request for acetaminophen measurement in patients with suspected acetaminophen overdose or those with unexplained elevated liver enzymes.

Moderate-to-severe elevations in aminotransferases are encountered in acetaminophen hepatotoxicity. Daily doses <4000 mg/dL are thought to be safe; however, the patient tolerance and response is variable; furthermore, 6% of prescriptions may be >4000 mg/day.

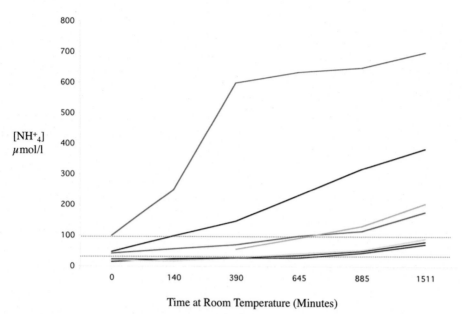

FIG. 8 Ammonia levels in whole blood samples (from 5 different normal volunteers). Ammonia levels increased over time in all samples; however, the rates were different between the different samples. *(Data from the author's laboratory.)*

The rise in aminotransferases is usually 2–3 days post the initial overdose, and thus, normal levels on presentation do not rule out toxicity. Cholestatic enzymes alkaline phosphatase and γGT and bilirubin and PT/INR all become elevated later eventually.

Acetaminophen is metabolized to *N*-acetyl-beta-benzoquinone imine (NAPQI) which leads to toxicity and cell death if not conjugated with glutathione to the nontoxic mercapturic acid. When the amount of NAPQI exceeds available glutathione, it accumulates. The use of *N*-acetyl cysteine stimulates glutathione production in capacity for conjugation with NAPQI and thus reduces hepatotoxicity. However, this has to be administered at appropriate time (Fig. 9), when liver enzymes become elevated signaling hepatocytes necrosis, it is often too late.

Biomarkers of liver injury and dysfunction

A group of biochemical tests in the assessment of liver injury and function is usually performed in the form of a profile. The mostly widely used combination includes total bilirubin concentration as a measure of hepatic conjugation and transport function and of the severity of jaundice, aminotransferase activity as a measure of the integrity of liver cells, alkaline phosphatase and gamma glutamyl transferase activities as an index of cholestasis, albumin levels and prothrombin time (as a measure of vitamin-K dependent synthesis of coagulation factors) as a measure of synthetic capacity, total globulin as a marker of chronic liver disease and a measure of severity, bile acids as more sensitive indices of hepatic transportation than bilirubin, alpha-fetoprotein in suspected hepatoma, alpha-1-antitrypsin in

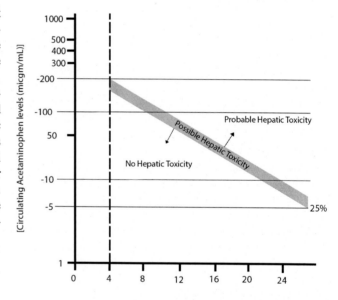

Hours after acetaminophen ingestion

FIG. 9 Rumack-Matthew nomogram guiding therapeutic intervention in patients with acetaminophen overdose. Plasma acetaminophen levels following ingestion and relationship with risk for acute liver damage with 25% of patients in the possible risk for hepatic toxicity. *(Figure modified from Rumack BH, Peterson RC, Koch GG, Amara IA. Acetaminophen overdose. 662 cases with evaluation of oral acetylcysteine treatment. Arch Intern Med. 1981;141(3 Spec No):380–385. https://doi.org/10.1001/archinte.141.3.380. PMID: 7469629.)*

acute liver disease and in emphysema, and ceruloplasmin in suspected live injury due to Wilson's disease.

Although measuring circulating albumin levels is considered a test of liver function where decreased synthesis in end-stage liver disease becomes obvious at advanced stag due to the albumin half-life of 21 days. Furthermore, prothrombin time is increased as a consequence of decrease in synthesis of coagulation factors (vitamin K dependent) liver synthesizes clotting factors I, II, V, VII, and X (coagulation factors half-life is about 24 h).

Albumin levels and coagulation factors are influenced by nonhepatic factors which require consideration. Circulating albumin levels are decreased due to loss into the urine in patient with glomerular proteinuria and nephrotic syndrome as well as in protein losing enteropathies and in malnutrition. Vitamin K deficiency causes prolonged prothrombin time. However, the two biomarkers are helpful in assessing liver reserve synthetic function.

Obstructive jaundice decreases the absorption of vitamin K, and thus increased prothrombin time. Lack of correction following parenteral administration of vitamin K suggests decreased hepatic cellular synthetic mass.

Although liver biopsy is the gold standard in the investigations of liver disease, its routine use is not practical and carries risks to the patient, which leads to complications (infection, injury, and mortality). Biochemical assessment of liver disorders is best described in terms of those helping in assessing (a) hepatocellular dysfunction and (b) in cholestasis.

The liver has large reserve capacity with synthetic capacity depending on liver mass which means that function tests are often within normal limits, and only become apparent at advanced disease status. Similarly, drainage depends on intactness of biliary ducts and lack of obstruction.

The etiology of the dysfunction is variable. It could be viral infection, autoimmune, metabolic, drug-induced, and other miscellaneous causes such as vascular occlusion, portal vein thrombosis, and polycystic liver disease among other miscellaneous causes.

Enzymes

Due to the complexity and wide extent of liver function, a single test does not represent the whole function and a profile is preferred when accessing liver disorders. Liver biochemical profile is often constructed and utilized on automated biochemical testing analyzers. Furthermore, the finding of abnormal results is not uncommon in patients not suspected of hepatic disease.

Increase in enzymes levels indicates either hepatocellular or cholestatic dysfunction. Classifying liver enzymes as part of "liver function rests" (LFTs) is a misnomer as they reflect cellular damage or cholestasis and not functions those of synthetic and excretory roles.

Several enzymes including aminotransferases (ALT and AST), lactate dehydrogenase (LDH), gamma glutamyl transferase (γGT), alkaline phosphatase (Alk Phos), and 5′nuceotidase (5′NT) are present at high concentrations inside hepatocytes and at sinusoidal membranes and that

detection of markedly elevated circulating levels are indicative of hepatic tissue leakage (injury).

The pathophysiology and the extent of enzymes elevation as well as their relative proportion are diagnostic and indicative of the pathology. Furthermore, the degree of enzyme elevation can be defined as either mild (<5× upper limit of normal (ULN), moderate 5–10×ULN), to severe >10 ULN.

In liver disease, transaminases (AST/ALT) are released into the circulation. The increased transaminases activity is sensitive but not specific index of liver damage, hepatitis (of any cause), toxic injury (including drug overdose), acute liver damage due to shock, severe hypoxia secondary acute circulatory and cardiac failure.

The extent of the enzymes' elevation although not accurate assessment of damage; however, they aid in the initial investigation. Furthermore, the relative ratios of the respective enzymes' levels are helpful. For instance, markedly elevated ALT is indicative of predominant hepatocellular pattern, a ratio of >2 but less than 5 is suggestive of a mixed hepatocellular and cholestatic involvement, whereas a ratio of <2 of the respective enzymes is indicative of primarily cholestatic disorder.

To correct for age, gender, and methods difference, enzyme ratios are best calculated as for example [(ALT/upper limit of normal ALT)/(Alkaline Phosphatase/upper limit of alkaline phosphatase)].

The small circulating amounts of normally intracellular enzymes (AST, ALT, LDH, alkaline phosphatase, γGT) present in plasma as a result of normal cell turnover. Increased amounts are a reflection of pathological damage to cells, increase in cell turnover, enzyme induction, obstruction to flow of exocrine secretion, and to decreased clearance from plasma. Therefore, their elevations are diagnostic rather than the cause of the disease. Additionally, several drugs, such as anticonvulsants, induce microsomal enzymes γGT and alkaline phosphatase elevation.

The lack of specificity of the enzymes to a particular tissue or cell type is overcome by combined analysis in a profile of two or more enzymes, or isoenzyme analysis, inclusion of metabolites in the profile. Additional contributors to specificity are the course and pattern of changes with time.

Alkaline phosphatase and γGT are markedly elevated in alcoholic hepatitis where AST and ALT are not as high as seen in viral hepatitis.

The ratio of AST to ALT of >2 is seen in alcoholic liver disease (more of the AST than ALT), whereas the ratio is much lower (<1) in viral hepatitis (more of the ALT than the AST) (see later).

Hepatocyte enzymes (transaminases (AST and ALT))

Aspartate transaminase (AST) is present in all cell types with both cytosolic (20%) and mitochondrial (80%) forms, and there are no organ-specific isoenzymes. The mitochondrial form is released except in cases of ethanol related severe cellular damage. With the mitochondrial form having half-life of several days (about 87 h) compared with 16–18 h for the cytoplasmic AST. The activity of AST is relatively predominant in zone 3 within the acinus (Fig. 2).

It is important to realize that declining aminotransferases in patients with acute liver failure likely indicate severe loss of liver tissue mass rather than an improving and resolving liver damage. At this stage, synthetic function tests of bilirubin and PT/INR provide better monitoring tests.

In patients with toxic or ischemic liver injury, there is markedly elevated transaminases often as high as >75 ULN with AST being predominant (being present in the mitochondrial-rich acinar zone 3). Lactate dehydrogenase (LDH) is severely elevated >10 ULN, which is in contrast to that seen in viral hepatitis. Therefore, the AST:LDH ratio of <1.5 helps differentiate ischemic from viral hepatitis. Alkaline phosphatase levels are often within the normal limits. There is mild elevation in bilirubin but often <3 mg/dL (51 μmol/L) and mild elevation of PT/INR values.

The activities of the two aminotransferases, AST and ALT, have become widely used in clinical practice. The relative activities of these enzymes in plasma and in various tissues are shown in Table 3.

AST is present in appreciable amount in red blood cells, and thus, hemolysis causes falsely high AST results.

Alanine aminotransferase (ALT) is found predominantly in hepatocytes (about 10 folds those in skeletal and cardiac muscle), therefore is of higher liver specificity compared to AST and elevated levels likely to represent hepatic involvement; it is however also present to a lesser degree in skeletal muscles, renal and cardiac tissue (Table 3). The half-life of ALT is 47 h compared with 17 h for total AST. Thus, in contrast to AST, significantly increased ALT levels indicate possible liver involvement. The enzyme is normally present

at about 30 IU/L in males and about 20 IU/L in females. The lower female range may be reflection of liver mass (or muscle mass).

ALT catalyzes the reaction between alanine and 2-oxoglutataret to form pyruvate and L-glutamine. The reaction is monitored by reducing pyruvate to L-lactate. NADH is used as H⁺ donner and reaction catalyzed by lactate dehydrogenase. The rate of NADH oxidation to NAD is monitored at 340 nm, and the decrease in absorbance is proportional to the ALT enzymatic activity. Pyridoxal phosphate is a cofactor for ALT, and a deficiency slows the reaction and gives a falsely low ALT activity. Widely used assays rely on the patient's pyridoxal phosphate status, whereas other reagent formulations are supplemented with pyridoxal phosphate and hence the reaction proceeds irrespective of the patient pyridoxal phosphate status. The latter assay formulation is preferred when the population being served has higher prevalence of nutritional deficiencies. The drawback is the lack of increased AST/ALT ratio often used in the investigation of alcoholic hepatitis as patients with chronic alcohol abuse are more likely to exhibit low pyridoxal phosphate levels and that ALT is more sensitive to pyridoxal phosphate compared to AST. Plasma pyridoxine binders in renal failure may cause falsely low values.

ALT has a longer half-life 42–48 h in liver damage, and thus, ALT is higher than AST after 1–2 day. Limited tissue distribution makes ALT more specific for liver.

Cholestatic enzymes (alkaline phosphatase, γ-glutamyl transferase, and 5′ nucleosidase)

Alkaline phosphates and γ-glutamyl transferase and 5′Nuclotidase are microsomal and sinusoidal enzymes present in liver and biliary tract. They are also found in pancreatic tissue, seminal vesicles, and kidneys. γ-Glutamyl transferase and 5′nuclotidase are predominantly elevated in hepatobiliary and cholestatic disease and are often used to characterize the bone or hepatic origin of an elevated alkaline phosphatase.

Alkaline phosphatase (ALP)

The alkaline phosphatases are widely distributed in liver, bone, small intestine, placenta, and kidney. In normal blood, the alkaline phosphatase activity is derived mainly from bone and liver, with small amounts from intestine. Placental alkaline phosphatase appears in the maternal blood in the third trimester of pregnancy.

Phosphatase activity under alkaline condition (alkaline phosphatase) cleaves p-nitrophenyl phosphate into phosphate and p-nitrophenol. The amount of p-nitrophenol released, measured by photometric recording of absorbance at 405 nm is directly proportional to the alkaline phosphatase activity. Importantly, magnesium and zinc are required for the reaction. In situation of hypomagnesemia (i.e., gastrointestinal

TABLE 3 Relative fold tissue distribution of AST and ALT in relation to plasma levels showing lack of tissue specificity.

AST	ALT	Tissue
8000	400	Heart
7000	3000	Liver
5000	300	Skeletal muscle
15	7	Erythrocytes
1	1	Plasma

ALT is also significantly present in the liver, myocardium and skeletal muscle, pancreas, spleen, and lung kidney tissue.
Modified from several sources including Vroon DH, Israili Z. Aminotransferases. In: Walker HK, Hall WD, Hurst JW, eds. *Clinical Methods: The History, Physical, and Laboratory Examinations*. 3rd ed. Boston: Butterworths; 1990. [chapter 99]. PMID: 21250265.

losses) and or chelation by EDTA contaminated blood sample collections, a reduced or often very low alkaline phosphatase activities are recorded. Alkaline phosphatase exhibits gender and age variations with slightly higher levels in males compared to females, and significantly high levels reflecting increased bone activity are seen in children and later in advanced ages.

Increases in alkaline phosphatase activity in liver disease are the result of increased activity of the enzyme in hepatocytes usually in response to cholestasis, either intra- or extrahepatic.

Raised alkaline phosphatase activity in the blood may also appear in bone disease. The source (liver versus bone) of elevated alkaline phosphate (sustained over at least two serial measurements) can be identified by electrophoresis, other methodologies include lectin binding ad heat inactivation.

The serum alkaline phosphatase activity is most widely used in liver disease to differentiate between hepatitis and cholestasis. The latter, even short of duration, results in increased enzyme activity of at least twice the upper end of the reference interval. High alkaline phosphatase activity may also occur in hepatic infiltrative diseases when space occupying (tumor) lesions are present and in cirrhosis.

Widely distributed in liver, bone, small intestine, placenta, and kidney, circulating alkaline phosphatase is derived mainly from bone and liver with small amounts form the intestine. Placental alkaline phosphatase appears during the third trimester of pregnancy. Elevated levels are associated with liver or bone disease. In liver, it is associated with cholestasis (2 ULN). High alkaline phosphatase levels are also found in infiltrating disease of the liver, i.e., by tumor. It is also elevated in cirrhosis.

Gamma glutamyl transferase (γGT)

This is a microsomal enzyme which is widely distributed in tissues including liver and renal tubules. The activity of γGT in plasma is raised:

A microsomal enzyme widely distributed in tissues including liver and renal tubules. Membrane bound enzyme in liver, prostate, kidney, pancreas, most plasma from liver. Synthesis induced by microsomal inducing drugs (ethanol, antiepileptics, cimetidine). It is raised in all forms of cholestasis; twofold higher in African Americans. 25%–50% higher in obese. In all forms of cholestasis, by ingestion of alcohol, even in the absence of recognizable liver disease. In acute hepatic damage in which changes in γGT activity parallel those of the transaminases. In a wide range of extrahepatic disorders. For this reason, it has not replaced the transaminases and alkaline phosphatase measurements in liver disease. Decreases after meals. 10% higher in smokers. Alcohol ingestion (in the absence of recognizable liver disease). In acute hepatic damage (levels parallel that of the transaminases). Wide range of extra hepatic disorders.

Serum GGT is raised in 75% of those who drink in excess of 60–70 g alcohol daily.

Its major role is probably in detecting alcohol abuse in the absence of liver disease. Serum γGT is raised in about 75% of those who drink in excess of 60–70 g of alcohol daily.

Enzymes (LDH)

Lactate dehydrogenase exists as a tetramer of H or M subunits, with different isoenzymes in different tissues. Isoenzymes 1 (H_4) and 2 (H_3M) predominant in cardiac muscle and 5 (M_4) in liver and skeletal muscle. LD_1 may be estimated by measuring β-hydroxy butyrate dehydrogenase.

5′-Nucleotidase (5′NT) enzyme

5′-Nucleotidase (5′NT) enzyme catalyzes the hydrolyses of nucleotides by removing 5′-phosphate of the pentose ring. It is present in the liver, intestine, brain, heart, pancreas, and blood vessels. In the liver, it is associated with canalicular and sinusoidal plasma membranes. Despite its distribution in other tissue, it is generally elevated in cholestatic hepatobiliary disease and is not elevated in bone disease. Thus, its measurement is helpful when investigating an isolated increase in alkaline phosphatase.

In contrast to alkaline phosphatase, levels are not influenced by gender or race, and is low in children increasing to a plateau at 50 years of age. Therefore, its measurement is helpful in children, and in pregnancy where physiological increase in alkaline phosphatase is not mirrored with 5′NT.

Syndromes of hepatic dysfunction and biomarkers

Biomarkers of liver disease can be described as those indicative of hepatocytes disease a, or cholestatic disease although the two are often overlap and are present together.

Liver dysfunction may present acutely, chronically, or may be acute on chronic liver dysfunction.

Acute liver dysfunction occurs over a period of less than 26-week duration. Intensive management improves survival.

Chronic liver disease describes a progressive deterioration of hepatic function of more than 6 months (as defined by reduce protein synthesis, reduced detoxification, impaired coagulation). It is a chronic continues process of inflammation leading to cirrhosis and fibrosis both being end stages of chronic liver disease.

Acute on chronic liver dysfunction is a serious condition with high degree of morbidly and mortality. It occurs in patients with existing chromic liver disease. Precipitating factors include alcohol or drug related injury, viral hepatitis, hypoxia, and infection.

Hepatocellular dysfunction

There is biological variability in liver enzymes AST and ALT the increase in strenuous exercise an increase of about

5% in AST and about 18% in ALT among hospitalized patients attributable to immobilization.

AST lacks tissue specificity, in addition to the liver, it is present in large amounts in RBC, skeletal muscle, kidney, and the brain. ALT is also present in skeletal muscle (Table 3).

Alkaline phosphatase is present also in bone, intestine, and placental tissue. γGT is more specific to the liver. Markers of liver function include bilirubin metabolism, proteins, and vitamin K-dependent clotting factors. Bilirubin elevation suggests impaired hepatic function, abnormal conjugation, and clearance as well as cholestatic obstruction. When assessing liver disease using enzymes, this selective or combined elevation as well as degree and extent of elevation is considered noting the change in enzyme levels overtime can also be helpful. Enzymes may reflect either cellular damage or cholestatic involvement often however it is a presentation of combined elevations.

To help understand the role of biochemical markers in the assessment of liver dysfunction, it is best to split into two components those of hepatocellular and cholestatic origin.

AST and ALT catalyze the transfer of alpha-amino group from aspartate and arginine respectively to and alpha-ketoglutaric acid forming acetoacetate and oxaloacetate both entering the citric acid cycle. The enzymes have no functional activity in plasma. Pyridoxal-5-phosphate is a cofactor required for both AST and ALT activity, although the deficiency is greater impact on ALT compared to AST. P-5-P is deficient in patient with alcoholic hepatitis (due to poor nutritional factors), and this explains the increased AST to ALT ratio observed in this patient population. Most laboratories, however, are adopting AST and ALT assays formulations that are supplemented with P-5-P and thus overcomes reduced enzymatic activities seen in alcoholic patients.

Liver enzymes AST and ALT are increased in response to hepatic injury. They are elevated in inflammation and in toxic injuries the extent of increase as well as its pattern reflects the cause. For instance, a marked increase with short duration are characteristic of toxic or ischemic injury compared with a gradual and prolonged increase seen in hepatitis due to infective agent, commonly viral hepatitis.

The extent of enzymes elevation can be classified into mild, moderate, and severe (<5 times the upper limit of normal, 5–10 the upper limit of normal, and >10 the upper limit of normal respectively). There is overlap in the AST and ALT levels that seen in patients with different causes for hepatitis (ischemic or toxic, alcoholic, or autoimmune). Highest sensitivity for AST and ALT in patients with acute injury is in the moderate range 200 IU/L for AST and 300 IU/L for ALT.

In ischemic or toxic liver injury, AST and ALT levels greater than 75 times the upper limit of normal are often seen where a rise in AST precedes that of ALT. AST is predominantly cytoplasmic, whereas ALT is predominantly (80%) mitochondrial.

In toxic/ischemic hepatitis, AST rises earlier than ALT due its cytoplasmic distribution. Levels decline rapidly compared with viral etiology, and total bilirubin rarely exceeds three times the upper limit of normal.

Declining enzymes levels are indicative of either resolution and recovery or significant hepatocytes cellular damage. The latter reflecting the ensued reduction in hepatic tissue mass. In the latter setting, high bilirubin levels and increased prothrombin time are observed. Compared to mild elevation in patients with viral hepatitis, LDH levels are markedly elevated in patients with toxic and ischemic damage.

Nonalcoholic fatty liver disease is a common cause of mild elevation of liver enzymes. γGT can be elevated three times ULN in the absence of alcohol consumption.

Short, intermediate, and long-term markers of hepatic function include Factor VII (half-life of 6 h) and thus changes quickly and PT (prothrombin time) thus useful for prognosis in acute liver disease. Similarly for prealbumin (half-life is <1 day) its influence is limited by the patient nutritional status and being a negative acute phase protein. Transferrin has a half-life of about 6 days and thus provides an intermediate timeframe measure of assessment, however limited by being a negative acute phase protein.

Many drugs cause elevation in liver enzymes either secondary to toxicity (transaminases) or to induced stimulation (cholestatic enzymes alkaline phosphatase, γGT and 5′NT). The drugs include antibiotics (Augmentin), macrolides (cholestatic pattern), ceftriaxone, anticonvulsants (cholestatic pattern), herbal supplements, statins, and antituberculosis medication.

For instance, 16% of patients on carbamazepine show evidence of hepatotoxicity with hepatocellular component (ALT ≥ 3 ULN and ratio of ALT:AST ≥ 5) and cholestatic pattern (Alkaline Phosphatase ≥ 2 ULN and ratio of ≤2).

Drugs with mixed hepatocellular and cholestatic involvement exhibit (ALT > 3 ULN and Alkaline phosphatase > 2 ULN and ratio = 2–5). The ratios are derived using the formula (ALT/ALT ULN) for ALT and (ALP/ALP ULN) for alkaline phosphatase.

Hepatitis

Inflammation of hepatocytes mostly due to viral infection (hepatitis A, B, C, or other less common viral subtypes). The infection episode can either be acute or chronic in nature lasting more than 6 months.

In acute damage to hepatocytes due to toxins, ischemia, infection, and injury, there is rapid onset of injury and rapid resolution. Peak AST, ALT often 100× normal. AST > ALT in the first 1–2 days. This episode is followed by a rapid fall, usually to normal levels by 8–10 days, AST takes longer than ALT. Prothrombin time (PT) markedly abnormal >15 s in 90% of cases and bilirubin minimally elevated 60 μmol/L (3.5 mg/dL) in 90% of cases.

Chronic hepatitis

This is a relatively more common than the acute form. It is present in 2%–3% of population. It often has no or nonspecific symptoms, e.g., fatigue. It is a major significant risk of progression to cirrhosis for HCV 20%–30%, hepatoma (1.5% per year once cirrhosis is present). Causes include chronic viral infection (mainly HCV 80%–90%), hemochromatosis, autoimmune chronic hepatitis, and among others. Minimally elevated ALT (1–4 ULN) 15%–25% have persistently normal and 60% intermittently normal ALT. AST normal more than ALT with AST/ALT ratio almost always low. There is normal bilirubin, albumin, prothrombin time a reflection of the large reserve capacity.

Two components are typically involved in chronic hepatitis inflammation and fibrosis. Inflammation damages cells, releases enzymes, and stimulates cytokines production. Fibrosis causes scarring, reduces portal blood flow, most predictor of progression to cirrhosis.

Viral hepatitis

The presence of circulating hepatitis B antigens and associated antibodies is the whole mark of the infection and of establishing the diagnosis. They appear 1–2 weeks of infection prior to clinical symptoms. The serological pattern is shown in Table 4.

The course being an immunologic pattern shown below with an average of 4–5 weeks of jaundice and elevated ALT levels. Peak AST and ALT are often 10–40 ULN (being >8 ULN in 95% of cases). Bilirubin is invariably increased with 30%–70% never become jaundiced. Prothrombin time (PT) is usually normal (14 s in 95%).

Alcoholic hepatitis

In alcoholic hepatitis, there are an average 4–5 weeks of jaundice and elevated ALT levels. Peak AST and ALT often <10 ULN (being <8 ULN in 95% of cases). Increased bilirubin levels are variable where in adult patients about 30%–70% never become jaundiced. See Table 5.

Autoimmune hepatitis

Inflammatory disorder with prevalence 1:5000–1:10,000 and more common in women. Jaundice and cirrhosis are found in 50% and 30% of patients, respectively, at diagnosis.

Aminotransferases are moderate to severe increased in the acute phase and decline to mild in the chronic state or when cirrhosis ensues.

Cholestatic picture predominates with elevation in alkaline phosphatase and γGT, and bilirubin. Alkaline phosphatase to AST ratio is often <3 calculated as [(Alk Phos/Alk Phos ULN)/(AST/AST ULN)]. Disproportionate elevations in alkaline phosphatase require investigation for primary biliary cholangitis.

Cholestatic hepatic dysfunction

Biochemical markers of cholestasis include alkaline phosphatase, bilirubin, and gamma glutamyl transferase (γGT). In the liver, alkaline phosphatase is present on the surface

TABLE 4 Summary of the presence of circulating HBsAg: Whole mark of HBV infection and established the diagnosis.

Course of infection	Serological markers			
	HBsAg	Anti-HBc (total)	Anti-HBc IgM	Anti HBs
Acute infection	+	+	+	−
Chronic infection	+	+	−	−
Resolved hepatitis B infection	−	+	−	+
Immunity from prior infection	−	−	−	+
Not immune or infected	−	−	−	−

Appears 1–2 weeks of infection prior to clinical symptoms. Viral hepatitis serology. This is often performed by immunology and microbiology laboratories.
Table modified from Prasidthrathsint K, Stapleton JT. Laboratory diagnosis and monitoring of viral hepatitis. *Gastroenterol Clin N Am.* 2019;48(2):259–279. https://doi.org/10.1016/j.gtc.2019.02.007. Epub 2019 Apr 1. PMID: 31046974.

TABLE 5 Pattern of enzyme biomarkers in viral, alcoholic, and in acute toxic hepatitis.

Biomarker/ hepatitis	Viral	Alcoholic	Toxic
ALT (fold increase)	>10	1–10	≫10
AST/ALT ratio	<1	>2	>1 early (<5 late)
Bilirubin (μmol/L)	60–22	40–220	<35

Modified from Kalas MA, Chavez L, Leon M, Taweesedt PT, Surani S. Abnormal liver enzymes: a review for clinicians. *World J Hepatol.* 2021;13(11):1688–1698. https://doi.org/10.4254/wjh.v13.i11.1688. PMID: 34904038; PMCID: PMC8637680.

of biliary tract. Cholestasis, obstruction of bile acids flow stimulates alkaline phosphatase release from cell surface.

Delayed and sustained elevation of alkaline phosphatase is due to its prolonged 1-week half-life.

Unlike the transaminases, the degree of alkaline phosphatase elevation is of no prognostic value.

The source of an elevated alkaline phosphatase can easily be ascertained by measuring the more liver specific γGT and or by performing isoenzyme electrophoresis. The sources for alkaline phosphatase are bone, liver, or from physiological sources such as placenta tissue during pregnancy or intestinal tumors (Regan isoform). Heat inactivation as well as lectin binding studies distinguishes bone from liver isoforms but are less widely used. Obstructive cholestasis due to metastatic liver disease, infiltrative disorders, lymphoma. Of note is that in some patients with those disorders, alkaline phosphatase is the only abnormality.

Alkaline phosphatase as well as gamma GT in female patients with autoimmune disorders measurement of high immunoglobulins, cholesterol antimitochondrial antibodies may indicate the presence of primary biliary cirrhosis. Patients with irritable bowel disease and a positive antineutrophil cytoplasmic antibodies may suggest the presence of primary sclerosing cholangitis.

γGT present in both hepatocytes and in biliary epithelial cells lining the biliary ducts. It is also present in renal tubules, pancreas, and intestine.

Microsomal enzyme induced by a number of drugs such as anticonvulsants, steroids (oral contraceptives), and alcohol. γGT is highly sensitive to stimulation compared to alkaline phosphatase with a ratio of γGT to alkaline phosphatase >2.5.

γGT is very sensitive; it is elevated in extra-hepatic disorders such as renal impairment and pulmonary disease. Levels are mildly elevated 2–3 ULN in half of patients with nonalcoholic fatty liver disease.

Hepatorenal dysfunction

Hepatorenal syndrome is a serious complication of hepatic cirrhosis leading to renal dysfunction. The reduction in glomerular filtration is secondary to functional circulatory changes affecting filtration. The degree of creatinine elevation is thought to be underestimated due to decreased haptic creatine, reduced muscle mass, increased tubular secretion of creatinine and technically falsely low creatinine estimation by the Jaffe (alkaline picrate method) in the presence of high bilirubin levels.

There is acute renal impairment with high serum creatinine in 19%–26% of patients with cirrhosis and in 32% of patients with severe alcohol-associated hepatitis.

Models for assessment of end stage liver disease (MELD)

A number of models are in use for the prediction of survival and assessment of prognosis in patients with various liver disorders. The models that are widely used include model for end-stage liver disease (MELD score), the Maddrey discriminant function (mFD), and the Glasgow alcoholic hepatitis score (GAHS), among others. The models utilize different clinical and laboratory findings to derive a risk score. The scores aid in patient management.

MELD score

The MELD score is the widely used in patients with chronic liver disease. The scores range from 6 to 40. The score contains the following: serum bilirubin and creatinine and INR and is calculated using the formula MELD $= 3.8*$loge (serum bilirubin [mg/dL]) $+ 11.2*$loge(INR) $+ 9.6*$loge(serum creatinine [mg/dL]) $+ 6.4$.

The mode was modified to include serum sodium as hyponatremia is a common complication in cirrhosis where mortality increased by 5% for each 1 mmol decrease in serum sodium levels between the 125 and 140 mmol/L range. The MELD-Na formula is calculated using the formula: MELD-Na $=$ MELD $+ 1.32 \times (137 - Na) - [0.033 \times MELD*(137 - Na)]$.

Modified Child-Pugh risk score

The Child-Pugh risk score uses clinical and laboratory findings. The score risk calculation includes the presence of ascites, the presence of encephalopathy, serum bilirubin and albumin levels, and prothrombin time (Table 6). Child-Pugh Class A (5–6 points) predicts 100% 1-year survival, class B (7–9 points) predicts 80% 1-year survival, and class C (10–15 points) predicts 45% 1-year survival.

Maddrey's discriminant function (mDF)

Maddrey discriminant function score is used in the assessment of severity of alcoholic hepatitis with a score of >32 implies severe liver disease with poor prognosis and represents a threshold for considering corticosteroid therapy. The model includes prothrombin prolongation and total bilirubin levels. The following formula is applied: Maddrey score $= 4.6 \times$ (prolongation of prothrombin time above control in seconds) $+$ Total bilirubin in mg/dL.

Glasgow alcoholic hepatitis score (GAHS)

The GAHS applies age and laboratory amusements of white blood cell count, prothrombin ratio, and serum urea and bilirubin (Table 7). GAHS score ≥9 is used as a threshold for initiating corticosteroid treatment.

The score is considered more accurate than mDF in the prediction of outcome from alcoholic hepatitis.

Hepatic fibrosis

Chronic injury and inflammation of the liver regardless of etiology leads to fibrosis. The degree of fibrosis, which may be reversible, increases with continued presence of injury

TABLE 6 Modified Child-Pugh risk score.

Parameter	Risk		
	1	2	3
Ascites	None	Slight	Moderate–severe
Encephalopathy	None	Slight–moderate	Moderate–severe
Bilirubin (mg/dL)	<2.0	2–3	>3.0
Albumin (g/dL)	>3.5	2.8–3.5	<2.8
Prothrombin time (prolonged in seconds)	1–3	4–6	>6.0

Child's Pugh Class A: 5–6 points, 1-year survival is 100%, Class B: 7–9 points, 1-year survival is 80%, and Class C: 10–15 points, 1-year survival is 45%.
Modified from Pugh RN, Murray-Lyon IM, Dawson JL, Pietroni MC, Williams R. Transection of the oesophagus for bleeding oesophageal varices. *Br J Surg.* 1973;60(8):646–649. https://doi.org/10.1002/bjs.1800600817. PMID: 4541913.

TABLE 7 Clinical and laboratory parameters applied in the Glasgow alcoholic hepatitis score.

Parameter	Factor		
	1	2	3
Age	<50	≥50	–
White blood cell count (10^9/L)	<15	≥15	–
Urea (mmol/L)	<5	≥5	–
PT ratio	<1.5	1.5–2.0	>2.0
Total bilirubin (μmol/L)	<125	125–250	>250

To convert BUN and bilirubin from convectional units to SI units multiply by 0.357 and 88.4 respectively.
Modified from Forrest EH, Morris AJ, Stewart S, et al. The Glasgow alcoholic hepatitis score identifies patients who may benefit from corticosteroids. *Gut.* 2007;56(12):1743–1746. https://doi.org/10.1136/gut.2006.099226. Epub 2007 Jul 12. PMID: 17627961; PMCID: PMC2095721.

and inflammation. Chronic liver disease due to hepatitis C and B infections and to nonalcoholic fatty liver disease is widespread which can result in liver fibrosis and progress to cirrhosis. Furthermore, advanced cirrhosis and fibrosis lead to liver failure and to hepatoma.

In patients with chronic liver disease, assessment of the degree of fibrosis predicts liver related morbidity and mortality. Fibrosis interferes with hepatic blood flow and thus leads to ischemia, impaired absorption, metabolism, detoxification, and secretory function of the liver.

As scarring and fibrosis worsens, portal vein pressure rises (portal hypertension) which may cause ascites (accumulation of abdominal fluid) fluid, dilated veins in the stomach and esophagus (varices), other findings, and hepatic function gradually worsens. A number of fibrosis risk scores assessment tests are in use (Table 8).

Assessment of the degree of fibrosis and cirrhosis is important in determining prognosis and in devising patient management protocol. For instance, patients with identified fibrosis require urgent attention to prevent progression to cirrhosis and both require screening for hepatocellular carcinoma. Although liver biopsy is the gold standard, it is invasive and carries risk of post procedure complications (pain, infection, bleeding, organ perforation). It also carries a risk of variation in interpretation influenced by the sample adequacy (only sampling small portion of the liver 1:50,000) and the semiquantitative nature of current histopathological examinations staging.

Noninvasive combination of biochemical markers is used to assess presence of and extent of fibrosis and as a guide for the ultimate invasive diagnostic liver biopsy. Due to the generally low prevalence of fibrosis, biomarkers, in the absence of clinical findings, have low positive predictive values. However, they have high negative predictive value for ruling out advanced fibrosis and cirrhosis.

Patients found to be at low risk for fibrosis are reassessed in 6-month intervals. Patients at intermediate or high risk for advanced fibrosis often require elastography and liver biopsy.

A number of biomarker sets are commercially available, and they include Fibrosis Score 4 (FIB-4) which consists of AST-Platelet Ratio index, and nonalcoholic fatty liver disease includes (see Table 8):

Of note, the majority of the scores were developed in patients with viral hepatitis to predict significant fibrosis or cirrhosis and to aid with decisions on available treatment therapies such as interferon.

The above three clinical scores (NFS, FIB-4, and APRI) are readily and freely available. The others carry propriety and royalty assignment when being used.

The FIB-4 score of <1.45 indicates low risk, >3.25 increased risk with in between being indeterminant. The findings of low risk indicate unlikely to develop advanced fibrosis.

Patients with high clinical suspicion or those that fall in the indeterminant range may require repeat assessment in 6 months

TABLE 8 Example blood-based biomarkers tests for detection of fibrosis in patients with chronic liver disease.

Test name	Biomarkers/parameters	Formula	Low risk	High risk
Fibrotest (FibroSure)	Alpha-2-macroglobulin, gamma GT, haptoglobin, bilirubin, apolipoprotein A1, and transpeptidase	4.467 log [Alpha-2-macroglubulin (g/L)] − 1.357 log [Haptoglobin (g/L)] + 1.017 log [gamma GT (IU/L)] + 0.0281 × [Age] + 1.737 log [Bilirubin (µmol/L)] −1.184 × [Apolipoprotein (g/L)] + 0.301 × B −5.54. Where B = 1 for male and B = 0 for female	<0.3	>0.7
FIB-4	Platelet count, AST, ALT, age	(Age×AST)/(Platelets×($\sqrt{}$ALT))	<1.45	>3.25
APRI (aspartate aminotransferase to platelet ratio index)	AST, platelet count	[(AST/ULN AST)×100]/platelets (10^9/L)	≤1.0	>1.0
Liver fibrosis panel (Hepascore)	Alpha-2-macroglubulin, gamma GT, Bilirubin, transpeptidase, hyaluronic acid	Hepascore = y/(y + 1), where y is obtained as follows. {y = exp[−4.185818 − (0.0249 × age (years)) + (0.7464 × gender) + (1.0039 × alpha-2-macroglobulin (g/L)) + (0.0302 × hyaluronic acid (µg/L) + 0.0691 × bilirubin (µmol/L) − (0.012 × gamma GT (U/L))]}. Where gender = 1 for male and gender = 0 for female	<0.4	≥0.5
NFS (nonalcoholic fatty liver disease (NAFLD)) Fibrosis Score	Glucose, platelet count, albumin, AST:ALT ratio, age, and BMI (F0 = no fibrosis, F1 = mild fibrosis, F2 = moderate, F3 = severe fibrosis, F4 = cirrhosis)	−1.675 + 0.037×age (y)+ 0.094×BMI (kg/m^2)+ 1.13×IFG/diabetes (yes=1, no=0)+0.99×AST/ALT ratio−0.013×platelet (×10^9/L) −0.66×albumin (g/dL)	<−1.455 (F0–F2)	>0.675 (F3–F4)
ELF (Enhanced Liver Fibrosis) score	N-terminal procollagen III peptide (PIIINP), metalloproteinase 1 (TMP-1)/ hyaluronic acid (HA)	2.494 + 0.846 ln (HA) + 0.735 ln (PIIINP) + 0.391 ln (TMP-1)	<9.8	>11.29

The names are proprietary and include various biomarkers. Different cut-offs for each score and for the different etiology, NAFLD, Hepatitis C, and Hepatitis B. Below cut-offs patient has low risk for significant fibrosis, advanced fibrosis, or cirrhosis (negative predictive values are high at >80%). A higher cut-offs above which the patient is considered high risk. The scores between the low and high cut-offs are considered indeterminate. NFS score of less than −1.455 predicts no advances fibrosis. Values in-between are indeterminant. Area under the receiver operator characteristics was >0.8 for predicting advanced fibrosis, 28% of patients may have indeterminate results. ELF, Enhanced Liver Fibrosis score developed by the European Liver Fibrosis group.
Modified from Lai M, Afdhal NH. Liver fibrosis determination. *Gastroenterol Clin N Am.* 2019;48(2):281–289. https://doi.org/10.1016/j.gtc.2019.02.002. Epub 2019 Apr 1. PMID: 31046975.

or use of combined testing scores and or imaging studies. High scores indicate high risk for fibrosis that need to be conformed with elastography and in some instances liver biopsy.

The ELF, Fibrotest (FibroSure), and hepatic scores, also known as combined biochemical panels, are commercially available.

The performance of the scores (e.g., Fibrotest—FibroSure) may be influenced by the presence of acute inflammation, sepsis, and extrahepatic cholestasis.

Knowing the constituents of the respective scores, it is important when accessing the utility of the scores for example, scores that include total bilirubin, elevated levels in Gilbert's syndrome do not reflect the risk for fibrosis.

Of note, those scores were developed assuming single liver disease, and since most patients will have more than one disease, patients with combined nonalcoholic fatty liver and cirrhosis may cause difficulty in interpretation. It is recommended that in patients with more than one liver disease a lower cut-off value for the score is applied. This however will likely lead to more liver biopsies.

About a third of patients 28%–30% fall in the indeterminant range of the different risk assessment models.

Blood biomarkers are more reliable and not influenced by BMI compared to radiological elastography procedures. Furthermore, combined biomarkers and electrography techniques have a high negative predictive value >85% for excluding advanced fibrosis and 40% to 70% positive predictive value for diagnosis advanced fibrosis or cirrhosis.

The availability of noninvasive blood tests has decreased the need for the invasive liver biopsy in a large proportion of patients.

Hepatic malignancy and malignancy-associated haptic dysfunction

Primary liver malignancies include hepatoma and cholangiocarcinoma. Malignancy-associated liver dysfunction includes secondary metastasis to the liver. Common cancers with hepatic metastatic involvement include breast, intestine, and lungs. Measurement of liver-specific tumor markers, as well as those associated with dysfunction and injury, is used in diagnosis and management.

Hepatoma

Hepatocellular carcinoma (HCC) common cancer (third most common). 80 cases/100,000 population per year in China. Relatively rare in Western world. Alfa-fetoprotein is elevated and may be in the thousands by the time clinical symptoms appear and the condition is discovered.

Alpha fetoprotein is mainly synthesized by the liver during fetal life and represent the main circulating protein in the fetus. Levels rapidly decline after birth, and in normal adult, it is present only in small amounts (<20 µg/L). Serum levels in adults of great use in the diagnosis of hepatocellular

carcinoma in which it is increased in 70%–90% of cases. Moderately elevated AFP levels may transiently be seen after acute liver injury. It is elevated in patients with cirrhosis.

Hepatocellular carcinoma is the most common hepatic malignancy. Dedifferentiation and transformation of regenerating cirrhotic hepatocytes, whereas patients with cirrhosis are at 10%–20% risk of developing hepatocellular carcinoma. It is rare in cirrhosis of autoimmune etiology compared to that of viral hepatitis. Screening is relevant and important as it takes a long time (about 20 years) to become malignant.

Bile duct malignancy

Cholangiocarcinoma represents less than 1% of all liver cancer. There are epithelial cell cancers that occur either intrahepatic (10% of cases), perihilar (50% of cases), or distal locations (40% of cases). Biliary obstruction is common in intrahepatic cholangiocarcinoma. Although most cholangiocarcinoma arises de novo with no risk identified, patients with cirrhosis and viral hepatitis B and C are shown to be at risk of developing cholangiocarcinoma. Similarly, patient with chronic inflammatory sclerosing cholangitis is at risk of developing particularly perihilar cholangiocarcinoma.

Markedly elevated CA 19-9 levels are seen in patients and are monitored for therapeutic response. In patients with primary sclerosing cholangitis, CA 19-9 level of 129 U/mL is a cut-off for indication of intrahepatic cholangiocarcinoma, without about 30% showing no evidence of malignancy. CA 19-9 level >1000 U/mL are indicative of advanced disease with metastasis involving the peritoneum. Patients negative for Lewis's antigen (among 7% of the population) levels of CA 19-9 are undetectable and thus misleading.

Inherited disorders

A number of inherited metabolic disorders exhibit abnormalities in liver enzymes. The reader is also referred to Chapter 12 on Metabolic disorders.

Hereditary hemochromatosis

Inherited disorder of iron metabolism, common autosomal recessive disorder (1:200 to 1:400 homozygous frequency). Single point mutation commonly C282Y and H63D among others results in iron deposition in the liver, pancreas, and heart. Patients will exhibit elevated serum iron, ferritin, and iron saturation (a reduction in iron binding capacity testing). Due to the high prevalence of the disorder, such iron studies should always be measured. High ferritin and transferrin saturation >45% are suggestive of HFE and are confirmed by genetic analysis for the mutation.

Wilson's disease

Wilson disease is an inherited disorder of copper metabolism characterized by mild elevation in liver enzymes. The prevalence is variable and range from 1:30,000 to 1:300,000 depending on the population and thus patients with abnormal and unexplained elevated liver enzymes should be screened for Wilson disease. The disorder is caused by mutations in the ATP7B alleles encoding the transmembrane copper-transporting ATPase which governs the excretion of copper into the bile. It also transports copper to apoceruloplasmin where the incorporation of six copper atoms forms ceruloplasmin, the major circulating copper containing protein. Late onset presentation of Wilson disease is seen in patients homozygous for an H1069Q mutation.

Serum and urinary copper levels are markedly elevated andserum ceruloplasmin (copper carrier protein) is reduced. The accumulation of copper in hepatocytes (confirmed by biopsy) leads to hepatocellular damage and inflammation with concomitant increase in liver enzymes.

Alpha-1-antitypsin deficiency

Alpah-1-antitrypsin (A1AT) is synthesized in the liver. The protein protects the lung tissue against attack by the enzyme neutrophil elastase. Point mutation results in its accumulation inside hepatocytes and low circulating levels. Normal wild-type allele is MM and has normal circulating levels of alpha-1-antitrypsin. The Z allele arises from a single amino acid Glu342Lys mutation, and the homozygous form is the most severe and is present in 1 in 25 patients of European descent. The milder form results from mutation Gluy264Val forming the S allele.

The deficiency is an autosomal codominancy inherited disorder with a likely underestimated prevalence of 3.4 million.

The disorder has multiple alleles (MM, MZ, and ZZ). Allele associated with liver damage is MZ allele. In the homozygous ZZ form, the large quantities of the mutated Z (abnormal folding) accumulate inside hepatocytes triggering hepatic injury and inflammation.

Elevated liver enzymes are seen in patients with A1AT. This may be suspected in patients presenting with emphysema in adulthood or with marked liver dysfunction in neonates.

Hepatic manifestation of accumulated A1AT is exacerbated by fat and alcohol. Although there is approved therapy (intravenous administration of plasma purified A1AT) in the lung variant of the disease, there is no currently approved therapy other than liver transplant in patients with advanced liver disease. Development of liver fibrosis is monitored using test described above (Table 6).

Liver transplant

The laboratory supports liver transplant program by, in addition to the measurement of the above markers of liver disorders, the determination of therapeutic levels of the commonly used immunosuppressants tacrolimus, sirolimus, everolimus, and cyclosporine. Those often given in combination therapy to reduce the individual drugs side effects and to effectively reduce risk of rejection and of drugs toxicity. Most clinical laboratories have developed those as profile group tests on liquid chromatography-mass spectrometry methods with rapid turnaround time often less than 24h.

Summary

- The acinus is the functional unit of the liver.
- Structural integrity of the liver is essential to its function (synthesis, secretion, conjugation, detoxification), although the liver has large reserve capacity as well as ability to regenerate. This contributes to the later presentations often encountered.
- Biochemical tests are designed to assess either hepatocellular injury or cholestatic disorder. The two disorders are often copresent. Enzymes markers of injury and cholestasis are AST, ALT and alkaline phosphatase, γGT respectively.
- The liver synthesize most blood proteins with the exception of immunoglobulins. Some of the proteins are termed acute phase proteins.
- Albumin is the major protein synthesized and secreted by the liver; accounting for about 50% of the total hepatic protein production and represents about 50%–60% of total serum proteins.
- The finding of hypoalbuminemia is therefore a feature of advanced chronic liver disease.
- Alpha-fetoprotein, a 70kDa glycoprotein is normally synthesized by liver during fetal life and is the predominantly circulating protein in fetal blood.
- The liver synthesizes 25-hydroxy vitamin D, insulin-like growth factor-I (IGF-1), angiotensinogen, and vitamin-K-dependent clotting factors.
- Disorders of bilirubin metabolism include those (a) affecting the conjugation process where unconjugated bilirubin exceeds the conjugation capacity of the liver (e.g., hemolysis), and (b) disorders affecting excretion of conjugated bilirubin (e.g., cholestasis and obstruction).
- Inherited disorders of bilirubin metabolism include those (a) affecting the conjugation process (Crigler-Najjar and Gilbert syndromes) and (b) those affecting excretion of conjugated bilirubin (Dubin-Johnson and Rotor syndromes).
- The liver is central to the synthesis and function of clotting factors, and that patients with chronic liver disease are at increased risk of bleeding and coagulopathy.
- Ten to twenty grams of daily nitrogenous was in the form of ammonia which is converted in hepatocytes to urea in the urea cycle and excreted into the urine.
- Increase in unconjugated bilirubin is secondary to excessive bilirubin production exceeding the liver conjugation ability as with hemolysis. It is also secondary to impaired bilirubin uptake and or conjugation.

- Biliary atresia is a serious condition in neonatal period due to bile duct obstruction. The prolonged jaundice is predominantly conjugated direct bilirubin, elevated bile acids, and presence of pale stool.
- Several enzymes (ALT, AST, LDH, γGT, Alk Phos, and 5′NT) are present at high concentrations inside hepatocytes and at sinusoidal membranes and that detection of markedly elevated circulating levels are indicative of hepatic tissue leakage (injury) and or to cholestatic induction.
- Biomarkers of liver disease can be described as those indicative of hepatocytes disease a, or cholestatic disease although the two are often overlap and are present together.
- The extent of enzymes elevation can be classified into mild, moderate, and severe (<5 times the upper limit of normal, 5–10 the upper limit of normal, and >10 the upper limit of normal respectively).
- Biochemical markers of cholestasis include alkaline phosphatase, bilirubin, and gamma glutamyl transferase (γGT).
- In ischemic or toxic liver injury, AST and ALT levels greater than 75 times the upper limit of normal are often seen where a rise in AST precedes that of ALT.
- Hepatorenal syndrome is a serious complication of hepatic cirrhosis leading to renal dysfunction. The reduction in glomerular filtration is secondary to functional circulatory changes affecting filtration.
- Chronic injury and inflammation of the liver regardless of etiology leads to fibrosis. The degree of fibrosis, which may be reversible. It increases with continued presence of injury and inflammation.
- Chronic liver disease leads to fibrosis. Several fibrosis scores are used to determine the risk for developing fibrosis. Risk assessment scores incude, NAFLD Fibrosis score (NFS) and Fibrosis-4-index among others.
- Primary liver malignancies include hepatoma and cholangiocarcinoma. Malignancy-associated liver dysfunction includes secondary metastasis to the liver.
- Alpah-1-antitrypsin (A1AT) is synthesized in the liver. The protein protects the lung tissue against attack by the enzyme neutrophil elastase.
- The laboratory supports liver transplant program by in addition to the measurement of the above markers of liver disorders the determination of therapeutic levels of the commonly used immunosuppressants.

Further reading

Lai M, Afdhal NH. Liver fibrosis determination. *Gastroenterol Clin North Am.* 2019;48(2):281–289.

Kalas MA, Chavez L, Leon M, Taweesedt PT, Surani S. Abnormal liver enzymes: a review for clinicians. *World J Hepatol.* 2021;13(11):1688–1698.

Kirk JM. Neonatal jaundice: a critical review of the role and practice of bilirubin analysis. *Ann Clin Biochem.* 2008;45(Pt 5):452–462.

Rhyu J, Yu R. Newly discovered endocrine functions of the liver. *World J Hepatol.* 2021;13(11):1611–1628.

Simonetto DA, Gines P, Kamath PS. Hepatorenal syndrome: pathophysiology, diagnosis, and management. *BMJ.* 2020;370:m2687.

Ye W, Rosenthal P, Magee JC, Whitington PF. Childhood Liver Disease Research and Education Network. Factors determining delta-bilirubin levels in infants with biliary atresia. *J Pediatr Gastroenterol Nutr.* 2015;60(5):659–663.

Hashim IA, Cuthbert JA. Elevated ammonia concentrations: potential for pre-analytical and analytical contributing factors. *Clin Biochem.* 2014;47(16–17):233–236.

Chapter 5

Bone metabolism and associated disorders

Introduction

This chapter describes the biochemistry and metabolism of bone, its disorders, and associated laboratory investigations. It comprises assessment of markers of bone resorption and formation, calcium, phosphate, and magnesium metabolism and their disorders.

In addition to providing structural and skeletal support and organ protection, bone exhibits many physiological roles. It is metabolically active playing vital roles in calcium, phosphate, and magnesium metabolism. It is also a major hydrogen ion buffering matrix. The clinical biochemistry laboratory is central to the investigation of bone metabolic disorders.

Bone structure and physiology

Bone tissue constitutes about 14% of adult body weight. It is metabolically active undergoing continued remodeling. The matrix is complex made up of organic (reprocessing 30% of bone content) and inorganic matrixes and provides an organized framework for deposition of hydroxyapatite which is a calcium phosphate $Ca_{10}(PO_4)6(OH)_2$ and constitutes 60% of the bone matrix, with water comprising 10% of bone content.

Compact bone tissue is well organized and represents 85% of bone content affording strength and structural support, and the remaining 15% are cancellous "spongy" in structure. The organic component representing 30% of bone structure contains mainly (90%) collagenous proteins and are predominantly type-I collagen in addition to other noncollagenous proteins such as osteocalcin. The inorganic material consists predominantly of calcium and phosphate ions (hydroxyapatite); however, significant amounts of bicarbonate, sodium, potassium, citrate, magnesium, fluoride, zinc, barium, and strontium are also present.

Bone contains about 1 kg of calcium and about 0.5 kg of phosphate and is thus considered a reservoir for circulating calcium. In addition to buffering acidosis (H^+ ions), bone tissue also absorbs toxins and heavy metals.

The composition of bone is variable and is influenced by age, nutrition, the presence of comorbidities, and by drugs such as bisphosphonates, steroids, and anticoagulants. Furthermore, bone pattern is influenced by the stress the bone is subjected to.

In addition to the local modulators such as cytokines, growth factors, alkaline phosphatase, acid phosphatase among others mediating bone metabolism, external modulators are important in both health and in disease. They include parathyroid hormone (PTH), 1,25 hydroxy vitamin D (1,25-(OH)$_2$ Vitamin D), calcitonin, glucocorticoids, androgens, and estrogens (discussed in detail later), as well as excercise and lifestyle.

Bone is considered a mineralized connective tissue with four types of cells, namely osteoclasts, osteoblasts, osteocytes, and lining cells (Fig. 1).

Homeostasis is maintained via a coupled processes of bone resorption and bone formation by osteoclasts and osteoblasts, respectively. Homeostasis is attained when the two processes are in balance, whereas imbalance leads to the various bone disorders discussed below.

Bone remodeling is a highly complex process and takes place in three phases; (a) phase 1 is initiation of bone resorption by osteoclasts, (b) phase 2 is transition phase from resorption to formation of new bone, (c) and phase 3 is bone formation by osteoblasts. Bone remodeling is important for the process of skeleton adaptation to mechanical use and for healing of fractures.

Resorption takes 7–10 days while formation takes 2–3 months. Cancellous bone makes up to 80% of surface area where bone remodeling takes place, and it is responsible for the 25% annual active and more rapid remodeling. Compact bone activity account for 2%–3% of the annual remodeling.

Osteoblasts

Osteoblasts comprise 4%–6% of bone cells and are responsible for bone formation which takes place in two phases. Initial phase is synthesis and secretion of organic matrix, namely collagen proteins (type-I collagen), noncollagen proteins (osteocalcin, osteonectin, ostopontin, and bone sialoprotein-II), and proteoglycan which all form the bone organic matrix, the second phase follows, that is mineralization which takes place in two steps, the vesicular phase where large matrix vesicles released from osteoblasts are deposited into the newly formed bone matrix. Due to its negatively charged sulfated proteoglycans, they immobilize calcium ions stored within the matrix vesicles.

Tutorials in Clinical Chemistry. https://doi.org/10.1016/B978-0-12-822949-1.00019-X

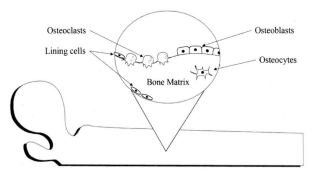

FIG. 1 Schematic diagram of bone showing osteoclasts, osteoblasts, osteocytes, and lining cells. *(Modified from Leeming DJ, Alexandersen P, Karsdal MA, Qvist P, Schaller S, Tankó LB. An update on biomarkers of bone turnover and their utility in biomedical research and clinical practice. Eur J Clin Pharmacol. 2006;62(10):781–792. https://doi.org/10.1007/s00228-006-0174-3. Epub 2006 Aug 16. PMID: 16912870.)*

Calcium is released from the proteoglycans, following degradation by osteoblasts enzymes, and cross-calcium channels formed by annexins. Similarly, phosphate containing compounds (organic phosphate) is released by the action of osteoblastic alkaline phosphatase releasing phosphate ions into the matrix vesicles. Calcium and phosphate ions inside the vesicles form the hydroxyapatite crystals.

The fibrillar phase is when supersaturation of calcium and phosphate ions leads to rupture and spread of the hydroxyapatite crystals to the surrounding matrix. Finally, mature osteoblasts either undergo apoptosis or become osteocytes or bone lining cells.

Bone lining cells

Bone lining cells are flat-shaped quiescent osteoblasts. They cover the bone surface where neither bone resorption nor formation is taking place. Although the function is not fully understood they prevent direct interaction between osteoclasts and bone matrix. However, they are responsible for removing nonmineralized collagen fibril and plays a role in stem cell differentiation. It is thought to play a role in osteoclast differentiation by producing osteoprotegerin (PG) and the receptor activator of nuclear factor kappa-β ligand (RANKL).

Osteocytes

Osteocytes are the most abundant representing 90%–95% of total bone cells and the long lived (up to 25 years) cells. They are located within the lacunae surrounded by mineralized bone matrix.

Due to its strategic location within the bone matrix, osteocytes are thought to play an important mechanosensitive function. It is thought to translate mechanical stimuli to biochemical signal, a process termed piezoelectric effect. The exact mechanism is not fully understood, but it has been shown that upon mechanical stimulation, osteocytes produce nitric oxide, ATP, calcium, and prostaglandins.

Once entrapped into the bone matrix several of the previously expressed osteoblast markers such as osteocalcin collagen type-I and alkaline phosphatase are downregulated.

Osteoclasts

Osteoclasts are responsible for bone resorption, and that their development and expression is complex with many ligands, cytokines, growth factors, RANKL, and macrophages-colony-stimulating factor (M-CSF) playing a role.

Osteoclasts exhibit four types of membrane domains namely, ruffled borders, the sealing zone both in contact with bone matrix, and the basolateral, and functional secretory domains not in contact with bone matrix. The domains are formed once the osteoclasts are in contact with the mineralized extracellular matrix.

The ruffled area releases tartrate-resistant acid phosphatase, cathepsin K, and matrix metalloproteinase-9 which in an acidic environment facilitates bone resorption in the lacuna. Endocytosis of the degradation products ensue and is transported to the functional secretory domain of the osteoclast plasma membrane.

Biomarkers of bone metabolism

A number of circulating and/or urinary biomarkers reflect the extent of bone resorption (osteoclastic activity) and bone formation (osteoblastic activity) and the remodeling process activities. Biomarkers are thus used to identify and to monitor bone disorders (Fig. 2).

Biochemical markers of bone metabolism express the balance between bone formation and bone resorption and detects pathological uncoupling of the two processes. Although bone histomorphometry is the gold standard for assessment of bone turnover, it is invasive, cannot be repeated many times (for serial determinations) in an individual, and requires specialist histopathological laboratory interpretation. Furthermore, bone turnover can also be quantified with calcium balance and kinetic studies, but they are time-consuming, use radioisotopes, and again need specialist interpretation.

Circulating and urinary biomarkers are noninvasive and reflect both acute and chronic changes. The biomarkers can be defined as either bone matrix-derived or cell-derived. The cell-derived biomarkers are bone alkaline phosphatase and osteocalcin by osteoblasts, and tartrate-resistant acid phosphatase by osteoclasts. Catabolic biomarkers are those representing osteoclastic bone resorption activity, namely c-terminal telopeptide (CTx), N-terminal telopeptide (NTx), and pyridinolines and deoxypyridinoline (PYD and DPD). Anabolic biomarkers representing bone formation due to osteoblastic activity are procollagen type I N-propeptide (PINP) and procollagen type-I C-propeptide (PICP) (Fig. 2).

Biomarkers playing a role in remodeling metabolic bone activity include lysozyme enzymes, citrate, lactate,

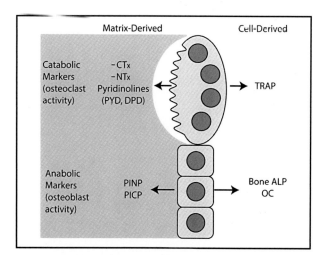

FIG. 2 Biomarkers of bone anabolic and catabolic activities. Normal levels indicate normal coupled metabolic activities. The relative change in biomarkers indicates uncoupled process in disease. Biomarkers are both osteoblasts and osteoclasts derived as well as bone matrix derived. Catabolic biomarkers: *CTx*, C-terminal telopeptide; *DPD*, deoxypyridinoline; *NTx*, N-terminal telopeptide; *PYD*, pyridinoline; *TRAP*, cellular acid phosphatase (tartrate resistant). Anabolic biomarkers: *ALP*, alkaline phosphatase (bone); *OC*, osteocalcin; *PICP*, procollagen type-I C-propeptide; *PINP*, procollagen type I N-propeptide. *(Reproduced with permission from Greenblatt MB, Tsai JN, Wein MN. Bone turnover markers in the diagnosis and monitoring of metabolic bone disease. Clin Chem. 2017;63(2):464–474. https://doi.org/10.1373/clinchem.2016.259085. Epub 2016 Dec 9. PMID: 27940448; PMCID: PMC5549920.)*

cytokines, prostaglandins, and growth factors. The biomarkers are influenced by mechanical stress and by metabolic demands on the bone.

Collagenous proteins

Type-I collagen is the most abundant protein component of bone. It is produced by osteoblasts. The three helical type-I procollagens are the building blocks of collagenous bone, and that the processing and cleavage of the collagen markers reflect the ongoing bone activity (Fig. 3).

Collagen propeptides

Type-I collagen propeptides are cleaved at both C-terminal (PICP) and N-terminal (PINP) during collagen build up (Fig. 3A). The cleaved C- and N-terminal collagen fragments cannot be reused. Therefore, they are markers of bone formation, and that increased levels indicate increased osteoblastic activity and thus increased bone formation.

Telopeptides

Telopeptides are components of incorporated collagen, and thus, their release denotes breakdown and bone resorption

(Fig. 3A) and that the rate of release is proportional to the rate of bone resorption activity. CTx is released following digestion by protease cathepsin K.

Assays for the N-terminal telopeptide are more specific compared to those for the CTx that suffer from cross-reactivities with other telopeptide variants. However, in general they have similar clinical utility. The molecules are cleared by the kidney and are thus measurable in both serum and urine samples. Serum CTx levels are often measured, whereas urinary NTx is preferred as serum NTx correlates poorly with antiresorptive therapy.

A cross-linked form of C-telopeptide is cleaved by matrix metalloproteinase and of trypsin digestion. It is distinct in that its release is thought to be associated with skeletal metastasis of solid tumors. It is difficult to measure and is not routinely available.

Pyridinoline and deoxypyridinoline

The pyridinolines and deoxypyridinoline are cross-linkers in formed collagen, linking type-I collagen "threads" at N and C terminal amino acid positions 103 and 1043, respectively, with covalent binding between lysine or hydroxylysine residues in the telopeptide region (Figs. 3B and 4) and their finding denotes breakdown of collagen and thus bone resorption.

About 30%–35% of the cross-linkers (pyridinoline and deoxypyridinoline) are cleared into the urine in free form, and the rest are bound to peptides or large protein complexes.

Biomarkers of bone formation

Biomarkers secreted by osteoblasts or in response to osteoblastic activity represent bone formation. They include osteocalcin, alkaline phosphatase (ALP), procollagen type I extension C- and N-peptides. Biomarkers are shown in Fig. 2 and listed in Table 1.

Alkaline phosphatase

Alkaline phosphatase, a cell surface membrane-bound enzyme attached to the cell membrane by means of a phosphatidyl-inositol-glycan anchor, catalyzes the hydrolysis of monophosphate esters at basic pH-releasing inorganic phosphate.

There are four isoenzymes of alkaline phosphatase depending on their tissue site of production. The sites are placental (also termed Regan isoenzyme), intestinal, germ cell, and a tissue nonspecific form produced in the liver, bone, and kidney. However, the major circulating forms in normal individuals are those of bone, liver, and kidney with the bone isoform contributing 40% of the total alkaline phosphatase plasma activity.

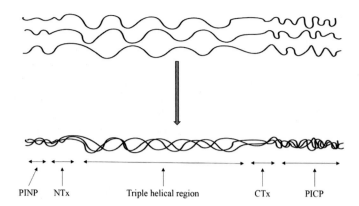

a) Collagen synthesis and metabolism

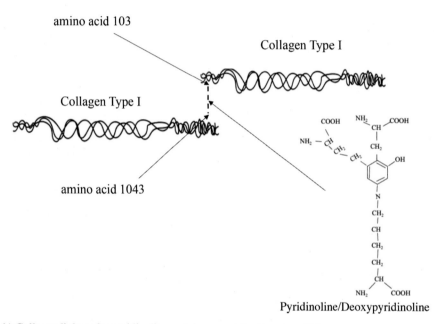

b) Collagen linkage by pyridinoline and deoxypyridinoline cross linkers

FIG. 3 (A) The three helical type-I procollagen and its fragments cleavage sites and associated fragments released. *CTx*, C-terminal telopeptide; *NTx*, N-terminal telopeptide; *PINP*, N-terminal propeptide; *PIPC*, C-terminal propeptide. Propeptides are released during collagen building and thus anabolic markers of bone build up (osteoblastic activity), whereas telopeptides (N- and C-terminal) are released during collagen breakdown and are thus catabolic makers of bone breakdown (osteoclastic activity), similarly (B) the telopeptide cross-linkers (pyridinoline and deoxypyridinoline) appear during bone resorption and thus a marker of catabolic activity (osteoclastic activity). *(Figures modified from several sources including Greenblatt MB, Tsai JN, Wein MN. Bone turnover markers in the diagnosis and monitoring of metabolic bone disease. Clin Chem. 2017;63(2):464–474. https://doi.org/10.1373/clinchem.2016.259085. Epub 2016 Dec 9. PMID: 27940448; PMCID: PMC5549920.)*

The bone and liver isoforms, product of the same genetic loci, exhibit posttranslational modification. Differences in glycosylation between bone and liver isoforms are utilized in chromatographic and lectin binding studies. Additionally, bone form is less stable at high temperature.

The enzyme contains two zinc (Zn^{2+}) and one magnesium (Mg^{2+}) metal ions in its active site, and they contribute to the allosteric conformational changes required for its enzymatic activity. Hypomagnesemia, often encountered in clinical practice, leads to falsely low alkaline phosphatase measured activity.

The possible contribution of the various circulating tissue specific forms contributes the poor diagnostic specificity and sensitivity of alkaline phosphatase and clinical correlation is often required. The finding of a normal γ-glutamyl transferase (GGT) suggests the elevated alkaline phosphatase is likely to be of bone origin.

Alkaline phosphatase activity correlates in a linear fashion with osteoblastic activity suggesting a role in mineralization. In invitro studies, alkaline phosphatase expression is induced by PTH, 1,25-(OH)$_2$ Vitamin D, glucocorticoids, steroid hormones, and growth factors.

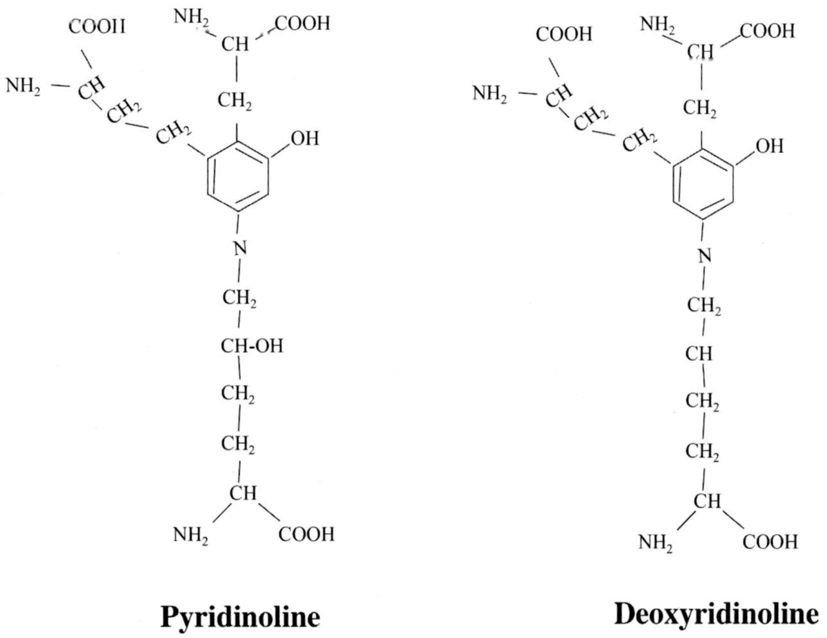

Pyridinoline   **Deoxyridinoline**

FIG. 4 Collagen linkers pyridinoline and deoxypyridinoline. *(Modified from Banse X, Devogelaer JP, Lafosse A, Sims TJ, Grynpas M, Bailey AJ. Cross-link profile of bone collagen correlates with structural organization of trabeculae. Bone. 2002;31(1):70–76. https://doi.org/10.1016/s8756-3282(02)00800-1. PMID: 12110415.)*

TABLE 1 Characterization and differentiation of alkaline phosphatase isoforms.

Isoform	Heat stability	Chromosome	Distribution	Chemical inhibition
Placental	Stable	2	Present at high concentration in placenta. Low in serum/some contribution from neutrophils	L-Phenylalanine, L-phenylalanine-glycine-glycine
Intestinal	Partially stable	2	Carbohydrate side chains do not terminate by sialic acid	L-Phenylalanine, L-phenylalanine-glycine-glycine
Germ cell	Stable	2	Germ cells, embryonal, some neoplastic tissue	L-Phenylalanine, L-phenylalanine-glycine-glycine
Liver/bone/kidney	Heat-labile. Rapidly inactivated at >65°C Liver form is slightly but significantly more stable than bone isoform.	1 (short arm)	Nonspecific tissue. Expressed in many tissues hence the designation but abundant in (bone, liver, kidney). Slight differences in electrophoretic mobility and heat stability between them due to difference in posttranslational modification.	L-Homoarginine

Modified from Sharma U, Pal D, Prasad R. Alkaline phosphatase: an overview. *Indian J Clin Biochem.* 2014;29(3):269–278. https://doi.org/10.1007/s12291-013-0408-y. Epub 2013 Nov 26. PMID: 24966474; PMCID: PMC4062654.

Bone-specific alkaline phosphatase has a half-life of 1–2 days, that sustained high levels indicate high bone turnover activity, and that levels correlate with both the number and differentiation state of osteoblasts.

Several methods are available to discriminate between the different alkaline phosphatase isoforms. Most widely used are electrophoresis where the isoforms separate into bone, liver, intestinal, and placental bands (Fig. 5). Other methods of differentiation are heat inactivation (bone isoform more heat labile compared with liver isoform (Table 1)), lectin binding studies, urea and guanidine denaturation, and neuraminidase pretreatment and by bone-specific immunoassay.

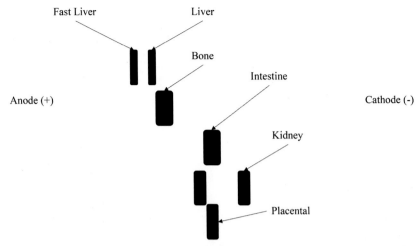

FIG. 5 Alkaline phosphatase isoenzymes by electrophoresis showing separation of the isoforms. The clinical interest is often the separation of bone and liver isoforms and although they migrate closely compared to the other tissue specific isoforms, the bone band often appears broader than that of the live, a fast and ultrafast liver forms may also be visible. *(Modified from The Helena Laboratories, SPIFE® Alkaline Phosphatase Isoenzyme Procedure. Helena Laboratories, Beaumont, TX, USA in use by the author's laboratory.)*

Data from normal subjects shows that bone alkaline phosphatase contributes about half the total alkaline phosphatase activity in adults. Physiologically elevated levels in seen in children (increased bone activity) and pregnant (placental origin) women.

Elevated serum levels are indicative of either bone or liver disorders. In liver, it suggests cholestatic liver disorder which can be confirmed by the presence of elevated gamma glutamyl transferase activity. Increased bone activity is either bone related disorders due to increased osteoblastic activity (bone formation) such as in Paget's disease, or secondary to disorders affecting calcium levels such as parathyroid disorders, vitamin D metabolism as well as in untreated celiac disease. Placental isoforms are elevated in seminomas.

Less common is reduced alkaline phosphatase levels seen in hypophosphatasia, menopausal women receiving estrogens therapy in osteoporosis, malnutrition, magnesium deficiency, hypothyroidism, severe anemia, children with achondroplasia, and men with recent heart surgery. Wilson disease and patients receiving oral contraceptives exhibit reduced alkaline phosphatase levels.

Bone-specific alkaline phosphatase

The finding of abnormal alkaline phosphatase levels either elevated or reduced require additional carful investigations. Some authors recommend algorithm that is driven by patient age at presentation.

Bone and liver forms (presenting the majority of circulating alkaline phosphatase) product of the same genes with little difference in posttranslational glycosylation. The latter is utilized in electrophoretic separation, and thus, separate identification of the relative contribution of the two forms to the total alkaline phosphatase activity.

Osteocalcin (OC)

This is a 49 amino acid (5–6kDa) molecule. It is a calcium binding protein. It is the most abundant noncollagen protein in bone. The majority is ossified within the bone matrix, with a small measurable fraction released into the circulation. It is bound to hydroxyapatite and that the binding affinity is enhanced by a posttranslational vitamin-K-dependent gamma carboxylation. Use of vitamin K antagonist (warfarin) reduced carboxylation and results in increased circulating osteocalcin levels.

Although it is secreted by mature osteoblast and thus considered a marker of bone formation, and that circulating levels correlate with direct histophotometric evidence of bone formation, it is also released from bone during bone resorption. Therefore, its value in assessing bone formation is limited.

Expression of osteocalcin is enhanced by $1,25\text{-}(OH)_2$ Vitamin D, vitamin K, thyroid hormones, glucocorticoids, insulin, estrogen, and growth factors. It is measured by immunoassay and increase levels are associated with bone mineralization. However, levels do not parallel alkaline phosphatase activity. Falsely elevated levels are encountered in renal dysfunction (impaired clearance). Osteocalcin is labile and storage and transportation at 4°C and measurement within 4h of collection has been recommended. Additionally, hemolysis enhances its degradation and thus, falsely low levels are obtained. The instability often molecule is attributed to the 6 C terminal amino acid sequence. Selective immunoassay for the N- or mid-molecule region may offer an alternative to intact osteocalcin assays.

Osteocalcin levels may vary depending on vitamin K status. Thus, vitamin K status must be assessed when osteocalcin is used to assess bone formation activity. Vitamin K administration induces increase in circulating osteocalcin with a decrease in urinary calcium excretion with a parallel decrease in urinary hydroxyproline excretion among fast losers of calcium. This is prominent in postmenopausal women compared with premenopausal.

Procollagen I extension N-peptides

Collagen type I is the major constituent of bone. Osteoblasts secrete type-I collagen (Fig. 3), the N- and C-terminals, termed propeptides are cleaved during collagen incorporation and appear in circulation and are thus markers of bone formation activities.

Pro-collagen I carboxy terminal (PICP), a 100 kDa and N-terminal (PINP), a smaller molecular weight. Measured by immunoassays, the finding of increasing levels in serum correlates with bone formation and mineralization.

They are trimers of the three collagen chains (Fig. 3). Although both fragments are similar, the N-terminal is more studied. Available assays measure either total forms (monomeric and trimeric) or just trimeric form termed intact-propeptide 1 N-terminal. The larger trimeric (intact form) is metabolized and cleared by the liver, whereas the smaller monomeric form is cleared by the kidney and thus accumulates in patients with reduced filtration rate. Thus, it suggests that elevated total propeptide levels (monomeric plus tetrameric) are higher compared with intact (tetrameric) levels in patients with impaired renal function.

Biomarkers of bone resorption

Biomarkers of bone resorption include circulating and urinary collagen cross-link molecules pyridinoline and deoxypyridinoline collagen cross-linkers, carboxy-terminal telopeptide (CTx) and N-terminal telopeptide (NTx), and urinary hydroxyproline and hydroxylysine glycosides.

The biomarkers are either nascent building material or those already incorporated and cannot be reutilized and thus markers of bone resorption. The various markers are of variable diagnostic utility and of value in monitoring progression of bone disease and in response to therapy.

The presence of renal and hepatic dysfunction as well as drugs intake, such as vitamin K, must be taken into consideration when using the bone markers.

Although 24 h urine collections are preferred, they are inconvenient and difficult to collect accurately. Urine sample is collected as second voided morning urine. Samples in three consecutive days are preferred to avoid variability. Samples can be pooled and measured as a single measurement.

Hydroxyproline

Hydroxyproline comprises about 13% of amino acids collagen content. It cannot be re-used in collagen synthesis and thus urine markers of collagen breakdown and bone resorption.

It has poor tissue specificity (collagen 10% of excreted amino acid, C1q hydroxyproline about 40%, dietary source, influenced by renal and hepatic dysfunction). Additionally, it has poor correlation with bone histomorphometry and calcium kinetics.

Hydroxylysine

Found in collagen in smaller amount than hydroxyproline. Hydroxylysine glycosides undergo posttranslational hydroxylation. Not reutilized in collagen synthesis and thus when present in urine it indicates collagen breakdown and bone resorption. Galactosyl-hydroxylysine is measured by HPLC. In osteoporotic women, it has equivalent predictive value to bone density. There is no significant correlation between hydroxylysine and hydroxyproline levels.

Collagen cross-link molecules

Adjacent collagen chains are stabilized by covalent cross-links, pyridinoline (cartilage). Deoxypyridinoline (collagen) accounts for 21% of total cross-links. They undergo posttranslational modification.

Cross-link molecules are only found in mature collagen and thus excretion reflects breakdown of mature collagen not and collagen synthesized but not incorporated into fibrils.

It is measured by HPLC (with fluorescence detection) or by immunoassays. The cross-link molecules are sensitive to UV light and protection from exposure to light is preferred. Excretion increases with age and is two to three folds greater in postmenopausal women. Excretion increases by 3 folds in patients with primary hyperthyroidism, 5 folds in thyrotoxicosis, and 12 folds in Paget's disease. Excretion falls following therapy, and there is positive correlation with bone density.

Carboxy- and N-terminal telopeptides

The carboxy- and N-terminal cross-linkers (CTx and NTx) are small molecular weight peptides (9–20 kDa), and therefore, their circulating levels are influenced by renal function. They are measured by immunoassays. Serum levels correlate with bone resorption indicated by densitometry.

Biochemical monitoring

A number of algorithms are in use to assess effectiveness of antiresorptive treatment. The biomarkers and sample type used in their measurement is summarized in Table 2.

For example, obtaining a baseline level for PINP and CTx, measured in 6 months following initiation of therapy and at 12 month a DXA bone scan performed that is as stated was the best predictor and is the endpoint.

TABLE 2 Biomarkers of bone resorption and formation and their sample type that are in clinical practice.

	Biomarker	Sample type
Bone formation	N-propeptide (PINP)	Serum
	Osteocalcin	Serum
	Alkaline phosphatase (total and/or bone)	Serum
Bone resorption	CTx (C-terminal telopeptide)	Serum/urine
	NTx (N-terminal telopeptide)	Serum/urine
	Deoxypyridinoline (DPD)	Urine
	Acid phosphatase (tartrate resistance)	Serum

Sheffield PINP monitoring algorithm for antiresorptive treatment where optimal treatment response with PINP is a decrease by 10 μg/L to below 35 μg/L. Optimal treatment response with CTx is a decrease by 100 ng/L to below 280 ng/L.

When using NTx (a cross-linked-N-telopeptide of type I collagen), NTx units = nM BCE (bone Collagen Equivalent)/mM Creatinine. Premenopausal reference interval being 17–94 nM BCE/mM creatinine and postmenopausal reference interval being 26–124 nM BCE/mM creatinine.

A decrease of 30%–40% from NTx baseline after 3 months of therapy is a typical response to antiresorptive therapy.

Osteocalcin levels vary with vitamin K status. Vitamin K administration increased osteocalcin. Levels in postmenopausal patients and decreased urinary calcium excretion among fast losers of calcium. This effect was not observed in premenopausal women. Therefore, knowing vitamin K status may be helpful when interpreting osteocalcin levels.

Metabolic bone disorders

Uncoupling of osteoblastic and osteoclastic activities leads to either increased bone resorption or formation. Decreased bone mass (Osteoporosis) is the most common disorder of metabolic bone disease where 1 in 2 women and 1 in 5 men are expected to experience an osteoporotic fraction in their lifetime with significant morbidity and mortality. The condition is asymptomatic until the patient presents with hip fracture or fractures following relatively mild trauma. Risk factors for osteoporosis include advanced age, menopause associated hormonal changes, prolonged steroids therapy, hyperthyroidism, and hyperparathyroidism.[1]

The following metabolic bone disorders will be discussed separately in details. They include osteoporosis (decreased bone mass of normal composition), osteomalacia (abnormal bone matrix due to failure of mineralization), Paget's disease (increased turnover irregular lamellae), renal osteodystrophy (secondary to vitamin D deficiency, and to secondary hyperparathyroidism), osteitis fibrosa cystica (secondary to primary hyperparathyroidism, bone cysts), and metastatic tumor (neoplastic infiltration with osteoclastic bone resorption).

Osteoporosis

Osteoporosis is characterized by abnormal increase in osteoclastic activity uncoupled to bone formation (osteoblastic activity). That is resorption exceeding formation leading to decreased bone density and therefore bone fragility and increased risk for bone fracture.

It is defined as bone mineral density (BMD) as 2.5 standard deviation (2.5SD) or more below the average bone mineral density value. Normal BMD is defined as T-score of −1.0 or higher. T-score of between −1.0 and −2.5 indicates osteopenia.

Peak bone mass is reached at about 20 years of age and that rate of bone loss at later years dictate risk for osteoporosis.

This is a growing health concern issue with the number of patients with osteoporosis in the United States alone is expected reach 71 million by year 2030. The epidemiology of osteoporosis reflects the importance of age and gender for example, 50% of women will have osteoporosis by 80 years of age. Risk factors also include, inactivity, nutritional low calcium intake, low vitamin D, hypogonadism, Cushing's syndrome, long-term steroid use, rheumatoid arthritis and inflammatory conditions, multiple myeloma, among others.

In inflammatory conditions, inflammatory cells migration to bone surface while producing inflammation mediators such as interleukin-6 and RANKL stimulating accumulation of osteoclasts and thus increased bone resorption.

Diagnosis is by radiological means. However, biochemical markers reveal the degree of bone resorption.

Biochemical investigation is appropriate in a patient with low bone density without an apparent cause (i.e., long-term glucocorticoids therapy). Secondary causes of osteoporosis (increased bone resorption) must be investigated. They include hyperparathyroidism. Hyperthyroidism, diabetes, cortisol abnormalities (excess and insufficiency), growth hormone abnormalities (excess and deficiency), hypogonadism, pregnancy, vitamin D deficiency, calcium deficiency, malabsorption syndromes, alcoholism, drugs (glucocorticoids, chemotherapeutics, immunosuppressants, antiepileptics, progesterone), multiple myeloma, idiopathic hypercalciuria, and immobilization. Similarly, bone infiltration by secondary tumor cells and in inflammatory arthritis leads to increased bone erosions and osteolytic legions. Bisphosphonate is the most widely used antiresorptive therapy.

The risk for osteoporotic fraction is increased in patients with chronic kidney disease, being twice as common in patients with eGFR <60 compared with those >60 mL/min with the hip being more involved than the spine. Hypocalcemia and increased PTH levels are common among patients with deteriorating kidney function leading to abnormal bone formation. Serum calcium does not appreciably decline until EGF is <20 mL/min/1.73 m^2.

Patients with impaired renal function have hyperphosphatemia due to reduced clearance. This leads to increased PTH levels. The latter remain normal until GFR is <45 mL/min/1.73 m^2. The accumulation or uremic toxins down regulates PTH receptors on osteoblasts leading to resistance to PTH and thus to bone fragility. Low vitamin D and 1,25 vitamin D in patients with renal disease does not become apparent until GFR is below 40 mL/min/1.73 m^2. All of those exchanges are associated with renal osteodystrophy which us associated with increased bone turnover. PTH levels >323 pg/mL are indicative of high bone turnover, while PTH <100 pg/mL is indicative of low bone turnover although PTH trend is more reliable indicator of bone turnover.

Therapeutic interventions are to reduce risk of fraction, and they include lifestyle changes as well as treatment of the associated caused such as nutritional deficiencies.

Biomarkers are used to monitor the response in bone formation (alkaline phosphatase and osteocalcin) and bone resorption (urinary calcium and telopeptides).

Rickets—Osteomalacia

Defective mineralization of the bone growth plate in the growing child is rickets and, in the adults, osteomalacia in the preformed osteoid.

With 50%–60% of bone tissue predominant calcium and phosphate and thus adequate availability of those is important. The disorder may be due to calcium insufficiency (calcinopenic osteomalacia) or to insufficient phosphate (phosphopenic osteomalacia). Reduced sun exposure and/or deficient dietary calcium collectively termed nutritional rickets.

For the calcinopenic form, it is a consequence of reduced availability of calcium secondary to vitamin D deficiency. Causes are those leading to vitamin D deficiency (poor intake, poor sun exposure, malabsorption, renal dysfunction).

In vitamin D-dependent rickets type I, 1,25-(OH)$_2$ Vitamin D levels are sufficient, but the active 1,25-(OH)$_2$ Vitamin D form is deficient (renal impairment results in reduced 1-alpha hydroxylase or to a rare genetic deficiency of the 1-alpha hydroxylase enzyme). This is in contrast to vitamin D-resistant rickets type II where both 25-OH and 1,25-(OH)$_2$ vitamin D forms are within the sufficient range and the disorder is due to defect in the 1,25-(OH)$_2$ vitamin D receptor (1,25-(OH)$_2$ vitamin D resistance).

Patients on anticonvulsants therapy exhibit reduced vitamin D levels due to the induced hepatic clearance and metabolism of 25-OH vitamin D.

In hypophosphatemic osteomalacia, the low plasma phosphate is the main cause, commonly associated with renal tubular dysfunction and assayed phosphaturia. Reduced plasma phosphate levels may be encountered in excessive intake of phosphate binders. Other causes of phosphaturia include (hereditary X-linked and autosomal hypophosphatemia rickets) malignancy (mesenchymal cell tumors, chemotherapeutic drugs). Renal tubular damage and thus impaired phosphate reabsorption in patients with Fanconi syndrome, Wilson's disease, cystinosis, heavy metal toxicity (lead), light chain deposition, and autoimmune SLE as well infection in interstitial disease.

Patients with hypophosphatemic rickets will often have sufficient vitamin D levels and are related to impaired phosphate renal tubular reabsorption.

Circulating FGF23 levels are elevated in patients with oncogenic osteomalacia and are associated with low 1,25-(OH)$_2$ vitamin D levels.

FGF23 produced primarily by bone but also by other tissue (thymus, heat, brain). Its production is stimulated by high phosphate levels, and it has a short half-life of 46 min. In its intact form regulates phosphate metabolism. At the renal tubules, it inhabits reabsorption of urinary phosphate by decreasing the expression of type II sodium-phosphate transporter. It also decreases transcription of 1-alpha hydroxylase thus reducing 1,25-(OH)$_2$ vitamin D synthesis and thus decreases phosphate renal and gastric absorption. Decreasing phosphate levels reduces FGF23 expression and thus levels.

Patients with renal tubular acidosis type I and II lead to osteomalacia, the exact mechanism is not fully understood, the acidosis inhibits 1-alpha hydroxylase activity, and that renal tubular reabsorption of phosphate is reduced.

Paget disease

The second more common bone disorder of the elderly, rarely before 35 years of age, affects slightly more men than women. There is geographical variation in prevalence ranging from 2.3% in the United States and 5.4% in United Kingdom. There is a strong genetic component, and mutations of the SQSTM1 gene have reported in up to 40% of patients with familial PDB and up to 10% of those with sporadic disease.

It is characterized by rapid bone turnover resulting in deformity of the affected areas with increase in the number and size of osteoclasts in those areas. The increased osteoclastic activity attracts osteoblasts that increases bone formation. The net effect being a localized area of increased bone turnover (resorption and deposition). This leads to disorganized architecture and associated structural weakness.

Although there is high calcium turnover as much as doubled even with little 10% skeleton involvement, extracellular calcium levels are not affected except in immobilized patients with active extensive disease, or to a concurrent primary hyperparathyroidism, the incidence of which is higher in patients with Paget's disease. There is high incidence of hypercalciuria and of renal stones among patients with Paget's disease.

Decline of the biomarkers following initiation of therapy is an indication of adequate response with the magnitude of reduction 10–15 days following initiation of therapy indicates long-term effect of therapy (bisphosphonates). Lack of early decline in the biomarkers level indicates the need for additional therapy. Decline in alkaline phosphatase is often measured in routine practice 3–6 months after initial to therapy with declining levels indicate response to therapy. The lower the decline in alkaline phosphate activity, the longer the period of remission. And suppression of alkaline phosphatase level well within the reference intervals remains the therapeutic target.

During the initial phase of the therapy while the osteoclastic-osteoblastic activity is still uncoupled, there might be increased calcium deposition into the bone. This results in transient hypocalcemia with increased PTH and $1,25\text{-}(OH)_2$ vitamin D activity leading to increased absorption of urinary calcium and intestinal calcium levels. This corrects the serum calcium level quickly; however, in patients (particularly the elderly and malnourished), they may be both calcium and vitamin D deficient and will require combined supplementation to avoid hypocalcemia. The patients will exhibit hypophosphatemia secondary to the increased PTH activity.

Lack of adequate response to bisphosphonate requires the use of newer therapy modalities such as denosumab the inhibitor of RANKL.

It could be isolated to one area of the bone or affecting multiple bones with the pelvis, vertebrae and the femur being the most affected. Patients presents with osteoarthritis, nerve entrapment, fracture secondary to the fragility of the affected bones.

Although diagnosis is achieved using plain radiographs or computed tomography in equivocal cases, all of the above described bone biomarkers are elevated (Table 3) and can be used to support diagnosis and monitor therapy. Although not all patients exhibit increasing alkaline phosphates levels that exceed the age adjusted upper limit of the reference intervals those increasing levels decline in response to bisphosphonate treatment. Interestingly, patients with skull involvement show the marked alkaline phosphatase activity. With the exception of few patients (10% with limited disease), patients exhibit elevated biomarkers of bone resorption (NTx and CTx) and formation (PINP).

Bisphosphonates are the treatment of choice, and they normalize biomarkers. Makers of bone formation, alkaline phosphatase and procollagen type-I amino terminal propeptide, whereas serum and urine C-terminal telopeptide and urine N-terminal telopeptide are markers of bone resorption. They correlate with bone activity as determined by scintigraphy indices. Additionally, there was no statistical

TABLE 3 Biomarkers of bone resorption and formation (osteoclastic and osteoblastic) activity in patients with primary and secondary bone malignancy and metastasis respectively.

Biomarker	Role
Bone formation biomarkers	
Alkaline phosphatase (bone isoenzyme)	Diagnosis and prognosis of bone metastasis in solid tumors. Risk of skeletal-related events. Prognosis during antiresorptive therapy. Prediction of response to treatment.
Procollagen I carboxyterminal propeptide (PICP)	Diagnosis of bone metastasis in prostate cancer. Prediction of response to atrasentan in prostate cancer.
PINP	Diagnosis of bone metastasis in breast and prostate cancer
Bone resorption biomarkers	
C-telopeptide (CTx)	Diagnosis of bone metastasis in prostate cancer. Prognosis of bone metastasis in breast cancer.
N-Telopeptide (NTx)	Diagnosis and prognosis of bone metastasis in prostate and lung cancer. Risk of skeletal-related events. Prognosis during antiresorptive therapy. Prediction of response to treatment.
Carboxyterminal telopeptide of type-I collagen (ICTP)	Diagnosis of bone metastasis in lung cancer. Prognosis of bone metastasis in breast cancer.
Tartrate-resistant acid phosphatase (TRACP)	Diagnosis of bone metastasis in breast cancer.
Pyridinoline	Prediction of response to atrasentan in prostate cancer.
Receptor activator or nuclear factor kB-ligand/osteoprotegerin (RANK/OPG)	Diagnosis of bone metastasis in solid tumors.
MicroRNAs (miRNAs)	Diagnosis of bone metastasis in breast cancer.

Modified from Clézardin P, Coleman R, Puppo M, et al. Bone metastasis: mechanisms, therapies, and biomarkers. *Physiol Rev.* 2021;101(3):797–855. https://doi.org/10.1152/physrev.00012.2019. Epub 2020 Dec 24. PMID: 33356915.

differences between the biomarkers. PINP, urinary NTx, and bonc alkaline phosphatase have higher correlation with scintigraphy at baseline.

Normal biomarker levels do not rule out the presence of Paget's disease.

Other biomarkers are relatively expensive and not routine offered by most clinical laboratories and are often referred to a reference laboratory, alkaline phosphatase widely available relatively less expensive is widely recommended. It has good correlation with Paget's and good correlation with the other bone biomarkers.

Renal osteodystrophy

Bone disorders are often encountered in patients with chronic kidney disease and those recovering renal replacement therapy (dialysis).

Reduced GFR $<50\,mL/min/1.73\,m^2$ results in mild hyperparathyroidism with elevated PTH secondary to the decreased ionized calcium, and to the reduced 1-alpha hydroxylase activity.

FGF23 contributes to the renal osteodystrophy where phosphate retention in renal failure stimulates FGF23 production, the latter inhibit 1-alpha-hydroxylase, further reducing the $1,25\text{-}(OH)_2$ vitamin D insufficiency. This leads to hypocalcemia and to secondary hyperparathyroidism.

Possible contributors to the metabolic bone disease in chronic kidney disease include the decline in Kloth protein expression (Kloth is a membrane protein expressed mainly in proximal and distal renal tubules), and the decline in expression leads to increase in FGF23 expression. The latter leads to increased urinary phosphate excretion by reducing phosphate reabsorption (phosphate retention in renal failure stimulates FGF23 production). Additionally, FGF23 inhibits 1,1lpah hydrolyze and thus reduces $1,25\text{-}(OH)_2$ Vitamin D synthesis, and similarly, increased phosphate inhibits 1-alpha hydroxylase enzyme activity in the kidney.

Accumulation of uremic toxins (indoxyl sulfate, *p*-cresyl sulfate) reduces the expression of PTH receptors in osteoblasts and is associated with bone resistance to PTH.

Sclerostin produced exclusively by osteocytes and binds to lipoprotein-reporter-related protein-5 (LRP-5) or 6 (LRP-6) and antagonizes the LRP5/6 mediated canonical wingless signaling (Wnt ligands, 19 ligands rich in cysteine residues and a molecular weigh about 40 kDa released as lipid modified glycoproteins), within the osteoblast, in effect inhibiting osteoblastic activity and promoting their apoptosis. It also stimulates osteocalcinogenesis via upregulation of RANKL production by osteocytes. This accumulates in renal failure and leads to bone resorption and has been the target of osteoporosis therapy (monoclonal therapy using romosozumab and blosozumab). DKK1 is a competitive inhibitor against Wnt3a, inhibiting the Wnt-mediated tissue repair process.

Hypocalcemia is common in patients with chronic kidney disease secondary to different factors including reduced $1,25\text{-}(OH)_2$ Vitamin D and impaired calcium renal tubular reabsorption. The hypocalcemia leads to increased PTH secretion and to abnormal bone remodeling. The total serum calcium concentration decreases following phosphate retention, decreased $1,25\text{-}(OH)_2$ Vitamin D (calcitriol) concentration, and resistance to the calcemic actions of PTH on bone during the process of CKD. Serum calcium typically remains normal until eGFR decreases to $20\,mL/min/1.73\,m^2$.

The decreased number and expression of CaSR in the hypertrophied parathyroid glands may be related to the proliferation of parathyroid tissue, resulting in inadequate suppression of PTH by calcium and high PTH even in the setting of hypercalcemia.

Phosphate retention begins early in CKD and plays a central role in the development of secondary hyperparathyroidism by inducing hypocalcemia, decreasing calcitriol synthesis, and increasing PTH gene expression. However, serum phosphate levels are not usually elevated in the early stages of CKD because of a reduction in renal proximal tubular phosphate resorption owing to increased levels of PTH and fibroblast-growth-factor (FGF)23.

Aluminum accumulation in bone has been reported in geographical areas with increased water aluminum content and dialysate water. This has been recognized and is now rare. In addition to being toxic to osteoblasts, aluminum inhibits mineralization at high dosage and accumulation in parathyroid glands results in reduced PTH synthesis.

Osteitis fibrosa cystica

Bone disorder is caused by excessive PTH in patients with primary hyperparathyroidism. It is an advanced manifestation of untreated hyperparathyroidism with incidence of about 15%. There is bone mass loss leading to weakened and deformed bone.

Osteogenesis imperfecta

A group of genetic disorders is leading to low bone mass and increased fragility. Several mutations in the collagen type I genes (COL1A1 and COL1A2) have been identified leading to decreased synthesis and release of type I procollagen.

Hypophosphatasia—Pseudohypophosphatasia

Autosomal recessive disorder, rare Paget-like skeletal disorder. An inborn error of metabolism that is characterized by reduced alkaline phosphatase levels. There is elevation in the pryrodal-5-pohosphate which is specific to hypophosphatasia. In contrast, pseudohypophosphatasia alkaline phosphatase is within normal limits.

The disorder is characterized by premature loss of deciduous teeth, or osteomalacia and dental problems in adults, and epileptic seizures in the most severe cases. It is caused by accumulation of inorganic pyrophosphate (PPi), abnormal metabolism of pyridoxal-50-phosphate (the predominant form of vitamin B6) and by hypomineralization of the skeleton and teeth featuring rickets and early loss of teeth in children.

Alkaline phosphatase product of the gene ALPL (alkaline phosphates liver) also known as (TNSALP—tissue nonspecific alkaline phosphatase) is produced in the skeletal, liver, kidney, and developing teeth. Isoforms arise following posttranslational modification. Subjects with hypophosphatasia have generalized deficiency of TNSALP activity and suffer from defective bone mineralization (rickets or osteomalacia), yet placental and intestinal ALP isoenzyme activity is normal. The most severe cases are lethal in infancy, with virtually complete absence of L/B/K ALP in all tissues.

Metastatic tumor

Effect of neoplasm on bone structure and activity is related to either tumors of the bone tissue or distant tumors metastasizing the bone. Hypercalcemia and pathological fractures are common features of bone associated malignancy.

Metastasis of neoplasm is inefficient profess in addition to the required transformation from epithelial to mesenchymal cell to be able to invade surrounding tissue and enter the microvasculature with only 0.02% of neoplasm entering the circulation produce clinical detectable metastasis. However, metastasis is responsible for 90% of cancer-associated mortality.

Bone is a common site for metastasis which occurs in in more than 1.5 million cancer patients worldwide (breast cancer most common about 73%, followed by prostate at 68%). Neoplastic infiltration with osteoclastic bone resorption.

Mixed connective tissue tumors with osteoclast-like giant cells and cartilaginous elements secrete ectopic FGF23 leading to tumor induced osteomalacia.

Plain X-ray is inadequate that will not correctly identify bone metastasis unless it exceeds 50% of an affected bone. Biomarkers of bone resorption and formation maybe used to assess the extent of bone metastasis and response to therapy; however, there significant inter- and intra-individual variability in the biomarkers that limits their value.

PINP is significantly elevated in patients with breast and prostate metastasis with detectable levels about 8 months prior to the first positive bone scintigraphy in patients with prostate malignancy metastasis.

Bone alkaline phosphatase concentration, at least 2.9-fold higher in patients with bone metastasis and that levels significantly correlated with extent of bone metastasis.

RANK/OPG levels are increased in patients with prostate cancer and metastasis to bone. The RANK to OPG ratio is increased in patients with osteolytic activity due to primary bone tumor and secondary metastasis originating in breast, renal, and lung tissue.

NTx a urinary marker of bone resorption is helpful. High levels are associated with prostate cancer and bone metastasis but not in lung metastasis.

Furthermore, patients with high baseline level and those are done decline in response to therapy are associated with poor outcome and prognosis.

NTx levels respond to targeted bone therapy and that reduced levels are associated with improved survival and outcomes (in a Zoledronic acid study).

Circulating microRNA forms (miRNAs) are increased in patients with increased bone activity doe to metastasis compared with normal subjects. They represent potential biomarkers in osteolytic bone metastasis; it is found to be increased in patients with breast cancer and metastasis to the bone.

The utility of the various biomarkers of bone resorption and formation in bone metastasis is shown in Table 3.

Endocrine and end organ dysfunction leading to metabolic bone disease

The pathophysiology of bone disorders is interlinked with endocrine disorders of the parathyroid and thyroid glands (affecting calcium and phosphate), renal dysfunction (affecting vitamin D, nitrogenous metabolites leading to renal osteodystrophy), among others (see later).

Therefore, assessment of disorders of those organs is integral to the investigation of bone pathology. The contributions of the above disorders are discussed separately.

Biochemical investigation of calcium, phosphate, and magnesium disorders

Biochemical investigation of metabolic bone disorders involves the assessment of bone activity (osteoblastic and osteoclastic activities) and assessing the coupled process using bone markers of resorption (NTx and CTx) and those of the formation building blocks (procollagen extension peptides). Increased activity using alkaline phosphatase levels and by assessing function or glands influencing bone metabolism that is the parathyroid gland (PTH), kidney (vitamin D activation), and malignancy-associated makers such as PTHrp.

First-line tests assess calcium status and include plasma albumin adjusted calcium and urinary calcium (assessing degree of urine calcium loss), phosphate, and alkaline phosphatase (indicative of osteoblastic activity). Additional (second line tests) which may be directed by the initial findings include, PTH, 25-hydroxycholecalciferol, 1,25 dihydroxycholecalciferol, magnesium and ionized calcium, urinary hydroxyproline, pyridinoline, and deoxypyridinoline, plasma osteocalcin and parathyroid hormone related protein (PTHrP).

To help understand the role of the various biomarkers, their respective biochemistry is discussed separately below.

Calcium metabolism

Assessment of calcium level and homeostatic dysfunction is one of the initial investigations in bone disorders.

Calcium is the most abundant cation in the human body. In an average 60 kg man, there will be 25,000 mmol (1 kg) of calcium with 99% of calcium is bound with phosphate in the crystalline structure of bone. Hydroxyapatite (calcium phosphate) $Ca_{10}(PO_4)6(OH)_2$ constitutes 65% of the matrix.

The extracellular fluid (ECF) contains 22.5 mmol of calcium with 9 mmol in the plasma. Within the ECF, calcium is present as free ionized calcium and protein bound calcium. It is the ionized calcium which is physiologically important, but most clinical chemistry laboratories will measure total calcium.

Normally, total circulating calcium levels in adults range between the serum 2.15 and 2.60 mmol/L (8.6–10.4 mg/dL; 4.3–5.2 mEq/L). Free or ionized calcium normal values range between 1.17 and 1.33 mmol/L.

The major calcium binding protein present in plasma is albumin and changes in albumin concentration will affect total calcium levels independently of the ionized calcium. A formula can be used to adjust the calcium measured for changes in albumin concentration.

Binding of calcium to proteins is dependent upon pH since the number of negative charges on proteins varies with hydrogen ion concentration. Acidosis increases ionized calcium, and alkalosis reduces ionized calcium.

About 45% of circulating calcium is bound to predominantly plasma proteins, mainly albumin. The reminder is a free ionized calcium (45%) form which is the readily available for cellular activity. A minor component (10%) of circulating calcium is complexed with anions such as phosphate and citrates.

Changes in circulating protein levels influence total calcium levels, whereas ionized calcium is not affected. Therefore, in patients with marked changes in protein concentration, hypoalbuminemia, hyperglobulinemia, in patients with hepatic and renal dysfunction.

Measured total calcium levels can be adjusted for changes in albumin concentration. The formula most widely used being total calcium plus 0.02 (40 − albumin level) when calcium is reported in mmol/L and plus 0.8 (4.0 − albumin level) when reported in mg/dL units.

Ionized calcium measurement requires careful sample collection and handling to maintain the acid-base status of the sample. This is necessary as changes in blood pH can alter the equilibrium constant of the albumin-ionized calcium binding. Acidosis causing a displacement of ionized calcium and alkalosis enhances its binding to albumin. Therefore, at altered acid base status and at extremes of albumin concentrations, measurement of ionized calcium is preferred.

Hypercalcemia

Defined as serum calcium >10.4 mg/dL (2.60 mmol/L) is a common finding the setting of ambulatory primary care (about 1%) and inpatient hospital population (about 1%–4%). The prevalence is variable and depends on the cause of the hypercalcemia. Primary hyperparathyroidism and malignancy represent about 90% of the causes of hypercalcemia.

Hypercalcemia due to hyperparathyroidism, most common among adults greater than 65 years old, has a prevalence of 1–7 cases per 1000 adults and an annual incidence ranging from 0.41 to 21.6 cases per 100,000. Primary hyperparathyroidism being the predominant cause in the general population with malignancy being the predominant cause among hospital population. The diagnosis of hypercalcemia is made when the albumin corrected calcium concentration is two standard deviations above the mean normal value in at least two samples that are at least 1 week apart over a period of 3 months. Symptomatic patients present with nausea, vomiting, mental disturbance, depression, polyuria, abdominal pain (peptic ulcer, renal colic), constipation, bone pain.

When investigating causes of hypercalcemia, it helps to define the cause as either PTH related or non-PTH hypercalcemia. The finding of an elevated PTH level or PTH level that is not appropriately suppressed in the presence of hypercalcemia indicates possible hyperparathyroidism. Additionally, mildly elevated calcium is often seen in patients with hyperparathyroidism this is in contrast to the markedly elevated calcium in patients with hypercalcemia of malignancy (non-PTH). Non-PTH-related hypercalcemia includes vitamin D toxicity, thyrotoxicosis (thyroid hormones stimulate RANK-ligand-mediated bone resorption), adrenal insufficiency, pheochromocytoma (part of the multiple endocrine neoplasia type II, some secrete PTH-related peptide, and/or directly stimulating bone resorption), certain drugs such as thiazide diuretics (in about 8% of patients, increased renal reabsorption of calcium resulting in hypercalciuria), and lithium (stimulating PTH secretion and thus increased renal calcium reabsorption), supplementation with calcium and vitamin D in patients with renal failure, and therapeutic recombinant PTH. A familiar form characterized by hypocalciuric hypercalcemia due to genetic abnormalities in calcium sensing and thus continued PTH action at the kidney with continued reabsorption of filtered calcium. Other causes of mild hypercalcemia include prolonged immobilization (prominent when there is high bone turnover such as in young persons) (Table 4).

TABLE 4 Classification, causes of hypercalcemia, and associated biochemical measurements.

Hypercalcemia causes	Disorders	Biochemical findings
PTH-related		
Hyperparathyroidism	Adenoma, hyperplasia, carcinoma, secondary, and tertiary hyperparathyroidism. Familial hypocalciuric hypercalcemia. Ectopic PTH	Elevated PTH (includes mildly elevated and within normal limits in the presence of hypercalcemia), i.e., inappropriate PTH levels for the calcium levels. Low urinary calcium in the presence of malignancy associated hypercalcemia (rare)
Non-PTH related		
Malignancy		
	Humoral hypercalcemia of malignancy. Osteolysis (bone metastatic involvement)	PTHrp (PTH-related peptide) [lung, esophagus, skin, cervix, breast, kidney]
Endocrine causes	Thyrotoxicosis Adrenal insufficiency Pheochromocytoma Vasoactive Intestinal Peptide (VIPoma)	Elevated thyroid hormones with suppressed TSH Elevated metanephrines Elevated VIP
Vitamin D related	Vitamin D intoxication Granulomatous disease (sarcoidosis, tuberculosis, histoplasmosis, etc.)	25(OH)D levels are markedly elevated 1,25-$(OH)_2$ Vitamin D levels elevated or within normal limits in the presence of suppressed PTH and PTHrp/ (Increased 1-alpha hydroxylation of 25-(OH) vitamin D) [lymphoproliferative and granulomatous]
Drugs		
	Lithium, thiazide diuretics, recombinant PTH, calcium, and antiacids	Lithium PTH
Other causes		
	Immobilization Renal dysfunction	Creatinine/BUN

Modified from Minisola S, Pepe J, Piemonte S, Cipriani C. The diagnosis and management of hypercalcaemia. *BMJ.* 2015;350:h2723. https://doi.org/10.1136/bmj.h2723. PMID: 26037642.

Hypercalcemia in malignancy is due to either production of PTH-related peptide (PTHrp) by the tumor, typically squamous carcinoma's, or infiltration by the tumors and local osteolysis, mostly seen in hematological malignancy. Additionally, malignant cells and granulomas overexpress 1-alpha hydroxylase which increases the conversion of 1,25-$(OH)_2$ vitamin D to the active form 1,25-$(OH)_2$ vitamin D (calcitriol) leading to increased intestinal absorption of calcium and the presence of hypercalcemia and hypercalciuria.

Investigations of hypercalcemia

Hypercalcemia is defined as serum calcium two standard deviations above the normal mean calcium levels in at least two samples at least 1 week part over a period of 3 months.[2] Normal calcium levels often range from 2.15 mmol/L (8.6 mg/dL) to 2.6 mmol/L (10.4 mg/dL).

Hypercalcemia is a common finding in ambulatory and hospitalized patients with primary hyperparathyroidism and malignancy accounting for 90% of all cases of hypercalcemia.

This as well as the causes of the remaining 10% require careful investigation.

The finding of hypercalcemia should be repeated in two different occasions within a period of 3 months mild increase in calcium over a very long time could be suggestive of the finding of hypercalcemia should be repeated in two different occasions within a period of three months mild increase in calcium over a very long time could be suggestive of primary hyperparathyroidism, whereas an acute rise in calcium levels over a short period of time is suggestive of malignancy as the cause. Therefore, clinical assessment guides the subsequent investigations for the hypercalcemia.

A stepwise diagnostic approach in the investigation of hypercalcemia is recommended (Fig. 6).

In outpatient settings, the finding of hypercalcemia needs to be confirmed by remeasuring serum calcium levels and correcting for albumin, or by measuring ionized calcium if available.

The finding of elevated PTH or unsuppressed PTH in the presence of hypercalcemia is indicative of primary

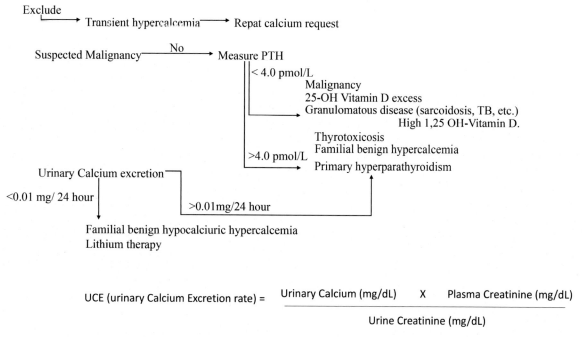

UCE (urinary Calcium Excretion rate) = $\dfrac{\text{Urinary Calcium (mg/dL)} \quad \text{X} \quad \text{Plasma Creatinine (mg/dL)}}{\text{Urine Creatinine (mg/dL)}}$

FIG. 6 Flow diagram showing a stepwise investigation of hypercalcemia. *(Modified from Tonon CR, Silva TAAL, Pereira FWL, et al. A review of current clinical concepts in the pathophysiology, etiology, diagnosis, and management of hypercalcemia. Med Sci Monit. 2022;28:e935821. https://doi.org/10.12659/MSM.935821. PMID: 35217631; PMCID: PMC8889795.)*

hypothyroidism and the finding of hypophosphatemia supports the diagnosis.

Finding of suppressed PTH in the presence of hypercalcemia indicates malignancy which is confirmed by the presence of elevated PTH-related peptide (PTHrp).

Increased 1,25-(OH)$_2$ vitamin D in the presence of hypercalcemia suppressed PTH, and PTHrp indicates the presence of granulomatous disease.

Reduced renal calcium clearance evident by calcium creatinine ratio less than 0.01 in the presence of hypercalcemia suggest the presence of familial hypocalciuric hypercalcemia.

Management of hypercalcemia includes establishing the cause, rehydrating with 0.9% sodium chloride, use of calcitonin (inhibits bone resorption and dresses renal tubular reabsorption—short lived, action onset within 2h and drug tolerance reached with 2days), phosphate, and glucocorticoids as well as bisphosphonates (inhibit osteoclast activity). Denosumab fully humanized monoclonal antibody binds to RANK-like ligands and inhibits the maturation, activation, and function of osteoclasts. Prednisolone inhibits 1-alpha hydroxylase and activates 24-hydroxylase thus directing vitamin D hydroxylation to the inactive 24,25 (OH)$_2$ vitamin D.

Other causes of hypercalcemia

Other causes of hypercalcemia include dehydration which can be considered as false hypercalcemia due to the increase in album and concentration ionized calcium is within normal range.

Prolonged immobilization leads to hypercalcemia secondary to increased bone resorption. It is more evident in young growing adults. Patients with acute renal failure secondary to rhabdomyolysis exhibits hypercalcemia in the presence of hyperphosphatemia.

Hyperparathyroidism

Primary hyperparathyroidism is the most common cause of hypercalcemia. Single parathyroid adenoma being the most common. Double adenomas are present in 15% of cases whereas multiglandular adenomas are present in 10%–15% of cases. Primary hyperparathyroidism has an estimated prevalence of 1–7 cases per 1000 adults. The incidence primary hyperparathyroidism is poorly defined showing a wide range from 0.41 to 21.6 cases per 100,000 person years. Hypercalcemia of malignancy is observed in 2.7% of patients with cancer in adults and much lower 0.5%–1% in children. Other causes of hypercalcemia include vitamin D excess, thyrotoxicosis, adrenal insufficiency pheochromocytoma. Drugs such as thiazide diuretics and lithium.

Primary hyperparathyroidism, 80%–85% is due parathyroid adenoma, 15% due to primary parathyroid hyperplasia, and <5% to parathyroid carcinoma.

Incidence of parathyroid adenomas peaks in the fifth and sixth decade of life being more common in females with 2:1 female-to-male ratio. Occurring more frequently in lower lobe, it can weigh from 300mg to several grams with size ranging from few millimeters to more than 10cm.

Parathyroid adenoma is found in both multiple endocrine neoplasia syndrome types 1 and 2 with type 1 being more common.

Secondary hyperparathyroidism mostly caused by chronic kidney disease. Hyperphosphatemia, hypocalcemia of renal disease as well as reduced 1,25-(OH)$_2$ vitamin D leads to increased PTH synthesis and release by the parathyroid. Additionally, impaired renal function leads to downregulation of the parathyroid and vitamin D and calcium sensing receptors. Parathyroid hyperplasia, bone disorders are the most clinical complication as well as cardiovascular disease.

Prolonged secondary hyperthyroidism leads to tertiary hyperparathyroidism evident in significant proportion of patients with chronic kidney disease who maintain increased levels of PTH fowling kidney transplant.

Hypercalcemia in the presence of inappropriately high or normal PTH

Clinical symptoms vary from mild to severe. Nonspecific symptoms of fatigue, mild depression, or cognitive impairment. Progressive and long-standing hypercalcemia leads to renal impairment, nephrolithiasis, gastrointestinal disturbances, nauseam peptic ulcer, pancreatitis, bone pain, secondary bone fractures, psychosis.

Parathyroidectomy: Symptomatic patients with or w/o osteoporosis, GFR <60 mL/min/1.73 m^2, Kidney stones, Hypercalciuria, <50 years old and calcium increased by 1 mg/dL above ULN. Note: PTH not included in the decision criteria. Required for discrimination between PHPT and other causes.

Assay performance is important for normo-calcemic hyperparathyroidism. Distinguish between parathyroid carcinoma and benign disease. Posttranslational modification (12–18 aa region) seen in carcinoma is detected by third generation assays gives lower value compared to second generation assays. Ratio > 1 suggestive of parathyroid carcinoma (lack of assay standardization, posttranslational modification present in healthy and patients with primary HPT or CKD).

Secondary HPT (elevated PTH in patients with chronic kidney disease, due to hyperphosphatasemia, hypocalcemia, low 1,25-(OH)$_2$ vitamin D and high FGF23). Detects renal osteodystrophy. C-terminal fragments accumulate.

PTH assays have evolved from that of the first generation detecting the 84 amino acid PTH molecule in addition to C-terminal fragments that accumulate in patients with renal impairment (carboxy terminal fragments accumulate in renal failure). Falsely elevated PTH levels in patients with renal impairment. A second generation assay developed (known as the Nichols institute intact PTH assays two set of antibodies are used as compared to the first generation assays that employed a single antibody set up,

the capture antibody is directed against the C-terminal and the detection (signal antibody was directed against the 1–34 amino acid terminal). Thus, only the intact molecule 1–84 is detected in theory; however, the assays took 24 h an improvement on the first assay that took 7 days (competitive assays). Successive improvements in the second generation assay lead to short incubation with results available within 20 min, commonly use assays, the finding of nearly intact PTH molecule (missing the 4–7 amino acids) but still detectable by the second generational assays and accumulated in patients with renal dysfunction. PTH was elevated out of proportion of bone disease in patients with elevated PTH and renal dysfunction, and this leads to the development of the third generational immunoassays targeted the 1–4 amino acids, and thus, in theory, only intact PTH is now measurable. However, although more accurate, they have not been shown to improve the diagnosis of bone disease in secondary hyperparathyroidism, similarly there does not seem to be a difference in the diagnostic sensitivity of primary hyperparathyroidism in patients with normal kidney function. That is second generation may be used in patients without renal dysfunction, second generation which suffered from interference of PTH fragments accumulating in patients with reduced glomerular filtration, to the third generational assays with improved performance but still has little advantage over the second generation assays. The generational assays are depicted in Fig. 7.

Humeral hypercalcemia of malignancy

Hypercalcemia in malignancy could be due to either production of parathyroid hormone related peptide (PTHrp) by the tumor. Another mechanism where are malignant cells and granulomas can overexpress 1-alpha hydroxylase and thus the over production of 1,25-(OH)$_2$ vitamin D (calcitriol), which results in increased intestinal absorption of calcium leading to both hypercalcemia and hypercalciuria.

Other endocrine causes

Patients with hypothyroidism may exhibit hypercalcemia secondary to increased bone resorption. This is thought to be mediated via RANK ligand stimulated by the increased thyroid hormones. Hypercalcemia secondary to pheochromocytoma is thought to be either related to production of PTHrp activity or to direct bone resorption.

Hypoparathyroidism

Hypoparathyroidism (HPT) is observed in auto-immune syndrome (APS-1), postthyroid surgery (0.6%–6.6%), in states of hypomagnesemia (magnesium required for PTH release and action), in patients with iron excess and tissue deposition (haemochromatosis), patients with copper excess (Wilson's disease), as well as in patients with metastatic infiltration by tumors. Hypoparathyroidim is

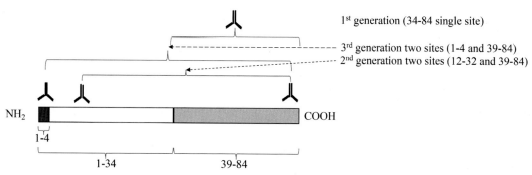

FIG. 7 Generational PTH assays targeted against different amino acid regions of the molecule. In the first generation assays, the polyclonal antibody is directed against the whole PTH molecule and found to cross-react with circulating PTH fragments, the second generation assays employs monoclonal antibodies (capture at the C-terminal and detector at the 1–34 amino acid terminal), this assay cross-react with nearly intact-PTH losing 4–7 N-terminal amino acids found to accumulate in patients with impaired renal function, the third generation assays employs two monoclonal antibodies one captured directed against the C-terminal portion of the molecule and the detection monoclonal antibody directed against the 1–4 N-terminal amino acids. The latter showed higher degree of specificity to the intact PTH molecule. *(Modified from Couchman L, Taylor DR, Krastins B, Lopez MF, Moniz CF. LC-MS candidate reference methods for the harmonisation of parathyroid hormone (PTH) measurement: a review of recent developments and future considerations. Clin Chem Lab Med. 2014;52(9):1251–1263. https://doi.org/10.1515/cclm-2014-0150. PMID: 24762644.)*

observed in certain genetic disorders such as DiGeorge syndrome (absent parathyroiud glands), genetic abnormalities in, calcium-sensing receptor, and in patients with familial hypoparathyroidism (mutation in the pre-proPTH gene).

Parathyroid hormone (PTH)

Chief cells of the gland secrete PTH as needed (few secretory granules for storage). Ionized calcium regulates PTH secretion. CaSR calcium-sensing receptor. The relationship is not linear. For any given ionized calcium concentration, PTH concentration is lower when the ionized calcium is rising than when it is falling suggesting that it is not the only control mechanism. The hormone exhibits diurnal variation with 50% nadir at 9 a.m., 50% peak at 2 a.m. This is helpful diagnostically, where measurement at 10 a.m. improves the test performance for hyperthyroidism (high PTH levels otherwise would be nadir in normal). The PTH is made up of 115 aa pre-pro-PTH. Hepatic and renal metabolism.

Molecular forms; 1–84 intact, smaller fragments with longer half-life 1–34 N biological activity, 7–84 mid molecule fragment (see Table 5). Accumulates in reduced GFR.

Transcribed as 119 amino acids long, pre-pro PTH, undergoes sequential cleavages to 90 amino acids pro-PTH and finally the format detected in circulation 84 amino acid PTH. The pre-pro and pro forms are not detectable by immunoassays.

Circulating intact 1–84 PTH is metabolized by the liver and kidney and cleared quickly from the circulation with 2–4-min half-life. Several molecular forms of PTH complicates its accurate measurement via interference in immunoassays and even LCMSMS (oxidized and phosphorylated forms),

PTH released in response to decreased ionized calcium, levels increases circulating calcium levels by stimulating bone resorption, reabsorption of renal filtered calcium, and stimulates 1-alpha hydroxylation of 25-(OH) vitamin D to the active 1,25-(OH)$_2$ vitamin D which facilitates renal and intestinal absorption of calcium.

It is of concern that PTH fragments accumulate in patients with impaired renal function and those interfere in the various immunoassays, and the very same patients they require assessment of renal osteodystrophy. It has been suggested that depending on the assay. Used, intact 1–84 PTH

TABLE 5 Molecular forms of PTH, their relative circulating concentration and half-life.

PTH molecule	Activity	Concentration	Half-life T1/2 (min)
Intact (1–84 aa)	Most (18%)	1–5 pmol/L	2.92 (±0.13)
C-PTH		5–20×intact PTH	Long
Mid-molecule		5–20×intact PTH	Long
7–84 aa	(44%–50%)	–	–

Modified from several sources including Henrich LM, Rogol AD, D'Amour P, Levine MA, Hanks JB, Bruns DE. Persistent hypercalcemia after parathyroidectomy in an adolescent and effect of treatment with cinacalcet HCl. *Clin Chem.* 2006;52(12):2286–2293. https://doi.org/10.1373/clinchem.2006.070219. Epub 2006 Nov 14. PMID: 17105782.

accounts for just 20% of the circulating forms in normocalcemic patients and a mere 5% of total PTH in patients with end-stage renal impairment.

The non-1–84 PTH fragments due to cleavage in the N-terminal 1–7 amino acids cross-react in the second generation assay and accumulate in patients with renal impairment representing up to 60% of the total immunoreactive PTH. This finding lad to the development of the third generation assays often termed "whole PTH assays."

PTH measurement

Ideal (to date) maker of metabolic bone disorders. Intact (1–84 amino acid) PTH is preferred. It is used in three scenarios: hyper and hypocalcemia investigation, secondary hyperparathyroidism (hypocalcemia, hyperphosphatasemia, vit D deficiency) (CKD, bariatric surgery), intraoperatively and postparathyroid surgery.

Immunoreactivity: first generation assays: Although using single polyclonal antibody that detects the 84 PTH molecule, it also cross-reacts against the C-terminal nonbioactive fragments that accumulate in patients with reduced renal clearance. The second generation assays, developed in collaboration with the Nichol's institute, and hence sometimes referred to as the Nichol's assays, employs two monoclonal antibodies, a capture antibody directed against the C-terminal half of the molecule 39–84 and a detection antibody directed against the first amino half 1–34. This is the most widely used assay in current practice with formulations in automated analyzers providing results within 20 min and thus facilitating intraoperative assessment of PTH levels (see later). The finding of elevated second generation PTH assay in some patients with renal dysfunction and are discordant with bone status suggested the presence of additional interference. The discovery of a nearly intact PTH variant with 4–7 amino acids missing but remained detectable in the third generation assays lead to the development of a third generation assays where the capture C-terminal antibody is the same, but the N-terminal detection antibody is specifically directed against the 1–4 amino acids. This facilitated the detection of only what is termed the biologically active 1–84 PTH, the nicked molecule is not biologically active.

However, there are difference in performance between the third and second generational assays in patients with normal renal function. The cleaved PTH molecule was found in 50% of uremic patients and up to 20% in normal individuals. Relative amount of C-terminal fragment to 1–84 is variable being higher in patients with CKD. Calcium concentration influences the relative ratio, being low ratio in hypocalcemia and high in hypercalcemia.

Automated immunoassays are widely used (9–18 min). There is, however, lack of standardization. Considerable assay variability. However, in most cases its used in trending fold increase above ULN. The lack of standardization, in primary hyperparathyroidism (not an issue precise concentration is irrelevant), second hyperparathyroidism (Renal) Rx at two to ninefold increase, and iPTH (third generation assay reflect therapy success better than second generation).

Biological activity: 1–34 aa and alpha helical structure. C-fragments do not bind PTH1R. Measurement by LCMSMS: Specific, Sensitive (pending), Influenced by the enrichment method (antibody used (C-Terminal)), requires Tryptic cleavage (arginine or lysine), i.e., 1–13 aa fragment denotes iPTH, 7–84 fragment not detected by LCMSMS.

There are plasma/serum differences (EDTA-plasma). CV biological: 20% in normal and 30% in CKD, thus the CD being 54% and 72% respectively.

There appear to be race-related stratification in circulating PTH levels as it is higher in AA. Similarly, PTH associated with BMI, PTH increase with age, 20% lower in Vit D sufficiency.

PTH assays are subject do interference by heterophile antibodies and human antimouse antibodies (HAMA). Elevated immunoglobulins in patients with autoimmune disorders and high autoantibodies such as rheumatoid factors are known as heterophile antibodies. Circulating antimouse antibodies (often seen in patients being treated by OKT3, an immunosuppressant drug used to treat acute transplant rejection). Use of HAMA blocking agents or the use of alternative assays that employs antibodies raised in other species such as rabbit and goat polyclonal antibodies.

LCMS-based quantitative PTH methods utilize immunoaffinity extraction with a C-terminal anti-PTH capture antibody immobilized onto a solid phase (beads or pipette tips). Nonspecific.

Binding removed following several washing cycles and the captured 1–84 PTH and related fragments digested using trypsin. Selected tryptic peptides are then quantified using LC-MS/MS.

Absolute quantification is carried out by preparation of calibration standards using recombinant human 1–84 PTH. Further analysis of PTH and related variants using high-resolution MS, without prior digestion, is necessary, but is especially challenging LCMS methods have the capacity to not only identify, but also quantify, PTH fragments. Reference materials for PTH fragments as well as PTH1–84 are therefore required.

Perioperative PTH measurement

Decline by at least 50% in PTH levels 10 min following resection indicates successful resection of parathyroid tissue.[3] Third generation assay performs better (as second generation detect C-terminal fragments (longer half-life), i.e., more rapid decline (more pronounced in CKD). In secondary hyperparathyroidism, it takes longer for PTH to drop 50% at 10 min for third gen assays, 15 min for second gen assay). PTH >15 pg/mL at 20 min postsurgery eliminated close monitoring of calcium for possible postsurgical hypoparathyroidism. Use the same assay for perioperative and postsurgical studies.

With the availability and use of intraoperative PTH the decision to conclude the parathyroid surgery following removal of one or more enlarged glands avoids subjectively and afforded an objective assessment of removal of the offending gland rather than reliance on visual appearance where a normal looking gland might be hyperfunctioning.

Klotho and fibroblast growth factor-23

Klotho and fibroblast growth factor-23 (FGF23) are expressed in many tissues including the kidney. Bone and the parathyroid. Via binding to its complex Klotho-FGF receptor 1-c splicing form (FGFR1c), FGF23 acts on the parathyroid gland to decrease PTH mRNA and thus circulating PTH levels. It also acts on the kidney proximal tubules to suppress phosphate reabsorption and on renal 1,25-$(OH)_2$ vitamin D synthesis.

In patients with chronic kidney disease, both PTH and FGF23 levels are increased. This may be a reflection of decreased renal clearance, secondary to hyperphosphatemia. It also suggests parathyroid resistance to FGF23 supported by finding of decreased Klotho-EGFR1c complex in parathyroid glands in patients with end-stage kidney disease.

Hypocalcemia

Hypocalcemia defined as calcium <7.2 mg/dL (1.80 mmol/L). It occurs in about 5%–8% of hospitalized patients mostly associated with low albumin levels.

Patients present with paresthesia, numbness, tingling, behavioral disturbance, tetany, convulsion, and cataracts in chronic hypocalcemia.

Causes of hypocalcemia include hypoparathyroidism, vitamin D deficiency, hypomagnesemia (reduced PTH activity). The investigation of hypocalcemia requires stepwise and systematic approach (Fig. 8).

Measurement of calcium

Total Calcium: o-cresolphthalein complexone (o-CPC) [in alkaline condition gives violet colored complex]. Protein binding: Albumin, Other proteins (immunoglobulins). Albumin (the most predominant) Adjusted Calcium (mg/dL) = Total Calcium + 0.8(4 − [albumin (g/dL]). Ionized calcium is measured using ion-selective electrode (ISE) and requires maintenance of the sample acid base status and rapid analysis.

Total calcium is widely and easily measured in automated chemistry analyzers and is component of both the basic and metabolic panel profiles. Total calcium reacts with o-cresolphthalein complexone in alkaline conditions giving a violet-colored complex, the intensity of which is proportional to the total calcium levels. Although the ionized form is the diffusible active form, it is analytically less convenient to measure requiring special sample precautions. Changes in blood pH alters the equilibrium constant of the albumin-ionized calcium fraction. Hydrogen ions displaces ionized calcium from protein binding and thus the sample acid-base status must be maintained to reflect

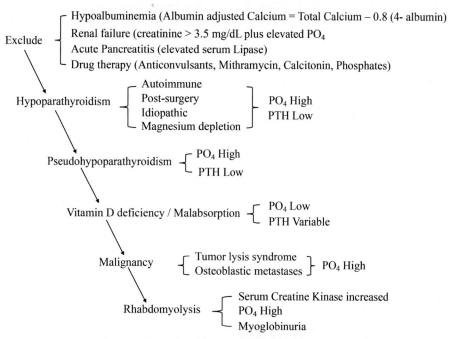

FIG. 8 Flow diagram showing stepwise investigation of hypocalcemia. (*Modified from various sources including Pepe J, Colangelo L, Biamonte F, et al. Diagnosis and management of hypocalcemia. Endocrine. 2020;69(3):485–495. https://doi.org/10.1007/s12020-020-02324-2. Epub 2020 May 4. PMID: 32367335.*)

circulating levels. Samples for ionized calcium are handled as for a blood gas specimen. A whole blood sample in the presence of heparin as anticoagulant, filling the tube to avoiding trapped air bubbles, and avoid delay in analysis by prompt transportation to the laboratory and analysis. Thus, measurement of ionized calcium is recommended when there are major changes in blood pH.

Phosphate homeostasis

Phosphorus being in its organic or inorganic form is a major constituent of all tissues and play vital roles in structure and in metabolism. It is incorporated into phospholipids of cell membranes and nucleic acids. Inorganic phosphate is a major constituent of hydroxyapatite of the bone serving as a body store for phosphate. It is present in phosphoproteins involved in metabolism in high-energy metabolism. Examples being ATP, creatine phosphate and in phosphoproteins involved in high energy metabolism such as muscle contraction, neurological functions, and electrolytes transport.

It is involved in many biochemical reactions and in cell signaling and metabolism examples being phosphate containing (ADP, NAD, cyclic-AMP, cyclic-GMP). It is involved in glucose phosphorylation by glucose-6-phospahte in glycolysis, in delivery of oxygen to tissue ion, and in the formation of erythrocytes 2,3-diphopsphglycerate. Phosphate has an important role as a urinary buffer in its HPO_4^{2-} form were advised to hydrogen ions in the urine.

A healthy adult will contain 630 g (22 mol) of phosphate 85% of which is present in the bone as hydroxyapatite, 10%–15% in skeletal muscle, and <1% in the extracellular fluid.

Dietary daily intake of phosphate is about 50 mmol with small intestinal absorption being higher in its soluble form (within meat) than in its insoluble form (within vegetables), with average absorption being 60%–70% of intake.

Plasma inorganic phosphate varies with diet, exercise, age and demonstrates a marked circadian rhythm. Large changes in PO_4 can be due to redistribution from the ECF to the ICF and vice versa. PO_4 changes may accompany calcium deposition or resorption of the bone. Direct control of plasma PO_4 is achieved mainly by the kidney, where tubular resorption is reduced by PTH. Eighty to ninety percent of phosphate filtered through the glomerulus is reabsorbed in the renal proximal tubules. The amount of phosphate absorbed exceeds the daily requirement and that serum phosphate level is maintained via homeostatic control of intestinal absorption and renal handling of phosphate excretion and reabsorption. Absorption of phosphate in the intestine is attained by either passive transport of phosphate across tide junctions between cells, and that the rate of absorption is directly proportional to the dietary phosphate contents. An active vitamin D-dependent absorption takes place via a sodium-phosphate call transporter expressed in the brush border of enterocytes. The active absorption component becomes important when dietary phosphate content is low. Intestinal absorption of phosphate is reduced in the presence of aluminum hydroxide containing antiacid, glucocorticoids, high magnesium, and in hypothyroidism.

Homeostatic regulation of circulating phosphate levels is influenced by phosphate movement between extraintracellular compartments. This transcellular movement is enhanced by respiratory alkalosis and by insulin.

Hormonal control of phosphate homeostasis is shown in Fig. 9. PTH has a phosphaturic effect by reducing the number of phosphate transporters in the proximal renal tubules. It stimulates the internalization and degradation of the sodium phosphate transporters.

The active form of vitamin D (1,25-(OH)₂ vitamin D) enhances intestinal absorption of phosphate by upregulating the sodium phosphate transporter. Its role in renal tubules remains unclear but shown to increase renal proximal transporters and thus reabsorption of phosphate.

FGF23 produced primarily by osteocytes and by osteoblast to a smaller extent is central to phosphate and calcium metabolism. Its expression is normally suppressed by phosphate regulating gene present on chromosome X. It has a net hypophosphatemic effect, where it inhibits renal tubular reabsorption of phosphate by suppressing the expression of the sodium phosphate transporters in the proximal renal tubules. Although 1,25-(OH)₂ vitamin D stimulates FGF23 synthesis, the latter enhances breakdown of 1,25-(OH)₂ vitamin D by stimulating CYP 24. FGF23 also inhibits PTH synthesis.

Total phosphate concentration in plasma is 3.9 mmol/L of which only 0.8–1.3 mmol/L is an inorganic phosphate. Ninety percent of the inorganic phosphate is present in a

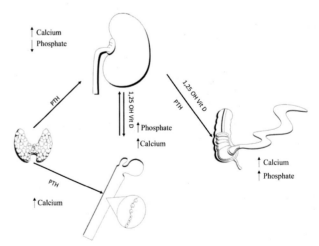

FIG. 9 Metabolism of calcium and phosphate via PTH and 1,25-(OH)₂ Vitamin D effect on the kidney, bone, and intestine. *(Modified from Leung J, Crook M. Disorders of phosphate metabolism. J Clin Pathol. 2019;72(11):741–747. https://doi.org/10.1136/jclinpath-2018-205130. Epub 2019 Aug 29. PMID: 31467040.)*

free form, 6% is complexed with calcium magnesium whereas, 10% is protein bound. Under normal acid base status, the majority of the free and organic phosphate is in the HPO_4^{2-} form compared to $H_2PO_4^-$ in a 4:1 ratio. The ratio decreases under acidic states and increases in alkaline states.

Hyperphosphatemia

The incidence of hyperphosphatemia among hospitalized patients without end-stage renal disease is reported to be about 12%. Among patients with renal disease who are on dialysis the incidence of hyperphosphatemia is 50%–74%.[4] Acute severe hyperphosphatemia when associated with symptomatic hypercalcemia can be life-threatening. Phosphate levels bind to calcium causing precipitation and deposition of calcium phosphate in soft tissues leading to calcification this may occur in any organ including the myocardium, lungs, liver, skin, cornea, and conjunctiva. Vascular calcification can produce a syndrome of systemic calciphylaxis.

Causes of hyperphosphatemia falls into the following categories, transcellular shift, decreased renal excretion, acute phosphate load, and artifactual hyperphosphatemia due to preanalytical and analytical factors (Fig. 10).

Preanalytical factors contributing to false hyperphosphatemia include hemolysis due to either poor sample collection or delayed sample processing due to intracellular phosphate leakage from erythrocytes.

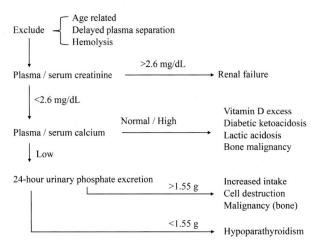

FIG. 10 Flow diagram of stepwise investigation of hyperphosphatemia. Reduced renal clearance, hypoparathyroidism, and increased intake and intracellular leakage are common causes. *(Modified from Leung J, Crook M. Disorders of phosphate metabolism. J Clin Pathol. 2019;72(11):741–747. https://doi.org/10.1136/jclinpath-2018-205130. Epub 2019 Aug 29. PMID: 31467040. García Martín A, Varsavsky M, Cortés Berdonces M, et al. Phosphate disorders and clinical management of hypophosphatemia and hyperphosphatemia. Endocrinol Diabetes Nutr (Engl Ed). 2020;67(3):205–215. [in English, Spanish]. https://doi.org/10.1016/j.endinu.2019.06.004. Epub 2019 Sep 26. PMID: 31501071.)*

The presence of excess immunoglobulins seen in patients with multiple myeloma, Waldenström's macroglobulinemia interfere with the phosphate phosphomolybdate complex formation, or possibly by phosphate binding to the negatively charged paraproteins. This is however not seen in all patients with multiple myeloma.

The most common cause of hyperphosphatemia is renal impairment. However, in early renal impairment, phosphate concentrations are often within normal levels by initial elevation of FGF23 which decreases proximal tubular reabsorption. Significant hyperphosphatemia is observed once the GFR is below 20%–30% of normal or below 30 mL/min. Reduced GFR leads to decreased secretion and increased retention of phosphate. Impaired renal synthesis of $1,25\text{-}(OH)_2$ vitamin D leads to secondary hyperparathyroidism seen in patients with kidney disease which results in increased osteoclastic bone resorption and the release of calcium and phosphate. Acidosis seen in patients with renal failure causes transcellular shift of phosphates from cells further contributing to hyperphosphatemia down an electronegativity gradient. This is also observed in patients with diabetic and lactic acidosis.

Excessive phosphate load due to either exogenous or indigenous sources leads to hypophosphatemia and hyperphosphatemia particularly when there is impaired phosphate excretion. Endogenous increase loads of phosphates are seen in patients with cumulative syndrome due to breakage of cells and leakage of phosphate into the circulation, in patients with rhabdomyolysis due to the high content of phosphate in muscles and with hematological malignancies lymphoblast a particularly high in phosphorus.

Exogenous sources of phosphates include ectopic skin applications or from sodium phosphate Animas widely used to treat constipation in both children and adults.

Tumor lysis syndrome is characterized by hyperphosphatemia and hyperkalemia. The hypophosphatemia may be present before chemotherapy due to spontaneous cell death.

Hyperphosphatemia is also seen in patients with vitamin D toxicity due to the increased intestinal absorption.

PTH has phosphaturic affect, and thus, hyperphosphatemia is seen in patients with hypoparathyroidism. Growth hormone and IGF-I increases renal phosphate reabsorption and thus elevated levels seen in patients with acromegaly exhibit mild hyperphosphatemia (Fig. 10).

Elevated thyroid hormones in thyrotoxicosis leads to hyperphosphatemia caused by increased tissue catabolism, bone resorption, elevated thyroid hormones in thyrotoxicosis leads to hyperphosphatemia caused by increased tissue catabolism, bone resorption, and renal phosphate reabsorption. Reduced PTH secondary to the ensued hypercalcemia contributes to the hyperphosphatasemia.

A rare loss of function mutation affecting FGF23 by your activity causes either a reduction in circulating intact levels or end organ resistance in hypophosphatemic familial tumoral calcinosis.

The most common cause of hyperphosphatemia is increased renal reabsorption and reduce glomerular preparation rate glomerular filtration rate. However, common causes being, artifactual hemolysis due to delayed sample separation, renal failure, physiological (pediatrics), increased intake of vitamin D, tissue damage (tumor lysis syndrome), malignancy, and in patients with GH excess.

Hypophosphatemia

Defined as serum phosphate less than 0.8 mmol/L with levels <0.3 mmol/L considered critically severe hypophosphatemia. Incidence among hospitalized patients is 2.2%–3.1%. The incidence is, however, much higher (29%–34%) among patients in the intensive care, 30% among patients with chronic alcoholism.

Among many factors (Fig. 11), hypophosphatemia is mainly due to either transcellular redistribution, most common cause in intensive care patients, decreased intestinal absorption, increased renal, and/or gastrointestinal losses.

Due to decreased intake, or to increased cellular uptake, high carbohydrate diet, therapeutic insulin intake, hungry-bone-syndrome, increased renal excretion, diuretic therapy, magnesium deficiency, Fanconi syndrome, hyperparathyroidism, alcoholism, enteral/parenteral nutrition in malnourished or alcoholic patient, and in patients in diabetic ketoacidosis. Redistribution of phosphate from extracellular space into the intracellular space is the most common cause of hypophosphatemia among intensive care patients.

False hypophosphatemia is observed in the presence of bilirubin levels and in presence of mannitol which binds molybdate.

Increased intracellular pH seen in respiratory alkalosis stimulates phosphofructokinase with increased glycolysis and utilization of phosphate into the intermediate; this leads to shift to phosphate from extracellular to intracellular and to hypophosphatemia.

It is seen in a patient with septicemia liver disease salicylate intoxication head injury heat stroke acute gout and in mechanically ventilated patients.

Administration of insulin and glucose causes a shift of phosphate from the extracellular space to the intracellular and that's a significant decrease in plasma phosphate concentration. Severe hypophosphatemia is seen in patient with nutritional deficiencies following refeeding the severe hypophosphatemia may precipitate cardiac failure and death.

Renal disease causes hyperphosphatemia; however, no phosphate levels are seen in up to 90% of patients in the early period of postrenal transplant and 6%–27% of patients have persistent low serum phosphate levels months or years later.

Primary hyperparathyroidism causes a reduction in the tubular maximum reabsorption of phosphate this leads to an initial increase in phosphate excretion and as a decrease in circulating phosphate levels; however, a steady state is reached and significant phosphate depletion is not seen; this explains the moderately low phosphate level seen in the presence of hypercalcemia secondary to hyperparathyroidism. Hyperparathyroidism secondary to vitamin D deficiency

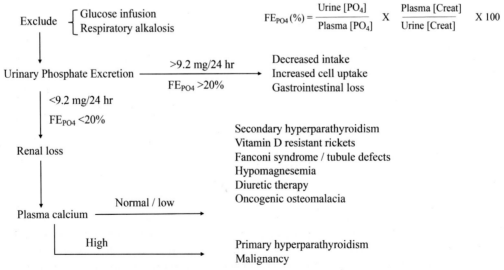

FIG. 11 Flow diagram of stepwise investigation of hypophosphatemia. Urinary phosphate loss is seen in hyperparathyroidism, and renal tubular defects, among other causes. Low urinary phosphate levels in the presence of hypophosphatemia suggest gastrointestinal loss and/or decreased intake. (*Modified from García Martín A, Varsavsky M, Cortés Berdonces M, et al. Phosphate disorders and clinical management of hypophosphatemia and hyperphosphatemia. Endocrinol Diabetes Nutr (Engl Ed). 2020;67(3):205–215. [in English, Spanish]. https://doi.org/10.1016/j.endinu.2019.06.004. Epub 2019 Sep 26. PMID: 31501071.*)

results in hypophosphatemia due to reduce intestinal absorption and to renal phosphate twisting by PTH. A number of rare genetic disorders associated with hypophosphatemia they include X linked hypophosphatemia rickets also known as vitamin D is resistant rickets.

Symptoms and signs of hypophosphatemia vary and are dependent on the severity and the chronicity of phosphate depletion. Moderate and mild hypophosphatemia usually has few clinical manifestations. Moderate and mild hypophosphatemia usually has few clinical manifestation clinical changes such as rickets or osteomalacia are often the only constitute consistent abnormality found.

Weather in patients with severe hypophosphatemia levels less than 0.3 million more per liter; a number of clinical features are seen the range from proximal myopathy tremor seizures confusion and cardiomyopathy congestive heart failure respiratory failure.

Methods of phosphate measurement

Total circulating inorganic phosphate is measured using ammonium molybdate method. Under acid conduction, phosphate binds to ammonium molybdate producing a colorless complex measured at 340 nm or at 600–700 nm after reduction to a colored blue complex. The absorbance at 340 nm is more prone to interference by bilirubin and lipidemia. A vanadate molybdate-based method and an enzymatic method are commercially available, but it's not widely used.

Magnesium metabolism

The second, next to potassium, and fourth most abundant cation in the intracellular compartment and whole body respectively. It is the most abundant divalent cation intracellularly, followed by calcium. The body content of magnesium is 21–28 g with 65% in bone bound to the surface of hydroxyapatite increasing the solubility of phosphorus and calcium, 34% intracellular compartment, and 1% is extracellular. The extracellular magnesium is bound to negatively charged proteins mainly albumin and molecules such as ATP. Normal circulating magnesium levels range from 0.7 to 1.1 mmol/L. It is present in free ionized form, bound to protein, or complexed with phosphates, citrates, bicarbonate, and sulfate. Under normal physiological conditions, 23%–31% is bound to protein, 5%–11% is complexed with an ounce, and 59%–72% is present in the free form.

Ionized magnesium is the biologically active form. When measuring total magnesium, significant changes in total proteins alters the proportion of free ionized magnesium and therefore measuring total magnesium may not represent magnesium status in nephrotic and protein losing enteropathies. Accurate measurement of ionized magnesium is performed by ion selective electrodes (ISE) and is dependent on using an ionophore specific for magnesium.

Magnesium is central to many biological functions. It is an essential cofactor for many enzymatic reactions such as alkaline phosphatase. It plays an important role in carbohydrate metabolism, insulin secretion, proteins, and nucleic acid synthesis. For instance, it is strongly bound to ATP forming a complex that is required for many rate limiting kinases.

Magnesium on influences potassium balance between intro and extracellular compartment by inhibiting potassium chloride "transporters." Magnesium competes with ionized calcium for cellular membrane binding sites and inhibits calcium activity.

Magnesium is central to calcitonin stimulation, parathyroid hormone secretion an action, alkaline phosphatase activity, osteoblast adhesion, and thus bone formation.

The main site for magnesium absorption is the small intestine, renal reabsorption, and negative feedback maintains magnesium homeostasis. High fat, protein, calcium, and phosphate dietary content as well as alcohol decrease the availability of magnesium in diet and reduce its ups and its absorption. Magnesium excretion is mostly vis the kidney and to smaller extent via the skin in sweat.

When using heparin as anticoagulant, it should be at low concentration as it interferes with ionized magnesium measurement, similarly silicon used in vacutainer coating causes falsely elevated ionized magnesium due to a surfactant effect which changes the selectivity of magnesium selective electrode.

Although assays for the measurement of ionized magnesium are commercially available, total magnesium measurement remains the mainstay in clinical laboratories. The need to maintain the acid-base status of the specimen, free ionized magnesium concentration is pH dependent and magnesium binding to protein is increased at increased pH, thus requirement for rapid measurements of ionized magnesium. Lack of standardization among commercial commercially available assays has made measuring ionized a magnesium less favorable.

Plasma levels not reliable indicator of body stores. However, persistent hypomagnesemia may indicate magnesium deficiency. Magnesium abnormality among 5%–10% of hospitalized patients.

Hypermagnesemia

Prevalence is 4%–5% among hospital population. Causes include decreased excretion due to renal failure, increased intake, oral antacid, intravenous magnesium therapy, e.g., in preeclampsia, cell release (in diabetic ketoacidosis), necrosis, and hemolysis.

Hypomagnesemia

The prevalence of hypomagnesemia is 4%–5% among outpatients and is higher up to 11% among hospital population.

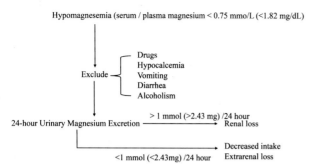

FIG. 12 Flow diagram of stepwise investigation of hypomagnesemia. The presence of high urinary magnesium supports renal loss, whereas low levels suggest reduced intake and/or impaired absorption as possible etiology of hypomagnesemia. *(Modified from Tucker BM, Pirkle JL Jr, Raghavan R. Urinary magnesium in the evaluation of hypomagnesemia. JAMA. 2020;324(22):2320–2321. https://doi.org/10.1001/jama.2020.18400. Erratum in: JAMA. 2021;326(20):2081. PMID: 33125046.)*

Causes of hypomagnesemia include decreased intake, gastrointestinal loss in diarrhea and reduced absorption and in reduced renal reabsorption in acute tubular necrosis and in patients with syndrome of inappropriate ADH secretion. An algorithm for the investigation of hypomagnesaemia is shown in Fig. 12.

Vitamin D

Vitamin D levels are routinely measured in the assessment of calcium homoeostasis. Vitamin D has been implicated in many metabolic pathways with vitamin D receptors expressed in nearly all cell types, at least at some stage of their development.

The vitamin D metabolites circulate in blood extensively bound to two liver-produced proteins, vitamin DBP and albumin. Approximately 85% of this binding is to DBP, 15% to albumin. Given the high affinity of these metabolites for DBP, and the abundance of DBP in normal individuals, free vitamin D metabolite levels are very low (approximately 0.03% of total for free 25-(OH) vitamin D and 0.4% of total for free 1,25-(OH)$_2$ vitamin D). Although the free form is the metabolically active, its measurement is very difficult due to the low concentration. It is however of value in conditions of marked changes in concentration of binding proteins., for instance both vitamin D binding protein and prealbumin are decreased in patients with chronic liver disease and in patients with nephrotic syndrome. Levels of vitamin D binding protein levels are elevated during third trimester of pregnancy.

Circulating 25-(OH) vitamin D in the blood is higher than those of any other vitamin D metabolite and that its level in blood is the best indicator of vitamin D nutritional status because of its relatively long half-life in the blood stream and first-order kinetics in which the rate of 25-(OH) vitamin D production is dependent on vitamin D levels.

Assays for the measurement of vitamin D include immunoassays, liquid chromatography-mass spectrophotometric assay, and competitive protein binding.

Immunoassays suffer from either interference by the different vitamin D forms and by the inability to detect low concentrations. The immunoassays suffer from cross-reactivity with 24,25-(OH)$_2$ vitamin D which can represent up to 10%–15% of circulating 25-(OH) vitamin D. Similarly, some of the 25 and 24,25-(OH)$_2$ vitamin D circulate at much high concentrations when compared to 1,25-(OH)$_2$ vitamin D levels. Sample extraction removing interfering vitamin D metabolites improved the assays specificity and performance; however, sample preparation is time consuming and not often performed.

LCMSM methods available for 25(OH) vitamin D measurements; they suffer from interference by C-3 epimers, and prior sample extraction is required.

In the competitive protein binding assay, the sample is incubated with ruthenium red-labeled DBP to which 25-(OH) vitamin D conjugated with biotin is then added to bind the free DBP. Streptavidin-coated beads are added to bind the 25-(OH) vitamin D biotin conjugate, the beads captured magnetically, and chemiluminescence induced. The concentration of 25-(OH) vitamin D in the sample is inversely proportional to the chemiluminescence signal.

Circulating 1,25-(OH)$_2$ vitamin D levels are 1:1000 fold lower than 25-(OH) vitamin D. It is measured by immunoassays, although the immunoassays are thought to underrecognize 1,25-(OH)$_2$ vitamin D compared to D$_3$. A recently available chemiluminescent assay uses ligand binding domain of vitamin D receptor (VDR) instead of vitamin D binding protein (DBP) and uses a detector monoclonal antibody that detects VDR conformational changes induced by ligand binding. The antibody is attached to magnetic beads. Following washing of unbound material, a detector second monoclonal antibody conjugated to a chemiluminescent label targeted against epitope on the ligand binding domain. The chemiluminescent signal is directly proportional to the concentration of the 1,25-(OH)$_2$ vitamin D levels.

Liquid chromatography-mass spectrometry (LCMS) is used in the measurement of 1,25-(OH)$_2$ vitamin D, however limitations exist due to its low concentration and to the poor ionization efficiency. The specificity limitation is addressed through prior sample preparation by immunoaffinity extraction using antibody to 1,25-(OH)$_2$ vitamin D. Lack of standard reference material for 1,25-(OH)$_2$ vitamin D limits the correlation and standardization of the different immunoassays and LCMS-based assays.

Similar to 25-(OH) vitamin D measurement issues, the presence of circulating C3 beta epimer of the 1,25-(OH)$_2$ vitamin D, and the dihydroxy metabolites 23,25-(OH)$_2$ vitamin D, 24,25-(OH)$_2$ vitamin D, 25,26-(OH)$_2$

vitamin D and the 4-beta,25(OH)$_2$ vitamin D all have the same molecular weight and *m/z* ratio and thus the need for sample preparation by prior separation of the 1,25-(OH)$_2$ Vitamin D before it can be relatively accurately measured. 24,25-(OH)$_2$ vitamin D is often measured as part of a multiprofile by LCMS for 25-(OH) vitamin D and 1,25-(OH)$_2$ vitamin D the C3-beta epimer of 24,25-(OH)$_2$ vitamin D.

Most of these assays used electron spray ionization (ESI) for ionization, triple-quadrupole instruments for MS, and nonspecific water loss transitions for monitoring. Derivatization is often employed to increase sensitivity for the less abundant metabolites in the profile, but PTAD derivatization of 25-(OH) vitamin D was found to interfere with the separation of C3-beta epi-25-(OH) vitamin D from 25-(OH) vitamin D.

A commercial immunoassay is available for the measurement of free 25-(OH) vitamin D. An LCMS method is also available for the measurement of saliva vitamin D which is in its free firm. One milliliter of saliva is deproteinized with acetonitrile, purified using a Strata-X cartridge, derivatized with PTAD, ionized by ESUI, and subjected to LCMS. The assays have a limit of detection of 2 pg/mL and normal salivary levels ranged from 3 to 15 pg/mL.

Summary

- Bone tissue constitutes about 14% of adult body weight. It is metabolically active undergoing continued remodeling.
- Hydroxyapatite is a calcium phosphate Ca$_{10}$(PO$_4$)(OH)$_2$ and constitutes 60% of the bone matrix.
- The organic component contains mainly (90%) collagenous proteins and are predominantly type-I collagen.
- Bone is considered a mineralized connective tissue with four types of cells, namely osteoclasts, osteoblasts, osteocytes, and lining cells.
- Osteoblasts comprise 4%–6% of bone cells and is responsible for bone formation.
- Bone lining cells cover the bone surface where neither bone resorption nor formation is taking place, however, they are responsible for removing nonmineralized collagen fibril and plays a role in stem cell differentiation.
- Osteocytes are the most abundant 90%–95% of total bone cells.
- Osteoclasts are responsible for bone resorption.
- Bone biomarkers reflect the remodeling process activities and thus are used to identify and monitor bone disorders.
- Biomarkers of bone resorption include circulating and urinary collagen cross-link molecules pyridinoline and deoxypyridinoline telopeptides, carboxy-terminal telopeptide (CTx) and N-terminal telopeptide (NTx), and urinary hydroxyproline and hydroxylysine glycosides, hydroxyproline, hydroxylysine, and carboxy- and N-terminal telopeptides.
- Biomarkers of bone formation include (alkaline phosphatase, osteocalcin, procollagen-I extension N-peptide, and procollagen I extension C-peptide).
- Metabolic bone disorders are mostly due to uncoupling of the osteoblastic and osteoclastic activity. They include, osteoporosis, osteomalacia and rickets, and Paget's disease, among other rare disorders.
- Osteoporosis is characterized by abnormal increase in osteoclastic activity uncoupled to bone formation. Bone density is ≪2.5 SD the average.
- Osteomalacia in adults and rickets in children are characterized by defective mineralization of the bone growth plate associate with hypocalcemia.
- Paget's disease is characterized by rapid bone turnover resulting in deformity of the affected areas with increase in the number and size of osteoclasts in those areas.
- Assessment of calcium, phosphate, magnesium, vitamin D levels, and their homeostatic dysfunction is one of the initial investigations in bone disorders.
- Parathyroid disorders play significant role in bone metabolism.
- Decline by at least 50% in PTH levels 10 min following resection indicates successful resection of parathyroid (ademona) tissue.
- Causes of hypocalcemia includes, hypoparathyroidism, vitamin D deficiency, and hypomagnesemia.
- Hyperphosphatemia is commonly due to reduced glomerular filtration rate, increased renal reabsorption (hypoparathyroidism), and to leakage from cells.
- Hypophosphatemia is mainly due to either transcellular redistribution, decreased intestinal absorption, increased renal, and/or gastrointestinal losses.
- Magnesium is central to calcitonin stimulation, parathyroid hormone secretion and action, alkaline phosphatase activity, osteoblast adhesion, and thus bone formation.
- Causes of hypermagnesemia include decreased excretion due to renal failure, increased intake, and due to cell release (e.g., in diabetic ketoacidosis, necrosis, hemolysis).

References

1. Greenblatt MB, Tsai JN, Wein MN. Bone turnover markers in the diagnosis and monitoring of metabolic bone disease. *Clin Chem.* 2017;63(2):464–474.
2. Minisola S, Pepe J, Piemonte S, Cipriani C. The diagnosis and management of hypercalcaemia. *BMJ.* 2015;350:h2723.
3. Rodgers SE, Lew JI. The parathyroid hormone assay. *Endocr Pract.* 2011;17(suppl 1):2–6.
4. Leung J, Crook M. Disorders of phosphate metabolism. *J Clin Pathol.* 2019;72(11):741–747.

Further reading

Appelman-Dijkstra NM, Papapoulos SE. Paget's disease of bone. *Best Pract Res Clin Endocrinol Metab.* 2018;32(5):657–668.

Clezardin P, Coleman R, Puppo M, et al. Bone metastasis: mechanisms, therapies, and biomarkers. *Physiol Rev.* 2021;101(3):797–855.

Sharma U, Pal D, Prasad R. Alkaline phosphatase: an overview. *Indian J Clin Biochem.* 2014;29(3):269–278.

Couchman L, Taylor DR, Krastins B, Lopez MF, Moniz CF. LC-MS candidate reference methods for the harmonisation of parathyroid hormone (PTH) measurement: a review of recent developments and future considerations. *Clin Chem Lab Med.* 2014;52(9):1251–1263.

Arceo-Mendoza RM, Camacho PM. Postmenopausal osteoporosis: latest guidelines. *Endocrinol Metab Clin N Am.* 2021;50(2):167–178.

Whyte MP. Hypophosphatasia—aetiology, nosology, pathogenesis, diagnosis and treatment. *Nat Rev Endocrinol.* 2016;12(4):233–246.

Haji SM, Chipchase A, Fraser WD, Gomez J. Retrospective evaluation of a local protocol used to enhance laboratory savings through minimizing the performance of alkaline phosphatase isoenzyme analysis. *Ann Clin Biochem.* 2019;56(2):298–301.

Bikle DD, Vitamin D. Assays. *Front Horm Res.* 2018;50:14–30.

Chapter 6

Diabetes mellitus and hypoglycemic disorders

Introduction

Glucose, a monosaccharide, a source of cellular energy, its circulating level is normally maintained within a narrow limit, with about 1%–2% intraindividual variability, to prevent hyperglycemia and hypoglycemia, both with unfavorable metabolic and pathological consequences.

Diabetes mellitus is a heterogeneous syndrome characterized by chronic hyperglycemia in which there is a fundamental defect in insulin secretion and or action. On the other hand, hypoglycemia is usually due to imbalance between glucose intake and utility. Causes of hypoglycemia include endocrine disorders, liver disease, gastrointestinal malabsorption, malignancy, insulinoma, drugs, and inborn errors of metabolism.

Uncontrolled or poorly controlled states of hyperglycemia in diabetes mellitus lead to complications such as nephropathy, neuropathy, retinopathy, and vascular circulatory disorders. Landmark clinical trials, namely the diabetes complication and control trial (DCCT) for type I DM and the United Kingdom prospective diabetes trial (UKPDS) for type II DM, have shown that glycemic control is vital to the prevention of complications and in some cases of reversal of early damage.

The clinical laboratory plays an important role in the diagnosis and management of glucose metabolic abnormalities.

This chapter describes glucose metabolism, the pathophysiology of diabetes mellitus, and the role of the clinical laboratory in the diagnosis and management of glucose homeostatic dysfunction.

Glucose metabolism

Carbohydrates have the empirical formula $(CH_2O)n$ where (n) equals 3 or more with glucose, a hexose (n equals 6). Hexoses also include D-Fructose and D-Galactose. Carbohydrates containing an aldehyde group are called aldoses, and those with acetone group are called ketoses (Fig. 1A and B). Glucose is an aldose, whereas fructose is a ketose. Those with free aldehyde or keto groups are reducing sugars and include glucose and lactose. Sucrose and maltose are nonreducing sugars. The reduction ability is characterized by the ability of the sugar to reduce copper (CU^{2+}) to CU^{3+}.

Those characteristics are helpful, for instance a positive reducing test will indicate the presence of either glucose or lactose, and that a corresponding lack for reaction with glucose oxidase (reagent in glucose test strip—see later) indicates that the reducing sugar is likely to be lactose.

Based on the number of the 5-carbon ring, carbohydrates are classified into monosaccharides (glucose, fructose, galactose), disaccharides (mono-mono linked by a glycosidic bond) include sucrose, lactose, and maltose, whereas polysaccharides (multiple 5-membered units) include starch.

Monosaccharides are glucose, fructose, and galactose (Fig. 1A and B). Disaccharides are sucrose, lactose, and maltose, whereas polysaccharides made up of series of monosaccharides (≫mono-mono) give rise to starch.

The disaccharides include maltose (two glucose molecules), lactose (glucose and galactose molecules), and sucrose (glucose and fructose molecules). Disaccharides and polysaccharides are converted enzymatically to monosaccharides for cellular utilization.

Glucose provides energy in the form of adenosine triphosphate (ATP) for cellular activity. One glucose molecule yields 36 ATPs (Table 1). The cellular uptake of glucose is through membrane receptors. There are five different receptors (membrane transporters), namely GluT-1 to GluT-5. These receptors have varied affinity with respect to tissue distribution. They are glycoproteins with molecular weight 55 kDa. GluT-1, GluT-3, and GluT-5 all have low Km (Michaelis constant (Km), an inverse measure of enzyme affinity for its substrate), whereas GluT-4 has intermediate Km and GluT-2 has high Km.

GluT-1, GluT-3 receptors are predominant in glucose-sensitive and insulin-dependent cells such as the brain and erythrocytes. They permit cellular uptake of glucose below the normal fasting range despite low levels of insulin and glucose. GlutT-2 receptors are predominant in cells involved in absorption of increasing glucose concentration intake that are independent of insulin, examples are small intestine, renal tubule, liver and pancreatic cells. GlutT-4 receptors are predominant in cells utilizing insulin-dependent uptake of glucose; examples are muscle and adipose tissue.

Tutorials in Clinical Chemistry. https://doi.org/10.1016/B978-0-12-822949-1.00017-6

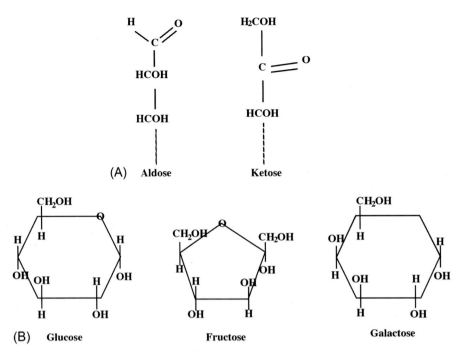

FIG. 1 (A and B) Carbohydrates skeleton structure indicating aldehyde group containing aldose and ketone group containing ketose as well as the monosaccharides glucose, fructose and galactose structures (building blocks for disaccharides) where maltose is made up of two glucose moieties, lactose is made up of a glucose and galactose moieties, whereas sucrose is made up of glucose and fructose moieties. Aldehyde group can be oxidized and thus aldose-containing sugars are reducing sugars. Reducing sugars include glucose, galactose, and fructose.

TABLE 1 Energy production in the form of ATP produced by glycolysis, tricyclic acid cycle (TCA), and electron transport chains (ETC) reactions.

Pathway	Site	Energy input	FADH₂	NADH	Substrate level phosphorylation	ATP count
Glycolysis	Cytoplasm	2 ATP	None	2 NADH	4 ATP	2 ATP
Pyruvate to acetyl-CoA	Mitochondria	None	None	2 NADH	None	None
TCA	Mitochondria	None	2 FADH₂	6 NADH	2 ATP	2 ATP
ETC	Mitochondria		2 FADH₂			4 ATP
ETC	Mitochondria			10 NADH		28 ATP

Modified from Dunn J, Grider MH. Physiology, adenosine triphosphate. [Updated 2022 Feb 17]. In: *StatPearls [Internet]*. Treasure Island, FL: StatPearls Publishing; 2022. Available from: https://www.ncbi.nlm.nih.gov/books/NBK553175/. Bonora M, Patergnani S, Rimessi A, et al. ATP synthesis and storage. *Purinergic Signal.* 2012;8(3):343–357. https://doi.org/10.1007/s11302-012-9305-8. Epub 2012 Apr 12. PMID: 22528680; PMCID: PMC3360099.

In glycolysis, glucose (6-carbon) is converted to two (3-carbon) pyruvate molecules. The initial step being phosphorylation to glucose 6-phospate. Pyruvate enters the tricarboxylic acid (TCA) cycle where it is metabolized to carbon dioxide and water. In this process, NADH and FADH₂ are generated and undergo oxidative phosphorylation in the mitochondria. Electron transfer from NADH and FADH₂ to a series of compounds to oxygen and water. TCA and oxidative phosphorylation yield 34 ATPs (Table 1). The oxidative

and ATP synthesis process is tightly coupled because the availability of ADP controls the rate of oxidation and oxygen availability regulates the rate of phosphorylation.

Anaerobic glycolysis occurs during states of oxygen deficiency. In this situation, glucose cannot be converted to pyruvate. Pyruvate is converted by lactate dehydrogenase to lactate. Only 2 mol of ATP are produced per mole of glucose. Lactate that is produced is transported to the liver where it is converted to glucose (in gluconeogenesis).

Excess glucose is stored inside cells as glycogen (high-molecular-weight polysaccharides). It is made up of several glucose units linked via 1,4 glycosidic bonds, with 1,6 branches occurring approximately every 10 units. Glycogenesis is enhanced by low cAMP and inhibited by high cAMP levels. cAMP levels are regulated by insulin which causes decreased cAMP levels.

In glycogenolysis, glycogen phosphorylase hydrolyzes the 1,4 glycosidic bond producing glucose-1-phospahte which is converted to glucose-6-phospahe and then to glucose (Fig. 2). In gluconeogenesis, glucose-6-phosphate is produced from amino acids, fatty acids, glycerol, and lactate. Pyruvate is an important intermediary in gluconeogenesis since it can be formed directly from lactate oxidation, and from alanine by alanine transaminase (ALT). Glycerol derived from hydrolysis of triglycerides enters the gluconeogenic pathway as glycerol-3-phosphate.

Postprandial glucose load results in hepatic glycogen, triglycerides, and fatty acids synthesis. The rest of the glucose passes to the peripheral tissues. During short-term fasting, glucose requirements are met by hepatic glycogen breakdown and gluconeogenesis from recycling lactate, pyruvate, and gluconeogenic amino acids. Longer-term fasting triggers free fatty acid oxidation as the major source of energy production. Mitochondrial fatty acid oxidation in the liver results in the production of acetyl CoA which ultimately leads to the production of ketone bodies (acetoacetate and 3-hydroxybutyrate). A lack of hepatic thiolase prevents any further hepatic oxidation, and these ketone bodies enter the circulation where they are available for oxidation by peripheral tissues in preference to glucose (reserving this for obligate glucose oxidizing tissues).

In diabetes, lack of insulin and or reduced activity impairs the above metabolic pathways where hyperglycemia presents as either ketotic or nonketotic respectively.

Hormonal regulation of glucose metabolism

A number of hormones regulate glucose metabolism include insulin, glucagon, growth hormone, and cortisol among others (see later). They act by either stimulating glucose uptake and storage of excess glucose or mobilize stored glucose with the end result being maintenance of blood glucose levels.

Insulin

Human insulin is a 51 amino acid yielding a molecular weight of 5805 Da peptide chain with two disulfide bonds (Fig. 3).

Insulin is synthesized within the endoplasmic reticulum of the β cells of the pancreatic islets of Langerhans. It is synthesized as a large precursor molecule called pre-proinsulin which is cleaved almost immediately to give a smaller peptide termed proinsulin (Fig. 3). Proinsulin is packed into granules by the Golgi apparatus and cleaved within the packing vesicles to produce insulin, the cleavage product (C-peptide) remains with the insulin granule and is secreted with it. Thus, insulin release is accompanied by an equimolar release of C-peptide. C-peptide has a longer half-life than insulin, 20 min versus 5 min for insulin, and its concentration is related only to endogenous insulin. Its estimation thus provides the best way to assess β cell

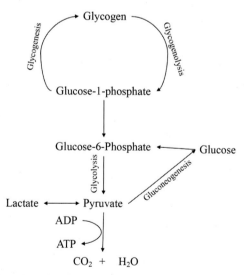

FIG. 2 Schematic diagram showing outlines of glucose metabolism. *(Modified from Rigoulet M, Bouchez CL, Paumard P, et al. Cell energy metabolism: an update. Biochim Biophys Acta Bioenerg. 2020;1861(11):148276. https://doi.org/10.1016/j.bbabio.2020.148276. Epub 2020 Jul 24. PMID: 32717222. Han HS, Kang G, Kim JS, Choi BH, Koo SH. Regulation of glucose metabolism from a liver-centric perspective. Exp Mol Med. 2016;48(3):e218. https://doi.org/10.1038/emm.2015.122. PMID: 26964834; PMCID: PMC4892876.)*

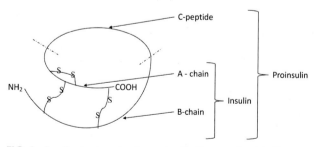

FIG. 3 Insulin structure showing proinsulin (intact molecule). Cleavage (-----) of C-peptide at positions Arg31Arg32 and Lys64AArg65 produces insulin. *(Modified from Mayer JP, Zhang F, DiMarchi RD. Insulin structure and function. Biopolymers. 2007;88(5):687–713. https://doi.org/10.1002/bip.20734. PMID: 17410596.)*

function as well as in the investigation of suspected exogenous insulin-induced hypoglycemia.

Several factors affect insulin secretion including glucose, glycogen, ketone bodies, fatty acids, amino acids, gut hormones, and vagal stimulation. Insulin secretion occurs in two phases. A "fast" phase where stored insulin granules are released and a slow phase of release of newly synthesized insulin. In the fasting state, basal insulin secretion is maintained by neuroregulation and euglycemia. Insulin action is central to the metabolism of carbohydrase, lipids, and proteins (Table 2).

Insulin secretion under normal physiological conditions is released in response to caloric intake and peaking at 30–45 min and subsequently returning to base level 1–3 h later. There is also a flat sustained basal insulin secretion at about 5–15 μU/mL thought to be in response to continued haptic gluconeogenesis which maintains glucose at about 4–5 mmol/L (80–90 mg/dL). In response to a glucose load (meal) which can increase glucose up to 7.5 mmol/L (135 mg/dL), a bolus insulin is released which returns glucose back to fasting levels. Thus, the two insulin release mechanisms maintain glucose levels within the narrow range of 3.5–7.5 mmol/L (63–135 mg/dL). The biological actions of insulin are shown in Table 2.

Insulin binds to its receptor and via series of phosphorylation and activates several intracellular proteins via protein-kinase B which leads to translocation of the glucose receptor GLUT-4 described earlier. Insulin also stimulates glycogen synthase and cell growth all leading to glucose uptake and utilization and thus normalization of blood glucose levels.

Loss of pancreatic β-cells function (due to autoimmune destruction) or to excessive metabolic load such as hyperglycemia, hyperlipidemia, hypoxia, reactive oxygen, etc. as well as toxins and pharmacological agents. Loss of β cells results in gradual loss of insulin production and release leading to unabated hyperglycemia.

Other glucose regulatory hormones

Several hormones in addition to the principal insulin play important roles in glucose regulation, they include glucagon, cortisol, growth hormone, insulin-liker growth factor-1 (IGF-1), catecholamines, gastrointestinal peptide (GIP), somatostatins, and thyroid hormones discussed below.

Glucagon

Synthesized in the α-cells of the pancreas in response to local changes in glucose, insulin, or amino acid concentrations. It is a single chain, 29 amino acids polypeptide, derived from a larger molecular weight precursor. It binds a G-protein-coupled receptor (glucagon receptor) predominantly expressed in the liver and to smaller extent in brain, heart, kidney, gastrointestinal, and adipose tissue.

Glucagon stimulates glucose production (in states of hypoglycemia) and thus counterbalances the effect of insulin. In normal metabolism, glucagon and insulin regulate systemic glucose levels.

Circulating glucagon levels are thus low in the prandial state (~10 pmol/L) and increase by two to threefold in response to long-term fasting or hypoglycemia.

At the hepatocytes, glucagon stimulates adenylate cyclase, cAMP production, and ultimately activation of pyruvate kinase-A, the net effect being increased in gluconeogenesis as well as glycogenolysis with the resultant increase in glucose levels.

In addition to gluconeogenesis and glycogenolysis, glucagon stimulates lipolysis and ketogenesis.

Glucagon secretion is stimulated by thyroid hormones, and high levels are seen in patients with thyrotoxicosis. The latter may contribute to the hyperglycemia seen in hyperthyroidism. Glucagon is elevated in patients with both types of diabetes mellitus, and it is suggested to be due to abnormal secretion of insulin and glucagon part of the bi-hormonal regulation theory for diabetes mellitus. Decreased insulin directly causes increased lipolysis, proteolysis, and decreased glucose utilization (Table 2), and that increased glucagon leads to glycogenolysis, ketogenesis, and gluconeogenesis. Therefore, it must be the dysregulation of both that leads to states of hyperglycemia in diabetes mellitus.

TABLE 2 Metabolic effects can be predicted if insulin is assumed to be the hormone of anabolism.

Carbohydrate metabolism	Lipid metabolism	Protein metabolism
↑ glucose transport	↑ fatty acid synthesis	↑ amino acid transport
↑ glycolysis	↑ triglyceride synthesis	↑ protein synthesis
↑ glycogenesis	↑ lipolysis by lipoprotein lipase	↓ protein degradation
↓ glycogenolysis	↓ lipolysis by tissue lipase	
↓ gluconeogenesis	↓ fatty acid oxidation	
	↓ ketogenesis	

Modified from Vargas E, Joy NV, Carrillo Sepulveda MA. Biochemistry, insulin metabolic effects. [Updated 2022 Sep 26]. In: *StatPearls [Internet]*. Treasure Island, FL: StatPearls Publishing; 2022. Available from: https://www.ncbi.nlm.nih.gov/books/NBK525983/.

There is inadequate suppression of postprandial glucagon in diabetics. Furthermore, exogenously administered insulin does not suppress portal vein glucagon levels. This leads to high glucagon to insulin ratio stimulating gluconeogenesis and glycogenolysis.

Additionally, suppression of glucagon may be an effective adjunct therapy in diabetes mellitus. Emerging glucagon-based therapies include glucagon-G receptor antagonists (in monoclonal antibody format) or those that are agonist to the glucagon-like peptide-1 (GLP-1) which is predominantly expressed in the intestinal L cells and activates GLP-1 receptor. The two (glucagon and glucagon-like peptide 1) are derived from the same precursor proglucagon.

Cortisol

Cortisol produced by the adrenal glands as part of homeostatic mechanism and in response to stress. It increases the rate of hepatic gluconeogenesis from proteins and amino acids and thus leads to a state of hyperglycemia.

Additionally, patients with diabetes (about 45% of patients) are widely known to exhibit diabetes-related stress that leads to increased cortisol production and loss of diurnal rhythm both contributing to the state of hyperglycemia and suboptimal diabetes control.

Furthermore, insulin resistance and impaired secretion occur in patients with elevated glucocorticoids. Diabetes mellitus is a frequent complication of Cushing's disease secondary to the hyperglycemia; furthermore, diabetes mellitus is difficult to control in those patients.

Epinephrine (adrenaline)

Adrenaline produced by the adrenal medulla mediates the counter regulatory mechanism in hypoglycemia. It is central to the fight-flight response where neuroglycopenia activates adrenaline and glucagon secretion.

Adrenaline raises glucose levels by inhibiting insulin secretion and by stimulating glucagon secretion and glycogenolysis and by inhibiting gluconeogenesis.

Furthermore, pharmacologically, epinephrine and glucagon contribute to the recovery from insulin induced hypoglycemia often encountered in patients with type I diabetes mellitus during intensive therapy.

Growth hormone (GH)

Growth hormone is a peptide hormone released by the anterior pituitary in response to stress. It raises circulating glucose levels by increasing rates of gluconeogenesis, glycogenolysis, and proteolysis.

Patients with excessive growth hormone production (e.g., pituitary tumors) exhibit insulin resistance. In contrast, patients with GH deficiency are insulin sensitive and are at risk of developing fasting hypoglycemia.

Thyroxine

Thyroid hormones influence glucose metabolism in a number of ways. For instance, they directly control insulin secretion by pancreatic cells by enhancing β-cells response to circulating glucose levels. Patients with hypothyroidism have reduced insulin secretion in response to glucose whereas, patients with thyrotoxicosis exhibit increased insulin clearance and degradation.

Thyroid hormones increase glucose absorption in the gastrointestinal tract by increasing gastrointestinal mobility. It increases gluconeogenesis in the liver by increasing the phosphoenolpyruvate carboxykinase activity which converts oxaloacetate to phosphoenolpyruvate (C4 to C3), being the committed step to gluconeogenesis. The increased hepatic glucose production increases insulin levels and glucose intolerance associated with peripheral insulin resistance.

Thyroid hormones induces lipolysis in adipose tissue and that the increased production of free fatty acids causes insulin resistance. Additionally, the increased lipolysis and ensued hepatic β-oxidation in the presence of insulin deficiency may lead to ketoacidosis.

Expression of GLUT4 gene in skeletal muscle is increased by thyroid hormones and thus results in increased glucose uptake by skeletal muscles.

Thyroid dysfunction and diabetes mellitus often coexist with both hypo- and hyperthyroidism being common in type II diabetes mellitus.

Insulin like growth factor-1 (IGF-1)

Insulin-like growth factors are proteins produced by the liver with structural homology with insulin, and their activity is regulated by their respective binding proteins. Generally, they promote tissue growth. Two IGFs are of physiological relevance, namely IGF-1 and IGF-2. They circulate bound to IGF binding proteins (IGF-BPs) with five different binding proteins identified, the most relevant being IGF-BP3.

Although GH, discussed above, mediates its action via IGF-1, the mechanism and action of IGF-1 in carbohydrate, lipid, and protein metabolism is distinct where it exhibits an insulin-like effect that reduces glucose levels.

Somatostatin

Somatostatin is a polypeptide hormone produced by the delta cells of the pancreas. It is also produced by the gastrointestinal tract, the hypothalamus, and central nervous system.

It is a pleotropic hormone with many functions but primarily inhibiting both insulin and glucagon release.

The hormone exhibits molecular heterogeneity with a small (14 amino acids long) and a larger (28 amino acid) form. The structural variants appear to express differential tissue specificity where the small molecular weight form acts on brain tissue and the higher variant acts on the gastro-intestinal tract. Somatostatin has a short half-life (1–3 min). It inhibits bile secretion, gastric acid secretion, pancreatic enzymes, cholecystokinin, and vasoactive intestinal peptide (VIP) synthesis. It also inhibits growth hormone, thyroid-stimulating hormone (TSH), prolactin, gastrin, insulin, glucagon, and secretin production.

The actions of somatostatin on those tissue are mediated by a G-protein coupled somatostatin specific receptors. Upon binding and activation of the receptors, there is a decrease in intracellular cyclic AMP and calcium and a concurrent increase in potassium efflux. The overall effect being a decrease in hormone secretion of the target tissue.

Excess somatostatin production in the neuroendocrine tumor syndromes in addition to the clinical presentation of cholelithiasis and steatorrhea (due to pancreatic insufficiency), pancreatic insulin production is inhibited by the high somatostatin levels leading to diabetes.

Pharmacologically, somatostatin analogues have been used in the management of malignancies which contribute to impaired glucose homeostasis such as insulinoma, growth hormone producing tumors, glucagonoma, pheochromocytoma, somatostatinoma, carcinoid tumors, many pituitary adenomas, VIPoma, and gastrinoma. Ultimately, surgical resection of these tumors is curative, but in advanced metastasis or nonsurgical candidates, medical treatment with somatostatin is the preferred treatment. Furthermore, somatostatin exhibits antiproliferative and antiangiogenesis activity and is used to arrest and reverse the neovascularization of the retina seen in diabetic retinopathy, which eventually leads to vision loss if untreated.

Glucose-dependent insulinotropic polypeptide (GIP)

Gastrointestinal hormones incretins include both glucose-independent insulinotropic polypeptide (GIP) and glucagon-like peptide-1 (GLP-1). They are produced by the gastrointestinal enteroendocrine K cells and L cells, respectively. They are rapidly produced in response to glucose, amino acids as well as by food ingestion. Therefore, they play important role in glucose homeostasis.

GIP and GLP-1 are responsible for up to 70% of insulin release after an oral glucose challenge, i.e., the incretin effect. Impairment or absence of the incretin effect is observed in type 2 diabetes.

Several GLP-1-based treatments have been developed and are now available for the management of type 2 diabetes.

Glucose metabolism dysfunction

Normally, fasting glucose levels is maintained at about 4.5–5.2 mmol/L (81–94 mg/dL) while postprandial glucose would normally not exceed 8–10 mmol/L (144–180 mg/dL).

Random nonfasting glucose levels above 11.1 mmol/L (200 mg/dL) are considered hyperglycemic, and levels blow 3.9 mmol/L (70 mg/dL) are considered hypoglycemic values.

Critically low and high glucose levels necessitating immediate medical intervention are often set at <2.2 mmol/L (<40 mg/dL) and >16.7 mmol/L (>300 mg/dL), respectively. Critical values appear on laboratory, and healthcare institutions critical values lists requiring immediate notification by the laboratory to the patient care area (within 30 min) and for the patient care area to record corrective action taken with 30 min of notification.

Metabolic basis of diabetes mellitus

Diabetes mellitus represents one of the largest epidemics the world has faced. It is a heterogenous syndrome characterized by chronic hyperglycemia in which there is a fundamental defect in insulin secretion and or action. It is a syndrome with several genetic, epigenetic, and multiple environmental influences such as nutrition, infection, and health style. The incidence of diabetes mellitus is rapidly increasing, and the condition often results in significant metabolic disorder with severe complications. The prevalence of diabetes expected to double from the current estimate of 29.1 million diabetic in the United States alone. Globally, the number of people with diabetes is estimated to be 642 million by year 2040.

Insulin deficiency or its dysfunction leads to state of hyperglycemia in two ways, first, impaired uptake of glucose into tissues and secondly promotes gluconeogenesis leading to hyperglycemia and diabetes mellitus.

Presenting features of diabetes mellitus

Hyperglycemia features tend to center on the osmotic effects of high glucose concentrations and the osmotic diuresis consequent to renal glucose excretion. Symptoms include polydipsia (thirst), polyuria and nocturia, and weight loss. Other hyperglycemic features include muscular cramps, paresthesia, and visual blurring (due to changes in lenticular osmotic potential).

Symptoms may develop gradually with features of complications of prolonged states of hyperglycemia appearing latter in the course of the disorder (see later) or acutely with diabetic ketoacidosis often seen in insulin deficiency type I diabetes.

Classification of diabetes mellitus

Historically, two major types of diabetes are described and have been differentiated either on the basis of age of presentation, as juvenile onset diabetes mellitus, and as maturity onset diabetes mellitus or on the basis of perceived insulin dependency as insulin-dependent diabetes mellitus (IDDM) or noninsulin dependent diabetes mellitus (NIDDM) respectively (Table 3).

TABLE 3 Types of diabetes mellitus (DM), biochemical and genetic characteristics.

DM type	Insulin level	Genetics	Etiology
Type I	Low	HLA	Autoimmune
LADA	Low	HLA + other genes	Autoimmune
Type II	High	Multiple SNPs	Nonautoimmune
MODY	High/ low	Autosomal dominant/ recessive	
Flatbush	High/ low	Unknown	
Lipodystrophy	High		
Secondary causes			
Cushing's	High	N/A	N/A
Pharmacological	Variable	N/A	N/A

HLA, human leukocyte antigens; LADA, latent autoimmune diabetes in adults; MODY, maturity onset diabetes in the young; SNPs, single nucleotide polymorphisms.
Modified from Hoogwerf BJ. Type of diabetes mellitus: does it matter to the clinician? *Cleve Clin J Med.* 2020;87(2):100–108. https://doi.org/10.3949/ccjm.87a.19020. PMID: 32015063.

Although still in common usage, such terminology is confusing, for instance, maturity onset diabetes is said to develop in teenagers occasionally (maturity onset diabetes in the young, MODY) and patients with severe noninsulin dependent diabetes mellitus often receive insulin as part of their therapy. The following classification as adopted by the American Diabetic Association is thus to be preferred.

Type I diabetes mellitus

Patients in this group represent (~5%–10%) of diabetic patients. This category is characterized by insulin deficiency due to destruction of the pancreatic β-cells. The cause of destruction is mostly autoimmune in nature and is associated with the human leukocyte antigens (HLA) system (Table 4); however, other idiopathic forms are present.

Features of type I are genetic predisposition with family history in 10% of cases. Peak onset being 5 years and early adolescence. The onset is often acute in nature, and that males and females are equally affected. The patients are often nonobese.

In early phase (1–5 years), some patients exhibit detectable but a much reduced insulin secretion and later no endogenous insulin secretion. It is a gradual loss of insulin that ranges from months to years. Patients are at risk of developing ketosis when insulin is withdrawn or under stress such as infections.

The demonstration of antiislet cell antibodies and their persistence in some cases (so-called type-Ib diabetes—associated with other endocrine autoimmune disorders and strongly familial) and the association of certain HLA haplotypes with higher risks of developing diabetes suggest an autoimmune basis for type I diabetes with damage to islet cells leading to an insulin deficiency state. Generally, cytoplasmic and complement-fixing antiislet cell antibodies are demonstrable at diagnosis, but later become undetectable.

Precipitating events may be environmental and could include viral infections which would account for the described associations of type I diabetes with Coxsackie B viral infections and mumps, and the increased incidence of type I diabetes in the winter months. Such viruses may express similar antigenic epitopes to islet β cells.

Measurement of C-peptide levels is used to assess pancreatic β-cell function. Level is low but may be detectable. Simultaneous measurement of glucose rules out low C-peptide secondary to hypoglycemia.

The diagnosis is confirmed by detecting antiglutamic acid decarboxylase (GAD) antibodies and or islet cell antibodies (ICA). However, those antibodies are present in about 2% of normal individuals. Those individuals, however, are at increased risk for future type I diabetes mellitus.

Furthermore, although those antibodies are initially present in >85% of patients with type I diabetes mellitus, their levels decline later on during the course of the disease and are undetectable by 10–15 years of disease.

Diabetes mellitus type I variants

Latent autoimmune diabetes in adults (LADA) The latent autoimmune diabetes in adults (LADA) is a variant that similarly exhibits inappropriately low insulin levels. It is autoimmune in nature and with the HLA system as well as novel genes The following have been associated with latent autoimmune diabetes of adults (LADA) DQA1*05-DQB1*0201 (OR 2.7), DQA1*03-DQB1*0401 (OR 1.6), DQA1*03-DQB1*0303 (OR 1.5), DQA1*0102-DQB1*0602 (OR 0.6), DRB1*0802-DQB1*0302 (OR 2.8), DRB1*0901-DQB1*0303 (OR 1.8), DRB1*03-DQB1*0201 (OR 3.7), DRB1*04-DQB1*0302 (OR 3.2) (Table 4). It is considered a rare variant of type I DM. The patient is nonobese presents early in a young adult, and the condition is suspected when an oral glucose lowering agent is needed to maintain normoglycemia. Autoantibodies are positive (similar to type I diabetes). Glutamic acid decarboxylase antibodies and islet cell antibodies are positive and the patient is started on insulin therapy.

Type II diabetes mellitus

Type II DM in its classic form is characterized by high but over time low insulin level. There is no autoimmune destruction of the β pancreatic islet cells. It is associated with

TABLE 4 HLA-associated relative risk for type I diabetes mellitus.

HLA genes	Association risk/protection	Race	Haplotypes and alleles	Function
HLA-DR HLA-DQ	Risk	European	DRB1*04:01/2/4/5-DQA1*03-DQB1*0302; DRB1*03-DQA1*05-DQB1*02; DRB1*04:05-DQA1*03-DQB1*02	Efficient presentation of autoimmunity-inducing peptides.
		African	DRB1*07-DQA1*03-DQB1*02; DRB1*09-DQA1*03-DQB1*03:02	
		Asian/far East	DRB1*04:05-DQA1*03-DQB1*04:01; DRB1*09-DQA1*03-DQB1*03:03; DRB1*08-DQA1*03-DQB1*03:02	
	Protective	European	DRB1*15-DQA1*01-DQB1*06:02; DRB1*15-DQA1*01-DQB1*06:01; DRB1*14-DQA1*01-DQB1*05:03; DRB1*07-DQA1*02-DQB1*03:03; DRB1*04:03-DQA1*03-DQB1*03:02	Inability to present critical antigen epitopes to T helper cells and competition for binding with risk haplotypes.
		African	DRB1*03-DQA1*04:01-DQB1*04:02; DRB1*08-DQA1*04:01-DQB1*03:01	
HLA-DP	Risk		DPB1*03:01	Efficient presentation of autoimmunity-inducing peptides.
	Protective		DPB1*04:02	Inability to present critical antigen epitopes to T helper cells and competition for binding with risk haplotypes.
Class I alleles	Risk		HLA-A*24; HLA-B*18; HLA-B*39:01; HLA-B*39:06	Efficient presentation of critical antigen epitopes to cytotoxic CD8+ T cells.

The HLA region on chromosome 6p21 accounts for approximately 50% of the familial aggregation of type-I diabetes mellitus. The strongest association is with HLA DR and DQ cell surface receptors that present antigens to T-lymphocytes. The highest risk haplotypes are the HLA Class II DR4-DQA1*03:01-DQB1*03:02 (DR4-DQ8 haplotype). DRB1*04:05 has an odds ratio (OR) of 11 and DRB1*04:01 an OR of 8. The second high-risk haplotype is DRB1*03:01-DQA1*05:01-DQB1*02:01 ("DR3-DRQ2" haplotype) and has an OR of 3.6. DR3 homozygotes HLA-DRB3*02:02 allele at significantly higher risk of developing type I diabetes than homozygous. Up to 90% of type I diabetics carry DR4-DQ8 or DR3-DQ2 and about 30% of patients carry both compared to 2% of the general population. The combination of those two haplotypes into the DR4-DQ8/DR3-DQ2 genotype confers the highest risk with an average OR of 16. The following have been associated with latent autoimmune diabetes of adults (LADA) DQA1*05-DQB1*0201 (OR 2.7), DQA1*03-DQB1*0401 (OR 1.6), DQA1*03-DQB1*0303 (OR 1.5), DQA1*0102-DQB1*0602 (OR 0.6), DRB1*0802-DQB1*0302 (OR 2.8), DRB1*0901-DQB1*0303 (OR 1.8), DRB1*03-DQB1*0201 (OR 3.7), DRB1*04-DQB1*0302 (OR 3.2).
Modified from Ilonen J, Lempainen J, Veijola R. The heterogeneous pathogenesis of type 1 diabetes mellitus. *Nat Rev Endocrinol.* 2019;15(11):635–650. https://doi.org/10.1038/s41574-019-0254-y. Epub 2019 Sep 18. PMID: 31534209. Chen W, Chen X, Zhang M, Huang Z. The association of human leukocyte antigen class II (HLA II) haplotypes with the risk of Latent autoimmune diabetes of adults (LADA): evidence based on available data. *Gene.* 2021;767:145177. https://doi.org/10.1016/j.gene.2020.145177. Epub 2020 Sep 28. PMID: 32998048.

multiple single nucleotide polymorphism (SNPs) without a specifically defined single SNP.

Characterized by a combination of insulin resistance and inadequate insulin secretion. It is more prevalent compared to type-I DM and is present in (∼90%–95%) of diabetic patients' population. There is a familial predisposition with family history in 30% of cases. Peak of onset is often at >40 years of age (but youth onset variants exist). Obese and nonobese-related forms are described, with obese patients usually hyperinsulinemic in comparison to normal weight nondiabetic subjects. Islet cell antibodies are often indemonstrable. Ketosis not provoked by insulin withdrawal but may occur with severe illness.

The pathogenesis of type II diabetes is complex and multifactorial. The evident genetic background of the disease as demonstrated by twin studies is polygenic with more than one gene being involved, and this genetic predisposition then interacts with environmental factors such as diet, obesity, etc. to lead to the disease phenotype. Two major pathologies can, however, be distinguished either or both of which may be operating in any individual with type II diabetes.

Around 75% of type II diabetics demonstrate a reduced insulin response to glucose loading in comparison to nondiabetic individuals. This may be related to a reduction in β cells mass with increased hyalinization of pancreatic islets.

Failure of either the insulin receptor or postreceptor effector pathways may explain many effects of type II diabetes. Insulin resistance need not be restricted to the glucose transport mechanism but could equally involve any other insulin modulated pathway, for instance insulin resistance of lipolysis may increase plasma lipids and explain the occasional hypertriglyceridemia of diabetes.

Many other metabolic disorders and or use of medication are associated with hyperglycemic states. They include pancreatic dysfunction, gluconeogenic hormonal dysfunction (elevated corticosteroids, glucagon, growth hormone, thyroid hormones (thyroxine and triiodothyronine), and catecholamines), drugs (diuretics, psychoactive agents, catecholaminergic, and analgesics), monogenetic disorders (Prader-Willi and Laurence-Moon-Biedl), genetic defects of ß-cell function, genetic defects in insulin action, and sepsis.

Other diabetes forms
Monogenic diabetes type

This is a much less common form of diabetes accounting for 1%–5% of the diabetes disorders. It is caused by mutation in a single gene out of over 40 candidates. Thus, it mostly affects the young (<25 years old). The term monogenic diabetes category includes (maturity onset diabetes of the young) MODY, neonatal diabetes mellitus, and syndromic diabetes. Those are highly penetrant variants with markedly impaired pancreatic β cell development and insulin secretion, leading to diabetes regardless of the risk factors seen in the classic type I and II.

Overlapping features with those of type I and II diabetes include, young onset, lean body mass (type I), and preserved pancreatic β cell function, and family history (type II). The variant requires genetic testing to establish the correct diagnosis as therapeutic intervention depends on the underlying etiology.

Maturity onset diabetes of the young (MODY)

Variants of type II include the maturity-onset diabetes of the young (MODY) as it is usually diagnosed in adolescence or early adulthood compared with type II DM. As the name implies it presents in the young occur at younger ages with lower BMI, lower hemoglobin A_{1c} and triglycerides have similar risk for microvascular complications. Insulin levels are variable but without autoimmune destruction. It is an autosomal recessive disorder. Two of the associated genotypes HFN4A and HNF1A respond to sulfonylurea therapy.

Neonatal diabetes mellitus (NTDM)

Neonatal diabetes mellitus term defines diabetes that is diagnosed within 6 months of age. It affects 1 in 90,000–260,000 live births with equal opportunity for being transient or permanent. The diabetes phenotype in NTDM results from inadequate insulin production presenting at the first week of life and usually resolve by 18 months, but

about 50% of patients relapse during early adulthood. There is often associated intrauterine growth retardation, failure to thrive, polyuria, and thus severe dehydration.

Among 60%–70% of the transient form there is overexpressed paternal genes on chromosome 6q24 resulting from paternally inherited duplication of that region of the chromosome. In the remaining 30%–40%, there is autosomal dominant mutation in the (potassium-ATP) K_{ATP} channel KCNJ11 and ABCC8 which are functionally less severe than those causing the permanent neonatal DM type.

Permanent form is associated with variants of the same genes ABCC8, KCNJ11, and INS as well as variants in the FOXP3 gene part of the IPEXC (immune dysregulation, poly-endocrinopathy, enteropathy, X-linked) syndrome.

Syndromic diabetes

Syndromic diabetes describes metabolic syndromes that are monogenic and include diabetes as one of their presentation and clinical features. They include Wolfram syndrome, insulin resistance syndrome, ketosis-prone diabetes, and lipodystrophy.

Wolfram syndrome

Wolfram syndrome, an autosomal recessive disorder, characterized by diabetes mellitus among other disorders. Two types of Wolfram syndrome (WS) corresponding to two causative genes have been identified (WFS1 and WFS2). This gene encodes a transmembrane protein, which is located primarily in the endoplasmic reticulum and ubiquitously expressed with highest levels in brain, and pancreas. Mutations in this gene are associated with Wolfram syndrome, also called DIDMOAD (Diabetes Insipidus, Diabetes Mellitus, Optic Atrophy, and Deafness).

Wolfram syndrome 1 (WS1), characterized by diabetes insipidus, DM, optic atrophy, and deafness, is a rare autosomal recessive disease caused by variants in the Wolframin ER transmembrane glycoprotein (*WFS1*). Severe cases with dominant heterozygous variants are also reported. Diabetes mellitus at early age (6 years) is often the patients' initial presentation. There are some *WFS1* mutations that cause isolated diabetes with significantly reduced penetrance or nonpenetrance for other WS-related features.

On the other hand, clinical features of Wolfram syndrome type II are similar to that of WS1 without diabetes insipidus and with the addition of peptic ulcer bleeding and defective platelet aggregation.

Insulin resistance syndrome due to insulin receptor defects

Genetic defects in the insulin receptor gene (*INSR*) result in several insulin resistance syndromes such as the Leprechaunism and Rabson-Mendenhall syndromes. It is an autosomal condition characterized by intrauterine and postnatal growth retardation, dysmorphic features, and impaired glucose tolerance.

The syndromes are distinguished from typical insulin resistance not only by their severity but by normal lipid profiles because the etiology is directly due to defects in insulin receptor signaling rather than obesity and its sequelae. The most common type is type A insulin resistance syndrome, which has autosomal dominant and autosomal recessive forms.

Lipodystrophy and associated diabetes

Individuals with lipodystrophy at risk of metabolic complications that include marked insulin resistance with no evidence of autoimmune component, nonalcoholic fatty liver disease, and dyslipidemia among others.

The monogenic lipodystrophy syndrome is a group of disorders featuring complete or partial lack of adipose tissue and adipose tissue-derived hormones, which results in insulin resistance and other metabolic complications.

Unlike insulin receptor defects syndrome described above, the lack of adipose tissue in lipodystrophy leads to dyslipidemia and insulin resistance due to fat in ectopic areas similar to the consequences of obesity.

Based on the loss of adipose tissue, this disease can be divided into congenital generalized lipodystrophy (CGL) and familial partial lipodystrophy (FPLD).

Congenital generalized lipodystrophy (CGL) is an autosomal recessive disease with variants in genes encoding 1-acylglycerol-3-phosphate O-acyltransferase 2 (AGPAT2) and Berardinelli-Seip congenital lipodystrophy 2 (BSCL2) account for most CGL cases, with rare cases being caused by variants in CAV1 and PTRF.

Familial partial lipodystrophy (FPLD) is mainly caused by variants in the lamin A/C (LMNA) or PPARγ (PPARG) genes. There are also other rarer forms caused by the variants PLIN1, AKT2, LIPE, CIDEC, and PCYT1A. Body fat deficiency in FPLD is found on limbs, buttocks, and hips. Patients with pathogenic variants of either LMNA or PPARG appear to benefit similarly from leptin replacement therapy.

Ketosis-prone diabetes variant (Flatbush diabetes)

A second variant Flatbush diabetes (Ketosis prone diabetes) is recognized as a separate entity. In sub-Saharan Africans, Asian and Indian population as Hispanic population, the clinical course resembles that of type II DM with higher degree of insulin loss and or action in target tissues. The mechanism responsible for the development of ketosis-prone diabetes as well as its remission remains unknown. Insulin levels are variable and have no autoimmune etiology and no associated genetic material identified as such.

Mitochondrial diabetes

Mitochondrial disorders represent consequences of respiratory chain dysfunction caused by mutations in the mitochondrial gene (mtDNA) or in the nuclear-encoded mitochondrial genes. The hallmark is a multisystem involvement. Mitochondrial diabetes, also known as maternally inherited diabetes and deafness (MIDD), is the most common mitochondrial genotype and is caused by a single nucleotide substitution m.3243A>G in the mitochondrial tRNA$^{Leu(UUR)}$ gene linked to a distinct clinical phenotype, that is maternally inherited diabetes and deafness.

Patients often present with diabetes in adulthood, but a greater proportion of mutated mitochondrial genomes in the affected tissues is associated with a younger age of diagnosis of diabetes.

The hearing loss associated with the m.3243A>G mutation is bilateral, sensorineural, and progressive, typically preceding the diagnosis of diabetes.

The penetrance of mitochondrial diabetes is estimated to be nearly 100% by the age of 70 years. Patients exhibit impaired insulin secretion, and insulin treatment is eventually required for most patients.

Gestational diabetes mellitus

The presence of hyperglycemia first detected during pregnancy is termed gestational diabetes. It is discussed in detail in Chapter 8 on obstetrics.

Patients with abnormal fasting or random glucose are subjected to glucose change test, where blood glucose is measured 1 h following a 50 g glucose challenge. The patient need not be fasting. Glucose levels above 7.8 mmol/L (140 mg/dL) are considered an impaired response and require confirmation with larger glucose load of 75 or 100 g. Blood samples are collected following 8–10 h fast, and at 1, 2, and/or 3 h following the glucose load. Two or more abnormal glucose levels confirm gestational diabetes (Table 5).

Those samples and often collected at an outpatient setting and sent to the clinical laboratory at the completion of the test. It is important that sample preservation guidelines are followed, that is use of glycolysis inhibitor tube additives (fluoride oxalate or citrate), immediate separation of plasma by centrifugation and immediate measurement of glucose levels.

Secondary diabetes

The term secondary diabetes refers to the presence of diabetes mellitus as a consequence of another disorders or use of medication interfering with insulin action. It encompasses effect of medication on insulin production and/or action such as steroids, pancreatitis and pancreatic cancer, Cushing's syndrome, acromegaly are common endocrine disorders causing secondary diabetes mellitus. Insulin levels are usually variable but often high in the presence of high glucocorticoids.

Loss of insulin secretion (tissue damage) is the primary cause for the development of diabetes mellitus in patients with hemochromatosis. Deposition of iron in tissue (including pancreatic tissue) is the likely cause for reduction in insulin secretion capacity. Insulin resistance is also common among patients with hemochromatosis.

TABLE 5 Diagnostic glucose and A1c values for diabetes mellitus, impaired glucose tolerance, and risk for diabetes.

Test	Normal	Impaired glucose tolerance (prediabetic)	Diabetes	Comment
Glucose (fasting)	70–99 mg/dL 4–5.5 mmol/L	≥100 mg/dL (5.6 mmol/L) <126 mg/dL (7.0 mmol/L)	≥126 mg/dL (7.0 mmol/L)	Fasting minimum 8 h (no caloric intake) water permitted
Glucose (random)	70–199 mg/dL 4–5.5 mmol/L		≥200 mg/dL (11.1 mmol/L)	Any time without regard to time since last meal
Glucose tolerance tests:				
Glucose tolerance test—75 g	Dose: 75 g. Samples: Fasting (minimum 8 h), and 2 h post dose.			
Glucose—Fasting	Normal: <100 mg/dL (5.6 mmol/L) Impaired: ≥100 (5.6 mmol/L) <126 mg/dL (7.0 mmol/L) Diabetes: ≥126 mg/dL (7.0 mmol/L)			
Glucose 2 h post 75 g	Normal: <140 mg/dL (7.8 mmol/L) Impaired glucose tolerance: ≥140 (7.8) <200 (11.1) Diabetes: ≥200 mg/dL (11.1 mmol/L)			
Gestational diabetes mellitus	Interpretation	Comment		
Glucose challenge test (50 g)	Normal response <140 (7.8 mmol/L)	Dose: 50 g. 1 h test. Patient need NOT be fasting		
	Abnormal response: >140 (>7.8 mmol/L)	Proceed to 100 g glucose tolerance test (GTT)		
2 h Glucose tolerance test—75 g (ADA) recommendation Dose: 100 g. Samples (n=3); Fasting, 1 h post dose, 2 h post dose	Normal response. GDM if any of the values below are met or exceeded			
Glucose—Fasting	<92 mg/dL (<5.1 mmol/L)			
Glucose 1 h post 100 g	<180 mg/dL (<10 mmol/L)			
Glucose 2 h post 100 g	<153 md/dL (<8.5 mmol/L)			
3 h Glucose tolerance test—100 g Dose: 100 g. Samples (n=4); Fasting, 1 h post dose, 2 h post dose, 3 h post dose	ADA guidelines. Normal response. GDM if any of the values below are met or exceeded	ACOG (O'Sullivan) Criteria guidelines. GDM if any of the values below are met or exceeded		
Glucose—Fasting	<95 (5.3 mmol/L)	<105 (5.8 mmol/L)		
Glucose 1 h post 100 g	<180 (10.0 mmol/L)	<190 (10.6 mmol/L)		
Glucose 2 h post 100 g	<155 (8.6 mmol/L)	<165 (9.2 mmol/L)		
Glucose 3 h post 100 g	<140 (7.8 mmol/L)	<145 (8.0 mmol/L)		
Glycohemoglobin (A1c)	Interpretation	Values (%)		
	Normal (nondiabetic)	<5.7%		
	At risk of diabetes (prediabetes)	5.7%–6.4%		
	Diabetes	≥6.5% 48 mmol/mol		
	Diabetes poor control	>7.0%		

ADA, American Diabetes Association. *ACOG (O'Sullivan)*, American College of Obstetrics and Gynecology criteria. WHO also define an "intermediate" category of individual with mild hyperglycemia following an oral glucose tolerance test (OGTT)—but not severe enough to be classified as diabetes. This category has been termed "impaired glucose tolerance." Such individuals would seem to be at higher risk of progressing to develop diabetes and diabetic complications, though the extent of this risk is controversial.
Modified from American Diabetes Association. 2. Classification and diagnosis of diabetes: *Standards of Medical Care in Diabetes-2019. Diabetes Care.* 2019;42(suppl 1):S13–S28. https://doi.org/10.2337/dc19-S002. PMID: 30559228.

However, the diagnosis may often be obvious following careful clinical assessment and laboratory testing.

Biochemical diagnosis of diabetes mellitus

Symptoms suggestive of diabetes mellitus (polyuria, polydipsia, lethargy, weight loss, etc.) and a random (regardless of time of preceding meal) blood glucose greater than or equal to 200 mg/dL (11.1 mmol/L) or higher, or a fasting blood glucose of 126 mg/dL (7.0 mmol/L) or higher are indicative of diabetes mellitus. Similarly, the finding of blood glucose of 200 mg/dL (11.1 mmol/L) or higher 2h following a 75 g glucose load are diagnostic of diabetes mellitus.

The above must be confirmed by repeat testing on a subsequent day. Repeat testing is not necessary in patients who have unequivocal hyperglycemia with acute metabolic decompensation.

Indeterminant glucose values indicate impaired glucose tolerance and the likelihood of progress to diabetes. Although A1c may be used in the diagnosis of diabetes mellitus where levels ≥6.5% are indicative of diabetes mellitus and levels <5.7% indicate normal glycemic status and low risk of diabetes mellitus, its utility has several limitations and it should be used with caution, for instance, in patients with red blood cells abnormalities and possible interference by hemoglobinopathies. Diagnostic criteria for diabetes mellitus are shown in Table 5.

Biochemical investigation in diabetes mellitus

Blood glucose levels, as shown above, are central to the diagnosis and management of patients suspected with diabetes mellitus. However, many other biomarkers are important in the management of diabetic patients.

Circulating biomarkers of support and relevance in the diagnosis and management of diabetes mellitus include insulin and C-peptide as a measure of pancreatic β-cell function. Low levels of the hormones in the presence of hyperglycemia are characteristic of type I diabetes mellitus, whereas in type II their circulating levels range from high (early in the disease) to low but detectable levels. Detection of circulating antiglutamic acid decarboxylase (GAD) antibodies is characteristic of type I diabetes mellitus.

Biomarkers include electrolytes (sodium, potassium, chloride, bicarbonate), urea (BUN), blood and urine ketones as well as arterial blood gases central to management of critically ill patient and at acute presentations (see "Treatment of diabetes" section).

Ketoacidosis

Patients with diabetes mellitus are at risk of developing diabetic ketoacidosis and hyperosmolar hyperglycemic syndrome. This is a life-threatening emergency and occurs in both type I and type II. The frequency of diabetic ketoacidosis has increased during the past decade, with more than 160,000 hospital admissions in 2017 in the United States. However, nonketotic hyperosmolar presentations are less common and represent less than 1% of all diabetes related hospital admissions.

In the pathogenesis of ketoacidosis, the relative presence of insulin to glucagon is key. In type-I diabetes mellitus, there is absolute insulin deficiency and increase in the counterregulatory hormones primarily glucagon but also catecholamines, cortisol, and growth hormone. This leads to marked increase in hepatic gluconeogenic enzymes fructose 1,6 bisphosphatase, phosphoenolpyruvate carboxykinase (PEPCK), glucose-6-phosphatase, and pyruvate carboxylase stimulated by the increase in the glucagon to insulin ratio and by an increase in circulating cortisol concentrations. The increased gluconeogenic and glycogenolysis activities and reduced glucose utilization (lack of insulin) all further exacerbate the hyperglycemia osmotic diuresis and thus hypovolemia (dehydration). Furthermore, in the adipose tissue, the combination of severe insulin deficiency with elevated counterregulatory hormone concentrations activates hormone sensitive lipase leading to an increase in circulating free fatty acids. The excess free fatty acids are oxidized to acetoacetate and β-hydroxybutyrate in hepatic mitochondria, resulting in increased ketone bodies and acidosis. This diabetic ketoacidosis does not occur to a large extent in type II diabetes where the relative insulin insufficiency prevents the marked increase in hepatic lipase activity and thus reduced free fatty acids and the ensued ketones production. Therefore, patients presenting with hyperglycemic hyperosmolar syndrome (HHS) have lower concentrations of free fatty acids, cortisol, growth hormone, and glucagon than do those presenting with diabetic ketoacidosis. The patients may have mild metabolic acidosis but due to the impaired renal function and dehydration.

Patients presenting with HHS have lower concentrations of free fatty acids, cortisol, growth hormone, and glucagon than do those presenting with diabetic ketoacidosis. Patients with HHS may have mild metabolic acidosis due to renal failure and dehydration. The hypovolemia encountered leads to reduced glomerular filtration rate and to osmotic diuresis resulting in sodium, potassium, calcium, magnesium, chloride, and phosphate loss. Additionally, the state of hyperglycemia and ketosis is exacerbated by the reduced renal clearance.

Diabetic ketoacidosis is defined by a triad of diagnosis of diabetes, metabolic acidosis, and the presence of ketones. Hyperosmolality (due to the ensued hyperglycemia and dehydration) and that clinical features include dehydration, air hunger with increased depth and rate of breathing (Kusmul breathing), and ketosis. The onset is slow (2–3 days or longer) with symptoms of increasing hyperglycemia. There is often associated anorexia and vomiting, and occasional severe abdominal pain.

Cerebral edema is common and serious complication in patients with concurrent ketoacidosis. Other causes of coma include lactic acidosis and uremia (in cases with advanced nephropathy).

Most patients present as stupor. Type I diabetes is present most commonly with ketoacidosis hyperglycemia. Type II diabetes with hyperglycemia may or may not be ketoacidosis. Biochemical abnormalities often encountered are shown in Table 6.

Nonketotic hyperglycemic states

The hyperosmolar, hyperglycemic nonketotic patient (often termed hyperosmolar nonketotic or HONK) tends to be present in a similar fashion to the ketotic though the history may be of a longer mean duration (~1 week), and the patient is often older. The major clinical feature is pronounced dehydration. Treatment is similar, but the common concurrence of hypernatremia means that rehydration with hypotonic saline is more often seen and since blood glucose concentrations are more likely to be extremely high it

is correspondingly more important than the restoration of normoglycemia not be rushed as too fast a fall in glucose concentration may have harmful osmotic effects on the central nervous system. Biochemical abnormalities often encountered are shown in Table 6.

Long-term complications of diabetes mellitus

Apart from the acute and life-threatening diabetic ketoacidosis and hyperglycemic hyperosmolarity syndrome, chronic complication of poorly controlled diabetes mellitus are profound and significant. Several long-term prospective landmark trials (e.g., DCCT and UKPDS) have assessed the effects of intensive diabetes therapy on the prevention and progression of chronic diabetic complications and validated the relationship between diabetes control and the development of complications secondary to diabetes mellitus and that patients with long term poor control are at risk of developing nephropathy, retinopathy, and neuropathy.

TABLE 6 Biochemical parameters in the diagnosis of patients with diabetic ketoacidosis and nonketoacidosis.

Parameter	ADA	UK	AACE/ACE
Hyperglycemia hyperosmolar (ketoacidosis)			
Plasma glucose (mmol/L)	>13.9 (<250 mg/dL)	>11 (>200 mg/dL)	NA
pH	7.25–7.30 (mild) 7.00–7.25 (moderate) <7.00 (severe)	<7.30 <7.0 (severe)	<7.3
Bicarbonate (mmol/L)	15–18 Mild 10–14.9 Moderate <10 severe	<15 <5 (severe)	NA
Anion gap (Na- (Cl + HCO$_3^-$))	>10 mild 10–12 moderate >12 severe	>16 severe	>10
Urine acetoacetate	Positive	Positive	Positive
B-hydroxybutyrate	NA	>3 (31 mg/dL) >6 severe (62 mg/dL)	≥3.8 (40 mg/dL)
Hyperglycemia hyperosmolar (non ketotic)			
Plasma glucose (mmol/L)	>33.3	≥30	
pH	>7.30	>7.30	
Bicarbonate (mmol/L)	>18	>15	
Urine acetoacetate	Negative/low positive	NA	
B-hydroxybutyrate (mmol/L)	NA	<3	
Serum osmolality (mOsmol/L)	>320	≥320	

As defined by the American Diabetes Association (ADA) (published year 2009 and updated 2019), the American Association of Clinical Endocrinologists (AACE), and the American College of Endocrinology (ACE) (published 2016) and that in use in the United Kingdom (UK) (published 2013). *NA*, not included in the respective guidance documents.
Modified from French EK, Donihi AC, Korytkowski MT. Diabetic ketoacidosis and hyperosmolar hyperglycemic syndrome: review of acute decompensated diabetes in adult patients. *BMJ.* 2019;365:l1114. https://doi.org/10.1136/bmj.l1114. PMID: 31142480.

Nephropathy

Diabetic nephropathy is a major cause of end-stage renal disease, and that hyperglycemia is central to the development of the renal structural changes seen in diabetic nephropathy.

It is characterized by proteinuria and gradual decline in glomerular filtration rate (often progressing over 10–20 years).

Although the progress of diabetic nephropathy is monitored by measuring urine albumin levels (microalbuminuria), it does not necessarily correlate with the severity or prognosis of nephropathy and indeed some patients with nephropathy do not develop significant proteinuria.

Histologically, glomerular lesions are the most consistent finding with diffused nodular mesangial expansion and thickening of the glomerular basement membrane. Glomerular expansion often occurs within 5 years of diabetes and progresses to glomerular membrane thickening which both correlate with albumin excretion rate.

Interstitial inflammation and expansion occur within the first 2 years eventually leading to tubular fibrosis. Renal vascular and interstitial damage is in part secondary to accumulation of advanced glycation end products and to the ensued oxidative stress.

Diabetic nephropathy is a progression from glomerular hypertrophy and increased permeability to development of nodules to interstitial and tubular damage. The increase in glomerular permeability is reversible in the early stages following intensive control of the hyperglycemia; however, over time the damage becomes irreversible.

Factors contributing to the pathology of diabetic nephropathy are many; they include phosphorylation of serine and/or threonine residue of intracellular proteins by protein kinase C enzymes thought to play a role in the pathogenesis in development of glomerular basement membrane hyperplasia. Oxidative stress due to increased production of superoxide dismutase and reactive oxygen species by renal mesangial cells during hyperglycemia leads to renal vascular damage.

Chronic inflammation with release of several inflammatory cytokines and TGF-β contribute to the pathogenesis of diabetic nephropathy, additionally, accumulation of advanced glycation end products, normally excreted into the urine induces expression of TGF-β and cytokines that leads to transformation of epithelial cells to myofibroblasts and the development of tubulointerstitial fibrosis.

Renal lesions in type II are more complex compared to those in type I. It is complicated by the high prevalence of nondiabetic superimposed and existing renal lesions and thus reflects the heterogeneity in type II DM with only 30% developing microalbuminuria, and only 50% of patients with proteinuria show typical diabetic glomerulopathy. There is tubular basement membrane thickening, advanced glomerular and tubular hyalinosis, atherosclerosis of large vessels and interstitial fibrosis, and widespread glomerular sclerosis.

The tubular interstitial lesions in addition to the hyperglycemia also reflect other causes such as aging arthrosclerosis and systemic hypertension characteristic of the time of presentation and of development of type II diabetes mellitus.

Renal biopsy is the gold standard in the differential diagnose of diabetic nephropathy; however, the majority of patients will not undergo diagnostic biopsies and hence the reliance on laboratory measurement of albumin excretion rate (AER) and early identification of microalbuminuria. It must be emphasized that although easy to perform, the diagnostic sensitivity is not as high as would expected. For example, in type 1 diabetes, diabetic nephropathy usually develops within 10–15 years after diagnosis, while microalbuminuria may occur as early as 2–5 years after diagnosis. Some patients with type 2 diabetes may already have microalbuminuria at the time of diagnosis secondary to other causes such as hypertension, but without diabetic nephropathy.

Furthermore, in patients with type-I diabetes mellitus, overt nephropathy usually occurs at 10–15 years after onset. During this phase, urinary albumin excretion rate is greater than 300 mg/24 h (200 μg/min), and if untreated, this stage is highly predictive of subsequent progress to renal failure.

It is important to note that despite the achievement of good diabetic control, few patients will progress to develop renal failure and that renal failure per se is a major risk factor for cardiovascular disease.

Retinopathy

Diabetic retinopathy is one of the common causes of irreversible visual impairment among adults with risk factors for development and progression being poor glycemic control, duration of diabetes mellitus, the presence of systemic hypertension, dyslipidemia, anemia, inflammation, and microalbuminuria.

Progressive changes in retinal microvasculature lead to increased vascular permeability, retinal hypoperfusion, and intraocular proliferation of retinal vessels with threat of sight loss.

Achieving diabetic control and frequent laboratory and clinical monitoring is thus essential to prevent sight loss.

Anemia mentioned above as a risk factor is thought to induce retinal hypoxia. In addition to nutrient and dietary deficiency seen in patients with diabetes mellitus, the anemia is often due to the coexistent diabetic nephropathy. Impaired renal function and reduced mass leads to reduced erythropoietin production and thus renal anemia exacerbating possible nutritional anemia.

Neuropathy

Most common troublesome complication of diabetes mellitus with significant morbidity and mortality. Responsible for 50%–75% of nontraumatic amputations. Most common form of neuropathy in the developed world.

The true prevalence is not known, and reports vary from 10% to 90% in diabetic patients, depending on the criteria and methods applied.

The major risk factors for the development and progression of diabetic neuropathy being poor glycemic control, duration of diabetes mellitus, the presence of systemic hypertension, dyslipidemia, anemia, inflammation, and microalbuminuria.

Recently, increased aortic stiffness has been identified as a prognostic marker of diabetic peripheral neuropathy.

Neurological complications occur equally in type I and type II diabetes mellitus. The loss of small fiber-mediated sensation results in loss of thermal and pain perception, whereas large fiber impairment results in loss of touch and vibration perception. Sensory-fiber involvement may also result in "positive" symptoms, such as paresthesia and pain.

Studies in type 1 diabetic patients show that intensive diabetes therapy retards but does not completely prevent the development of diabetic peripheral neuropathy. In the UKPDS trial, the intensive therapy in diabetes management showed a lower rate of impaired vibration perception threshold, 31% in intensive therapy and 52% when conventional therapy was used.

Hyperglycemia induces superoxide and peroxynitrite ions; additionally, antioxidants are reduced. This increased oxidative stress induces nerve damage in diabetic neuropathy. Furthermore, advanced glycation end products formed in nonenzymatic addition of glucose or saccharides to proteins and lipids and nucleotides leads to intracellular and extracellular protein cross-linking and protein aggregation.

There is deficiency in nerve growth factor and neuropeptides substance P and calcitonin gene-related peptide. All of those abnormalities contribute to the development of diabetic neuropathy.

Maternal/fetal complications in gestational diabetes mellitus

Gestational diabetes mellitus (GDM) is when a pregnant woman without previously diagnosed diabetes develops chronic hyperglycemia during gestation and that it often resolves following partition. According to the most recent (2017) International Diabetes Federation (IDF) estimates, GDM affects about 14% of pregnancies worldwide, representing approximately 18 million births annually.

The complications associated with gestational diabetes affects two individuals, the mother, the fetus, and the newly born. Approximately 60% of women with a past history of GDM develop type II diabetes mellitus with a yearly risk of conversion of ~2%–3%.

In the unborn fetus, the increased transport of glucose, amino acids, and fatty acids across the placenta stimulates fetal production of insulin and insulin-like growth factor-1 (IGF-1). The outcome of this increased glucose uptake is fetal overgrowth and in macrosomia at birth which is a risk for shoulder dystocia. Caesarian section being common delivery form in pregnancies with gestational diabetes mellitus.

The development of gestational diabetes mellitus is often on the background of an existing and or developing maternal insulin resistance, more often a partially additive component during pregnancy. The latter (lack of insulin signaling) is associated with a number of factors such that overweight, obesity and excessive weight gain during pregnancy, gestational weight gain, diet style and micronutrients deficiency, ethnicity, family history of insulin resistance and or diabetes, and advanced maternal age are all risk factors for gestational diabetes.

In obesity where the increased number of adipose tissue macrophages produce inflammatory cytokines (IL-6, TNF-α, and IL-1 α), this low-grade inflammation impairs insulin signaling and thus inhibits insulin release by β cells. There is also downregulation of insulin receptor tyrosine kinase activity, increasing serine phosphorylation of the inulin receptor S-1 which leads to its degradation.

The rate of glucose uptake is reduced by 54% in gestational diabetes. The failure in insulin signaling results in inadequate glucose receptor (GLUT4) translocation, i.e., lack of glucose entry into cells.

Saturated fatty acids increase intracellular diacylglycerol within myocytes, activating protein kinase C and inhibiting tyrosine kinase, and IRS-1 (insulin receptor and PI3K (insulin being the main ligand)). This impaired glucose tolerance is secondary to impaired pancreatic β-cell and or to insulin resistance.

Heart failure in patients with diabetes mellitus

Heart failure is common among patients with diabetes mellitus with prevalence of 9%–27% and leads to serious complications and mortality. Following the recent reclassification of heart failure, diabetes has been identified as risk factor for heart failure and all diabetics are in stage A of heart failure classification (that is at risk of developing heart failure). There has recently been campaigns to increase awareness and development of recommendation for the routine assessment for heart failure among diabetics.

The risk of developing heart failure among DM type I is higher than in type II. Furthermore, the risk of developing advanced heart failure, and hospitalization and associated mortality is two to six folds that of type 2 or those without diabetes. Additionally, child onset type-I is at higher risk of developing heart failure than those with type-I onset at adulthood.

Biochemical measurement of B-type natriuretic peptides (NTproBNP or BNP) at least annually has been recommend among asymptomatic patients. Patients with diabetes mellitus are more likely to be cared for in general practice, where the diagnosis of heart failure might not be so obvious. High-sensitivity troponins also offer a risk assessment for the extent of cardiac failure.

See Chapter 7 on cardiac biomarkers for more details.

Treatment of diabetes

The basis of treatment is to provide insulin to counter the hyperglycemia and to rehydrate the patient while replacing sodium and potassium (although prior treatment potassium may be normal or even elevated in the ensued acidosis, insulin therapy increases potassium tissue uptake). Insulin/dextrose is often used to treat hyperkalemia. Therapy should be monitored by means of regular plasma potassium and glucose measurements and blood gases.

The two main aims of diabetic therapy are to prevent short- and long-term complications associated with hyperglycemia. Landmark trials (DCCT and UKPDS) have shown that adequate control defined as A1c less than 6.5% is associated with reduced incidence of complications.

Biomarkers in diabetes management

Central to the management of diabetes mellitus is assessment of glycemic control.

Hemoglobin A1c (A1c), fructosamine, and glycated albumin provide important evidence for the average circulating glucose levels over time. The latter as described above correlates with development and progression of diabetes complications.

Glucose measurement

Glucose levels are measured in whole blood, plasma, and or serum. Differences exist between glucose concentrations as estimated in whole blood or plasma and venous or capillary samples. Capillary glucose concentrations are ~8% higher than in venous, and plasma glucose concentrations are about 10%–15% higher than in whole blood sample.

It is important to maintain the sample stability as glucose degradation takes place in vitro, and glucose in blood tube is lost via glycolysis (cell uptake and utilization). Rate of glycolysis is 5%–7% (~10 mg/dL (0.6 mmol/L)) per hour and varies with glucose concentration, and is influenced by ambient temperature (increases with temperature), the number of white blood cell (leukocytes count), and infection (e.g., sepsis), etc. Use of preservatives such as fluoride (sodium) or citrate (sodium) inhibits glycolysis and thus preserves sample glucose content during storage and transportation. Plasma should be transported without delay and plasma separated immediately from cells by centrifugation upon receipt into the laboratory.

The measurement of blood glucose level is central to both diagnosis and to management of diabetes. Glucose measurement must be performed in an accredited laboratory and that analytical imprecision must be <3.3% (that is at least half its biological variability of 5%–7%).

There are several methods for the measurement of glucose (Figs. 4–6). They include enzymatic glucose oxidase, hexokinase, glucose dehydrogenase methods, and the nonenzymatic colorimetric (*o*-toluidine) methods.

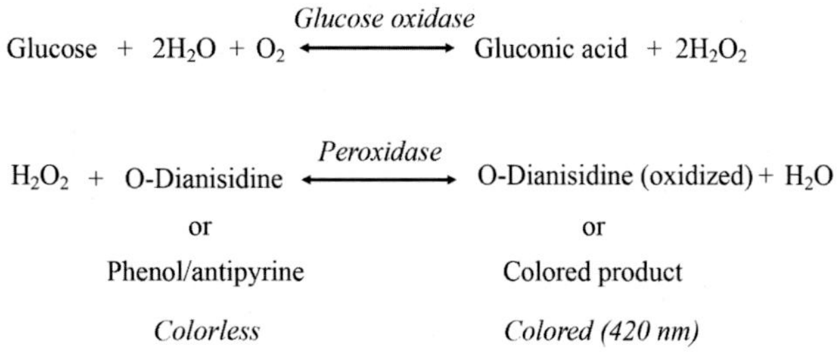

$$\text{Glucose} + 2H_2O + O_2 \xleftrightarrow{\text{Glucose oxidase}} \text{Gluconic acid} + 2H_2O_2$$

$$H_2O_2 + \text{O-Dianisidine} \xleftrightarrow{\text{Peroxidase}} \text{O-Dianisidine (oxidized)} + H_2O$$

or   or

Phenol/antipyrine   Colored product

Colorless   *Colored (420 nm)*

FIG. 4 Glucose oxidase-based reactions in the measurement of glucose. The oxidation of colorless substrate by hydrogen peroxide (H_2O_2) produced in the initial peroxidase step is oxidized to a colored product the concentration of which is proportional to the glucose concentration. *(Modified from Galant AL, Kaufman RC, Wilson JD. Glucose: detection and analysis. Food Chem. 2015;188:149–160. https://doi.org/10.1016/j.foodchem.2015.04.071. Epub 2015 Apr 23. PMID: 26041177.)*

$$\text{Glucose} + \text{ATP} \xleftrightarrow{\text{Hexokinase}} \text{Glucose-6-phopsphate} + \text{ADP}$$

$$\text{Glucose-6-phosphate} \xleftrightarrow{\text{G-6-PD}} \text{6-phosphoglucanate}$$

NAD/ NADP   NADP / NADPH

240 nm

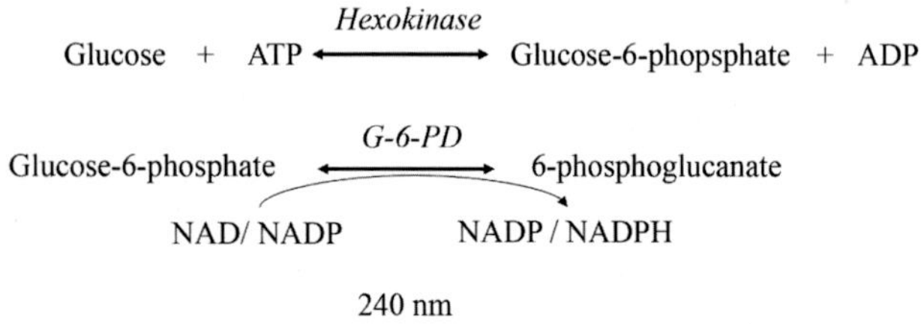

FIG. 5 Hexokinase-based reactions in the measurement of glucose. The reaction includes the enzyme glucose-6-phophate dehydrogenase (G-6-PD) which converts the substrate glucose-6-phophate to 6-phosphoglucanate. NAD/NADP is reduced to NADH/NADPH. The latter is monitored by recording absorbance at 240 nm and is proportional to the glucose concentration. *(Modified from Galant AL, Kaufman RC, Wilson JD. Glucose: detection and analysis. Food Chem. 2015;188:149–160. https://doi.org/10.1016/j.foodchem.2015.04.071. Epub 2015 Apr 23. PMID: 26041177.)*

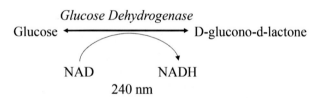

$$\text{Glucose} \xleftrightarrow{\text{Glucose Dehydrogenase}} \text{D-glucono-d-lactone}$$

NAD   NADH

240 nm

FIG. 6 Glucose dehydrogenase-based reaction in the measurement of glucose concentration. The reduction of NAD to NADH is monitored by recording absorbance at 240 nm. The concentration of NADH is proportional to the glucose concentration. *(Modified from Galant AL, Kaufman RC, Wilson JD. Glucose: detection and analysis. Food Chem. 2015;188:149–160. https://doi.org/10.1016/j.foodchem.2015.04.071. Epub 2015 Apr 23. PMID: 26041177.)*

Glucose measurement methods principles in common use are shown in Figs. 4–6. The majority of automated chemistry analyzers employ hexokinase method, as they are relatively cheaper. Point of care devices and strips and cartridge-based methods often employ the more rapid and specific glucose oxidase methods.

The use of point of care devices (employing glucose oxidase) in critically ill patients have recently been cautioned. The rationale being critically ill patients are likely to experience hypovolemia, reduced peripheral circulation (figure prick blood collection sites) and may exhibit states of variable blood pO_2 levels and often critically ill patients with $pO_2 > 70–100$ mmHg. To this effect, use of nonoxygen sensitive devices be used to use minimize the oxygen tension effect on glucose testing. Errors of up to 15% or more lead to the use of oxygen-insensitive methods in critically ill patients with >70–100 mmHg or with unpredictable pO_2 levels.

Glucose oxidase (GOX) methods are extremely specific for glucose but impacted by O_2 content dissolved in sample with hyperoxia (>100 mmHg) results in falsely low glucose. In contrast, hypoxia ($pO_2 < 44$ mmHg) leads to falsely high glucose.

Glucose-1-dehydrogenase (GDH)-based methods are not affected by O_2 concentration but, in patients receiving pyrroloquinoline quinone (PQQ) coenzyme therapy, this catalyses the enzymes GDH and glucose oxidase rerndering the reagent enzymes nonglucose specific reacting with other sugars and can thus cause falsely elevated glucose results.

Drugs interfere with glucose measurement, for instance ascorbic acid leads to falsely low glucose levels when using the glucose oxidase and glucose dehydrogenase-based methodologies. Acetaminophen causes falsely low glucose results when using glucose oxide oxidase and glucose-6-dehrogenase methods.

Patients with marked hypertriglyceridemia and hyperproteinemia (e.g., paraproteinemia) are at risk of having falsely hypoglycemia when using point of care devices due to plasma size exclusion effects and thus lower water content.

Glucose levels are slightly higher in arterial samples, compared to capillary samples and compared to venous samples in this order. The distribution is further reduced due to increased glucose utilization and poor tissue perfusion in critically ill patients.

In general, samples used for the measurement of glucose must be rapidly handled and preserved to reduce ongoing invitro glycolysis which leads to falsely low samples glucose levels. Blood is collected using glycolysis inhibitors as tube additives (e.g., fluoride oxalate).

The management of hyperglycemia is complicated by changes in inpatient conditions, diet, and drugs regimens as well as comorbidities and presence of other disorders. A blood glucose target of 140–180 mg/dL (7.8–10.0 mmol/L) for inpatients glycemic management is a common goal. Tighter glycemic control may be required with glucose targeted at 110–140 mg/dL (6.1–7.8 mmol/L), however care must be taken to avoid significant and recurrent hypoglycemia. Tight and intensive glucose management leads to reduced morbidity and mortality among critically ill patients. Electronic continuous glucose monitoring (see later) helps overcome some of the above variations. Several device options are available and are in current clinical use.

Point of care testing

Conventional point of care testing (POCT) is widely used in critical care units facilitating rapid availability of essential laboratory test results and thus facilitating rapid and appropriate therapeutic interventions. Point of care glucose monitoring refers to use of nonlaboratory devices in the measurement of glucose levels. Samples applied are often whole blood (venous, capillary heal, and figure prick). Transdermal continuous measuring devices measuring glucose in interstitial fluid are increasingly being used and are integral to the use of wearable insulin pumps.

The methods in general utilize glucose oxidase or glucose dehydrogenase enzymes with amperometric or photometric readout of reaction. This may be different from glucose methods on automated laboratory-based analyses.

However, the accuracy of their performance in critically ill patients has been questioned by various regulatory agencies and have resisted certification of the devices for use in critically ill patients. The problem being that most of the instruments were not validated for use in critically ill patients. The studies on tight glycemic control on improved outcomes and reduced mortality were performed on blood gas analyzers.

Differences in peripheral blood circulation and thus glucose levels between peripheral interstitial, and venous blood glucose may be at such variance as to cause mismanagement and thus pose risk to patients.

Factors commonly thought to impact analytical accuracy of these values that are prevalent in critically ill patients include poor blood flow to peripheral capillaries due to shock and/or vasopressor use, fluid overload or anasarca, and decreased hemoglobin concentration/hematocrit, as well as medications and oxygen supplementation in use in critically ill patients.

Critical care areas continue to use point of care devices for glucose measurement and that few studies have shown that its use remains safe and that only rarely that a significant difference (one patient experienced under treatment for hyperglycemia and should have received two additional units of rapid acting insulin when based on venous blood glucose levels) that may have led to inappropriate management.

Frequent measurement of glucose by POCT devices is used to minimize hyperglycemia, hypoglycemia and marked variation in glucose levels. Both hyperglycemia and hypoglycemia among critically ill patients have been associated with increased overall mortality and that hyperglycemia has been most associated with impaired immune function, impaired wound healing, and increased overall morbidity in critically ill patients.

Continuous glucose monitoring (CGM)

Continuous monitoring of body glycemic status is achieved by use of electronic sensor device inserted under the skin in subcutaneous interstitial tissue (upper arm, or abdomen). The device is currently approved for use by patients with type-I diabetes mellitus. The sensor measures interstitial glucose levels at few minutes intervals. Glucose is widely distributed in blood, intracellular fluid, interstitial fluid, tears, saliva, urine, and vitreous humor (in postmortem studies). Blood being the main sample in the diagnosis of diabetes mellitus.

Glucose values are transferred to an electronic readout device (or mobile reader or to an application on a mobile phone) that allows the patients to continually monitor their glucose levels with alarms when glucose levels exceed low and high set limits. The results may also be transmitted to a care provider (medical or not). The performance of those devices needs to be checked at least twice a day using a figure prick sample to validate readings obtained using the continuous glucose meter.

Although those are meant for continued monitoring, there is currently one CGM device that is approved for treatment decisions (Dexcom G5). Others require a confirmed figure stick blood test before treatment is instituted.

The devices are integral part of an automated insulin administration based on interstitial glucose levels "artificial pancreas." A closed loop system includes a CGM device as well as an insulin pump, which would allow for the improvement in blood glucose monitoring and insulin therapy administration in an all-in-one system. However, it is recommended that figure prick blood is used to validate the therapeutic corrections when using the automated insulin therapy.

In patients with type I diabetes mellitus, it is recommended that four glucose measurements are performed per day and more frequently in patients with concurrent illness. With continuous glucose monitoring, more frequent glucose levels are obtained (every 5 min) facilitating closer monitoring of fluctuations in glucose levels and ability for early intervention.

Imitations of interstitial glucose monitoring device are the physiological lag between blood and interstitial glucose that can last anywhere between 4 and 27 min affecting accuracy of measurement and thus placing the patient in risk of inappropriate insulin therapy. Appropriate calibrations of the CGM device with blood glucose readings are known to help minimize the lag time.

Glycated hemoglobin (A1c)

Hemoglobin A1c is a glycated form of hemoglobin (it is formed by a nonenzymatic chemical process where glucose binds to hemoglobin and not by an enzymatic glycosylation). The first step in the chemical reaction is the formation of an aldimine which is unstable (labile). This undergoes what is termed Amadori rearrangements which offer stability and commit the reaction to the stable glycated hemoglobin (Fig. 7). In normoglycemia, the percentage of hemoglobin that is glycated is less than 5.8%. The higher the glucose concentration and the longer hyperglycemia persists leads to higher percentage of glycated hemoglobin. Under normal red blood cell lifetime of 120 days, the percentage of glycated hemoglobin represents the integrated glucose levels over the receding 6–8 weeks. This is helpful, as glucose levels change in response to recent dietary and medications intake prior to sample collection. A normal glucose level during diabetes clinic visit may give a false reassurance of adequate management. Approximately half of the glycation occurs in the preceding 30 days. Forty percent between 31 and 90 days and 10% after 90 days. The half-life of the RBC mean survival is 120 days; thus A1c reflects a weighted mean glycaemia over the preceding 2–3 months in the absence of blood loss or hemolysis.

Several methods are avaiable for the measurement of A1c, they include chromatography and immunoassay based assays. Laboratories must use A1c assays that are certified by the NGSP as traceable to DCCT reference, and that laboratories should participate in proficiency testing programs. It is important to note that A1c methods are subject to interference by hemoglobin variants and discrepant results must be investigated for possible interference (see later).

Results of the DCCT and UKPDS trials have verified the close relationship between glycemic control measured by A1c and the risk for diabetes-related complications. A1c has been widely accepted as the standard used to measure glycemic control over the previous 3-month period and that

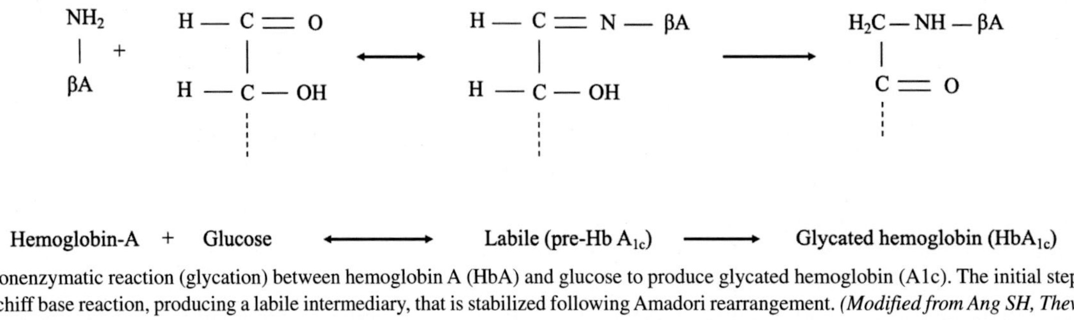

FIG. 7 Nonenzymatic reaction (glycation) between hemoglobin A (HbA) and glucose to produce glycated hemoglobin (A1c). The initial step is a rapid aldimine Schiff base reaction, producing a labile intermediary, that is stabilized following Amadori rearrangement. (*Modified from Ang SH, Thevarajah M, Alias Y, Khor SM. Current aspects in hemoglobin A1c detection: a review. Clin Chim Acta. 2015;439:202–211. https://doi.org/10.1016/j.cca.2014.10.019. Epub 2014 Oct 22. PMID: 25451954.*)

it correlates with patients' risk for developing diabetes-related complications such as retinopathy, nephropathy, and neuropathy. A1c measurement is required in the assessment of glycemic control in patients with diabetes mellitus. It provides an objective assessment of glycemic control in patients where frequent glucose values are variable and control status is difficult to assess clinically. Additionally, it has been approved for use in diagnosis of diabetes mellitus in patients with variable glucose values. Risk of developing diabetic complications, their progression, and improvement has been associated with A1c levels. For instances in patients with nephropathy and microalbuminuria, lower A1c levels are associated with more favorable renal outcomes. Similarly, for risk of development of diabetic retinopathy it is associated with both the duration of diabetes and the degree of A1c levels. Furthermore, as shown in the DCCT study, a 21% reduction in the risk of the composite primary cardiovascular disease outcome per 10% lower mean A1c is observed.

The frequency of A1c measurement varies from 3 to 4 times a year for patients with type I diabetes and twice a year for patients with type II. In general, while in patients with good control, A1c measurements at 1–2 times a year is appropriate and more frequently in those with difficult to control diabetes. A1c should be maintained at <7%, and that treatment regimen should be reevaluated if A1c is >8%.

Average glucose levels based on glycated hemoglobin (A1c) results

Professional societies support the reporting of estimated glucose concentrations in mg/dL or mmol/L from A1c results. This helps patients compare the glucose values with those reported in term of their periodic (less frequent) A1c testing. The patients are likely to have frequent glucose results obtained by home monitoring devices (fingerpick) or be continuous glucose monitoring or by laboratory-based methodologies on venous blood (Table 7). The relationship between A1C and eAG is described by the formula $28.7 \times A1C - 46.7 = eAG$.

Factors that affect interpretation of A1c results (interference—hemoglobinopathies)

Normal hemoglobin is made up of two α and two β subunits (97%). Other minor hemoglobin components are formed by posttranslational modification of HbA. They include hemoglobin's A1a, A1b, and A1c, with A1c being the most abundant hemoglobin variant component. Hemoglobin A1c is measured either by chromatographic methods (HPLC, electrophoresis) or by immunoinhibition (immunoassay) methodologies. Most methods in routine use are now standardized and are traceable to glycohemoglobin standardization program methodology. The National Glycohemoglobin Standardization Program (NGSP) was established in

TABLE 7 Estimated average glucose values using glycated hemoglobin (A1c) results.

A1C (%)	eAG (mg/dL)	(mmol/L)
6	126	7.0
6.5	140	7.8
7	154	8.6
7.5	169	9.4
8	183	10.1
8.5	197	10.9
9	212	11.8
9.5	226	12.6
10	240	13.4

The following formula is applied. $28.7 \times A1C - 46.7 = eAG$. Modified from Nathan DM, Kuenen J, Borg R, et al. Translating the A1C assay into estimated average glucose values. *Diabetes Care.* 2008;31(8):1473–1478. https://doi.org/10.2337/dc08-0545. Epub 2008 Jun 7. Erratum in: *Diabetes Care.* 2009;32(1):207. PMID: 18540046; PMCID: PMC2742903.

1996 to standardize A1c results to those of the DCCT and UKPDS trials that defined the relationship between A1c and vascular complications.

The four most commonly used methods to measure A1c are ion-exchange high-performance liquid chromatography (HPLC), boronate affinity HPLC, immunoassay, and enzymatic assays. Chromatographic methods employ separation of hemoglobin variants (including A1c) based on their charge and peaks quantified spectrophotometrically. The percentage of A1c is calculated using the ratio of A1c to total HbA and expressed as a percentage.

The methods are subject to interference by hemoglobin variants leading to either over or under estimation of A1c values. Genetic variants (e.g., HbS trait, HbC trait), elevated fetal hemoglobin (HbF) and chemically modified derivatives of hemoglobin (e.g., carbamylated Hb in patients with renal failure) can affect the accuracy of A1c measurements. However, the degree of interference is variable between the different methods and can lead to falsely low or falsely high A1c results. Patients heterozygous for HbS and HbC are at lower risk of interference when compared with those homozygous for the disorders. Interference often suspected when the A1c result is not consistent with blood glucose results and course of the disease. Interference from common A1c variant and the different methods for A1c commonly used for the measurement of A1c is shown in Table 8. Patients with red blood cell disorders (e.g., hemolytic anemia) or patients receiving blood transfusions have a short RBC half-life and thus unsuitable for A1c determination. For those patients, measurement of glycated albumin may be a possible alternative (see later).

TABLE 8 Interference from common hemoglobin variants on A1c measurements from commonly used methods.

Method	Interference (yes/no)					
	HbC trait	HbS trait	HbE trait	HbD trait	Elevated HbF	Carb Hb
Abbott Architect c Enzymatic	No	No	No	No	–	–
Alere Nycocard	No	No	a	a	b	–
Alere Afinion	No	No	No 16	No 16	b	–
Arkray ADAMS A1c HA-8180V Variant Mode (Menarini)	No	No	–/no/yes	–/yes/no	No <30%	–
Arkray ADAMS A1c HA-8180T	No	No	No	No	–	–
Arkray ADAMS A1c HA-8190V Variant Mode	No	No	No	No	No	–
Arkray The Lab 001 (POC)	No	Yes	No	No	No <42%	–
Beckman A1c, Advanced B93009 Online. Application on DxC 700 AU	No	No	No	No	–	–
Beckman A1c Advanced B00389 Manual Application on DxC 700 AU	No	No	No	No	–	–
Beckman A1c on Unicel DxC	No	No	No	No	–	–
Bio-Rad D-100	No	No	No	No	No ≤20%	–
Bio-Rad D-10 (short Program)	No	No	No	No	–	No
Bio-Rad Variant II A1c (NU)	No	No	No	No	No <10%	No
Bio-Rad Variant II Turbo (270-2415/2417)	No	No	Yes	Yes	No <5%	No
Bio-Rad Variant II Turbo 2.0	No	No	No/yes	No	No <25%	No
Diazyme Direct Enzymatic A1c	No	No	No	No	–	No
JEOL BM Test A1c on JCA-BM 6010/C	No	No	No	No	No <15%	–
Menarini HA-8160 (Diabetes Mode)	No	No	Yes	Yes	–	No
Menarini HA-8160 (Thalassemia Mode)	–	–	No	–	–	–
Ortho-Clinical Vitros	No	No	No	No	b	–
Pointe Scientific Hemoglobin A1c	No	No	No	No	b	–
Polymer Tech Systems A1cNow	Yes	Yes	No	No	b	–
Roche Cobas Integra Gen2	No	No	No	No	b	No
Roche Tina-quant II on Hitachi	No	No	No	No	b	No
Roche Cobas c513	No	No	No	No	b	–
Roche b 101	Yes/no	No	Yes	No	No <9.5%	–
Sebia Capillarys 2 Flex Piercing	No	No	No	No	No ≤15%/≤23%	No
Sebia Capillarys 3 Tera	No	No	No	No	No ≤23%	No
Siemens Advia A1c (original version)	Yes	Yes	a	a	b	–
Siemens Advia A1c (new version)	No	No	No	No	b	–
Siemens Atellica A1c	No	No	No	No	b	–
Siemens DCA 2000/DCA Vantage	No	No/yes	No/yes	No	No <10%	No
Siemens Dimension	No	No	No	No	b	–
Tosoh G7 Variant Mode	Yes/no	No	Yes	No	No ≤30%	No

TABLE 8 Interference from common hemoglobin variants on A1c measurements from commonly used methods—cont'd

Method	Interference (yes/no)					
	HbC trait	HbS trait	HbE trait	HbD trait	Elevated HbF	Carb Hb
Tosoh G8 Variant Mode Depends on software version	Yes/no	Yes/no	Yes/no	Yes/no	No ≤30%	No
Tosoh GX (orig. version)	Yes	Yes	Yes	Yes	–	–
Tosoh GX V1.22	Yes	Yes	No	Yes	–	–
Tosoh GX V1.24	No	No	No	No	–	–
Tosoh G11 Variant Mode (orig. version)	Yes	No	No	No	–	–
Tosoh G11 Variant Mode	No	No	No	Yes/no	–	–
Trinity (Primus) Boronate Affinity HPLC	No	No	No	No	No <15%	No

[a]In the absence of specific method data, it can generally be assumed that immunoassay methods do not have clinically significant interference from HbE and HbD because the E and D substitution are distant from the N-terminus of the hemoglobin beta chain.
[b]In the absence of specific method data, it can generally be assumed that both immunoassay methods and boronate affinity methods exhibit interference from HbF variant when present at levels >10%.
Many other publications have been reviewed. Only those with conclusions that are reasonably supported by data are included. For ion-exchange HPLC methods, interference from Hb variants and adducts may be dependent on the lot of reagents used. All entries in were based on published information. In addition, if a product insert indicates clearly that there is inference from a particular factor, then the interference is entered as "yes" and the product insert is cited. –, Not yet evaluated.
Modified from NGSP: A1c Assay Interferences. A1c methods: Effects of Hemoglobin Variants (HbC, HbS, HbE and HbD traits) and Elevated Fetal Hemoglobin (HbF). Updated June 2022. http://www.ngsp.org/interf.asp. Accessed 26 November 2022.

Over the past several years, there has been expanded use of point of care (POC) assays to measure A1c. Advantages of POC testing include fingerstick sampling in the provider's office and immediate patient and provider feedback leading to timely adjustments in the treatment regimen.

Results of the DCCT and UKPDS trials verified the close relationship between glycemic control measured by A1c and the risk for diabetes-related complications. A1c has been widely accepted as the standard used to measure glycemic control over the previous 3-month period and correlates with patients' risk for developing diabetes-related complications. As a general rule, for every 1% change in A1c, it is associated with an approximate 30 mg/dL (1.7 mmol/L) change in estimated average glucose.

Interestingly, significant racial and ethnic differences seem to exist in A1c readings for a given average glucose value. For example, Caucasians have been reported to have an absolute A1c reading approximately 0.1%–0.4% lower for the same average glucose levels when compared to other ethnicities such as Hispanics, Africans, or Asians. The reasons for these differences remain unclear.

Conditions leading to prolonged or decreased turnover of RBC life lead to prolonged or shortened exposure to circulating glucose and thus to false high and low A1c results respectively.

Any condition that shortens erythrocyte survival or decreases mean erythrocyte age (e.g., recovery from acute blood loss, hemolytic anemia) will falsely lower A1c test results regardless of the assay method used. Patients receiving blood transfusion, A1c results are uninterpretable; conflicting results some indicated falsely high A1c thought to be due to prolonged preservation of the transfused blood while others showed decreased values thought to be associated with dilutional effect.

Iron deficiency anemia, folate and B12 deficiency are associated with falsely elevated A1c, and correction of the anemia corrects A1c values. The exact mechanism is not known but thought to be related to decreased cell turnover.

Iron deficiency anemia, a major public health problem in developing countries, is associated with higher A1c and higher fructosamine. Consistent with these observations, iron replacement therapy lowers both A1c and fructosamine concentrations in diabetic and nondiabetic individuals.

Furthermore, A1c, but not glycated albumin, is increased in late pregnancy in nondiabetic individuals owing to iron deficiency. Insight into the mechanism was recently obtained by the observation that malondialdehyde, which is increased in patients with iron deficiency anemia enhances the glycation of hemoglobin. Alternative measures of glycemic assessment (e.g., continuous glucose monitoring) must be used in the presence of significant iron deficiency anemia, at least until the iron deficiency has been successfully treated.

Chronic renal failure develops in many diabetic patients. The role of glycemic control and the value of A1c in diabetic subjects with renal disease are controversial.

While interference from carbamylated Hb can be evaluated, the role of renal anemia, erythropoietin intake, and other factors in chronic renal failure is more difficult to evaluate.

Recent reports suggest A1c underestimates glycemic control in diabetic patients on dialysis, and that glycated albumin is a better indicator of glycemic control. Further studies are needed to clarify the role of A1c in diabetic patients with chronic renal failure.

Hypertriglyceridemia, uremia, high bilirubin >20 mg/dL are all associated with falsely elevated A1c. High dose vitamin C causes inhibition of glycation and causes a falsely low A1c when measured by electrophoresis. Drugs such as salicylate or lead poisoning result in falsely elevate A1c.

However, the degree of interference is variable between the different methods and can lead to falsely low or falsely high A1c results. Patients heterozygous for HbS and HbC are at lower risk of interference when compared with those homozygous for the disorders.

Genetic variants (e.g., HbS trait, HbC trait), elevated fetal hemoglobin (HbF) and chemically modified derivatives of hemoglobin (e.g., carbamylated Hb in patients with renal failure) may interfere with measurement of A1c.

The interference (positive or negative) depends on the methodology being used for A1c determination (e.g., immuno-based, ion-exchange chromatography, electrophoretic, etc.) and also on the hemoglobin variant. A recent review published on the National Glycohemoglobin Standardization Program (NGHSP) website is shown in Table 8. However, interpretation is complicated by the differences in the criteria applied for classification of significant interference between the different published studies.

It is important that when selecting an A1c assay methodology, laboratories consider the characteristics of their patient population (e.g., high prevalence of hemoglobinopathies or renal failure).

Glycated proteins—albumin (fructosamine)

Fructosamines are glycated proteins with the predominant protein being albumin. Nonenzymatic reaction between sugar and proteins.

Given the limitations with A1c measurements described above, few other alternative biomarkers of glycemic control have been used. They include fructosamine (glycated plasma proteins), glycated albumin, 1,5-anhydroglucitrol (1,5AG), as well as the continuous glucose monitoring.

Albumin, the predominant circulating protein, has a half-life of 21 days (shorter than of 120 days of hemoglobin), and thus, it provides an integrated glucose assessment over a 2–3-week period. It's utility is however influenced by disorders affecting albumin levels such as reduced synthesis in patients with chronic liver disease, in protein losing enteropathies (gastrointestinal disorders), and in kidney disease (nephrotic syndrome and proteinuria). Thyroid hormones stimulate albumin degradation. Albumin is a negative acute phase protein where reduced levels occur in inflammatory conditions and in sepsis.

Glycated albumin is typically reported as a percentage of total albumin. Interestingly, it performs better than A1c in patients with end-stage renal disease where A1c underestimates glycemic control.

Given the common variability in albumin and protein levels, its measurement is reserved for when A1c may be inaccurate, or to assess recent changes in glycemic control. The correlation between estimated average glucose, A1c, and fructosamine is shown in Table 9.

A1c results from patients with HbSS, HbCC, and HbSC must be interpreted with caution given the pathological processes, including anemia, increased red cell turnover, and transfusion requirements, that adversely impact A1c as a marker of long-term glycemic control. Alternative forms of testing such as fructosamine or glycated albumin should be considered for these patients.

1,5-Anhydroglucitol (1,5-AG)

1,5-Anhydroglucitol is a naturally occurring dietary polyol (e.g., glucitol, xylitol, and maltitol food sweetners). Renal absorption of 1,5-AG is competitively inhibited by glucose; thus, there is an inverse relationship between serum 1,5-AG and glycemic control. In the presence of high serum glucose (thus glucose filtrate), there is a reduction in serum 1,5-AG. It is thus a marker of glycemic control although over the preceding 48h and up to 2 weeks. It is helpful in detecting postprandial

TABLE 9 Correlations between estimated average glucose, A1c, and fructosamine levels.

Glucose (average) (mg/dL)	A1c (%)	A1c (mmol/mol)	Fructosamine (μmol/L)
97	5	31	131
126	6	42	203
154	7	53	273
183	8	64	345
212	9	75	417
240	10	86	487
269	11	97	559
298	12	108	631

(A1c = 0.017 × fructosamine level (μmol/L) + 1.61).
Modified from Radin MS. Pitfalls in hemoglobin A1c measurement: when results may be misleading. *J Gen Intern Med.* 2014;29(2):388–394. https://doi.org/10.1007/s11606-013-2595-x. Epub 2013 Sep 4. PMID: 24002631; PMCID: PMC3912281.

hyperglycemia and glucose variability. It is particularly helpful when A1c targets have been achieved, but there remains a need to assess the degree of postprandial hyperglycemia. Clearly, it depends on renal function and thus not reliable in patients with renal impairment producing falsely high 1,5-AG levels. Similar in pregnancy where there is altered renal glucose reabsorption threshold, leading to falsely low 1,5-AG serum levels. Falsely low levels are encountered in patients with low calorie intake or in chronic liver disease.

Although fructosamine, glycated albumin, 1,5-AG, and continuous glucose monitoring have been shown to correlate with mean glucose levels, it is important to remember that only A1c has been validated as a measure of both long-term glycemic control and risk for development of complications. Therefore, A1c remains the gold standard to measure average glycemic control.

Microalbumin (albuminuria)

Microalbuminuria denotes albumin concentration that is not detectable by urine strip test. Defined as excretion of 30–300 mg/24 h or 30–300 mg/g creatinine or 20–200 μg/min on two of three urine collections. The term microalbuminuria is a "misnomer," it denotes low amount of albumin and not a "small" albumin variant. Annual testing for microalbuminuria should be performed in patient without clinical proteinuria.

Albumin:creatinine ratio (ACR)

Diabetes mellitus is the leading cause of end-stage renal disease. Albuminuria is the hallmark of impaired kidney function in patients with diabetes mellitus. It is used to detect signs of diabetic nephropathy and monitor the course of the disease and response to therapy and diabetes control.

Microalbuminuria (albumin 30–300 mg/g) is an independent risk factor for the decline in renal function as well as cardiac morbidity and mortality. It is defined as albumin levels that are below the detection of urinary protein dipstick test, that is <300 mg/day. Microalbuminuria is defined as 30–300 mg/day (Table 10).

However, collection of timed urine collections (e.g., 24 h) is often inaccurate and cumbersome. The measurement of albumin in a random (spot) urine sample corrected for creatinine is a preferred alternative. Urine concentration is variable throughout the day and is influenced by patient hydration status and thus indexing measured analyte to creatinine concertation corrects for such variabilities.

Albumin measurement has a higher sensitivity for low levels of proteinuria when compared to total protein measurement.

ACR values vary by time of day and that a confirmatory sample be performed using a subsequent early morning sample when the ACR is between 3 mg/mmol and 70 mg/mmol in the initial detection of albuminuria.

ACR <10 mg/g (<1.1 mg/mmol) is considered normal, and ACR 10–29 mg/g (1.1–3.3 mg/mmol) is considered mildly increased. ACR values 30–300 mg/mmol are considered moderately increased, whereas ACR levels >300 considered severely increased and within the detection limit of urinary protein dipstick classified as proteinuria (Table 10).

The assays used for microalbuminuria employ antibodies directed against human albumin. The assays are nephelometric or turbidimetric in design. Polyethylene glycol (PEG) enhanced immunoturbidimetric assays offer higher degree of sensitivity and is widely used.

Diabetic nephropathy develops over a longtime before overt evidence of kidney disease is recognized. However, subtle increase of albumin excretion in urine (microalbuminuria) is an early indication of ongoing disease and early sign of an impending overt disease. Intervention does not just halt progression of kidney damage but may also reverse some of the damage that had occured.

Microalbuminuria can be detected within the first 10 years prior to overt clinical presentation. Periodic monitoring 2–3 times per year of urine albumin levels in patients with diabetes mellitus is thus recommended as early damage can be detected early and appropriate therapeutic intervention instituted including tighter glycemic control.

TABLE 10 Diagnostic microalbumin levels for different sample collection types.

	mg/24 h	Microgram/minute	Microgram/mg creatinine
Normal	<30	<20	<30
Microalbuminuria	30–300	20–200	30–300
Clinical albuminuria	>300	>200	>300

Modified from Kamińska J, Dymicka-Piekarska V, Tomaszewska J, Matowicka-Karna J, Koper-Lenkiewicz OM. Diagnostic utility of protein to creatinine ratio (P/C ratio) in spot urine sample within routine clinical practice. *Crit Rev Clin Lab Sci.* 2020;57(5):345–364. https://doi.org/10.1080/10408363.2020.1723487. Epub 2020 Feb 14. PMID: 32058809. Papadopoulou-Marketou N, Chrousos GP, Kanaka-Gantenbein C. Diabetic nephropathy in type 1 diabetes: a review of early natural history, pathogenesis, and diagnosis. *Diabetes Metab Res Rev.* 2017;33(2). https://doi.org/10.1002/dmrr.2841. Epub 2016 Oct 4. PMID: 27457509.

Other biochemical investigations

Ketone bodies include: acetone, acetoacetate, and β-hydroxybutyrate are qualitatively screened for or measured using urine or blood samples respectivley. Urine and blood qualitative strips detect acetone and acetoacetate but not β-hydroxybutyrate (which is the predominant metabolite early in diabetic ketoacidosis presentation). This may lead to misclassification of early presenters as nonketotic hyperglycemia. Lack of insulin results in increased lipolysis, increased fatty acids and production of ketone bodies. Ketones lead to metabolic acidosis. Patients require close biochemical monitoring for blood Na, K, Cl, bicarbonate, urea (BUN), and creatinine. It is important to note that alkaline picrate methods for measurement of creatinine is affected by ketones and falsely elevated creatinine results are obtained. Enzymatic methods for creatinine are not affected by ketones and similarly for uric acid.

Diabetic dyslipidemia is characterized by elevated LDL-c, hypertriglyceridemia, and low HDL-c. All adults with diabetes mellitus should receive annual lipid profile (total cholesterol, LDL-c, HDL-c, and triglycerides levels) measurement. Individuals at low risk, where LDL-c < 100 mg/dL (2.6 mmol/L) and HDL-c > 45 (1.15 mmol/L) in men, and 55 (1.4 mmol/L) in females, are screened less frequently.

Although there is little value in routinely measuring insulin levels in the diagnosis of diabetes mellitus where the differentiation between diabetes type I and type II is based on clinical presentation and subsequent course, in rare instances it is useful to identify patients with absolute requirements for insulin prior to switching to oral agents, to assist patients in obtaining insurance coverage for continuous subcutaneous infusion pumps, and for the assessment of insulin resistance in the evaluation of patients with polycystic ovary syndrome.

Population screening for diabetes: Mellitus

Population screening for diabetes has been performed as part of health awareness fairs and health promotions, examples during celebrations of world diabetes day. Screening is recommended because, the onset of type II DM occurs ~4–7 years before clinical diagnosis, onset of complications may begin several years before clinical diagnosis, and that patients with type II may not be diagnosed (in the United States, ~30% of type-II are not diagnosed). Screening is recommended for those at risk (≥45 years old, BMI ≥ 25 kg/m^2).

Screening children is at age 10 years and every 2 years in overweight individuals with two other risk factors (family history, race/ethnicity, and signs of insulin resistance). In patients with fasting blood glucose < 100 mg/dL (5.6 mmol/L) and or 2 h < 140 mg/dL (7.8 mmol/L), repeat testing can be delayed up to 3 years.

Instruments often used in screening initiatives are those of point of care testing (used outside healthcare facility in the field). They have limitations stated above with regards to hematocrit, operator techniques as in sample volume application and proper strip use and instrument calibration.

Most glucose screening activities are opportunistic (health fairs, annual physical exam, preemployment exams, etc.). There are no clear guidelines on active screening, however those at risk, patients >65 years old, >45 with one or more risk factor (e.g., BMI ≥ 25, hypertension, vascular disease, hyperlipidemia, polycystic ovary syndrome, previous gestational diabetes, autoimmune disorders, and on certain drugs, e.g., steroids, β-blockers), and patients <45 years old with two or more risk factors should be screened. Random or preferably fasting glucose measurements are performed, and repeat confirmation of abnormal result using a confirmed fasting sample unless symptoms are present.

Use of abnormal glucose values obtained on whole blood capillary samples using a glucose meter must not be used to label the diagnosis of diabetes mellitus, and that the abnormal glucose values must be confirmed by two laboratory measurements unless unequivocal symptoms are present. Urine testing for diagnosis is not recommend.

Hypoglycemia

Hypoglycemia is usually due to imbalance between glucose intake, endogenous glucose production, and glucose utilization. Hypoglycemia is defined as circulating glucose levels less than 45 mg/dL (2.5 mmol/L), with levels less than 40 mg/dL (<2.0 mmol/L) considered critical requiring immediate notification and corrective action.

Glucose is maintained by hepatic gluconeogenesis from protein metabolism (alanine and glutamine), glycerol (from fats), lactate and pyruvate. Ketone bodies (obtained following fatty acids oxidation) provide source of energy for the brain and for the gluconeogenic pathway.

Hypoglycemia can be due to increased glucose utilization in states of hyperinsulinism for instance, secondary to maternal diabetes, in patients with islet cell adenoma, nesidioblastosis, neonatal idiopathic hyperinsulinism, surreptitious insulin administration (C-peptide levels are relatively and inappropriately low in surreptitious administration).

Hypoglycemia can be secondary to impaired glycogen metabolism due to the various glycogen storage disorders (glycogen synthase deficiency) and impaired glycogenolysis (hepatic glycogen storage disorders), impaired ketogenesis and ketone bodies utilization, carnitine-mediated defects, (carnitine palmitoyl transferase deficiency), β-oxidation defects with short-, medium-, and long-chain acyl CoA dehydrogenase deficiency, enoyl CoA hydratase deficiency, ketone body utilization defects, reduced gluconeogenesis, interference with glucose homeostasis, other causes include endocrine disorders, liver disease, gastrointestinal surgery, insulinoma, malignancy (due to tumor production of IGFs and associated with tumor burden), drugs, and iatrogenic and idiopathic in nature.

Excessive glucagon secretion is seen in patients with pancreatic tumor, in the carcinoid syndrome and as part of neuroendocrine neoplasm and hepatocellular carcinoma. Patients being investigated for hypoglycemia often have glucagon measured as part of a metabolic hypoglycemic profile that incudes insulin and C-peptide levels often as part of a mixed-meal test in patients with suspected post-prandial hypoglycemia.

Onset of hypoglycemia is rapid with characteristic symptoms due to either neuroglycopenia or the increased catecholamine release brought about by the developing hypoglycemia. Such symptoms include altered behavior, pallor, anxiousness, sweating, and palpitations.

The etiology of hypoglycemia is best defined by the age of the patient at presentation. For instance, in adults, drugs (insulin dosage in relation to dietary caloric intakes), insulinoma, malignancy, and starvation, and possible inborn errors. For the latter, however, adults with managed inborn errors of metabolism who have survived into adulthood are obviously at risk of hypoglycemia secondary to the primary inborn errors in metabolism.

In neonates, the etiology is likely to be due to reduced glycogen stress (intrauterine growth retardation), infants of diabetic mothers (state of maternal hyperglycemia, suppressed or inadequate neonatal insulin response), and inborn errors of metabolism. Biochemical investigations of hypoglycemia include insulin, C-peptide, free fatty acids, amino acids, organic acids, and drug measurements.

Age-related reference intervals are required to aid with the interpretation of hormones for instance glucagon levels as they are markedly elevated in the neonatal period (up to 8 times the upper limit in adults) this is due to reduced glycogen stores and to feeding patterns.

Neonates and children are at risk of hypoglycemia because they have increased glucose utilization rate per kg body weight relative to adults, they also have little glycogen stores which are quickly depleted (after a 12–14h fast) compared to adults. The muscles also contain little precursors for gluconeogenesis. All of this makes neonates prone to hypoglycemia hence more common in neonates and children than in adults.

When investigating causes of hypoglycemia in neonates, blood samples would ideally be collected during the hypoglycemic episode. The following biochemical tests are performed and include glucose, lactate, free fatty acids, 3-β hydroxybutarate, alanine and carnitine, insulin, c-peptide, cortisol, urine organic acids, pyruvate, and acetoacetate measurements. Laboratory findings associated with hypoglycemia are summarized in Table 11.

TABLE 11 Common age-related causes of hypoglycemia and associated biochemical findings.

Patients	Increased utilization:	Impaired glycogenolysis	Impaired ketogenesis	Impaired gluconeogenesis	Organic and amino aciduria
Adult	High insulin High C-peptide	Hepatic dysfunction	Hepatic dysfunction	Hepatic failure	Patients with neonatal disorders reaching adulthood on maintenance therapy
Neonate/childhood	High insulin Low free fatty acids (<0.8 mmol/L) High C-peptide	High lactate	High free fatty acids. Low ketone bodies Variable carnitine	High lactate Hypopituitary (Low TSH, T4, GH, cortisol)	Variable GC and LCMSMS profile abnormalities

Patient presentation lead investigation:	
	Investigation:
Ill on presentation	Review of medications (drugs: insulin, alcohol, cibenzoline, gatifloxacin, pentamidine, quinine, indomethacin, etc.) Critical illness: Sepsis Organ failure: Hepatic, renal, cardiac Hormone deficiencies: Cortisol, glucagon, and epinephrine (in insulin deficiency diabetes) Nonislet cell tumors
Healthy on presentation	Endogenous hyperinsulinism: Insulinoma, nesidioblastosis, insulin autoimmune hypoglycemia, antibodies to insulin, antibodies to insulin receptor, post gastric bypass, etc. Factitious/accidental insulin use

Modified from several sources including Cryer PE, Axelrod L, Grossman AB, et al. Evaluation and management of adult hypoglycemic disorders: an Endocrine Society Clinical Practice Guideline. *J Clin Endocrinol Metab.* 2009;94(3):709–728. https://doi.org/10.1210/jc.2008-1410. Epub 2008 Dec 16. PMID: 19088155.

Summary

- Glucose, a monosaccharide, a source of cellular energy, its circulating level is maintained within a narrow limit, with about 1%–2% intraindividual variability, to prevent both hyperglycemia and hypoglycemia.
- A number of hormones regulate glucose metabolism include insulin, glucagon, growth hormone, cortisol, IGF-1, thyroid hormones, among others.
- Carbohydrates with free aldehyde or keto groups are reducing sugars and include glucose and lactose.
- Insulin is synthesized within the endoplasmic reticulum of the β cells of the pancreatic islets of Langerhans.
- Glucagon is synthesized in the α-cells of the pancreas in response to local changes in glucose, insulin, or amino acid concentrations.
- Cortisol increases the rate of hepatic gluconeogenesis from proteins and amino acids and thus leads to a state of hyperglycemia.
- Fasting glucose is maintained at about 4.5–5.2 mmol/L (81–94 mg/dL), whereas postprandial glucose normally does not exceed 8–10 mmol/L (144–180 mg/dL).
- Random nonfasting glucose levels above 11.1 mmol/L (200 mg/dL) are considered hyperglycemic and are suggestive of diabetes mellitus.
- Diabetes mellitus, a heterogenous syndrome characterized by chronic hyperglycemia, is a fundamental defect in insulin secretion and or action.
- Patients with type-I diabetes mellitus represent (∼5%–10%) of diabetic patients.
- Type II DM in its classic form is characterized by high but low over time insulin level. There is no autoimmune destruction of the β pancreatic isle cells.
- Several variants of type I and II diabetes mellitus are described.
- The presence of hyperglycemia first detected during pregnancy is termed gestational diabetes.
- Uncontrolled or poorly controlled states of hyperglycemia in diabetes mellitus lead to complications such as nephropathy, neuropathy, retinopathy, and vascular circulatory disorders.
- Heart failure is common among patients with diabetes mellitus with prevalence of 9%–27% and leads to serious complications and mortality. Periodic screening using BNP or NTproBNP is recommnded.
- Proper sample handling is required to minimize invitro glucose consumption and thus falsely low glucose results.
- Several enzymatic methods (glucose oxidase, hexokinase, etc.) are used in the measurement glucose. The methods are subject to interference in critically ill patients and by other hexoses (galactose) in the hexokinase method.
- Hemoglobin A1c is glycated hemoglobin (it is a chemical process where glucose binds to hemoglobin and not an enzymatic glycosylation).
- A1c levels provide an assessment of the average blood glucose levels over the preceding 2–3 months.
- Glycated albumin provides an integrated glucose level over a 2–3-week period.
- Albuminuria is the hallmark of impaired kidney function in patients with diabetes mellitus.
- Hypoglycemia is defined as circulating glucose levels less than 45 mg/dL (2.5 mmol/L) and the etiology is often guided by the age of the patient at presentation.
- Causes of hypoglycemia include endocrine disorders, liver disease, gastrointestinal surgery, insulinoma, malignancy, drugs, and inborn errors of metabolism.

Further reading

Niswender KD. Basal insulin: physiology, pharmacology, and clinical implications. *Postgrad Med.* 2011;123(4):17–26.

Nathan DM, DCCT/Edic Research Group. The diabetes control and complications trial/epidemiology of diabetes interventions and complications study at 30 years: overview. *Diabetes Care.* 2014;37(1):9–16.

UK Prospective Diabetes Study (UKPDS) Group. Intensive blood-glucose control with sulphonylureas or insulin compared with conventional treatment and risk of complications in patients with type 2 diabetes (UKPDS 33). *Lancet.* 1998;352(9131):837–853.

Hoogwerf BJ. Type of diabetes mellitus: does it matter to the clinician? *Cleve Clin J Med.* 2020;87(2):100–108.

Jia Y, Liu Y, Feng L, Sun S, Sun G. Role of glucagon and its receptor in the pathogenesis of diabetes. *Front Endocrinol (Lausanne).* 2022;13:928016.

Plows JF, Stanley JL, Baker PN, Reynolds CM, Vickers MH. The pathophysiology of gestational diabetes mellitus. *Int J Mol Sci.* 2018;19(11).

Ekanayake PS, Juang PS, Kulasa K. Review of intravenous and subcutaneous electronic glucose management systems for inpatient glycemic control. *Curr Diab Rep.* 2020;20(12):68.

Lebovitz HE, Banerji MA. Ketosis-prone diabetes (Flatbush diabetes): an emerging worldwide clinically important entity. *Curr Diab Rep.* 2018;18(11):120.

Kaminska J, Dymicka-Piekarska V, Tomaszewska J, Matowicka-Karna J, Koper-Lenkiewicz OM. Diagnostic utility of protein to creatinine ratio (P/C ratio) in spot urine sample within routine clinical practice. *Crit Rev Clin Lab Sci.* 2020;57(5):345–364.

Chapter 7

Lipids metabolism and cardiac biomarkers

Introduction

This chapter describes lipids metabolism and dysfunction and their laboratory investigation. It also discusses cardiac biomarkers and their utility in the assessment of acute coronary syndrome and in patients congestive heart failure.

Lipids and cardiovascular disease risk

The relationship between lipids and risk for cardiovascular atherosclerotic disease is well stablished with several pathogenesis and risk models described.

Lipoprotein particles (with variable sizes and density secondary to the relative triglycerides and cholesterol contents) are present in the circulation. They originate from dietary cholesterol and triglycerides transported from the intestinal and from the liver and from endogenous hepatic de novo synthesis (Fig. 3).

Very low-density lipoprotein particles (VLDL) contain most of the triglyceride in plasma whereas low-density lipoprotein (LDL) particles contain most of the cholesterol. In addition to few chylomicrons, they all contain Apo B which aid in their solubility and entry into tissue.

Circulating LDL and small (<70 nm) Apo B lipoproteins and VLD and their remnant particles flux freely across endothelial barrier and interact with extracellular structures such as proteoglycans and become retained in the extracellular matrix.

According to the "response-to-retention" model of atherosclerosis, the retention of Apo B-containing lipoprotein particles in the subintimal arterial wall provokes a complex inflammatory process that initiates the formation of an atheroma. Over time and as more and more lipoprotein particles become retained in the artery wall the initial atheroma gradually enlarges, leading to the formation of an increasingly larger and more complex atherosclerotic plaques.

Normally >90% of circulating plasma Apo B-containing lipoproteins are actually LDL particles and that at any LDL concentration, the likelihood of the LDL particles being retained in the artery wall is small; however, as additional LDL particles become entrapped and retained overtime, this leads to the development and growth of atherosclerotic plaques with intravascular ultrasound studies consistently demonstrate that the rate of atherosclerotic plaque progression is directly proportional to the absolute plasma LDL levels.

Plaque burden is determined not just by its LDL and Apo B concentrations (among other Apo B-containing lipoproteins), but also by the length of exposure. Therefore, a person's total atherosclerotic plaque burden is approximately proportional to his or her cumulative exposure to LDL and other Apo B-containing lipoproteins, and it can be approximated by multiplying a person's age by the LDL concentration to obtain an estimate of cumulative LDL exposure determined in either mg-years (age LDL-C measured in mg/dL) or mmol years.

The accumulated threshold for cumulative LDL exposure required to develop an atherosclerotic plaque burden large enough to increase the risk for acute cardiovascular syndrome is about 5000 mg years or 125 mmol years.

It is thus clear that reducing the levels and minimizing cumulative exposure to LDL and Apo-B-containing lipoprotein is the goal to reduce risk of atherosclerotic plaque accumulation and thus leading to substantial reduction in lifetime risk of experiencing a cardiovascular event.

Lipids and lipoproteins

Lipids are a heterogeneous group of substances which have in common their low solubility in water and being more readily soluble in organic solvents but are diverse in their structures with little functional relationship with each other.

They are broadly divided into sterols (which include cholesterol), fatty acids (which include triglycerides), phospholipids, C-20 eicosanoids (which include prostaglandins), sphingolipids, and lipoproteins (which include chylomicrons, VLDL, ILDL, LDL, and HDL) (Table 1).

The principal lipids are cholesterol and triglycerides. They differ markedly in their structure and their clinical and diagnostic importance. The lipids are dynamic in nature with variable size and constituents.

Cholesterol

Cholesterol is the predominant sterol and may exist as free cholesterol or as esterified with a fatty acyl group. It is an essential component of cell membranes where it is present

Tutorials in Clinical Chemistry. https://doi.org/10.1016/B978-0-12-822949-1.00010-3

TABLE 1 Major classes of lipids, their structure and function.

Lipid classes	Contents	Function
Cholesterol		Precursor of adrenal and gonadal steroids and bile acids, vitamin D. Structural component of membrane
Triglycerides	Fatty acids	Energy
	Glycerol	Energy
Phospholipids		Structural component membrane
Eicosanoids		Multifunctions: coagulation, reproduction, vascular
Sphingolipids		Blood groups, central nervous system
Lipoproteins	Major apolipoprotein	
	Chylomicrons	Contains B-48
	VLDL	Contains B-100
	ILDL	Contains B-100
	LDL	Contains B-100
	HDL	Contains A-I and A-II

HDL, high-density lipoprotein; *IDL*, intermediate density lipoprotein; *LDL*, low-density lipoprotein; *VLDL*, very low-density lipoprotein.
Modified from Feingold KR. Lipid and lipoprotein metabolism. *Endocrinol Metab Clin N Am.* 2022;51(3):437–458. https://doi.org/10.1016/j.ecl.2022.02.008. Epub 2022 Jul 4. PMID: 35963623. Feingold KR. Introduction to lipids and lipoproteins. 2021 Jan 19. In: Feingold KR, Anawalt B, Blackman MR, et al., eds. *Endotext [Internet].* South Dartmouth, MA: MDText.com, Inc.; 2000. PMID: 26247089.

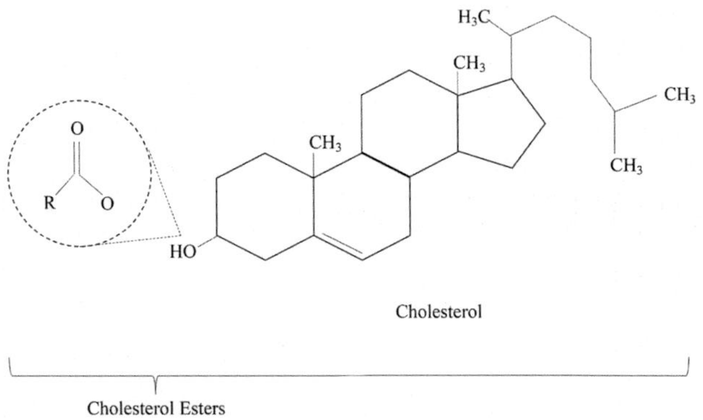

FIG. 1 Cholesterol and cholesterol esters chemical structure. *(Modified from Fahy E, Subramaniam S, Brown HA, et al. A comprehensive classification system for lipids. J Lipid Res. 2005;46(5):839–861. https://doi.org/10.1194/jlr.E400004-JLR200. Epub 2005 Feb 16. Erratum in: J Lipid Res. 2010;51(6):1618. PMID: 15722563.)*

Dietary fats are hydrolyzed in the intestine to free fatty acids and triglycerides. Triglyceride-rich lipoproteins constitute chylomicrons, whereas triglycerides of endogenous origin circulate in hepatically derived VLDL (Figs. 2 and 3).

Triglycerides taken in the diet are hydrolyzed by pancreatic lipase into its monoacylglycerol and free fatty acids constituents. Those are emulsified by luminal bile acids and absorbed by enterocytes. They are resynthesized into triglycerides and stored into chylomicrons which enter the circulation.

Adipose and muscle tissue rich in lipoprotein lipase takes up chylomicrons and metabolize triglycerides. The small number of remaining chylomicrons is taken up by hepatocytes where their triglycerides content is metabolized into fatty acids.

During fasting states, albumin bound plasma fatty acids are the main sources of hepatic triglycerides where it is taken up by hepatocytes and converted into triglycerides. Plasma insulin levels are low during fasting states, and fatty acid levels increase following increased lipolysis in white adipose tissue. In the fed state, glucose is converted to fatty acids in hepatocytes (de novo lipogenesis).

Hypertriglyceridemia is common in clinical practice with prevalence about 10% among adults. However, the prevalence of severe hypertriglyceridemia is defined as triglycerides >10 mmol/L (>885 mg/dL) and is low ranging from 0.1% to 0.2%.

as free cholesterol and unesterified form. It is the precursor of steroid hormones (adrenal and gonadal steroids).

Cholesterol although present in the diet, the major source is hepatic de-novo synthesis from acetate. The rate determining step of its synthesis is the conversion of 3-hydroxy-3-methylglutaryl-coenzyme A to mevalonate, a step catalyzed by the enzyme 3-hydroxy-3-methylglutaryl-coenzyme A (HMG-CoA) reductase. The enzyme is the target of the statin cholesterol lowering drugs.

Metabolically, it is the backbone of steroids synthesis and a structural component of cellular membranes influencing the stability of phospholipids (Fig. 1).

Triglycerides and fatty acids

Composed of three fatty acid molecules esterified with glycerol. They represent the major storage form of fatty acids and serve as the major energy store in mammals.

Lipoproteins

Macromolecular complexes of lipid and protein. They are the large triglyceride-rich lipoproteins. Chylomicrons and VLDL (very low-density lipoproteins), small cholesterol-rich lipoproteins LDL (low-density lipoprotein), and HDL (high-density lipoprotein). Despite such classification, it must be emphasized that lipoprotein sizing and composition does not represent a series of discrete groups but a

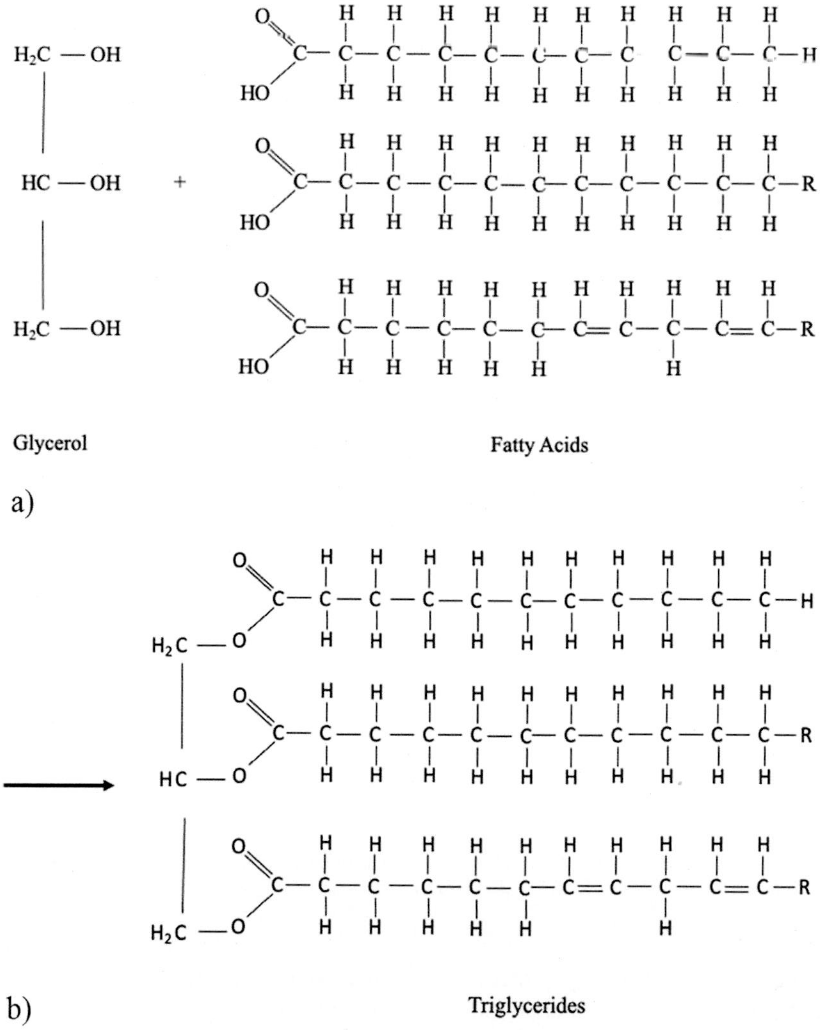

FIG. 2 Triglycerides chemical structure. Triglycerides composed of glycerol and three free fatty acids (saturated and unsaturated), and they are often >16C in length. *(Modified from Fahy E, Subramaniam S, Brown HA, et al. A comprehensive classification system for lipids. J Lipid Res. 2005;46(5): 839–861. https://doi.org/10.1194/jlr.E400004-JLR200. Epub 2005 Feb 16. Erratum in: J Lipid Res. 2010;51(6):1618. PMID: 15722563.)*

spectrum. It is dynamic in nature, and its solubility is enhanced by binding to apoproteins forming lipoproteins (Lipids + Apolipoproteins = Lipoproteins).

All lipoproteins have a water-soluble surface layer, the so-called amphipathic shell, consisting of phospholipids, apolipoproteins, and free cholesterol. Within this is contained a polar core rich in cholesteryl ester and triglyceride.

Lipids represent hydrophobic molecules that must be carried in a hydrophilic environment, thus they are stabilized as lipoproteins.

Chylomicrons

Produced in the small intestine, they are hydrolyzed by lipoprotein lipase in the capillary bed and the resulting smaller triglyceride depleted remnants removed by hepatic uptake. During hydrolysis, surface components are transferred to HDL particles.

Formed in the intestine, chylomicrons are the largest among the lipoproteins with molecular weight ranging 50,000–1,000,000 (kDa). They contain dietary fats with triglycerides constituting 95% of content. The major protein component is Apo B-48. It also contains Apo A-I and A-II and acquires Apo E and Apo D from HDL-cholesterol.

Very low-density lipoprotein (VLDL)

Produced by the liver, their ultimate fate is either hepatic uptake or conversion to LDL.

The major content is endogenously synthesized lipids and represents the largest among those with molecular weight 10,000–80,000 kDa. Apo B-100 is the predominant protein but also contain Apo CI, -II,-III. Apo E is acquitted from circulating HDL-cholesterol. Although similar to chylomicrons, predominantly containing triglycerides, it differs in that the triglycerides are endogenous and not dietary source.

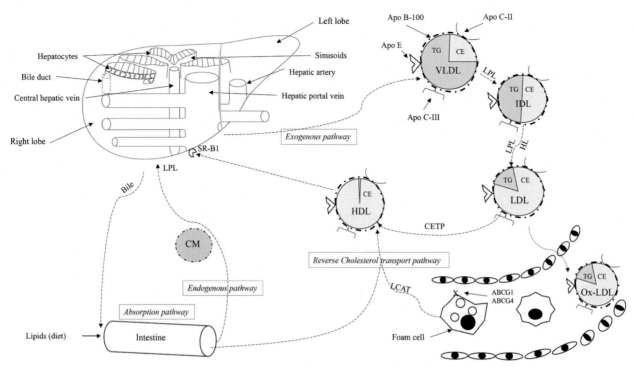

FIG. 3 Lipids metabolism and transformation of the various lipid molecules. They are dynamic in nature.

(Apo B-100), Apo-E, Apo C-II, Apo C-III, SR-B1: scavenger receptor B1. *CE*, cholesterol esters; *CETP*, cholesterol ester transport protein; *CM*, chylomicrons; *HDL*, high-density lipoprotein; *HL*, hepatic lipase; *IDL*, intermediate density lipoproteins; *LCAT*, lecithin cholesterol transferase; *LDL*, low-density lipoprotein; *LPL*, lipoprotein lipase; *Ox-LDL*, oxidized LDL; *TG*, triglycerides; *VLDL*, very low-density lipoprotein. *(Modified from Mehta A, Shapiro MD. Apolipoproteins in vascular biology and atherosclerotic disease. Nat Rev Cardiol. 2022;19(3):168–179. https:// doi.org/10.1038/s41569-021-00613-5. Epub 2021 Oct 8. PMID: 34625741.)*

During its transition to low-density lipoprotein, an intermediate form (IDL) with molecular weight 5000–10,000 kDa appears in circulation containing relatively more cholesterol esters and less triglycerides, and that contains mainly apoproteins B-100, C, and E.

Intermediate density lipoprotein (IDL)

Produced by lipolysis of VLDL by lipoprotein lipase, they can be either cleared by hepatic uptake or converted to LDL by further removal of triglyceride and transfer of surface components to HDL.

Low-density lipoprotein (LDL)

Produced, though direct synthesis may rarely occur, from VLDL via IDL removal is by peripheral or hepatic uptake by ligand-receptor or scavenger pathways.

The major cholesterol containing and circulating lipoprotein with predominately cholesterol esters. The major protein is B-100. Its molecular weight is 2300 kDa and represents the end product of VLDL metabolism.

Although there are analytical methods for direct measurement of LDL-cholesterol, LDL-cholesterol has histori-

cally been estimated by calculating total cholesterol minus HDL-cholesterol.

High-density lipoprotein (HDL)

Produced as nascent particles by the liver and small intestine. Surface components (mainly Apo C) are acquired from VLDL and chylomicrons during their hydrolysis by lipoprotein lipase. The fate of these particles is obscure, but they are thought to play a role in reverse cholesterol transport to the liver. They appear to be inversely associated with atherogenesis.

This is the smallest of the lipoproteins with molecular weight ranging between 200 and 400 kDa. The HDL component may be classified into three components (HDL2, HDL3, and pre-beta-HDL) based on molecular weight, apoprotein contents and electrophoretic mobility, although not routinely measured separately, the classification helps with understanding the variable contents and metabolic action pre-β-HDL (molecular weight 70 kDa) predominantly contains Apo AI, and phospholipids, and is a substrate for ATP-binding cassette transporter AI, which exports circulating free cholesterol from peripheral cells and macrophages, HDL3 (molecular weight

200 kDa) formed from pre-β by acquiring more free cholesterol and is a substrate for lecithin cholesterol acyl transferase (LCAT). Thus, esterifies free cholesterol which cause increase ion the size of the particle facilitating uptake of more free cholesterol leading to the formation of the larger particle HDL2 (molecular weight 400 kDa). HDL2 predominantly contains Apo AI, where Apo AI and II predominates in HDL3.

Lipoprotein lipase (LPL)

Lipoprotein lipase (LPL) is present in cells that either stores triglycerides, i.e., adipose tissue and or uses it as energy source (skeletal and cardiac muscle). LPL is anchored on the endothelial cell on the luminal side by becoming attached to glycans and captures triglyceride-rich lipoprotein particles as they pass through.

Activated LPL together with heparan sulfate proteoglycans is anchored onto the luminal side of capillary endothelial cells by glycosylphosphatidylinositol-anchored HDL-binding protein. VLDL and chylomicrons newly synthesized have low surface pressure and readily binds to LPL and ApoC-II and are displaced as surface pressure increases with lipolysis. LPL is inhibited by ApoC-II and ApoC-I as well as by angiopoietin-related proteins 3, 4, and 8. Apo A-V is another LPL cofactor. Those components are of interest as therapeutic targets.

Apolipoproteins

Apolipoproteins are structural components of plasma lipoproteins they render the lipoproteins soluble, and as such influence the pathophysiology of atherosclerosis. There are a number of apolipoproteins (Apo A, B (B-48, B-100), Apo C (I, II, III), D, E). Apo B (100 and 48), Apo A (I), Apo C (II, III), Apo E, and Apo (a) are the most clinically relevant (Table 2). The insoluble apolipoproteins act as the skeleton backbone on which lipids (triglycerides and cholesterol esters), free cholesterol phospholipids aggregate to from lipoprotein particles. Additionally, they maintain the structural integrity, and facilities transfer lipids into tissues. They facilitate by acting as cofactors for lipoprotein lipase facilitating binding to its active site. Apolipoproteins C-II, C-III, and E participate in triglyceride-rich lipoprotein metabolism. Apolipoprotein (a) covalently binds to Apo B-100. Apo B and Apo (a) individually and collectively play central and highly specialized roles in the metabolism of lipoproteins. In addition to their catalytical activities, they represent structural ladder/backbone for the lipids to build on and organize.

Recent advances in cardiovascular therapeutics have led to the development of novel agents that target specific apolipoproteins to reduce the risk of atherosclerotic cardiovascular disease.

They are characterized either exchangeable (soluble) or nonexchangeable (insoluble) (Table 2). The insoluble (e.g., Apo B100, B-48) are not found freely in plasma and not exchangeable between the various lipoproteins.

Apo A-I

ApoA-I is a 243 amino acid long. It is primarily associated and is a major structural component of HDL and thus plays an important role in reverse cholesterol transport mechanism. It is synthesized by hepatocytes and intestine. It is degraded by the cubilin system if not utilized.

Apolipoprotein A-I provides the scaffolding for HDL build up and thus play an important role in reverse cholesterol transport (Fig. 3).

Lipid-free ApoA-I stimulates the reverse cholesterol pathway facilitating transfer of free cholesterol and phospholipids into nascent HDL. LCAT transfers fatty acyl chains to free cholesterol relocating the newly formed cholesterol esters from surface to core of the HDL particle. Both ApoA-I and ApoC-I are potent activators of this process.

Mature HDL interacts with ABCG1/4 and SR-B1 (Fig. 3) mediating passive cholesterol efflux from the foam cell, in addition to a passive concentration driven cholesterol efflux.

Hepatic uptake of mature HDL via SR-B1 receptor completes the revers cholesterol transport cycle. There is a close relationship between ApoA-I and HDL-cholesterol levels. Furthermore, HDL-cholesterol is inversely related to cardiovascular risk.

Ratio of ApoB to ApoA has a high population-attributable risk and odds ratio for estimating the risk of coronary artery disease compared with traditional lipids markers (tot Chol, non-HDL chol).

ApoB-100

Important structural component of VLDL, IDL, LDL, and Lp(a). A 4536 amino acid product of the APOB gene, its level is highly regulated given its important structural role.

Apo B-100 is the major structural component of very low-density lipoprotein (VLDL), intermediate density lipoprotein (IDL), low-density lipoprotein (LDL), and apolipoprotein (a). B-48, a truncated form of B-100, is the major structural component of chylomicrons.

Synthesized by the liver and its production is constitutively expressed, that is its production depends on the liver fat content. In low lipid states ApoB-100 is directed toward degradation, in high lipid states, triglycerides are added to forming pre-VLDL, which is further added triglycerides forming VLDL, and the latter is secreted into the extracellular environment and that triglycerides are delivered to those

TABLE 2 Apolipoproteins characteristics and function.

Apo-lipoprotein	Site of production	Mol. wt.	Solubility	Associated with	Role
A-I	Livre, small intestine	29	Soluble	HDL, CM	Major apolipoprotein found in HDL. Cofactor for lecithin cholesterol acyltransferase (LCAT). Deficiency of Apo A-I associated with premature cardiovascular disease. Hypoalphalipoproteinemia (Tangier disease) rare
A-II		17		HDL	LPL-regulator, LCAT and CETP cofactor
A-IV		44		Chylomicron, HDL	LCAT activator
A-V		41		Chylomicron, VLDL, HDL	LPL activator, chylomicron assembly
C-I		7		Chylomicron, VLDL, HDL	
C-II	Liver, small intestine, macrophages, adipose tissue	9	Soluble	Chylomicron and VLDL (also in IDL and HDL). Activates LPL	LPL activator
C-III	Liver, small intestine	9	Soluble	VLDL, Chylomicrons, HDL	Hepatic synthesis, LPL inhibitor, VLDL assembly
B-100	Liver	500	Insoluble	VLDL, IDL, LDL, Lp(a)	Synthesized in the liver. Major structural protein for VLDL, LDL. Interacts with LDL receptors Apo B & E playing a role in catabolism of LDL
B-48	Small intestine	240	Insoluble	Chylomicron and remanent particles	Synthesized in the intestine. Major structural protein for chylomicrons
a	Liver	200–800 (variable glycosylation)	Soluble	Forms disulfide bridges with LDL Apo B100 forms Lp(a).	Contains Apo B-100 and Apo-(a) as its major protein component. High degree of homology with plasminogen but does not possess fibrinolytic activity. Its presence is associated with increased risk of coronary artery disease
D		33		HDL, VLDL, IDL, LDL. Increased lipoprotein lipase activity	Transport of small lipophilic molecules
E	Liver, brain	34	Soluble	All except LDL CM, VLDL, IDL, HDL	Control removal of chylomicrons and VLDL
M		26		HDL (5%)	Transport of small lipid. Antioxidative effect of HDL. Role in cholesterol metabolism

CETP, cholesterol ester transfer protein; *CM*, chylomicrons; *HDL*, high-density lipoprotein; *IDL*, intermediate density lipoprotein; *LCAT*, lecithin cholesterol acyl transferase; *LDL*, low-density lipoprotein; *LPL*, lipoprotein lipase; *VLDL*, very low-density lipoprotein.
Modified from Mahley RW, Innerarity TL, Rall SC Jr, Weisgraber KH. Plasma lipoproteins: apolipoprotein structure and function. *J Lipid Res*. 1984;25(12):1277–1294. PMID: 6099394. Dominiczak MH, Caslake MJ. Apolipoproteins: metabolic role and clinical biochemistry applications. *Ann Clin Biochem*. 2011;48(Pt 6):498–515. https://doi.org/10.1258/acb.2011.011111. Epub 2011 Oct 25. PMID: 22028427.

use its energy or storage in skeletal and cardiac muscle and adipose tissue. Lipoprotein lipase hydrolyzes triglyceride and converts VLDL to IDL which contains equal amounts of triglycerides and cholesterol esters. IDL is further metabolized by lipoprotein lipase and hepatic lipase to form remnants with ApoB-100. The remnants are taken up by the liver via LDL receptor.

Measurement of ApoB-100 predicts the risk of atherosclerotic cardiovascular disease and that its levels correlate with LDL-C and non-HDL-C. A cluster of ApoB-100 structural basic amino acids (3359–3362) anchors the LDL particle to proteoglycans in the arterial intima leading to retention and to the initiation of further deposition, inflammation, and development of atheroma. The entrapped LDL particles are oxidization of the lysyl residues of ApoB-100 and phospholipids content.

Circulating ApoB-100 correlate with LDL and non-HDL cholesterol. With ApoB-100 being a more accurate cardiovascular risk maker than LDL or non-HDL cholesterol (evidence for nondiscordance studies).

Tracking longitudinal changes in ApoB-100 levels in response to lipid-lowering therapies can be useful in clinical practice, particularly when discordance between LDL cholesterol and ApoB-100 exists. In addition to the above, Apo B has been used in diagnosis of dyslipidemia, for instance ApoB-100 levels <120 mg/dL considered normal and ≥120 mg/dL being abnormal. This is measured in combination with total cholesterol, triglycerides, and determining the ratio of cholesterol to ApoB-100 and triglycerides to ApoB-100.

ApoB-48

Truncated form of ApoB100 (about 48% of the size of ApoB-100). Associated with chylomicron and thus responsible for absorption of dietary fat. It is 2152 amino acids long, synthesized in the small intestine and is a major structural component of chylomicrons.

In the fed state with high triglycerides, ApoB-48 is lapidated by MTP forming nascent chylomicrons, whereas unlipidated ApoB-48 is degraded. A constitutive mechanism similar to that seen on ApoB-100.

ApoA-IV is added to the nascent chylomicrons. Lipoprotein lipase degrades CM to form, CM remnants. The decrease in triglycerides in CM dose not result in LDL formation as in VLDL above, but the remnants are taken up by hepatocytes via Apo E.

ApoB-48 lacks the C-terminal LDL-R binding domain and thus unlike ApoB-100 cannot interact with the LDL-receptor.

Chylomicrons also contribute to atherosclerotic cardiovascular disease via promotion of inflammation following sequestration into the arterial subendothelial space.

Apolipoprotein C-II

Primary role in triglycerides metabolism. Produced by hepatocytes and in the intestine with adipose tissue and macrophages minor sites, a 79 amino acid lipoprotein associated with triglycerides rich chylomicron, VLDL, IDL, HDL. It is considered a lipoprotein lipase c-factor as it facilitates entry of triglycerides into the LPL active site.

It inhibits binding of the lipoproteins to the LPL receptor by displacing Apo CII for their surfaces. It also impairs Apo E-mediated hepatic uptake and thus clearance. It promotes LDL retention and aggregation in subendothelial space and thus promotes inflammation and atherosclerosis.

Expression of LPL is highest in tissue that use triglycerides as main source of energy (skeletal and cardiac muscle) or for storage (adipose tissue).

ApoC-II is an essential LPL cofactor facilitating entry of triglycerides into LPL active site and thus triglycerides hydrolysis. Interestingly, in triglyceride-rich particles, the surface tension is low facilitating rapid anchorage of ApoC-II and LPL, whereas the surface tension increases expelling LPL and ApoC-II as triglycerides are hydrolyzed and their content decrease.

ApoC-III

ApoC-III is 79 amino acids long predominantly produced by the liver and intestine. Similar to ApoC-II, it is associated with chylomicrons, VLDL, IDL, HDL, and to a lesser degree LDL.

Apo CIII inhibits TRL remnant uptake in the liver by displacing apolipoprotein E (ApoE) from the lipoprotein surface and preventing it from interacting with the LDL receptor (LDLR) and LDL-related protein 1 (LRP1) on hepatocytes. ApoC-III displaces ApoC-II from its binding and thus inhibits LPL-driven lipolysis. It also inhibits ApoE (see later)-mediated hepatic clearance of triglyceride-rich lipoproteins remnants. ApoC-III promotes atherogenesis by promoting LDL retention and aggregation in the subendothelial space and by promoting inflammatory cascade in arterial wall.

Apo E

Produced primarily by the liver and brain, by adrenal gland, kidney, spleen, and adipose tissues to lesser degree. It is a large molecule compared to CI and CII a with 299 amino acids. It is associated with CM, CM remnants, VLDL, IDL, and HDL. ApoE binds to hepatic LDL, LRP1, and VLDLR receptors with high affinity (20 fold higher than that of ApoB100) promoting the rapid uptake and thus clearance of the triglycerides rich lipoproteins and their remnants.

ApoC-III has been shown to displace ApoE from triglycerides rich lipoproteins and also blocks the triglyceride-rich lipoprotein from binding to hepatocytes.

ApoE has several isomers, and the presence of ApoE-e4 isomer has been found to be a strong risk factor for extracellular deposition of amyloid-B in the brain and the late onset sporadic Alzheimer's disease.

Apo (a)

It is produced by the liver with structural homology to plasminogen. Soluble covalently binds to ApoB100 of an LDL-like particle to form Lp(a). It is casually associated with atherosclerosis, several mechanisms have been postulated from its structural similarly to plasminogen promoting thrombosis, to its promoting endothelial inflammation and dysfunction. An elevated circulating Lp(a) is considered a risk factor for calcific aortic stenosis. It is an independent risk factor for atherosclerotic cardiovascular disease and calcific aortic stenosis.

The addition of Lp(a) to quantitative risk assessment in primary prevention enhances cardiovascular risk prediction by improving discrimination and net reclassification index.

Structural characteristics and function of apolipoproteins are shown in Table 2.

The molecular contains Kringle IV and V common to plasminogen, relevant is that variation in the number of Kringle IV type 2 copies is responsible for size heterogeneity of Apo(a) isoforms.

Lipoprotein metabolism

VLD is synthesized in hepatocytes from ApoB-100 and excreted into the circulation where it is converted by lipoprotein lipase to intermediate density lipoprotein and further metabolized by LPL and hepatic lipase low-density lipoprotein (LDL). The relative content of cholesterol esters increasing in the process (see Fig. 3). LDL binds to intimal proteoglycans and is retained in the arterial wall. Oxidation of retained LDL leads to inflammation and the recruited monocytes transform into macrophages and take up oxidized-LDL in unregulated fashion leading to foam cell formation. The latter further amplifies the inflammatory response eventually leading to ischemic injury and formation of atherosclerotic plaques. The latter leads to further ischemia and tissue damage and thus to more plaques which result in obstruction of blood flow and hypoxia further expanding the ischemic injury. The triglyceride-rich VLDL and IDL passes through the endothelial barrier.

Endogenous pathway (Fig. 3) describes the hepatic formation of the lipoproteins VLDL and LDL transporting and distributing endogenously synthesized lipids. The exogenous pathway (Fig. 3) describes metabolism of dietary triglycerides and lipids mediated by chylomicrons which are taken up by lipoprotein lipase-containing tissue and hepatocytes.

Reverse cholesterol transport

Nascent HDL is converted to mature HDL by lecithin cholesterol acyltransferase (LCAT) which converts free cholesterol to cholesterol esters (CE) sequestered into the core of the HDL particle.

Apo A-I interacts with ATP-Binding cassette transporters present in hepatocytes, intestine, and foam cells. Nascent HDL is converted to mature HDL by lecithin cholesterol acyltransferase (LCAT) which converts free cholesterol to cholesterol esters. This process by continued removal of free cholesterol from the surface of the particle forces a unidirectional reaction facilitating uptake of free cholesterol and its efflux from foam cells. Mature HDL particles deliver its cholesterol ester contents to hepatocytes via hepatic SR-B1 receptor (scavenger receptor B1) (Fig. 3).

Apo B-100 particles incorporate triglycerides (TG) forming the triglycerides rich VLDL. Lipoprotein lipase metabolizes VLDL producing IDL. The latter is further metabolized to LDL by lipoprotein lipase (LPL) and hepatic lipase (HL) forming cholesterol-rich LDL. Apo B-100-specific amino acid facilitates interaction with proteoglycans and cause retention of LDL particles in arterial wall. The retained LDL particle is oxidized secondary to the imitated localized immune and inflammatory response. Monocytes transformed into macrophages uptake the oxidized-LDL via the SR-B1 receptor but appears to be in unregulated form leading to the formation of foam cells. The latter amplifies the inflammatory response ultimately leading to the formation of atherosclerotic plaque.

In the reverse cholesterol transport pathway, mature HDL particles interact with foam cells via its surface ATP-binding cassette transporter subfamily G member 1 and member 4 (ABCG1, ABCG4) and SR-B1 and mediates efflux of cholesterol from foam cells.

Exogenous pathway

The exogenous pathway in lipoprotein metabolism describes the handling of dietary lipids (free cholesterol, fatty acids, and mono-triglycerides).

Cholesterol is esterified into cholesterol ester and fatty acids (with $\geq$C14) and triglycerides are incorporated into chylomicrons. ApoB-48 synthesized in enterocytes is essential component of chylomicron for its sections (other apolipoproteins are also present Apo AI, Apo AII, and ApoA-IV) all with phospholipids constitute the surface of the chylomicrons. There is only one ApoB-48 per each chylomicron. As such, formed chylomicrons enter the circulation via the lymphatic system.

Chylomicrons undergo modification while in the circulation acquiring Apo CII, C-III, and ApoE and phospholipids from HDL. Acquisition of ApoC-II is central to the action of lipoprotein lipase downstream in adipose tissue, vascular endothelium, muscle. Extracellularly, LPL hydrolyzes triglycerides releasing fatty acids where they are taken up by tissue and either converted back to triglycerides or consumed as energy source. As triglyceride hydrolysis continues, this causes a reduction in the size of the chylomicrons and the excess surface components (ApoC-II, free cholesterol, and phospholipids) are transferred to HDL. The remaining chylomicron remnant (the product when all of the Apo CII is exhausted), and thus, no further triglyceride hydrolysis. The remnants have high content of cholesterol esters and ApoE normally cleared rapidly by hepatocytes where hepatic lipase further catabolizes remaining triglycerides.

The cholesterol esters reaching the liver in the chylomicron ruminant is reutilized into formation of bile acids or membranes or is secreted as VLDL and the attached ApoB-48 undergoes degradation.

A small fraction of the generated fatty acids remain the circulation bound to albumin and transported to hepatocytes and other tissues. The remnants deliver the remaining triglycerides and all of the cholesterol to the liver.

Endogenous pathway

The endogenous lipoprotein metabolism pathways describe hepatic synthesis of lipids.

Triglycerides are produced either de novo or taken up from plasma derived from chylomicron remnants. Those are secreted with ApoB-100 (Fig. 3) in the form of VLDL. ApoC-I, II, III, and ApoE are also present and probably acquired from HDL in the circulation. The action of lipoprotein lipase, triglycerides are hydrolyzed producing gradually increasing cholesterol ester and ApoE rich remnants surface components transferring back to HDL. The remnants form IDL, half are taken up by the liver and the other undergoes further hydrolysis by hepatic lipase to form LDL.

LDL, the major cholesterol carrying lipoprotein, accounts for 70% or more of the total plasma cholesterol. LDL receptors are present on hepatocytes as well as on peripheral tissue. Approximately 50% of the LDL is taken up by the liver, and thus, the major determinant of circulating level of LDL is the number of LDL receptors. They recognize both aopoB-100 on LDL and ApoE on remanent particles and on HDL. The LDL receptor is recycled, and the lipoproteins are degraded.

Cholesterol released is available for further metabolic transformation as well as to regulate the transcription and in translation of the HMG-CoA reductase and the LDL receptor genes. The cholesterol is re-esterified by the acylcoenzyme A cholesteryl transferase (ACAT) and stored or may be utilized for bile acids, steroids, or membrane synthesis.

Biochemical investigation of lipid disorders[1]

Population screening

The frequency of lipids measurement with different recommendations. If no cardiovascular risk, most suggest once every 5 years and yearly if there is low risk since lipids do not vary significantly from year to year. However, in patients with high risk for coronary vascular disease, yearly assessment of lipid levels is warranted (Table 3).

There is significant difference between fasting and nonfasting cholesterol levels HDL-cholesterol. This will improve compliance for screening and facilitates more screening. Elevated triglycerides (>400 mg/dL (4.52 mmol/L)) on a nonfasting sample should be repeated in a confirmed fasting specimen collection (triglycerides can increase by as much as 20% in nonfasting state). Triglycerides <150 mg/dL (91.70 mmol/L) are considered normal, 150–199 mg/dL (1.70–2.24 mmol/L) is borderline high, and >500 mg/dL (5.64 mmol/L) is considered very high. In addition to cardiovascular risk, the latter is a risk for pancreatitis.

The prevalence of secondary hypertriglyceridemia is low (about 1.8% in one study). Excessive alcohol intake, hepatic dysfunction is common cause of secondary hypertriglyceridemia. It is also common in in type II DM (with triglycerides level as high as 20 mmol/L observed at type of DM diagnosis).

Triglycerides are measured in patients suspected of cardiovascular disease risk and patients being considered for lipid lowering drugs and monitored for response to therapy.

Triglycerides are elevated if >2.3 mmol/L and markedly elevated if >5.6 mmol/L. Five millimoles per liter carry a probable increased risk of pancreatitis; 10 mmol/L carry a high risk of pancreatitis; and 20 mmol/L carry a very high risk of pancreatitis.

All lipid components vary significantly with age. The age at which screening should occur is also debatable and differ between the different societies' guidelines, however, for men 20–35 years and for women 20–45 years if at increased risk for coronary heart disease.

Lipid values associated with high cardiovascular risk include total cholesterol ≥240 mg/dL (≥6.20 mmol/L), LDL-cholesterol >160 mg/dL (4.13 mmol/L), and triglycerides >200 mg/dL (2.35 mmol/L) or a decreased HDL-cholesterol <40 mg/dL (<1.03 mmol/L).

HDL-cholesterol levels are inversely associated with cardiovascular risk. Values <40 mg/dL (1.03 mmol/L) predict an increase in atherosclerotic events for each 1 mg/dL

TABLE 3 Lipid target goals for patients on treatment and as defined by their cardiovascular risk.

	Risk category	Risk factors[a]/10-year risk[b]	Treatment goals		
			LDL-C (mg/dL)	Non-HDL-C (mg/dL)	ApoB (mg/dL)
Extreme risk	AACE	• Progressive ASCVD after achieving an LDL-C <70mg/dL • Established clinical cardiovascular disease in patients with DM, CKD ¾, or HeFH • History of premature ASCVD (<55 male, <65 female)	<55	<80	<70
	EAS	No recommendation made	–	–	–
Very high risk	AACE	• Established or recent hospitalization for ACS, Coronary, carotid or peripheral vascular disease, 10-year risk >20% • Diabetes or CKD ¾ with 1 or more risk factor(s) • HeFH	<70	<100	<80
	EAS	• Established ASCVD • Severe CKD (GFR <30) • DM with target organ damage or major risk factor	<70	<100	<80
High risk	AACE	• >2 risk factors and 10-year risk 10%–20% • Diabetes or CKD ¾ with no other risk factors	<100	<130	<90
	EAS	• Diabetes, moderate CKD (GFR 30–50), 10-year risk 5%–10%, Familial hypercholesterolemia	<100	<130	<100
Moderate risk	AACE	<2 risk factors and 10-year risk <10%	<100	<130	<90
	EAS	10-year risk 1%–5%	< 115	–	–
Low risk	AACE	No risk factors	<130	<160	NR
	EAS	10-year risk <1%	< 115	–	–

Guidelines differ between the various societies. Abbreviations: ACS, acute coronary syndrome; ASCVD, atherosclerotic cardiovascular disease; CKD, chronic kidney disease; DM, diabetes mellitus; HDL-C, high-density lipoprotein cholesterol; HeFH, heterozygous familial hypercholesterolemia; LDL-C, low-density lipoprotein cholesterol; NR, not recommended.

[a] Major independent risk factors are high LDL-C, polycystic ovary syndrome, cigarette smoking, hypertension (blood pressure ≥140/90mmHg or on hypertensive medication), low HDL-C (<40mg/dL), family history of coronary artery disease (in male, first-degree relative younger than 55 years; in female, first-degree relative younger than 65 years), chronic renal disease (CKD) stage 3/4, evidence of coronary artery calcification and age (men ≥45; women ≥55 years). Subtract 1 risk factor if the person has high HDL-C.

[b] Framingham risk scoring is applied to determine 10-year risk.

Modified from Jellinger PS, Handelsman Y, Rosenblit PD, et al. American Association of Clinical Endocrinologists and American College of Endocrinology guidelines for management of dyslipidemia and prevention of cardiovascular disease. *Endocr Pract.* 2017;23(suppl 2):1–87. https://doi.org/10.4158/EP171764.APPGL. PMID: 28437620.

(0.02 mmol/L) reduction is estimated that coronary risk increases by 2%–3%. Additionally, an increase in 13 mg/dL (0.33 mmol/L) is associated with a 30% reduction in mortality.

Cardiovascular risk reduction is the mainstay of the various cholesterol levels and management guidelines. Dyslipidemia being an important risk factor for coronary artery disease and stroke with strong relationship between high LCD-cholesterol lower level of HDL-cholesterol and increasing risk for coronary heart disease.

Diagnosis and confirmation of lipid disorders relies on the measurement of serum cholesterol, triglycerides, HDL cholesterol, LDL cholesterol, and lipoprotein. Overnight (10–12 h) fasting is required to confirm an initial finding of hypertriglyceridemia but is not required for the assessment of cholesterol status.

Patients with very low LDL cholesterol measurement of ApoB helps establish if the patient has hypobetalipoproteinemia. Similarly in patients with low HDL cholesterol levels, measurement of serum ApoA-I is helpful.

Very high levels of lipoprotein a (Lp(a)) can contribute to high LDL-cholesterol levels and therefore in patients with elevated total cholesterol as well as elevated LDL-cholesterol of at least 190 mg/dL or higher, measurement of Lp(a) is required. Estimation of Lp(a) cholesterol is obtained by multiplying Lp(a) levels by 0.3 in men and 0.25 in women when reported in mg/dL.

Laboratory tests include

Total cholesterol, LDL-cholesterol, triglycerides, and HDL-cholesterol. In patients with high coronary vascular disease risk, measurement of lipoprotein (a), apolipoprotein B, and apolipoprotein A1 are warranted. The latter are performed in patients suspected of inherited familial hypercholesterolemia (high LDL-cholesterol levels).

Apolipoprotein (proteins within lipid particles) in addition to proving an accurate measure of the lipids, they inform on the type of dyslipidemias.

Total cholesterol

Total cholesterol is measured enzymatically using cholesterol esterase which converts cholesterol esters to cholesterol. The latter is oxidized by cholesterol oxidase to produce cholest-4-en-3-one and hydrogen peroxide and the corresponding ketone product. Hydrogen peroxide reacts with 4-aminoantipyrine in the presence of phenol forming a colored product quinonimine dye which is recorded at 500 nm. The color intensity correlates with cholesterol concentration, and the assay is precise and accurate which has been traceable to CDC reference methods. Possible interference is by bilirubin, ascorbic acid and hemoglobin. The method is usually linear to 600–700 mg/dL (15.5–18.0 mmol/L).

The reaction sequence is as follows:

$$Cholesterolesters + H_2O \xrightarrow{\text{Cholesterylester Hydrolase}} Cholesterol + Fatty\,acids$$

$$Cholesterol + O_2 \xrightarrow{\text{Cholesterol Oxidase}} Cholest\text{-}4\text{-}en\text{-}one + H_2O_2$$

$$2H_2O_2 + 4\;aminophenazone + Phenol \xrightarrow{\text{Peroxidase}}$$
$$4\text{-}(p\text{-benzoquinone-monoimino})\text{-phenazone} + 4H_2O$$

HD-cholesterol

The original methods for the determination of HDL are cumbersome involving density gradient ultracentrifugation which are not amenable to routine analysis. Current assays termed homogenous assays are enzymatical based and apply the same enzymatic reaction on total cholesterol measurement, but using a scavenger in the last step.

Several methodological approaches have been adopted, and they include antibody four reagents method, polyethylene glycol-modified enzymes, synthetic polymer detergents, antibodies, and use of catalase.

The method in use by the authors laboratory applies the polyethylene glycol methods where in this method a magnesium/dextran sulfate solution is first added to the specimen to form water-soluble complexes with non-HDL cholesterol fractions. These complexes are not reactive with the measuring reagents added in the second step.

With addition of reagent 2, HDL-cholesterol esters are converted to HDL-cholesterol by PEG-cholesterol esterase. The HDL-cholesterol is acted upon by PEG-cholesterol oxidase, and the hydrogen peroxide produced from this reaction combines with 4-amino-antipyrine and HSDA under the action of peroxidase to form a purple/blue pigment that is measured photometrically at 600 nm (secondary wavelength = 700 nm). When the cholesterol measuring enzymes are modified with PEG, they are preferentially more reactive with HDL-cholesterol than the other cholesterol fractions. This is an endpoint reaction that is specific for HDL-cholesterol.

Low serum concentrations of HDL-cholesterol are associated with increased risk for CHD. Coronary risk increases markedly as the HDL concentration decreases from 40 to 30 mg/dL. A low HDL-cholesterol concentration is considered to be a value below 35 mg/dL, and high HDL, >60 mg/dL. HDL-cholesterol values are also used in the calculation of LDL-cholesterol (see LDL below).

Direct HDL method. HDL is measured directly in serum. The basic principle of the method is as follows.

The ApoB-containing lipoproteins in the specimen are reacted with a blocking reagent that renders them nonreactive with the enzymatic cholesterol reagent. The ApoB-containing lipoproteins are thus effectively excluded from the assay, and only HDL-cholesterol is detected under the assay conditions.

The method in use by the authors laboratory uses dextran sulfated α-cyclodextrin, in the presence of Mg^{2+}, which forms complexes with ApoB containing lipoproteins, and polyethylene glycol-coupled cholesteryl esterase and cholesterol oxidase for the HDL-cholesterol measurement. The following enzymatic reaction follows, and the appearance of the quinonimine dye is monitored by recording absorbance at 600 nm.

$$\text{HDL-Cholesteryl esters} \xrightarrow{\text{PEG-Cholesteryl Esterase}}$$

$$\text{HDL -Unesterified cholesterol} + \text{Fatty acids}$$

$$\text{HDL-Unesterified cholesterol}$$

$$+ O_2 \xrightarrow{\text{PEG-Cholesterol Oxidase}} \text{Cholestenone} + H_2O_2$$

$$H_2O_2 + \text{4-aminophenazone} + N\text{-ethyl-}N\text{-}$$

$$(\text{3methylphenyl})\text{-}N\text{-succinyl ethylene diamine}$$

$$+ H_2O \xrightarrow{\text{Peroxidase}} \text{Qunoneimine dye} + H_2O$$

Non-HDL-cholesterol

This is simply a derivation using the formula (total cholesterol − HDL-cholesterol). It has been shown to correlate better to Apo B in some epidemiological studies than LDL-cholesterol and this may be related to the fact that VLDL on its own carries an atherosclerotic risk. Its derivation does not require fasting as it does not include triglycerides.

LDL-cholesterol

LDL-cholesterol levels continue to be estimated by subtracting values from HDL-cholesterol from that of measured total cholesterol, in a Friedewald formula (LDL-cholesterol = (Total cholesterol) − (HDL-Cholesterol) − (Triglycerides/5)) or using (Triglycerides/2.2) when reporting lipids in mmol/L. The formula assumes that moist of the triglycerides are in the VLDL and that there is a molar ratio of 5:1 of triglycerides to cholesterol in the VLDL fraction. The formula is applicable when triglycerides levels are less than 400 mg/dL (4.5 mmol/L) since at this level the VLDL contains higher proportion of triglycerides, and thus, it will overestimate the VLDL component and underestimates LDL-cholesterol calculated component.

Due to the variability in triglycerides content, the error in LDL-cholesterol estimation is thought to be >10% ion 30% of patients with plasma triglycerides 200–300 mg/dL (2.3–3.4 mmol/L) and in >40% of patients with triglycerides of 300–400 mg/dL (3.4–4.5 mmol/L).

However, specific enzymatic methods for the measurement of LDL are now widely available that are less cumbersome and available for most automated chemistry analyzers, i.e., can be measured in nonfasting samples (no need to minimize triglycerides levels). The tolerance for triglycerides in the direct measurement method is being 1000 mg/dL.

Similar to the HDL and total cholesterol methods, several are available, however, homogenous assays are more widespread used in clinical practice. They utilize surfactants, solubilization, and use of catalase enzyme in the multienzymatic reaction steps.

In the authors laboratory, the assay in use applies homogeneous enzymatic colorimetric assay where cholesterol esters and free cholesterol in LDL are measured using cholesterol enzymatic method using cholesterol esterase and cholesterol oxidase in the presence of surfactants which selectively solubilize only LDL. The enzyme reactions to the lipoproteins other than LDL are inhibited by surfactants and a sugar compound. Cholesterol in HDL, VLDL, and chylomicron is not determined. The enzymatic reactions are as follows. The color intensity of the dye is directly proportional to the cholesterol concentration and is measured photometrically at 700/600 nm.

$$\text{LDL-Cholesterol esters} + H_2O \xrightarrow[\text{Detergent}]{\substack{\text{Cholesterol} \\ \text{Esterase}}} \text{LDL}$$

$$\text{-Cholesterol} + \text{free fatty acids}$$

$$\text{LDL-Cholesterol} + O_2 \xrightarrow{\substack{\text{Cholesterol} \\ \text{Oxidase}}} \text{Delta-4}$$

$$\text{-cholestenone} + H_2O_2$$

$$2H_2O_2 + \text{4-aminoantipyrine} + N\text{-ethyl-}N\text{-}$$

$$(\text{3-methylphenyl})\text{-}N\text{-succinylethylenediamine} +$$

$$H_2O + H + \xrightarrow{\text{Peroxidase}} \text{Red-purple pigment} + 5H_2O$$

Triglycerides

Triglycerides are measured using enzymatic method. Triglycerides in the sample are hydrolyzed to glycerol and fatty acids by lipoprotein lipase. Glycerol and NAD^+ generate dihydroxyacetone and NADH in the presence of glycerol dehydrogenase. WST8 is reduced to formazan dye by diaphorase and NADH through oxidation-reduction reaction. The color intensity of the formazan is proportional to triglyceride concentration and calculated by measuring at a wavelength of 460 nm.

$$\text{Triglycerides} \xrightarrow{\text{Lipoprotein Lipase}} \text{Glycerol} + \text{Fatty acids}$$

$$\text{Glycerol} + NAD^+ \xrightarrow{\text{Glycerol Dehydrogenase}} \text{Dihydroacetone}$$

$$+ \text{NADH}$$

$$\text{NADH} + \text{WST8} \xrightarrow{\text{Diaphorase}} NAD^+ + \text{Formazan dye}$$

Another assay format employs a series of coupled reactions in which triglycerides are hydrolyzed to produce glycerol. Glycerol is then oxidized using glycerol oxidase, and H_2O_2, one of the reaction products, is measured as described above for cholesterol. Absorbance is measured at 500 nm. The reaction sequence is as follows:

$$\text{Triglycerides} + 3H_2O \xrightarrow{\text{Lipase}} \text{Glycerol}$$
$$+ \text{Fatty acids}$$

$$\text{Glycerol} + \text{ATP} \xrightarrow{\text{Glycerokinase}} \text{Glycerol-3-phosphate}$$
$$+ \text{ADP}$$

$$\text{Glycerol-3-phosphate} + O_2 \xrightarrow{\text{Glycerophosphate Oxidase}}$$
$$\text{Dihydroxyacetone phosphate} + H_2O_2$$

$$H_2O_2 + \text{4-aminophenazone} + \text{4-chlorophenol} \xrightarrow{\text{Peroxidase}}$$
$$\text{4-}(p\text{-benzoquinone-monoimino})\text{-phenazone}$$
$$+ 2H_2O + HCL$$

Apolipoproteins

Apolipoproteins are measured using immune-based assays. The methods employ anti-Apo B antibodies that react with the antigen in the sample to form antigen/antibody complexes which, following agglutination, the reaction is measured turbidimetrically. The primary measuring wavelength is 340 nm, and the secondary wavelength is 700 nm.

Apo B

Measured in assessment of risk for atherosclerotic cardiovascular disease as well as in monitoring response to therapy. Its levels correlate highly with LDL-Cholesterol and non-HDL Cholesterol levels. Several studies have shown that Apo B is a more accurate risk predictor than LDL-cholesterol and non-HDL cholesterol, particularly in cases where there is discrepancy in the LDL and ApoB values.

Normal Apo B levels (<120 mg/dL) or elevated ≥120 mg/dL plus total cholesterol, triglycerides, total cholesterol to Apo B ratio and triglycerides to Apo B ratio have been applied to diagnose one of the six atherogenic Apo B dyslipidemias.

Dyslipidemia investigation

When investigating patients with dyslipidemia, visual assessment of separated serum/plasma and particularly following storage at 4°C may reveal the patient dyslipidemia (Fig. 4).

Diagnosis and confirmation of lipid disorders relies on the measurement of serum cholesterol, triglycerides, HDL

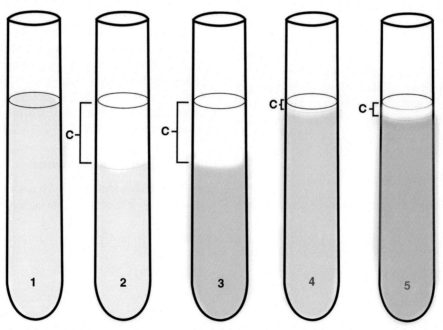

FIG. 4 Schematic drawing showing serum/plasma appearance among patients with dyslipidemia following an overnight storage at 4°C. Sample (1) represents clear serum/plasma indicating predominant LDL-cholesterol and normal triglycerides levels (Fredrickson-Levy and Lees (FLL) classification-IIa). Sample (2) represents a marked milky top layer of chylomicron (C) and a clear serum/plasma bottom layer, likely to exhibit normal or slightly elevated LDL-cholesterol and a markedly elevated triglycerides level (FLL classification-I). Sample (3) represents a marked top milky layer of chylomicron (C) and a markedly opaque bottom layer representing high degree of lipemia. The sample will exhibit normal to slightly elevated LDL-cholesterol and a markedly elevated triglyceride level [chylomicron and VLDL (very low-density lipoproteins)] (FLL classification-V). Samples 4 and 5 show relatively small chylomicron (C) top layer (slightly thicker in sample 5) and different degree of opaqueness (representing lipemia) in the lower serum/plasma layer (more turbid/lipemic in sample 5). The samples will exhibit elevated triglycerides and VLDL and elevated LDL-cholesterol. Respective triglycerides levels being higher in sample 5 (FLL classification-III) and cholesterol lower in sample 4 (FLL classification-IIb). *(Courtesy Quispe R, Hendrani AD, and Baradaran-Noveiry B, et al. Characterization of lipoprotein profiles in patients with hypertriglyceridemic Fredrickson-Levy and Lees dyslipidemia phenotypes: the Very Large Database of Lipids Studies 6 and 7. Arch Med Sci. 2019;15(5):1195–1202. https://doi.org/10.5114/aoms.2019.87207. Epub 2019 Aug 22. PMID: 31572464; PMCID: PMC6764300.)*

cholesterol, LDL cholesterol, and lipoprotein. Overnight (10–12 h) fasting is required to confirm an initial finding of hypertriglyceridemia but is not required for the assessment of cholesterol status.

Patients with very low LDL cholesterol measurement of ApoB help establish if the patient has hypobetalipoproteinemia. Similarly in patients with low HDL cholesterol levels measurement of serum ApoA-I is helpful.

Very high levels of lipoprotein a (Lp(a)) can contribute to high LDL-cholesterol levels and therefore in patients with elevated total cholesterol as well as elevated LDL-cholesterol of at least 190 mg/dL or higher, measurement of Lp(a) is required. Estimation of Lp(a) cholesterol is obtained by multiplying Lp(a) levels by 0.3 in men and 0.25 in women when reported in mg/dL.

Biochemical assays in the investigation of dyslipidemia include total cholesterol, HDL-cholesterol, LDL-cholesterol, apolipoproteins A-1 and B, Apolipoprotein E phenotypes, and Lp(a).

In addition to available direct measurement of LDL-cholesterol levels, the levels can be calculated using the formulae (calculated LDL-cholesterol = Total cholesterol − HDL-cholesterol − (Triglycerides/5) mg/dL). The formula known as the Friedewald formula is not reliable when triglycerides concentrations are >400 mg/dL or in the presence of chylomicrons or IDL seen in dysbeta-lipoproteinemia.

Lipoprotein phenotyping by electrophoresis partitions lipids into; α band (HDL-cholesterol), β-band (LDL-cholesterol), broad β band (IDL-cholesterol), pre-β band (VLDL-cholesterol), and chylomicrons at the point of application. With the availability of advanced technologies, the electrophoretic procedure is not widely used.

Classification of dyslipidemia

Dyslipidemias is classified as either primary or secondary.

Primary dyslipidemias

Primary hyperlipidemias may be classified either by phenotype or genotype. There are six types of phenotypes of primary dyslipidemia disorder, and these are defined on lipoprotein phenotype alone, not on etiology (Table 4).

Familial disorders

In addition to routine biochemical measurements for total cholesterol, triglycerides, HDL-cholesterol, and either measured or calculated LDL-cholesterol, genetic analysis is becoming available in the diagnosis of lipid disorders. Current focus is on patients with elevated LDL cholesterol with sequencing of the LDLR, APOB, and PCSK9 genes.

Familial combined hyperlipidemia hypercholesterolemia

Familial combined hyperlipidemia is characterized by high triglycerides >200 mg/dL (>2.26 mmol/L) and LDL-C above the 90th percentile value >170 mg/dL (>4.4 mmol/L), but rarely exceeding 225 mg/dL (5.82 mmol/L). Isolated increase in cholesterol or triglycerides is seen in about 15% of patient with premature coronary vascular disease. Apo B levels are greater than 120 mg/dL (>2.34 mmol/L) and a decreased HDL-C < 40 mg/dL (<1.03 mmol/L).

Associated genetic linkage studies show independent determinants, and that DNA sequencing shows large effect variants in genes encoding the LDL receptor and lipoprotein lipase in some patients.

Familial hypercholesterolemia

Familial hypercholesterolemia is an autosomal dominant disorder with high risk of premature cardiovascular disease and

TABLE 4 Primary dyslipidemia phenotypes and associated lipid abnormalities.

Phenotype	Lipid abnormality	Diagnostic criteria
Type I:	Elevated chylomicrons	TG/TC ratio > 10 and VLDL-C < 90th percentile
Type II a:	Elevated LDL	LDL-C > 90th percentile, V2LDL-C < 90th percentile, and VLDL-C/TG < 0.3
Type II b:	Elevated LDL and VLDL	LDL-C, VLDL-C > 90th percentile, and VLDL-C/TG < 0.3
Type III:	Elevated LDL and chylomicron remnants	VLDL-C/TG > 0.3, TG > 130, and LDL-C < 90th percentile
Type IV:	Elevated VLDL	VLDL-C > 90th percentile, LDL-C < 90th percentile, and VLDL-C/TG < 0.3
Type V:	Elevated chylomicrons and VLDL	TG/TC ratio > 10 and VLDL-C > 90th percentile

Modified from Quispe R, Hendrani AD, Baradaran-Noveiry B, et al. Characterization of lipoprotein profiles in patients with hypertriglyceridemic Fredrickson-Levy and Lees dyslipidemia phenotypes: the Very Large Database of Lipids Studies 6 and 7. *Arch Med Sci.* 2019;15(5):1195–1202. https://doi.org/10.5114/aoms.2019.87207. Epub 2019 Aug 22. PMID: 31572464; PMCID: PMC6764300.

characterized by elevated LDL-Cholesterol $\geq$190mg/dL ($\geq$4.91 mmol/L). Clinical phenotype includes corneal arcus and tendon xanthoma. The prevalence is 1:250 of the population and in 1% of patients with premature cardiovascular disease.

Associated genetic findings are mutations in the LDLR, APOB, or PCSK9 genes in the proband or first-degree relative. Severely affected heterozygotes or familial homozygote hypercholesterolemia LDL apheresis may be necessary to correct LDL-Cholesterol levels compared with statin therapy in heterozygous familial hypercholesteremia.

Sitosterolemia hypercholesterolemia

Sitosterolemia is a potential cause of elevated LDL cholesterol levels. It is a rare autosomal recessive disorder with defects in the ABCG5 and ABCG8 genes and is associated with marked intestinal hyperabsorption of cholesterol, Beta-sitosterol, and campesterol.

LDL-cholesterol may be normal or elevated, whereas plasma Beta-sitosterol and campesterol levels above the 99th percentile values of 8.0mg/dL (0.019 mmol/L) and 10.0mg/dL (0.025 mmol/L) respectively.

Inhibition of cholesterol absorption by ezetimibe and dietary modifications are the treatment of choice.

Hypercholesterolemia secondary to lysosomal acid lipase deficiency

Deficiency of lysosomal acid lipase causes LDL cholesterol elevation due to lack of intracellular cholesterol ester on the triglycerides hydrolysis in hepatocytes and macrophages. Patients will have elevated LDL cholesterol greater than 225mg/dL and decreased HDL cholesterol less than 40mg/dL.

The disorder is associated with LIPA mutations, commonly c.894G.A; p.Ser275_Gln298del. The disorder is treated with sebelipase enzyme replacement therapy.

Cerebrotendinous xanthomatosis

A rare autosomal recessive disorder and characterized by markedly elevated plasma cholesterol levels greater than 50mg/dL (>0.012 mmol/L). This is secondary to the deficiency of sterile 20 market markedly elevated plasma cholesterol levels greater than 5mg/L. This is secondary to the deficiency of sterile 27 hydroxylase activity and the defect in the CYP to 7A1 gene.

Classification of inherited lipid disorders

Polygenic (common) hypercholesterolemia

Mild to modernity severity. Heterogeneous etiology including genetics and environment. LDL is increased, as is total cholesterol. This disorder carries an increased atherogenic risk. Physical signs are rare (corneal arcus and xanthelasma). Inheritance is complex.

Familial combined hyperlipidemia (FCH)

Moderate elevation of total cholesterol and/or triglyceride seen reflecting a rise in LDL and/or VLDL. Lipoprotein phenotype is not consistent within or between individuals. The disorder carries an increased atherogenic risk. Physical signs are rare. Inheritance is complex.

Familial hypercholesterolemia (FH)

Moderate to severe elevation of total cholesterol reflecting a rise in LDL concentration. Caused by a reduced expression of functional LDL receptors secondary to a gene defect. LDL receptor gene is codominant and maximally expressed; thus, heterozygotes for an LDL receptor defect are receptor deficient, while homozygotes are receptor negative. Affects 0.2% of population. Associated with a greatly increased risk of atherogenicity. Physical signs are pathognomonic and include tendon xanthomata, subperiosteal deposits, and premature corneal arcus.

Remnant hyperlipidemia (type III)

As for WHO phenotypic classification, an elevation of IDL and chylomicron remnants. Such particles depend on the binding of Apo E to the LDL receptor for clearance. The Apo E2 variant only binds very poorly. One percent of population are homozygous for Apo E2. Two percent of these individuals develop remnant hyperlipidemia when subjected to a secondary stress requiring increased remnant particle clearance to cope with it. Such stresses include hypothyroidism, diabetes or most commonly obesity. Physical signs are pathognomonic including striate xanthoma of the palmar skin creases and tuberous xanthoma. The condition carries an increased atherogenic risk.

Familial hypertriglyceridemia

Mild to moderate severity. Reflecting an elevation in VLDL. Severe forms reflecting an elevation of VLDL and chylomicrons are rare. As well as an elevation in triglyceride there may well be a mild elevation in total cholesterol due to the cholesterol content of VLDL and chylomicrons. The atherogenicity of the condition is variable and controversial. Physical signs include eruptive xanthomata on extensor surfaces.

Inheritance is usually dominant, but penetrance and phenotype may vary widely. Hypertriglyceridemia associates with pancreatitis, hepatosplenomegaly, and peripheral neuropathy.

Hyperchylomicronemia syndrome

Elevated chylomicron concentrations underlying a severe hypertriglyceridemia secondary to a reduced lipoprotein lipase activity. This may be caused by: LPL deficiency, a defect in the LPL gene may lead to the production of an inactive or less active enzyme, Apo CII deficiency, Apo CII is an obligate activator of LPL. An absence of Apo CII can lead to a reduced or absent LPL activity. Inheritance is autosomal recessive. Physical signs include eruptive xanthomata and retinal lipemia.

Secondary (acquired) dyslipidemias

Secondary causes of lipid disorders are seen in patients with chronic inflammation, diabetes, hypothyroidism, renal disease, and liver disease. Biochemical assessment of these disorders is high sensitivity C-reactive protein (hsCRP), glucose, creatinine, liver enzymes, alkaline phosphatase, and thyroid stimulating hormone tests, respectively.

Hyperlipidemia is also seen with aging, obesity, increased intake of saturated fat trans fats, sugars and alcohol as well as certain medication such as glucosteroids, amiodarone protease inhibitors, anabolic steroids, and immune suppressants.

Secondary causes of hyperlipidemias include hypothyroidism (elevated triglyceride and/or cholesterol) due to reduced metabolism (cholesterol levels rise with TSH where 12% of patients with biochemical evidence of hypothyroidism exhibits elevated cholesterol levels), diabetes mellitus (elevated triglyceride infrequently and/or cholesterol), alcohol abuse (elevated triglycerides), obstructive jaundice (elevated cholesterol) due to cholestasis, severe acute hepatitis (elevated triglyceride), nephrotic syndrome (elevated triglyceride and cholesterol), and in renal failure (elevated triglyceride).

Drugs causing hypertriglyceridemia include diuretics, beta blockers, estrogens, progestogens, retinoids, and corticosteroids.

Therapeutic interventions and biochemical monitoring

A number of large studies have looked at the association between plasma lipids (Table 5) and cardiovascular atherosclerosis and cardiovascular mortality. Similarly, several trials showed that by reducing plasma cholesterol and triglycerides while increasing HDL concentrations, the risk of cardiovascular disease is reduced.

TABLE 5 Levels of lipid fractions and associated risk and desired action.

Lipid biomarker	Measured level	Risk	Action items
Total cholesterol	<200 mg/dL (<5.2 mmol/L)	Low	Repeat within 5 years
LDL-cholesterol	<130 mg/dL (3.4 mmol/L)		
HDL-cholesterol	≥40 mg/dL (≥1.0 mmol/L)		
Triglycerides	<150 mg/dL (<1.7 mmol/L)		
Total cholesterol	200–239 mg/dL (5.2–6.2 mmol/L)	0–1 risk factor	Re-evaluate in 1 year
LDL-cholesterol	130–159 mg/dL (3.4–4.1 mmol/L)		
HDL-cholesterol	≥40 mg/dL (1.0 mmol/L)		
Triglycerides	150–199 mg/dL (1.7–2.2 mmol/L)		
Total cholesterol	≥200 mg/dL (6.2 mmol/L)	≥2 risk factors	Initiate therapy
LDL-cholesterol	130–159 mg/dL (3.4–4.1 mmol/L)		
HDL-cholesterol	<40 mg/dL (<1.0 mmol/L)		
Triglycerides	≥200 mg/dL (≥2.2 mmol/L)		
Total cholesterol	>240 mg/dL (6.2 mmol/L)		Lipoprotein analysis

Modified from Jellinger PS, Handelsman Y, Rosenblit PD, et al. American Association of Clinical Endocrinologists and American College of Endocrinology guidelines for management of dyslipidemia and prevention of cardiovascular disease. Endocr Pract. 2017;23(suppl 2):1–87. https://doi.org/10.4158/EP171764. APPGL. PMID: 28437620. Catapano AL, Graham I, De Backer G, et al. 2016 ESC/EAS guidelines for the management of dyslipidaemias. Eur Heart J. 2016;37(39):2999–3058. https://doi.org/10.1093/eurheartj/ehw272. Epub 2016 Aug 27. PMID: 27567407.

Data from the Framingham study shows risk rises most rapidly for increasing plasma cholesterol in the presence of other risk factors such as smoking and hypertension.

A number of lipid management approaches and therapeutic drugs and interventions are available and are beyond the scope of this book. In summary, they include lifestyle changes including diet reduce risk of cardiovascular event, and for many patients, this is insufficient and may require medication to reach favorable lipid levels. Drug therapies include bile acid sequestrant block enterohepatic circulation of bile salts. Cause increased expression of LDL receptor within liver and lower LDL-cholesterol. Indicated for treatment of hypercholesterolemia, they can cause an increased synthesis of VLDL and rise in triglyceride concentrations and must not be used in patients with hypertriglyceridemia.

HMG CoA Reductase Inhibitors (Statins), of the rate limiting enzyme for cholesterol biosynthesis and promote the expression of LDL receptors in the liver and thus enhances the uptake and clearance of circulating LDL-cholesterol. Although they reduce LDL concentration they do not affect triglyceride metabolism and may be safely used in the hypertriglyceridemia patient. Fibrates activate lipolysis causing a reduction in LDL and VLDL concentrations while elevating HDL-cholesterol. They can be used to treat pure hypercholesterolemia but are of most use in the treatment of mixed hyperlipidemias, patients receiving both HMG-CoA inhibitors and fibrates are at increased risk for myositis.

Omega-3 fatty acids (e.g., Lovaza, Omtryg) inhibit hepatic triglycerides synthesis and increases lipoprotein lipase activity increasing triglycerides and chylomicron clearance.

Therapeutic modalities are often lifelong and take at least 6 months from initiation to reduce risk for cardiovascular disease.

Laboratory monitoring

During the first year of hyperlipidemia therapy (e.g., statins), hepatic and muscle aminotransferases and creatine kinase enzymes, respectively, are measured at baseline, and at 3, and 12 months following initiation of statin therapy. Risk of hepatic damage is high if aminotransferases are more than 3 times upper limit of normal requiring clinical assessment for dosage adjustment or discontinuation. Elevated creatine kinases are seen in patients with myopathy.

Cardiovascular risk assessment

Multisociety guidelines are published on cardiovascular risk calculation. The estimated ASCVD risk score.

Patients at risk of cardiovascular disease are those with dyslipidemia (elevated LDL) diabetes.

In the general population without identifiable risk, the 10 year risk score for cardiovascular disease is calculated using eASCVD risk assessment equation. No additional investigation is required in patients with values <7.5%. Similar those with values <3 and only one risk factor, no further investigation or intervention is needed. However, patients with >20% require lipid lower drugs. In patients with rick score >7.5%, an alert is sent to perform PCE calculation.

Patient's 10-year ASCVD risk is estimated at an initial visit to establish a reference point. Ten-year risk for ASCVD is categorized as, <5% (Low-risk), 5%–7.4% (borderline risk), 7.75%–19.9% (intermediate risk), and those with >20% as (high risk).

Compliance with medication and follow-up remains an issue in clinical practice.

ApoB measurement in risk assessment

ApoB is a more accurate risk assessment biomarker for atherogenic risk factor than LDL and HDL cholesterol. Effectively, it represents the total number of LDL and VLDL particles.

Since ApoB45 is in triglycerides and ApoB-100 is in LDL, a measure of each atherogenic molecule represents either triglycerides or LDL. This is a more accurate measure of risk than measuring LDL-C or non-HDL-C. Additionally, it is a more accurate measure of the adequacy of therapy than LDL-C or bon-HDL-C.

ApoB can be measured relatively easily and is available automated system and reliably particularly at low concentrations than LDL-C or non-HDL-C. It is suggested that ApoB should be the primary marker for monitoring response to therapy (responds better than LDL-C).

Lipoprotein (a) (Lp(a))

Lp(a) has a similar atherogenic risk similar to that of LDL-C (pro-atherogenic). It is the same size and density as LDL. It is composed of one molecule of ApoB is covalently attached to apolipoprotein (a).

It carries oxidized phospholipids and thus promotes foam cell formation, inflammation, and thrombosis.

It exhibits homology to plasminogen and exhibits possible inhibition of fibrinolysis.

Lpa has size heterogeneity with molecular weight ranges from 30 to 800 kDa. The variability in the number of Kringle IV2 repeats is thought to contribute to the considerable variability in Apo(a) size.

Risk enhancers include high sensitivity C-reactive protein (hsCRP) ≥2.0 mg/L, Lp(a) >50 mg/dL (>1.78 μmol/L), ApoB >−130 mg/dL, and Ankle-brachial index (ABI) <0.9. About 20%–30% of patients have elevated Lp(a) above the level associated with increased risk for cardiovascular event.

Lp(a) should be measured at least once in a lifetime as it is a genetic condition. It should be measured in patients with strong family history of ischemic heart disease, patients on statins but remains hypercholesterolemic, and in patients with intermediate risk. Lp(a) will be counted with calculated LDL as well as measured LDL since Apo Lp(a) is similar size to LDL and contains cholesterol as LDL.

A monoclonal antibody-based sandwich assay for Lp(a) is described with Kringle IV domain 9 and Kringle IV domain 2 monoclonal antibodies directed against capture (IV-2) and detection (IV9) allows detection of all Lp(a) isoforms.

Statins lower overall cholesterol but not Lp(a) genetic condition. They actually increase the expression of Lp(a). Estrogens lower Lp(a) by about 20% (i.e., affects women and has a potential thromboembolic disease). Niacin lowers Lp(a) by about 20%–30% but has gastrointestinal side effects and limited data for improved outcomes. Apheresis (every 2 weeks) helps reduce Lp(a) by about 30%.

Novel antisense oligonucleotide targets Apo(a) mRNA in hepatocytes. The therapy is currently in phase 3 clinical trials.

Calculated LDL-cholesterol

LDL-cholesterol is the main target for therapy as the relative risk of major vascular events and all-cause mortality are reduced by 22% and 10%, respectively, for each 1 mmol/L (39 mg/dL) reduction in LDL-cholesterol. Therefore, accurate determination of LDL-cholesterol is essential to assessing risk of atherosclerotic cardiovascular disease and in monitoring response to therapy.

LDL-cholesterol can be obtained via either direct measurement and by calculation using a number of available formulas (Table 6).

The accurate LDL measurement method is labor-intensive requiring ultracentrifugation, an automated easy to perform measurement is available on automated analyzers; this however suffers from few limitations. The assays lack standardization and, thus incommutable, varying significantly among the different manufactures, more evident when triglycerides exceeds 2.0 mmol/L. Each direct chemical assay uses proprietary chemicals in an attempt to block non-LDL lipoproteins and facilitate measurement of LDL-C.

LDL-C values obtained via direct chemical assays vary significantly among different manufacturers, most prominently among patients with hypertriglyceridemia (>2 mmol/L), mixed dyslipidemia, and diabetes mellitus.

Calculated LDL-C values may be affected by the biological variability of triglycerides levels and by the variability of direct HDL-C assays among the different manufacturers.

Several formulas are in use and some are under validation are available for the calculation of LDL-cholesterol. The most widely used formulae is the Friedewald formula. The formula, LDL-C = Total cholesterol − HDL-Cholesterol − Triglycerides/5 if reported in mg/dL or (triglycerides/2.2) if reported in SI mmol/L. The triglyceride factors and estimation of VLDL-Cholesterol have limitations at low VLDL-C levels and at high triglycerides levels where the formula is not valid when triglycerides exceed 400 mg/dL (10.3 mmol/L).

Another formula increasing being applied is the Martin/Hopkins equation, where LDL-C = TC-HDL-C − Triglycerides/adjustable factor. The formular applies barebone correction faction for triglycerides in an attempt to account for the interindividual differences in triglycerides to VLDL-C ratio.

TABLE 6 LDL-cholesterol formulas in use.

Nomenclature	Formula	Comments
Friedewald equation	LDL-C = TC − HDL-C − TRG/5 OR (TRG/2.2) when all parameters reported in. SI mmol/L units	Triglyceride <400 mg/dL
Martin-Hopkins equation	[LDL-C] = TC − HDL − TRG/Adjustable Factor	Triglycerides <400 mg/dL Adjustable factor is an estimate of triglycerides to VLDL-C ratio. Depends on non-HDL-C and triglycerides values
Hattori formula	LDL-C = 0.94 TC − 0.94 HDL-C − 0.19	
NIH Equation 2	$LDL\ C = \dfrac{TC}{0.948} - \dfrac{HDL\ C}{0.971} - \left(\dfrac{TG}{8.56} + \dfrac{[TG*non\ HDL]}{2140} - \dfrac{TG^2}{16,100} \right) - 9.44$	Triglycerides <800 mg/dL.

HDL, high-density lipoprotein; LDL-C, low-density lipoprotein; TC, total cholesterol; TRG, triglycerides.
Modified from Martins J, Rossouw HM, Pillay TS. How should low-density lipoprotein cholesterol be calculated in 2022? Curr Opin Lipidol. 2022;33(4): 237–256. https://doi.org/10.1097/MOL.0000000000000833. PMID: 35942811.

Another reported formula is the "Hattori" formula, where LDL-C = 0.94 TC − 0.94HDL-C − 0.19 triglycerides.

The Martin/Hopkins formula appears to perform better low LDL-C <1.8 mmol/L. It is especially useful in patients with low LDL-C levels <1.8 mmol/L (<70 mg/dL) and high triglyceride levels between 1.7 and 4.5 mmol/L (150–399 mg/dL) and is reliable in the nonfasting state.

It is reportedly more accurate in patients with diabetes mellitus, familial combined hypertriglyceridemia and in those tanking proprotein convertase subtilisin/kexin type 9 (PCSK9) inhibitors.

Recently, a new formular "NIH formula" is described. LD-C = [TC/0.948 − HDL-C/0.971 minus (TG/8.56 plus [TG × non-HDL-C]/2140 minus TG^2/16,100) minus 9.44] is derived and reported to before better with triglycerides up to 800 mg/dL compared with the Friedewald 400 mg/dL.

Cardiovascular disease

Cardiovascular disease is the leading cause of death globally, and this is responsible for 45% of all deaths worldwide according to the World Health Organization. Furthermore, acute coronary syndrome and congestive heart failure being the most common presentations to emergency departments.

Chest pain suspected of acute coronary syndrome represents about 10% of emergency department presentations.

The clinical biochemistry laboratory plays an important role in the management of patients with both acute and chronic myocardial dysfunction via measurement of biomarkers for the diagnosis, risk stratification, and management of patient suspected of cardiovascular disease.

Cardiac biomarkers[2,3]

Biomarkers released from myocardial tissue following injury or overload include troponins (troponin T and I), cardiac enzymes (CK (MB), LDH and AST), and natriuretic peptides (NTproBNP and BNP). Availability highly specific and sensitive cardiac biomarkers, namely troponins and natriuretic peptides, have rendered the measurement of cardiac enzymes (CKMB, LDH, and AST) obsolete. However, some see a benefit in continued availability of CKMB measurement (see later).

Although extremely valuable, the increased use of high sensitivity assays is associated with increased risk of false positive results reported at 1% compared with the conventional biomarker CK-MB at 0.04% as an example. A recent survey showed only 41% of hospitals used high sensitivity troponins and that <10% implemented a 0/1 h or 0/2 h protocols (see later).

Troponins

Cardiac troponin complex consists of three isoforms, namely troponin "C" which binds calcium, troponin "I" which inhibits the ATPase activity of actomycin, and troponin "T" which interacts with tropomycin (Fig. 5). The troponins mediate the interaction between actin and myosin in cardiac muscle and thereby facilitate myocardium contractions.

Troponin "C" is also present in skeletal muscle whereas troponin "T" and troponin "I" are specific to cardiac muscles. It is this degree of specificity that affords cTnT and cTnI biochemical utility in the detection of myocardial injury ("suffix C" denotes cardiac source).

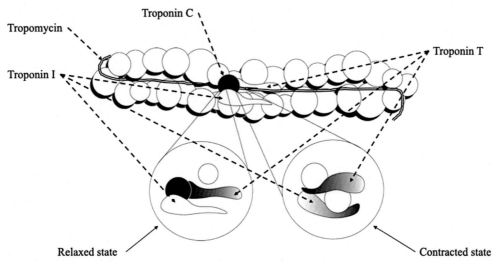

FIG. 5 A segment of sarcomere showing troponin complex troponin T (tropomycin), troponin C (calcium binding), troponin I (inhibitory). The respective arrangement with each other and with tropomycin is shown for the relaxed and contracted states. *(Modified from Gomes AV, Potter JD, Szczesna-Cordary D. The role of troponins in muscle contraction. IUBMB Life. 2002;54(6):323–333. https://doi.org/10.1080/15216540216037. PMID: 12665242. Marston S, Zamora JE. Troponin structure and function: a view of recent progress. J Muscle Res Cell Motil. 2020;41(1):71–89. https://doi.org/10.1007/s10974-019-09513-1. Epub 2019 Apr 27. PMID: 31030382; PMCID: PMC7109197.)*

Troponin measurements

Advancement in troponin assays over recent years has made them central to the diagnosis and management of acute coronary syndromes and myocardial infarction particularly in patients with non-ST elevation myocardial infarction (NSTEMI). Improvement in assay sensitivity from the contemporary assays to those of high sensitivity with circulating troponin levels detectable in normal individuals.

Leading analytical considerations are those of limit of detection, limit of blank, functional sensitivity (also termed limit of quantification), and the 99th percentile of a "healthy" reference population. The assays are now able to reproducibly measure within high degree of precision troponin values consistently in >50% of the general healthy population (Fig. 6).

Analytical consideration

The lowest assay signal (background signal) generated, usually in the presence of a zero-calibrator or the assay diluent buffer, is termed the limit of blank (LoB) and provides an indication for the background noise characteristics of the assay. However, the ability to measure the biomarker level in a sample with the lowest concentration is termed limit of detection (LoD). The latter alone is not helpful unless it is assessed in terms of the assay reproducibility at that low concentration defining the limits of its operational characteristics. An imprecision of less than 10% is considered an acceptable performance and that low biomarker levels detected with less than <10% imprecision is classified as the assay true functional sensitivity or limit of quantification (LoQ).

Often quoted (see later) is the assay performance at the 99th percentile, this describes the absolute value of the biomarker (in this case troponin) corresponding to the 99th percentile value found in the normal healthy population and is used as a cut off for troponin assays provided that performance is at <10% imprecision. Additionally, preferred assays are those that where at least 50% of values below the upper 99th percentile of the normal population are measurable. Although guidelines recommend an imprecision of <10% at the 99th percentile, imprecisions between 10% and 20% are considered clinically acceptable, with imprecision >20% being too variable to be of clinical value.

The percentage of measurable troponin with the 99th percentile normal range defines the generational sensitivity of the assay. Those that detected <50% were contemporary sensitivity assays, 50%–75% were the first generational high sensitivity assays, and 75%–95% were the second generational assays, those >95% are the third generational assays with the latest generation high-sensitivity assay detecting 99%–100% of values among normal population (Fig. 6).

When the distance (ratio) between the limit of detection and the value of the 99th percentile is <1 this is a clinically useful high sensitivity assays, and when the ratio is ≥10 is extremely high sensitive assays, with ≥20 representing an ultra-sensitive assay. This helps identify patients within the normal reference intervals driven by the fact that patients at the higher end further away from the LoQ but within the 99th percentile at higher risk of adverse events than those at lower values. This is important when deriving rule-out and risk assessment algorithms in emergency departments and at presentations. This also led to the avoidance of the use of the 99th percentile as cut-off value and relying on the LoQs and includes shorter time intervals to monitor that is within the 1–2 h following presentation in contrast to the 3, 6, and even longer hours following baseline sample at presentation. This approach allowed the use of acute coronary syndrome rule-out protocols (Fig. 7).

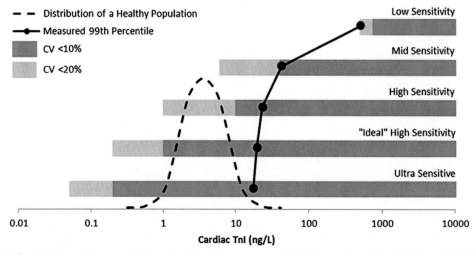

FIG. 6 Sensitivity of cardiac troponin I assays. The impact of improving assays sensitivity from contemporary to high sensitivity. The graph indicates the detection at the 99th percentile and associated assay imprecision. *(Modified from Conrad MJ, Jarolim P. Cardiac troponins and high-sensitivity cardiac troponin assays. Clin Lab Med. 2014;34(1):59–73, vi. https://doi.org/10.1016/j.cll.2013.11.008. Epub 2014 Jan 14. PMID: 24507787.)*

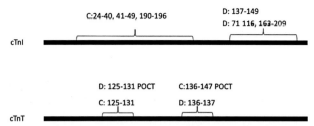

FIG. 7 Capture and detection epitope regions for troponin T (cTnT) and troponin I (cTnI) by various commercially available assays. *(Modified from Contemporary cardiac troponin assays: Analytical characteristics. https://www.ifcc.org/media/479434/contemporary-cardiac-troponin-i-and-t-assay-analytical-characteristics-designated-by-manufacturer-v052022.pdf. Accessed 22 February 2023. Point-of-care cardiac troponin I and T assays: Analytical characteristics designated by manufacturers. https://www.ifcc.org/media/479438/point-of-care-cardiac-troponin-i-and-t-assay-analytical-characteristics-designated-by-manufacturer-v052022.pdf. Accessed 22 February 2023.)*

TABLE 7 Characteristics and operational differences between contemporary and high-sensitivity troponin assays.

	Contemporary troponin T	High sensitivity troponin T
Lower decision limit	<0.01 ng/mL	<6 ng/L
Differences between successive samples	N/A	3, 7, 12 ng/L
Critical value	≥0.01 ng/mL	≥52 ng/L
AMI Rule-out protocol	6 and 8 h	1 and 3 h

AMI, acute myocardial infarction (assays characteristics in the author's laboratory).

The improved imprecision (<10% CV) for most assays allow their use in serial measurements which are integral part of the rule-out/rule-in protocols for successive measurers within the at admission (time 0) and at 1 h postadmission time frame (Fig. 9).

The use of high-sensitivity troponin assays led to the identification of previously unrecognized myocardial injury in a range of clinical conditions.

Despite harmonization between troponin assays, there is till lack of standardization across the commercially available troponin assays.

The clinical need as well as the expectation of improved performance of troponins assessed at the 99th percentile has contributed to the development of high-sensitivity troponin assays also known as fifth generation troponin assays. Professional societies have over the time advocated an imprecision of less than 10% CV at the 99th percentile. This led to the development of troponin assays measuring down to 0.01 ng/mL in the fourth generation assays. Unitage and numeric values changed in the further improved 5th generation troponin assays (Table 7).

Improvements from 10% CV at the 99th centile for the conventional assays to high sensitivity troponin assays (hsTn) with the ability to detects levels below 99th centile of values among normal individuals (at least >50% of detectable normal). This assay characteristic is considered a performance indicator. Although a performance of 10% at the 99th centile has been required, this resulted in improvement in performance of commercially available assays, assays with performance between 10% and 20% are unlikely to impact clinical decision.

Rise or fall in troponin levels (with one point at least above the 99th centile) is diagnostic of myocardial infarction.

Outlier troponin results have been reported for some assays, and they often represent false and irreproducible results that may lead to excessive additional investigations, and delays in diagnosis. The exact nature of the outlier remains unclear. However, interferences from heterophilic antibodies, biotin, rheumatoid factors, although the impact is often predictable (decrease or increase in values), unpredictable and irreproducible outliers remain problematic.

Sample type (serum versus plasma), presence of fibrin clots and the impact of centrifugation speed, reagents lot number (affects both quality control and patient samples), pack size reagent volume, larger volumes have higher outlier rates (may be related to frequency of calibration, etc.).

Several assays are commercially available for the measurement of troponin "T" and troponin "I". Troponin "T" is available by one major manufacturer namely "Roche Diagnostics" and in some "Siemens Medical Solutions" platforms, whereas troponin "I" measurement is available in all the clinical laboratory instruments manufacturers. Several versions and generations of the troponin's assays are available, and over the time, they have gradually improved sensitivity with third and fourth generation assays exhibiting what is termed high-sensitivity troponins assays.

This high sensitivity facilitates measurement of troponins in healthy individuals, and as such, they provide a very sensitive marker of early significant myocardial injury. Due to the high sensitivity and improve performance of the troponin assays, they have become integral to the diagnosis of acute coronary syndrome and acute myocardial infarction. Several rule out protocols using timed troponins measurements are in routine practice where undetectable level of high sensitivity troponin at presentation has a high negative predictive value and that's allow for rule out of acute myocardial infarction in patients with acute chest pain using a 0 and 1 h and a 0 and 3 h algorithms (Fig. 9).

Assays termed contemporary (or fourth generation) report troponin values to two decimal points in micrograms per liter. Whereas those termed fifth generation affords

TABLE 8 Examples of commercially available laboratory-based instruments for the measurement of high-sensitivity troponin T (hsTnT) or troponin-I (hsTnI).

Instrument/ test	A	B	C	D	E	F	G
hsTnT	X						
hsTnI		X	X	X	X	X	X
LoD	5	1.7	2.3	17	12	1.3–3.2	20
LoQ 10% (ng/L)	6	4.6	5.6	50	34	2.9–4.9	35
99th centile (ng/L)	F: 14 M: 22 Overall: 19	F: 17 M: 35 Overall: 28	F: 14.9 M: 19.8 Overall: 17.9	Overall: 56	Overall: 34	Overall: 19	Overall: 40

Assay characteristics published by the respective manufacturers. *F*, female; *LoD*, limit of detection; *LoQ*, limit of quantitation; *M*, male. A: COBAS, Elecsys, Troponin T Gen 5, Roche diagnostics, IN, United States, B: Abbott (ALINITY and ARCHITECT), Abbott Diagnostics, IL, United States, C: Beckman Coulter (ACCESS and DXI), Beckman, D: Siemens (DIMENSION), Siemens Medical Solutions USA, PA, United States, E: Ortho Clinical Diagnostic (VITROS ECi), New York, United States, F: bioMerieuX S.A., VIDAS HS, Mercy L'Etoile, France, and G: Tosho, AIA 3G, Tosho Corporation-Bioscience Division, Tokyo. Japan. Modified from High sensitivity cardiac troponin I and T assays. Analytical characteristics designated by the manufacturers v052022. https://www.ifcc.org/media/479435/high-sensitivity-cardiac-troponin-i-and-t-assay-analytical-characteristics-designated-by-manufacturer-v052022.pdf. Accessed 20 February 2023.

high-sensitivity degree of measurements and that results are reported as whole numbers in nanograms per liter. Examples of commercially available laboratory-based troponin assays are shown in Table 8. It is important to note that there is lack of standardization, lack of correlation, and thus lack of commutability and transferability between troponin T and troponin I assays and between 4th and 5th generation assays.

High-sensitivity troponin assays have until recently been confined to the clinical laboratory, with the advent of new recently point of care testing laboratories. The laboratory-based methods often employs 9 and 18 min assay incubation cycle time culminating in about 25–30 min results turnaround from receipt of the sample by the laboratory. Point of care devices offer results within 10 min at the bedside.

Natriuretic peptides

Natriuretic peptide originally isolated from porcine brain and later isolated from human myocardium. It is synthesized by myocardial tissue and is present within both atrial and ventricle tissues. The peptide is produced in its pre-pro form before being cleaved into BNP and NTproBNP (Fig. 8).

Natriuretic peptides consist of three structurally similar peptides. The atrial natriuretic peptide (ANP), B-type (Brain type) natriuretic peptide (BNP), and C-type natriuretic peptide. They are released secondary to increased wall stretching due to volume overload or stress in heart failure. In general, natriuretic peptides play a critical role in maintaining homeostasis in the cardiovascular system acting as counterregulatory hormones for volume and pressure overload.

NTproBNP half-life is prolonged at 1–2 h compared with BNP 20 min. Hence, NTproBNP is often measured as surrogate markers of BNP.

Circulating levels are raised in heart failure and in conditions associated with intravascular volume overload and increased central venous pressure.

Natriuretic peptides, as the name implies, acts on glomerular to stimulate sodium secretion with associated water loss and hence leading to reduction in circulatory volume.

Elevated levels are used in the diagnosis of congestive heart failure and in patient risk assessment for heart failure.

In the Breathing Not Properly (BNP) study, using plasma level of 100 pg/mL as cut-off, with sensitivity of 90%, specificity of 76% and, diagnostic accuracy of 81%. Its measurement is superior to clinical assessment alone.

Testing for natriuretic peptides in the emergency department setting improves the evaluation and treatment of patients with acute dyspnea, and that levels correlate with symptoms, and reduced the time to discharge and thus total cost of treatment. Furthermore, both BNP and NTproBNP levels provide additional information for risk stratification and for prognosis.

There is evidence that plasma BNP or NTproBNP testing can be helpful to guide therapy in patients with mild-to-moderate heart failure and that plasma BNP levels fall rapidly in patients on diuretic therapy. However, routine testing for therapeutic decision on patients with acute or chronic heart failure is not recommended, and that the frequency of monitoring remains unclear.

However, in patients with diabetes mellitus, the professional societies (cardiac, endocrine and diabetes) recommend annual monitoring for patients at risk of developing heart failure (see later).

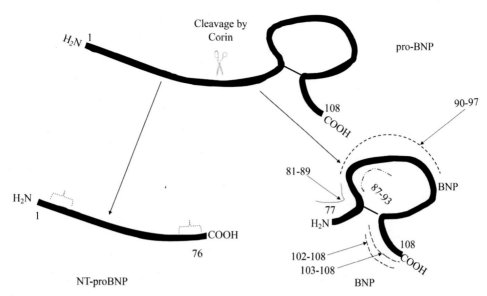

FIG. 8   Natriuretic peptides proBNP and its cleavage product NTproBNP and BNP. Capture and detection epitope amino acids regions are indicated. *BNP*, B-type natriuretic peptide; *NTproBNP*, N-terminal proBNP. *(Modified from Semenov AG, Katrukha AG. Analytical issues with natriuretic peptides— has this been overly simplified? EJIFCC. 2016;27(3):189–207. PMID: 27683533; PMCID: PMC5009944.)*

The structure of BNP and NTproBNP is shown in Fig. 8. Both active BNP and inactive NTproBNP generated from the cleavage of pro BNP, and therefore, they are secreted into the bloodstream in equal concentrations.

They are elevated due to systolic and or diastolic dysfunction, left ventricular hypertrophy, valvular heart disease, ischemia or combinations of these factors. The performance in the diagnosis of heart failure is superior to individual history and physical examinations, chest X-ray, and other laboratory findings. They are used in the diagnostic algorithm for heart failure particularly in patients with unremarkable echocardiogram.

Diagnostic cut-off values for BNP and NTproBNP for the diagnosis of congestive heart failure in an acute and nonacute setting have been established (Table 9). BNP levels <100 pg/ mL rules out heart failure irrespective of patient age, whereas for NTproBNP, age-related thresholds are in use. For those aged less 50 years threefold is <450 pg/mL and doubles to <900 pg/mL for the age 50–75 years, and <1800 pg./mL for patients >75 years old. The notion being NTproBNP is a low molecular fragment, and its circulating concentration is influenced by glomerular filtration rate which declines with age. Overall, a NTproBNP levels <125 pg/mL regardless of age rules out heart failure (Table 9).

Several assays for the measurement of BNP and NTproBNP are commercially available (Table 9).

Point of care testing (POCT) methodologies

A number of POCT devices are commercially available for the measurements of troponin T and troponin I as well as for the natriuretic peptides NTproBNP and BNP. The performance of various commercially available point of care devices is summarized by the IFCC committee on clinical application of cardiac Biomarkers (Table 10).

POCT is applicable in early decision, in a busy high index of suspicion area of low risk patients, who can be safely discharged from the emergency department. Although recent studies showed comparable performance of the POCT assays with laboratory-based assay, the studies were often conducted using stored serum samples and not the would be utilized whole blood sample.

The measurement of troponin T is limited to few manufactures (Table 10). Roche Diagnostics are the main manufacturer with availability on their platforms as well as on few other selected platforms. This limited availability has allowed standardization by default of the various published studies using troponin T. The assays employ two monoclonal antibodies directed at different epitopes on the troponin T molecule. Sandwich assay utilizing two monoclonal antibodies to human cardiac troponin recognizes two epitopes amino acids (125–131 and 136–147) (Fig. 7).

Venous or arterial whole blood sample collected in the presence of anticoagulant (sodium/lithium heparin) or without anticoagulant if tested within on minute of collection (i.e., non clotted sample). Some assays have neither not validated the use of oxalate, citrate, or EDTA as anticoagulants or that they interfere in the assay. However, plasma sample obtained following centrifugation may be acceptable for some but not all available assays. Although those assays are designed for near patient use, capillary blood sample collected by finger stick (often the case in point of care devices (e.g., glucose)), they require blood sample collected by venipuncture.

TABLE 9 Performance characteristics of commercially available laboratory-based assays for the measurement of natriuretic peptides (BNP and NTproBNP).

Instruments	A	B	C	D	E
BNP				X	X
NTproBNP	X	X	X		
LLD (pg/mL)	5	11	<20	1.7	1
LoQ (pg/mL)	50 at CV <20%.	20		20	1
AMR (pg/mL)	10–35,000	20–30,000			1–5000
CRR	10–70,000				1–10,000
Diagnostic threshold (pg/mL) <50 years old 50–70 years old <75 years old >70 years old >75 years old	<125 (All patients age, <450 for >75 years old: Exclude) <450[a] <900[b] <1800[d]	125[c] 450[e]	125[c] 450[e]	100	<100
Sensitivity (%)	83	91.5	93.7	85	82
Specificity (%)	83	76.9	85	92	98
Imprecision (%)	5.2	4.0	5.1	4.2	5.8
RCV (%)	30.1	29.6	30.8	80.1	80.1

RCV, relative change value, calculated by combining both published analytical and biological variations (see Chapter 16 on laboratory management for details). A: Roche NTproBNP, Roche Diagnostics, IN, United States, B: NTproBNP II, VITROS, Ortho Clinical Diagnostics, Rochester, NY, United States, C: BioMerieux/Vidas/NTproBNP bioMerieux Inc., MO, United States, D: BNP, Abbott Diagnostics, IL, United States, E: Beckman Coulter Triage-QUIDEL, Quidel Cardiovascular Inc., San Diego, CA, United States. Diagnostic threshold based on age (yrs; years); (a) <50 yrs, (b) 50–70 yrs, (c) <75 yrs, (d) >70 yrs, and (e) >75 yrs.
Modified from IFCC BNP, NT-proBNP, and MR-proBNP assays analytical characteristics designated by the manufacturer v052022. https://www.ifcc.org/media/479433/bnp-nt-probnp-and-mr-proanp-assays-analytical-characteristics-designated-by-manufacturer-v052022.pdf. Accessed 20 February 2023. From Biomarkers for the diagnosis of heart failure in people with diabetes article: a consensus report from diabetes technology society. *Prog Cardiovasc Dis.* [article submitted for publication].

Several point of care assays are commercially available for the measurement of cTnI (Table 10) with analytical time less than 10 min. Contemporary point of care troponin assays compare well with laboratory-based assays and are best suited for rule-in acute myocardial infarction within 3–6 h of presentation, however up to 6 h sampling may be required to comfortably rule-out infarction.

Most assays employ two monoclonal antibodies specific to the troponin (I or T) located on an electrochemical sensor fabricated on a silicon chip. The detector antibody is conjugated with an enzyme (e.g., alkaline phosphatase, peroxidase) and directed against separate region of the troponin molecule. The assays do not exhibit significant cross-reactivity with cardiac troponin C or the other cardiac troponin (I versus T depending on the manufacturer).

As for natriuretic peptides, several point of care devices are commercially available (Table 11) for the determination of BNP (most of available assays) and limited NTproBNP assays.

In the BNP assay, venous whole blood sample collected in the presence of anticoagulant into EDTA as anticoagulant (or separated plasma following centrifugation). The assays have an analytical measurement range of 5–500 pg/mL. Criteria for 100 pg/mL are applied, where values <100 pg/mL indicates patients without congestive heart failure. The assays employs a fluoresce immunoassay assays utilizing monoclonal and polyclonal antibodies directed against BNP.

The Quidel test is two site-immuno-enzymatic (sandwich) assay. Employing a mouse monoclonal antihuman BNP alkaline phosphatase conjugated and a paramagnetic particle coated with mouse monoclonal antibody. BNP bins to the paramagnetic antibody and (capture) and detected suing the alkaline phosphatase conjugated antibody. A chemiluminescent substrate (Lumi-Phsoi 530) is added, and light generated measured using a luminometer. Signal production is directly proportional to the BNP concentration in the samples. The assay offers acceptable imprecision at about 4.1% at BNP 77 pg/mL.

Alere (Triage Cardio3 Panel) offering combined measurement of creatinine Kinase MB, troponin I, and B-type natriuretic peptide. Using EDTA whole blood or separated plasma samples.

TABLE 10 Example point of care (near patient testing) devices for the qualitative or quantitative determination of troponin I or T.

Instrument	I	J	K	L	M	N	O	P	Q	R	S	T#	U	V
TnT												X (HS)	X (C;	X (C)
TnI	X (Q-LF)	X (Q-LF)	X (C)	X (C)	X (C)	X (C)	X (C)	X (HS)	X (HS)	X (HS)	X (HS)			
LoD	1.5	1.5	0.07 ng/mL							2.33	0.03 ng/mL	1.2–1.6		
LoQ 10% (ng/L)	N/A	N/A	0.1 ng/mL	0.06 µg/L	0.027 µg/L	0.21 µg/L	0.1 µg/L	15	5.8–6.2 (Whole blood)	14	0.06 ng/mL	6.7 (at 20%)	0.026 µg/L	0.04–0.2
99th centile (ng/L)	(Qualitative) >1.5 ng/mL +ve result	(Qualitative) >1.5 ng/mL +ve result	0.08 ng/mL	Overall: 0.07 µg/L	Overall: 0.023 µg/L	Overall: <0.10 µg/L	Overall: 0.08 µg/L	F: 20.3 M: 29.7 Overall: 27.9	F: 14.4 M: 27.7 Overall: 20.5	Overall: 29	0.07 ng/mL	F: 18.5 M: 27.1 Overall: 22.9 (ng/L)	Overall: 0.017 µg/L	NP

Some are designed for high sensitivity (HS) testing, and some remained in contemporary (C) troponin reporting levels. Two of the assays are based on lateral flow and offer qualitative (positive/negative) results. Assay characteristics shown are published by the respective manufacturers. Abbreviations: TnT, troponin T; TnI, troponin I; LoD, limit of detection (the lowest concentration that can theoretically be distinguished from blank); LoQ, limit of quantitation (the lowest concentration that can reliably be measured with an imprecision less than 10%), the 99th percentile: This is the upper limit at the 99th percentile of normal subjects without heart disease. Those parameters are required to satisfy the required assay sensitivity (Required sensitivity being ≤10% at the 99th percentile, and ≥50% measurable concentration is ≥ limit of detection (LoD) for both male and female). Sample type, plasma, serum, and whole blood samples are in use with plasma (lithium heparin) being the preferred sample. C, contemporary troponin assays; HS, high-sensitivity troponin; NP, not performed; Q-LF, qualitative lateral flow assay. I: LifeSign MI, Princeton BioMeditech Corp., NJ, United States, J: instant View, Alfa Scientific Designs, CA, United States, K: iSTAT: Abbott Park, IL, United States, L: STRATUS CS Acute Care, Siemens Medical Solutions, United States, M: AQT90 FLEX, Radiometer (TnI), Denmark, N: RAMP, Response Biomedical, Canada, O: i-STAT, Abbott Diagnostics, United States, P: PATHFAST, LSI Medience, Japan, Q: TriageTrue, Quidel/Alere, CA, United States, R: Mitsubishi Chemical Medience Corp., PATHFAST Cardiac Troponin I, Polymedco, LLC, NY, United States, S: Siemens Healthcare, Stratus CS Acute Care, Siemens Medical Solutions, PA, United States, T#: Atellica VTLi, Siemens Medical Solutions, United States, U: AQT90 FLEX, Radiometer (TnT), Denmark, and V: Cobas h 232, Roche Diagnostics, United States. Troponin values obtained by high sensitivity (fifth generation assays) are reported in whole numbers in ng/L. The values are not interchangeable but roughly 17× values obtained by the contemporary assays (for troponin T). Modified from the published assays characteristics, International Federation of Clinical Chemistry and Laboratory Medicine—Clinical Applications of Cardiac Bio-Markers Updated Tables (https://www.ifcc.org/media/477653/point-of-care-cardiac-troponin-i-and-t-assay-analytical-characteristics-designated-by-manufacturer-v012019.pdf). From Cullen L, Collinson PO, Giannitsis E. Point-of-care testing with high-sensitivity cardiac troponin assays: the challenges and opportunities. Emerg Med J. 2022;39(11):861–866. https://doi.org/10.1136/emermed-2021-211907. Epub 2022 Jan 11. PMID: 35017187; PMCID: PMC9613856.

TABLE 11 Examples commercially available point of care devices (assays) for the determination of BNP and NTProBNP.

Instrument	POCT			
Characteristics	A	B	C	D
BNP	X	X		
NTproBNP			X	X
LLD (pg/mL)	5	15		34
LoQ (pg/mL)	5	15	48	57
AMR (pg/mL)	5–5000	15–5000	20–35,000	18–35,000
CRR	5–5000	15–5000		
Diagnostic threshold (pg/mL) <50 years old 50–70 years old <75 years old >70 years old >75 years old	100	<100	<125[a]	<125[a] <450[b]
Sensitivity (%)	80	74.2	88	95.4
Specificity (%)	98	91.5	87	90.7
Imprecision (%)	9.1	11.1	15	10.3
RCV (%)	83	84.9	49.5	39.4

A: Triage BNP (Beckman Coulter) QUIDEL Cardiovascular Inc., CA, United States (limited availability as the assay is being transitioned to Beckman from QUIDEL), B: iSTAT POCT Abbott, Diagnostics, IL, United States, C: Triage NTproBNP, Alere San Diego, Inc., CA, United States, D: RAMP NTproBNP Response, Response Biomedical, BC, Canada. *AMR*, analytical measurement range; *CRR*, clinical reportable range; *LLD*, lower limit of detection; *LoQ*, lower limit of quantitation; *RCV*, relative change value calculated using published data on biological and analytical variability (see Chapter 16 on Aspects of Laboratory Management). Diagnostic threshold based on age (yrs; years); (a) <75 yrs, (b) >75 yrs.
Modified from IFCC BNP, NT-proBNP, and MR-proBNP assays analytical characteristics designated by the manufacturer v052022. https://www.ifcc.org/media/479433/bnp-nt-probnp-and-mr-proanp-assays-analytical-characteristics-designated-by-manufacturer-v052022.pdf. Accessed 20 February 2023. From published data on biological and analytical variabilities.

Algorithms in acute coronary syndrome

Acute coronary syndrome usually caused by decreased coronary artery perfusion due to stenosis or distal mobilization of the thrombus to sudden and total occlusion of the coronary artery by thrombosis. The syndrome ranges from minor ischemia, ischemia, and some degree of tissue necrosis, to marked tissue necrosis. Biomarkers are indicative of tissue injury due to either ischemia and or necrosis. Cardiac troponins are sensitive and specific markers of myocardial ischemia and necrosis. Heart failure is the end stage of a wide range of cardiovascular disorders that results in the limitation of the heart's ability to contract or relax. The major biomarkers of heart failure are the natriuretic peptides reflecting the hemodynamic changes associated with heart failure. Cardiac biomarkers are thus indicative of myocardial ischemia, injury, necrosis, heart failure, as well as inflammation.

Protocol for the use of high-sensitivity troponin T (fifth generation assays) in use by the authors' laboratory. The protocol was developed to aid in early identification of patients with acute coronary syndrome (ACS) and the safe disposition of patients without ACS (Fig. 9).

Heart failure

Heart failure, a recognized clinical syndrome, is recently defined as "structural and or functional abnormalities of the heart with signs or clinical symptoms supported by an elevated natriuretic peptide and or pulmonary or systemic congestion."

Globally, heart failure remains a leading cause of morbidity and mortality. Using left ventricular ejection fraction, heart failure is defined as ejection fraction ≤40%. Patients with heart failure but with normal ejection fraction (considered to be ≥50%) represents about 50% of the patient population.

Abnormal values undergo echocardiography and receive collaborative care between primary care physicians and specialist cardiologist.

Three plausible arguments for the measurement of natriuretic peptides in diabetes, 1) they are elevated prior to

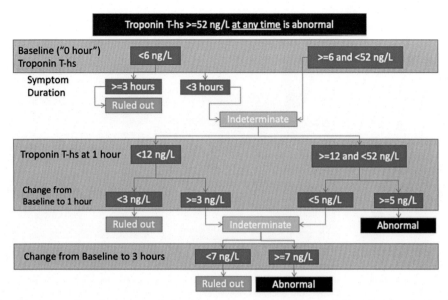

FIG. 9 Algorithm describing process for patients suspected of acute coronary syndrome. The protocol allows for rule out at time 0, 1, and 3 h. *(Modified from the authors' laboratory. From Vigen R, Kutscher P, Fernandez F, et al. Evaluation of a novel rule-out myocardial infarction protocol incorporating high-sensitivity troponin T in a US hospital. Circulation. 2018;138(18):2061–2063. https://doi.org/10.1161/CIRCULATIONAHA.118.033861. PMID: 30372140.)*

echocardiogram evidence of heart failure, b) heart failure is a complication of diabetes, and that the prevalence is reported to be between 9% and 27% among diabetics, c) effective treatment for heart failure (SGLT2i, ACEi, etc.) is available that arrests progression of preclinical heart failure and decrease cardiovascular morbidity and mortality.

The commonest causes include ischemic heart disease, myocardial infarction, hypertension, cardiac valvular disease, diabetes mellitus, genetic familial cardiomyopathies, autoimmune, amyloidosis, drugs such as alcohol, cocaine, methamphetamines, stress-induced cardiomyopathy, sarcoidosis, hemochromatosis (iron overload).

The degree of dysfunction is described by four stages A through D. Stage A describes patients at risk of developing heart failure (stage A) they are without current or prior symptoms or signs of heart failure and without cardiac changes or elevated biomarkers. Patients in stage B are asymptomatic with biochemical evidence (BNP, NTproBNP) of heart failure (overload). Stage A are those at risk of heart failure, stage B is pre-HF, and patients in stage C are symptomatic with biochemical evidence of heart failure. Patients in stage D are in advanced heart failure (Fig. 10).

Heart failure and diabetes mellitus

All patients with diabetes are at risk of developing heart failure and are classified as being in heart failure stage A (Fig. 10).

Among patients with diabetes, the probability of developing frank stage C after 5 years has been reported to be 36.9% compared to 16.8% in the nondiabetic.

Five-year survival in patients with stage A is 97%, stage B 96%, stage C 75%, and stage D 20%. This rapid decline thus requires early identification and initiation of therapy to manage each stage and to delay or prevent progression of preclinical disease to stage C and D heart failure.

The incidence of heart failure among diabetics is reported to be 2.5% per 100 person-year compared to 1.5% per 100 person-year in the nondiabetic population and that the risk is higher among patients with type-I diabetes mellitus than among those with type-II diabetes mellitus. Risk factors among diabetics include female gender, cumulative hyperglycemia, hypertension, hyperlipoidemia, obesity, and smoking. Additionally, the risk of developing advanced heart failure, hospitalization, and mortality is two to six folds in patients with diabetes type II compared to nondiabetic patients. There also appear to be race related component where blacks are at twofold higher risk of developing heart failure compared to nonblacks.

Heart failure may develop in diabetic patients in the absence of hypertension, coronary heart disease, or valvular heart disease and thus a significant cardiovascular complication in among the 9%–27% of diabetic patients. Furthermore, the relationship between diabetes and heart failure is bidirectional where more than 60% of patients with heart failure exhibit a degree of insulin resistance and that heart failure may be the first presentation of cardiovascular complication among patients with diabetes mellitus.

The pathogenesis of heart failure is distinct from that in atherosclerosis. In diabetic cardiomyopathy, there is cardiac hypertrophy and myocardial stiffness unrelated to coronary artery disease, atherosclerosis, or hypertension. Early

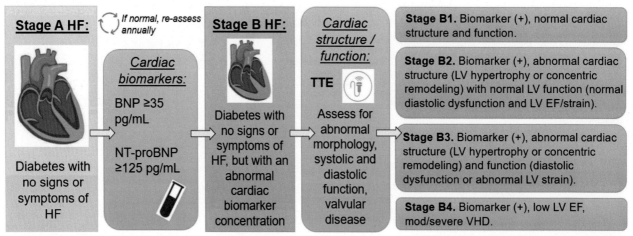

FIG. 10 Early stages of heart failure A and B. Patients with diabetes mellitus are at risk and are thus in stage A. Those in stage B are asymptomatic but with biochemical evidence of heart failure. Assessment of cardiac biomarkers and trans-thoracic echocardiogram to identify subclinical heart failure (Stage B) and subcategories of Stage B in PWD at high risk for developing heart failure. Cardiac structure and function parameters include the following: morphology=LV mass, LV wall thickness, relative wall thickness, LA volume; systolic function=LV EF, LV global longitudinal strain; diastolic function=E/e' (a noninvasive estimate of LA filling pressure and diastolic function), septal e' (the early diastolic wave on the septal side of the mitral annulus), lateral e' (the early diastolic wave on the lateral side of the mitral annulus), TR velocity, estimated PASP. Abbreviations: *BNP*, brain natriuretic peptide; *E/e'*, early mitral inflow velocity/mitral annular early diastolic velocity; *EF*, ejection fraction; *HF*, heart failure; *LA*, left atrium; *LV*, left ventricle; *NTproBNP*, N-terminal prohormone of brain natriuretic peptide; *PASP*, pulmonary artery systolic pressure; *PWD*, persons with diabetes; *TR*, tricuspid regurgitation; *TTE*, trans-thoracic echocardiogram; *VHD*, valvular heart disease. *(Figure courtesy of Ambarish Pandey MD, UT Southwestern Medical Center, Dallas, TX, USA.)*

features are those of cardiac fibrosis, left ventricular hypertrophy and subclinical diastolic dysfunction eventually progressing to systolic dysfunction and hence symptoms of heart failure.

In their recent guidelines (2022), the American Heart Association, American College of Cardiology Foundation, and the Heart Failure Society of America recommended annual screen using natriuretic peptides (NTproBNP or BNP) in high-risk diabetic patients. Annual screen at 5 years post-diagnosis in patients with type I and then annually, and annually for patients with type II diabetes anytime of diagnosis. Additionally, screening patients >30 years old that have type I diabetes mellitus and at any age for patients with type II.

Patients at high risk in stage A heart failure include, diabetes mellitus, obesity, hypertension, hyperlipidemia, diabetic kidney disease, coronary artery disease, male gender, and social determinants of health. In those patients, if the initial NTproBNP <125 pg/mL (BNP <100 pg/mL), repeat testing in 1 year and if values are >125 pg/mL (BNP >100 pg/mL), the patient is subjected to imaging and cardiac assessment of ejection fraction, etc. Similarly, in patients with stage B heart failure with clinical evidence of structural heart disease (LV systolic dysfunction, LV diastolic dysfunction, LV hypertrophy, chamber enlargement, valvular disease, increased filling pressure or elevated biomarkers), the patient is frequently monitored and subjected to imaging and cardiac assessment of ejection fraction, etc. In those patients, in addition to diagnosis and identification, measurement of natriuretic peptides (NTproBNP, BNP) levels are used to guide management, and to predict progression.

Identification of patients at high risk for heart failure (stage A), and or those with stage B (without symptoms but with either structural/functional cardiac abnormalities or elevated cardiac biomarkers) would facilitate earlier application of effective strategies to prevent or delay the progression to advanced heart failure such as optimizing use of RAAS inhibitors and b-blockers or earlier initiation of other therapies such as sodium glucose cotransporter 2 (SGLT2) inhibitors (SGLT2i).

Functional limitations of cardiac biomarkers (troponins and natriuretic peptides)

Whereas natriuretic peptides (NTproBNP and BNP) are indicators of cardiac myocyte stretch and wall stress and have strong mechanistic link to heart failure, troponins (T or I) are markers of myocardium injury, and their release is common to many pathology (Table 12) and thus exhibits poor specificity when used in screening.

The assays for both troponins and natriuretic peptides are immuno-based and are thus subject to the common interference encountered with such assays. For instance, in the presence of circulating human antimouse antibodies (HAMA) and or heterophile antibodies, falsely high or inaccurate results are obtained. Samples suspected of interference must be tested for the presence of HAMA using blocking reagents as well as performing serial dilutions

TABLE 12 Nonacute myocardial infarction (AMI) causes and conditions associated with circulating troponin levels elevation.

Cardiac cause	Tachycardia and arrhythmia
	Aortic valve disease
	Cardiomyopathy
	Acute heart failure
	Blunt cardiac injury
	Chest compression
	Myocarditis
	Cardiac tumors
	Infiltrative disease
Systemic causes	Hypertension
	Sepsis
	Renal failure
	Stroke
	Diabetic ketoacidosis
	Subarachnoid hemorrhage

Modified from Akwe J, Halford B, Kim E, Miller A. A review of cardiac and non-cardiac causes of troponin elevation and clinical relevance Part II non cardiac causes. *J Cardiol Curr Res.* 2018;11(1):00364. 10.15406/jccr.2018.11.00364.

measurements which identifies the presence of interference of HAMA and heterophile antibodies.

Sample hemolysis (the presence of free hemoglobin) interferences with the chemiluminescence detection signal of the assays causing quenching of the signal and thus often falsely low values. Free hemoglobin >0.1 g/dL is reported to cause falsely low troponin T results in most assays. Sample hemolysis is avoided through staff training and avoidance of using small needle and established catheters and intravenous lines etc.

In assays that employ avidin-biotin as part of their formulation, biotin intake (>5 mg/day) will cause interference leading to falsely low results. Although modification of those assay formulation by some manufacturers have removed the interference, however for those assays with biotin interference abstinence from biotin intake for >8 h allow for its clearance from circulation and removes the interference.

Heart failure management drugs Sacubitril and Valsartan are inhibitors of neprilysin, a neutral endopeptidase (degrades natriuretic peptides, vasoactive neurohormones, bradykinin, angiotensin II, and adrenomedullin), and thus prevents the degradation of natriuretic peptides and the neurohormones also contributing to their production.

As stated, use of neprilysin inhibitors inhibits the degradation of natriuretic peptides. This leads to accumulation of BNP (the biologically active component), and thus, interpretation of response to therapy becomes complex. There is a modest and chronic elevation of BNP and a reduction in NTproBNP levels. BNP is the target of neprilysin, while NTproBNP is eliminated by a different mechanism.

With the increasing use of sacubitril/valsartan, there is debate on whether NTproBNP is preferred over BNP. However, the mechanism of changes in natriuretic peptides as a result of neprilysin inhibition is complex.

For instance, there is a slight sustained elevation of BNP and a reduction in NTproBNP levels in response to therapy correlates with improvements in left ventricular systolic and diastolic function as well as decreases in left ventricular and left atrial volumes particularly when measured within 8–10 weeks of initiation of therapy. As for BNP, knowing the baseline steady-state level while using the same assay formulation can aid with BNP interpretation.

However, overall, during treatment both BNP and NTproBNP predict the risk of major adverse outcomes in patients treated with the angiotensin receptor-neprilysin inhibitors.

Other biomarkers associated with heart failure

Troponins as described above are markers of cardiac injury. Sustained elevation (as compared to a rise and fall in acute myocardial infarction) of troponins is seen in patients with cardiac failure.

Diabetes mellitus associated biomarkers

Although urine albumin and A1c are established biomarkers of diabetes control they are as such also risk factors for complications such as heart failure. Additionally, at A1c >7%, the rate of heart failure is highest among young patients with diabetes mellitus.

Similar to screening for chronic kidney disease (at 5 years) postdiagnosis of type I diabetes mellitus and every year in patients with type II diabetes mellitus; however, natriuretic peptides (NT-proBNP and BNP) correlate better than urine albumin. In one study, albumin clearance rate (ACR > 30 mg/g creatinine) minimally added information to that already provided by NTproBNP.

One area of concern remains is the lack of consensus on NTproBNP threshold. Several cohorts reported different NTproBNP thresholds based on statistical correlation based on outcomes. For instance, in the EXAMINE cohort HR 3.27 for NTproBNP 154.1–420.4 pg/mL, the CAVAS cohort, HR 5.4 for NTproBNP ≥125 pg/mL, and in the Thousand and 1 Study cohort HF 41 per 1000 person-years if NTproBNP >300 pg/mL, and 10 per 1000 person-years if NTproBNP <150 pg/mL.

Biomarkers of inflammation is use in assessment of the acute coronary syndrome

Several biomarkers appear in the literature with potential for the management and prognosis assessment in patients with acute coronary syndrome. However, they lack diagnostic specificity and sensitivity and may not be available for routine clinical use.

High sensitivity C-reactive protein (hsCRP)

Positive acute phase marker wild widely used in routine clinical practice. However, it is neither specific nor sensitive for cardiac injury compared to troponins. Circulating levels >5 mg/L have prognostic value and is a predictor of acute coronary syndrome with elevated levels correlating with higher risk of future cardiovascular morbidity and mortality. In patients with IHD, 1SD increase in CRP is associated with 45% increase in relative risk of nonfatal MI or sudden cardiac death over 2 years of follow-up. High sensitivity C-reactive protein assays are available on automated clinical chemistry analyzers.

The assay is based on enhanced immunoturbidimetric assay with 5 mg/L as the limit of quantification. Regular sensitivity CRP assays are not appropriate for use in ACS, with a higher limit of quantification that are used in the investigation of acute phase responses, inflammatory disorders, and rheumatological disorders.

Homocysteine

It is a marker of CVD risk assessment. Increased levels are independently associated with increased rates of all-cause and cardiovascular-related mortality. The levels are reported correlate with the degree of coronary calcification (an indication of atherosclerotic vesicles plaques). Elevated in renal disease. Elevated levels are also independent risk factor.

Copeptin

Copeptin is the C-terminal of the pro-arginine vasopressin. It is detected within 4 h following onset of ACS symptoms. Although it has been recommended by the European society of cardiology for a combined use with troponins for the early rollout of acute myocardial infarction, it is a nonspecific prognostic marker and that is elevated in renal disease and in patients with lower respiratory tract infection. High sensitivity assay format does not seem to increase the diagnostic or prognostic value already provided by troponin assays in patient suspected of having myocardial infarction in the emergency department. Furthermore, the ideal cut-off level remains to be defined.

Interleukin-6

A number of highly sensitive but not specific biomarkers of inflammation have been proposed as helpful or value in the assessment and prognosis of patient with acute coronary syndrome.

IL-6 is a sensitive marker of inflammation and has been shown to offer both risk stratification and prognostic value in patients with acute myocardial infarction. IL-6 levels independently related to adverse cardiac events in this regard the use of IL-6 receptor antagonist has been proposed to improve the inflammatory response and endothelial cell activation postpercutaneous coronary intervention.

Other biomarkers of inflammation with possible prognostic values have been proposed; however, their value remains debatable; they include soluble CD40 ligand, involved in inflammation and thrombosis, Galectin-3 (Gal-3), an inflammatory marker related to myocardium inflammation and fibrosis, interleukin-37 (IL-37), inflammatory cytokine with elevated baseline levels associated with poor outcome in ACS, cardiac myosin-binding protein-C (cMyC), a cardiac-specific myosin binding protein appears in the circulation following myocardial necrosis earlier than high sensitivity to pony however its diagnostic accuracy is similar to that of troponin, cystatin-C (cys-C) (elevated levels is seen in patients with impaired coronary perfusion, lipoproteins associated phospholipase A2 (an inflammatory marker with the risk protection for cardiovascular outcomes), pregnancy-associated plasm protein-A (PAPP-A), a high molecular weight zinc binding metalloproteinase cardiac specific elevated in patients with acute coronary syndrome. It's an independent risk factor for all-cause mortality or cardiovascular events.

Biomarkers of historical interest

The quest for the ideal cardiac biomarker has been and continues to be an active research and clinical assessment arena. Some assays although considered obsolete by many continue to be available and in use by some, hence their inclusion in this chapter.

Myoglobin and CK-MB

The third universal definition of myocardial infarction refers to do utility of biomarker troponins performance at the 99th percentile as a decision value for acute myocardial infarction.[4] There is no mention of the earlier myoglobin and CK-MB isoform markers previously the most widely used markers. CKMB has retained a degree of utility in some institutions as an indication of reinfarction or in detecting a new infarct postcatheterization.

Amyloid heart disease

Transthyretin amyloid cardiomyopathy (ATTR-CM) is an underrecognized cause of heart failure (HF) in patients >60 years old. It arises from deposition of misfolded transthyretin or misfolding of immunoglobulin light-chain aggregates and involves the heart in 50%–75% of cases. Diagnosis is via imaging studies; however, new recommendations for treatment include screening for serum and urine monoclonal light chains.

Summary

– The relationship between lipids and risk for cardiovascular atherosclerotic disease is well stablished with several pathogenesis and risk models described.
– Very low-density lipoprotein particles (VLDL) contain most of the triglyceride in plasma whereas low-density lipoprotein (LDL) particles contain most of the cholesterol.
– The rate of atherosclerotic plaque progression is directly proportional to the absolute plasma LDL levels.
– The principal lipids are cholesterol and triglycerides. They differ markedly in their structure and their clinical and diagnostic importance. The lipids are dynamic in nature with variable size and constituents.
– Cholesterol although present in the diet, the major source is hepatic de-novo synthesis from acetate.
– Composed of three fatty acid molecules esterified with glycerol. They represent the major storage form of fatty acids and serve as the major energy store in mammals.
– Lipoproteins are macromolecular complexes of lipid and protein. Lipids + Apolipoproteins = Lipoproteins.
– VLDL: Produced by the liver, their ultimate fate is either hepatic uptake or conversion to LDL, IDL: Produced by lipolysis of VLDL by lipoprotein lipase.
– LDL: Produced, though direct synthesis may rarely occur, from VLDL via IDL removal is by peripheral or hepatic uptake by ligand-receptor or scavenger pathways.
– HDL: Produced as nascent particles by the liver and small intestine.
– Lipoprotein lipase (LPL) is present in cells that either stores triglycerides, i.e., adipose tissue and or uses it as energy source (skeletal and cardiac muscle).

– Primary hyperlipidemia may be classified phenotypically by the WHO system or according to the underlying genetic defect.
– Cardiac troponin complex consists of three isoforms namely, troponin "C" which binds calcium, troponin "I" which inhibits the ATPase activity of actomycin, and troponin "T" which interacts with tropomycin.
– Natriuretic peptides consist of three structurally similar peptides. The atrial natriuretic peptide (ANP), B-type (Brain type) natriuretic peptide (BNP), and C-type natriuretic peptide.
– Acute coronary syndrome usually caused by decreased coronary artery perfusion.
– All patients with diabetes are at risk of developing heart failure and are classified as being in heart failure stage A.

References

1. Schaefer EJ, Geller AS, Endress G. The biochemical and genetic diagnosis of lipid disorders. *Curr Opin Lipidol.* 2019;30(2):56–62.
2. Wang XY, Zhang F, Zhang C, Zheng LR, Yang J. The biomarkers for acute myocardial infarction and heart failure. *Biomed Res Int.* 2020;2020, 2018035.
3. Garg P, Morris P, Fazlanie AL, et al. Cardiac biomarkers of acute coronary syndrome: from history to high-sensitivity cardiac troponin. *Intern Emerg Med.* 2017;12(2):147–155.
4. Thygesen K, Alpert JS, Jaffe AS, et al. Third universal definition of myocardial infarction. *J Am Coll Cardiol.* 2012;60(16):1581–1598.

Suggested reading

Mehta A, Shapiro MD. Apolipoproteins in vascular biology and atherosclerotic disease. *Nat Rev Cardiol.* 2022;19(3):168–179.

Volpe M, Battistoni A, Rubattu S. Natriuretic peptides in heart failure: current achievements and future perspectives. *Int J Cardiol.* 2019;281:186–189.

Kontos MC, Turlington JS. High-sensitivity troponins in cardiovascular disease. *Curr Cardiol Rep.* 2020;22(5):30.

Collinson PO, Saenger AK, Apple FS, on behalf of the IFCC C-CB. High sensitivity, contemporary and point-of-care cardiac troponin assays: educational aids developed by the IFCC Committee on Clinical Application of Cardiac Bio-Markers. *Clin Chem Lab Med.* 2019;57(5):623–632.

Goetze JP, Bruneau BG, Ramos HR, Ogawa T, de Bold MK, de Bold AJ. Cardiac natriuretic peptides. *Nat Rev Cardiol.* 2020;17(11):698–717.

Chapter 8

Obstetrics, fetal, and neonatal disorders

Introduction

This chapter describes the clinical biochemistry laboratory role in support of two individuals, the mother and her baby. From pregnancy to obstetric and fetomaternal care, to investigation of infertility and malignancy.

Pregnancy

Conception is suspected when menstrual period is missed. For women of productive age with regular menstrual cycles, a period that is ≥ 1 week late is presumptive evidence of pregnancy, and a confirmatory serum or urine pregnancy test is required (see later).

A viable and normal course of pregnancy is considered to last about 266 days from the time of conception or 280 days from the first day of the last menstrual period if periods occur regularly, every 28 days.

Delivery prior to 37 weeks of gestation is considered preterm, whereas delivery post 42 weeks is considered postterm. The delivery date is estimated based on the last menstrual period and could vary by up to 2 weeks (earlier or later).

Pregnancy test (human chorionic gonadotropin, hCG)

Successful conception is confirmed biochemically by a detectable and rising level of human chorionic gonadotropin (hCG) produced by the developing syncytiotrophoblastic cells of the placenta.

Physiologically, hCG stimulates the corpus luteum to produce progesterone which maintains the pregnancy by stimulating thickening of the uterine lining to support embryo implantation.

Positive hCG urine results are obtained on the second week after missed period when urine hCG levels exceed 20 IU/L. However, blood assays with a detection sensitivity of at least 5 IU/L are positive for hCG earlier at 8–11 days postconception (third week from the last menstrual period). Gestational sac in the uterus is seen with ultrasonography typically at about 4–5 weeks of pregnancy and typically corresponds to a serum hCG level of about 1500 IU/L.

hCG is a 37.9 kDa, glycoprotein heterogeneous molecule. It is present as a heterodimer of α and β subunits (intact heterodimer form), free beta subunit, nicked (by human leukocyte esterase) and partially cleaved forms, as well as hyperglycosylated forms.

It shares a single gene (c:6) product (α) with TSH, LH, and FSH. The hCG β subunit confers specificity.

It exhibits molecular heterogeneity with various forms appearing in circulation and in the urine (Fig. 1). The c-terminal is cleaved to create core fragments composed of two pieces of β-subunits held by disulfide bridges. Urine contains mainly intact, core and nicked fragments. Some of the forms are specific to certain disorders and thus offer a diagnostic advantage. Furthermore, those forms exhibit different reactivity among different assays. Some assays recognize the last 30 amino acids, whereas some recognize the 1st to 115 amino acids region.

Levels of βhCG correlate with gestational age (Table 1), and it can be used to determine whether a fetus is growing normally. The best approach is to compare two serum βhCG values, obtained 48–72 h apart and measured by the same assay. Doubling in the βhCG values in a singleton pregnancy every 1.4–2.1 days during the first 60 days (7.5 weeks) indicates a normal course of pregnancy. Levels begin to decline between 10 and 18 weeks.

hCG is cleared from circulation following hepatic metabolism, hepatic clearance being $2\,mL/min/m^2$ and renal clearance at $0.4\,mL/min/m^2$, of about 20% of the hormone. The β subunit is degraded in the kidney producing a core fragment detected in the urine pregnancy test. Urine contains mainly hyperglycosylated hCG, intact hCG, core-hCG, and nicked fragments (Fig. 1).

Commercially available immunoassays detect hCG forms as either, βhCG, total hCG comprising (βhCG and Intact-hCG), and intact hCG only (Fig. 1). The assays are standardized against the third international reference material (IRP 75/537).

Several commercials over the counter point of care urine pregnancy test are available; however some do not detect the major urine hyperglycosylated hCG variant and thus produce an early false negative result. The hyperglycosylated form being predominant during the first 3 weeks of gestation (Table 1). It contains larger and complex N- and O-linked carbohydrate oligosaccharides compared to the other βhCG moieties.

Tutorials in Clinical Chemistry. https://doi.org/10.1016/B978-0-12-822949-1.00014-0

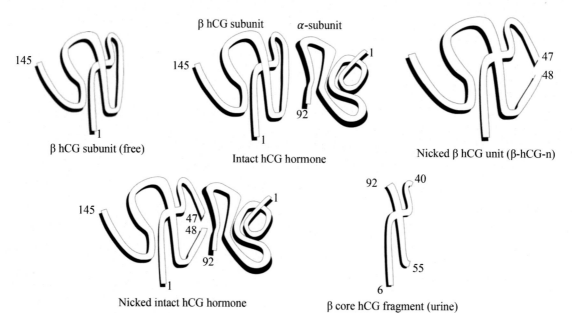

FIG. 1 Molecular forms of hCG. Subunits as well as posttranslational cleavage forms. *(Modified from Cole LA. hCG, five independent molecules. Clin Chim Acta. 2012;413(1–2):48–65. https://doi.org/10.1016/j.cca.2011.09.037. Epub 2011 Oct 18. PMID: 22027338.)*

TABLE 1 The relative proportion of hyperglycosylated hCG in urine during pregnancy by gestational weeks.

Gestational age (weeks)	Total hCG (median) (mIU/L)	Hyperglycosylated hCG (%) (median ± SD)	Highest proportion (%) of hyperglycosylated form
Blood (plasma)			
3	12	90 ± 11	100
4	72	54 ± 27	81
5	521	42 ± 27	69
6	1879	29 ± 38	67
7	16,049	16 ± 13	29
8	47,641	7 ± 13	20
9	64,150	5.1 ± 4.4	9.5
10	102,750	4.3 ± 3.1	7.4
11	95,650	2.3 ± 1.5	3.8
Urine			
3	13	83 ± 92	100
4	139	72 ± 51	100
5	902	38 ± 46	84
6	2730	22 ± 25	47
7	7500	15 ± 13	28
8	16,650	13 ± 10	23
9	50,458	8.2 ± 8.5	16.7
10	81,625	5 ± 6	11
11	19,130	4.2 ± 3.8	8

Modified from Cole LA. Hyperglycosylated hCG, a review. *Placenta*. 2010;31(8):653–664. https://doi.org/10.1016/j.placenta.2010.06.005. Epub 2010 Jul 8. PMID: 20619452.

Quantitative serum hCG assay for confirmation of pregnancy gives information on prognosis and that serial measurements assesses viability of pregnancy and time for ultrasonography as stated above. Blood hCG levels peaks at 100,000 IU/L normally reached at 8–10 weeks of gestation. Higher and earlier hCG levels require clinical assessment for suspected molar pregnancy.

Following delivery (partition) hCG levels decline to undetectable levels by 7–60 days.

Serial measurements are helpful in assessment of effectiveness of curettage can be assessed by monitoring its clearance half-life ($t_{1/2} = 0.693/k$, where $k = \ln[hCG_1] - \ln[hCG_2]/(time_1 - time_2)$).

Discordant hCG results (false positive or false negative) may occur due to interference by heterophilic antibodies (see later), immunoscintigraphic reagents, rheumatoid factors, biotin therapy. Some assays are prone to antigen excess "hook effect," where the high concentration of hCG exceeds the analytical measuring range of the assay and assay reagents are overwhelmed by the hCG levels giving a falsely low or negative results. Additionally, some assays are sensitive to matrix effects (hyperviscosity syndromes, serum, plasma, hypovolemia) which may result in −2% to 13% change in measured hCG concentration.

In summary, there are important limitations with regard to measurement of hormones. hCG levels can be below the detection limit of the assay, for instance for a positive urine result, a value has to be above 25 IU/L in serum before it can be detected in urine. Similarly, levels for hCG can be extremely high reaching about 100,000 IU/L during normal pregnancy, and much higher ($\gg$100,000 IU/L) in patients with hederiform and ectopic pregnancy. Such high levels may exceed the assay capacity leading to a falsely low hCG due to the antigen excess phenomena (hook-effect). Serum assays have a detection limit of 5 IU/L. The different hCG forms are variably detected by different commercially available immunoassays measuring either βhCG, total hCG (β subunit plus intact hCG), and intact hCG only (see earlier).

Ectopic pregnancy

Implantation taking place outside the uterus termed ectopic pregnancy. The most common (95%) of the ectopic pregnancy occurs in the fallopian tube. There is risk of tube rupture if not treated with risk of severe intra-abdominal bleed.

Serial determination of hCG helps identify the presence of ectopic pregnancy. In normal developing pregnancy, hCG rate of increase doubles every 2 days (48 h). In ectopic pregnancy, the rate of increase is much lower.

Detection by transvaginal ultrasound is possible when βhCG is above 1000 IU/L where absence of visible embryonic sac within the uterus confirms suspicion for ectopic pregnancy.

Use of methotrexate (folate antagonist) is preferred to surgical intervention when βhCG is less than 5000 IU/L.

hCG levels in nonpregnant patients

Circulating hCG levels increase with age with pituitary being the plausible sources in nonpregnant female. It thus recommended that the serum hCG cutoff be increased from 5 IU/L to 14 IU/L for patients over the age of 55 years. Additionally, increasing detectable hCG levels in nonpregnant female require evaluation for malignancy (ovarian, bladder, testicular) when hCG is persistently detectable.

Interference in immunoassays

In additions to differences in assay immunoreactivity due to molecular heterogeneity described above, a major source of possible interference is that of circulating human-antimouse antibodies (HAMA) and of heterophile antibodies.

Heterophile antibodies are seen in patients with autoimmune disorders (rheumatoid arthritis, etc.) The antibodies interfere in the assay although the mode of interference in the case of heterophile antibodies is not clear, whereas for HAMA interference is observed in immunoassays that utilize mouse monoclonal antibodies. The presence of circulating human antimouse antibodies will cross react with the assays mouse monoclonal reagent antibias and participate in the reaction, often producing a false positive result. Sample treatment with HAMA blocking tubes (proprietary commercial martial most likely contain mouse sera that will adsorb circulating HAMA). Following sample treatment, a repeat analysis often provides reliable results having removed/blocked the interfering antibodies.

Another cause of interference is biotin. Circulating biotin levels (in patients taking large dose supplements) can interfere with avidin-biotin-based immunoassays (see Chapter 17).

Biochemical/physiological variability during pregnancy

Pregnancy is associated physiological adaptation affecting every organ in the body. It is accompanied by marked hormonal changes that supports the developing fetus, with significant metabolic, hemodynamic, and immunological changes. It is a major endocrine event, and the metabolic changes seen in pregnancy are relatively short lived and return to normal postpartum.

Cardiac output increases by 30%–50%, at about 6 weeks' gestation peaking between 16 and 28 weeks (usually at about 24 weeks). It remains near peak levels until after 30 weeks. Renal glomerular filtration rate (GFR) increases by 30%–50% and peaks between 16 and 24 weeks of gestation and remains at that level until nearly term, when it may decrease slightly. It roughly parallels changes with cardiac output. Furthermore, renal plasma flow increases in proportion to the GFR and as a result, blood urea nitrogen (BUN) decreases, usually to <10 mg/dL (<3.6 mmol/L), and creatinine levels decrease proportionally to 0.5–0.7 mg/dL (44–62 µmol/L). However, patients with impaired renal function prior to pregnancy often experience deterioration in renal function with increase in creatinine and urea levels.

The renal tubular reabsorption threshold alters in pregnancy, for instance, threshold for glucose reabsorption from glomerular filtrate changes from 90 (5 mmol/L) to 180 mg/dL (10 mmol/L) in pregnancy.

Total blood volume increases proportionally with cardiac output, but the increase in plasma volume is greater (close to 50%, and usually by about 1600 mL for a total of 5200 mL) than that in red blood cell (RBC) mass (about 25%); thus, hemoglobin (Hb) is lowered by dilution, from about 13.3 to about 12.1 g/dL. This dilutional anemia decreases blood viscosity. With twins, total maternal blood volume increase is higher at about 60%. White blood cell count (WBC) increases slightly to 9000–12,000/mcL. Marked leukocytosis (≥20,000/mcL) occurs during labor and during the first few days postpartum.

Requirement for iron increases by a total of 1 g (the growing fetus and placenta use about 300 mg, and an increased maternal RBC mass requires 500 mg, and there are about 200 mg lost in excretion) during pregnancy. Iron supplementation is thus required.

Changes in maternal lung function includes increase in tidal and minute volume and thus respiratory rate increasing blood pH. This is in part due to increasing progesterone levels signaling the brain to lower carbon dioxide (CO_2) levels. The maternal lung function changes are secondary to the enlarging uterus interfering with lung expansion. Oxygen consumption increases by about 20% to meet the increased metabolic needs of the fetus, placenta, and several maternal organs.

Maternal gastrointestinal motility decreases in response to the elevated progesterone levels which cause relaxation of gastrointestinal smooth muscle.

Increased pigmentation of maternal skin late in pregnancy is due to the increased circulating melanocyte-stimulating hormone (MSH), produced by the placenta.

The pituitary gland enlarges by about 135% during pregnancy. The growth in pituitary size may exceed the blood supply leads to infraction (Sheehan's syndrome—see later).

Maternal plasma prolactin level increases by 10-fold secondary to an increase in thyrotropin-releasing hormone production, stimulated by estrogen. The primary function of increased prolactin is to ensure lactation. The level returns to normal postpartum, even in women who breastfeed.

hCG has thyrotrophic effect stimulating the thyroid to secrete thyroid hormones, thyroid hyperplasia, and increased vascularity. However, true hyperthyroidism occurs in only 0.08% of pregnancies.

Estrogen stimulates hepatocytes, causing increased thyroid-binding globulin levels; thus, although total thyroxine levels may increase, levels of free thyroid hormones remain within normal limits.

Pregnant patients are at risk of thyroid dysfunction, and that preexiting thyroid dysfunction needs to be closely monitored to maintain euthyroid status of the mother. However, this is complicated by the physiological changes described above where the increasing hCG levels have thyrotropic activity leading to suppression in TSH level during the first and second trimesters (Fig. 2). To avoid misinterpretation of thyroid function test, gestational age appropriate reference intervals are required. The changes in TSH are different between singleton and twin pregnancies (Fig. 2).

Additionally, the markedly increased thyroxin binding globulin (TBG) during pregnancy and the decreased serum albumin levels influence the measurement of thyroid hormones. Total thyroid hormones will be elevated due to the marked increase in TBG levels, and the low albumin may interfere in some of the free thyroid home assays due to the albumin effect on the free-bound equilibrium and assay reaction methodologies.

Total proteins and albumin levels are reduced by about 15%, in contract to alpha-1-antitrypsin, fibrinogen, and ceruloplasmin which all increase by two to three folds. Similarly, aspartate transaminase (AST) and alkaline phosphatase enzymes levels increase by 2–3 folds by the third trimester. Contribution from placental tissue contributes to the total alkaline phosphatase levels seen in pregnancy. This is observed in alkaline phosphatase isoenzymes analysis.

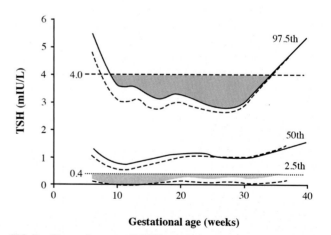

FIG. 2 Changes in maternal TSH levels during pregnancy by gestational weeks. TSH is suppressed during the first trimester secondary to the thyrotrophic effect of hCG that peaks during that period. Values are established from singleton (*solid lines*) and twin pregnancy (*dashed lines*). *Modified from Dashe JS, Casey BM, Wells CE, et al. Thyroid-stimulating hormone in singleton and twin pregnancy: importance of gestational age-specific reference ranges. Obstet Gynecol. 2005;106(4):753–757. https://doi.org/10.1097/01.AOG.0000175836.41390.73. PMID: 16199632.)*

Fasting triglycerides levels are two to three folds higher by the third trimester of pregnancy; however, changers in cholesterol, phospholipids, and nonesterified fatty acids are less apparent. Initially during pregnancy, an increase in LDL cholesterol and HDL cholesterol is observed for at least 10 weeks in pregnancy before leveling. Pregnant patients also exhibit state of insulin resistance secondary to the increase in estradiol and progesterone.

The above changes render the pregnant patient at risk for gestational diabetes.

Gestational diabetes describes diabetes mellitus diagnosed for the first time in the second and third trimester. Patients are often asymptomatic and thus screening is important. Patients with gestational diabetes mellitus are at risk of developing hypertension, preeclampsia, fetal macrosomia, and fetal dystocia.

Disorders in pregnancy

Disorders associated with pregnancy include gestational diabetes mellitus, preeclampsia, premature rupture of membrane (PROM), antiphospholipid syndrome, among increased risk for a number of autoimmune disorders.

Gestational diabetes mellitus

Gestational diabetes mellitus describes diabetes in a pregnant woman without a previous diagnosis of diabetes mellitus. Gestational diabetes is diagnosed in the second and third trimester, whereas diabetes diagnosed in the first trimester is often considered type 2. Gestational diabetes is distinct from type 1 and 2 diabetes mellitus. The prevalence of gestational diabetes ranges from 1% to 25% (median 9%).

Additionally, mothers with gestational diabetes are at high risk of developing type II diabetes mellitus in subsequent years. Patients are often asymptomatic and thus screening is important. Patients with gestational diabetes are at risk of developing fetal macrosomia.

Fetal macrosomia is associated with high risk for cesarean section delivery, shoulder dystocia, and injury due to the large size fetus. This is secondary to excessive circulating maternal glucose. Fetal hyperinsulinemia secondary to the maternal hyperglycemia alters lung surfactant synthesis, predisposing to fetal respiratory distress syndrome.

Similarly, complication of gestational diabetes mellitus is fetal hypoglycemia secondary to the high insulin levels. The newborn is at risk of neonatal hypoglycemia secondary to the hyperinsulinemia in the newborn period released in response to the uterus maternal hyperglycemia during fetal life and thus following delivery and the abrupt drop of glucose at delivery, and once fetal glucose stores are exhausted, neonatal hypoglycemia develops.

There is discrepancy among the different studies and professional societies guidelines and different protocols preferences are taking place. However, two approaches are in use. A two-step approach in which the pregnant patient (at about 24–28 weeks' gestation) receives a 50-g glucose challenge. The patient need not be fasting. Blood sample is collected at 1-h postchallenge and glucose level measured. Glucose level above 140 mg/dL (7.8 mmol/L) is considered abnormal and requires confirmation using a 2- or 3-h glucose tolerance test.

In the follow-up confirmation glucose tolerance test, the fasting patient (often >8 h overnight fast) consumes 100 g or 75 g glucose load and blood samples collected for glucose measurement at times 0 (just prior to dose), and at 1, 2, and or 3 h postdosage. There are various glucose thresholds proposed by the different societies (Tables 2 and 3), but in general gestational diabetes is diagnosed when at least two abnormal glucose values are obtained as defined by the cutoffs in Tables 2 and 3.

In the one-step approach, performed during 24–28 weeks' gestation, screening and diagnosis are combined into a single 75 g glucose tolerance test. Following an overnight fast, the patient consumes 75 g glucose load and blood samples are collected at time 0 (just prior to dose), and at 1 and 2 h post dose (Table 2). The one step requires only on glucose value to be abnormal.

Target glucose levels have been defined by several organizations as shown in Tables 2 and 3. Most guidelines recommend screening using the one stop approach 6–12 weeks' postpartum with repeat screening 1–3 years afterward.

TABLE 2 Glucose threshold values for the diagnosis of gestational diabetes mellitus.

Time post glucose load (hours)	One step glucose tolerance test (mg/dL) (≥1 value exceeded) (75 g glucose load)	Carpenter-Coustan criteria (mg/dL) (≥2 values exceeded) (100 g glucose load)	National Diabetes Data Group criteria (≥2 values exceeded) (100 g glucose load)
Fasting	92	95	105 mg/dL
1 h	180	180	190 mg/dL
2 h	153	155	165
3 h	N/A	140	145

The glucose load is taken in the morning following an overnight (at least 8 h not exceeding 14 h) fast and following >3 days of unrestricted normal diet and physical activity.
Modified from Szmuilowicz ED, Josefson JL, Metzger BE. Gestational diabetes mellitus. *Endocrinol Metab Clin N Am.* 2019;48(3):479–493. https://doi.org/10.1016/j.ecl.2019.05.001. Epub 2019 Jun 18. PMID: 31345518; PMCID: PMC7008467.

TABLE 3 Professional societies protocols for the diagnosis of gestational diabetes mellitus following meal are different from those shown in Table 2.

Guideline	Fasting (mg/dL)	1h post intake (mg/dL)	2h post intake (mg/dL)
ADA	≤95	<140	<120
Endocrine Society (United States)	≤95	NA	<120
NICE (post 75 g glucose)	<100	NA	<140

ADA, American Diabetes Association; *NICE*, National Institute for Health and Care Excellence (United Kingdom); *NA*, not applicable.
Modified from American Diabetes Association. 14. Management of diabetes in pregnancy: *Standards of Medical Care in Diabetes-2020*. *Diabetes Care*. 2020;43(suppl 1): S183–S192. https://doi.org/10.2337/dc20-S014. PMID: 31862757. Szmuilowicz ED, Josefson JL, Metzger BE. Gestational diabetes mellitus. *Endocrinol Metab Clin N Am*. 2019;48(3):479–493. https://doi.org/10.1016/j.ecl.2019.05.001. Epub 2019 Jun 18. PMID: 31345518; PMCID: PMC7008467. National Institute for Health and Care Excellence (NICE). Diabetes in Pregnancy: Management From Preconception to the Postnatal Period. NICE Guideline [NG3]. 2017. https://www.nice.org.uk/Guidance/NG3. Liu B, Cai J, Xu Y, et al. Early diagnosed gestational diabetes mellitus is associated with adverse pregnancy outcomes: a prospective cohort study. *J Clin Endocrinol Metab*. 2020;105(12):dgaa633. https://doi.org/10.1210/clinem/dgaa633. PMID: 32898218.

TABLE 4 Biomarkers and hematological indices associated with preeclampsia.

Biomarker	Preeclampsia-associated findings
Proteinuria (Protein:creatinine ratio)	≥30 mg/mmol (0.3 mg/mg)
Creatinine	≥90 μmol/L (≥1.1 mg/dL)
AST or ALT	>2 ULN
Platelet count	<100,000 plt/μL

ALT, alanine transaminase; *AST*, aspartate transaminase; *ULN*, upper limit of normal.
Modified from Report of the American College of Obstetricians and Gynecologists' Task Force on hypertension in pregnancy. *Obstet Gynecol*. 2013;122(5):1122–1131. https://doi.org/10.1097/01. AOG.0000437382.03963.88. PMID: 24150027.

Increased red blood cell turnover during pregnancy results in reduced A1c during pregnancy by about 0.5%. The use of A1c is thus unreliable for assessment of diabetes control and of assessment of risk for complications, in contrast to postprandial glucose which has a better prediction for GDM complications.

Preeclampsia

Preeclampsia is a pregnancy associated multisystem dysfunction. The disorder is thus defined as new onset hypertension (systolic blood pressure sustained at ≥140 mmHg or diastolic blood pressure sustained at ≥90 mmHg or both), and proteinuria or end organ dysfunction after 20 weeks' gestation (Table 4). It complicates about 4.5% of pregnancies. There is variable degree of placental perfusion with release of placental soluble factors. The latter lead to maternal endothelial injury with resultant multiorgan injury and hypertension.

End organs affected include the brain (severe headache, visual disturbances, eclamptic seizures), the liver (epigastric pain, abnormal liver enzymes and function tests), the kidney (proteinuria, abnormal kidney function tests), hematological; system (hemolysis, thrombocytopenia, coagulopathy), the lungs (low oxygen saturation, pulmonary edema), the placenta (fetal growth restriction).

The ensued maternal complications lead to restriction in fetal growth and development and contributes to fetal demise and stillbirth.

There are no specific biochemical tests to diagnose preeclampsia; however, the laboratory plays a supportive role in the assessment of material organ function as renal function and associated proteinuria. Twenty-four hour urinary protein excretion ≥300 mg is diagnostic of preeclampsia and random urinary protein creatinine ratio >0.63 is indicative of a 24 h urinary protein >300 mg.

Risk for preeclampsia include prior history of preeclampsia (8 times increase in risk), with chronic hypertension (5 times higher risk), pregestational diabetes (3.7 times high risk), maternal age <17 years (about 3 times higher risk), multifetal pregnancy (about 3 times higher risk), family history of preeclampsia (3 times), antiphospholipid syndrome (2.8 higher risk), SLE (2.5 higher risk), assisted reproduction (1.8), chronic kidney disease (1.8 higher), maternal age >40 years (1.5 times higher).

Research biomarkers for preeclampsia include circulating placental growth factor (PIGF) a preangiogenic protein, secreted by the placenta increases with advancing gestation before decreasing toward term and is decreased in patients with preeclampsia. Circulating placental soluble fms-like tyrosine kinase-1 (sFlt-1) increases toward term in healthy pregnancy is elevated in patients with preeclampsia the finding of low PIGF and high sFlt-1 concentration predate the clinical diagnosis of preeclampsia by some weeks enabling the potential use as diagnostic adjuncts.

Premature rupture of membrane

Preterm (premature) rupture of membrane (PROM), evident by breakage of the amniotic sac, prior to 37 weeks' gestation. Approximately 3%–12% of births worldwide are product of preterm delivery. This represents a major factor contributing to the perinatal morbidity and mortality.

Detection of amniotic fluid in vaginal secretions is an indication of leakage of the amniotic sac. This is detected and confirmed biochemically by measuring alpha-fetoprotein and insulin like growth factor binding protein-1 (IGFBP-1) in vaginal secretions.

Virginal swab (for few seconds) is obtained and applied to a test reagent strip containing antibodies directed against the amniotic fluid proteins (AFP and IGFBP-1). A positive test indicates leak of amniotic fluid. Patients with false positive results are often found to be at term which may indicate the near delivery and physiological leakage of the membrane without gross rupture.

Several commercial assays are available as point of care tests. Amniotic fluid AFP and IGFBP-1 are present at high concentration, and therefore, an important characteristic of the assays is the required wide detection concentration range as well as high sensitivity (low detection limit). For instance, one of the assays in use by the authors laboratory has an analytical measurement range of 150–200,000 ng/mL for AFP and from 5 to 400,000 ng/mL for IGFBP-1. A wide detection ranges particularly for a point of care test without the provision for manual sample dilution or preparation prior to testing. This is important as such high levels may lead to antigen excess "hook effect" producing a falsely negative result. The assay has negative predictive value of 99% and a positive predictive value of 85%.

Another marker of amniotic fluid leak, placental alph-1-microglobulin protein (PAMG-1), is commercially available (AmioSure, QIAGEN).

PAMG-1 concentrations in the amniotic fluid fall into 2000–25,000 ng/mL range compared with up to 0.22 ng/mL cervical and vaginal secretions of pregnant women without complications in pregnancy and in vaginitis and nonsignificant presence of blood, up to 3 ng/mL. The test is lateral flow based. A sample taken by vaginal swab is placed into a vial with a solvent. The solvent extracts the sample from the swab for 1 min, after which the swab is disposed, and the sample extract applied to the test strip. Two visually observed lines indicate a positive finding for amniotic fluid and PROM.

Antiphospholipids syndrome

The antiphospholipid syndrome is an autoimmune systemic disorder characterized by circulatory (arterial, venous, or small vessel) thrombosis and/or recurrent early pregnancy loss, fetal loss, or pregnancy morbidity.

The patient exhibits persistent circulating antiphospholipid antibodies (lupus anticoagulant, anticardiolipin, anti-β2-Glycoprotein I antibodies).

Phospholipids on cell membrane are classified according to their charge. Negatively charged phospholipids

include cardiolipin, phosphatidylserine, phosphatidylglycerol, phosphatidylinositol, and phosphatidic acid. Neutral phospholipids include phosphatidylethanolamine, phosphatidylcholine, and sphingomyelin.

The antibodies to those phospholipids include IgG, IgM, and IgA. Antibodies against the phospholipids are either cofactor-dependent or independent with the cofactors being phospholipids binding proteins and include among those mostly coagulation and fibrinolysin: β2-GPI, prothrombin, protein C, protein S, kininogen, thrombomodulin, annexin A5, factors XI and XII, prekallikrein, oxidized-LDL, and thromboxane A2.

The degree of risk associated with antiphospholipid antibody depends on the characteristics of the antiphospholipid antibody profile and on the presence of additional thrombotic risk factors.

Antiphospholipid antibodies are attributed to recurrent pregnancy loss in about 19% of patients with about 16.8% of those the predominant antibody being antiphosphatidylethanolamine IgM.

Clinical obstetrics presentation associated with the antiphospholipid syndrome is ≥1 fetal loss at ≥10 weeks of gestation, ≥3 early pregnancy loss at <10 weeks gestation, preeclampsia/placental insufficiency occurring ≤34 weeks gestation.

The antiphospholipid syndrome is also associated with coagulopathy (deep venous thrombosis, stroke, and thrombotic microangiopathy). The criteria for the classification of antiphospholipid syndrome are shown in Tables 5 and 6.

Differentiating between antiphospholipid syndrome and coagulopathy as a cause of recurrent fetal loss is important for patient management. The classification criteria for the antiphospholipid syndrome are shown in Table 5.

TABLE 5 Points score and weights of the global antiphospholipid syndrome score (GAPSS).

Marker	Antibody	Criteria	Points
Anticardiolipin	IgG or IgM	+	5
Anti-β2-glycoprotein 1	IgG or IgM	+	4
Antiphosphatidylserine-prothrombin complexes	IgG or IgM	+	3
Lupus anticoagulant		+	4
Hyperlipidemia		+	3
Arterial hypertension		+	1

(+) indicates a positive test or a positive clinical finding.
Modified from Sciascia S, Sanna G, Murru V, Roccatello D, Khamashta MA, Bertolaccini ML. GAPSS: the Global Anti-Phospholipid Syndrome Score. *Rheumatology (Oxford)*. 2013;52(8):1397–1403. https://doi.org/10.1093/rheumatology/kes388. Epub 2013 Jan 12. PMID: 23315788.

TABLE 6 Revised Sapporo classification criteria for antiphospholipid syndrome.

Criteria	Definition	Comment
Laboratory	Two positive tests, at least 12 weeks apart	
Lupus anticoagulant	Prolonged PL-dependent coagulation test: aPTT, dRVVT recommended	Failure to correct on mixing with normal platelet-poor plasma and correction with adding excess PL
Anticardiolipin IgG, IgM	≥40 MPL or GPL units	aβ2GPI-dependent ELISA
Anti-β2 glycoprotein I IgM, IgG	≥99th percentile	Standard aβ2GPI ELISA
Clinical: Vascular		
Thrombosis:	Any tissue or organ	Confirmed by imaging, ultrasound, or histopathology No significant inflammation in vessel wall
Arterial	≥1 arterial thrombosis	
Venous	≥1 venous thrombosis	
Microthrombi	≥1 small vessel thrombosis	
Clinical: Obstetric		
Pregnancy loss:		
Early	≥3 preembryonic or embryonic loss <10 weeks	Consecutive Anatomic, hormonal, and chromosomal abnormalities excluded
Late	≥1 fetal death ≥10 weeks	Normal morphology
Pregnancy morbidity:	≥ premature birth ≤34 weeks due to eclampsia, severe preeclampsia, or severe placental insufficiency	

Modified from Sammaritano LR. Antiphospholipid syndrome. *Best Pract Res Clin Rheumatol.* 2020;34(1):101463. https://doi.org/10.1016/j.berh.2019.101463. Epub 2019 Dec 19. PMID: 31866276, and other sources.

Laboratory investigation of infertility

The laboratory support for the investigation and management of infertility is by providing appropriate test menu and turnaround time. For example, βhCG (start in an emergency presentation with abdominal pain) and urgent estradiol (E2) when supporting in vitro fertilization and stimulation programs. Other primary tests in the investigation of infertility include follicle stimulating hormone (FSH), luteinizing hormone (LH), prolactin, and thyrotropin (TSH), testosterone and sex hormone binding globulin (SHBG) among others and are discussed in detail in their relevant sections. The investigation of infertility in male and female patients is different (see later).

A stepwise approach to biochemical investigation of infertility is preferred. Initially, a male patient with normal semen analysis (viability and mobility) outcomes indicates that no endocrine investigation is required. Similarly, no additional biochemical testing is required in a female patient with normal menses and a normal mid-luteal progesterone level.

Secondary biochemical testing for infertility in the male patient suspected of hypogonadism include measurement of FSH, LH, PRL, and testosterone. The findings of an elevated FSH levels in the presence of low or low-normal testosterone levels indicate primary testicular dysfunction.

The findings of a low low-normal testosterone in the presence of inappropriately low low-normal gonadotrophins suggest secondary hypopituitary cause or a tertiary hypothalamic cause.

The finding of hyperprolactinemia is indicative of either prolactinoma or secondary to stalk compression (obstruction of dopamine flow) as a cause for the infertility or hypothyroidism. The latter is confirmed by finding an elevated TSH in the presence of low free thyroid hormones.

When investigating female infertility, the finding of an appropriately elevated luteal phase progesterone in the presence of regular menses indicates ovulatory cycle. Profile of circulating maternal hormones during follicular, ovulatory, and luteal phase of menstrual cycle is shown in Fig. 3.

Samples for progesterone measurement have to be collected at mid-cycle (day 21); some laboratories collect samples at day 20, 21, and 22 for average values. This is however impractical for most.

In patients with amenorrhea, measurements of human chorionic gonadotrophin (βhCG) confirm pregnancy as the most common cause for amenorrhea. Measurements of gonadotrophins (FSH and LH) and of prolactin and of estradiol are performed. The finding of elevated gonadotrophins in the presence of low estradiol suggests primary gonadal dysfunction, whereas the finding of an inappropriately low gonadotrophins in the presence of low estradiol suggests secondary causes of hypothalamic-pituitary dysfunction.

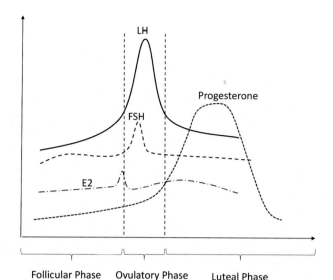

Follicular Phase   Ovulatory Phase   Luteal Phase

FIG. 3 Profile of circulating maternal hormones during follicular, ovulatory, and luteal phase of menstrual cycle. *(Modified from Baker FC, Driver HS. Circadian rhythms, sleep, and the menstrual cycle. Sleep Med. 2007;8(6):613–622. https://doi.org/10.1016/j.sleep.2006.09.011. Epub 2007 Mar 26. PMID: 17383933.)*

Discordant LH and FSH elevation with marked LH elevated levels is suggestive of polycystic ovary. Similarly, the finding of elevated FSH is indicative of gonadal failure and the menopause.

FSH is produced in a pulsatile fashion, whereas in the premenopausal period, a change in the frequency as well as the amplitude of the FSH peaks, and this is often difficult to identify clinically as it requires frequent sampling, an FSH value greater than 30 U/L is suggestive of ovarian failure and the menopause (FSH >30 IU/L and E2 <200 pmol/L (54.5 ng/L) suggests primary ovarian failure), LH >15 IU/L and normal FSH suggests polycystic ovary syndrome. Measurement of estradiol is not helpful in this case.

Hyperprolactinemia leads to infertility by suppressing gonadal androgens. Hyperprolactinemia can be due to pituitary tumor (prolactinoma) or secondary to stalk compression by a space occupying lesion restricting dopamine flow to the lactotrophs. Very high level of prolactin is often suggestive of an adenoma, whereas moderately elevated levels are seen in patients with stalk compression.

Prolactin is also elevated in hypothyroidism and in patient with renal dysfunction which can be investigated by measuring TSH and creatinine respectively. Physiological causes of hyperprolactinemia need to be ruled out such as stress where a repeat measurement yields a near normal level. False hyperprolactinemia due to macroprolactin is investigated following sample treatment with polyethylene glycol.

The presence of hirsutism in patient being investigated for infertility suggests imbalance between androgens and estrogens. This can be due to gonadal tumors, abnormal steroidogenesis due to genetic disorders, malignancy, and/or medication. Patients with late onset congenital adrenal hyperplasia present with hirsutism. The finding of an elevated 17-hydroxy progesterone is suggestive of the disorder. The following biochemical tests are performed; hCG, FSH, LH, PRL, E2, testosterone, SHBG, 17-OH-Progesterone.

Laboratory support for in vitro fertility units includes availability of appropriate and timely test menu. Estradiol is used to monitor treatment efficacy and avoiding hyperstimulation syndrome. LH Follicular growth and oocyte maturation. A rapid (within 2–4 h) estradiol measurement is required for support of IVF unit.

Investigation of amenorrhea

Baseline biochemical investigations which may be helpful include measurement of circulating follicle stimulating hormone (FSH), luteinizing hormone (LH), prolactin (PRL), thyroid-stimulating hormone and free thyroxine (TSH, FT4), estradiol, and progesterone. Testosterone, sex hormone binding globulin (SHBG), androstenedione, dehydroepiandrosterone sulfate (DHEAS), 17α-hydroxyprogesterone are added in the presence signs of androgen excess.

Lack of sexual maturation in a 12–13 years old girl may be simple delayed puberty but physical examination or karyotype may point to Turner's syndrome.

Anosmia may be indicative of isolated gonadotrophin deficiency. A GnRH test may be helpful in cases of delayed puberty where a high LH:FSH ratio in response to the challenge indicates imminent puberty.

Although hyperprolactinemia can be associated with amenorrhea, care should be exercised in interpreting these results as many exogenous factors may contribute to increased prolactin secretion. The mechanism whereby prolactin induces amenorrhea is thought to be by a short feedback loop to the hypothalamus inhibiting gonadotrophin secretion.

In patients suspected with anorexia nervosa, GnRH challenge test shows a prepubertal pattern gradually reverting to postpubertal on increasing weight loss.

Clomiphene citrate challenge is used to stimulate the estrogen secretion by the ovary and thus to assess ovarian reserve.

Many women may be cycling regularly but have difficulty in conceiving, and among those, male problems will exclude 50% of the patients. If the patient is menstruating regularly, a serum progesterone level around 21 days from the start of the last period will help in deciding whether she is ovulating. A level in excess of 30 nmol/L (950 ng/dL) may be suggestive of ovulation.

An unruptured follicle will also luteinize to produce an increase in progesterone synthesis. Mechanical problems, e.g., nonpatent fallopian tubes, may be the cause of the infertility. These require surgical intervention.

Primary amenorrhea

Causes of primary amenorrhea are usually genetic or anatomical in nature. However, causes of secondary amenorrhea (see below) may also present as primary.

Common causes and their frequency include: gonadal dysgenesis (turner syndrome) (43%), Mullerian agenesis (15%), acute and chronic illness (14%), polycystic ovary syndrome (7%), delayed puppetry and isolated gonadotrophin-releasing hormone deficiency (5%), and weight loss (anorexia nervosa) (2%).

Secondary amenorrhea

Causes of secondary amenorrhea include pregnancy (the most common cause), in primary ovarian failure, menopause physiological, premature ovarian failure (as for primary amenorrhea), in hypogonadotrophic hypogonadism (as for primary amenorrhea), vascular (Sheehan's Syndrome), pituitary surgery, in excess sex steroid production, polycystic ovarian disease, congenital adrenal hyperplasia, virilizing tumors, androgen administration, e.g., anabolic steroids, and estrogen producing tumors.

Female infertility

Female patients with regular menses may only require progesterone measurement to assess ovulatory cycle.

Pregnancy is the most common cause of suspected infertility, measurement of serum or urinary hCG confirm pregnancy. Blood measurement is more sensitive where elevated levels are detected at 1–2 weeks post conception, whereas for urine hCG to be detected levels have to exceed 25 IU/L which is often at 4–6 weeks of gestation. Furthermore, the detection I urine is governed by the urine concentration, an early morning urine sample provide the best sample option.

Measurements of hCG, FSH, LH, prolactin, and estradiol will often identify the cause. FSH levels >30 IU/L and E2 below 200 pmol/L (58 ng/mL) are indicative of primary ovarian failure,

Among patients with regular menses, almost all are ovulatory, however only 60% of patients with hyperandrogenism and regular cycles are ovulatory. Therefore, confirmation of ovulatory cycle is required. This is done by measuring mid-luteal phase progesterone. Levels >30 nmol/L confirm an ovulatory cycle; however, lower levels may also be seen in ovulatory cycles and that a single measurement of >−15.9 nmol/L has a sensitivity of 89.6% and a specificity of 98.4% for predicting ovulation.

Other biochemical investigation in women, are FSH, LH, SHBG, testosterone, free testosterone, prolactin, follicular phase 17-hydroxy progesterone, and serum anti-Mullerian hormone.

Progesterone >30 nmol/L collected during mid-luteal phase (days 20–21) indicates adequate ovulatory cycle, and low levels are suggestive of deficient luteal phase. In patients with oligomenorrhea, elevated FSH (above 30 IU/L) suggests ovarian failure. Although elevated LH level relative to FSH are observed in patients with polycystic syndrome, radiological examinations (ultrasound) often confirm the clinical suspicion. Normal TSH levels rules out hypothyroidism as a cause of infertility (Fig. 4).

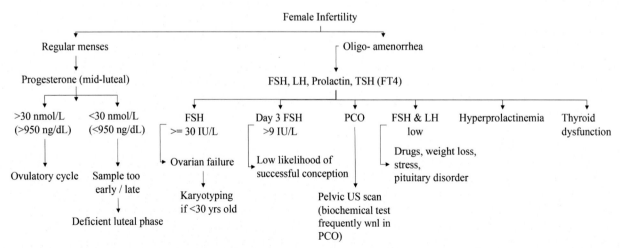

FIG. 4 Flow diagram in the investigation of female infertility. *PCO*, polycystic ovary syndrome. *(Modified from Thurston L, Abbara A, Dhillo WS. Investigation and management of subfertility. J Clin Pathol. 2019;72(9):579–587. https://doi.org/10.1136/jclinpath-2018-205579. Epub 2019 Jul 11. PMID: 31296604.)*

Progesterone

Progesterone is a C21 compound with 315 Da molecular weight. It is produced by a stimulated corpus luteum in a viable pregnancy. There is little change in progesterone levels during the first 8–10 weeks of gestation with levels declining with failing pregnancy. A single measurement showing a value >79.5 nmol/L (>2500 ng/dL) excludes ectopic pregnancy with 97.5% sensitivity. Progesterone levels <15.9 nmol/L (<500 ng/dL) indicate nonviable pregnancy with 100% sensitivity.

Progesterone day 19–24 (median day 21) levels can be used as indicator of ovulation status. Values <10 nmol/L (<314 ng/dL) suggest anovulatory cycle, values 10–30 nmol/L (315–950 ng/dL) suggest deficient luteal phase, whereas values >30 nmol/L (>950 ng/dL) suggest ovulatory cycle. The progesterone values are wise and are method dependent.

Anti-Mullerian hormone (AMH)

Anti-Mullerian hormone, a glycoprotein, is produced by the granulosa cells of the small growing ovarian follicles.

Its circulating level is a reflection of ovarian reserve and is often measured to that regard. Additionally, as its concentration do not vary during the menstrual cycle it is preferred over FSH in the assessment of follicular protentional in response to ovarian stimulation.

Prolactin

Prolactin is produced by the pituitary lactotrophs. The hormone is synthesis and release is under negative feedback inhibition by dopamine. The monomeric form has a molecular weight of 23,000 Da. It exhibits molecular heterogeneity (monomeric, dimeric, and large aggregates often to antiprolactin antibody). The latter often termed macroprolactin. The molecular heterogeneity affects immunoassays to variable degree.

Mild elevation in prolactin levels can be due to stress (phlebotomy, hospital, and clinic environment), and mildly elevated levels need to be confirmed by repeat testing. Markedly elevated prolactin >2000 mIU/L (>77 ng/mL) is often indicative of microadenoma and/or stalk compression, whereas values above >4000 mIU/L (>154 ng/mL) are suggestive of a macroadenoma (Table 7). Of analytical importance is the possibility of macroprolactin. This causes falsely elevated levels in most immunoassay analyzers. Repeat sample analysis is following polyethylene glycol (PEG) precipitation.

Inhibin

A glycoprotein produced by the growing follicles. It is a dimer of a common alpha subunit and specific beta subunit. Two different beta subunits are present β-A and β-B. In the

TABLE 7 Possible causes of hyperprolactinemia as suggested by the degree of prolactin elevation.

Circulating prolactin levels	Pathology	Physiological causes
>700 mIU/L (>27 ng/mL)	Hyperprolactinemia	Psychological stress Repeat measurement. Initial falsely high levels may be associated with stress. Drugs (e.g., neuroleptics) Macroprolactin
700–4000 mIU/L (27–154 ng/mL)	Microadenoma Primary hypothyroidism Renal impairment Polycystic ovary syndrome Drug therapy	Pregnancy/lactation Hypothalamic stalk compression
>4000 mIU/L (>154 ng/mL)	Macroadenoma	Pregnancy/lactation

Modified from Cortet-Rudelli C, Sapin R, Bonneville JF, Brue T. Etiological diagnosis of hyperprolactinemia. *Ann Endocrinol (Paris)*. 2007;68(2–3):98–105. https://doi.org/10.1016/j.ando.2007.03.013. Epub 2007 May 23. PMID: 17524347.

dimeric inhibin A, it comprises an α-subunit and β-A subunit, whereas inhibin B comprises an α-subunit and a β-B subunit.

In the luteal phase, inhibin A inhibits FSH secretion. The level of inhibin A then declines as the corpus luteum involutes.

Inhibin A exhibits paracrine activity promoting follicle growth, and that elevated levels of inhibin A as well as estradiol are reraised from the dominant developing follicle. It is measured as part of the fetal risk assessment screens (see above).

Investigation for polycystic ovary syndrome and congenital adrenal hyperplasia

Anovulatory women, a common cause of pregnancy, is eliminated first (pregnancy test), elevated LH (secondary to increased GnRH pulsatility) is suggestive of polycystic ovary syndrome (PCOS). Raised androgens suggest possible PCOs or congenital adrenal hyperplasia (CAH). In patients with hyperprolactinemia, LH is reduced secondary to reduced GnRH pulsatility, and reduced estradiol.

17-Hydrozxyprogesterone is measured in patients suspected of late onset congenital adrenal hyperplasia. 17-OH progesterone is measured during follicular phase should be assessed in women with hyperandrogenisms. Short synacthen test may be required to improve the diagnostic sensitivity of 17-hydroxytprogesterone.

Estradiol

Although immunoassay-based methods for the measurement of estradiol are widely available, they suffer from few limitations. For instance, the assays are not reliable for estradiol concentrations <300 pmol/L (<81.3 pg/mL). The assay is also not reliable in pregnancy due to interference by elevated endogenous sex hormone binding globulin (SHBG) which compromises the steroid antibody reaction in some assays. Subjecting the sample to solvent extraction prior to measurement by immunoassay has been suggested at least in samples from pregnant patients.

Hirsutism

Patients are presenting with hirsutism which is prepubertal and pubertal excessive hair growth distributed in sexual areas (not general body hair growth which may be due to racial genetic factors (hypertrichosis). In addition to measurement of gonadotrophins, hCG and gonadal hormones (testosterone, and E2). The presence of late onset congenital adrenal hyperplasia needs to be ruled out by measuring 17-OH progesterone. Measuring 17-hydroxy-progesterone following ACTH stimulation improves the diagnostic sensitivity of 17-hydroxy-progesterone.

Hirsutism is due to increased free testosterone in epidermal tissue. The balance between free and bound testosterone and SHBG binding is helpful in the investigation.

Testosterone

Testosterone is measured either as total testosterone (free plus bound testosterone) or that free testosterone fraction is directly measured or following equilibrium dialysis. Direct measurement of free testosterone is inaccurate in female sera due to interference by SHBG. Prior sample treatment by solvent extraction reduces the interference.

Sex hormone binding globulin (SHBG)

Sex hormone binding globulin (SHBG) has a molecular weight of 80,000 Da. It binds testosterone, estradiol among other steroid hormones and in addition to facilitating transport, it also acts as a storage pool for those hormones. It is thus measured in the estimation of free hormones (testosterone) and the calculation of the free androgen index.

Its production is regulated by balance between circulating androgens and estrogens, thyroid hormones, insulin, and dietary factors. Its level is increased in hyperthyroidism, hypogonadism, androgen insensitivity, hepatic cirrhosis in men, hyperprolactinemia, drug therapy.

SHBG levels are affected by steroids (causes SHBG elevation), conditions of protein losing enteropathies (nephrotic syndrome, gastrointestinal dysfunction), and reduced synthesis by hepatocytes due to chronic liver disease.

Menopause

The menopause represents a state of ovarian depletion of oocytes. Physiologically, at 20 weeks of gestation, the female fetus ovary contains about 7 million oocytes, decreasing to 1 million at birth and to about 200,000 oocytes by end of puppetry and only about 350 follicles ovulate during reproductive years.

Most women will experience menopause between the ages of 45 and 55 with only 1% undergoing menopause before the age of 40 (premature). Premature ovarian failure associated with genetic predisposition (fragile X syndrome), obesity, dieting, excessive exercise, fibrosis, and endometriosis. It is also a high risk for osteoporosis and bone fracture.

Estrogens are essential in maintenance of lipid and glucose homoeostasis. They also promote protein synthesis; similarly, progesterone promotes synthesis of proteins supporting the uterus, ovary, mammary gland and brain function. Decline in estrogen and progesterone with elevated somatropins (FSH and LH) are signatures of the disorder. Prior to the absolute decline and deficiency of the steroids, there are observed changes in their circadian and cyclical rhymes.

FSH levels >25 IU/L on two occasions, 4 weeks apart indicates premature ovarian insufficiency. The causes include autoimmune, Cushing' syndrome although rare cause of menstrual disturbances, overt thyroid dysfunction leads to menstrual and ovulatory disturbances and infertility.

Ovarian reserve capacity refers to number of oocytes remaining within the ovaries and is a measure of fertility potential. Routine measurement is not advocated as they do not predict fertility related time to conception, time to menopause and thus measurement as part of health screen is not recommended.

Serum anti-Mullerian hormone is a useful marker of ovarian reserve and levels correlate with total antral follicle count. AMH levels <5.4 pmol/L predicts for a low response during IVF treatment and >25 pmol/L predicts a high response. Serum AMH levels are also increased in polycystic ovary syndrome (PCOS).

FSH levels >89.9 IU/L during early follicular phase is reflective of reduced ovarian reserves, although it is a relatively late feature.

Microbiological investigations for chlamydia, trichomonas, and gonorrhea are frequent causes of tubal subfertility.

Use of appropriate reference intervals for laboratory test at the menopause is sparse. In addition to the expected changes in steroid hormones and associated pituitary glycohormones, menopausal women exhibit higher HDL cholesterol, lower creatinine, glucose, uric acid, urea, alkaline phosphatase, aspartate aminotransferase, creatine kinase, and gamma glutamyl transferase. Laboratory support for the hormonal replacement therapy in the menopause includes measurement of FSH and LH.

Male infertility investigation

Semen analysis should be performed at least after 2–5 days of sexual abstinence, due to the high variability in results; usually, two samples are required to confirm an abnormal result.

With a mild abnormal result repeated 12 weeks to allow for cycles of spermatogenesis, whereas fewer abnormality (azoospermia) the test is repeated sooner.

No endocrine testing is required in a male patient with normal sperm analysis (count, motility, and viability) testing.

In patients with leukocytospermia, urine microscopy and culture are performed. Similarly, postejaculation semen samples should be assessed for retrograde ejaculation.

Normal semen analysis is those of semen volume ≥ 1.5 mL, pH ≥ 7.2, sperm counts ≥ 15 million spermatozoa per mL, with $\geq 40\%$ being motile, $\geq 58\%$ live spermatozoa, and $\geq 4\%$ normal morphology.

Patients with oligospermia (<15 million), severe oligospermia (<5 million), and azoospermia (no sperm) require endocrine investigation by measuring FSH and LH and 10 a.m. fasting testosterone levels. For levels <5 million, chromosomal analysis for Y microdeletions is performed.

Antisperm antibodies are assessed in samples of azoospermia (low motility <40%). Other biochemical investigations include SHBG, albumin, iron studies for hemochromatosis.

In patients with evidence for hypogonadism, measurement of LH, FSH, prolactin, and testosterone is required.

Hyperprolactinemia causes infertility by suppressing gonadotrophins. The finding of hyperprolactinemia may be primary to a prolactinoma, secondary to stalk compression (preventing dopamine from reaching and inhibiting the pituitary lactotrophs), or due to hypothyroidism or renal dysfunction.

The finding of elevated FSH in the presence of low or low normal testosterone levels suggests primary testicular failure. Similarly, when both testosterone levels are low with relatively low or low normal gonadotrophins (FSH/LH), it suggests the presence of hypothalamic-pituitary disease (Fig. 5).

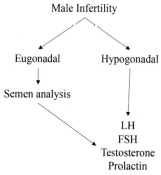

FIG. 5 Flow diagram for the investigation of male infertility. In eugonadal male, only semen analysis is required. Hormonal measurements are not required expect in clinically suspicious for hypogonadal states. *(Modified from Thurston L, Abbara A, Dhillo WS. Investigation and management of subfertility. J Clin Pathol. 2019;72(9):579–587. https://doi.org/10.1136/jclinpath-2018-205579. Epub 2019 Jul 11. PMID: 31296604.)*

Malignancy

Malignancy complicating pregnancy is fortunately rare affecting 1 in 1000–1500 pregnancies. Diagnosis and management require multispecialty support with the clinical laboratory playing a central role. Reference intervals for laboratory analytes are different in pregnancy and influences both tumor-associated and tumor-derived biomarkers. For instance, hemoglobin and hematocrit are physiologically lower (but low values in malignancy carry a poor outcomes), alkaline phosphatase physiologically higher due to placenta sources (elevated in metastatic liver disease), and lactate dehydrogenase physiologically higher (elevated in hematological malignancies and levels correlate with tumor burden). Similarly circulating albumin level are physiologically; lower in pregnancy secondary to volume overload, is reduced in malignancy as part of the cachexia and low level is associated with poor outcome in malignancy.

Tumor-derived markers such as CA125 is elevated in with wide variation during the first trimester before returning to normal range by the second and third trimester. Rising again immediately prior to delivery.

hCG is markedly elevated during pregnancy, similarly AFP is elevated. In contrast, CEA and CA19-9 levels are not affected by pregnancy.

Fetomaternal biochemistry

This section describes the role of the clinical chemistry laboratory in the assessment of fetal and neonatal health.

Fetal risk assessment for aneuploidy

The clinical laboratory plays a role in the assessment of risk for fetal aneuploidy via measurement of circulating markers of risk in maternal serum. With the advent of cell free DNA and noninvasive prenatal testing, some of the biochemical testing is becoming less widely used. To this effect, they are summarized below.

Maternal serum biomarkers

Maternal serum is used for screening purpose, and those positive findings are confirmed by radiological examinations or by amniocentesis amniotic fluid collection and analysis.

The abnormalities screened include neural tubular defects, Down's syndrome, and Trisomy 18. The maternal biomarkers commonly used to assess risk for the above disorders are alpha-fetoprotein (AFP), human chorionic gonadotrophin-beta (βhCG), unconjugated estratriol (uE3), and dimeric inhibin A (DIA), and pregnancy associated plasma protein-A (PAPP-A).

AFP is elevated in Anencephaly, Congenital nephrosis, Cystic hygroma (common in Turner's syndrome), Duodenal atresia, Encephalocele, Esophageal atresia, Fetal blood contamination, fetal demise, Gastroschisis, Hydrocephalus, Meckel's syndrome, Meningomyelocele (open spina bifida), Necrosis of fetal liver secondary to herpesvirus infection, Normal pregnancy, Nuchal bleb, Omphalocele, Rh isoimmune disease, Sacrococcygeal teratoma, Spontaneous or impending abortion, Trisomy 13, Twins and other multiple gestations, Underestimated gestational age.

Reduced AFP levels are seen in Down's syndrome, fetal demise, Molar pregnancy, Normal pregnancy, Overestimated gestational age, Pseudocyesis (imaginary pregnancy), Spontaneous abortion, and Trisomy 18. Screening is either performed during the second trimester or combined at the first and second trimester (Tables 8 and 9) (Figs. 6–8).

AFP, uE3, and PAPP-A are decreased in patient carrier of a Down's syndrome infant, whereas hCG and dimeric inhibin-A are elevated. The markers are variable for the other commonly tested for aneuploidy (trisomy 13 and 18).

AFP increases with gestational age and is higher in black patients. A correction factor is applied for insulin-dependent (IDDM) diabetics but does not include gestational diabetes mellitus. Multiples of the median (MoM)'s values decrease with increasing maternal age and MoM's are increased in patients with twin pregnancies (but not doubled).

Confirmatory testing for screen positive cases for fetal anomalies

Positive screen for neural tubular defects used to be confirmed by measurement of amniotic fluid AFP and or acetylcholinesterase levels. Advancement in imaging technique and the associated risk with amniocentesis, this is no longer offered for neural tubular defects.

TABLE 8 The different screening modalities, trimester and tests included, single assessment and combined trimester screens.

Test modality	Biomarkers	Trimester
Dual	AFP + tot. hCG	Second
Triple	AFP + tot. hCG + uE3	Second
Quadruple (QUAD)	AFP + tot., βhCG + uE3 + DIA	Second
Combined	NT + PAPP-A + free βhCG	First
Integrated serum	PAPP-A + QUAD	First (PAPP-A) and Second (QUAD)
Integrated-NT	NT + PAPP-A + QUAD	First (NT + PAPP-A) and Second (QUAD)

AFP, alpha-fetoprotein; *DIA*, dimeric inhibin-A; *MA*, maternal age; *NT*, nucltraslucency; *PAPP-A*, pregnancy associated plasma protein-A; *Total hCG*, total human chorionic gonadotropin; *uE3*, unconjugated estratriol. Modified from Wald NJ, Rodeck C, Hackshaw AK, Walters J, Chitty L, Mackinson AM. First and second trimester antenatal screening for Down's syndrome: the results of the Serum, Urine and Ultrasound Screening Study (SURUSS). *J Med Screen.* 2003;10(2):56–104. https://doi.org/10.1258/096914103321824133. Erratum in: *J Med Screen.* 2006;13(1):51–52. PMID: 14746340.

Karyotyping of chromosomes from cells in amniotic fluid or chorionic villus samples is performed to confirm positive screens for 13, 18, and 21 aneuploidies.

Reporting and risk calculation

Fetal risk assessment report includes concentration of analyte, calculation of the multiples of the median (MoM), estimated risk of disease if abnormal.

The calculated for risk assessment is influenced by and corrected for IDDM, the presence of twins, and age.

The following priory risks are noted; Family history for; Open neural tube defect, first-degree relative (parent, sibling) 26.7, second-degree relative (aunt, uncle, niece, nephew) 3.7, third-degree relative (first cousin) 1.4, parent with scoliosis 5, sibling with hydrocephalus 20, sibling with tracheoesophageal fistula or cleft lip/palate 3, sibling with exstrophy of bladder 6, sibling with diaphragmatic hernia 8, sibling with renal agenesis 4. Maternal factors are: insulin-requiring diabetes mellitus 4, and valproate therapy 20.

Cell-free DNA

About 10% of circulating cell free DNA in maternal serum is placental in origin and can be used as a proxy for the fetus. Testing often performed much earlier at 10-week gestation compared to the conventional maternal biomarkers.

TABLE 9 Clinical and biochemical makers applied in screening for fetal anomalies.

Test/parameter	False positive rate (%)	DSDR (%)
Maternal age (at delivery) ≥35 years	5	20
AFP	5	21
Second trimester screening		
MA+AFP	5	36
MA+AFP+Total hCG	5	62
MA+AFP+Total hCG+uE3	5	58 (66)
MA+AFP+βhCG+uE3	5	52
MA+AFP+Total hCG+uE3+DIA	5	75
First trimester screen		
NT+PAPP-A+βhCG	5	85
Integrated screen (first and second trimester screens combined)		
(NT+PAPP-A)+(AFP+Total hCG+uE3+DIA)	5	94

AFP, alpha-fetoprotein; *DIA*, dimeric inhibin-A; *DSDR*, Down's syndrome detection rate; *MA*, maternal age; *NT*, nucltraslucency; *PAPP-A*, pregnancy associated plasma protein-A; *Total hCG*, total human chorionic gonadotropin; *uE3*, unconjugated estratriol.
Modified from; Knight GJ, Palomaki GE, Neveux LM, Fodor KK, Haddow JE. hCG and the free beta-subunit as screening tests for Down syndrome. *Prenat Diagn.* 1998;18(3):235–245. PMID: 9556040. Haddow JE, Palomaki GE, Knight GJ, Foster DL, Neveux LM. Second trimester screening for Down's syndrome using maternal serum dimeric inhibin A. *J Med Screen.* 1998;5(3):115–119. https://doi.org/10.1136/jms.5.3.115. PMID: 9795869.

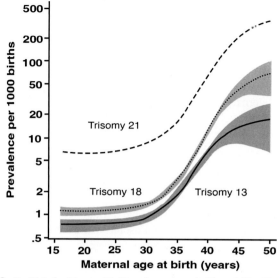

FIG. 7 Risk for trisomy 21 (Down's syndrome), 18, and 13 with maternal age. *(Modified from Savva GM, Walker K, Morris JK. The maternal age-specific live birth prevalence of trisomies 13 and 18 compared to trisomy 21 (Down syndrome). Prenat Diagn. 2010;30:57–64. https://doi. org/10.1002/pd.2403.)*

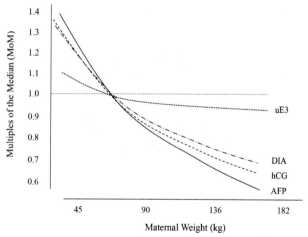

FIG. 8 Impact of maternal weight on the calculated multiple of the median (MoM). *(Modified from Reynolds TM, Vranken G, Van Nueten J. Weight correction of MoM values: which method? J Clin Pathol. 2006;59(7):753–758. https://doi.org/10.1136/jcp.2005.034280. Epub 2006 Apr 7. PMID: 16603647; PMCID: PMC1860422.)*

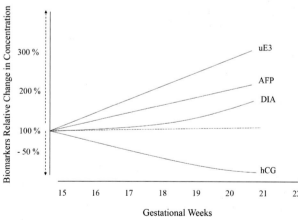

FIG. 6 Relative values of aneuploidy risk biomarkers in maternal serum with time *(AFP, alpha-fetoprotein; DIA, dimeric inhibin A; hCG, human chorionic gonadotropin; uE3, unconjugated estratriol). (Modified from Shaw SW, Lin SY, Lin CH, et al. Second-trimester maternal serum quadruple test for Down syndrome screening: a Taiwanese population-based study. Taiwan J Obstet Gynecol. 2010;49(1):30–34. https://doi. org/10.1016/S1028-4559(10)60005-8. PMID: 20466289.)*

Assessing the relative genomic contribution of chromosomes 13, 18, 21 in relation to other autosomes suggesting a high chance of a trisomy and is the basis of identifying aneuploidy for the three common abnormalities. As a consequence of the improved performance (compared to the traditional biomarkers in maternal serum), the additional to reduction in false detection rate is the reduction in invasive confirmatory amniocentesis performed (Table 9).

Where some healthcare systems have adopted a switch from biomarkers to noninvasive prenatal testing (NIPT), others adopted a more transitional process were patient identified at high risk (i.e., $\geq 1:150$) based on the biomarkers are offered NIPT. The cost benefit of the two approaches are not yet known.

Maternal plasma collected by centrifugation (whole blood collected in lithium heparin anticoagulated sample). DNA is extracted using DNA extraction reagents/columns. Sequencing, amplification, reads and comparison with sequencing libraries are applied. A sample-specific-derived normalized chromosome value of greater than 4 is considered significant for the aneuploidy (13, 18, or 21). Some healthcare systems will assess the normalized chromosome value (NCV) for the X-chromosome when there is clinical suspicion for Turner's syndrome or there is consent for provision of gender.

Biochemical aspects of neonatology

Immediately following delivery, the clinical laboratory participates in the care of the neonate. The clinical biochemistry support extends to the newborn where few common physio-pathological disorders are encountered and are discussed below. For instance, appropriate precautious of samples volume and quality, availability of relevant test menu, and the application of appropriate test reference intervals, cord blood gases in the assessment of hypoxia during delivery, electrolytes, and intermediary metabolites in the assessment of organ prematurity, among others.

Assessment of newborn

A neonate is an infant less than 28 days old with day of birth being day 1 of age. Preterm (premature) newborn with gestational age of 36 weeks and 6 days or less. Low birth weight is birth weight less than 2500 g, very low birth weight is less than 1500 g.

A normal newborn of uncomplicated pregnancy often does not require more than a heal prick blood sample 4–5 days of life for the routine newborn blood screening programs (often in force in many countries).

Preanalytical factors

Neonates may undergo multiple laboratory testing and thus requires a relatively (to body weight) large amount of blood volume. Total blood volume of neonate is about 275 mL. A premature weighing less than 1 kg will have total blood volume of about 80 mL.

Therefore, frequent blood withdraw for laboratory testing can render the neonate anemia. Laboratories should employ instruments that use small volume of blood sample, perform most of the prioritized test on less than 500–600 µL, facilitate point of care testing, and limit test to essential biochemical tests. Provision of appropriate test menu, turnaround and results reported with appropriate age stratified reference intervals.

Care should be taken to minimize risk of infection and trauma and to avoid repeated collections because of an inadequate or hemolyzed poor quality sample. Hemolyzed sample renders unsuitable for potassium, AST, magnesium, zinc, LDH, etc. measurements, and that markedly hemolyzed sample is unsuitable for bilirubin measurement essential in the investigation of neonatal hyperbilirubinemia. The finding of significant direct bilirubinemia is indicative of biliary atresia that requires immediate medical and surgical intervention. The use of assays that are tolerant of hemolysis. An example being measurement of direct bilirubin. The widely used diazo chemical method is more prone to interference by hemolysis, whereas the vanadate method can tolerate hemolysis up to a 1000 level allowing reporting of important direct bilirubin result (see later).

Capillary blood sample collection

During early life, most biochemical tests are performed using blood samples obtained by heel prick often collected by trained laboratory phlebotomy personnel care.

Sample quality is important where heel prick may represent more of a tissue extract, and ample is this at high risk of hemolysis given the massaging and heel worming and pressure required.

Urine collections and volume

Urine volume is very low early in life and thus a small loss in time urine collection will lead to significant error. Urine volumes by age are shown in Table 10.

Appropriate reference interval

The growing and developing newborn requires age-related laboratory test reference intervals. The values are likely to alter with age and with maturity.

For instance, in addition to pregnancy-related changes in thyroid hormone function tests and the need for gestational-related reference intervals for TSH discussed above, and there is a similar need in the newborn where circulating TSH levels are markedly elevated immediately at birth and decline within the 6–8 weeks. Similarly, thyroid hormone levels are elevated and decline to adult ranges within 6–8 weeks (Table 11).

Although the direct development of age-related appropriate reference intervals is cumbersome, statistical manipulation of the large laboratory data available in electronic health records are used to establish age and population related reference intervals. Hoffmann's approach and various modifications where cumulative frequency of the laboratory data are calculated following repeated removal of the top

TABLE 10 Age-related urine volumes.

Age	Urine volume
Fetus (feta age)	
20 weeks	4 mL/h
25 weeks	13 mL/h
30 weeks	27 mL/h
35 weeks	39 mL/h
38 weeks	45 mL/h
Newborn	**(mL per 24 h)**
Full term <2 days	15–60
>2 days to <2 months	300
2 months	250–450
6–8 months	400–500
1–2 years	500–600
2–4 years	600–750
5–7 years	650–1000
8–15 years	700–1000
Adult	1200 (female)–1600 (male)

In addition to age, urine volumes vary with gender, diet, exercise, environment, and habits. Neonates produce small urine volumes and thus appropriate sample handling, prioritization of tests, and use of appropriate testing technologies are important aspects of the neonatal care laboratory. Modified from several sources and Valentin J. Basic anatomical and physiological data for use in radiological protection: reference values: ICRP Publication 89: approved by the Commission in September 2001. *Ann ICRP.* 2002;32(3–4):1–277. https://doi.org/10.1016/S0146-6453(03)00002-2.

TABLE 11 TSH and FT4 in the newborn showing gradual change to adult normal values.

Test date	TSH (mIU/L)	FT4 pmol/L (ng/dL)
Day <1	8.04	51.2 (3.9)
Day 9	2.71	35.9 (2.8)
Day 60	1.37	20.5 (1.6)

Appropriate dereference intervals must be applied to avoid misinterpretation and inappropriate management. Modified from the author's laboratory.

and bottom 10–205 (outliers) and the upper and lower limits at the 2.5th and 97.5th percentiles, respectively, determined at the points of line inflection of the cumulative frequency plot (Fig. 9). This mathematical indirect approach avoids the need for blood samples collected from normal neonates for the purpose of establishing laboratory test reference intervals.

Jaundice

About 30%–70% of infants will develop jaundice (plasm bilirubin >80 μmol/L (>4.7 mg/dL)) appearing on the second day of life and usually resolves by day 10 or longer in breast feeding baby. This jaundice is termed physiological jaundice and is predominantly unconjugated. It is a reflection of increased bilirubin load from ineffective erythropoiesis, shortened red blood cell lifespan, deficient glucuronyl

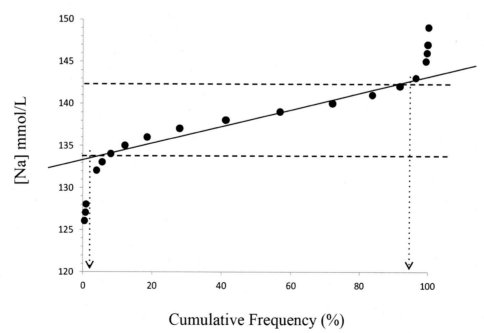

FIG. 9 Cumulative frequency approach for the determination of sodium upper and lower reference intervals. The curve indicates a reference intervals of 134–142 mmol/L for plasms sodium. *(Data obtained from the author's laboratory.)*

transferase (first few days of life), and to increased intestinal absorption due to meconium β-glucuronidase. Exposure to breast milk (pregnanediol, nonesterified fatty acids (NEFA), and other inhibitors of conjugation) leads to physiological jaundice.

Bilirubin is the major metabolite of heme in hemoglobin, myoglobin, and cytochromes. One gram of hemoglobin yields 35 mg/dL (600 μmol/L) of bilirubin.

There are four bilirubin fractions. Unconjugated bilirubin (alpha), mono-conjugated bilirubin (β), di-conjugated bilirubin (γ), and albumin bound bilirubin (δ).

Conjugated and unconjugated bilirubin are metabolized and are removed from plasma mainly by the liver. Therefore, hyperbilirubinemia is a reflection of an imbalance between production and excretion of bilirubin. Hyperbilirubinemia is observed hepatocellular disorders (reduced conjugation), hemolytic diseases (increased production), and cholestasis (decreased removal).

Determining bilirubin fractions (conjugated and unconjugated) helps in the differential diagnosis and in delivery of apocopate therapy and in monitoring response to therapy.

Physiological jaundice is that occurring within few days of birth (peak 3–5 days) and may last up to less than 2 weeks. Total bilirubin does not exceed 5 mg/dL (85.5 μmol/L) (90% unconjugated).

In addition to contribution of breast feeding, neonates at risk of prolonged physiological jaundice are those who are premature, with, hemolysis, polycythemia, meconium retention and intestinal obstruction and infection, dehydration, hypoxia, and hypothyroidism.

Persistent and increasing jaundice after 14 days of life, as well as the presence of early <24 h, total bilirubin >300 μmol/L (>17.5 mg/dL), and of conjugated >25 μmol/L (>1.5 mg/dL) require investigation for possible hepatobiliary abnormalities.

Unconjugated bilirubin crosses the blood brain barrier and at risk of causing kernicterus (chronic bilirubin encephalopathy) if exceeds 340 μmol/L (19.9 mg/dL) or if increasing rapidly at a rate > 8.5 μmol/L/h (>0.5 mg/dL/h). The risk increases in babies >37 weeks' gestation.

Preterm infants are at increased risk of kernicterus because of the hypoalbuminemia and thus reduced amount to bind the unconjugated bilirubin, and that they are more prone to hypoxia which impairs the effectiveness of the blood-brain barrier and the impaired albumin binding in acidosis and hypoxia.

Pathological jaundiced is that hyperbilirubinemia occurring early following birth at least <24 h, and that total bilirubin is >300 μmol/L (>17.5 mg/dL), and there is rapid increase >8.5 μmol/L/h (>0.5 mg/dL/h), and jaundice that is prolonged more than 14 days, and if conjugated bilirubin exceeds 25 μmol/L (1.5 mg/dL) (Table 12).

Measurement of bilirubin

Several methods are available for the measurand and assessment of hyperbilirubinemia. Lack of standardization as well as presence of interfering substances leads to variability among bilirubin results obtained by the different methodologies (see Table 13).

Colorimetric diazo method

The diazo method (described in 1883 by Ehrlich and modified in 1938 by Jendrassik and Grof) are still widely used. Bilirubin reacts with a diazotized (3,5-dichlorophenyl diazonium) reagent formed by the substitution of 2,4 dichloroaniline for sulfanilic acid forming azobilirubin. Absorbance recorded at 660/570 nm. In the total bilirubin method by the diazo method there is no interference by hemolysis up to 1000 mg/dL and lipemia up to an index of 1000.

TABLE 12 Type of bilirubin (bilirubin fraction), its pathophysiology, and laboratory investigation.

Predominant bilirubin type	Condition/disorder	Investigation/pathology
Unconjugated	Breast feeding	Normalize after cessation
	Hypothyroidism	TSH/Free T4
	Crigler-Najjar (I: complete enzyme deficiency, II: partial enzyme deficiency)	Glucuronides in bile, glucuronyl transferase activity
	Gilbert's syndrome	Decreased uptake by hepatocytes
	Sepsis	Decreased uptake by hepatocytes. Blood culture
	Hemolysis (hereditary, acquired), Ineffective erythropoiesis, rapid turnover of increased RBC mass	Hematological indices
	Glucose-6-phosphate dehydrogenase deficiency	RBC glucose-6-phosphate dehydrogenase activity

TABLE 12 Type of bilirubin (bilirubin fraction), its pathophysiology, and laboratory investigation—cont'd

Predominant bilirubin type	Condition/disorder	Investigation/pathology
Conjugated	Biliary atresia	Radiological exam
	Intrahepatic cholestasis	g-GT, total bile acids, genetic tests for familial syndrome
	Rhesus isoimmunization	Hematological indices of hemolysis, reduced haptoglobin
	Alpha-1-antitrypsin deficiency	α-1-antitypsin
	Galactosemia	RBC galactose-1-phosophate uridyl transferase
	Tyrosinemia I	Plasma amino acids analysis. Urine succinyl acetone, Serum AFP elevated
	Dubin-Johnson and Rotor's syndrome	50 direct fraction. In Dubin-Johnson syndrome: Total urinary coproporphyrin excretion is normal but 80% is coproporphyrin I (in normal subjects 75% of urinary porphyrins are coproporphyrin III). In Rotor syndrome: Total urinary coproporphyrins are increased to 250%–500% of normal with approximately 65% being coproporphyrin I.
	Cystic fibrosis	Immunoreactive trypsin, genetic testing
	Total parenteral nutrition	Normalize after stopping
	Hypopituitarism	TSH, FT4, cortisol
	Extra- and intrahepatic obstruction (stones, malignancy, strictures)	Alkaline phosphatase, γ-glutamyl transferase, tumor makers
Mixed conjugated/ unconjugated	Infection	Serology tests and microbiological culture
	Many of the above may experience combined conjugated and unconjugated forms during the disorder	

TABLE 13 Examples of commercially available methods for the measurement of bilirubin fractions.

Methods	Chemic reaction	Bilirubin fraction	Limitations
Chemical-spectrophotometric	Diazo reagent	Direct., conjugated reacts rapidly. The Bc assay measures only conjugated bilirubin using direct spectrophotometry, whereas the direct bilirubin assays measures conjugated bilirubin, delta bilirubin, and some unconjugated bilirubin using the diazo chemical reaction. As a result, Bc levels will usually be lower than the direct bilirubin levels from the same sample.	Overestimates direct fraction as other components also react (delta—albumin bound)
	Indirect	Unconjugated fraction	Requires addition of accelerator (e.g., Na benzoate, caffeine)
Enzymatic	(Bilirubin oxidase)	Bilirubin oxidized to biliverdin.	Little cross-reactivity with delta fraction
Dual spectrophotometric method	Dry slide	Measures both conjugated and unconjugated	

Continued

TABLE 13 Examples of commercially available methods for the measurement of bilirubin fractions—cont'd

Methods	Chemic reaction	Bilirubin fraction	Limitations
Multiwavelength absorbance	Calculates bilirubin concentration	In blood gases instruments using whole blood sample	
Enzymatic	Vanadate oxidase	Total and direct bilirubin	High degree of tolerance for sample hemolysis and lipemia. Helpful in direct bilirubin (in biliary atresia)
Transcutaneous bilirubin methods	Transcutaneous bilirubin concentration	Transmitted light is reflected, and multiple spectrophotometric readings taken and mathematically calculate bilirubin	Mathematical calculation influenced by skin thickness, melanin, and hemoglobin concentration. Used in babies >35 weeks gestation and >24 h of age to identify those at risk of severe hyperbilirubinemia. Values >250 μmol/L (14.6 mg/dL) require confirmation using a laboratory-based method.

Bc, bilirubin conjugated, assay using film technology (ortho clinical disgnostics, CA).
Modified from Ngashangva L, Bachu V, Goswami P. Development of new methods for determination of bilirubin. *J Pharm Biomed Anal.* 2019;162:272–285. https://doi.org/10.1016/j.jpba.2018.09.034. Epub 2018 Sep 18. PMID: 30273817. Rabbani T, Guthery SL, Himes R, Shneider BL, Harpavat S. Newborn screening for biliary atresia: a review of current methods. *Curr Gastroenterol Rep.* 2021;23(12):28. https://doi.org/10.1007/s11894-021-00825-2. PMID: 34817690; PMCID: PMC8651301.

In the direct bilirubin assay, conjugated bilirubin reacts directly with the diazo reagent (thus the designation of conjugated bilirubin as "directly reacting" or "direct" bilirubin). Acidified sodium nitrite produces nitrous acid, which reacts with sulfanilic acid (in acidic solution) to form a diazonium salt. The diazotized sulfanilic acid then reacts with bilirubin to form isomers of azobilirubin. In the direct bilirubin assay, only conjugated bilirubin is converted by the diazotized sulfanilic acid. The intensity of the red color of azobilirubin is measured photometrically and is proportional to the direct (conjugated) bilirubin concentration.

In the direct bilirubin assays, hemolysis (H) index interference at 30 units, which equates to 30 mg/dL (18.6 μmol/L) and lipemia at an index of 100 (there is however poor correlation between the turbidity index "L" and triglycerides concentration).

In a typical automated diazo method, serum/plasma is incubated with diazo reagent at approximately pH 1.7–2.0 to form a diazonium salt. The resulting product then reacts with bilirubin to form isomers of azobilirubin.

In the direct bilirubin assays, conjugated bilirubin is the predominant form converted by the diazotized sulfanilic acid (approximately 5% of unconjugated bilirubin may react as well). The intensity of the red color of azobilirubin is measured photometrically at approximately 600 nm and is proportional to conjugated bilirubin concentration.

Unconjugated bilirubin reacts with diazo reagents following the addition of accelerants (e.g., caffeine, sodium benzoate, or methanol), thus allowing for the determination of the concentration of total sample bilirubin. The difference represents the unconjugated bilirubin fraction.

Measurements allows for the estimation of the concentration of unconjugated bilirubin hence the designation of this difference as "indirect" bilirubin.

The enzymatic vanadate oxidase method

Under acidic condition (pH 2.9), bilirubin is oxidized by vanadate to produce biliverdin. In the presence of a detergent, both conjugated and unconjugated bilirubin moieties are oxidized. The reaction is monitored by recording a decrease in absorbance at 450/546 nm.

For both total and direct bilirubin, there is no interference from either hemolysis up to 1000 mg/dL nor triglycerides up to up to 2000 mg/dL. This is advantageous when measuring direct bilirubin in neonates. In neonates, the capillary samples are often of poor quality and high degree of hemolysis. Thus, in the vanadate method the higher degree of tolerance for hemolysis allows for reliable measurement of direct bilirubin essential for the detection of biliary atresia.

$$\text{Bilirubin} + \text{Surfactant} + \text{VO}^{3-} \rightarrow \text{Biliverdin}$$

Congenital bilirubin abnormalities

Biliary atresia

Biliary atresia is the primary cause of extrahepatic biliary disease in neonates. It affects approximately 1 in 8000–18,0000 live births and account for most of the pediatric liver transplant worldwide. There is no recognized screening program for biliary atresia in place.

Suspected in an increasing and sustained conjugated hyperbilirubinemia and pale stool. Initially latent with visible symptoms develop after the first week of life. Surgical intervention involves the Kasai portoenterostomy which directly connects the intestines to the liver to restore bile flow. A critical factor predicting surgical outcomes is the time at which the operation is performed. Procedures performed before 30–45 days of life (often requiring detection within the preclinical phase) have the greatest chances of delaying or avoiding liver transplant.

The onus is thus on the clinical laboratory identify those patients in timely manner this involves two issues, one is the derivation of age specific reference intervals and second, the use of a reliable bilirubin assays that are not influenced by interferences. Common interference being hemolysis, lipemia, and certain medications.

The nature of sample collection (often a heel prick) has a higher degree of hemolysis compared to venous blood sample. The use of bilirubin methods, e.g., vanadate enzymatic method with higher tolerance for hemolysis, is thus preferred (Table 13).

Patients appear normal at birth, there is hepatomegaly without splenomegaly. Jaundice is not obvious when serum bilirubin levels are below 5 mg/dL and thus do not appear jaundice despite elevate fractionated bilirubin. Secondly, those appearing jaundiced may commonly be due to physiological jaundice or that due to breast feeding, for instance up to 15% of neonates appear jaundiced at 14 days because of breast feeding. There is also interindividual variability in visually defining jaundice, this improves when total bilirubin levels exceed 12 mg/dL.

Obstruction of bile flow to the intestine leads to pale stool. This is often detected using a stool color card. More recently, the availability of phone application using phone camera to compare stool color.

Use of fractionated bilirubin (conjugated and unconjugated) as well as ratio of conjugated bilirubin to total bilirubin ratios not used since ratios ≤0.2 are common among infants at 24–48 h of life.

A two-step screening approach using fraction bilirubin in the neonatal period 24–48 h and at 2 weeks of life had a sensitivity of 100%, specificity of 99.9% and positive predictive value of 5.9%–18.2%. In addition to early detection of biliary atresia, this helped early identification of other liver disorders such as alpha-1-antitrypsin and Alagille syndrome (bile accumulation due to few bile ducts).

Assays for direct (conjugated) bilirubin vary among manufacturers, and thus, each laboratory must derive the appropriate reference intervals for their patient's population. Furthermore, there appear race differences that must be accounted for, for instance a higher positive rate with the initial test at 24–48 h of life in Black infants versus infants

from other races. Thus, infants with elevated initial levels are retested by 2 weeks of life.

Use of bile acids has been advocated but is limited by the availability of reliable methods. Those reliably measuring serum taurocholate and adopting a cut-off of 0.63 μmol/L, and this test had a sensitivity of 79.1% and specificity of 62.5% for biliary atresia.

Although the cost-effectiveness of newborn fractionated bilirubin screening remains unknown, a number of screening program are already in place. For example, infants with initial levels exceeding the laboratory's 97.5th percentile value are considered positive, and a repeat testing is performed by 2 weeks of life. Infants with repeat fractionated bilirubin levels >1 mg/dL are urgently referred for further evaluation. Infants with a normal level, or a level ≤1 mg/dL and less than or equal to the initial level are not evaluated further for biliary atresia. However, in infants with a level greater than the initial level but ≤1 mg/dL in stage 2 undergo repeat testing in 1 week and are referred if the levels do not decline.

In contrast to direct bilirubin and conjugated bilirubin (Bc) levels of unconjugated bilirubin will not vary across sites and a standard reference interval of 0.0–0.2 mg/dL can be used.

It must be stated that conjugated bilirubin (Bc) is not equivalent direct bilirubin as the latter also contains delta bilirubin and thus overestimates conjugated bilirubin. Direct bilirubin levels vary across analyzers, depending on slight variations in reaction conditions such as temperature, pH, and time. Important reasons for identifying the type of assay is that direct bilirubin assays require reference intervals to be derived. Furthermore, the ratios of conjugated bilirubin (Bc) or direct bilirubin to total bilirubin are not used as they may miss many infants with biliary atresia.

Use of age-appropriate reference intervals for bilirubin fractions improve their diagnostic utility. Liver enzymes elevated and pattern difficult to distinguish from neonatal hepatitis. It is very important to make the diagnosis promptly so that surgical correction (hepatoportoenterostomy procedure) best results if performed before 8 weeks of age.

Inherited disorders of bilirubin metabolism

Crigler-Najjar hyperbilirubinemia

A mild form of hyperbilirubinemia with unconjugated bilirubin not exceeding 340 μmol/L (19.9 mg/dL). The disorder is secondary to reduced conjugation enzyme UDP-glucuronyl transferase activity. In type II variant, the activity is reduced whereas in type I, the enzyme activity is completely deficient. Hyperbilirubinemia is significantly reduced by phenobarbital therapy.

Dubin-Johnson and Rotor syndromes

In this disorder, there is benign conjugated hyperbilirubinemia. The liver size and liver enzymes are within normal limits. The extent of jaundice is enhanced by stress, intercurrent illness, and fasting. Analysis of the ABCC2 gene allows for the definitive diagnosis of Dubin-Johnson syndrome.

Other congenital disorders presenting with neonatal jaundice include hypothyroidism and alpha-1-antitrypsin deficiency.

Congenital hypothyroidism

Neonates with congenital hypothyroidism exhibit prolonged neonatal jaundice. Liver dysfunction and hyperbilirubinemia resolves within 6 weeks following imitation of thyroid replacement.

Alpha-1 antitrypsin deficiency

Alpha-1-antitrypsin deficiency expresses either ZZ or SZ phenotypes. The incidence is 1:2000, and there is prolonged neonatal jaundice with variable presentation from mild liver dysfunction resolving over time to rapid progressive liver failure requiring transplant. The presentation is undisguisable from that of biliary atresia.

Enzyme levels are variable as it is an acute phase response protein; however, levels <1.1 g/L during the first week of life are suggestive of possible deficiency. However, phenotyping is required to establish the diagnosis.

Hypoglycemia

The fetus receives maternal glucose supply via the placenta, following birth neonatal glucose drops as low 1.7 mmol/L (30.6 mg/dL) within 1–2 h of life. Glucose levels correct quickly following feeding.

Newborns are susceptible due to low glycogen stores and inadequate supplementation and to increased requirements, and that few newborns develop hypoglycemia defined as plasma glucose <2.5 mmol/L (<45 mg/dL), particularly among premature infants.

It is important to identify neonates at high risk of developing hypoglycemia so that immediate intervention is available.

Neonates at risk of developing hypoglycemia are neonates of mothers with impaired glucose homeostasis, maternal diabetes, and gestational diabetes, on oral hypoglycemic drugs, neonates with identified abnormalities during fetal life (e.g., hydrops fetalis), at birth (prematurity, small for gestational age as they have reduced glycogen reserve at birth and little adipose tissue. This is further exacerbated by increased energy demand in the rapid extrauterine growth period.), polycythemia, hypopituitary, isolated ACTH deficiency, cortisol deficiency secondary to congenital adrenal hyperplasia, or those who suffered perinatal hypoxia/ischemia hypoxia, hypothermia, heart failure.

State of neonatal hyperinsulinism is the primary cause of hypoglycemia in neonates of mothers with gestational diabetes. Hypoglycemia develops as early as 1 h of age and often by 12 h of age. The hypoglycemia is transient and resolves within the first 24–72 h of life.

Hyperinsulinemia is seen in neonates with islet cell hypertrophy (Beckwith-Wiedemann syndrome) in about 30%–50% of casers. The hypoglycemia is often transient and resolves within few days. The condition prevalence is around 1:15,000.

Persistent hyperinsulinemia is when plasma glucose ≤3.0 mmol/L (54 mg/dL) and can only be maintained by continuous glucose infusion at high rate (>10 mg/kg/min). Insulin and c-peptide are elevated without ketonuria. Glucose levels are ≤2.5 mmol/L (45 mg/dL) when measured using blood gases analyzer (glucose method on the blood gas analyses employs glucose-specific glucose oxidase enzyme which is often substituted by the less specific hexokinase on automated laboratory-based chemistry analyzers).

Familial or sporadic congenital hyperinsulinism of infancy with unregulated insulin secretion by pancreatic beta islet cells is encountered and is secondary to defective glucose uptake and phosphorylation (impaired K/ATP channels).

Activating mutation of glutamate dehydrogenase is activated by leucine. Therefore, affected neonates ae likely to develop hypoglycemia prior to and postfeeding. This is often accompanied by hyperammonemia possibly due to increased glutamate dehydrogenase activity and to increased hepatic synthesis. The disorder responds to diazoxide treatment and thus must be ruled out before proceeding to other causes.

Other inedited metabolic causes of neonatal hypoglycemia are glycogen storage disease, fatty acid oxidation defects, galactosemia, and organic acidemias. Biochemical screening followed by confirmatory and additional teste guided by clinical presentation often identifies the disorder.

Neurological manifestation is the mainstay neonatal hypoglycemia, with irritability, sweating, lethargy, poor feeding, hypothermia and hypotonia, apnea, stupor, coma, and seizures.

Hyperglycemia

Hyperglycemia is defined as glucose >8.0 mmol/L (>144 mg/dL). It important to note that glucose concentrations are 10%–15% higher in arterial blood compared to venous, and that capillary samples are somewhat in-between.

Risk factors for hyperglycemia are immaturity, low birth weight for gestational age, sepsis, stress, glucose infusion (>6 mg/kg/min), steroids, intralipid, drugs such as theophylline. Hyperglycemia leads to hypovolemia secondary to hyperglycemic diuresis.

Neonatal diabetes is very rare at 1:300,000–500,000 live births. Insulin levels are low. In addition to hyperglycemia, and ketoacidosis, there is severe dehydration, failure to thrive. Ketoacidosis progresses to coma. It is not an autoimmune disease as in childhood, but rather a consequence of heterogeneous genetic defects impairing pancreatic islet cell development.

Possible causes are increased pancreatic beta cell apoptosis or islet cell dysfunction. Forty to fifty percent of cases persist through life with impaired insulin production in response to hyperglycemia, the other half 50%–60% is transient severe nonketotic hyperglycemia, insulin concentration is low or undetectable. This resolves spontaneously with 50% of cases recurrence during childhood and adolescence.

Electrolytes

Neonates at risk of fluid loss and thus to hypovolemia, electrolytes imbalance. Hyponatremia is common due to renal sodium loss whereas, hypernatremia is a reflection of dehydration or of iatrogenic causes.

Although hypokalemia is related to tubular dysfunction, diuretic therapy or to gastrointestinal dysfunction, hyperkalemia is often artifactual due to poor sample collection practices. Iatrogenic causes and endocrine causes must be considered. Additionally, hypocalcemia and hypomagnesemia increase the risk of cardiac arrhythmias in the setting of hyperkalemia.

Acid base status

Blood gases abnormalities are common in neonates due to immaturity. Blood gases disorders can be metabolic or respiratory in nature. The etiologies include maternal drugs (causing respiratory depression in the newborn), analgesics, sedatives, general anesthesia during labor will all cross the placenta and suppress the patient respiratory center. Prematurity is associated with reduced lung surfactant and may further contribute to the respiratory component. Impaired renal handling of bicarbonate and metabolic waste in premature newborn contributes to the metabolic component of acid base status.

The increased partial pressure of oxygen upon birth causes a reduction in erythropoietin synthesis and to the observed physiological neonatal anemia with hemoglobin levels falling to a nadir of 8–10 g/dL during the 8–10 weeks of life, and this may be even lower in preterm infants (7–8 g/dL).

The clinical biochemistry laboratory plays a significant role in assessment of acid-base status thru measurement of arterial and arterialized blood gases. However, in unit, point of care pulsometry provides alternative to arterial oxygen saturation blood gases measurement.

Cord blood gases

Cord blood gases are measured as indication of the neonate oxygenation status during the delivery process. This intrapartum acid status is important in establishing the link between postdelivery neonatal condition and intrapartum events. It is often used as a surrogate maker of in the investigation of postpartition neurological deficit or abnormalities.

The measurement is affected by sampling factors such as delays in collection, storage, and handling. The main emphasis to maintain the acid-base status of the blood is to reflect that in the immediate cord blood.

Marked acidemia indicates significant hypoxia in the intrapartum period, and that the finding of a normal pH values practically excludes causal relationship between subsequent development of brain damage and the intrapartum period and events.

Blood pH is derived from the pCO_2/HCO_3^- Henderson-Hasselbalch equation. Thus, when metabolic acidemia is present, the timing of the hypoxic insult cannot be established. This is contrast to the presence of a respiratory component of hypoxic insult as the respiratory comment cannot last more than 20–30 min. The pH value before the acute insult can be estimated by reducing the respiratory component. First subtracts the value of the normal neonatal pCO_2 (50 mmHg) from the pCO_2 value obtained in the blood gas analysis to establish the excess in CO_2. Given that every 10 mmHg of the pCO_2 reduces the pH by 0.08, the excess pCO_2 is divided by 10 and multiplied by 0.08. The resultant respiratory acidosis component is added to the measured pH to establish the mixed acidosis level.

Given the accepted prevalence of cerebral palsy of 2 per 1000 normally grown term infants, an obstetric service with 15,000 deliveries per year will have 30 annual cases with 25 expected to be delivered without hypoxic event.

Circulation is reversed where the umbilical vein carries oxygenated blood to the fetus and the two umbilical arteries carry deoxygenated blood in the opposite direction, from the fetus to the placenta.

Given the variability among studies on the stability and appropriateness of the various collection practices, e.g., time delay in collection, need to clamp the cord, venous versus arterial collections, the following are recommendations of the American College of Obstetricians and Gynecologists for umbilical cord blood gas sampling, cord blood segment is immediately clamped after birth (if the neonate appears vigorous the clamped cord segment can be discarded), blood sample is obtained using a heparinized syringe, although institutions may elect to collect one sample type (venous or arterial), the use of paired sampling of the artery and vein may prevent a dispute over the accuracy of arterial sampling, blood is collected within 60 min from birth, and blood gases measured within 60 min of sample collection.

Neonatal anemia

Anemia (hemoglobin <13.0 g/dL) can occur before birth (fetomaternal hemorrhage, immune hemolysis, infection, and congenital disorders) or at delivery during the first 24 h (rupture of umbilical cord, obstetric complication, hemorrhage, infraction), and post 24 h of life (iatrogenic blood loss (repeated blood collections)), internal hemorrhage, red cell membrane disorders, abnormal hemoglobin, e.g., alpha thalassemia, glucose-6-phosphate-dehydrogenase (G6PD), and pyruvate kinase G6PD deficiency.

At full-term birth newborn hemoglobin levels are relatively high at 15.0–22.5 g/dL and gradually fall to 11.0 g/dL by 2 months of age and normalizes to 13.0 g/dL after 6 years of age secondary to increased erythropoietic activity.

During fetal life HbF predominates, it is produced in the liver and has a higher affinity to oxygen compared to HbA to capture maternal oxygen. As the bone marrow becomes the main site of erythropoiesis, a gradual shift from HbF to HbA (alpha 2, beta2) begins at about 34 weeks gestation. At full term, 20% of circulating HbA and by age 6 month HbF makes up less than 1% of total hemoglobin.

Frequent and repeated blood samples collection for testing is the most common contributor to neonatal anemia.

Electrolytes and plasma volume

During fetal life, the fetus plasma volume and electrolytes are well controlled by maternal homoeostatic mechanism. This is lost at birth and the neonate as well as the caretaker assume that role. At birth, 75% of body weight is water with 45% being extracellular and 30% intracellular. The relative distribution remains the same in premature infants but with higher total water content by weight being 85% in preterm. A loss of 5%–10% of body weight (isotonic fluid loss) due to increased glomerular filtration rate.

Hyponatremia <130 mmol/L is either associated with renal immaturity or because of an iatrogenic cause of fluid management. It is either due to reduced extracellular sodium or secondary to excessive body water overload. It is often encountered in premature infants due to reduced renal tubular reabsorption and loss of sodium into the urine. Congenital disorders include congenital adrenal hyperplasia leading to reduction in aldosterone and mineralocorticoids synthesis, depending on the enzyme deficiency (21-hydroxlase the more common) leading to salt losing crises with virilization in affected females causing ambiguous genitalia. The extent of sodium deficit is estimated using the formula:

$$\text{Sodium deficit} = (135 - \text{measured sodium})$$
$$\times 0.7 \times \text{body weight in kg}.$$

The fractional excretion of sodium (FENa) due to the immature renal tubular reabsorption is calculated using the sodium fractional excretion formula:

$$\text{FENa} = (\text{Urine Na} / \text{Urine creatinine})$$
$$\times (\text{Plasma creatinine} / \text{plasma Na}) \times 100.$$

Metabolic bone activity

Disturbances in calcium magnesium and phosphate are common in premature neonates. The disturbances are associated with the exaggerated response to the transition from intrauterine environment to neonatal life.

During fetal life, the placenta actively transfers calcium and phosphate from maternal circulation, and they accumulate in the developing fetus particularly during the third trimester. It is mediated by fetal PTHrp and not by maternal PTH and 1,25-$(OH)_2$ vitamin D which do not cross the placenta. The accumulation is required to support the mineralization of the growing fetal skeleton. At birth, the placental supply of calcium and phosphate is lost, and neonatal calcium drop to <1.75 mmol/L (7 mg/dL) within the first 24–48 h of life and gradually increasing to 2.2–2.6 mmol/L (8.8–10.4 mg/dL) as the neonate processes both PTH and 1,25-$(OH)_2$ vitamin D and initiates own intestinal absorption.

The incidence of hypocalcemia is 30%–90% and is exaggerated by the hypoalbuminemia during neonatal period where total calcium is low (a decrease of 0.02 mmol/L (0.08 mg/dL)) for every drop of 1 g of albumin. This relationship, however, does not hold in premature infants. The biologically active ionized calcium is about 1.2 mmol/L.

Factors contributing to early (24–48 h) hypocalcemia are preterm infants, diabetic mothers (associated with hypomagnesemia), low nutritional intake in infant, more evident in formula milk where absorption of phosphate is low compared to breast feeding.

Hypermagnesemia is rare in neonates, but high levels are seen in infants of mothers who received magnesium sulfate in the treatment of eclampsia. Renal impairment leads to hypermagnesemia due to impaired execration.

Inborn errors of metabolism

This is discussed in detail in Chapter 12 on common and rare metabolic disorders. Newborn with failure to thrive, neuropathy and dysmorphia require investigation for inborn errors of metabolism. Samples during the clinical episode (seizures, hypoglycemia, etc.) are best when investigating inborn errors of metabolism prior to the institution of therapeutic interventions. The initial samples, as well as those symptomatic following initiation of feeding, are valuable and are often available stored in the laboratory usually within 48 h of collection.

Sepsis

Neonatal sepsis accounts most common cause of morbidity and mortality. The incidence ranges from 1 to 5 cases per 1000 live births among preterm neonates and 1–2 per 1000 live births in full-term newborn. In addition to the microbiological (culture) and hematological investigation including complete blood count and neutrophile (WBC count <5000–7500/mm^3) applied as a cut-off for neonatal sepsis, leukopenia has a low sensitivity (29%) but high specificity (912%) for neonatal spies, additionally absolute neutrophil counts (ANC) and immature neutrophils to total neutrophil ratio has a high negative predictive value for sepsis where ratio of 0.16 in uninfected newborn in the first 24 h. Gradually decreasing within the next 5 days to 0.12 (age-related ANC counts), whereas a ratio >0.2 supports neonatal sepsis.

Lactate levels >2.0 mmol/L are indicative of metabolic acidosis seen in sepsis. The higher the lactate level the higher the risk for sepsis and for its complication with levels >4.0 mmol/L associated with poor outcome. Samples for lactate measurements should be transported to the laboratory immediately (preferable on ice) and separated from cells and processed within 15 min of collection.

Assessment of renal function

Accurate assessment of kidney function in the preterm infant is important. In addition to their relatively low GFR compared to full-term neonate, infants are at higher risk acute kidney injury.

Limited by inherent bias due to maternal factors such as hypertension where up to 80% of preterm neonates were product of hypertensive pregnancy.

In neonates, serum creatinine is low due to low muscle mass (derived from creatine in muscle) additionally circulating maternal creatinine in neonatal blood lasts for 2 days following partition.

In low gestational age neonates (age <34 weeks' gestation), the process of nephrogenesis is not complete and the kidney is not fully developed.

Markers in use include cystatin C (independent of muscle mass), neutrophil gelatinase-associated lipocalin (NGAL), kidney injury molecule-1 (KIM-1), and osteoprotegerin (OPN). With the exception of serum cystatin-C and NGAL to some extent, the other biomarkers are not currently available in routine analysis.

Neutrophil gelatinase-associated lipocalin (NGAL)

NGAL is responsible for kidney development converting embryonic mesenchymal cells into epithelial cells forming tubules and complete nephron. It is produced by leukocytes, loop of Henle, and collecting ducts. Expressed by tubular epithelial cells in response to tubulointerstitial damage during the course of acute kidney injury and that levels correlate with degree of injury damage and the increase precedes decline in kidney function. It is sensitive to damage of the loop of Henle and the distal tubule.

It is closely associated with acute kidney injury and several studies showed early detection of acute kidney injury following a number of invasive procedures (e.g., cardiovascular invasive procedures (hemodynamic changes affecting renal blood flow), use of radiology contrast medium), and in the early detection of acute kidney injury in the high risk preterm underdeveloped kidney.

Urine and serum levels are elevated in AKI with urinary NGAL elevated early in AKI. Serum and urine cut-off values with associated sensitivities and specificities are shown in Table 14.

Cystatin-C

Cystatin-C, a 122 amino acid cysteine proteinase inhibitor protein with molecular weight, 13 kDa. It is present on the surface of all nucleated cells, a product of a general housekeeping gene expressed at constant rate. It is freely filtered at the glomerulus with no tubular reabsorption. This renders it an ideal marker of GFR. Cystatin-C is more reliable for the assessment of kidney function compared to creatinine.

TABLE 14 Cut-off values associated with severe acute kidney injury.

Biomarker	Urine	Serum
Cystatin-C (mg/L)	0.03–0.08	0.63–1.03 (adult)
NGAL (ng/mL)	12 (95% sensitivity) 580 (95% specificity)	79 ng/mL (95% sensitivity) 364 ng/mL (95% specificity)
	8.34–128.8 ng/mg creatinine	
KIM-1 (ng/mL)	<1	
	0.08–2.39 (ng/mg creatinine)	

KIM-1, kidney injury molecule; NGAL, neutrophil gelatinase-associated lipocalin.
Modified from various sources including Schrezenmeier EV, Barasch J, Budde K, Westhoff T, Schmidt-Ott KM. Biomarkers in acute kidney injury—pathophysiological basis and clinical performance. Acta Physiol (Oxf). 2017;219(3):554–572. https://doi.org/10.1111/apha.12764. Epub 2016 Aug 25. PMID: 27474473; PMCID: PMC5575831. Albert C, Zapf A, Haase M, et al. Neutrophil gelatinase-associated lipocalin measured on clinical laboratory platforms for the prediction of acute kidney injury and the associated need for dialysis therapy: a systematic review and meta-analysis. Am J Kidney Dis. 2020;76(6):826–841.e1. https://doi.org/10.1053/j.ajkd.2020.05.015. Epub 2020 Jul 15. PMID: 32679151; PMCID: PMC8283708.

It is completely metabolized in renal tubules. It thus overcomes the limitation of serum creatinine (low muscle mass, maternal creatinine, metabolism, and interference by neonatal hyperbilirubinemia in pediatrics). It is measured using immunoassay and this not interfered by some high circulating intermediate metabolites.

Urinary cystatin-C is inversely proportional to renal volume (determined by radiological measurements using echo ultrasound) and thus reflects the degree of nephrogenesis (nephron formation) in neonates. Combined with renal volume assessment can help identify neonates with initial kidney impairment.

KIM-1

Kidney injury molecule-1, is a transmembrane, mucin-containing T-Cell immunoglobulin, a transmembrane protein. It is not detected in normal in healthy kidney nor in the urine; however, it is upregulated and appears in the urine of patients with dedifferentiated proximal tubule epithelial cells following ischemic or toxic injury. It is a good predictor of injury damage prior to reduction in kidney function. Normally, levels are below 1 ng/mL and are elevated up to 3–7 ng/mL in patients with ischemic kidney injury.

Uromodulin

Uromodulin (also known as the Tamm-Horsfall protein) is a glycoprotein. It is produced in the tubular cells of the thick ascending limb and the early distal tubule and released into the tubular lumen where it forms a layer on the tubular cell surface. It is the most abundant protein in urine and is thought to provide protection of tubular cells from ascending urinary tract infections involved in chronic pyelonephritis and urolithiasis. Reduced urinary and serum concentrations of uromodulin are found in patients with interstitial fibrosis or tubular atrophy in the course of chronic kidney disease. Uromodulin has been suggested as a surrogate biomarker for the number of intact nephrons, which indicates renal mass rather than kidney function. Uromodulin concentrations gradually decrease with worsening kidney function.

Summary

- Conception is suspected when menstrual period is missed.
- Successful conception is confirmed biochemically by a detectable and rising level of human chorionic gonadotropin (hCG) produced by the developing syncytiotrophoblastic cells of the placenta.
- Levels of β-hCG correlate with gestational age and that serial measurements assesses viability of pregnancy.

- Discordant hCG results (false positive or false negative) may occur due to interference by heterophilic antibodies.
- Implantation taking place outside the uterus termed ectopic pregnancy.
- Serial determination of hCG helps identify the presence of ectopic pregnancy.
- Circulating hCG levels increase with age with pituitary being the plausible sources in nonpregnant female.
- Increased red blood cell turnover during pregnancy results in reduced A1c during pregnancy by about 0.5%.
- The use of A1c is thus unreliable for assessment of diabetes control and of assessment of risk for complications, in contrast to postprandial glucose which has a better prediction for GDM complications.
- Gestational diabetes mellitus (GDM) describes diabetes diagnosed in the second and third trimester.
- Antiphospholipids antibodies are attributed to recurrent pregnancy loss.
- Detection of amniotic fluid in vaginal secretions by measuring alpha-fetoprotein and insulin like growth factor binding protein-1 (IGFBP-1) confirms premature rupture of membrane.
- The antiphospholipid syndrome is characterized by the presence of moderate to high titers of antibodies against cardiolipin and beta-2 glycoprotein-I.
- A stepwise approach to biochemical investigation of infertility is preferred.
- In patients with amenorrhea, measurements of human chorionic gonadotrophin (β-hCG) confirm pregnancy as the most common cause for amenorrhea.
- The findings of a low low-normal testosterone in the presence of inappropriately low low-normal gonadotrophins suggests secondary hypopituitary cause or a tertiary hypothalamic cause.
- AMH levels <5.4 pmol/L predict for a low response during IVF treatment and >25 pmol/L predict a high response.
- No endocrine testing is required in a male patient with normal sperm analysis (count, motility, and viability) testing.
- Pregnancy is the most common cause of suspected infertility.
- Cord blood gases are measured as indication of the neonate oxygenation status during the delivery process.
- The growing and developing newborn requires age-related laboratory test reference intervals. The values are likely to alter with age and with maturity.
- NGAL is closely associated with acute kidney injury.
- Cystatin-C is more reliable for the assessment of kidney function compared to creatinine.
- Urine volume is very low early in life, and thus, a small loss in time urine collection will lead to significant error urine.

Further reading

Szmuilowicz ED, Josefson JL, Metzger BE. Gestational diabetes mellitus. *Endocrinol Metab Clin N Am.* 2019;48(3):479–493.

Chappell LC, Cluver CA, Kingdom J, Tong S. Pre-eclampsia. *Lancet.* 2021;398(10297):341–354.

Rabbani T, Guthery SL, Himes R, Shneider BL, Harpavat S. Newborn screening for biliary atresia: a review of current methods. *Curr Gastroenterol Rep.* 2021;23(12):28.

Dogan S, Sel G, Arikan II, et al. Accuracy of the 24-h urine protein excretion value in patients with preeclampsia: correlation with instant and 24-h urine protein/creatinine and albumin/creatinine ratios. *J Obstet Gynaecol.* 2019;39(8):1075–1080.

Nada A, Bonachea EM, Askenazi DJ. Acute kidney injury in the fetus and neonate. *Semin Fetal Neonatal Med.* 2017;22(2):90–97.

Sammaritano LR. Antiphospholipid syndrome. *Best Pract Res Clin Rheumatol.* 2020;34(1):101463.

Mahany EB, Randolph Jr JF. Biochemical and imaging diagnostics in endocrinology: predictors of fertility. *Endocrinol Metab Clin N Am.* 2017;46(3):679–689.

Mack LR, Tomich PG. Gestational diabetes: diagnosis, classification, and clinical care. *Obstet Gynecol Clin N Am.* 2017;44(2):207–217.

Mak RH, Abitbol CL. Standardized urine biomarkers in assessing neonatal kidney function: are we there yet? *J Pediatr (Rio J).* 2021;97(5):476–477.

Gil MM, Galeva S, Jani J, et al. Screening for trisomies by cfDNA testing of maternal blood in twin pregnancy: update of The Fetal Medicine Foundation results and meta-analysis. *Ultrasound Obstet Gynecol.* 2019;53(6):734–742.

Carlson LM, Vora NL. Prenatal diagnosis: screening and diagnostic tools. *Obstet Gynecol Clin N Am.* 2017;44(2):245–256.

Doret M, Cartier R, Miribel J, et al. Premature preterm rupture of the membrane diagnosis in early pregnancy: PAMG-1 and IGFBP-1 detection in amniotic fluid with biochemical tests. *Clin Biochem.* 2013;46(18):1816–1819.

Chapter 9

Neurological disorders

Introduction

The clinical biochemistry laboratory plays a significant role in the investigation of neurological dysfunction. Several biochemical analysis ranging from routine electrolytes and osmolality, blood gases, hematology indices, blood and cerebrospinal fluid glucose, renal and liver tests, C-reactive protein, B12, folate, vitamins, serum protein electrophoresis, thyroid function tests, toxicology, paraneoplastic autoimmune antibodies, cerebrospinal fluid proteins and oligoclonal bands, porphyria testing, to specialized genetic testing are performed. Whereas the majority of initial tests are performed within the laboratory, a significant number of esoteric tests may be sent to a specialized reference laboratory.

Neurological disorders can be broadly described as (a) intrinsic neurologic disease such as spinal muscular atrophy, myasthenia gravis (acetylcholine receptor antibodies), (b) malignancy-associated paraneoplastic syndrome, (c) metabolites-associated includes drugs (neurometabolic, toxic metabolites, organs dysfunction, drugs and their metabolites) and heavy and trace elements (lead, copper, aluminum, cobalt, mercury), nutritional (vitamins), and (d) infectious disease (bacterial, viral, fungal) encephalitis.

Clinical presentations

Clinical presentation is either acute presenting over hours to days, subacute (weeks to months), or chronic (over a year) (Fig. 1). They vary from mild peripheral neuropathy or central encephalopathy (presenting with altered mental status), tremors or seizures to severe movement disorders and encephalopathy including coma and death. The impact ranges from reversible to minor and permanent neurological deficits modulated by the etiology, the nature of the metabolites involved, and the associated pathology.

The majority of neurological disorders are diagnosed clinically, and the laboratory provides confirmation and support for monitoring and assessment of prognosis. For many of the disorders, the clinical chemistry laboratory is central to their diagnosis.

Neurological disorders

The main categories of neurological disorders are vascular, infectious, neoplastic, degenerative, psychogenic, genetic (congenital), autoimmune, endocrine, toxicological (drugs), metabolic, and traumatic causes (Table 1). Neurological disorders present as either peripheral neuropathy, encephalopathy, or as movement disorders. Clinical presentation, causes, and biochemical investigations are discussed separately.

Peripheral neuropathy

Peripheral neuropathy is commonly encountered in clinical practice. The prevalence in the general population is reported to be between 1% and 4%. It is a spectrum of disordered affecting the peripheral nervous system. The common pattern affected being, distal sensory polyneuropathy (DSP). This is a nerve length-dependent peripheral nerve injury where clinical symptoms (sensory loss, pain, or gait stability in severe cases) may begin at the toe and gradually increase up the leg to the knee and the hand. A less common neuropathy pattern is that of "mononeuritis multiplex," a patch pattern that is nonlength dependent involving multiple individual nerves.

Among the different causes of peripheral neuropathy (Table 1), diabetes mellitus is the most common disorder leading to peripheral neuropathy accounting for 50% of cases with DSP being the most common. The prevalence, which changes with duration of diabetes, is higher among patients with type II diabetes (6100 per 100,000 person years) compared to those with type I (2800 per 100,000 person years). Risk factors being the duration of diabetes and the cumulative hyperglycemia exposure. The clinical laboratory plays a major role in the management of diabetic neuropathy by measuring glycated hemoglobin (A1c) levels.

A1c is a major predictor of diabetic neuropathy as it reflects the cumulative degree of glycemia exposure. However, other factors such as hypertension, hypertriglyceridemia, low levels of high-density lipoprotein (HDL), and

Tutorials in Clinical Chemistry. https://doi.org/10.1016/B978-0-12-822949-1.00005-X

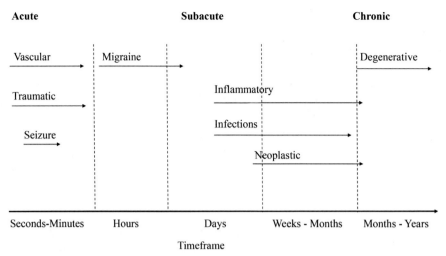

FIG. 1   Type and time course of neurological disorders. The disorders may present acutely, subacutely, or chronically in nature. *(Modified from Milligan TA. Diagnosis in neurologic disease. Med Clin North Am 2019;103(2):173–190. https://doi.org/10.1016/j.mcna.2018.10.011. Epub 2018 Dec 17. PMID: 30704675.)*

TABLE 1 Metabolic contributors to the neurological presentation (encephalopathy and peripheral neuropathy).

Cause	Example	Presentation
Toxicology	Drugs, alcohol, carbon monoxide	Encephalopathy Subacute/acute
Infection	Meningitis/encephalitis, sepsis	Encephalopathy. Acute
Trauma	Trauma, vascular injury (stroke), space-occupying lesion	Encephalopathy. Acute
Malignancy	Primary/secondary	Encephalopathy, neuropathy. Subacute
Autoimmune	Paraneoplastic, hypothyroid, degenerative (Alzheimer, Parkinson, Creutzfeldt-Jacob disease)	Encephalopathy, peripheral neuropathy Subacute/chronic
Organ dysfunction	Hepatic failure, renal failure, cardiovascular failure	Encephalopathy Subacute/chronic
Nutritional	Deficiency: Thiamine (B1), niacin (B2), B5, B12, folate, vitamin E, pyridoxine, copper	Peripheral neuropathy, encephalopathy Subacute/chronic
Endocrinological	Diabetes (hypo/hyperglycemia) Hypohypernatremia Hypohypercalcemia Hypophosphatemia	Encephalopathy, peripheral neuropathy Acute/subacute
Metabolic	Porphyria, amyloidosis, mitochondrial, and glycogen storage disorders	Peripheral neuropathy, encephalopathy Acute

Modified from Fernández-Eulate G, Carreau C, Benoist JF, Lamari F, Rucheton B, Shor N, Nadjar Y. Diagnostic approach in adult-onset neurometabolic diseases. J Neurol Neurosurg Psychiatry. 2022;93(4):413–421. https://doi.org/10.1136/jnnp-2021-328045. Epub 2022 Feb 9. PMID: 35140137; PMCID: PMC8921565.

truncal obesity, all being constituents of insulin resistance and metabolic syndrome, contribute to the risk of developing diabetic neuropathy.

Although the pathogenesis is multifactorial and some remains debated, certain elements are clearly involved. For instance, the glycation of structural and functional proteins results in the formation of advanced glycation end products (AGEs). The latter results in the production and release of inflammatory cytokines and free radicals which causes nerve injuries.

In Schwann cells, distal root ganglion (DRG), and axons, glucose, and fatty acids are metabolized for energy producing NADH and FADH$_2$ by glycolysis and by β-oxidation of fatty acids where one molecule of acetyl CoA is produced by each fatty acid oxidation cycle. Acetyl CoA enters the tricarboxylic acid (TCA) cycle to produce NADH and FADH$_2$.

In states of hyperglycemia, the transport mechanism of acetyl CoA to the TCA cycle is overwhelmed and acetyl-CoA is converted to acylcarnitine. Thus, acetyl carnitine production increases in states of hyperglycemia and of increased long-chain fatty acids. Acetyl carnitine is toxic to both Schwann cells and dorsal root ganglia (DRG) neurons.

Mitochondrial oxidative phosphorylation utilizes NADH and $FADH_2$ to generate ATP. Low amounts of free radicals are generated in the enzymatic processes and are effectively neutralized by cellular superoxide dismutase, glutathione, and catalase antioxidants. Overwhelming production of oxygen-reactive species due to the increased fatty acids β-oxidation in response to accompanying hyperlipidemia, to the production of advanced glycation end products, and to mitochondrial failure leads to metabolic and oxidative damage of Schwann cells, DRG neurons, and axons.

In the presence of hypercholesterolemia and an abundance of reactive oxygen species, LDL-cholesterol is oxidized. The latter binds to oxidized LDL receptor 1 (LOX1) and toll-like receptor 4 (TLR4) activating caspase-3 and nuclear DNA degradation leading to additional inflammation and reactive oxygen and to continued insult and nerve damage.

The above metabolic derangement is complicated by microcirculatory dysfunction seen in long-standing and poorly controlled diabetes, with reduced blood supply to peripheral neurons.

It must be stated that factors other than hyperglycemia such as dyslipidemia, insulin resistance, and chronic inflammation contribute to the pathophysiology of diabetic neuropathy, particularly in patients with type II diabetes mellitus.

Schwann cells are thus affected by chronic hyperglycemia and features of demyelination are seen in severe cases. The consequent loss of Schwann cells impairs the cytoskeletal structure of nerve axons and thus impairing its function (e.g., axonal firing). Affected sensory neurons develop hyperexcitability and can generate action potentials in the absence of a stimulus (spontaneous activity) as well develop an altered stimulus-response function.

Although diffused diabetic neuropathy occurs, it involves in addition to the DSP, autonomic axons such as in cardiac autonomic neuropathy, gastrointestinal dysmotility, and impotence. Diabetic peripheral neuropathy is the most common and is diagnosed by a process of elimination after other etiologies have been ruled out. Clinical findings of diabetic neuropathy are those of loss of sensation to pinprick, temperature (cold), vibration, numbness, tingling, pain and weakness, and unsteadiness. Approximately 30%–50% of patients with diabetic neuropathy develop neuropathic pain.

Those sensations begin at the toes (distally) and spread proximally until the knees before extending to the upper limbs. Pinprick and temperature sensations are mediated via small nerve fibers, whereas vibration sensation and proprioception are mediated by large nerve fibers. Loss of ankle reflexes occurs early in diabetic neuropathy; thus, an initial examination should include reflex testing. Small fibers are involved early during the course before extending to large fibers, however, involvement of large fibers does not always occur.

The landmark Diabetes Control and Complications Trial (DCCT) and the United Kingdom Prospective Diabetes Study (UKPDS) trials have clearly shown that improved glycemic control contributes to the prevention of and progression of diabetic neuropathy. Diabetes professional societies recommend screening for diabetic peripheral neuropathy for all patients with diabetes at diagnosis and annually for patients with type II and five years after diagnosis and then annually for patients with type I.

Furthermore, although hyperglycemia is clearly associated with peripheral neuropathy, the degree of diabetic control is less evident in type II than in type I DM. The current approaches to the management of diabetic neuropathy focus on improving glycemic control (mainly in patients with type I diabetes mellitus), lifestyle modifications (mainly in patients with type II diabetes mellitus), and management of neuropathic pain.

Although achieving the A1c goal of <6% has little effect on diabetic neuropathy, it increases mortality in patients with type II diabetes mellitus and therefore it is not recommended but rather good glycemic control is targeted. Tight glycemic control has a large impact on the prevention of diabetic neuropathy, this is however not statistically apparent in patients with type II, although likely to be relevant.

In addition to the assessment of diabetes control using A1c, other laboratory assessments in diabetic patients with neuropathy include measurement of B12 levels (methylmalonic acid with or without homocysteine can provide additional information in patients receiving metformin), thyroid function tests, and serum protein electrophoresis plus immunofixation to evaluate for a monoclonal gammopathy.

Multiple myeloma is also associated with peripheral neuropathy but is considered underreported. This may be a consequence of the need for higher sensitivity methods such as immunofixation often following a subjective reflex protocol from serum protein electrophoresis, and mild cases may initially be missed. In this pathology, peripheral nerves can be damaged by either immunological targeting of the myelin by paraproteins, by deposition of light chains amyloid and cryoglobulins, or by direct infiltration. Additionally, the hyperviscosity due to hyperproteinemia reduces peripheral blood flow and causes neuropathy.

First-line and second-line treatments for painful diabetic neuropathy include several drug classes, such as anticonvulsants (gabapentin or pregabalin), serotonin and noradrenaline reuptake inhibitors (SNRIs; duloxetine or venlafaxine) and tricyclic antidepressants (amitriptyline, nortriptyline, desipramine, or imipramine), and use of opiates (e.g., tramadol, tapentadol, and oxycodone). Although there is evidence of the efficacy of opioids for pain relief, these drugs are associated with a high risk of addiction and safety concerns. The laboratory plays a role in monitoring compliance and usage (diversion) of drugs by monitoring the urinary presence of the prescribed drugs and their metabolites as evidence of compliance.

Amyloidosis

Amyloidosis is characterized by the deposition of aggregated free light chains on nerves and organs.

Diagnosis is often delayed due to the heterogenous clinical presentation (systemic component and extent of organ involvement) complicated by misleading investigational findings. However, accurate and timely diagnosis of amyloid neuropathy significantly impacts the outcomes with new gene-silencing treatments for hereditary transthyretin amyloidosis becoming available.

Neurological presentation is typically sensory polyneuropathy, focal neuropathy (such as carpal tunnel syndrome), or autonomic neuropathy.

The condition is either hereditary or acquired. Light chains multiple myeloma deposition is the most acquired form whereas autosomal dominant mutation in the transthyretin (TTR) (prealbumin) gene is the most common hereditary form.

Laboratory investigations include protein and urine electrophoresis and immunofixation to paraproteins. In patients with amyloid light chain-amyloidosis, the sensitivity of serum protein electrophoresis for detecting a monoclonal protein is 66%, but this increases to over 90% if reflexed to serum electrophoresis with immunofixation and Bence Jones protein testing on urine. Serum-free light chain assay has a sensitivity of 88%. However, the absolute values and ratios need to be interpreted with caution in patients with impaired renal function.

Amyloidosis is a histological diagnosis and imaging studies are required to assess the extent of amyloidosis (amyloid deposits in the body).

Alcoholic neuropathy

Alcoholic myopathy is characterized by muscle weakness, tenderness, and swelling in patients with alcohol abuse disorder. It is present in 0.5% to 2.0% of alcoholics with an estimated prevalence of 20 cases per 100,000 patients. The prevalence is difficult to ascertain as the concurrent presence of liver cirrhosis may contribute to the myopathy. The neurological effect of alcohol depends on the blood alcohol concentration (Table 2).

In an acute setting of alcohol level of 0.08 g/dL, rhabdomyolysis accompanied by pain and biochemical evidence of muscle injury (elevated creatine kinase, AST, and LDH enzymes and myoglobin) is often seen. In contrast, in

TABLE 2 Neurological effects in relation to blood alcohol levels.

Blood alcohol level (mg/dL)	Neurological symptoms
10–40	Mild euphoria, relaxation, and increased social interactions
50–70	Euphoria with loss of inhibition. Some impairment of motor skills in some individuals (in Germany, the legal limit for driving is 50 mg/dL)
80	The legal limit for driving in the United States. Some impairment of driving skills may be present in some individuals
80–120	Moderate impairment to significant impairment of motor skills. Emotional swings and depression may be observed in some individuals
120–150	Motor function, speech, and judgment are all severely affected. Staggering and slurred speech may be observed
150–200	Symptoms of intoxication. May have a severe visual impairment
200–300	Vomiting, incontinence, symptoms of alcohol intoxication
300–400	Signs of severe alcohol intoxication. Stupor, blackout, and total loss of consciousness
400–500	Potentially fatal and patient may be comatose
>500	Highly dangerous/fatal blood alcohol level

Modified from Dasgupta A. 1. Alcohol a double-edged sword: health benefits with moderate consumption but a health hazard with excess alcohol intake. In: Alcohol, Drugs, Genes and the Clinical Laboratory, Academic Press, 2017:1-21, ISBN 9780128054550, https://doi.org/10.1016/B978-0-12-805455-0.00001-4.

chronic alcoholic myopathy, patients present with progressive proximal muscle weakness over weeks to months, pain, muscle twitching, and tightness.

Chronic alcohol consumption often leads to protein-calorie malnutrition and is related to the severity of the alcoholic liver disease. Nutritional deficiencies include folate, thiamine, vitamin B6, zinc, iron, and vitamin D. In addition, chronic alcohol consumption decreases muscle protein synthesis and increased protein degradation.

Blood ethanol levels provide an accurate assessment of alcohol levels. However, ethanol intoxication is not detected until 6–8 h post-ingestion. Urine and breath are alternative sample types, with breath tests often used in nonclinical settings. Influenced by the analytical assay limit of detection, however, blood alcohol levels >5 mg/L reflect recent alcohol intake.

Alcohol is metabolized by alcohol dehydrogenase to acetaldehyde which is in turn is metabolized to acetate. The latter is oxidized to carbon dioxide and to acetyl CoA in the brain and peripheral tissue. Minor metabolites of alcohol metabolism are ethyl glucuronide (EtG) (0.02% to 0.06 %) and ethyl sulfate (EtS) (0.01% to 0.016%). Those minor metabolites appear after 45 min of alcohol ingestion and remain in circulation for up to 8 h (in the case of ethyl glucuronide) longer than ethanol and twice as long as ethanol for ethyl sulfate.

EtG is detectable in urine for up to 24 h following ingestion of small quantities and up to 130 h following excessive alcohol intake.

Alcohol metabolites, ethyl glucuronide, and ethyl sulfate metabolites are indicators of acute and short-term alcohol exposure (−2 weeks or longer) detectable up to 36 h in blood and up to 5 days in urine post alcohol ingestion. They are thus biomarkers of short-term biomarkers of alcohol ingestion. Urinary levels are influenced by the degree of diuresis and urine concentration. Intake of large volumes of fluids dilutes the urine and could lead to false negative results. Results are thus considered valid for an appropriate urine concentration, that is, a urinary creatinine >20 mg/dL (1.8 mmol/L).

Carbohydrate-deficient transferrin is an indirect biomarker of alcohol consumption. Transferrin, a main transporter of Fe^{3+}, is synthesized by hepatocytes. A 670 amino acids glycoprotein with several amino acid substitutions results in many genetic variants. It has two N-linked oligosaccharidosis chains (Asn432, and 630). Similarly, variations in the oligosaccharide chains result in different glycoforms. The oligosaccharide chains can be bi-, tri-, and tetra-antennary with each antenna terminated by sialic acid, and the total number of sialic acids provides the basis for the glycoforms nomenclature. The total transferrin measured in circulation comprises 80% tetrasialotransferrin, 14% pentasialotransferrin, 4% trisialotransferrin, <2% disialotransferrin, and 1% hexasialotransferrin.

The total circulating concentration of transferrin is 2.0–3.5 g/L. The concentration of disialotransferrin was shown to increase in response to chronic heavy alcohol consumption and decrease again on abstinence with a half-life of about 10 days. The elevated disialotransferrin is accompanied by an increase in asialotransferrin (carbohydrate-deficient transferrin, (CDT)). The latter is thus used as a marker of sustained alcohol intake.

Alcohol intake (>50–80 g per day) over at least 1 to 2 weeks results in the loss of the carbohydrate side chains of transferrin. The resultant carbohydrate-deficient transferrin (CDT) is thus a specific but not highly sensitive biomarker of excessive and pronged alcohol ingestion. Its circulating levels (proportion of carbohydrate-deficient transferrin to normally glycosylated transferrin) correlate with drinking pattern. Levels >1.7% indicate chronic and excessive

alcohol consumption. It is measured using a combination of affinity chromatography and mass spectrometry or by immunoturbidimetric and nephelometric methods. Capillary electrophoresis is used. A recent IFCC working group identified the anion-exchange HLPC method as the candidate reference measurement procedure. The test is not valid in patients with congenital disorders of glycosylation.

Phosphatidyl ethanol (PEth) is an abnormal phospholipid that is produced following exposure to cellular membrane phospholipids (particularly red blood cells). It is a group of glycerol phospholipids with fatty acids of various lengths and degrees of saturation resulting in over 48 identifiable species. The main form PEth 16:0/18:1 produced following alcohol ingestion is measured. It is detectable in circulation within 30 min of alcohol intake with peak levels reaching 90 to 120 min. PhEth accumulates in blood in frequent alcohol consumption and can last up to 12 days after a one-time alcohol intake. It is thus used to differentiate and determine current intake and abstinence. Similarly, it can be used to distinguish patients consuming >60 g ethanol daily and those with lower consumption (Table 3).

Other nonspecific markers of alcohol intake include hepatic microsomal enzymes gamma-glutamyl transferase (γGT) which is induced by alcohol, and elevated levels are seen up to 2–3 weeks post-injection. It is nonspecific as it is also elevated in cholestatic liver disease and is induced

TABLE 3 Alcohol consumption biomarkers and their detection window at the shown cut-off values.

Biomarkers of alcohol consumption	Cut-off value	Detection timeframe
Ethanol	<5 mg/dL	1–12 h (blood or urine)
Ethyl glucuronide	≥100 ng/mL	1–5 days (urine) 36 h (blood)
Ethyl Sulfate	≥100 ng/mL (≥80 ng/mL in chronic liver disease)	1–5 days (urine) 36 h (blood)
Carbohydrate deficient transferrin	≥1.7%	2–3 weeks or longer (serum)
Phosphatidyl ethanol	≥20 ng/mL (moderate consumption) ≥200 ng/mL (heavy/chronic consumption)	1–2 weeks

Modified from various sources and Andresen-Streichert H, Müller A, Glahn A, Skopp G, Sterneck M. Alcohol biomarkers in clinical and forensic contexts. Dtsch Arztebl Int 2018;115(18):309–315. https://doi.org/10.3238/arztebl.2018.0309. PMID: 29807559; PMCID: PMC5987059.

by a number of therapeutic drugs. The increased activity of the enzymes aspartate-aminotransferase (AST) and alanine aminotransferase (ALT) is increased (AST/ALT>2).

An increase in mean corpuscular volume (MCV) of red blood cells and above all of gamma-glutamyl transferase activity (GGT) may also be a sign of harmful alcohol consumption and alcohol-induced hepatic injury.

Furthermore, it takes several weeks after termination or reduction of alcohol consumption before they return to normal (γGT: 2–6 weeks; AST/ALT: 2–4 weeks; MCV: 8–16 weeks [12]). A disadvantage of indirect alcohol biomarkers is their low specificity (Table 3).

Medication-induced neuropathy

Peripheral neuropathy is a common complication of chemotherapeutic agents' usage where chemotherapy drugs damage the sensory, motor, autonomic, or cranial nerves in approximately 30%–60% of patients with cancer.

The neuropathy appears immediately after initiation of chemotherapy (e.g., oxaliplatin causes transient sensory neuropathy secondary to nerve hyperexcitability within hours of infusion). Chemotherapeutic drugs exhibit a phenomenon called "coasting" which describes persistent and progressive worsening of symptoms over time even after the completion of chemotherapy.

The prevalence of chemotherapy-induced peripheral neuropathy (CIPN) is dependent on the type of malignancy, drug regimen, cumulative doses, duration, synergistic neurotoxicity from prior chemotherapy, co-morbidities, and other risk factors. The reported prevalence varies among several studies. Commonly 68% of patients in <1 month, 60.3% in three months, and 30% of patients in 6 months following chemotherapy.

Encephalopathy

Encephalopathy is a general term encompassing altered brain function. Clinical presentation ranges from confusion states, dementia, and delirium to loss of consciousness and coma. It can occur either acutely (within hours) or subacutely (over weeks or months) or chronically (over years) (Fig. 1). The cause is either direct damage to the brain architecture or by toxic compounds interfering with brain function. For the latter, metabolic encephalopathy which constitutes 75% of encephalitis, contributors include toxin (drugs, carbon monoxide), uremic and hepatic metabolites (e.g., ammonia and bilirubin), vitamins deficiency (thiamine B1 and B6, folate), extremes levels (high or low) of glucose, sodium and/or calcium levels, and cardiovascular circulatory failure (hypoxia and ischemia) and infective encephalitis as in sepsis.

Early identification of metabolic causes of encephalopathy is required as most of the neurological dysfunctions are reversible if corrected early. Examples of the common metabolic contributors are shown in the following Table 1.

In addition to the global cognitive presentation above, other global neurological signs include generalized seizures and tremors. This is in contrast to the focal signs of localized dysfunction, such as areas affecting speech, vision, or swallowing difficulties.

Movement disorders

Movement disorders represent neurological disorders that present as either excessive movement (hyperkinesia) or a paucity of movements that may be either voluntary or involuntary (excessive or slow movement). It is a reflection of cerebellar disease, basal ganglia, or their connection. Movement disorders are further described as ataxia, dystonia, and tremor.

Ataxia

Ataxia describes a lack of co-ordinated movements produced by dysfunction of the cerebellum or cerebral pathways. The causes of ataxia are either acquired or genetic. The most common acquired cause of ataxia is chronic alcohol consumption, above therapeutic levels of antiepileptic dosages, cerebrovascular disease, cancer, and multiple sclerosis.

Several autosomal dominant genetic mutations have been reported, the most common being Friedreich ataxia (excessive iron accumulation in mitochondria is a feature of the condition), ataxia telangiectasia due to mutation in the ATM gene, fragile X-associated tremor/ataxia syndrome, isolated vitamin E-deficiency associated ataxia, and apolipoprotein.

Dystonia

Longer duration of muscle contraction involving simultaneous contraction of both agonist and antagonist muscles known as dystonia, leading to torsion postures of the body muscles. The condition is seen in patients with Wilson's disease, dopa-responsive dystonia, and in dystonia Oppenheim.

Tremor

The most common among movement disorders. It presents as rhythmic oscillation of part of the body. It can be essential as in Parkinsonism or secondary to thyrotoxicosis, toxins, and drugs. Physiological tremors are observed in states of anxiety and stress.

Causes of neurological dysfunction

Many disorders can lead to neurological dysfunctions. Causes of neurological dysfunction include metabolic disorders, drugs and toxins, nutritional disorders, malignancy, and autoimmune disorders (Table 1). Those where biochemical tests are central to the diagnosis are discussed in the following section.

Metabolic and toxicological (drugs) causes

Encephalopathy and neuropathy may be the main clinical presentation associated with metabolic components as a cause. For instance, high levels of circulating toxins (ammonia) and urea in hepatic and renal failure, respectively, and of drugs and their metabolites.

Organs-failure-associated neuropathies

Accumulation of intermediate metabolites such as ammonia and urea leads to a variable degree of encephalopathy. Those are elevated in patients with liver and renal impairment or as a consequence of the combine hepatorenal syndrome.

Hepatic encephalopathy

The liver has a large reserve capacity, however, in end-stage liver disease high circulating ammonia levels lead to hepatic encephalopathy. The etiology of liver failure can either be acute or chronic and is discussed in detail in the chapter on the liver.

In the acute setting of presentation and management, measurement of drugs such as acetaminophen facilitates immediate intervention as required.

In chronic liver disease, the presence of a portosystemic shunt facilitates the entry of ammonia, produced in the gut from deamidation, into the systemic circulation. The poor correlation between the degree of encephalopathy and ammonia levels does not support its measurement in management. The presence of other abnormal liver function tests supports the diagnosis. Hyperbilirubinemia and hypoalbuminemia are the hallmarks.

Renal encephalopathy

Accumulation of high urea levels in patients with renal dysfunction leads to neurological presentations of confusion, irritability, fatigue, etc., although the mechanism is unknown.

Accumulation of phosphate, organic acids, and calcium (secondary to renal tertiary hyperparathyroidism) in cerebrospinal fluid as well as the presence of inflammatory cytokines may be contributing factors to neuropathy in renal failure. Removal of those metabolites by dialysis as monitored by the reduction in circulating levels leads to improvement in the symptoms of neuropathy.

Cardiorespiratory failure

Carbon monoxide poisoning is a common accidental cause of poisoning (common during winter as faulty heating devices in vehicles/homes). It is odorless and colorless. The atmospheric concentration of carbon monoxide is <0.001% except in urban areas and those with high levels of pollution.

Carboxy hemoglobin levels are elevated with values >10% consistent with clinical neurological sequelae ranging from confusion, paralysis, and coma.

Neurological symptoms appear when 20%–30% of total hemoglobin is bound to carbon monoxide presenting with headache and nausea. Coma occurs when 50%–60% is bound. Heavy smokers and patients living in areas of high air pollution may have levels of 5%–15%. Blood gases including carboxyhemoglobin are performed to confirm clinical suspicion and monitor response to oxygen therapy.

Elevated arterial pCO_2 levels are seen in patients with COPD and acute respiratory failure. The clinical presentation correlated with the levels of pCO_2 (severity of hypercapnia) and ranged from headache, drowsiness, confusion, and coma. The latter at pCO_2 levels >9 kPa (>67.5 mmHg). The pathogenesis is not fully known but may be related to CO_2 causing pH imbalance within the CSF.

On the other hand, hypoxia as a result of either respiratory or circulatory failure leads to ischemia, cells, necrosis, and apoptosis. The clinical presentation is variable and depends on the degree as well as the duration of hypoxia resulting in reversible to permanent neurological damage. Measurement of arterial blood gases will exhibit reduced pO_2 levels.

Neurotoxicity of drugs and their metabolites

Alcohols (ethanol/methanol/ethylene glycol)

Alcohols are the most common cause of altered mental status and central nervous system depression. They include ethanol, methanol, and ethylene glycol. Methanol and ethylene glycol are metabolized by alcohol dehydrogenase into formic acid (in the case of methanol) and to glycolic acid and oxalic acid (in the case of ethylene glycol).

Methanol and ethylene glycol can result in death, and some survivors are left with blindness, renal dysfunction, and chronic brain injury. However, even in large ingestions, a favorable outcome is possible if the patient arrives at the hospital early enough and the poisoning is identified and appropriately treated in a timely manner.

Ethanol levels are easily and directly measured by routine clinical chemistry analyzers, however, measurement of methanol and ethylene glycol requires specialized instruments such as gas chromatography-mass spectrometry. However, suspicion for the presence of nonethanol alcohol is suspected from initial biochemistry results. The presence of a high anion gap, unaccounted for osmotic gap, metabolic acidosis, and undetectable ethanol directs investigation towards methanol and ethylene glycol. The sample is immediately sent to a reference laboratory for urgent determination and empirical therapy (blocking of alcohol dehydrogenase by either fomepizole or ethanol) and supportive therapy, and sodium bicarbonate is instituted and reviewed following the availability of methanol and ethylene glycol results.

The following criteria are often used to initiate antiethylene glycol therapy, suspected ethylene glycol ingestion (include prior history of ingestion), arterial pH < 7.3, serum bicarbonate < 20 mmol/L, osmolal gap > 10 mOsmol/L, and/or presence of oxalate crystalluria.

Since rapid measurement of ethylene glycol level is usually not readily available, the osmolal gap serves as a rapid surrogate test. The formula commonly used to calculate serum osmolality is osmolality (serum) = (2 × serum sodium) + (glucose/18) + (blood urea nitrogen/2.8). If ethanol is present in the blood, then the formula becomes osmolality (serum) = (2 × serum sodium) + (glucose/18) + (blood urea nitrogen/2.8) + (ethanol/3.7). An osmolal gap of > 10 mOsmol/L is considered a significant gap. However, the limitation is that it is insensitive in late presentations, as most of the parent alcohol has already been metabolized.

Opiates

Excessive opiate use leads to respiratory depression and unconsciousness. This is often in the form of accidental, iatrogenic, or suicidal overdose or commonly due to the use of illicit drugs.

Measurement of urinary opiates will help elucidate the cause and confirm the clinical findings of pinpointed pupils.

Administration of Naloxone reverses the neurological presentation. Although the mechanism of action is not fully understood, it is thought to act as a competitive antagonist of the mc, k, u, and alpha opiates receptors.

Neurometabolic disorders (inborn error of metabolism-associated neuropathies)

This describes neuropathy secondary to inherited metabolic disorders. About a third of the identified metabolic disorders present with some degree of neuropathy ranging from acute and chronic encephalopathy, movement disorders (myopathy, ataxia), and or behavioral abnormalities.

Developmental delay and psychomotor retardation are the most common and often progressive in nature. Acute presentation is seen in patients with amino acids and organic acids disorders, fatty acid oxidation, and mitochondrial respiratory chain defects.

Progressive psychomotor dysfunction (ataxia, myopathy, seizures) is often seen in patients with lysosomal storage disorders. Intermittent ataxia is seen in urea cycle defects, branched-chain amino acids defects (maple syrup urine disease (MSUD)), and organic acidemias.

Patients with inborn errors of metabolism will often present early in childhood, however, for some disorders, the presentation may appear late into adulthood and may be precipitated by an episode of acute illness.

Acute neurological presentations include seizures in amino acids disorders (such as maple syrup urine disease, nonkenotic hyperglycinemia), and in organic acids, fatty oxidation defects, biotin metabolism defects, and hereditary fructose intolerance, pyruvate metabolism defects, and mitochondrial reparatory chain defects.

Progressive neurological presentation is that of ataxia encountered in galactosidases, GM2 gangliosides, Niemann-Pick type C, abetalipoproteinemia, and mitochondrial electron chains defects, etc. Glycogen storage diseases are associated with generalized myopathy and muscle weakness, and rhabdomyolysis.

Patients present with developmental delay and psychomotor retardation. However, routine screening for inborn errors of metabolism in a child was developmental delay has a diagnosis yield of about 1%–5%, biochemical tests are required for suspected metabolic disorders in neuropathy.

Biochemical investigation

The biochemical investigations in patients suspected of neurometabolic disorders are best performed in a stepwise fashion.

Initial investigation

Initial biochemical laboratory investigation includes measurement of glucose, liver enzymes and bilirubin, arterial blood gases, electrolytes, ammonia, lactate, muscle enzymes (creatine kinase, lactate dehydrogenase), myoglobin, urine amino acids and organic acids, reducing substances, mucopolysaccharides screens.

Follow-up and expanded biochemical investigation

Based on findings during the initial investigation and directed by clinical course follow-up, advanced laboratory investigations include urinary organic acids, plasma carnitine and acyl carnitine profile, plasma very-long-chain fatty acids, red cell plasmalogens, plasma and urinary pipecolic acid, serum copper, ceruloplasmin, 24-h urinary copper, serum uric acid, urine uric acid/creatinine ratio, urine myoglobin, blood lipid profile and lipoproteins, cerebrospinal fluid lactate, oligoclonal bands, C-peptide, cortisol, and IGF-1 in patients with hypoglycemia as well as molecular genetic studies. Although several generic disorders exhibit ataxia and or polyneuropathy, diagnosis is often clinical with little or no diagnostic biochemical tests, but the latter are often supportive of the clinical findings and in patient management.

When an inborn error of metabolism is suspected in a patient with metabolic acidosis and an increased anion gap, and a plasma lactate level within the normal range, the patient is investigated for possible organic acidurias.

In patients with hypoglycemia and elevated lactate and pyruvate levels, the presence of glycogen storage disorders is suspected. Investigation of possible pyruvate dehydrogenase or decarboxylase deficiencies is helpful In general, urine and blood screen for organic acid disorders in patients with neuropathy is helpful.

Glucose metabolism

Hypoglycemia (regardless of the cause) leads to neurological manifestations from mild apathy and confusion to coma. With sequelae ranging from none to permanent neurological damage.

The brain has 1–2 g of glucose in the form of glycogen that is consumed within 30 min in states of hypoglycemia. Thus, hypoglycemia can cause neurological dysfunction quickly. 15% of patients with diabetes mellitus will have one episode of hypoglycemia. Additionally, those with insulinoma may present with epilepsy and neurological dysfunction before their diagnosis. Due to the recurrent and periodic nature of the disease; similarly, due to a lack of ketones when insulin is high. Ketones provide an insufficient alternate source of energy, particularly during long episodes of hypoglycemia.

Glucose measurement is easily performed at the bedside (point of care testing of capillary blood) and that a finding of low glucose confirms the clinical suspicion and management is immediately instituted and a blood sample sent to the laboratory for confirmation (limitations of the capillary POCT measurement may be lead to false hypoglycemia (see Diabetes mellitus chapter for causes of hypoglycemia)).

Similarly, hyperglycemia in uncontrolled diabetes mellitus (ketotic or nonketotic depending on the relative amount of insulin), and in iatrogenic intravenous administration, causes hyperosmolality (increased osmolality) with CNS dehydration.

Coma develops in patients with diabetic ketoacidosis when hyperglycemia, acidosis, dehydration, and severe shock ensue. The treatment as well as the state of hyperglycemia leads to cerebral edema if not managed appropriately.

Electrolytes dysfunction

Hyponatremia (sodium <120 mmol/L) whatever the cause leads to cellular swelling as fluid moves along a concentration gradient. When sodium levels fall rapidly, this overwhelms the adaptative capacity of the cells and leads to cerebral edema. Demyelination due to rapid central edema presents with quadriparesis, dysphagia, dysarthria, diplopia, and altered mental status.

Similarly, hypernatremia (sodium >150 mmol/L) causes fluid loss and cellular shrinkage, the rate of change is as important and elicits the clinical presentation. Hypernatremia occurs in states of dehydration, hypotonic fluid loss, dehydration, diarrhea, hyperglycemia, and diabetes insipidus with restricted fluid intake.

In addition to dehydration, the presence of hypercalcemia (calcium >14 mg/dL (>3.5 mmol/L)) decreases neuronal excitability. Clinical presentations range from fatigue and headache to muscle weakness and confusion.

Glycogen storage disorders

Glycogen storage disorders (Table 4) include hexosaminidase deficiency characterized by the accumulation of glycosphingolipids within neural cells. There is a spectrum of presentation; infantile presenting with myoclonic seizure, juvenile (dementia, seizures, and ataxia), childhood (muscle wasting and weakness), and adult (dementia).

Amino acid disorders

Amino acid disorders are many (Table 5) and represent a significant contributor to neurological disorders. Disorders are those due to enzyme delicacies and or organ handling and metabolism. For instance, defects in renal and gastric handling of neural amino acids may result in neurological symptoms. For instance, in Hartnup disease, there is reduced tryptophan levels (due to impaired absorption resulting in low production of nicotinamide (niacin) required for the synthesis of nicotinamide adenine dinucleotide (NAD+). This leads to neurological symptoms such as cerebellar ataxia, dysarthria, seizures, headache, dizziness, or psychiatric symptoms such as anxiety, rapid mood changes, and delirium).

Adrenoleukodystrophy

X-linked recessive generic disorder of the peroxisomal fatty acid oxidation. Resulting in the accumulation of very long fatty acid chains in the adrenal gland, myelin, and Leydig cells of the testes. Sensorimotor peripheral neuropathy, ataxia, and memory loss may also be present are the presenting feature including those associated with adrenal insufficiency. There is biochemical evidence for hypoadrenalism, the presence of high levels of very long-chain fatty acids, in both circulation and accumulation in adrenal tissue. The genic disorder is known due to a mutation in the gene ABCD1 (encoding peroxisomal transporter protein) (Table 5).

Mucopolysaccharidosis

A mucopolysaccharidosis is a group of inherited metabolic disorders of mucopolysaccharides (dermatan and heparan sulfates). The latter accumulates in neuronal cells leading to dysfunction and damage. Several disorders have been described (Table 6).

Porphyria

There are four porphyria disorders exhibiting acute neurovisceral presentation. They are acute intermittent porphyria (AIP), variegate porphyria (VP), hereditary coproporphyria, and aminolaevulinic acid (ALA) dehydratase deficient

TABLE 4 Glycogen storage disorders presenting with neurotological dysfunction.

Disorder	Enzyme	Gene	Clinical presentation
GSD type 2: Pompe's disease	Acid alpha-glucosidase	GAA (AR)	Myopathy, hypotonia, hepatomegaly, hear defects
GSD type 3: debrancher deficiency	Glycogen debranching enzyme	AGL (AR)	Hypoglycemia, hepatomegaly, myopathy, cirrhosis
GSD type 4: Andersen's disease	Glycogen branching enzyme	GBE1 (AR)	Hepatomegaly, liver dysfunction, cirrhosis, myopathy
GSD type 5: McArdle's disease	Muscle glycogen phosphorylase	PYGM (AR)	Neuromuscular presentation
GSD VI: Tarui disease	Phosphofructokinase	PFKM (AR)	Exercise intolerance. Rhabdomyolysis. Abdominal pain/vomiting with exercise. Hemolytic anemia
GSD type 9a: phosphorylase kinase deficiency	Phosphorylase kinase deficiency	PHKA2 (X linked recessive)	Cirrhosis
GSD X	Phosphoglycerate mutase	PGAM2 (AR)	Exercise intolerance. Rhabdomyolysis
GSD XI	Lactate dehydrogenase	LDHA	Exercise intolerance. Rhabdomyolysis
GSD XIII	B-enolase	ENO3 (AR)	Exercise intolerance. Rhabdomyolysis
GSD XIV (CDG type It)	Phosphoglucomutase-1	PGM1 (AR)	Exercise intolerance. Rhabdomyolysis
Phosphoglycerate kinase deficiency	Phosphoglycerate kinase-1	PGK1 (XLR)	Exercise intolerance. Rhabdomyolysis. Seizures

Modified from Tarnopolsky MA. Myopathies related to glycogen metabolism disorders. Neurotherapeutics 2018;15(4):915–927. https://doi.org/10.1007/s13311-018-00684-2. PMID: 30397902; PMCID: PMC6277299 and Lilleker JB, Keh YS, Roncaroli F, Sharma R, Roberts M. Metabolic myopathies: a practical approach. Pract Neurol 2018;18(1):14–26. https://doi.org/10.1136/practneurol-2017-001708. Epub 2017 Dec 9. PMID: 29223996.

porphyria. They exhibit a triad of abdominal pain, neuropsychiatric symptoms, and neuropathy, and patients often present with abdominal pain, nausea, vomiting, and constipation.

The VP and CP present similarly to AIP but with the additional light hypersensitivity skin lesion in the presence or absence of neurological symptoms.

Acute porphyria is often induced by drugs (e.g., steroids (contraceptives), anticonvulsants (carbamazepine and phenytoin), alcohol, and endogenous steroids (puppetry and menstrual cycle)).

The heme synthesis pathway (Fig. 2) begins in hepatocytes following the formation of δ-aminolaevulinic acid (ALA). δ-aminolaevulinic acid is neurotoxic and its accumulation secondary to the metabolic bloc in heme synthesis (Fig. 2) elicits the autonomic, peripheral, and central nervous system symptoms.

The pathophysiology of symptoms is possibly related to free radicals generation, competition with gamma-aminobutyric acids (GABA) binding sites, impaired mitochondrial function, and inability to maintain Na/K ATPase function leading to neuronal membrane instability.

Lead poisoning can also present with a similar neurologic phenotype as can hereditarytyrosinemia type B (see later).

In patients with AIP, about 10% to 40% exhibit neuropathy attacks and that can present anytime ranging from 3 to 75 days into the attack. Pain reaches intensity at 2 to 4 weeks.

Muscles predominantly affected (80%) are the proximal muscles where symptoms are in the upper limbs in 50% of patients. Complex partial seizers occur in 5% of patients and some may develop absence myoclonic jerks and tonic-clonic seizures. Patients (up to 70%) develop encephalopathy and 20%–58% of patients develop neuropsychiatric symptoms during the acute attack. The neuropsychiatric symptoms may initially present as minor behavioral changes, such as anxiety, impatience or insomnia, severe depression, anhedonia, grandiose delusions, and severe psychotic episodes, resembling symptoms more typically associated with schizophrenia.

Laboratory finding in support of acute porphyria is the finding of markedly elevated urinary porphobilinogen (PBG). The sample is tested for delta aminolaevulinic acid (ALA). This is elevated in patients with ALA dehydrates deficiency acute porphyria. Total porphyrins are also measured.

The sample is subjected to protoporphyrin fluorescence emission scanning. Protoporphyrin is fluorescent

TABLE 5 Biochemical investigations in patients presenting with neuropathy and suspected of inborn error of metabolism.

Metabolite	Abnormality	Disorder
Blood		
Plasma amino acids	High glycine	Non-ketotic hyperglycinemia
	Low serine	Serine biosynthesis defects
	High phenylalanine	Phenylketonuria (PKU)
	High-branched chain amino acids	Maple syrup urine disease (MSUD)
Uric acid	Low	Molybdenum cofactor deficiency
Copper and ceruloplasmin	Low	Menkes disease
Homocysteine	High	Methylene tetrahydrofolate reductase (MTFHR) deficiency, Disorders of vitamin B12 metabolism
Plasma VLCFA	High	Peroxisomal disorders
Isoelectric focusing of silaotransferrins	Abnormal transferrin glycoforms	Congenital disorders of glycosylation
Urine		
Organic acids	Specific organic acids	Organic acidemias (methylmalonic acid in methylmalonic aciduria and disorders of vitamin B12 metabolism)
Sulfite and sulfocysteine	High	Sulfite oxidase and molybdenum cofactor deficiency
Guanidinoacetic acid	High	GAMT deficiency
	Low	AGAT deficiency
Creatine	Low	GAMT and AGAT deficiency
	High	
α-aminoadipic semialdehyde	High	Pyridoxine dependency, sulfite oxidase, and molybdenum cofactor deficiency
CSF		
Glucose	Low CSF-Blood glucose ratio (<0.4)	GLUT1 deficiency
Lactate	High	Mitochondriopathies
Amino acids	High glycine	Non-ketotic hyperglycinemia
	Low serine	Serine biosynthesis defects
GABA	High	GABA transaminase deficiency
Glutamine	Low	Congenital glutamine deficiency
Pyridoxal 5′-phosphate	Low	PNPO deficiency, pyridoxine-dependent epilepsy
Methylene tetrahydrofolate reductase	Low	MTFHR deficiency
Biogenic monoamine metabolites	Abnormalities in the levels of 3 O-methyldopa, L-Dopa, 5-hydroxytryptophan, 5-hydroxy-indole acetic acid, homovanillic acid, 3-hydroxy-4-methoxy propylglycol	Neurotransmitter disorders, homovanillic acid, and 5-hydroxy-indole acetic acid low in PNPO deficiency and PDE
Methylation pathway metabolites	Low methionine	5 MTFHR deficiency, acquired or congenital cerebral folate deficiency, cerebral folate transporter defect

Modified from Sharma S, Prasad AN. Inborn errors of metabolism and epilepsy: current understanding, diagnosis, and treatment approaches. Int J Mol Sci 2017;18(7):1384. https://doi.org/10.3390/ijms18071384. PMID: 28671587; PMCID: PMC5535877.

TABLE 6 Mucopolysaccharidosis. Enzymes defects, metabolites detected in urine, and clinical presentations.

MPS	Defective enzymes (biochemical metabolite)	Clinical syndrome
MPS IH (Hurler syndrome) MPS IS (Scheie syndrome) MPS IH/S (Hurler-Scheie syndrome)	Alpha-L-iduronidase (Dermatan sulfate, heparan sulfate)	Corneal clouding, Stiff joints, dysostosis multiplex, coarse facies, coarse hair, macroglossia, organomegaly, intellectual disability with regression, valvular heart disease, hearing and vision impairment, inguinal and umbilical hernia, sleep apnea, hydrocephalus. Onset at 1st year (in IH), >5 years (in IS), 3–8 years (in IH/S)
MPS II (Hunter syndrome)	Iduronate sulfate sulfatase (Dermatan sulfate, heparan sulfate)	Similar to Hurler syndrome but milder and with no corneal clouding. In mild form, normal intelligence. In severe form, progressive intellectual and physical disability, death before age 15. Onset 2–4 years
MPS III (Sanfilippo syndrome)	(Heparan sulfate)	Similar to Hurler syndrome but with severe intellectual disability and mild somatic manifestations onset at 2–6 years
Type IIIA	Heparan N-sulfatase	
Type IIIB	Alpha-N-acetylglucosaminidase	
Type IIIC	Acetyl CoA: alpha-glucosaminide acetyltransferase	
Type IIID	N-acetylglucosaminine-6-sulfatase	
MPS IV (Morquio syndrome)	Keratin sulfate; in IVB, also chondroitin 6-sulfate	Similar to Hurler syndrome but with severe bone changes including odontoid hypoplasia; possibly normal intelligence. Onset at 1–4 years
Type IVA	Galactosamine-6-sulfate sulfatase	
Type IVB	Beta-galactosidase	
MPS VI (Maroteaux-Lamy syndrome)	N-Acetylgalactosamine-4sulfatase (arylsulfatase B) Dermatan sulfate	Similar to Hurler syndrome but with normal intelligence. Onset is variable but can be similar to Hurler syndrome
MPS VII (Sly syndrome)	Beta-glucuronidase (Dermatan sulfate, heparan sulfate, chondroitin 4-sulfate, chondroitin 6-sulfate)	Similar to Hurler syndrome but with greater variation in severity. Onset at 1–4 years
MPS IX (hyaluronidase deficiency)	Hyaluronidase	Bilateral soft-tissue periarticular masses, dysmorphic features, short stature, normal intelligence. Onset at 6 months

Modified from Marion RW, Paljevic E. The glycogen storage disorders. Pediatr Rev. 2020;41(1):41–44. https://doi.org/10.1542/pir.2018-0146. Erratum in: Pediatr Rev. 2020 Feb;41(2):99. PMID: 31894075 and Hicks J, Wartchow E, Mierau G. Glycogen storage diseases: a brief review and update on clinical features, genetic abnormalities, pathologic features, and treatment. Ultrastruct Pathol 2011;35(5):183–96. https://doi.org/10.3109/01913123.2011.601404. PMID: 21910565.

with a maximum emission spectrum of 624 nm. A plasma sample fluoresce emission peak at ≥624 nm is consistent with protoporphyrin and thus with variegate porphyria (Fig. 2, Table 7). If both urine and blood studies are negative or inconclusive for the determination of the acute presentation, fecal porphyrin analysis is performed to distinguish between hereditary coproporphyria and acute intermittent porphyria. The presence of hereditary coproporphyria is confirmed when the ratio of coproporphyrin III to coproporphyrin I is above 1.5, and if the ratio is below 1.5 the presence of acute intermittent porphyria is suspected.

Technical considerations: urine, blood, and fecal samples are often required in the investigation of porphyria. Ideally, samples are collected during the neurovisceral attack and presentation.

Urine samples are often the starting point of investigation in a patient presenting with an acute neurovisceral attack. Urine samples should be protected from light and sent to the clinical laboratory for analysis.

Samples (urine, blood, fecal) collected during remission are usually within normal limits for the three autosomal dominant porphyrias. However, the plasma emission spectrum for variegate porphyria in the blood remains unchanged during remission. Testing for metabolic pathway enzymes and genetics testing is recommended during periods of remission. This is indicated in patients with a past history of suspicious neurovisceral attack s and those patients at risk of the disorders.

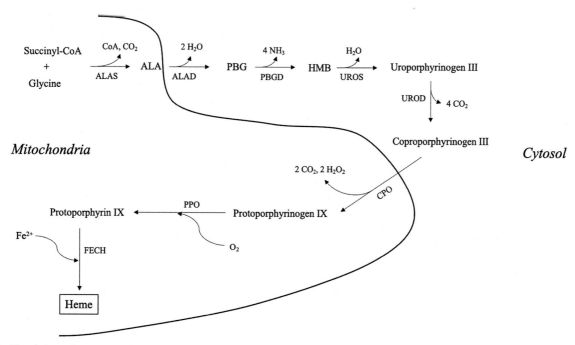

FIG. 2 Hepatic heme (iron protoporphyrin IX) synthesis metabolic pathway. *ALAS*, delta-aminolaevulinic acid synthase; *ALA*, aminolaevulinic acid; *ALAD*, aminolaevulinic acid dehydratase; *PBG*, porphobilinogen; *PBGD*, porphobilinogen deaminase; *HMB*, hydroxymethylbilane; *UROS*, uroporphyrinogen III synthase; *UROD*, uroporphyrinogen decarboxylase; *CPO*, coproporphyrinogen oxidase; *PPO*, protoporphyrinogen oxidase; *FECH*, ferro-chelatase. *(Adapted from Puy H, Gouya L, Deybach JC. Porphyrias. Lancet 2010;375(9718):924–37. https://doi.org/10.1016/S0140-6736(09)61925-5. PMID: 20226990.)*

TABLE 7 Types of porphyria, their clinical presentation, mode of inheritance, enzymatic deficiency.

Acute intermittent porphyria	Acute	Hepatic	AD	Neuro	Porphobilinogen deaminase (HMBS)
Variegate porphyria	Acute/and or cutaneous	Hepatic	AD	Neuro	Protoporphyrinogen oxidase (PPOX)
Hereditary coproporphyria	Acute and or cutaneous	Hepatic	Ad	Neuro	Coproporphyrinogen oxidase (CPOX)
Aminolaevulinic acid dehydratase deficient porphyria	Acute	Hepatic	AR	Neuro	
Porphyria cutanea tarda	Cutaneous		AD	Hepatic	Uroporphyrinogen 5-Aminolevulinic acid dehydratase (ALAD)en decarboxylase (UROD)
Hepato-erythropoietic porphyria	Cutaneous		AR	Hepatic and bone marrow	Uroporphyrinogen decarboxylase (UROD)
Congenital erythropoietic porphyria	Cutaneous	Marrow	AR		Uroporphyrinogen III synthase (UROS)
Erythropoietic protoporphyria	Cutaneous	Marrow	AR		Ferrochelatase (FECH)
X-linked erythropoietic protoporphyria	Cutaneous	Marrow	X-linked		ALA synthase 2†(ALAS2)

Adapted from O'Malley R, Rao G, Stein P, Bandmann O. Porphyria: often discussed but too often missed. Pract Neurol 2018;18(5):352–358. https://doi.org/10.1136/practneurol-2017-001878. Epub 2018 Mar 14. PMID: 29540448.

Usually, an acute attack leads to the identification of the proband case, with asymptomatic carriers of the genetic mutation in their families identified through the screening.

Hyponatremia (sodium less than 125 mmol/L) is often (40% to 90% of patients) encountered in patients presenting with acute porphyria. The hyponatremia is secondary to either the accompanying inappropriate antidiuretic hormone production (syndrome of inappropriate (ADH)) and/or a combination of increased renal and gastrointestinal loss. Although symptomatic hyponatremia is observed at a sodium of 125 mmol/L and seizures develop at a sodium of 112 mmol/L. Furthermore, the hyponatremia threshold when neurological symptoms appear may be lower in patients with porphyria. The attack could be extremely severe leading to quadriplegia and respiratory failure.

Heme is the essential prosthetic group for hemoglobin, myoglobin, respiratory cytochromes, cytochrome P450, catalase, peroxidase, tryptophan pyrrolase, and nitric oxide synthase. Heme synthesized in the bone marrow is incorporated into hemoglobin whereas heme produced in the liver is incorporated into cytochromes in the endoplasmic reticulum. Rapid synthesis of heme by hepatocytes supports the rapid turnover of cytochromes rapidly consumed in detoxification and several pathways.

Glycine and succinyl co-enzyme A condense in the presence of ALAS to form aminolaevulinic acid, the latter is converted to porphobilinogen (PBG) by ALA dehydratase and to hydroxymethylbilane by UROS, a cytosolic enzyme, catalyzes the formation of uroporphyrinogen III from hydroxymethylbilane. Only the type III isomers are precursors of heme (Fig. 2).

Defects in four steps lead to acute porphyria driven by the accumulation of ALA and PBG. Hereditary coproporphyria and variegate porphyria (termed hepatic porphyria) arise due to defects in CPO and PPO enzymes. Neurovisceral attacks are similar to that seen in acute intermittent porphyria and the cutaneous presentation are similar to that seen in porphyria curtana tarda (PCT) with the cutaneous symptoms more common in variegate porphyria comparted to hepatic coproporphyria.

Plasma and urinary PBG levels are elevated during an acute attack. Fecal porphyrin levels are predominantly elevated in coproporphyrin (HCP) (predominantly coproporphyrin III), whereas in VP (both coproporphyrin III and protoporphyrin are equally increased or protoporphyrin) while they are normal or only slightly elevated in AIP.

The fecal coproporphyrin III/I ratio is sensitive for the diagnosis of HCP, even in the asymptomatic stages of the disease. Erythrocyte PBG deaminase activity is normal in HCP and VP, and usually deficient in AIP.

Plasma porphyrin concentrations are increased in VP, seldom increased in HCP (unless there are cutaneous manifestations), and are normal or only slightly increased in AIP. A specific feature of VP is a plasma porphyrin fluorescence maximum at neutral pH of ~626 nm, which is believed to represent protoporphyrin bound covalently to plasma proteins.

Fluorometric scanning of plasma is rapid compared to extensive extraction and HPLC analysis of fecal porphyrins for identifying and detecting asymptomatic patients with VP. This plasma fluorescence scanning is also useful for rapidly differentiating VP from PCT, which displays a fluorescence peak at ~620 nm.

Circulating and urinary aminolaevulinic acid (ALA) is elevated in nonporphyria disorders (lead poisoning, and hereditary tyrosinemia type 1) disorders with similar neurological manifestations.

VP and HCP are autosomal dominant with variable penetrance and similar to AIP most heterozygous carriers remain asymptomatic. The prevalence of variegate porphyria is 1.3 per 100,000, compared to 1–9 in 1,000,000 for AIP and 0.2 per 100,000 for HCP.

The lack of phenotypic penetrance in gene carriers for AIP requires a high index of suspicion at initial presentation. Acute porphyria should be suspected in patients with unexplained abdominal pain and investigated by urgent quantitative assessment of urinary ALA and PBG using samples collected during the attack. An increase in urinary PBG confirms the clinical suspicion of AIP, HCP, or VP, and in very rare cases ADP.

If PBG urine excretion is increased, generally 50–200 mg/day (normal range ≤4 mg/day) during acute AIP attack. Urinary excretion of ALA is usually about half that of PBG (expressed as mg/day). Urinary ALA and PBG can remain elevated for prolonged periods between acute attacks, especially in AIP.

However, samples of plasma, erythrocytes, and feces should also be obtained before treatment with hemin. This approach facilitates rapid initial diagnosis of AIP, HCP, and VP, and for subsequent biochemical differentiation of these conditions.

Biochemical diagnosis of ADP includes the demonstration of markedly deficient erythrocyte ALA dehydratase activity, marked elevation in urinary ALA and coproporphyrin III and erythrocyte zinc protoporphyrin, with little or no increase in urinary porpholobilinogen. Erythrocyte ALA dehydratase activity is approximately half-normal in both parents.

Although biochemical measurements can strongly suggest ADP, the diagnosis must be confirmed by DNA studies.

Lead poisoning is identified by increased blood lead levels. Patients with hereditary tyrosinemia type I may also have ALAD inhibition and increased excretion of ALA. Succinyl acetone, a structural analog of ALA and a potent ALAD inhibitor, accumulates due to an inherited deficiency of fumaryl acetoacetate hydrolase. A diagnosis of tyrosinemia can be made by demonstrating succinyl acetone in urine by measuring ALAD activity in normal blood after the addition of a patient's urine.

Wilson's disease

Inherited disorder of copper elimination leads to the accumulation of copper in neural tissue. It is autosomal recessive. Mutation in the gene is responsible for the P-type ATPase enzyme. The latter binds to copper and facilitates its entry into the hepatocytes.

Intestinal absorption is normal. Elimination is by binding to ceruloplasmin in the Golgi apparatus and delivery to the plasma. The other is via exertion into the bile. Mutation in the P-type ATPase leads to accumulation of the free copper in the liver, brain, eye, bone, and kidney leading to the observed neuropathy. Nearly all patients with Wilson's associated neuropathy will have a Kayser-Fleischer ring at the end of the cornea.

Menkes disease

Menkes disease is a genetic disorder affecting copper uptake in the intestine resulting in copper deficiency. It is a congenital X-linked disorder with an incidence of about 1:100,000 live births. A defect in the transport protein mediating copper uptake from the intestine is encoded by the *ATP7A* gene. Copper deficiency is characterized clinically by fragile, abnormally formed hair, depigmentation of the skin, muscle weakness (myeloneuropathy), neurologic abnormalities, edema, hepatosplenomegaly, and osteoporosis. The neurologic manifestations include ataxia, neuropathy, and cognitive deficits that can mimic vitamin B12 deficiency. A variant of the *ATP7A* gene results in severe copper deficiency with progressive neurologic deterioration and death during early childhood

Abetalipoproteinemia

Patients with abetalipoproteinemia present with failure to thrive in infancy and steatorrhea and progressing with age to cerebral ataxia, dysarthria, tremors and involuntary movements, and peripheral neuropathy and may develop retinitis pigmentosa.

Abetalipoproteinemia is an autosomal recessive disorder characterized by the deficiency of beta-containing lipoproteins. This is caused by a mutation in the MTTP gene (microsomal triglycerides transfer protein) essential for the hepatic synthesis of beta-lipoproteins.

The condition impairs the absorption of fat-soluble vitamins (K, A, E, and D) and is possibly secondary to vitamin E deficiency. Anemia, and red blood cell acanthocytosis. Abnormal liver enzymes due to fatty liver

Nutrition-associated neuropathies

Vitamins and micronutrient deficiency lead to neurological presentations. Neurological disorders such as myopathy and ataxia present either in acute or chronic form. The biochemical investigation includes an assessment of thiamine status, folate, B12, vitamin E, as well as trace elements. There are risk factors for nutritional deficiencies; they include old age, eating disorders, malabsorption syndromes, alcohol abuse, pregnancy, liver and pancreatic dysfunction, gastrointestinal disorders, long-term use of total parenteral nutrition, as well as social determinants.

Nutritional neuropathy manifestation includes acute, subacute, or chronic in nature. They can either be axonal, demyelinating, or myeloneuropathy (combined myelopathy and peripheral neuropathy) seen in B1w2 and copper deficiencies.

Thiamine B1

Thiamine (vitamin B1) is a cofactor for the red blood cell transketolaminase where the reduced activity of the RBC transketolaminase activity supports thiamine deficiency. Thiamine deficiency is often seen in patients with alcohol abuse, nutritional insufficiency secondary to malabsorption, anorexia nervosa, hyperemesis gravidarum, and in patients on total parenteral nutrition (TPN).

Recommended daily allowance (RDA) for thiamine ranges from 1.0 mg in young healthy adults to 1.5 mg for athletes and patients with higher metabolic needs as seen during pregnancy, systemic infections, and in certain cancers where a higher daily intake is required.

Neuropathy due to thiamine deficiency, known as beri-beri, was the first clinically described deficiency syndrome in humans. Patients present with ataxia, eye movement disorder, and confusion being the whole mark of Wernicke-Korsakoff encephalopathy. Serum thiamine levels are variably influenced by dietary intake and therefore do not reflect body store status. However, measurements of erythrocyte transketolase activity or thiamine pyrophosphate are preferred. Testing is performed before thiamine supplementation.

However, clinically the diagnosis is often made by a process of elimination in the presence of chronic liver disease and alcoholism. It is important to note administration of glucose in the malnourished patient results in the refeeding syndrome and thus reduced thiamine levels exacerbating the encephalopathy. Giving thiamine before glucose prevents the refeeding syndrome.

Vitamin B12 deficiency

Vitamin B12 (cobalamin) is obtained from food intake and despite B12 fortification in diets, deficiency occurs and is observed in 5% to 20% of the elderly and in states of increased utilization such as in pregnancy. Recommended daily intake for vitamin B12 is 2.4 mcg.

Dietary B12 is released from food by gastric acid and pepsin. Free B12 binds to an intrinsic factor, and it is the B12-intrinsic factor complex that is absorbed in the terminal ileum. Deficiency of B12 can thus be secondary to intrinsic factor deficiency. The latter is seen in pernicious anemia. A common cause of B12 deficiency. It is an autoimmune disorder characterized by the destruction of the gastric mucosa. Patients exhibit circulating parietal cell and intrinsic factor antibodies leading to impaired B12 absorption. Pernicious anemia is common among blacks and northern Europeans.

Vitamin B12 deficiency results in neurological as well as hematological abnormalities. The onset of symptoms is insidious with a continuum of peripheral neuropathy symmetrical uncomfortable tingling paresthesia initially in the feet but later involving the hands progressing to ataxia, optic neuropathy, myelopathy, and encephalopathy due to white matter degeneration.

Measurement of B12 levels helps confirm clinical suspicion and also helps distinguish it from clinically similar cryptogenic sensory polyneuropathy.

In the presence of anemia (macrocytic), high mean corpuscular volume (MCV) (>100), hypersegmented neutrophils, few neutrophils exhibit >5 lobes, neuropathy (described above), B12 levels <200 pg/mL confirms B12 deficiency.

However, B12 levels up to 300–400 pg/mL may also harbor deficiency in some patients. In those patients with hematological and clinical indices and low normal B12 levels, measurement of methylmalonic acid (MMA) and homocysteine levels improves the diagnostic sensitivity. Elevated MMA and homocysteine levels confirm the clinical suspicion of B12 deficiency. False positive MMA and homocysteine are seen in patients with renal impairment and those with hypovolemia. Additionally, isolated homocysteine elevation may also be seen in hypothyroidism, deficiency of folic acid and pyridoxine and in elderly patients, and in those smoking.

Detection of circulating antiintrinsic factor antibodies (high specificity, low sensitivity) as well as antiparietal cell antibodies (high sensitivity, low specificity) help conform the diagnosis of pernicious anemia.

The pathophysiology is not clear, but since B12 is a cofactor in the conversion of homocysteine to methionine and of methylmalonyl-CoA to succinyl-CoA it is plausible that impaired synthesis of methionine leads to the depletion of s-adenosylmethionine required for myeline synthesis and in the formation of tetrahydrofolate a precursor of purine and pyrimidines (DNA synthesis).

Vitamin B12 levels are easily measured and early correction of B12 deficiency improves prognosis, and the neurological damage can be reversed.

And that major residual disability remains in patients presenting late with advanced disease. Common therapeutic supplementation is 1000 mcg intramuscularly daily for 5–7 days, followed by monthly 1000 mcg intramuscular injections among other approaches, however, periodic monitoring of B12 levels is required to help avoid inappropriate levels.

Vitamin E deficiency

Vitamin E (α-tocopherol) is one of the fat-soluble vitamins (K, A, and D). Vitamin E deficiency is rare as it is abundantly present in the diet. The recommended dietary daily intake is 15 mg of the biologically active form of vitamin E (alpha-tocopherol).

Dietary vitamin E is incorporated initially into dietary chylomicrons before being transferred to chylomicron remnants and to very low-density lipoprotein (VLDL) via alpha-tocopherol transfer protein (TTP) when it is passively absorbed in the intestine. Bile acids, fatty acids, and monoglycerides are required for absorption.

Therefore, most vitamin E deficiencies occur in patients with fat malabsorption or due to a rare autosomal transport protein deficiency due to autosomal recessive mutation in the α-tocopherol transfer protein gene located on chromosome 8q13. Similarly, vitamin E and other fat-soluble vitamins deficiency are encountered in abetalipoproteinemia a rare autosomal dominant disorder due to mutations in the microsomal triglycerides transfer protein. This results in fat malabsorption.

α-tocopherol deficiency is also observed in patients with malnutrition, chronic alcohol abuse, or renal patients receiving long-term dialysis.

Vitamin E is an antioxidant and scavenger of free radicals and plays a role in marinating cell membrane structure and antioxidant status. Los of those protective activities in states of vitamin E deficiency is postulated to contribute to the neurological manifestations.

Alpha-tocopherol is stored in adipose tissue and symptoms of vitamin E deficiency take 5 to 10 years to manifest and symptoms appear and progress slowly.

Clinical features of vitamin E deficiency mimic Friederich's ataxia and include ataxia, loss of deep tendon reflexes, and loss of proprioception and vibration. Other findings include anemia, dysarthria, nystagmus, ophthalmoparesis, pigmented retinopathy, head titubation, decreased sensation, and proximal muscle weakness. Pes cavus, and scoliosis may also be present.

Vitamin E deficiency is easily confirmed by measuring circulating α-tocopherol levels. Levels <5 mcg/mL (<11.6 mcmol/L) are consistent with deficiency, however, levels may be normal even when deficiency is present particularly in patients with dyslipidemia. The ratio of total serum α-tocopherol to the total serum lipid concentration has been suggested to improve vitamin E status assessment. Ratio of serum α-tocopherol to total lipids (<0.8 mg/g total lipids) is a better indicator of deficiency in adults with hyperlipidemia. Deficiency is corrected with supplementation often with vitamin A.

Folate deficiency

Folate deficiency is a risk factor for neuropathy. Patients exhibit slowly progressive and sensory-dominant patterns, which was different from thiamine-deficiency neuropathy. The risk of peripheral neuropathy among adults increased as serum folate decreased, and even insufficient serum folate of 6.8 to 13.5 nmol/L appeared to be important. In the developing fetus, folate deficiency increases the risk for neural tubular defects. Folate deficiency has been reported during pregnancy, in pediatric and geriatric patients where there is increased demand for folate, and in conditions such as hemolysis, leukemia, and exfoliative dermatitis which are associated with rapid cellular proliferation. Jejunum disease and short-bowel syndrome cause malabsorption, and bacterial overgrowth, as well as drugs such as alcohol, anticonvulsants, oral contraceptives, and folate antagonists (methotrexate, trimethoprim, and pyrimethamine), have been shown to cause folate deficiency.

Other vitamins

Deficiency in niacin (vitamin B3) and pantothenic acid (vitamin B5) is associated with peripheral neuropathy. Supplementation of niacin with statins has been shown to reduce the risk of peripheral neuropathy in patients with dyslipidemia and on statin therapy.

Vitamin B5 is an obligatory cofactor for acetyl-coenzyme A. The latter is necessary for myelin synthesis and of the neurotransmitter acetylcholine. Symptoms of deficiency include headache, fatigue, irritability, insomnia, nausea, vomiting, numbness and burning sensation in hands and feet, and muscle cramps. Supplementation in patients with diabetic neuropathy improves symptoms.

Vitamin B6

Vitamin B6 encompasses six interconvertible pyridine compounds. They are pyridoxine, pyridoxamine, and pyridoxal, and their 5'-phosphorylated forms pyridoxine 5'-phosphate, pyridoxamine 5'-phosphate, and pyridoxal 5'-phosphate. It is an essential vitamin with pyridoxal 5'-phosphate being the biologically active compound serving as a cofactor for over 140 enzymatic reactions. It is thus central to the maintenance and proper functioning of many pathways including those of synthesis, degradation, and amino acids and their interconversion, neurotransmitter metabolism, amine biosynthesis, lipid metabolism, heme synthesis, nucleic acid synthesis, and protein and polyamine synthesis among several.

Vitamin B6 (pyridoxine) is readily and adequately available in diets and that deficiency is rare. The recommended daily requirement is 1.3 mg with an upper limit of 100 mg.

Following absorption, pyridoxine is converted to the major metabolite pyridoxal phosphate, a co-factor in several metabolic pathways.

Pyridoxal 5'-phosphate is a coenzyme in the synthesis of neurotransmitters (D-serine, D-aspartate, L-glutamate, glycine, γ-aminobutyric acid (GABA), serotonin, epinephrine, norepinephrine, histamine, and dopamine).

Levels of pyridoxal 5'-phosphate are tightly regulated and abnormal levels (low or high) leads to many disorders. Vitamin B6 is unique among vitamin disorders in that neuropathy can present is both states of deficiency or excess.

Vitamin B6 deficiency (deficiency of pyridoxal 5'-phosphate) leads to epileptic encephalopathies. Deficiency is most often encountered in patients receiving B6 antagonist medications (isoniazid phenelzine, hydralazine, penicillamine). Deficiency is also encountered during excessive metabolic needs as in pregnancy and during lactation.

Inherited metabolic disorder of pyridoxine deficiency is seen in infancy. VitB6-dependent epileptic encephalopathies (B6EEs) are a clinically and genetically heterogeneous group of rare inherited metabolic disorders. They are characterized by recurrent seizures in the prenatal, neonatal, or postnatal period, which are typically resistant to conventional anticonvulsant treatment.

In addition to seizures, children affected with B6EEs may also suffer from developmental and/or intellectual disabilities, along with structural brain abnormalities. Five main types of B6EEs are known to date that are PN-dependent epilepsy due to ALDH7A1 (antiquitin) deficiency (PDE-ALDH7A1), hyperprolinemia type 2, PLP-dependent epilepsy due to PNPO deficiency, hypophosphatasia, and PLPBP deficiency.

Clinical presentation is that seizures in infants (with inborn errors deficiency of pyridoxin) and of neuropathy in adults.

Neuropathy symptoms include numbness, paresthesia, a length-dependent polyneuropathy with decreased distal sensation (initial burning pain in the feet ascending to affect the legs and hands), reduction of deep tendon reflexes, ataxia, and mild distal weakness.

Whereas, vitamin B6 (pyridoxal 5'-phosphate) excess leads to motor and sensory neuropathies. Excess levels are due to either dietary sources or to a genetic abnormality.

Vitamin B6 toxicity is secondary to excessive supplementation. Symptoms of toxicity include sensory ataxia, areflexia, and impaired cutaneous sensation. Patients often complain of burning or paresthesia.

Circulating pyridoxal phosphate can also be measured in the blood to confirm clinical suspicion of either deficiency or toxicity. The reference range for pyridoxal phosphate (PLP), the biologically active form of vitamin B6, is 5–50 μg/L. <3.4 mcg/L deficiency, 3.4–5.1 mcg/L marginal, >5.1 mcg/L is adequate.

Trace elements

Neuropathy is encountered in patients with deficiency or excess circulating and tissue levels of various trace elements such as selenium, manganese, and copper.

Selenium

Selenium an ultra-trace element (with recommended daily dosage of 20 mcg in children rising to 55 mcg in adults) plays important roles in many metabolic pathways. Optimal levels of selenium are narrow with a risk for toxicity if supplemented in patients with normal or high selenium intake.

Selenium is essential with over 30 seleno-proteins including glutathione peroxidase important in antioxidant defense, and iodothyronine deiodinase 2 (three forms), which play a role in the production of thyroid hormones. Severe selenium deficiency is associated with skeletal muscle dysfunction and cardiomyopathy, mood disorders, and impaired immune function.

Clinical manifestations of selenium toxicity include nausea, emesis, diarrhea, hair loss, nail changes, mental status changes, visual loss, and peripheral neuropathy. Magnetic resonance imaging (MRI) of the brain in patients with selenium toxicity may indicate abnormalities resembling the reversible posterior encephalopathy syndrome.

Manganese

Manganese toxicity is seen in workers exposed to manganese dust in welding or steel industries and individuals drinking well water with high manganese concentration. High manganese levels are neurotoxic primarily affecting the extrapyramidal parts of the brain with symptoms similar to Parkinson's disease. They include ataxia, loss of coordination and balance, confusion, headache, and vomiting. Serum and whole-blood manganese measurements are used to investigate suspicion of toxicity. Patients on long-term parenteral nutrition require monitoring for possible manganese toxicity, particularly in patients with cholestasis and decreased manganese excretion.

Copper

Copper is an essential trace element present at 62 to 140 mcg/dL in circulation. It plays a significant role in metabolism and is an important cofactor of metalloenzymes including superoxide dismutase, cytochrome oxidase, and tyrosinase with roles in many metabolic pathways including hematopoiesis and protective antioxidative reactions.

Rich sources of copper are seafood, nuts, wheat, and grains. The adult daily recommended dosage is 900 mcg.

Following solubilization by gastric acid, dietary copper is absorbed by the intestine. Two mechanisms of copper absorption are present: a predominant active absorption when dietary copper levels are low and a passive diffusion absorption mechanism when dietary copper levels are high. In the circulation, absorbed copper binds to plasma proteins and via the portal vein, reaches the liver where it is incorporated into ceruloplasmin, the format reaching cells. Excess copper is excreted into the bile.

Common causes of copper deficiency include gastric surgery (reduced gastric acid) and excessive dietary zinc intake (or in dental creams). For the latter mechanism, both zinc and copper bind to metallothionines, and copper has a higher binding affinity compared to zinc. In the presence of excess zinc, metallothionine production is upregulated and the high avidity of copper displaces zinc from the upregulated metallothionines in enterocytes. Zinc is then absorbed into the blood and the complex copper-metallothionine remains in enterocytes and is shed into the feces during the normal sloughing of cells.

Copper deficiency is when plasma copper levels are <40 mcg/dL and plasma ceruloplasmin level is <13 mg/dL.

Copper deficiency is best recognized in malabsorption syndrome, inflammatory bowel disease, gastric acid deficiencies, and genetically in Menkes disease characterized by the inability to transport copper across the intestinal barrier due to a mutation in the *ATP7A* gene.

Copper is absorbed in the proximal small intestine, primarily in the duodenum, and to a lesser extent in the stomach and more distal small intestine. Thus, impaired intestinal and or gastric absorption leads to copper deficiency. Additionally, copper deficiency is encountered secondary to excess intake of zinc (see later). Copper deficiency can also be seen in association with excess iron consumption.

Copper deficiency is a known cause of hematologic abnormalities where copper deficiency hinders iron transport and utilization at several key points and impairs heme synthesis leading to sideroblastic anemia and neutropenia, however, the contribution of the deficiency to neurological abnormalities was later attributed to peripheral neuropathy, myelopathy, or a myeloneuropathy to copper deficiency.

Patients present with gait difficulty and lower limb paresthesia, loss of proprioception and vibration due to dorsal column dysfunction and sensory ataxia, upper motor neuron signs (bladder dysfunction), brisk knee jerks, and extensor plantar reflexes. A motor neuron disease-like presentation has also been reported.

In copper deficiency serum copper, ceruloplasmin and urinary excretion of copper are low. Zinc levels are often high. Ceruloplasmin is an acute-phase reactant protein and thus in inflammatory states elevated and normal levels are misleading.

In patients with copper toxicity (e.g., Wilson's disease), the development of neurodegenerative disorders such as Parkinson's and Alzheimer diseases are associated with the copper accumulation and toxicity.

It is an autosomal recessive genetic disorder due to mutations in the intracellular copper transporter ATP7B gene. Prevalence is about one case in 30,000 live births in most populations. The mutation leads to impaired biliary copper excretion.

An excessive amount of copper accumulates in the liver (hepatolenticular degeneration), brain (neuropsychiatric dysfunction), and eye (green-to-brownish ring (Kayser-Fleischer ring) surrounding the colored part of the eye leading to abnormalities in eye movements and restricted ability to gaze upwards), manifestations are common.

Neuro-psychiatric disorders present in 18% to 73% of patients and are often the initial features in young adults with Wilson disease. Symptoms include clumsiness, tremors, difficulty walking, speech problems, impaired thinking ability, depression, anxiety, and mood swings.

Nearly all (98%) of patients with Wilson disease with neurologic manifestations have Kayser-Fleischer rings. Furthermore, neurologic symptoms may be very subtle or may be rapidly progressive, leading to severe disability over the course of months.

Common neurological manifestations include (dysarthria (85% to 97%), gait abnormalities/ataxia (30% to 75%), dystonia (11% to 69%), tremors (22% to 55%), and Parkinsonism (19% to 62%)). In patients with marked hepatic cirrhosis, neurologic manifestations may be mistaken for hepatic encephalopathy.

Laboratory investigations include liver tests (enzymes, and bilirubin), full blood count, serum ceruloplasmin and copper levels, and a 24-h urinary copper excretion. The outcomes may be sufficient to make a diagnosis of Wilson disease, but few patients will have indeterminate results that will require a liver biopsy with copper quantitation and histologic evaluation and or molecular testing for ATP7B mutations.

Bariatric surgery (iatrogenic nutritional neuropathy)

Bariatric surgery is an effective often last resort in patient weight management. Neuropathies secondary to bariatric surgery occur and may cause complications ranging from diffuse encephalopathy to peripheral neuropathy to myopathy. Peripheral neuropathy is the most common and may affect up to 16% of patients with three dominant patterns. Sensory predominant (acute, subacute, and chronic), mononeuropathy, and radiculoplexopathy with sensory and mono-neuropathy being the most common.

Although the effect of bariatric surgery may be complicated by malnutrition and restricted dietary intake either before or following the surgical intervention and the onset of symptoms may vary from months to years and may be subacute to insidious.

Following bariatric surgery, the most encountered nutrient deficiencies are thiamine, vitamin B12, vitamin E, vitamin D, and copper.

Laboratory assessment of thiamine, B12, and copper is required at baseline metabolic assessment for patients undergoing bariatric surgery, particularly patients (commonly encountered) who were on weight management dietary restriction before surgery. Periodic laboratory assessment of thiamine, vitamin B12, vitamin E, vitamin D, and copper is essential in ascertaining the adequacy of post-surgical nutritional supplements and appropriate adjustments to prevent peripheral neuropathy developed post-bariatric surgery.

Infection-associated encephalopathy

Infection-associated encephalopathy is associated with reduced oxygen and blood flow, edema, accumulation of toxins, and inflammatory markers that cause neurological deficits.

Meningitis

Meningitis, inflammation of the meninges, secondary to viral or bacterial infection. Bacterial meningitis although relatively uncommon in the developed world remains a significant burden in developing nations. Viral meningitis is more common and is associated with aseptic culture.

Comparative measurements of cerebrospinal fluid (CSF) and plasma total proteins and glucose levels are essential in the biochemical investigation of the etiology of meningitis (Table 8). CSF total protein is elevated compared to serum and glucose levels are within the 60% cutoff. Bacterial meningitis will exhibit much higher CSF total proteins levels and markedly reduced glucose compared to that in plasma often with a ratio of $\leq 40\%$.

Other markers are those of CSF lactate, and interleukin 6. Lactate and Il-6 are higher in bacterial and fungal infection compared to that due to viral infection similar to proteins, but glucose is lower than 60% to that of blood in patients with bacterial and fungal infection.

Microscopy and microbiological culture confirm the source of infection. White blood cell counts are elevated in both bacterial and viral meningitis.

Sepsis-associated encephalopathy

This clinical entity describes the neurological manifestation of systemic sepsis. Clinical presentation ranges from delirium to coma. The incidence is 50% and varies from 8% to more than 70% of septic patients admitted to the intensive care units and is associated with high mortality. Furthermore, long-term cognitive and functional outcomes are poor. The pathophysiology includes neuro-inflammation, ischemia, vascular changes, and metabolic failures.

Autoimmune encephalopathy

Autoimmune encephalitis is a clinical presentation with a high index of suspicion necessitating frequent and extensive laboratory investigations. The majority of immunology

TABLE 8 Laboratory findings in cerebrospinal samples from patients with infection and traumatic injuries.

Dysfunction	Appearance	Cell count (/uL)	Protein, mg/dL (g/L)	Glucose, mg/dL (mmol/L)	Glucose CSF/Plasma ratio
Bacterial infection (acute)	Turbid	1000–10,000 (polymorphonuclear cells)	100–500 (10–50)	<40 (<2.2)	Low
Tuberculosis	Opaque	100–600 (lymphocytes, mixed cells)	Increased	Low	Low
Viral infection	Clear	5–300 (rarely >1000) (lymphocytes)	Normal/mildly increased	Normal	Normal/low
Fungal infection	Cloudy	40–400 (mixed cells)	Increased	Low	Low
Subarachnoid hemorrhage	Xanthochromic	Increased (slight)	Increased	Normal	Low
Normal	Clear	0–4 (lymphocytes)	23–38 (2.3–3.8)	50–80 (2.8–4.4)	0.6

Adapted from Thomson RB Jr, Bertram H. Laboratory diagnosis of central nervous system infections. Infect Dis Clin N Am 2001;15(4):1047–71. https://doi.org/10.1016/s0891-5520(05)70186-0. PMID: 11780267.

tests are often referred to outside specialized laboratories with significant costs.

It is as common as infectious encephalitis with an estimated prevalence of 13.7 per 100,000. This noninfectious autoimmune-mediated inflammatory condition targets the brain parenchyma and often involves cortical or gray matter with or without the involvement of the white matter, or meninges and spinal cord.

Autoimmune causes

In antibody-mediated encephalopathy, there are two types of antibodies: (a) Antibodies to intracellular proteins that are associated with malignancy, and that (b) against extracellular domains of neural cell surface proteins. The latter causes encephalitis compared to these against intracellular proteins.

The antibodies involved are often in response to a T-cell-mediated immunity against a neoplasm with a secondary response against the nervous system. Common antibodies found were against neuronal surface or synaptic antigens. Examples are N-methyl-D-aspartate receptor (NMDAR)-antibody and leucine-rich glioma inactivated (LGI1)-antibody.

The paraneoplastic syndrome occurs in <1% of malignancies and can present much earlier than the cancer is diagnosed. More than 25% of the syndrome presents with sensory and autonomic neuropathies and Lambert-Easton myasthenic syndrome. The most common underlying malignancy (50%–75%) is patients with small cell carcinoma of the bronchus. These markers despite their association with a particular cancer type are not reliable in determining the origin of cancer.

Memory loss, behavioral disturbances, and seizures are the often clinical presentation that initiates serological testing for antibodies and associated antigens. The target

antigens tested for and their associated malignancy are; Hu (Bronchial small cell carcinoma), Ma2 (testicular tumor), collapsing response mediator protein-5 (lymphoma) and small cell lung carcinoma, and nonneuronal nuclear 3 (small cell lung carcinoma). The extracellular circulating receptor antibodies tested for include those directed against; voltage-gated channel, glutamine receptor 1,2 subunits (in SCLC, breast thymoma), gamma-aminobutyric acid-B-receptor (in SCLC), Glutamic acid decarboxylase receptor, and N-methyl-D-aspartate receptor (in ovarian teratoma, and rarely testicular teratoma or SCLC).

Paraneoplastic encephalitis is confirmed following the detection of the specific antibodies above. Other antibodies causing encephalopathy include antithyroglobulin and anti-thyroid peroxidase antibodies in patients with Hashimoto's thyroiditis. Those antibodies are often performed at a reference laboratory, at high expense and thus review for improved utilization is warranted (Table 9).

Systemic lupus erythematosus (SLE)

Systemic lupus erythematosus (SLE) is a chronic autoimmune disease that can affect any organ, including the nervous system. Estimates of the incidence and prevalence of neurologic and psychiatric symptoms among patients with SLE vary greatly with various studies reporting that approximately one-third to one-half of SLE patients report neurologic or neuropsychiatric symptomatology.

Sarcoidosis

Sarcoidosis is characterized by noncaseating granulomatous inflammation, affecting multiple systems throughout

TABLE 9 Clinical and laboratory findings associated with various autoimmune encephalitis.

Anatomical classification of autoimmune encephalitis	Corresponding clinical syndromes	Possible associated antibodies
Limbic encephalitis	Cognitive, psychiatric, and epileptic presentation	Hu, CRMP5/CV2, Ma2, NMDAR, AMPAR, LGI1, CASPR2, GAD65, GABABR, DPPX, mGluR5, AK5, Neurexin-3α antibodies
Cortical/subcortical encephalitis	Cognitive, seizure presentation	PCA-2 (MAP1b), NMDAR, GABA A/B R, DPPX, MOG antibodies
Striatal encephalitis	Movement disorder presentation	CRMP5/CV2, DR2, NMDAR, LGI1, PD10A antibodies
Diencephalic encephalitis	Autonomic, sleep disorder presentation	Ma 1–2, IgLON5, DPPX, AQP4 antibodies
Brainstem encephalitis	Cognitive, movement disorder, Cranio-bulbar presentation	Ri, Ma 1–2, KLHL11, IgLON5, DPPX, AQP4, MOG, GQ1b antibodies
Cerebellitis or cerebellar degeneration	Ataxic presentation	Hu, Ri, Yo, Tr, CASPR2, KLHL11, NIF, mGluR1, GAD65, VGCC antibodies
Meningoencephalitis	Cognitive, seizure, meningeal presentation	GFAP antibody or seronegative AE
Encephalomyelitis	Movement disorder presentation including PERM and SPS; Spinal, Opticospinal presentation	GAD65, amphyphysin, glycine receptor, PCA-2 (MAP1B), GABA A/B R, DPPX, CRMP5/CV2, AQP4, MOG antibodies
Possible associated peripheral syndromes		
Neuropathy/neuronopathy	Ataxic, Sensoriomotor presentation	Hu, PCA-2 (MAP1B), CRMP5, Amphiphysin, CASPR2, CASPR1, CONTACTIN1, NIF155 antibodies
Autonomic neuropathy/ganglionopathy	Autonomic presentation	Hu, CRMP5, antiganglionic AChR antibodies
Neuromuscular junction dysfunction	Myasthenic presentation	VGCC, AchR antibodies
Myopathy	Motor presentation	Striational antibodies

AchR, Acetyl choline receptor; AE, autoimmune encephalitis; AK5, Adenylate kinase 5 Ab; AMPAR, α-amino-3-hydroxy-5-methyl-4-isoxazolepropionic acid receptor; AQP4, aquaporin-4; CASPR, Contactin-associated protein-like; CRMP5, Collapsin response mediator protein 5; DPPX, Dipeptidyl-peptidase-like protein 6; GABAR, gamma-amino butyric acid receptor; GAD65, glutamic acid decarboxylase 65; GFAP, glial fibrillary acidic protein; GQ1b, ganglioside Q1B antibody; IgLON5, immunoglobulin-like cell adhesion molecule 5; KLHL11, Kelch-like protein 11; LGI1, Leucine-rich glioma inactivated; mGluR1, metabotropic glutamate receptor 1; mGluR5, metabotropic glutamate receptor; MOG, myelin oligodendrocyte glycoprotein; NIF, neuronal intermediate filament; NMDAR, N-methyl-D-aspartate receptor; PCA2, Purkinje cell cytoplasmic Ab type 2; PERM, progressive encephalomyelitis with rigidity and myoclonus; SPS, stiff-person syndrome; VGCC, voltage gated calcium channel.
Modified from Abboud H, Probasco JC, Irani S, Ances B, Benavides DR, Bradshaw M, Christo PP, Dale RC, Fernandez-Fournier M, Flanagan EP, Gadoth A, George P, Grebenciucova E, Jammoul A, Lee ST, Li Y, Matiello M, Morse AM, Rae-Grant A, Rojas G, Rossman I, Schmitt S, Venkatesan A, Vernino S, Pittock SJ, Titulaer MJ; Autoimmune Encephalitis Alliance Clinicians Network. Autoimmune encephalitis: proposed best practice recommendations for diagnosis and acute management. J Neurol Neurosurg Psychiatry 2021;92(7):757–768. https://doi.org/10.1136/jnnp-2020-325300. Epub 2021 Mar 1. PMID: 33649022; PMCID: PMC8223680.

the body. It exhibits neurological manifestations in about 5%–15% of cases. The neurological presentation includes cranial neuropathies, meningeal disease, parenchymal disease, spinal cord involvement, vasculopathy, and peripheral nervous system disease.

Celiac disease

Celiac disease is a chronic immune-mediated enteropathy disorder where dietary gluten triggers an inflammatory response. There is a genetic predisposition to the disease and clinical presentation is variable. The manifestation, in addition to intestinal inflammation, is secondary to side effects such as iron-deficiency anemia, osteoporosis, dermatitis hypertiformis, and neurologic disorders. Gluten ataxia usually has an insidious onset with a mean age at onset of 53 years.

Patients presenting with neurological symptoms without gastrointestinal symptoms. Due to active case findings, presenting symptoms have changed to that of the extraintestinal component. Manifestations include a broad spectrum of musculoskeletal and neurological (about 6% of patients exhibit peripheral neuropathy and ataxia). Patients with ataxia often present with difficulty with arm and leg control, gait instability, poor coordination, loss of fine motor skills such as writing, problems with talking, and visual issues. Other neurological symptoms include encephalopathy, myopathy, myelopathy, ataxia with myoclonus, and chorea.

Termed gluten neuropathy, it is sporadic and idiopathic neuropathy in the absence of an alternative etiology and in the presence of serological evidence of gluten sensitivity.

A third of patients will have evidence of enteropathy on biopsy, but the presence or absence of enteropathy does not predetermine the effect of a gluten-free diet therapeutic intervention.

Peripheral neuropathy is in the form of tingling, numbness, and pain initially in the hands and feet.

Patients with gluten ataxia also often show oligoclonal bands in cerebrospinal fluid, evidence of perivascular inflammation in the cerebellum as well as anti-Purkinje cell antibodies.

Adherence to a strict gluten-free diet results in clinical improvement in both gluten neuropathy and gluten ataxia. The manifestations may, however, exist in the presence of antigluten antibody alone without evidence of enteropathy. Those patients equally benefit from a gluten-free diet.

Endocrine disorders associated with neurological presentations

Patients with endocrine-related disorders (Table 10) may exhibit some degree of neurological dysfunction in the form of peripheral neuropathy and or encephalopathy.

Hypothyroidism leads to carpel tunnel syndrome secondary to the deposition of mucopolysaccharides. Similarly, growth hormone excess leads to edema swelling of the median nerve leading to carpel tunnel syndrome or secondary to associated diabetes in acromegaly.

Hyperthyroidism leads to peripheral neuropathy seen more often in patients presenting with thyroid storm.

Malignancy-associated causes

Paraneoplastic syndrome

Paraneoplastic syndrome affects <1% of patients with cancer. However, neuropathy and cancer are more common, they may be co-present by chance. Thus, a well-characterized criterion for paraneoplastic syndrome is necessary. Additionally, paraneoplastic disorders (e.g., peripheral; neuropathy) may develop before cancer detection or during cancer (Table 11).

Paraneoplastic syndromes are widely and increasingly encountered in patients with malignancy. The cause is an immune response against neural proteins expressed by

TABLE 10 Metabolic disorders associated with peripheral neuropathy and associated biomarkers.

Metabolic disorder	Biomarker/Investigation
Diabetes	Glucose (fasting, random, tolerance test, A1c) Hypo/hyperglycemia
Renal dysfunction	eGFR, creatinine, urea, electrolytes
Herpetic dysfunction	Bilirubin, ammonia, albumin, liver enzymes
Endocrine	Thyroid hormones (FT4, T3, TSH)
Paraproteinemia (multiple myeloma)	Protein electrophoresis (serum and urine) plus immunofixation. Bence Jones protein Antinuclear antibodies (ANA), antineuronal antibodies, antiganglioside antibodies, myelin, and connective tissue antibodies.
Nutritional deficiencies/factors	Vitamins (B1, B3, B5, B6, B12, E, folic acid, pyridoxine), hypophosphatasemia, copper deficiency
Infection. Viral	Microbiology tests and culture, viral serology (HIV)
Inborn errors of metabolism	Porphyria, mitochondrial disorders, amyloid disorders, Refsum disease, Fabry disease, Tangier disease (Metabolites plus molecular generic tests)
	Other inherited biochemical disorders include fatty acid oxidation disorders, Carnitine palmitoyltransferase II deficiency, very-long-chain acyl-Coenzyme A dehydrogenase deficiency, multiple acyl-Coenzyme A dehydrogenase deficiency, disorders of purine metabolism, myoadenylate deaminase deficiency, and mitochondrial disorders
Paraneoplastic disorders	Malignancy, carcinoma, lymphoma. Malignancy-associated proteins and antibodies
Drugs/toxins	Drugs levels measurement and toxicology screens

Modified from Barrell K, Smith AG. Peripheral neuropathy. Med Clin North Am 2019;103(2):383–397. https://doi.org/10.1016/j.mcna.2018.10.006. Epub 2018 Dec 17. PMID: 30704689.

tumors, and testing for paraneoplastic antibodies, a series of antibodies thought to be an autoimmune response to neuronal antigens expressed on cancer cells, is widely employed in the investigation of patients presenting with neurological symptoms and suspected of malignancy. The incidence of their presence is reported to be variable (0.5%–1% of all cancer patients) and their elevation is one of the diagnostic criteria of paraneoplastic syndrome.

TABLE 11 Classification of paraneoplastic cancers neuropathy and associated antibodies.

Neuropathy	Malignancy	Reported case number	Abs and other biomarkers	Other criteria for definite paraneoplastic	Comments
Neuronopathies					
Sensory neuronopathy	SCLC 80%—HL and other carcinomas	>500	Hu, CV2/CRMP5, other onconeural	–	One case with Ma2 Abs and NHL
Lower motor neuron disease	SCLC-HL-carcinoma	<20 cases	Hu with SCLC only	some improved with tumor treatment	Rare cases of Ma2 Abs
Mixed sensory and motor	SCLC-70%	>200	Hu	–	According to the presentation, may be confused with different forms of axonal sensory-motor neuropathy
Autonomic neuropathy	SCLC 70%—HL and other carcinomas	SCLC<200 Other <10	Hu, (ganglionic AChR) Some with HL improved with immunotherapy		Frequently associated with SSN and antiHu Abs
Sensory-motor neuropathies without gammopathy					
Axonal	Carcinoma and HL	Rare	Usually none	Some improved with tumor treatment	Rare cases with Yo or Ma2 Abs
Axonal and demyelinating	SCLC and thymoma	<50 with CV2/CRMP5 AB	CV2/CRMP5		Frequently associated with CN5 involvement with CV2/CRMP5 Abs
Demyelinating (CIDP)	Carcinoma and NHL	<50	Rarely CV2/CRMP5	Some improved with tumor treatment	With NHL, neurolymphomatosis is the differential diagnosis
Vasculitic neuropathy	SCLC, NHL, and other carcinomas	<50	Rarely Hu	Some improved with treatment	
Sensory-motor neuropathies with gammopathy					
Axonal sensory and painful	AL amyloidosis and myeloma	>500	Free light chains		Multisystemic organ involvement
Demyelinating	Waldenströ¨em	>500	AntiMAG IgM k		Mostly sensory and distal, tremor
	NHL	<10	Antiganglioside IgM		CANOMAD or neuropathy according to Abs activity
	Osteosclerotic myeloma and plasmacytoma (POEMS)	>400	IgG I VEGF		multisystemic organ involvement
Vasculitic neuropathy	type I cryoglobulinemia lymphopathy	>200	Cryoglobulin and low complement level		Mostly sensory and multisystemic organ involvement
Neuromyotonia	Thymoma (SCLC and NHL) 30%	<100	Caspr2 and Netrin 1 receptor		Insomnia, delirium with Morvan syndrome. Myasthenia gravis frequent

Abs, antibodies; *CANOMAD*, chronic ataxia neuropathy, ophthalmoplegia associated with IgM monoclonal gammopathy; *HL*, Hodgkin's lymphoma; *NHL*, non-Hodgkin's lymphoma; *POEMS*, polyneuropathy-organomegaly-endocrinopathy-M component-skin changes; *SCLC*, small cell lung cancer; *VEGF*, vascular endothelial.
Modified from Antoine JC, Camdessanché JP. Paraneoplastic neuropathies. Curr Opin Neurol 2017;30(5):513–520. https://doi.org/10.1097/WCO.0000000000000475. PMID: 28682959.

A panel of antibodies is often tested for. Often single, dual, or multiple antibodies may be detected.

In patients with carcinoma, the presence of antiHu, antiCV2/CRMP5 as well as seronegative neuropathies are common. Paraneoplastic syndrome is most common in patients with lymphomas, monoclonal gammopathy, AL amyloidosis, POEMS syndrome, type I cryglubuniameia, and antimyelin-associated glycoproteins and Waldenström's syndrome.

The antibodies encountered and their target antigens and associated malignancy are summarized in Table 12.

The antibodies react with the neural cell surface or synaptic proteins leading to limbic and encephalitis presentations. The common (classic) paraneoplastic syndromes include encephalomyelitis, limbic encephalitis, subacute cerebellar degeneration, opsoclonus myoclonus, sensory neuropathy, chronic gastrointestinal pseudoobstruction, Lamberty-Eaton myasthenic syndrome, and dermatomyositis.

TABLE 12 Onconeuronal antibodies and associated paraneoplastic syndromes.

Antibody	Main tumor	Neurological syndrome
Hu (ANNA1)	Small cell lung cancer	Encephalomyelitis, limbic encephalitis, brainstem encephalitis, paraneoplastic cerebellar degeneration, sensory neuropathy, gastrointestinal pseudo-obstruction
CV2 (CRMP5)	Small cell lung cancer, thymoma	As above plus, chorea, optic neuropathy, isolated myelopathy, and mixed neuropathies
Amphiphysin	Breast and small cell lung cancer	Stiff-person syndrome, myelopathy and myoclonus, encephalomyelitis, sensory neuropathy
Ri (ANNA2)	Breast and small cell lung cancer	Brainstem encephalitis, opsoclonus myoclonus
Yo (PCA1)	Ovary, breast	Paraneoplastic cerebellar degeneration
Ma2	Testicular	Limbic and brain stem encephalitis
Tr	Hodgkin's	Paraneoplastic cerebellar degeneration

Modified from Graus F, Dalmau J. Paraneoplastic neurological syndromes. Curr Opin Neurol 2012;25(6):795–801. https://doi.org/10.1097/WCO.0b013e328359da15. PMID: 23041955; PMCID: PMC3705179.

Testing for antiaquaporin AQP4 is important in the differential diagnosis of multiple sclerosis particularly if optic neuritis, myelitis, and/or brainstem encephalitis are present.

NMDAR-IgG and VGKC-complex IgG testing help discriminate between patients with encephalitis who are likely to respond to immunotherapy.

The identification of the antibodies as well as their association with varied neurological disorders have highlighted the value of diagnostic laboratory testing. In AQP4 and NMDAR encephalomyelitis, a direct pathogenic role of the respective antibodies is highly likely, and that therapeutic and prognostic implications are known.

Antibodies to AMPAR, GABABR, GABAAR, glycine receptors, mGluR5, and DPPX in encephalitis; ITPR1, Homer-3, CARP, PKCγ, and ARHGAP26 in cerebellitis (termed "Medusa head ataxia"); MUSK and LRP-4 in myasthenia gravis; and CASPR2 in neuromyotonia. Moreover, antimyelin oligodendrocyte glycoprotein antibodies are associated with myelitis and optic neuritis in the absence of antiAQP4 antibodies.

N-methyl-D-aspartate receptors (NMDARs) and the voltage-gated potassium channel (VGKC) complex proteins LGI1 and CASPR2 are target antigens in limbic encephalitis.

Multiple sclerosis

Multiple sclerosis is the most common inflammatory condition of the central nervous system. Antibodies detected in CSF (oligoclonal bands). Oligoclonal bands are detected in the CSF of 95% of patients with multiple sclerosis.

Its progressive gradual incidence correlates with distance from the equator (Fig. 3).

Cerebrospinal fluid (CSF) proteins

The cerebrospinal fluid contains proteins that are either ultrafiltrate of plasma (the majority excluded by the blood-brain barrier) or are due to intrathecal synthesis. The amount, as well as the composition of CSF proteins, are of diagnostic value. Protein concentrations are high during infancy and decrease over time. Due to its large molecular weight, circulating immunoglobulins do not cross the blood-brain barrier (BBB) and thus the presence of increased concentrations of immunoglobulins, usually IgG, in CSF is clinically significant only if its origin as leakage from the blood can be excluded. The integrity of the BBB should be assessed before estimating intrathecal IgG synthesis. The combined determination of the IgG Index and or IgG$_{loc}$ virtually eliminates the possibility of false-positive interpretations due to BBB leakage.

Detection of intrathecal synthesis of immunoglobulin is indicative of either cerebral infection, hemorrhage, or to inflammatory multiple sclerosis. Oligoclonal bands are

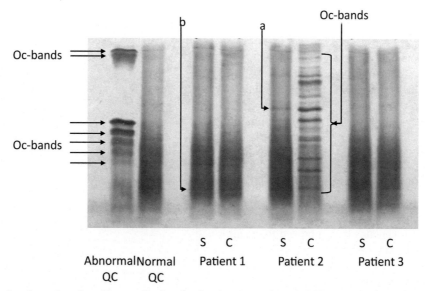

FIG. 3 Isoelectric focusing electrophoresis and immunoblotting showing the pattern of matched CSF and serum samples from patients being investigated for oligoclonal bands (multiple sclerosis). The abnormal quality control sample shows several oligoclonal bands (Oc-bands) when compared to the negative normal control. Matched CSF (C) and serum (S) samples from patient 1 showed few corresponding bands (B) in both CSF and serum samples (indicating the serum source of the CSF bands due to impaired blood-brain barrier). This is in contrast to patient 2 where several oligoclonal bands appear in the CSF and that are absent in the serum (with the exception of one band (A)) this pattern indicates intrathecal synthesis of immunoglobins and diagnostic of multiple sclerosis. Patient 3 samples show a normal pattern with no bands in CSF samples. *QC*, quality control sample. *(Adapted from the author's laboratory.)*

observed in the electrophoretic separation of CSF samples and immunostaining for IgG (Fig. 3).

Indices are used to evaluate the permeability of the blood-brain barrier and to estimate the extent of intrathecal local IgG synthesis (IgG$_{loc}$) and include:

Albumin index (AI)

This is derived by measuring both serum and CSF albumin levels (AI=Albumin in CSF/Albumin in serum (both in mg/dL) × 1000). Values for AI <9.0 indicate an intact BBB and that IgG index determination accurately represents intrathecal synthesis. However, if the AI >9.0, the IgG index calculation is invalid and the alternative IgG$_{loc}$ equation (see later) provides a better estimate of intrathecal IgG synthesis.

CSF: Serum IgG index

This is a measure of the degree of intrathecal IgG synthesis. Three formulas are in use and are helpful to varying degrees.

IgG index can simply be derived as IgG Index = ([IgG]$_{CSF}$ × [Alb]$_{Serum}$)/([IgG]$_{Serum}$ × [Alb]$_{CSF}$). A value <0.66 indicates a lack of intrathecal IgG synthesis.

Another equation is IgG local synthesis (IgG$_{loc}$) calculated as follows:

IgG$_{loc}$=[Q$_{IgG}$ − 0.8[Q$_{Alb}^2$ + (15×10^{-6})]$^{1/2}$ + 1.8×10^{-3}] × [IgG]$_{Serum}$. (where Q$_{IgG}$=[IgG, mg/dL]$_{CSF}$/[IgG, mg/dL]$_{Serum}$). Values <0.0 mg/dL suggest absent intrathecal IgG synthesis.

The IgG synthesis rate equation (IgG$_{sr}$) for the assessment of intrathecal IgG synthesis in the presence of a moderately impaired blood-brain barrier is shown below.

IgG$_{sr}$ = [[IgG]$_{CSF}$ − ([IgG]$_{Serum}$/369) − ([Alb]$_{CSF}$ − ([Alb]$_{Serum}$/230)([IgG]$_{Serum}$/[Alb]$_{Serum}$)(0.43))] × 5. A synthesis rate of −9.9 to 3.3 mg/day suggests a lack of intrathecal IgG synthesis. Although the equation overcomes some degree of BBB impairment, it cannot be relied on to yield only true-positive results in the presence of BBB damage.

The presence of oligoclonal bands in the CSF, in the absence of such bands in serum from the same individual, is diagnostic of intrathecal immunoglobulin (IgG) synthesis. In active disease, oligoclonal bands are present in the CSF of 95% of multiple sclerosis cases.

However, it is important to note that oligoclonal bands (o-bands) are seen also in a variety of other chronic inflammatory disorders of the central nervous system (CNS). They include cerebral syphilis infection, subacute sclerosing panencephalitis (SSPE), trypanosomiasis, Guillain-Barre syndrome, AIDS, Lyme disease, cysticercosis, and adrenoleukodystrophy (ALD).

Pheochromocytoma

Tumors of the adrenal medulla are termed pheochromocytomas (brown-black colored cells when reacting with dichromate). They are chromaffin cell tumors derived from the neural crest.

Epinephrine and norepinephrine are converted to metanephrine and normetanephrine by catecholamine-o-methyltransferase (COMT). Common to the production of catecholamines are extra-adrenal paragangliomas which are neural crest tumors.

The tumors are rare but must be considered in patients with hypertension, autonomic disturbances, panic attacks, and adrenal incidentalomas, or in Familia disease featuring predisposing to the development of pheochromocytoma (Table 13).

Incidence 2–9.1 per million persons. Many of the tumors are benign, clinically silent, and detected at autopsy.

Despite the fact that the pretest prevalence of pheochromocytoma is very low about 0.5% among those tested because of hypertension, and 4% in patients with adrenal incidentalomas, testing is essential as surgical removal is successful in 90% of cases whereas if left untreated is fatal. Furthermore, advances in genetics had improved the management of familial pheochromocytoma and the surgical procedure for preserving normal adrenal cortical tissue in patients with bilateral adrenal tumors.

Most pheochromocytomas are sporadic. Familial predisposition is seen mainly in patients with multiple endocrine neoplasia type II (MEN II), von Hippel-Lindau disease, neurofibromatosis type 1, and familial carotid body tumors. Family members develop these tumors at a higher frequency and a younger age than members of families with other mutations.

Genetical, pheochromocytomas arise sporadically or in the familial MEN type 2 syndrome associated with RET mutation, neurofibromatosis type 1, and the VHL gene mutation syndrome (Hippel-Lindau).

First-line investigation in patients suspected of pheochromocytoma is plasma or urine-fractioned metanephrines. Elevated levels confirm the diagnosis. Dopamine is usually part of the test profile, but if not few patients with dopamine-only tumors as well as those with small tumors (<1 cm) secreting low metanephrines will be missed as hormone levels correlate with the size of the tumor. Plasma metanephrines have a diagnostic sensitivity ranging from 89.5% to 100% and specificity ranging from 79.4% to 97.6%. This is compared with 85.7% to 97.1%, and from 68.6% to 95.1% when measured in urine, respectively (Table 14).

TABLE 14 Performance characteristics of catecholamines metabolites in the diagnosis of pheochromocytoma.

Catecholamine	Sensitivity	Specificity
Plasma metanephrine	99	89
Plasma catecholamine	85	80
Urinary catecholamine	83	88
Urinary metanephrine	76	94
Urinary vanillylmandelic acid	63	94

The sensitivities of tests of plasma metanephrines or plasma and urinary catecholamines were determined, respectively, as the percentage of patients with pheochromocytoma who had positive test results for normetanephrine or metanephrine or norepinephrine or epinephrine. The specificities of tests of plasma metanephrines or plasma and urinary catecholamines were determined as the percentage of patients without pheochromocytoma who had negative test results for both normetanephrine and metanephrine or both norepinephrine and epinephrine. The sensitivities and specificities of tests of urinary metanephrines reflect tests of urinary total metanephrines (that is, the combined sum of free plus conjugated normetanephrine and metanephrine).
Modified from Pacak K, Linehan WM, Eisenhofer G, Walther MM, Goldstein DS. Recent advances in genetics, diagnosis, localization, and treatment of pheochromocytoma. Ann Intern Med 2001;134(4):315–29. https://doi.org/10.7326/0003-4819-134-4-200102200-00016. PMID: 11182843.

Periodic post-surgical follow-up is required. Plasma and urinary fractionated metanephrines should be performed within the first month postoperatively, at 6 months, at one year, and yearly.

Upper limits for normal levels being, normetanephrine 0.47 nmol/L (children), 1.05 nmol/L (>60 years old), metanephrine at 0.45 nmol/L, and 3-methoxytyramine at 0.10 nmol/L.

Several physiological and pharmacological factors can elevate catecholamines leading to false positive results.

Plasma normetanephrine >2.5 pmol/mL or metanephrine levels >1.4 pmol/mL (that is more than 4- and 2.5-fold above the upper reference limits) indicate the presence of a pheochromocytoma with 100% specificity. Such levels can be reached in patients with monoamine oxidase deficiency.

TABLE 13 Hereditary pheochromocytoma associated with MEN II.

Syndrome	Gene	Frequency of pheochromocytoma, %
Multiple endocrine neoplasia type II	RET oncogene	30–50
von Hippel-Lindau disease	von Hippel-Lindau tumor suppressor gene	15–20
Neurofibromatosis type 1	Neurofibromatosis type 1	1–5
Familial carotid body tumors	Paraganglioma	

Modified from Pacak K, Linehan WM, Eisenhofer G, Walther MM, Goldstein DS. Recent advances in genetics, diagnosis, localization, and treatment of pheochromocytoma. Ann Intern Med 2001;134(4):315–29. https://doi.org/10.7326/0003-4819-134-4-200102200-00016. PMID: 11182843.

At a 2% pretest probability of pheochromocytoma and at a specificity of 89%, a positive result on an initial test of plasma metanephrines increases the probability of pheochromocytoma to nearly 16%.

Metanephrines are produced continuously by pheochromocytoma and thus normal plasma levels of normetanephrine and metanephrine in repeat testing exclude pheochromocytoma, even if results of the first test or other tests are positive.

The clonidine suppression test is useful for distinguishing between high levels of plasma norepinephrine caused by release from sympathetic nerves and those caused by release from a pheochromocytoma.

A decrease of more than 50% in plasma norepinephrine levels or a decrease after clonidine administration to less than 2.96 nmol/L indicate normal responses, whereas consistently elevated concentrations before and after clonidine administration indicate a pheochromocytoma.

The glucagon stimulation test can be useful when high plasma levels of normetanephrine or metanephrine are noted and plasma catecholamine levels are normal or moderately elevated. A greater than threefold increase in norepinephrine levels 2 min after intravenous administration of glucagon indicates a pheochromocytoma, however, a negative test result does not exclude pheochromocytoma.

False positive results are seen in patients taking diuretics or tricyclic antidepressants.

Neuroblastoma

In contrast to pheochromocytoma, neuroblastoma belongs to the extra-adrenal paraganglia tumors. It is derived from the primordial neural crest cells and tumors may develop at any site within the sympathetic nervous system.

It is the most common extracranial solid tumor in children accounting for nearly 10% of children's cancers, the incidence of neuroblastomas is estimated at 10.5 cases per million children.

The most common primary site is the adrenal gland and most tumors arise in the abdomen. The median age at diagnosis is 17 months with most diagnoses made below 5 years of age. Clinical presentation depends on the site of the tumor, for instance, neurological symptoms secondary to spinal cord involvement, abdominal mass and pain, and respiratory distress.

The tumor is heterogenous in its course, some regress spontaneously without treatment whereas others metastasize, are aggressive, and have a poor prognosis.

Diagnosis is established via biopsy of the primary tumor or the metastatic soft tissue lesions. Diagnosis is also reached following bone marrow involvement and elevated urinary catecholamines (see later) if a biopsy of the tumor is risky and not possible. Disease staging is achieved via CT or MRI imaging using MIBG (meta-iodobenzylguanidine) scans and that therapy is guided by disease stage and risk.

Neuroblastomas synthesize excess catecholamines norepinephrine, norepinephrine, and dopamine. Little is stored inside the cells and the majority is metabolized to 4-hydroxy-3-methoxyphenylhlycol (MHPG) by catechol-o-methyltransferase (COMT) and monoamine oxidase (MAO). The MHPG is further metabolized in the liver to vanillylmandelic acid (VMA) by hepatic alcohol dehydrogenase and that dopamine is metabolized to homovanillic acid (HVA) by COMT and MAO within the neuroblastoma. The latter HVA and VMA are used in the biochemical diagnosis and monitoring of neuroblastoma. When combined, diagnostic sensitivity and specificity are 60% to 100% and >99% respectively. Approximately 90% of patients with neuroblastoma express elevated HVA and VMA levels.

Low levels of urinary VMA and VMA/HVA ratios or high levels of dopamine/VMA and dopamine/HVA ratios are associated with unfavorable features and poor prognosis in patients with aggressive neuroblastoma.

Elevated dopamine, norepinephrine, HVA, and VMA, have been used in early detection in screening programs for neuroblastoma. Other biomarkers used in clinical practice but are not specific for neuroblastoma include chromogranin A, neuron-specific enolase (NSE), lactate dehydrogenase (LDH), and ferritin.

High pressure liquid chromatography (HPLC) with electrochemical detectors has been widely used in the determination of urinary HVA and VMA, recently several LCMSMS based methods have been developed allowing the simultaneous determination of both biomarkers' epinephrine and dopamine.

Neuroblastoma patients with tumor stages 1, 2, and 4S (localized) have low circulating ferritin, LDH, NSE compared with elevated levels in patients with stages 3, and 4 (distant metastasis) with poor prognosis

Genetic predisposition and chromosomal aberrations have been linked to the staging and severity of neuroblastoma. Approximately 20% of patients present amplification of the MYCN locus located on chromosome 2p24, and the degree of amplification strongly correlates with advanced disease stage and poor outcome. Aggressive forms are also associated with deletion of the distal part of chromosome 1 (1p loss), a gain of the long arm of chromosome 17 (11q gain), and a loss of a part of the long arm of chromosome 11 (11q loss).

The optimal treatment strategy is driven by the pretreatment risk to this effect the international neuroblastoma risk group staging system was developed and applied (Table 15).

POEMS

POEMS (polyneuropathy, organomegaly, endocrinopathy, monoclonal gammopathy, and skin changes) syndrome is characterized by the presence of a monoclonal plasma cell disorder, peripheral neuropathy, and one or more of the following features, osteosclerotic myeloma, Castleman disease

TABLE 15 International neuroblastoma risk group staging system (INGSS).

Risk group for treatment	INRGSS	IDRFs in primary tumor	Distant metastases	Age (months)	Histological category	Grade of differentiation	MYCN status	Genomic profile	Very low
Very-low	L1	Absent	Absent	Any	GNB nodular, NB	Any	–	Any	Any
	L1 or L2	Any	Absent	Any	GN, GNB intermixed	Any	–	Any	Any
	MS	Any	Present	<12	Any	Any	–	Favorable	Any
Low	L2	Present	Absent	<18	GNB nodular, NB	Any	–	Favorable	Any
	L2	Present	Absent	≧18	GNB nodular, NB	Differentiating	–	Favorable	Any
	M	Any	Present	<18	Any	Any	–	Any	Hyperdiploid
Intermediate	L2	Present	Absent	<18	GNB nodular, NB	Any	–	Unfavorable	Any
	L2	Present	Absent	≧18	GNB nodular, NB	Differentiating	–	Unfavorable	Any
	L2	Present	Absent	≧18	GNB nodular, NB	Poorly differentiated, undifferentiated	–	Any	Any
	MS	Any	Present	12–18	Any	Any	–	Favorable	Any
	MS	Any	Present	<12	Any	Any	–	Unfavorable	Any
High	L1	Absent	Absent	Any	GNB nodular, NB	Any	+	Any	Any
	L2	Present	Absent	≧18	GNB nodular, NB	Poorly differentiated, undifferentiated	+	Any	Any
	M	Any	Absent	12–18		Any	–	Unfavorable	And or diploid
	M	Any	Present	<18		Any	+	Any	Any
	M	Any	Present	≧18		Any	Any	Any	Any
	MS	Any	Present	12–18		Any	–	Unfavorable	Any
	MS	Any	Present	<18		Any	+	Any	Any

IDRF, image-defines risk factors; L, localized; M, metastasis; MS, distant metastasis to the skin; GN, ganglioneuroma; GNB, ganglioneuroblastoma.
Modified from Monclair T, Brodeur GM, Ambros PF, Brisse HJ, Cecchetto G, Holmes K, Kaneko M, London WB, Matthay KK, Nuchtern JG, von Schweinitz D, Simon T, Cohn SL, Pearson AD; INRG Task Force. The International Neuroblastoma Risk Group (INRG) staging system: an INRG Task Force report. J Clin Oncol. 2009;27(2):298–303. https://doi.org/10.1200/JCO.2008.16.6876. Epub 2008 Dec 1. PMID: 19047290; PMCID: PMC2650389 and Nakagawara A, Li Y, Izumi H, Muramori K, Inada H, Nishi M. Neuroblastoma. Jpn J Clin Oncol 2018;48(3):214–241. https://doi.org/10.1093/jjco/hyx176. PMID: 29378002.

(angiofollicular lymph node hyperplasia), increased levels of serum vascular endothelial growth factor (VEGF), organomegaly, endocrinopathy, edema, typical skin changes, and papilledema

Vascular endothelial growth factor (VEGF) is a critical modulator of angiogenesis (the growth of new blood vessels). In mammals, there are five members of the VEGF family, each arising from different genes, with VEGF-A being the most well-studied. VEGF-A promotes angiogenesis by inducing migration of endothelial cells, promoting mitosis of endothelial cells, and upregulating matrix metalloproteinase activity. VEGF-A is regulated by hypoxia, with increased expression when cells detect an environment low in oxygen. Physiologically, VEGF induces new blood vessel formation during embryonic development, after tissue injury, and in response to blocked vessels.

An elevated concentration of vascular endothelial growth factor (VEGF) may be consistent with a diagnosis of POEMS. Although the pathologic role of VEGF in POEMS is unclear, it is useful as a diagnostic marker and for assessing response to therapy.

Decreasing concentrations of VEGF over time in a patient with POEMS syndrome may be consistent with therapeutic response.

Elevated circulating concentrations of vascular endothelial growth factor (VEGF) may be observed in a variety of disease states, especially those associated with angiogenesis. Elevated concentrations of VEGF must be interpreted within the clinical context of the patient.

Normal concentrations (≤ 96.2 pg/mL) of VEGF do not exclude the diagnosis of POEMS.

VEGF has limited stability. Following centrifugation, plasma must be either immediately frozen or refrigerated. Samples can only be stored at refrigerated temperatures for 24 h, after which time samples must be frozen. Storage of plasma for any length of time at room temperature renders the sample unacceptable. The presence of bevacizumab in patient serum interferes with the detection of VEGF. Caution should be taken while interpreting the results of patients receiving bevacizumab therapy.

New biomarkers in neurological disorders

Several new biomarkers are being proposed in the investigation of patients with psychological stress and traumatic brain injury.

Traumatic brain injury biomarkers

Traumatic brain injuries are associated with mortality and long-term poor residual functional outcomes some are nonreversible. The initial insult is often nonreversible, however, secondary injuries occurring following the initial insult are those secondary to hypoxia and or to hypotension and thus expanding the overall affected area.

Intrathecal expression of inflammatory proteins, biomarkers of apoptosis, oxidative stress, all of those leading to impairment in the blood-brain barrier and brain edema, and intracranial hypertension.

Biomarkers in CSF are used to assess ongoing neuronal damage, and the presence of subarachnoid hemorrhage, and may be predictive of increased morbidity and mortality following traumatic and nontraumatic acute brain injury. Examples of tentative biomarkers and utility are indicated in Table 16.

Biomarkers of phycological stress

The utility of measuring several biomarkers in the identification and monitoring of psychological stress is being

TABLE 16 Tentative biomarkers in the investigation and assessment of various neurological symptoms.

Neurological symptoms	Tentative biomarkers
Inflammation	Procarboxypeptidase U, TAFI, proCPB2, Matrix metalloproteins (MMP-9), CRP, Apo-E, S-100Beta, MBP, tau-fraction, albumin, IgG, transferrin, MMP-2
Apoptosis	NLRP1, ASC, Caspase 1, Caspase-3, cytochrome C, sFas, Caspase-9, ASC, Clusterin, NLRP1, UCH-L1, MAP-2, SBDP150, SBDP145, SBDP120, MBP, S-100β, NALP-1, Alpha-2 spectrin, c-tau
Neurodegeneration	Alpha-synuclein, UCH-L1, AB-amyloid 1–42, tau protein, Beta-amyloid peptide 1–41
Primary brain injury (neuron cell cytoskeleton)	BDNF, S-100β, UCH-L1, MAP-2, SBDP150, SBDP145, SBDP120, MBP, H-FABP, tau protein, NSE, glial fibrillary acidic protein, Apo-E, Albumin, IgG, Transferrin, NMP, AB-amyloid 1–42
Energy	NSE, Ab42, MBP, GFAP, Sulfonylurea receptor-1
Redox (oxidative stress)	Peroxiredoxin, (Prdx) VI

Apo-E, apolipoprotein E; *ASC*, apoptosis-associated speck-like protein containing a caspase recruitment domain; *BDNF*, brain-derived neurotrophic factor; *CRP*, C-reactive protein; *C-tau*, cleaved tau protein; *H-FABP*, heart-type fatty acid binding protein; *MAP-2*, microtubule-associated protein; *MBP*, myelin basic protein; *MMP*, matrix metalloproteinase; *NALP1*, Nacht leucine-rich-repeat protein-1; *NSE*, neuron-specific enolase; *UCH-L1*, ubiquitin C-terminal hydrolase; *S-100β*, S-100 beta; *SBDP*, spectrin breakdown products; *TAFI*, thrombin activatable fibrinolysis inhibitor. Modified from Santacruz CA, Vincent JL, Bader A, Rincón-Gutiérrez LA, Dominguez-Curell C, Communi D, Taccone FS. Association of cerebrospinal fluid protein biomarkers with outcomes in patients with traumatic and non-traumatic acute brain injury: systematic review of the literature. Crit. Care 2021;25(1):278. https://doi.org/10.1186/s13054-021-03698-z. PMID: 34353354; PMCID: PMC8340466.

examined. Biomarkers including catecholamines, prolactin, cortisol, and alpha salivary amylase were found to correlate with stress. During stress, alpha salivary alpha-amylase changes and correlates with blood pressure, heart rate, and plasma catecholamines. Amylase peaks 10–15 min after stress is induced. This is thought to be related to the association of norepinephrine and amylase. It is important to note that the elevation of certain biomarkers such as cortisol and catecholamines leads to hypertension which is an individual marker of stress.

Summary

- The clinical biochemistry laboratory plays a significant role in the investigation of neurological dysfunction.
- Neurological presentation is either acute, subacute, or chronic in nature.
- Presentation varies from mild peripheral neuropathy to severe movement disorders and encephalopathy including coma and death.
- Diabetes mellitus is the most common disorder leading to peripheral neuropathy accounting for 50% of cases.
- Encephalopathy ranges from confusion states, dementia, and delirium to loss of consciousness and coma.
- Movement disorders present as ataxia, dystonia, or tremors.
- Carbon monoxide poisoning is a common accidental cause of poisoning.
- Alcohols are the most common cause of altered mental status and central nervous system depression.
- Third of the identified metabolic disorders present with some degree of neuropathy ranging from acute and chronic encephalopathy, movement disorders (myopathy, ataxia), and or behavioral abnormalities.
- Multiple myeloma is also associated with peripheral neuropathy but is considered underreported.
- Amyloidosis is characterized by the deposition of aggregated free light chains on nerves and organs.
- Peripheral neuropathy is a common complication of chemotherapeutic agents.
- About a third of the identified metabolic disorders present with some degree of neuropathy.
- There are four porphyria disorders exhibiting acute neurovisceral presentation. They are acute intermittent porphyria (AIP), variegate porphyria (VP), hereditary coproporphyria, and aminolaevulinic acid (ALA) dehydratase deficient porphyria.

- Wilson's disease is an inherited disorder of copper elimination it leads to the accumulation of copper in neural tissue.
- Menkes disease is a genetic disorder affecting copper uptake in the intestine resulting in copper deficiency.
- Vitamins and micronutrient deficiency lead to neurological presentations.
- Neuropathy is encountered in patients with deficiency or excess circulating and tissue levels of various trace elements such as selenium, manganese, and copper.
- Infection-associated encephalopathy is associated with reduced oxygen and blood flow, edema, accumulation of toxins and inflammatory markers that cause neurological deficits.
- Autoimmune encephalitis is a clinical presentation with a high index of suspicion necessitating frequent and extensive laboratory investigations.
- Patients with endocrine-related disorders may exhibit some degree of neurological dysfunction in the form of peripheral neuropathy and or encephalopathy
- Paraneoplastic syndrome affects <1% of patients with cancer. However, neuropathy and cancer are more common, they may be co-present by chance.
- Traumatic brain injuries are associated with mortality and long-term poor residual functional outcomes some are nonreversible.

Further reading

Hwang N, Chong E, Oh H, et al. Application of an LC-MS/MS Method for the Simultaneous Quantification of Homovanillic Acid and Vanillylmandelic Acid for the Diagnosis and Follow-Up of Neuroblastoma in 357 Patients. *Molecules.* 2021;26(11).

Christopher R, Sankaran BP. An insight into the biochemistry of inborn errors of metabolism for a clinical neurologist. *Ann Indian Acad Neurol.* 2008;11(2):68–81.

Santacruz CA, Vincent JL, Bader A, et al. Association of cerebrospinal fluid protein biomarkers with outcomes in patients with traumatic and non-traumatic acute brain injury: systematic review of the literature. *Crit Care.* 2021;25(1):278.

Tarnopolsky MA. Myopathies related to glycogen metabolism disorders. *Neurotherapeutics.* 2018;15(4):915–927.

Nakagawara A, Li Y, Izumi H, Muramori K, Inada H, Nishi M. Neuroblastoma. *Jpn J Clin Oncol.* 2018;48(3):214–241.

Barrell K, Smith AG. Peripheral neuropathy. *Med Clin North Am.* 2019;103(2):383–397.

Antoine JC, Camdessanche JP. Paraneoplastic neuropathies. *Curr Opin Neurol.* 2017;30(5):513–520.

O'Malley R, Rao G, Stein P, Bandmann O. Porphyria: often discussed but too often missed. *Pract Neurol.* 2018;18(5):352–358.

Chapter 10

Plasma and body fluids proteins

Introduction

Most circulating major proteins are produced by the liver except for immunoglobulins produced by lymphocytes and apoproteins by enterocytes and other tissues. This chapter describes proteins in body fluids, namely, plasma, cerebrospinal fluid, peritoneal, pleural, and joint fluids, and urine, their relative distribution, function, associated disorders, and diagnostic utility.

Plasma proteins

Plasma contains many proteins with a wide range of sizes, shapes, and abundance all contributing to a total protein concentration of about 80 g/L (8.0 g/dL) with albumin being the most abundant protein at about 45 g/L (4.5 g/dL).

Plasma is made up of 91%–92% water and 8%–9% of particulates including proteins. The terms plasma and serum are often used interchangeably, however, in serum the clotting factors have been consumed and thus fibrinogen and clotting factors are not detectable in serum. Plasma is obtained in the presence of anticoagulant tube additives such as heparin (sodium, or lithium salt), ethylenediaminetetraacetic acid (EDTA) (potassium, sodium, or citrate salts), and oxalate (sodium, fluoride salts). The difference in total measured protein concentrations between serum and plasma due to the presence of coagulation factors in the latter is small and clinically negligible.

In the clinical laboratory, direct photometric measurements are made of total proteins and of albumin concentrations. However, reported total globulins are deduced by subtracting albumin from total protein measurements. Specific globulins including immunoglobulin concentrations may individually be measured using protein-specific and sensitive immuno-based turbidimetric and nephelometric methods (see Chapter 17).

Electrophoresis

When separated and visualized by electrophoresis, serum proteins separate (based on their net charge mass ratio) into a predominant and fast-moving albumin (preceeded by a faint prealbumin band), and five slower-moving globulin groups, namely, alpha 1 (α_1), alpha 2 (α_2), beta 1 (β_1), beta 2 (β_2), and gamma (γ) globulin regions. Each globulin region is heterogeneous in its protein content (see later). For instance, prealbumin (often a faint band) migrates anodally to the albumin band, alpha-1 antitrypsin and alpha-1 glycoprotein migrate within the alpha 1 region, alpha 2-macroglobulin and haptoglobin migrate within the alpha 2 regions, and beta lipoproteins migrate within the beta 1 and 2 regions whereas the immunoglobulins span the beta-gamma globulin electrophoretic regions (Fig. 1).

Although abnormalities in the electrophoretic pattern (relative band concentrations) are indicative of various pathologies such as a low albumin band and high alpha 2 and beta 1, 2 bands characteristic of patients with nephrotic syndrome (loss of albumin in urine and hyperlipidemia), and the finding of low albumin in the presence of polyclonal gammopathy with beta-gamma bridging is indicative of chronic liver disease (reduced albumin synthesis, generalized increase in immunoglobulins including IgA which spans the beta-gamma region), similarly an increase in the alpha 2 regions reflects elevated haptoglobin and ceruloplasmin in inflammatory conditions as they are both positive acute-phase reactants, additionally, alpha-2-macroglobulin is increased in nephrotic syndrome and in liver cirrhosis.

The essential purpose of protein electrophoresis is the identification of a monoclonal component (i.e., multiple myeloma) usually observed in the gamma globulin but may also appear in the proximity of the beta region and rarely as far as the alpha 2 region (see later).

Electrophoresis is performed using serum as a sample not plasma to avoid confusion with the large fibrinogen band in the beta-gamma region with a possible paraprotein.

Prealbumin

Also known as transthyretin, prealbumin is a 55-kDa homotetramer, synthesized in the liver and present in serum and cerebrospinal fluid (CSF). Normal circulating levels range from 150 to 300 mg/L and from 200 to 400 mg/L in adults and children, respectively. It has a short half-life of 18 to 24 h.

Prealbumin has a short half-life and its hepatic synthesis is dependent on amino acids nutrient supply making it a suitable candidate for the assessment of nutritional status. Healthcare regulatory agencies (The Joint Commission among others) mandate clinical screening for nutritional

Tutorials in Clinical Chemistry. https://doi.org/10.1016/B978-0-12-822949-1.00012-7

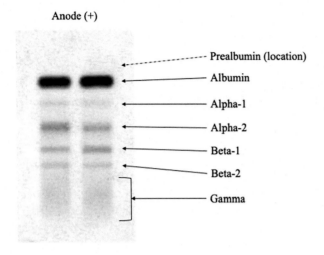

Anode (+)

- - - Prealbumin (location)
— Albumin
— Alpha-1
— Alpha-2
— Beta-1
— Beta-2
— Gamma

Cathode (-)

FIG. 1 Serum proteins separated by electrophoresis on agarose gel and stained with Coomassie brilliant blue. Serum proteins migrate and separate into the above regions. Albumin (anodal migration), alpha-1 (alpha-1 antitrypsin, alpha-1-acid glycoprotein, alpha-1 lipoprotein, and alpha-1 fetoprotein), alpha-2 (haptoglobin, alpha-2 macroglobulin, ceruloplasmin), beta-1 (transferrin, beta-lipoproteins, C4 complement, hemopexin), beta-2 (C-reactive protein, C3, fibrinogen), and gamma globulins (immunoglobulins). The degree of band intensity reflects the relative concentration of the protein. Prealbumin runs ahead of the albumin band. Its low concentration and short half-life render it difficult to view. A smear observed in front of the albumin band may be due to the bilirubin (in states of hyperbilirubinemia) and or to drugs bound albumin. *Courtesy of the author's laboratory.*

deficiency within 24h of hospitalization. Additionally, its pre-operative level is a strong predictor of postsurgical outcomes and has become a modifiable risk factor for postsurgical outcomes. Measurement of prealbumin has been used to assess the need for pre-surgical need for parenteral nutrition. In patients where levels of prealbumin and albumin can be solely attributed to nutritional status (that is in the presence of confounding factors such as inflammation), a recommendation for the delay in elective surgical procedures to improve nutrition is suggested to improve postoperative outcomes.

Prealbumin levels less than 186 mg/L are one of the criteria for instituting perioperative (7–15 days before and 3 days afterward) parenteral nutritional support.

Although prealbumin and albumin have been used as markers of nutritional assessments, their levels are markedly influenced by the presence of inflammatory conditions. Prealbumin is a negative acute-phase reactant protein with decreasing levels at the expense of the upregulation and synthesis of the "positive" acute-phase proteins. Thus, for it to be of value in the assessment of nutritional status, the patient must exhibit a state of homeostasis for its optimal use, that is, does not have any protein-losing enteropathy, reduced synthesis in chronic liver disease, or catabolism in inflammatory conditions.

Prealbumin facilitates systemic amyloid deposition whereas in the brain it has an antiamyloidogenesis effect.

It is expressed in retinal epithelium where it is complexed with retinol-binding protein which binds retinol (vitamin A). It is also expressed in the pancreatic alpha (glucagon) cells in the islet of Langerhans, however, its pancreatic function remains unknown but is thought to play a role in glucose homeostasis via regulating the expression of glucagon. Prealbumin binds and transports about 20% of thyroid hormones.

Albumin

Prealbumin, a precursor for albumin synthesized by hepatocytes, is cleaved in the endoplasmic reticulum into proalbumin, the most abundant intracellular form of albumin before it is transformed into albumin in the Golgi apparatus and released into the circulation as albumin.

Albumin is a single polypeptide chain with 583 amino acids giving a molecular weight of 68 kDa. Its average half-life in circulation is 21 days. It is the predominant circulating protein representing 55%–65% of total plasma proteins and about 40% being intravascular.

About 14 g per day are synthesized at a synthesis rate of 200 mg/day/kg. Albumin content in a 70-kg man's body is about 300 g.

It is secreted into vascular space and is not stored by the liver with about a 4% degradation rate. Albumin is metabolized by most organs, 40%–60% in muscle and skin, <15% in the liver, 10% degraded by the kidney, 10% leaks into the gastrointestinal tract, and less than 20 mg/day is lost in the urine.

Albumin has many important roles, in addition to being a reservoir of the amino acids pool, it transports many proteins and molecules where binding to albumin renders them often soluble and facilitates their delivery to their respective receptors and sites of action; examples are unconjugated bilirubin, calcium, long chain fatty acids, drugs, thyroid hormones, steroids, among others. Albumin with its net negative charge acts as a buffer binding hydrogen ions. It binds free radicals and thus plays a role as an antioxidant. Albumin also, due to its size, predominance, and negative charge, contributes about 80% of the plasma oncotic pressure (colloidal osmotic pressures) collectively with globulins producing about 25 mmHg (3.33 kPa) facilitating retention of fluid within the extravascular space. However, interestingly, in analbuminemia reported in about 20 families worldwide with albumin levels being less than 10% of normal, the patients are clinically normal with mild edema and dyslipidemia (see later).

Hypoalbuminemia is defined as less than 35 g/L (3.5 g/dL) with clinically significant levels at less than 20 g/L (2.0 g/dL). Low albumin levels indicate poor outcomes and predict morbidity and mortality regardless of the cause.

Causes of hypoalbuminemia include redistribution of albumin due to altered capillary permeability, physiological volume overload during pregnancy, decreased protein intake (malnutrition, malabsorption), excessive loss (nephrotic syndrome, protein-losing enteropathies, burn exudates), and decreased synthesis (chronic liver disease) and in malignancy due to increased metabolism and cachexia. Low albumin levels are an indicator of poor prognosis and more than one of these causes may be present.

Albumin is a negative acute-phase protein. It is reduced by 5–10 g/L within one week in patients with sepsis, infection, and trauma. This could be due to reduced hepatic synthesis by interleukins 1, and 6, as well as tumor necrosis factor-alpha during infection. Synthesis is reduced secondary to a reduction in energy as well as in amino acid supply. Hypoalbuminemia is seen exaggerated by increased leakage into interstitial space. Movement of albumin from intravascular to interstitial space is about ten times the amount of synthesized albumin, transcapillary escape is the most likely cause for observed hypoalbuminemia in inflammation and in sepsis. During major surgery, transcapillary escape as well as reduced lymph flow are the major contributors to the observed hypoalbuminemia. Hypoalbuminemia in pregnancy is associated with volume overload.

In edema, water passes from the intravascular to the extravascular space, and the ensuing circulatory volume depletion results in secondary hyperaldosteronism with sodium and water retention leading to a further reduction in albumin concentrations in all forms of edema. Edema primarily due to hypoalbuminemia usually only occurs when circulating albumin levels fall below 20 g/L (2.0 g/dL). Measurement of albumin in patients with edema of unknown origin may be helpful and when albumin concentration is below 20 g/L, then hypoalbuminemia itself is the likely cause.

Whereas hypoalbuminemia is a common finding, hyperalbuminemia is rare and is found only in patients with severe dehydration.

Albumin is measured either using a colorimetric assay (Bromo-Cresol Green/Purple) or by immunological assays (nephelometry and turbidimetry) depending on the albumin concentration.

Albumin is routinely measured in the assessment of liver function where normal level makes the diagnosis of cirrhosis unlikely. Levels are reduced in patients with viral hepatitis suggesting severe hepato-cellular damage or other complications. Albumin is measured to adjust measured calcium in patients with marked changes in albumin levels (about 50% of circulating calcium bound to albumin). It is also measured when monitoring patients receiving albumin replacement and or total parenteral nutrition therapy.

Bis-albuminemia describes the presence of two distinct albumin bands visible on protein electrophoresis. It has no known clinical significance. Nearly in all cases, one of the bands represents the original albumin and the other is either a product of congenital mutations. There are over 80 alleles for albumin giving rise to bis-albuminemia with many isotypes. Bis-albuminemia may also be acquired. The latter is often transient and is seen in patients on high-dose beta-lactam antibiotics, with diabetes mellitus, pancreatic pseudocyst, nephrotic syndrome, Waldenström's macroglobulinemia, and multiple myeloma. Albumin has a single free thiol in position Cys34 that undergoes varying (30%–70%) levels of cysteinylation.

Analbuminemia is a rare family disorder first described in 1954 and affects less than 1 in one million. About 20 families have been described in the literature, and the condition apart from a confusing protein electrophoretic pattern (often wrongly attributed to a technical error with several samples repeated), is benign. Albumin levels are very low, less than 0.5 g/L (a tenth of normal), and with little edema. There is often mild edema and dyslipidemia with marked hypertriglyceridemia. Interestingly, hyperlipidemia is not associated with increased atherosclerosis and infused albumin although reduced the observed minor ankle edema, and mild hypocalcemia during infusion, the infused albumin has an extended half-life of about 50 to 60 days.

Pseudo-analbuminemia due to the presence of a slow-moving albumin variant in the alpha-1 region has been reported.

Total globulins

They represent all of the nonalbumin and prealbumin proteins in serum. Although respective proteins can specifically be measured (see respective section), their collective concentration is often calculated collectively by subtracting measured albumin from measured total protein concentrations [Total protein] − [Albumin] = [Total Globulins] which acts as a screening test to detect abnormally increased immunoglobulins.

Electrophoretic regions (alpha to gamma) and their respective proteins are discussed separately in detail in the following sections.

Alpha-1 (α1) globulins

Proteins migrating within the alpha-1 region include alpha-1-antitrypsin (constituting about 90% of the band intensity), alpha-1 lipoprotein, alpha-1-acid glycoprotein, and alpha-1 fetoprotein. A haze stain at the leading edge of this band may be due to high-density lipoprotein (HDL).

α-1-Antitrypsin (AAT)

Alpha-1-antitrypsin (AAT) is the major component of the electrophoresis α-1-globulin fraction. It is a 52-kDa glycoprotein with over 80% of it synthesized by hepatocytes. Other minor sources of production include monocytes, macrophages, pancreas, lung alveolar cells, enterocytes, endothelium, and by some cancer cells. It has a circulating half-life of 4–5 days. Produced at 34 mg/kg/day, it has a plasma concentration of 1–2 g/L and is measured by immune-based assays (turbidimetric or nephelometric).

It is a positive acute-phase reactant increasing by about 45 folds during inflammation. Despite its nomenclature, it provides more than 90% of the antiproteinase activity in serum and its specific substrate is serine proteinase elastase. In addition to its antiproteinase activities, it possesses multiple antiinflammatory activities where it reduces the expression of proinflammatory cytokines (IL-6, TNF-alpha, IL-1beta) without interfering with the release of antiinflammatory modulating cytokines IL-10, and IL-1 receptor antagonist.[1]

The alpha-1-antitrypsin band is decreased in patients with alpha-1-antitrypsin deficiency or decreased production of globulin in patients with severe liver disease.

Deficiency of AAT results in neonatal hepatitis (liver cirrhosis in early childhood), and in severe pulmonary emphysema in adults. The presence of an abnormal allele of α_1-antitrypsin is associated with emphysema, juvenile cirrhosis, or neonatal jaundice.

As AAT constitutes the majority of the alpha-1 region, findings of decreased levels in electrophoresis should trigger nephelometric or turbidimetric measurements to confirm the deficiency followed by the analysis of the genotyping or phenotyping.

Deficiency of AAT is underrecognized with less than 2% of individuals detected and that diagnostic delay ranges from 7 to 10 years. Severe deficiency mainly affects Caucasian individuals with a prevalence of 1:2000 to 1:10000 with a fifth of the prevalence among Latin America and very low among Africans and Asians.

The AAT gene is located in chromosome 14 and is activated by inflammatory markers in response to infection and inflammation, namely, lipopolysaccharides, IL-1, IL-6, TNF-alpha, and by oxidative stress. The gene has two alleles transmitted in an autosomal codominant Mendelian inheritance. Normal alleles are designated M and are present in 85%–90% of individuals. This genotype is MM. The most common deficiency alleles are designated S and Z and their prevalence among Caucasians is 5%–10% and 1%–3%, respectively. Consequently, the alleles variability are either normal MM (in 89%–95%), MS, SS, MZ, SZ, and ZZ five deficiency genotype present in the remaining 5%–15% with a relative distribution of 80%, 60%, 55%, 40%, and 15%, respectively (Table 1).

AAT levels <35% of the mean value of 50 mg/dL as measured by nephelometry is considered as severe deficiency and is often associated with the ZZ genotype and less frequently with Z or S types. The majority (96%) seen in clinical practice are homozygous ZZ type.

Interestingly, the presentation of AAT deficiency is markedly variable. Although a high percentage will develop chronic obstructive airway disease (COPD) or liver cirrhosis, few individuals suffer from panniculitis or vasculitis. Some will have a combination of the different presentations and a third of patients with AAT deficiency will exhibit minor or no symptoms. This variability suggests the association or environmental factors or other genetic predispositions. For instance, liver involvement is associated with

TABLE 1 Genotype, phenotype, and tissue distribution of alpha-1-antitrypsin.

AAT (mg/dL)	Genotype	Prevalence	Risk for lung disease	Risk for liver disease
100–220	MM	85%–90%	Normal	Normal
10–40	ZZ	96% of AAT deficiency	Very high 60% develop emphysema at 35–45 years	Increased Cirrhosis: (intrahepatic cholestasis): Childhood-adolescent: 2.5% Adult: (chronic hepatitis): 10% (<50-years old), 20%–40% >50-years old Hepatocellular carcinoma: 2%–3%
45–80	SZ		High risk of COPD	Some risks of liver disease
66–120	MZ		Increased COPD risk if smoke	Nonsmokers are not at risk for COPD Heavy smokers, alcohol use, or hepatitis C at risk of end stage liver disease
70–105	SS		Risk for COPD unknown	Normal
100–180	MS		Patients' genetic carriers of the S mutation. There is no known risk for lung or liver disease. S mutation causes a moderate reduction in AAT. Can contribute to AAT disease if the patient has another low AAT disease mutation (e.g., SZ)	

Modified from multiple sources; Strnad P, McElvaney NG, Lomas DA. Alpha₁-Antitrypsin Deficiency. N Engl J Med. 2020 Apr 9;382(15):1443–1455. https://doi.org/10.1056/NEJMra1910234. PMID: 32268028 and Köhnlein T, Welte T. Alpha-1 antitrypsin deficiency: pathogenesis, clinical presentation, diagnosis, and treatment. Am J Med. 2008 Jan;121(1):3–9. https://doi.org/10.1016/j.amjmed.2007.07.025. PMID: 18187064.

hepatitis B and C viral infection, chronic inflammatory conditions, use of nonsteroidal antiinflammatory drugs, alcohol abuse, hepatotoxic drugs, and hemochromatosis. Similarly in the case of lung presentation, smoking, environmental pollution, and respiratory infections are strong contributing factors.

The electrophoretic pattern shows AAT as the predominant band, however, alpha-1-lipoproteins and alpha-1 acid glycoproteins are present but their large carbohydrate and lipid contents interfere with staining, and this appears faint.

The initial measurement of AAT by nephelometric or turbidimetric base methods using either serum or plasma. Levels <1 g/L are analyzed by qualitative isoelectric focusing and immunoblotting and or by genotyping analysis.

However, if an MM variant was detected and the levels were <0.9 g/L or an MZ/MS variant is identified with a level <0.7 g/L, DNA sequencing is performed. If an SS or ZZ phenotyping is found, then genotyping is performed to exclude the possibility of a null mutation.[2]

α-1 Acid glycoprotein (Orosomucoid)

α-1 Acid glycoprotein is synthesized in hepatocytes, granulocytes, and monocytes. It has a molecular weight of 40 kDa. Its concentration in circulation is 0.5 to 1.2 g/L. It binds lipophilic compounds such as progesterone and many drugs. It is a sensitive positive acute-phase reactant. During inflammation, concentration increases by a factor of 3 in 24–48 h. It has a half-life of 5 days.

It helps identify in vivo hemolysis when measured with haptoglobin where increased levels with concomitant slight in vivo hemolysis indicate acute-phase reaction. It helps in differentiating acute from recurring inflammations, and in indicating the presence of tumor lysis syndrome. It is measured by immuno-based (turbidimetric or nephelometric) assays.

Alpha-1 antichymotrypsin

Alpha-1 antichymotrypsin is a 66-kDa serine protease inhibitor of several serine proteases including pancreatic chymotrypsin, leukocytes cathepsin G, mast cell, human glandular kallikrein 2, kallikrein 3, pancreatic cationic elastase with the strongest association found with cathepsin G contained in neutrophil granules released at the site of inflammation where it kills degrades pathogens, remodels tissues and activate proinflammatory cytokines. Excessive prolonged cathepsin G activity due to deficient chymotrypsin leads to tissue damage.

It consists of 423 amino acids but the high degree of glycosylation produces the apparent molecular weight ranging from 55 to 66 kDa. Glycosylation is not required for serine protease inhibitory activity. It is a positive acute-phase reactant. Expression is upregulated by inflammatory cytokines. It has a half-life of 2 days. Normal circulating levels range

from 0.3 to 0.6 g/L. Its level increases 2–3 folds during an acute-phase response. Deficiency and polymorphism in the chymotrypsin genes have been linked to Alzheimer's disease among other amyloid deposition disorders.

There is no clinical utility in the measurement of antichymotrypsin except in research into Alzheimer's disease research among other myeloid-associated deposition diseases. It is complexed to PSA and interference in the measurement of total PSA and free PSA and the assay's ability to detect complex PSA form must be known.

Alpha 1-fetoprotein

Alpha 1-fetoprotein has a molecular weight of 69 kDa. It has a half-life of 3.5 days. It is produced by the liver and is the predominant protein during the fetal life produced by the fetal liver and the yolk sac with levels detectable in maternal circulation. In normal adults, circulating levels are <7.5 µg/L. It is considered a tumor maker (see chapter on malignancy) markedly elevated in hepatoma and few gastrointestinal tumors.

Alpha-1 lipoprotein

Alpha-1 lipoprotein comprises ApoA-I giving it a high and variable molecular weight at 180–360 kDa. It represents high-density lipoprotein (HDL) and is a cholesterol transporter delivering cholesterol to hepatocytes. Normal levels are about 110 to 205 mg/dL and levels are elevated in dyslipidemia.

Alpha-2 (α2) globulins

Proteins migrating within the alpha-2 region include haptoglobin, alpha-2 macroglobulin, and ceruloplasmin.

α-2 Macroglobulin

α-2 Macroglobulin is a large protein with a molecular weight of 725 kDa. It is a tetramer of 190 kDa identical units and is retained in plasma in protein-losing states.

It is a broad-spectrum endopeptidase inhibitor. It inhibits virtually any proteinases present in plasma regardless of their specificity. It transports cytokines, insulin, growth hormone, and transforming growth factor-β. It is increased in nephrotic syndrome and states of elevated estrogen levels. It is decreased during acute-phase response, pancreatitis, and in patients with prostatic carcinoma.

It is a metalloprotein; a major zinc-binding plasma protein. Although zinc is not required for binding to proteinases but required for binding to the inflammatory cytokine IL-1β.

It has two identical but independent proteinase binding sites. The main function of α-2 macroglobulin is the inhibition of proteinases released during tissue injury and inflammatory markers at the site of inflammation, thus protecting the tissues from excessive and uncontrolled proteolytic activity. However, it does not inactivate the proteinases but hinders the access of large molecular weight substrates to the proteinase's active site which is acting as entrapment rather than inhibition.

The α-2 macroglobulin complex is cleared by hepatocytes from the circulation, whereas within tissues is removed by fibroblasts, monocytes and macrophages, and syncytiotrophoblasts.

Haptoglobin

Haptoglobin is synthesized primarily by hepatocytes. It is also synthesized in the lung, spleen, kidney, thymus, and heart to a lesser extent. It is a glycoprotein dimer of two alpha and two beta subunits linked by disulfide bonds.

There are three gene products with different molecular weights, binding affinities, and clearance. The three phenotypes are Hp 1-1, Hp 2-1, and Hp 2-2. Haptoglobin is an essential hemoglobin transporter and a positive cute phase reactant with levels increasing in response to elevated IL-1 and IL-6.

Haptoglobin plays an important role in hemoglobin metabolism. The biological importance of haptoglobin is in the binding of free hemoglobin released following red cell destruction. Free hemoglobin is detrimental in that it scavenges nitric oxide required for the regulation of smooth muscle relaxation, platelet activation, and aggregation as well as for the expression of endothelial adhesion molecules.

The antioxidant properties of haptoglobin are via binding to free hemoglobin-containing iron which produces free radicals. The half-life of free hemoglobin is 5 days compared to a few minutes (<10 min) of haptoglobin-hemoglobin complex.[3]

Hemoglobin is enzymatically degraded in the liver and haptoglobin is released from hepatocytes about three days later. The high-affinity complex formation and rapid hepatic uptake and removal from circulation (hence reduced circulating haptoglobin levels in states of intravascular hemolysis) conserves iron released in hemolysis and prevents its renal loss in the form of hemoglobinuria.

Heme moiety is degraded by heme oxygenase-I to iron, CO, and biliverdin. The latter is converted to bilirubin by biliverdin oxidase, iron stimulates ferritin synthesis and binds ferritin (Fig. 2).

The haptoglobin-hemoglobin binding is irreversible. The complex binds to CD163 receptors and is internalized and degraded by tissue macrophages. Haptoglobin-hemoglobin complexes deposit in hepatocytes. Decline in free haptoglobin level is indicative of intravascular hemolysis.

In addition to its role in the hemoglobin metabolism described, haptoglobin plays an immunological role via suppressing lymphocytes and viral hemagglutination. It is suggested to play a role in autoimmune disorders, allergies, and angiogenesis.

Haptoglobin level is commonly measured on an automated immunoassay analyzer using turbidimetric or nephelometric methodologies. Semi-quantitatively, it can be estimated following the electrophoretic separation of serum proteins during protein electrophoresis where it makes up most of the alpha-2 electrophoretic region.

When using immune-based methods, the antibody must recognize all three haptoglobin variants as well as those bound to hemoglobin.

Haptoglobin levels below 25–28 mg/dL had 83% to 91.8% and 96% to 98.4% sensitivity and specificity, respectively, for detecting intravascular hemolysis.

Although decreased haptoglobin levels are seen in patients with hemolysis, decreased synthesis is seen in patients with hemodilution, following blood transfusion, in liver cirrhosis, ovarian carcinoma, pulmonary sarcoidosis, and in states of high estrogen levels (i.e., in pregnancy).

Elevated levels are seen in patients on corticosteroids and androgens. High levels are seen in chronic inflammation,

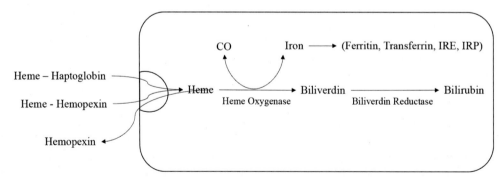

FIG. 2 Heme metabolism and reutilization by hepatocytes. Heme-bound haptoglobin and hemopexin are taken up by hepatocytes. Heme is dissociated from bound protein which is either degraded (haptoglobin) or released into the circulation (hemopexin). Heme is degraded to iron and biliverdin by hemoxygenase. Iron is recirculated into the general pool in the reticuloendothelial tissue. The presence of high intracellular iron suppresses the iron response elements (IRE) and iron regulatory proteins (IRP) leading to the upregulation of ferritin synthesis and downregulation in transferrin receptor expression on the surface of hepatocytes, respectively. *Modified from Delanghe JR, Langlois MR. Hemopexin: a review of biological aspects and the role in laboratory medicine. Clin Chim Acta. 2001 Oct;312(1-2):13–23. https://doi.org/10.1016/s0009-8981(01)00586-1. PMID: 11580905.*

and a low haptoglobin in patients with C reactive protein (CRP) above 5 mg/dL is seen in patients with active intravascular hemolysis. This haptoglobin response however is variable and requires clinical correlation when interpreting laboratory results.

Haptoglobin is not detectable in newborns less than 3-months old and within the first 10 days following a liver transplant.

Reduced haptoglobin is observed in both intravascular and extravascular hemolysis and therefore cannot be used to differentiate between the two. Although haptoglobin measurement is used to assess the presence of in vivo hemolysis, in vitro hemolysis also interferes with haptoglobin measurement at a hemolysis index of 10 equivalent to about 10 mg/dL of free hemoglobin levels, which is within the normal range of up to 15 mg/dL.

A haptoglobin complex is formed with hemoglobin and is removed rapidly. Low levels of haptoglobin are found in hemolytic conditions.

As haptoglobin is a strong positive acute-phase reactant (elevated as part of the acute-phase response) and levels may be reduced despite the acute-phase response when accompanied by hemolysis (hemolysis mediated reduction in levels).

Ceruloplasmin

Migrates in the alpha-2 region, it is a large carrier protein with a molecular weight of 160 kDa and a half-life of 4.5 days. The protein binds up to 90% of copper; each molecule binds six copper atoms whereas albumin carries the remaining 10% with less avidity (i.e., albumin donates copper more readily). The amount of copper associated bound to ceruloplasmin is approximately 3.15 μg of copper per mg of ceruloplasmin.

Its level is decreased in Wilson's disease due to hepatocellular degeneration. It has a ferroxidase redox antioxidant capacity by oxidizing Fe^{2+} to Fe^{3+}. Similar to haptoglobin, ceruloplasmin is a positive acute-phase reactant increasing in inflammatory states.

Levels are low in Wilson disease, however, similar to haptoglobin in intravascular hemolysis, this may be difficult to realize in patients with hepatic inflammation. However, inflammation may be sufficient to increase ceruloplasmin levels.

Measured using immune-based assays (immunoturbidimetry or nephelometry), the assays will measure both apo- and holo-ceruloplasmin forms (bound and unbound) and thus overestimates the level of functional ceruloplasmin.

The functional oxidase assays are a more reliable measure of ceruloplasmin activity, however, the assays are technically difficult to perform and not amenable to automated analyzers. The functional assay measures copper-containing active ceruloplasmin. It will also facilitate accurate estimation of nonceruloplasmin bound copper and thus indicates a possible early copper deficiency in treated patients.

Other non-Wilson causes of reduced ceruloplasmin include chronic liver disease, protein-losing enteropathies, intestinal malabsorption, and nephrotic syndrome as well as malnutrition.

Reduction in ceruloplasmin gradually leads to the accumulation of iron in hepatocytes. As the ferroxidase activity oxidizes Fe^{2+} to Fe^{3+}. Oxidation of iron is required for binding to transferrin.

The antioxidant properties of ceruloplasmin are attributed to its sequestering of free copper ions and its ferroxidase activity (oxidizing Fe^{2+} to Fe^{3+}) inhibiting the participation of Fe^{2+} in free hydroxyl radicals production. Ceruloplasmin is also thought to inhibit myeloperoxidase.

Concentration of copper not bound to ceruloplasmin is determined as follows: [Nonceruloplasmin-bound copper = total serum copper (in μg/dL) − 3.15×ceruloplasmin (in mg/dL)] with values <15 μg/dL considered normal. Alternatively, [nonceruloplasmin-bound copper = total serum copper (in μmol/L) − 0.049×ceruloplasmin (in mg/L)] with levels <1.6 μmol/L considered normal.

One limitation of this calculation is the lack of a standardized reference method for ceruloplasmin. Moreover, several routinely available assays for ceruloplasmin cross-react with apoceruloplasmin and thus result in falsely high values.

There is an association between high ceruloplasmin levels and the incidence of heart failure and the rate of increase correlates with the degree of heart failure. This may reflect the degree of inflammatory status in patients with cardiac failure or to the role of ceruloplasmin in the increase in its nitric oxide oxidase activity. Ceruloplasmin via its nitric oxide oxidase activity reduces the amount of nitric oxide available, where nitric oxide has a protective role in ischemic and heart failure, thus enhancing oxidative stress in the heart.

Wilson disease is a rare congenital disorder (1 in 30,000 individuals) associated with mutations in the gene on chromosome 13 encoding for cellular adenosine triphosphatase (ATPase) (ATP7B) with more than 500 mutations having been detected and over 300 causing disease, resulting in impairment of ATP7B function and intracellular copper accumulation.

Beta globulins

When using high-resolution electrophoresis, the beta globulin band separates into two distinct regions, beta-1 and beta-2.

Beta-1 (β1) globulins

Proteins migrating in the beta-1 region include transferrin, C4, lipoproteins, and hemopexin.

Transferrin

Transferrin is synthesized predominantly by hepatocytes. In addition to plasma, it is present in cerebrospinal fluid, amniotic fluid, bile, lymph, and in breast milk. It has an 8 days half-life with circulating levels ranging from 2 to 3 g/L. It is the principal Fe^{3+} transport in plasma, often saturated at 30%–40%. Correlates with total iron binding capacity. Levels less than 0.1 g/L are associated with anemia, infection, and growth retardation.

It is a glycoprotein with 79 kDa with different numbers of terminal sialic acid moieties (tri-tetra-penta-sialo forms) being the most predominant. Alcohol interferes with glycosylation and carbohydrate-deficient transferrin is used as a marker for alcohol intake greater than 80 g per day (increased carbohydrate-deficient transferrin). Glycosylated transferrin returns to normal levels two weeks following cessation of alcohol.

Transferrin is involved in the transport of iron (in a redox-inactive form) with binding influenced by in vitro pH, temperature, and chloride ions, the latter slows iron release at neutral pH. Transferrin with its bound iron binds to transferrin receptors on actively dividing cells (two distinct types, transferrin R1 and R2) (transferrin R1 is present in RBCs, hepatocytes, blood-brain barrier, and monocytes. Transferrin R2-alpha is present in the liver, whereas transferrin R2-beta is present at a lower level and in a variety of cell types). The complex transferrin-receptor is internalized and taken up by endosomes where a high hydrogen ion concentration promotes iron release.

Additionally, the acidic environment causes confirmational changes stabilizing the transferrin having lost its iron (apo-transferrin) which is released back to the circulation binds free iron (following gastrointestinal absorption or hemoglobin breakdown) and the cycle continues. One transferrin molecule can participate as many as 100 times. Rapidly dividing cells can express transferrin receptor at 100,000 receptors per cell.

Atransferrinemia

This is a rare hereditary condition presenting with anemia, iron overload, growth retardation, and increased infections. Nonhereditary atransferrinemia is encountered in patients with circulating anti-transferring immunoglobulin, nephrotic syndrome, and erythroleukemia (a subset of acute myeloid leukemia). It is worth noting that therapeutic apoferritin was used in iron overload to minimize ischemic reperfusion injury related to the binding of free iron and thus limiting oxidative stress. It is a negative acute-phase protein down regulated in inflammatory conditions. Hyperglycemia (diabetes mellitus) and glycation impairs iron binding by transferrin.

Transferrin is increased in iron-deficiency anemia, and this is evident by the increase in the beta-1 band in patients with iron-deficiency anemia.

Transferrin is a negative acute-phase reactant. It is also decreased in liver disease and in protein-losing enteropathies.

Complements (C4)

Although predominantly within the beta-1 region, complements C3, C4, and C5 span both beta-1 and beta-2 regions.

The complements are labile and this affects both antigenic and functional assays.

Functional assays evaluate classical pathway activation where serial dilution of sample incubated with antibody sensitized to sheep erythrocytes. CH50, which is the reciprocal of the dilution of 50% hemolysis substituting for rabbit antibody-sensitized erythrocytes, measures the alternative pathway.

Nephelometric and turbidimetric assays have excellent concordance with hemolytic assays with the added benefit of speed and automation. Detection depends on the specificity of the antibody used. Some detect whole proteins, others detect proteolytic fragments.

Samples for the measurement of C4 are transported in ice, immediately centrifuged, and stored frozen at −70°C until analysis.

β-lipoproteins

Beta-lipoprotein consists predominantly of low-density lipoprotein (LDL) and associated ApoB100 (about 0.7–0.9 g/L), and transferrin. VLDL usually appears in the pre-beta zone (at the alpha 2 beta 1 interface). The region also contains hemopexin. LDL and VLDL are discussed in detail in Chapter 7 on lipids testing.

Hemopexin

Hemopexin is synthesized by hepatocytes and it is a single polypeptide chain containing 439 amino acids. It is a 60-kDa glycoprotein with carbohydrates constituting 20% of its molecular weight. It binds heme and is commonly used to assess the severity of intravascular hemolysis as its concentration begins to decline when the hemoglobin binding capacity of haptoglobin is exceeded.

Free hemoglobin in patients with intravascular hemolysis binds to circulating hemopexin. A hemoglobin binding capacity of 1 g/L has been reported for patients with wild-type hemopexin form and a slightly reduced capacity at about 0.7 g/L in rare phenotypes (2-2 or 2-1). Haptoglobin, hemopexin, transferrin, and ferritin all play important roles in iron metabolism (see Fig. 2).

Heme (iron-protoporphyrin IX) is lipophilic and binding to hemopexin and haptoglobin renders it water soluble with reduced oxidative reactivity and facilitating its circulation and delivery to the liver. It maintains heme in a soluble state and thus acts as an antioxidant. Heme is a byproduct of the degradation of heme-containing molecules such as hemoglobin, myoglobin, peroxidases, neutrophil myeloperoxidases, and cytochrome enzymes. In normal individuals, about 10% of intravascular hemolysis occurs as part of normal red blood cell turnover. It noncovalently binds a single hcmc molecule, one to one ratio, a binding that is clinically significant once haptoglobin has been depleted.

The carbohydrate component does not participate in heme binding. Barrier tissues, namely, neurons of the peripheral nervous system, human retinal photoreceptors and ganglion cells, and ovary are sites of minor production. It is a positive acute-phase protein stimulated by interleukin-6.

Heme-bound hemopexin enters the hepatocytes by receptor-mediated endocytosis. Heme is degraded by heme oxygenase and its iron is reutilized (Fig. 2). Heme-free hemopexin is released into the circulation; this is in contrast to haptoglobin which is degraded once internalized and bound heme is removed.

Hemopexin also binds to methemalbumin (heme bound to circulating albumin) and to porphyrins (when elevated, for instance, in patients with acute porphyria).

Hemopexin is measured using antibody-based turbidimetric and nephelometric methods. Normal levels range from 0.4 to 1.5 g/L. Measurement is not affected by in vitro hemolysis unlike in haptoglobin.

Low circulating hemopexin levels are seen in patients with in vivo hemolysis. Hemopexin is detected in urine normally at about 2 mg/L with increased levels seen in patients with diabetic nephropathy.

Circulating hemopexin decreases once haptoglobin heme binding capacity has been exceeded. That is in severe intravascular hemolysis. The half-life of hemopexin is about 7 days whereas the half-life of the heme-hemopexin complex is about 7–8 h compared with the few minutes (<10 min) for the heme-haptoglobin complex. Therefore, due to the long half-life, low hemopexin values indicate the presence of severe hemolysis. Furthermore, the long half-life makes it a better index of chronic hemolysis compared to haptoglobin. Hemopexin is never totally depleted even in massive hemolysis.

In contrast to potassium, lactate dehydrogenase, free hemoglobin, and methemalbumin, hemopexin and haptoglobin are not influenced by in vitro hemolysis.

Beta-2 (β2) globulins

Proteins migrating in the beta-2 region include C-reactive protein, fibrinogen (when using plasma, it is missing in serum sample), C3 complement, and beta-2 microglobulin.

β-2 Microglobulin

Serum β_2-microglobulin (B2M) is a polypeptide with a molecular weight of 11.9 kDa forming the single beta chain of the human leukocyte antigen (HLA) class I molecule. It arises from the HLA system on the surface of myeloid and lymphoid cells. Serum levels are low 1–2 mg/L and increased in myelo- and lympho-proliferative conditions. In patients with myeloma, β_2-microglobulin can be used to assess prognosis and monitor response to therapy. B2M

is present in the cell surface of most nucleated cells. It is detected in the circulation, urine, and synovial and cerebrospinal fluids.

Two hundred milligrams are synthesized daily. Normal circulating levels are 1.5 to 3 mg/L. It is filtered through the glomerular membrane due to its small molecular weight. However, filtered amounts are metabolized in the renal tubule with very little appearing in the urine (few micrograms).

In renal dysfunction, circulating levels accumulate and are raised to 65 to 100 mg/L (>60 folds) due to reduced filtration and reduced catabolism. Circulating levels are inversely proportional to the glomerular filtration rate. Accumulation of B2M in renal failure contributes to the formation of B2M amyloids. Additionally, advanced glycation products modified B2M are also observed.

Fibrinogen

Fibrinogen is an essential component of coagulation, it is a fibrin precursor, and has a large molecular weight (340 kDa). A predominant fibrinogen band is observed in plasma samples at 1.5–4.5 g/L. The band migrates in the beta-globulin electrophoretic region. The fibrinogen band can be confused for a monoclonal abnormality that fails immunofixation and can lead to unnecessary laboratory investigation and repeat analysis. It is, for this reason, a serum sample devoid of clotting factors (fibrinogen) is used in protein electrophoresis analysis.

C-reactive protein (CRP)

C-reactive protein (CRP) is a major acute-phase reactant. CRP may span the beta-2 and gamma regions. It has a molecular weight of 111 kDa and is normally <5 mg/L in circulation. However, it is markedly elevated in infections, inflammatory disease, and in malignant neoplasms. Circulating CRP levels in patients with bacterial infections are up to 10 times higher than those seen in patients with viral infections. Its half-life is short <1 day and persistent elevations indicate ongoing infection and inflammatory response. During the acute phase, CRP rises rapidly and is detectable within 6–8 h reaching a peak at 24–48 h. It is routinely measured using an immuno-based assay (turbidimetric or nephelometric) and often by particle-enhanced immunoturbidimetry facilitating enhanced sensitivity (i.e., high sensitivity CRP assays).

Acute-phase reactants

Acute-phase proteins are those where their circulating levels alter in response to inflammation, infection, trauma, etc. These are mediators of the body's response. The proteins have specific roles and functions related to the acute-phase response. Acute-phase reactants are produced by hepatocytes at the expense of prealbumin and albumin and stimulated by interleukin-6 and other proinflammatory cytokines.

Changes in circulating concentrations of the specific proteins in the alpha and beta regions are of both diagnostic and prognostic value. In the "Acute Phase Reaction," e.g., after trauma or infection, there are increases in the plasma concentration of C-reactive protein (CRP), α_1-antitrypsin, α_1-acid glycoprotein, haptoglobin, ceruloplasmin, complements (C3, C4), and fibrinogen (termed positive acute-phase proteins), but a fall in the plasma concentration of albumin and transferrin (termed negative acute-phase response proteins). For instance, those neutralizing inflammation causative agents (CRP, cytokines, and complement cascades) and those that limit the damage caused by the ensuing inflammatory responses by inactivating proteases as well as scavenging reactive oxygen species include alpha-1 antitrypsin, alpha-1 antichymotrypsin, and alpha-2 macroglobulin, as well as haptoglobin, ferritin, ceruloplasmin, and hemopexin, respectively.

Each protein shows a characteristic pattern of change. The increase in serum CRP concentration may be used to monitor the acute-phase response.

Gamma (γ) globulins

Although describing serum protein electrophoresis is helpful in the discussion and description of serum proteins, much of the clinical interest in serum protein electrophoresis is focused on the gamma zone of immunoglobulins in the investigation of monoclonal gammopathies (multiple myeloma).

This electrophoretic mobility area includes the immunoglobulins IgG, IgA, IgM, IgD, IgE, and C-reactive protein (CRP). Virtually, all γ-globulins are immunoglobulins, but not all immunoglobulins are γ-globulins; some are found in α_2 and β positions (e.g., IgA). A generalized increase in gamma globulins occurs in chronic inflammatory states and some autoimmune diseases.

Immunoglobulins

Immunoglobulins have a Y-shaped basic structure containing two heavy and two light chains in each unit. There are two antibody-combining sites per unit, at the ends of the arms of the Y.

Heavy chains determine the Ig class. α, γ, μ, δ, and ε heavy chains occur in IgA, IgG, IgM, IgD, and IgE, respectively. Light chains are of two types, k or λ. In a single molecule, the light chains are of the same type but not both in each immunoglobulin molecule, although the immunoglobulins class as a whole, contains both types.

Immunoglobulins are produced by plasma cells. One individual cell produces one protein. An increase in several immunoglobulin proteins is a generalized polyclonal response whereas, an increase in only one immunoglobulin is considered a monoclonal response seen in a number of conditions including clonality in multiple myeloma,

TABLE 2 Immunoglobulins, function, and tissue distribution.

Ig Class	Function
IgG	Protects tissue spaces. Prevents bacterial infection
IgA	Mucosal defense against viral and other infections. Particularly GI and respiratory tracts
IgM	Usually first to be synthesized. Attacks particulate antigens in circulation
IgD	Present on the surface of β lymphocytes. Likely involved in antigen recognition
IgE	Involved in allergic response at cell surfaces

Modified from Schroeder HW Jr, Cavacini L. Structure and function of immunoglobulins. J Allergy Clin Immunol. 2010 Feb;125(2 Suppl 2):S41–52. https://doi.org/10.1016/j.jaci.2009.09.046. PMID: 20176268; PMCID: PMC3670108.

lymphoma, and in oligoclonal bands seen in chronic viral infections such as HIV and CMV infections, often in a polyclonal background pattern.

During an infection, IgM production occurs rapidly within 2–3 days of onset and eventually is replaced by an increasing IgG response with the same specificity to the infective agent within 5–7 days with a more rapid IgG response in subsequent infection (memory response) accompanied by a moderate increase in IgM levels (Table 2).

Functions of immunoglobulins

See Table 2.

IgG subclasses

Immunoglobulins are characterized by the five different classes described above, however, IgG is further divided into four subclasses, namely, IgG 1, IgG 2, IgG 3, and IgG4.

Total immunoglobulins

A general increase in immunoglobulins observed on electrophoresis is usually polyclonal, e.g., during an infectious disease. In certain conditions, although there is a general response, one or more Ig classes predominate, e.g., IgA in alcoholic cirrhosis, and IgM in primary biliary cirrhosis.

A monoclonal increase in immunoglobulin is observed as a paraprotein. A tumor of a single immunoglobulin-producing cell will eventually result in a large population of cells producing identical Ig molecules (plasma cell dyscrasia).

In the presence of a suspected monoclonal band in the electrophoretic pattern, the monoclonal band is measured semi-quantitatively using a densitometric scan of the gel (Fig. 3). The electrophoretic pattern is repeated and subjected to immunofixation to confirm the presence of the

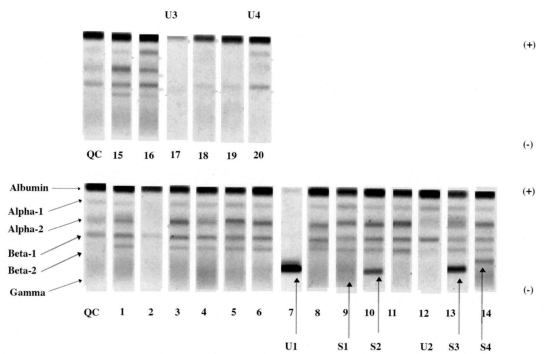

FIG. 3 Protein electrophoresis of serum (S) and urine (U) samples from patients being investigated for monoclonal gammopathy. QC: Quality control sample of a normal sample to ascertain the adequacy of both protein separation and staining. Samples 1, 3–6, 8–11, and 13–16 are serum samples while the remaining are urine (U) samples. U1: Urine sample with a marked monoclonal band in the cathodal region with a faint albumin band at the anodal region. Sample U2: Urine sample from a patient with nephrotic syndrome. Pattern showing marked albumin band (albuminuria) and bands in the alpha 1 and 2 and beta 1 and 2 regions consistent with generalized glomerular protein loss into the urine (proteinuria). U4 is a similar pattern (to U2) but with a lower degree of proteinuria. Sample U3 is a urine sample from a normal individual. Faint albumin is often seen following an adequate concentration of normal urine samples. Serum (S) samples S1, S2, S3, and S4 indicate abnormalities showing distinct monoclonal bands. In the S1 sample, the bands are faint bi-clonal bands. Bands observed on the electrophoretic gel are confirmed and identified by immunofixation (examples are shown in Fig. 4 below). *Courtesy of the author's laboratory.*

paraprotein as well as to determine the isotype of the paraprotein.

When a monoclonal band is identified in the serum immunofixation, a urine sample (either random) or timed following a 24 h collection is obtained and subjected to electrophoresis and immunofixation to investigate the presence of free light chains (kappa/lambda) (Bence Jones protein) or the presence of monoclonal overflow into the urine.

It is often essential to concentrate urine before electrophoresis due to the low urine protein concentration. It is important to note that urine strip tests for albumin and protein will often not detect excess light chains. Deposition of light chains in the kidney leads to nephrotic syndrome and renal dysfunction.

In about 5% of cases, two paraproteins may be detected. This is referred to as bi-clonal gammopathy. A patient may also have nonsecretory myeloma, as in the case of a plasma cell neoplasm in which the clonal cells are not either producing or secreting M proteins.

The most commonly observed paraprotein is IgG followed by IgA, light chain, and rarely IgD and IgE.

Abnormalities in protein distribution and pattern separation reflect abnormalities in protein. However, the patterns are not specific to a particular abnormality, for instance, a decrease in albumin levels is indicative of either reduced synthesis in chronic liver disease, urinary losses due to renal dysfunction, as well as secondary to volume redistribution and capillary leakage seen in inflammatory conditions and in sepsis. Additionally, albumin is a negative acute-phase protein, that is, its level declines in acute-phase response.

In immunofixation electrophoresis where only free kappa or free lambda light chains are detected and an apparent band in the SPEP pattern may suggest the presence of either IgD and/or IgE monoclonal antibodies, substituting antiIgA, IgG, and IgM for IgD and IgE confirms the findings.

Tests have been developed to specifically quantify the heavy and its associated light chains (i.e., IgA kappa or lambda, similarly for the other immunoglobulins). Measuring a specific heavy-light isotype is used to monitor monoclonal components migrating within the beta and alpha region replacing the need for IFEs.

Consideration when interpreting protein electrophoresis and immunofixation patterns include false fibrinogen seen as a discrete band when electrophoresis is performed on plasma instead of serum specimen. This fibrinogen band is seen between the beta and gamma regions. The beta-2 band is mostly composed of complement proteins. If the electrophoresis is repeated after the addition of thrombin, this band should disappear. In addition, immunofixation would be negative for a distinct monoclonal band.

A distinct but faint band may be visible at the point of application typically present in all samples performed at the same time, this is an artifact and may be related to sample storage. It must be noted that a low concentration of a paraprotein may not be readily detected by serum electrophoresis.

In patients with intravascular hemolysis, the release of free hemoglobin in circulation binds to haptoglobin. The hemoglobin-haptoglobin complex may appear as a large band in the alpha-2 area. This pattern often triggers an immunofixation study which should be negative for monoclonal bands often suspected as IgA migration extending to this region. In patients with iron deficiency anemia, concentrations of transferrin may be high, which may result in a band in the beta region with negative immunofixation studies. Patients with nephrotic syndrome exhibit low albumin and total protein and increased alpha-2 and beta components (often due to hypertriglyceridemia) and bands in either of these regions may mimic a monoclonal band.

Paraproteins may form dimers, pentamers, polymers, or aggregates with each other resulting in a broad smear rather than a distinct band. In light chain myeloma, light chains are rapidly excreted in the urine and no corresponding band may be observed in serum. In some patients with IgD myeloma, the paraprotein band may be very faint.

Although monoclonal gammopathy is the major reason for performing protein electrophoresis, polyclonal gammopathy may be observed in some patients. This is a nonspecific increase in gamma globulins often associated with infection and or liver cirrhosis. In addition to the polyclonal hypergammaglobulinemia, a low albumin band due to significant hypoalbuminemia with a prominent beta-2 band and beta-gamma bridging is a characteristic feature of liver cirrhosis or chronic liver disease.

Hypogammaglobulinemia may be congenital or acquired. Among the acquired causes are multiple myeloma and primary amyloidosis. Pan-hypogammaglobulinemia can occur in about 10% of cases of multiple myeloma. Most of these patients have Bence Jones protein in the urine but lack intact immunoglobulins in the serum.

Bence Jones proteins are monoclonal free kappa or lambda light chains in the urine. Detection of Bence Jones protein may be suggestive of multiple myeloma or Waldenström's macroglobulinemia. Pan-hypogammaglobulinemia can also be seen in 20% of cases of primary amyloidosis.

A clear band is not seen in cases of heavy chain disease presumably due to the tendency of these chains to polymerize or due to their high carbohydrate content. Heavy chain diseases are rare B-cell lymphoproliferative neoplasms characterized by the production of a monoclonal component consisting of monoclonal immunoglobulin heavy chain without an associated light chain. The heavy chain is often truncated or incomplete. In mu-heavy chain disease, patients often exhibit symptoms secondary to chronic lymphocytic leukemia, multiple myeloma, or lymphoproliferative disease, and a localized band is found in only 40% of cases with only a third of patients with mu-heavy chain disease having chronic lymphocytic leukemia. Pan-hypogammaglobulinemia is a prominent feature in those patients.

Capillary zonal electrophoresis

Recent development in automation led to capillary zone electrophoresis consisting of multiple capillary electrodes allowing for rapid analysis of large volumes of samples.

Immunotyping

Immunotyping is identical to immunofixation described above but uses capillary electrophoresis (Fig. 5). Samples are pre-incubated with antiimmunoglobulin antibodies (anti-IgG, IgA, and IgM, IgD, IgE and antifree light chains, kappa and lambda). Samples are then analyzed using capillary electrophoresis in the normal manner. The presence of a monoclonal band will appear as a subtraction (disappearance) of the peak seen in the nonincubated sample (Fig. 5). This is in contrast to the additional and apparent band seen in immunofixation.

Paraproteinemia (monoclonal gammopathy)

Multiple myeloma accounts for the majority of paraproteinemia. Diagnosis requires the presence of paraproteins in serum or urine and/or plasma cell infiltrate in the bone marrow and/or radiological evidence of bone lesions. Serum total protein may be increased and there may be apparent pseudohyponatremia.

The relative prevalence of monoclonal types is that IgG is most common (around 60%), less common IgA (around 25%), and rarely IgD, M, or E. In only 80% of cases of myeloma is a serum paraprotein detected and approximately 20% have light-chain (Bence Jones protein) excess only. The presence of a paraprotein is usually accompanied by suppression of the other immunoglobulins (immunoparesis).

In 70% of myeloma, light chains are made in excess over heavy ones because of their low molecular weight (20,000) and hence, they are excreted in the urine. They may form amyloid deposits in the kidney.

Other causes of malignant paraproteinemia include macroglobulinemia (IgM only), heavy chain disease, and malignancy of the lymphoreticular system.

Benign paraproteinemia is usually associated with conditions normally producing a polyclonal response, e.g., autoimmune disease or cirrhosis, but may be present with no associated pathology.

Heavy chain multiple myeloma involves the finding of truncated heavy chains for either IgA, IgG, or IgM without the corresponding light chains. This is often missed in protein electrophoresis and careful examination of the pattern is required. Corresponding free light chains are not detected and are often mistaken for analytical error with the antikappa and or antilambda antibodies. Clinical findings of organomegaly, adenopathy, oropharyngeal infiltration, or swelling in the presence of immunofixation findings confirm the diagnosis.[4]

Patients with inflammatory conditions (infection, sepsis), acute or chronic, lead to an increase in many proteins reflected in increased alpha-1, beta, and polyclonal increase in gamma globulins as well as a decrease in albumin reflecting cachexia, redistribution, and or increased protein catabolism.

A discrete band demonstrates the presence of a monoclonal (M) band indicative of the clonality of plasma cells (Figs. 4 and 5). 5%–20% of patients will exhibit no M band and often in the presence of hypogammaglobulinemia. Difficulties arise in the detection of an M band when levels are either low or the band is comigrating within an elevated gamma or beta globulin region. This is often encountered when there is IgA or IgD paraproteinemia as these often migrate within the beta region. False positive M band detection is seen in patients being infused with therapeutic monoclonal antibodies, often within two days of infusion. For instance, daratumumab reported as IgG kappa and detected within the gamma region (Fig. 6).

Therefore, multiple myeloma patients receiving antiCD38 humanized monoclonal antibody (daratumumab) may exhibit an IgG kappa band on the electrophoretic gels (Fig. 6). This may be confused and misinterpreted as a pathological monoclonal IgG kappa band in addition to the original patient monoclonal band (that is a bi-clonal gammopathy) or if the original multiple myeloma monoclonal band is an IgG kappa and comigrating with the daratumumab (IgG kappa), this leads to an overestimation of the semi-quantitation of the monoclonal band, although the contribution is often small and <0.3 g/dL and often clinically insignificant given the semi-quantitative nature of the estimation of the monoclonal band size.

The measurement of the amount of immunoglobulins is important in the management of multiple myeloma; sustained and increasing levels indicate progressive disease and or resistance to therapy. Similarly, declining levels suggest improvement and response to therapy. Monoclonal bands are semi-quantified from scanning densitometric analysis of the bands as a percentage of the total protein measurement of the sample. This is termed semi-quantitative as it is often 70% of that obtained by nephelometric measurements. Although the latter is automated and more precise, it does not distinguish between the functional normal immunoglobulin and that of the clonal format. This renders it unreliable in the assessment and monitoring of levels of the monoclonal band.

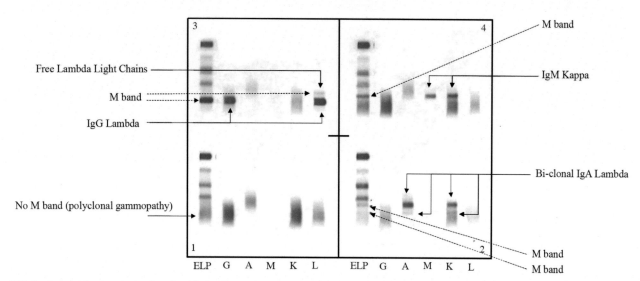

FIG. 4 Immunofixation electrophoresis of four different samples (1–4). Samples were immuno-stained with antibodies directed against IgG, IgM, and IgA heavy chains and against free kappa and free lambda light chains. There were no clear distinct bands in sample 1 corresponding to those in the ELP lane. This is in contrast to samples 2, 3, and 4 with clear and distinct bands corresponding to those observed in the ELP lanes. In sample 2, the additional bands were identified as bi-clonal IgA lambda bands (may also represent aggregate or dimers—dissociates upon treatment with β2-mercaptoethanol), for sample 3, the bands were identified as IgG lambda and an anodal light chain band without a corresponding heavy chain as free lambda light chains, and IgM kappa distinct monoclonal band in sample 4. *Courtesy of the author's laboratory.*

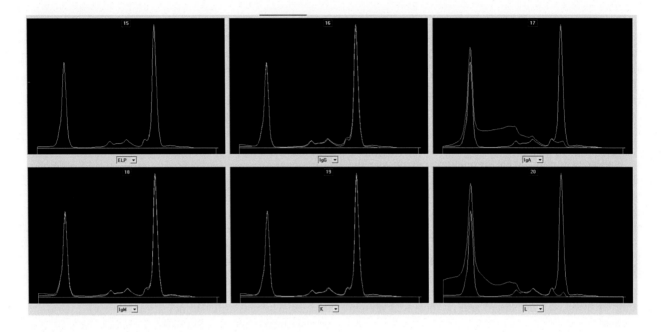

(A)

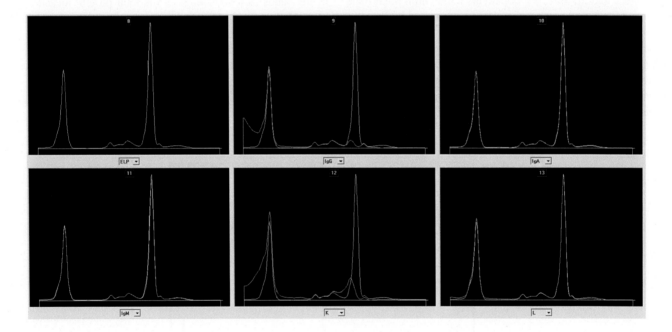

(B)

FIG. 5 Immunotyping showing subtraction of peak following sample incubation with anti-IgG, anti-IgM, anti-IgA, and antifree kappa and antifree lambda. (A) The original peak (in *brown* tracing) was lost following incubation with anti-IgA (heavy chain) and free kappa light chains indicating that the monoclonal band observed represents IgA kappa. (B) The observed additional band (*brown* tracing) was lost when the sample was incubated with anti-IgG heavy chain antibodies and antikappa light chain antibodies. This indicates that the monoclonal band observed represents the IgG kappa monoclonal component. *Courtesy of the author's laboratory.*

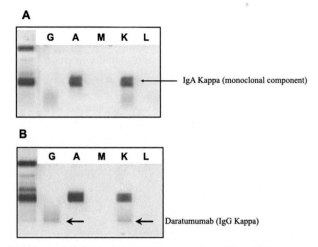

FIG. 6 Immunofixation of sample from a patient with multiple myeloma typed as IgA kappa monoclonal band (A). The patient was placed on ant-CD38 (daratumumab) therapy. Daratumumab is detected as an IgG kappa is observed in addition to the patient IgA kappa monoclonal band (B). *From the authors laboratory and modified from Vakili H, Koorse Germans S, Dong X, Kansagra A, Patel H, Muthukumar A, Hashim IA. Complete depletion of daratumumab interference in serum samples from plasma cell myeloma patients improves the detection of endogenous M-proteins in a preliminary study. Diagnostics (Basel). 2020 Apr 14;10(4):219. https://doi.org/10.3390/diagnostics10040219. PMID: 32295157; PMCID: PMC7235820.*

The performance of both electrophoretic densitometry-based and immune-based measurement of monoclonal components is poor at levels <1 g/dL, particularly in the presence of comigrating polyclonal immunoglobulins. This is similar for those migrating within the beta region contaminated by proteins in that electrophoretic region. Current developments using liquid chromatography-mass spectrometric methods (LCMSMS) offer improved measurements of monoclonal components.

Of concern is the difficulty in detecting low levels of monoclonal component comigrating within normal proteins of the respective electrophoretic region. A serum protein electrophoretic pattern will indicate a negative result, which shows a positive monoclonal band present when subjected to immunofixation. The latter should be performed in the presence of an apparently normal electrophoretic pattern when there is a high index of clinical suspicion.

In patients classified as having MGUS, 1% of IgM will develop into multiple myeloma and 0.5% per year will progress to malignancy. The risk of progression to multiple myeloma is determined by the level of the immunoglobulin, the abnormality in the free kappa/lambda, and the degree of bone marrow involvement.

The criteria (CRAB) in multiple myeloma (calcium >11 mg/dL, renal dysfunction with creatinine >2 mg/dL, anemia with hemoglobin <10 g/dL (or <2 g/dL from baseline), and the presence of bone disease with ≥1 lytic lesion) distinguishes multiple myeloma from monoclonal gammopathy of undetermined significance (MGUS). The finding of <10% plasma cells in bone marrow, an M band less than 3 g/dL and the absence of CRAB, and serum free light chains ratio less than 100, suggest MGUS and is considered a precursor for multiple myeloma.

Measurement of light chains (kappa and lambda) often quantitatively by nephelometry and determining the ratio of kappa and lambda helps detect unbalanced ratios and the presence of light chain disorders. The mean normal kappa/lambda ratio is 0.9 (ranging from 0.25 to 1.65). Free light chain measurement helps detect light chain multiple myeloma, light chain deposition disease, light chain amyloidosis, and nonsecretory multiple myeloma.

Although protein electrophoresis and immunofixation are designed for the detection of the suspected presence of monoclonal components, abnormalities of the electrophoretic pattern become a reflection of many systemic disorders. For example, low albumin occurs in patients with renal dysfunction, protein-losing enteropathies, and in patients with chronic liver disease due to reduced synthesis. In patients with renal dysfunction, the concomitant elevation in alpha and beta region proteins suggests the presence of nephrotic syndrome due to the increased lipoproteins migrating in the beta-alpha-2 regions. Inflammatory conditions lead to elevation in alpha and beta regions of positive acute-phase proteins. Similarly, cholestatic liver disease (biliary cirrhosis and obstruction) leads to elevated lipoproteins in the beta-alpha-2 regions. Polyclonal diffused increase in gamma globulins reflects a polyclonal response to infections. More specifically, the presence of beta-gamma bridging is indicative of liver cirrhosis (due to the associated increase in IgA spanning the beta-gamma region).

Split albumin bands reflect the presence of bis-albuminemia. It has no clinical significance and may indicate binding to drugs or the presence of albumin variants. A small number of families reported having familial analbuminemia. That is the absence of a detectable albumin band. Albumin is often very low <0.5 g/dL. The patients may exhibit mild edema and dyslipidemia. A decrease in the alpha-1 band densitometric measurement indicates possible alpha-1-antitrypsin deficiency. This is because the protein is the predominant component of the alpha-1 electrophoretic region. Patients with clinical findings of emphysema or acute liver disease require accurate and specific measurement of alpha-1-antitrypsin and identification of genetic isotype (see above).

Several forms of monoclonality are present and require careful investigation. They include monoclonal gammopathy-associated proliferative glomerulonephritis, C3 nephritis, bone-associated osteoporosis and fractures, dermatological-associated vasculitis (cryoglobulin), Schnitzler syndrome, necrobiotic xanthogranuloma and scleromyxedema, and neurological associated MGUS neuropathies.

Schnitzler syndrome occurs in middle age and is characterized by intermittent fever, myalgia, neutrophilic urticarial eruption, pruritus, bone pain, and generalized lymphadenopathy. IgM or IgG is often detected.

POEMS (*polyneuropathy, organomegaly, endocrinopathy, monoclonal protein, skin changes*) syndrome occurs mostly in the fifth and sixth decade of life. Detected paraproteinemia is associated with edema, thrombocytosis, chronic inflammatory demyelinating polyneuropathy, and peripheral neuropathy. The syndrome is characterized by positive bone marrow biopsy for plasma cells, elevated plasma vascular endothelial growth factor (VEGF), and the presence of IgA or IgG lambda. The paraprotein presence is mandatory for the diagnosis.

Immunoglobulin deficiency (decreased levels)

Decreased immunoglobulin levels may be physiological as in premature neonates due to delayed transfer of immunoglobulin across the placenta during fetal life. Primary immunoglobulin deficiency is rare (e.g., infantile sex-linked agammaglobulinemia), however, secondary immunoglobulin deficiency is more common and is secondary to chronic illnesses (diabetes, renal impairment, nephrotic syndrome, and protein-losing enteropathies) and medication (long-term steroids therapy). The most common immunoglobulin deficiency is IgA deficiency.

IgA deficiency

IgA accounts for about 13% of plasma immunoglobulins. It exists in monomeric, dimeric, and tetrameric forms. It protects the skin and mucosa against microorganisms which in combination with lysozyme has antibacterial and antiviral activities. It also binds microbial toxins and food antigens in the gastrointestinal tract. It is the predominant immunoglobulin in body secretions (colostrum, saliva, and sweat). IgA molecular forms in body secretion are predominantly in dimeric form with an additional secretory component containing one joining chain (J chain). IgA levels are increased in chronic liver disease, chronic infections, autoimmune disorders (rheumatoid arthritis, systemic lupus erythematosus), and sarcoidosis.

Decreased synthesis occurs in congenital deficiency and increased losses occur in protein-losing enteropathies and loss via skin and burns. Physiologically, low IgA levels in neonates are due to delayed IgA synthesis.

Levels are measured by immunoturbidimetry. The presence of polyethylene glycol in the reagents improves assay sensitivity (due to water displacement and thus improved antibody-antigen concentrations).

Allergy testing

Immunoglobulin E

Immunoglobulin E is produced by mast cells in response to allergic reactions and is often measured as part of the allergic reaction. However, it is nonspecific where elevated levels can neither confirm nor exclude allergy. Although increased concentrations suggest an atopic state, normal values do not exclude allergic response. Additionally, IgE concentrations can be increased in nonallergic states such as parasite infections, Churg-Strauss vasculitis, and certain immune deficiencies such as hyper IgE syndrome, IgE myeloma, Hodgkin lymphoma, and in atopic dermatitis. Therefore, normal IgE levels should not be used in isolation to rule out a topic allergy. Measurement of allergen-specific IgE in the presence of clinical suspicion is more appropriate. Different cut-off levels for IgE have been proposed in children and in adults to improve total IgE sensitivity, with children having lower cut-off values.

Inhalants and food panels

Allergen-specific IgE testing often termed radioallergosorbent testing (RAST) is no longer in use. The testing is targeted towards either inhalants or food-type allergens and specific testing is directed by clinical examination and findings.

Cryoglobulins

Immunoglobulins that precipitate at low temperatures and dissolve back into the serum when the temperature is increased are termed cryoglobulins. They are classified based on their type and clonality and persistent circulating levels results in cryoglobulinemia.

Three types are defined. Type I; a single monoclonal immunoglobulin usually an IgG or IgM (simple cryoglobulinemia). Type II; polyclonal immunoglobulins with one or more monoclonal immunoglobulins, commonly a monoclonal IgM and polyclonal IgGs (mixed cryoglobulinemia, when separated nonprecipitate alone), seen in HCV hepatitis. HCV genome acting as an antigenic determinant for the IgG. The IgM often has rheumatoid factor activity and binds to the Fc region of the IgG antibody. Type III is made up of only polyclonal IgMs and IgGs (mixed polyclonal cryoglobulinemia). Commonly found at low levels in normal individuals.

The classification aids in the management and etiology of the disorder. Type I accounts for 10%–15% of symptomatic vasculitis often associated with multiple myeloma, lymphoma, and monoclonal gammopathy of undetermined significance (MGUS). Mixed cryoglobulinemia represents 80%–85% and is associated with infectious diseases notably chronic hepatitis C viral infection, B-cell malignancies, and autoimmune disorders.

Investigating the presence of cryoglobulinemia requires careful sample handling. To avoid premature precipitation, the sample is collected, kept transported, and centrifuged warm at 37°C. A thermos maintained at 37°C is provided by the clinical laboratory for the transportation of the sample. Following centrifugation, the sample is stored at 4°C for up to 8 days to ensure detection of delayed cryoprecipitation. Confirmation is obtained when cryoprecipitate redissolves on warming the sample to 37°C.

The type of cryoglobulin is determined by immunoelectrophoresis with immunofixation for quantification. Levels above 50 mg/L are considered abnormal, whereas, the concentration does not correlate with disease severity, high levels are encountered in symptomatic patients.

In hepatic involvement in mixed cryoglobulinemia (type II), 50%–70% have elevated transaminases and alkaline phosphatase often secondary to hepatitis C infection (less commonly hepatitis B).

Hypogammaglobinemia may be seen due to cryoprecipitation. Similarly, interference in protein measurement and in erythrocytes sedimentation rate determination is encountered.[5]

Amyloidosis

Amyloidosis is a group of disorders characterized by mainly extracellular deposition of abnormally folded proteins in various tissues leading to respective organ failure. The folding of the protein into beta-pleated sheets renders the protein mostly hydrophobic, insoluble, nonfunctional, and resistant to degradation. The disorder is both rare and heterogenous with about 36 proteins identified.

Some are amenable to treatment and thus it is important to identify treatable forms to prevent end organ damage.

In addition to the protein component, amyloid deposits include apolipoprotein E and glycosaminoglycans. The International Society of Amyloidosis defines amyloid to be mainly extracellular deposits of fibrillar protein that are recognized by their affinity to Congo red and showing yellow-green birefringence under polarized light.

Nomenclature is defined as A for amyloid, followed by the type that is AL, the most common type (amyloid derived from immunoglobulin light chain).

Amyloid deposits may be localized and present in a single organ (19 protein types exclusively associated) or systemic affecting various organs and tissues throughout the body. With few proteins associated exclusively with systemic presentation many exhibits mixed presentations (Table 3).

Hereditary amyloidosis, although individually rare, collectively constitute about 10% of all systemic forms with the transferrin variant being the most common (ATTRv). The latter is being recognized as the cause of underdiagnosed cardiac failure and polyneuropathy.

The presence of amyloidosis should be suspected in patients with nondiabetic nephrotic proteinuria, heart failure with preserved ejection fraction, nondiabetic neuropathy, or unexplained gastrointestinal symptoms and splenomegaly. Although diagnosis is based on the detection of tissue deposits, the clinical chemistry laboratory helps in the identification of associated causes such as multiple myeloma, etc.

Additionally, amyloid typing by mass spectrometry, considered, the method of choice, allows for both wide-range identification of proteins and the discovery of unsuspected amyloid forms.

Currently, amyloid typing by mass spectrometry is recommended for samples where histological examination of tissue was either negative or equivocal.

TABLE 3 Amyloid types, associated proteins, and most common tissue involvement.

Amyloid protein	Precursor protein	Deposition	Target tissues/organ
AL, AH	L light and H heavy Ig	S, L	All organs except the central nerve system
AA	Apo	S	All except central and peripheral nerve system
ALECTR2	Leukocyte chemotactic factor 2	S	Kidney>liver
ATTRv	Transthyretin (variant)	S	Heart, peripheral nerve system
AFib	Fibrinogen A alpha chains	S	Kidney
Apolipoproteins (AI, II, CII, CIII)	Apolipoprotein variants	S	All organs
ALys	Lysozyme variants	S	Kidney
AGel	Gelsolin variants	S	Peripheral nerve system, cornea, kidney, heart
AB2Mv	B2 microglobulin variant	S	Autonomic nerve system

The distribution in urogenital (renal parenchyma) is in the following prevalence, AL (86%) >AA (7%) >ALECT2 (3%)>AFib (1%). The distribution in heart involvement is AL, ATTR, and AL (less common hereditary variants of AApoAI, AFib, ALys, and AGel). In the peripheral nervous and autonomic system, amyloidosis is a rare cause of peripheral neuropathy (3%): ATTRv most common>AL (17%–35%)≫AGelv (AApoAI, AFib, and AB2Mv). In gastrointestinal amyloidosis (AL>AA>ALECT2). In hepatic involvement, systemic is frequent AL (62%) > ALECT2 (25%) >AApo AI (7%) > AA (4%) > ATTR (2%) > ALys (1%), whereas in lung involvement, systemic is frequent AL (80%) >ATTR>AA>AApoAIV>AB2M. *L*, localized; *S*, systemic.
Modified from Picken MM. The pathology of amyloidosis in classification: a review. Acta Haematol. 2020;143(4):322–334. https://doi.org/10.1159/000506696. Epub 2020 May 11. PMID: 32392555.

Alzheimer's disease evaluation

Dementia is a prevalent condition affecting an estimated 2.4 to 4.5 million individuals in the USA with Alzheimer's disease (AD) being the most common cause of dementia. Laboratory support in the investigation and assessment of cognitive impairment and of dementia in adult including for Alzheimer's disease include measurement of the following.

Cerebrospinal fluid (CSF) β-amyloid (1–42) (Aβ42) usually assessed with Tau protein (total and phosphorylated) valuable in the differential diagnosis of Alzheimer's disease and other cognitive disorders. Tau protein (total) is associated with neurodegeneration and with neuronal and axonal damage. Aβ42 levels inversely correlate with amyloid burden and that the ratio of Aβ42 to other Aβ isoforms (Aβ40 or Aβ38) strongly correlate with a clinical diagnosis of Alzheimer's disaese. The ratio remains unchanged between the proderemal and demented stages in non-Alzheimer's patients. The measurement of those proteins are becoming increasingly available on automated laboratory analyzers.

Urinary proteins

Proteins in urine are characterized by their low concentration beyond detection for most except for albumin in normal subjects. Proteinuria is the whole mark of kidney dysfunction.

The glomerular membrane is impermeable to large molecular weight proteins and thus their presence in urine is indicative of glomerular damage. Significant proteinuria is also attributable to tubular interstitial dysfunction.

Urinary proteins are a mixture of low and high-molecular-weight proteins with 30% originating from glomerular filtrate and 70% being intrinsic to the kidney. Depending on the technology, over 150 proteins have been identified. Proteins are a reflection of both systemic and renal dysfunction.

Normally, very little proteins are detected with levels being less than 200 mg/g creatinine. However, "physiological" proteinuria is encountered following extraneous exercises, changes in postures in orthostatic proteinuria, and during febrile episodes. This proteinuria is transient and resolves following recovery from febrile illness, from strenuous exercise, and when the urine sample is collected first in the morning after getting up.

Low molecular weight proteins ≤5 kDa (size of insulin) are freely filtered with permeability inversely related to molecular size.

Low molecular weight proteins such as alpha-1 and beta-2 microglobulins, cystatin C, retinol-binding protein (RBP), and hormones, among other biomarkers will appear in the glomerular ultrafiltrate, about 9.6 g daily. However, on active receptor-mediated reabsorption by the proximal tubules, the proteins are metabolized and do not appear in the circulation. Overflow of low molecular weight proteins (following excess filtration and levels exceeding the reabsorptive capacity) appear in the urine in the absence of tubular dysfunction.

Although the larger size of albumin and its negative charge precludes it from being filtered through the glomerulus, very few amounts pass through. The small amount is reabsorbed by both the proximal and distal tubule. However, significant albuminuria is present in rare tubular reabsorption dysfunction in the presence of a normal glomerular function.

Pathological proteinuria is a reflection of a spectrum spanning from impaired filtration restriction and sieving effect at the glomerular levels to that of impaired tubular reabsorption. This spectrum can be identified following analysis of urinary proteins albeit with considerable overlap.

When investigating proteinuria, urinary dipstick (coulometric) widely used, is based on the protein error of indicators where the protein (anionic albumin and transferrin) causes a shift in pH. The latter leads to color changes in the indicator, the degree of which correlated with protein concentration. The relative affinity for H^+ by the different proteins and thus impact on indicator color change contributes to the differential in detectability (Table 4).

Thus, the screening urine dipstick will detect macroalbuminuria (levels >150 mg/L or >30 mg/g creatinine). The detection depends on the urine concentration, a diluted urine sample may provide a false negative result. Early morning urine sample provides the optimum concentrated samples and is devoid of orthostatic proteinuria. Interestingly, it is the level of albuminuria below the detection limit of the dipstick (<200 mg/L) that defines "microalbuminuria.". The latter, a misnomer for low albumin levels in microamounts, is accurately measured using a methodology offering higher sensitivity, that is, antibody-based immunoturbidimetric or immunonephelometric method.

TABLE 4 Detection limit of various proteins. This depends on their respective anionic change and thus impacts H^+ buffering and the protein error of indicators.

Protein	Limit of detection (mg/L)
Albumin	150
Transferrin	200
IgG	500
Beta-2-microglobulin	600
Light chains	1000

Modified from Schroeder HW Jr, Cavacini L. Structure and function of immunoglobulins. J Allergy Clin Immunol. 2010 Feb;125(2 Suppl 2):S41–52. https://doi.org/10.1016/j.jaci.2009.09.046. PMID: 20176268; PMCID: PMC3670108.

Similarly, low molecular weight proteins (alpha 1, beta 2 microglobulin, retinol-binding protein, and cystatin C) measurement requires the use of highly sensitive antibody-based immunoassays. It is worth noting that, the normally acidic protein favors the measurement of alpha-1 micro-globulin and RBP to that of beta-2 microglobulin due to the instability of the latter in acidic urine.

There remains debate over the accuracy of random early morning urine collection over a 24 h urine collection when determining total urinary protein concentration, although the latter is preferred and recommended for management decisions; it suffers from inaccuracy of collection and inconvenience.[6]

Urinary protein contents are expressed in terms of selectivity. For instance, the finding of predominant large molecular weight proteins suggested nonselectivity. Highly nonselective proteinuria is seen in glomerulonephritis and in patients with steroid-resistant nephrotic syndrome.

Selective proteinuria (as in minimal change disease). This discribes increased selective permeability to albumin without marked increase in other high molecular weight proteins such as $\alpha2$ macroglobulin and immunoglobulins). This is used to differentiate minimal change disease from focal segment glomerulosclerosis where it is low. However, albuminuria may be seen in membraneous nephropathy and in early stages of focal segmented glomerulosclerosis. The albumin/total protein ratio is inversely proportional to the severity of tubular interstitial disease.

In addition to diagnostic and discriminatory utility, the urinary makers provide prognostic values for disease progression. Low molecular weight proteins predict tubulointerstitial damage rather than impaired reabsorption due to glomerular overflow proteinuria (Table 5).

Analytical aspects

Urinary biomarkers are those reflecting urogenital disease as well as a systemic disease. Variability in urine concentration is minimized by indexing protein determination to urine creatinine. Sample concentration is required to visualize proteins (as proteins are low in concentration). Each type of proteinuria is characterized by a typical urine protein electrophoresis pattern.

Total urinal protein is measured by chemical or colorimetrical means using Biuret or by chemical turbidimetric-based assays.

More than 1500 unique proteins are identifiable when using electrophoretic and liquid chromatography-mass spectrometry which affords both sensitivity and unique identification.

Urine proteins are stable when stored at 4°C for ≤3 days, for ≤6 h when stored at room temperature, and for long term when stored at frozen at $\leq-20°C$. The use of preservatives is avoided as they affect protein and cause protein damage and thus impact the ability of their measurement.

TABLE 5 Proteins and their selectivity index influencing their appearance in urine.

Biomarker	Selectivity
Albumin	High degree of selectivity (glomerular)
IgG	High degree of selectivity (glomerular)
Transferrin	High degree of selectivity (glomerular)
$(IgG_u \times Tf_s)/(IgG_s \times Tf_u)$	Minimal change proteinuria. SI: ≤1.0 (selective) SI: 0.11–0.2 (moderate selectivity) SI: ≥0.21 (unselective, i.e., steroid-resistant nephrotic syndrome)
Alpha-1-microglobulin/ Creatinine ratio	$\alpha1$-microglobulin: Creatinine ratio=120 mg/g Distinguishes dent disease from other forms of CKD. (Sensitivity 86%, Specificity 95%) Increased production indicates significant tubulointerstitial damage
Albumin/Total protein ratio	Distinguishes glomerular from tubular: 0.40 mg/mg cut-off ratio (Sensitivity: 75%, Specificity: 73%) Patients with glomerular disease: >0.6 mg/mg Post glomerular hematuria ratio: >0.55 mg/mg (higher values suggest glomerular hematuria)
Beta-2-microglobulin	$\beta2$ microglobulin fractional excretion $\geq0.35\%$ discriminates between isolated glomerular proteinuria and mixed glomerular and tubular proteinuria
$\beta2$ microglobulin/RBP	$\beta2$ microglobulin/RBP ratio >3 mg/g and an RBP/Creatinine >4 mg/g (3–3.8 times more likely steroid nonresponsive nephrotic syndrome)

Modified from Bökenkamp A. Proteinuria-take a closer look! Pediatr Nephrol. 2020 Apr;35(4):533–541. https://doi.org/10.1007/s00467-019-04454-w. Epub 2020 Jan 10. PMID: 31925536; PMCID: PMC7056687 and Picken MM. The pathology of amyloidosis in classification: a review. Acta Haematol. 2020;143(4):322–334. https://doi.org/10.1159/000506696. Epub 2020 May 11. PMID: 32392555.

Urinary proteins

A small amount of protein (<150 mg/d) is excreted normally in the urine of healthy individuals consisting primarily of albumin, low molecular weight proteins, immunoglobulins, and to a lesser extent, proteins derived from the urinary tract itself.

Proteinuria (i.e., >150 mg protein excreted in the urine/day) can be subdivided into four major types:

Glomerular proteinuria

Glomerular proteinuria most commonly results from increased glomerular permeability. The underlying causes include diabetes mellitus, immune complex disease, systemic lupus erythromatosis (SLE), and glomerulonephritis.

Proteinuria is further classified into two distinct types: *Selective* (characteristic of early nephrotic syndrome) and here the urinary protein electrophoresis is characterized by the presence of predominantly albumin and transferrin. *Nonselective* (more plasma proteins enter the urine as the glomerulus loses its ability to restrict plasma proteins from the urine based on their size) and here urine protein electrophoresis approaches to and resembles serum protein electrophoresis indicating nonselective proteinuria.

Tubular proteinuria

Tubular proteinuria results from defective reabsorption of filtered proteins in a variety of renal tubular pathology. Low molecular weight proteins that are usually reabsorbed within the kidney tubules are excreted into the urine. Urinary protein electrophoresis will typically demonstrate a faint albumin band, a prominent alpha-$_2$-band, and a prominent beta-band.

Overflow proteinuria

Overflow proteinuria describes excess filtration of plasma proteins at amounts that exceed the reabsorption capacity of the nephron. It results from urinary excretion of the increased serum levels of low molecular weight proteins (e.g., acute-phase reactants) that occur in some conditions (e.g., septicemia and multiple myeloma).

Para-proteinuria

Overflow monoclonal components are detected in the urine. Free light chain detection and quantification are helpful for prognosis and for monitoring disease progression. Intact as well as free light chains are detectable. Free lambda light chains detected carry a poor prognostic value for tubular renal damage compared to kappa. Due to the difficulty with accurate 24 h urine collections, random urine and values corrected using creatinine are used. The use of serum-free light chain assays has led to a reduction in the use of urine samples for the diagnosis of multiple myeloma.

Uromodulin

Uromodulin (also known as the Tamm-Horsfall protein) is a glycoprotein. It is produced in the tubular cells of the thick ascending limb and the early distal tubule and released into the tubular lumen where it forms a layer on the tubular cell surface. It is thought to protect tubular cells from ascending urinary tract infections involved in chronic pyelonephritis and urolithiasis. Reduced urinary and serum concentrations of uromodulin are found in patients with interstitial fibrosis or tubular atrophy in the course of chronic kidney disease. Uromodulin has been suggested as a surrogate biomarker for the number of intact nephrons, which indicates renal mass rather than kidney function. Uromodulin concentrations gradually decrease with worsening kidney function.

Cerebrospinal fluid (CSF) proteins

Biochemical analysis for CSF includes those for investigation of infection, hemorrhage, malignancy, neurological dysfunctions, multiple sclerosis, and biomarkers of traumatic brain injury. The content of the CSF fluid is a mixture of ultrafiltrate of blood and intrathecal synthesis.

In traumatic brain injuries, intrathecal expression of inflammation-related proteins, as well as apoptosis, and associated oxidative stress collectively and ultimately leads to brain edema, intracranial hypertension, and to impaired blood-brain barrier (see chapter on neurology for more details).

CSF proteins

CSF intrathecal proteins originate from the choroid plexus. Serum proteins are excluded from CSF by the blood-brain barrier. Physiologically, intrathecal protein concentration is higher in infants than in children and in the latter is higher than that in adults.

CSF total protein is markedly elevated in bacterial and fungal meningitis infection and moderately elevated in patients with viral meningitis. The ratio of CSF to plasma glucose levels helps discriminate viral infection from other infective causes. The ratio of CSF to plasma glucose, normally about 60%–70% is markedly reduced in patients with bacterial and fungal meningitis compared to those with viral causes. Furthermore, CSF lactate helps in the discrimination with markedly elevated levels in patients with bacterial and fungal infections.

In inflammatory central nervous system disorders (CNS) (infectious or autoimmune in nature), the contribution from serum proteins via impaired (nonintact) blood-brain barrier limits the diagnostic utility of CSF protein contents. The presence of increased concentrations of immunoglobulins, usually IgG, in CSF, is clinically significant only if its origin as leakage from the blood can be excluded.

The integrity of the blood-brain barrier (BBB) should be assessed before estimating intrathecal IgG synthesis. The combination of the IgG index and IgG$_{loc}$ virtually eliminates the possibility of false-positive interpretations of increased BBB synthesis of IgG due solely to the presence of BBB damage.

The indexing calculations are useful in assessing the integrity of the BBB, in detecting intrathecal synthesis of immunoglobulins, and in reliable detection of the presence of oligoclonal bands (*Oc-bands*).

Indices are used to evaluate the permeability of the blood-brain barrier (BBB) and to estimate the extent of intrathecal local IgG synthesis [IgG(loc)] and include albumin index, IgG index, IgG synthesis rate (SR), and localized IgG(loc).

Albumin index

The albumin index is calculated following the measurement of albumin levels in both CSF and serum corresponding samples. It is used to assess the intactness of the blood-brain barrier. If the index is low (<9.0), this indicates an intact blood-brain barrier, and the IgG index formula may be used to calculate intrathecal IgG levels. However, if the albumin index is high (>9.0), that is the presence of an impaired blood-brain barrier, the use of the IgG synthesis rate provides a better estimate of intrathecal IgG production.

Albumin index $(AI) = Q_{Alb} \times 1000$, where $Q_{Alb} = [Alb]_{CSF}/[Alb]_{Serum}$, and both $[Alb]_{CSF}$ and $[Alb]_{Serum}$ are measured in or converted to units of mg/dL.

Albumin index values <9.0 indicate an intact blood-brain barrier. When the albumin index is normal (<9.0), the IgG index provides a reliable estimate of intrathecal IgG synthesis, whereas if the albumin index (AI) is >9.0, the IgG(loc) equation provides a better estimate of intrathecal IgG synthesis than the IgG synthesis rate (SR).

IgG index

IgG index is not only used to estimate intrathecal IgG production, but also to correct for blood-brain barrier intactness using albumin. Serum and CSF IgG and albumin levels are obtained, and the index is calculated as shown below. Normal values, that is, no intrathecal synthesis, and the presence of an intact blood-brain barrier is <0.66. Higher values indicate intrathecal synthesis corrected for instance of the blood-brain barrier. The calculation can be an absolute value, or rate value, or using a coefficient quotient.

IgG Index (absolute):

$$IgG\ Index = \left([IgG]_{CSF} \times [Alb]_{Serum}\right) / \left([IgG]_{Serum} \times [Alb]_{CSF}\right)$$

Normal values: IgG Index: <0.66.

IgG synthesis rate

$$IgG_{SR} = \left[\begin{array}{c} [IgG]_{CSF} - \left([IgG]_{Serum}/369\right) \\ -\dfrac{\left([Alb]_{CSF} - \left([Alb]_{Serum}/230\right)\right)}{\left([IgG]_{Serum}/[Alb]_{Serum}\right)(0.43)} \end{array}\right] \times 5$$

Normal values: −9.9 to 3.3 mg/day. IgG synthesis rate is unreliable to yield only true-positive results in the presence of blood-brain barrier damage.

IgG Localized:

$$IgG(loc), mg/dL =$$

$$\left[Q_{IgG} - 0.8\left[Q_{Alb}{}^2 + \left(15 \times 10^{-6}\right)\right]^{1/2} + 1.8 \times 10^{-3}\right] \times [IgG]_{Serum}$$

Where $Q_{IgG} = [IgG, mg/dL]_{CSF}/[IgG, mg/dL]_{Serum}$.
Normal values: <0.0 mg/dL.

Immunoelectrophoretic analysis

When matched CSF and serum samples are subjected to immunoelectrophoretic analysis (Fig. 7), the presence of oligoclonal bands (o-bands) (i.e., the presence of two or more immunoglobulin bands) is observed frequently in the CSF of individuals with multiple sclerosis (MS).

The presence of oligoclonal bands in the CSF, in the absence of such bands in serum from the same individual, is diagnostic of intrathecal immunoglobulin (IgG) synthesis. In active disease, oligoclonal bands are present in the CSF of 95% of multiple sclerosis cases.

However, it is important to note that oligoclonal bands (o-bands) are seen also in a variety of other chronic inflammatory disorders of the central nervous system (CNS). They include cerebral syphilis infection, subacute sclerosing panencephalitis (SSPE), trypanosomiasis, Guillain-Barre syndrome, AIDS, Lyme disease, cysticercosis, and adrenoleukodystrophy (ALD).

Beta-2-Transferrin

Also termed CSF-transferrin, in the cerebrospinal fluid, sialic acid moieties are cleaved from transferrin by cerebral neuraminidases. This causes a decreased negative charge on the transferrin molecule (β2-transferrin) and reduces its mobility in agarose gel-based electrophoretic media.

Addition of transferrin-specific antiserum that reacts with both β1-transferrin and β2-transferrin demonstrates the presence of these two transferrin variants when stained with Coomassie brilliant blue dye (Fig. 8).

CSF and nasal or ear fluid contaminated with CSF due to trauma to the blood-brain barrier demonstrate two bands, β1-transferrin and β2-transferrin, while serum demonstrates only a single β1-transferrin band. β2-transferrin is relatively specific for CSF and is used to detect CSF rhinorrhea and otorrhea.

β2-transferrin is helpful in the diagnosis of cerebral spinal fistula. Detectable β2-transferrin in circulation with levels 1 to 2 ng/mL suggests a successful ventriculoperitoneal shunt. The detection is used to assess the functional status of the shunt with the surgical change of the CSF physiological absorption site from arachnoid granulations to the peritoneum. Measurement of β2-transferrin is limited by the presence of sample hemolysis. Measurement of beta-trace protein, a low molecular weight (~25 kDa) monomeric

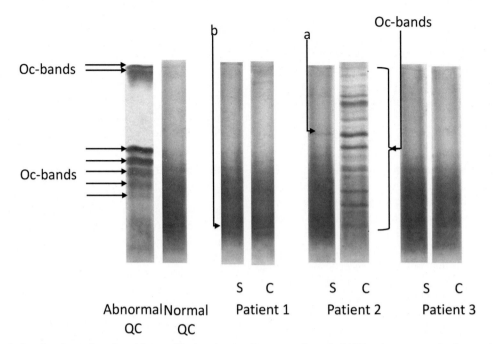

FIG. 7 Isoelectric focusing electrophoresis and immunoblotting showing the pattern of matched CSF and serum samples from patients being investigated for oligoclonal bands (multiple sclerosis). The abnormal quality control sample shows several oligoclonal bands (Oc-bands) when compared to the negative normal control. Matched CSF (C) and serum (S) samples from patient 1 show few corresponding bands (B) in both CSF and serum samples (indicating serum source of the CSF bands due to impaired blood-brain barrier). This is in contrast to patient 2 where several oligoclonal bands appear in the CSF and that are absent in the serum (except for one band (A)). This pattern indicates intrathecal synthesis of immunoglobins and is diagnostic of multiple sclerosis. Patient 3 samples show a normal pattern with no bands in CSF samples. *Courtesy of the author's laboratory.*

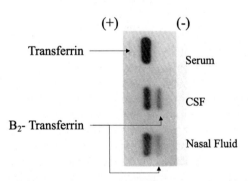

FIG. 8 Nasal fluid positive for beta-2-transferrin suggesting CSF source. *Modified from Normansell DE, Stacy EK, Booker CF, Butler TZ. Detection of beta-2 transferrin in otorrhea and rhinorrhea in a routine clinical laboratory setting. Clin Diagn Lab Immunol. 1994 Jan;1(1):68–70. https://doi.org/10.1128/cdli.1.1.68-70.1994. PMID: 7496925; PMCID: PMC368198.*

glycoprotein, in circulation is used to indicate CSF leakage and impaired blood brain barrier. The protein is measured by immunoassay.

Pleural and peritoneal fluid proteins

Biochemical measurements in pleural and peritoneal fluids include total protein, albumin, electrolytes, lipids, tumor markers, LDH, glucose, pH, amylase, adenosine deaminase and lysozyme, prealbumin, beta-2-microglobulin, ferritin, urea, inflammatory cytokines, among others. Some of the assays are well recognized with available quality control material and matrix validate commercial assays, whereas some analytes, for example, tumor markers remain exceptional as well as for research use applications.

Protein measurement is to determine the nature of exudate versus transudate. This is important in elucidating the cause as well as directing therapeutic intervention.

Pleural fluid

Pleural fluid is an ultrafiltrate of plasma. Less than 10 mL is produced daily in each pleural cavity. The fluid accumulates if production is increased or drainage (removal) is reduced.

Decreased removal of pleural fluid is secondary to impaired lymphatic drainage and/or decreased pressure in pleural space. Increased production of pleural fluid is secondary to elevated hydrostatic pressure, a decrease in colloid osmotic pressure, and to increased permeability of capillary vessels.

Congestive heart failure is the most common precipitant of pleural effusion, whereas other less common causes include cirrhosis, nephrotic syndrome, ovarian hyperstimulation, post-thoracic and abdominal surgery, and myxedema.

Exudate exhibits higher levels of LDH, protein, and cholesterol compared with transudate.

As per Light's criteria, total protein >30 g/L, pleural fluid to serum total protein ratio >0.5, LDH pleural fluid

TABLE 6 Sensitivity, specificity, positive (PPV), and negative (NPP) predictive values of biomarkers indicative of transudate.

Analyte	Cut-off (transudate)	Sensitivity	Specificity	PPV	NPP
Protein (PF)	>30 g/L	89	91	96	80
Pleural fluid/serum ratio	>0.5	90	98	99	82
LDH (PF)	>200 U/L	71	100	100	61
PF:serum ratio	>0.6	86	98	99	77
Light's criteria for any of the above:	99	98	99	98	
Cholesterol	(1.2–1.55 mmol/L) 45–60 mg/dL	73–96	81–100		

PF, pleural fluid.
Modified from Porcel JM, Light RW. Pleural Fluid Analysis: Are Light's Criteria Still Relevant After Half a Century? Clin Chest Med. 2021 Dec;42(4):599–609. https://doi.org/10.1016/j.ccm.2021.07.003. PMID: 34774168.

levels ≥200 U/L, and LDH pleural fluid serum ratio >0.6 supports the presence of exudate (Table 6).

Modification of the Light's criteria by either increasing the pleural fluid to serum protein ratio and or LDH ratio, as well as absolute LDH values resulted in significantly improved specificity.[7]

Peritoneal fluid proteins

Peritoneal fluid is the fluid in the cavity space between the wall of the abdomen and organs. Analysis of ascetic fluid post paracentesis is of diagnostic value in patients with new onset ascites. Causes of interest are those of suspected infection (bacterial peritonitis) and of suspected malignancy. Microbiology culture for bacteria and hematological cell count provide higher diagnostic value compared to biochemical tests. Polymorphonuclear cells >250 per mm^3 should receive antibiotic therapy before culture results are available.

Determining the source of bacterial infection as being either spontaneous or due to secondary peritonitis is difficult, however, two findings of the following three suggest secondary bacterial peritonitis or perforation peritonitis, that is a total protein >10 g/L, glucose <2.8 mmol/L (<50 mg/dL), and lactate dehydrogenase (LDH) above the upper limit of normal for blood.

Microscopic cytology often reveals the presence of malignancy in 75% of malignancy-associated ascites. However, cytology is negative in hepatic metastasis, and only 10% of hepatocellular carcinoma are positive cytology. This is in contrast to patients with ovarian carcinoma with frequently positive cytology.

Fluid is inspected for appearance, a clear straw color suggests the common etiology of cirrhosis, blood contaminated is usually due to traumatic tap which will clot on standing, and unclotted hemolyzed sample may indicate pancreatitis or malignancy, tuberculosis infection, intestinal infarction, or a recent abdominal trauma.

Of interest is that in a hemolyzed ascitic fluid, a red blood cell count >10,000 mm^3 is only seen in 8.3% of patients with carcinoma, and 22% of overall is malignancy related. In other words, low RBC counts in a blood-stained fluid are highly suggestive of malignancy.

Turbid appearance is due to either chylous high triglycerides (seen in 20%–30% of patients with cirrhosis) or bacterial infection or high neutrophils. The frequency of malignancy in chylous ascitic fluid is high at about 80%. Chylous ascites are due to high triglyceride levels (>200 mg/dL) secondary to traumatic injury or obstruction.

Joint synovial fluid analysis

The clinical laboratory will occasionally receive a joint fluid sample analysis. In addition to microbiological analysis (microscopic and staining) for infective agents, biochemical analysis is those for uric acid (urate) in patients suspected of gout, or other crystals.

The synovial fluid is named due to its resemblance to egg white, with a clear yellow, transparent, and viscous fluid. The fluid originates from plasma filtrate (by the joint capillary net) and diffuses to the joint cavity. Local synthesis of hyaluronic acid gives its viscous fluidity. Fluid accumulation results in clinically apparent effusions and swelling. Two types of conditions affecting the joints are inflammatory and noninflammatory.

Appearance

The turbid appearance of joint fluid suggests cellularity and suggests inflammatory and infective conditions. Slight turbidity can result from red and white blood cells, floating small fragments of the synovial membrane, and cartilage or fibrous tissue contributing to the turbid appearance. Significant turbidity can be due to frank pus.

Many infections yield less turbid fluids and often noninfective inflammatory conditions such as crystals synovitis or rheumatoid disease can exhibit marked turbidity. Monosodium urate crystals lead to a milky white appearance. Similarly, for calcium pyrophosphate dihydrate (apatite) crystals. Cholesterol crystals may also give a yellow-creamy appearance.

Metal fragments from older joint prostheses may produce a grayish hue, and fragments of ochronotic cartilage may result in salt and pepper appearance. Fibrin in rheumatoid, an inflammatory condition, may contribute to cloudiness.

Microscopic analysis is preferred to identify cellular and crystals, bacterial, cellular, and other particulates contributing to the sample turbidity.

The use of saline solution at a concentration of 0.3% is a preferred diluent as it promotes osmotic rupture of contaminant red cells. Synovial fluid cell counts should be performed as soon as possible after aspiration, although accurate results can be obtained 24 h later if the fluid is stored refrigerated in the presence of EDTA.

Normal synovial fluid has a low cell count (<100 cells/μL (mean 35 cells/μL)). At the upper end of the scale, a count of 50000 cells/μL has been considered to be the cut-off between inflammatory and septic arthritis.

Synovial fluid glucose is interpreted with concurrent plasma glucose level (because there is a delay in the diffusion of glucose to the joint cavity the synovial fluid and serum samples should be taken at a time when serum glucose is expected to be stable). Noninfectious highly inflammatory synovial fluid exhibits a low glucose level (≤ 40 mg/dL) or even lower than the simultaneous blood glucose. High synovial fluid lactate levels are suggestive of septic arthritis.

The identification of monosodium urate crystal is the definitive diagnosis of gout. Monosodium urate and calcium pyrophosphate dihydrate crystals are associated with noninflamed arthropathy.

All monosodium urate crystals are strongly birefringent and are clearly distinguished using compensated polarized light microscopy, whereas calcium pyrophosphate dehydrate crystals are only weakly birefringent.

Calcium oxalate crystals have been identified in synovial fluid from the joints of patients receiving periodic hemodialysis and in those with hyperoxalemia. Other crystals encountered include cholesterol crystals found in the chronic effusion and corticosteroid crystals.

Alpha defensin

Prosthetic joint infection is the indication for over 14% revision of total hip and up to 25% of total knee arthroplasties and carries significant morbidity and mortality. Different treatment options are available and therefore early and reliable detection of infection is essential to guide management.

Infection is empirically defined by the presence of one of the major or three of the minor criteria established by professional societies. The major criteria include sinus tract communicating with the joint, or a single isolated pathogen from two or more samples from the prosthetic joint, whereas the minor criteria include elevated serum ESR and CRP, elevated synovial fluid white cell count, or positive leukocyte esterase test strip, elevated synovial polymorphonuclear percentage, isolated microorganism in a periprosthetic sample, and/or positive histological analysis of periprosthetic tissue. However, limitations of the various criteria parameters remain, for example, the sensitivity and specificity of CRP for prosthetic joint infection are 82% and 77%, respectively. Similarly, the sensitivity of the aspiration culture is only 72%.

Alpha-defensin is a cysteine-rich antimicrobial peptide produced by neutrophils in response to infection. It disrupts the synthesis of bacterial cell walls. It appears to be specific to activated neutrophils in response to infection and is not elevated in noninfection inflammatory arthritis (e.g., in gout).

The peptide may be measured quantitatively using laboratory-based enzyme-linked immunosorbent assay (ELISA) or with a lateral flow point of care device. The laboratory-based assays although often performed as an esoteric test with at least 24–48 h turnaround time are more accurate in diagnostic sensitivity and specificity 96% and 97%, respectively, compared with 86% and 96%, for the point of care lateral flow assay (results available in <10 min). Despite the low sensitivity of the lateral flow test, it remains a candidate for intraoperative confirmation for infection.

False positive results are seen in patients with metalloids (adverse tissue reaction and crystals deposition disease). Measurement of synovial fluid CRP has been suggested to improve α-defensin performance (reduce false positive). Negative CRP values (<3 mg/L) in the presence of a positive α-defensin indicates aseptic inflammation. A positive CRP confirms periprosthetic infection.

Summary

- Most plasma proteins are produced by the liver except for immunoglobulins produced by lymphocytes and apoprotein by enterocytes and other tissue.
- Plasma contains many proteins making up about 80 g/L (8.0 g/dL) with albumin being the most abundant at about 45 g/L (4.5 g/dL).
- Serum is obtained when the clotting factors have been consumed. Plasma is obtained in the presence of anticoagulant tube additives.
- Electrophoresis is performed using serum as a sample and not plasma to avoid confusion with a large fibrinogen band in the beta region with a possible paraprotein.

- Except for albumin, all proteins are classified by their zone of mobility in electrophoresis.
- Prealbumin has a short half-life and its hepatic synthesis is dependent on amino acids nutrient supply making it a suitable candidate for the assessment of nutritional status.
- Albumin's average half-life in circulation is 21 days. It is the predominant circulating protein that represents 55%–65% of total plasma proteins.
- Low albumin levels indicate poor outcomes and predict morbidity and mortality regardless of the cause.
- Bis-albuminemia describes the presence of two distinct albumin bands visible on protein electrophoresis.
- Total globulin is calculated collectively by subtracting measured albumin from measured total protein concentrations.
- Alpha-1-antitrypsin is the major component of the electrophoresis α 1-globulin fraction.
- The alpha-1-antitrypsin band is decreased in patients with alpha-1-antitrypsin deficiency.
- The half-life of free hemoglobin is 5 days compared to a few minutes (<10 min) of the haptoglobin-hemoglobin complex.
- Ceruloplasmin binds up to 90% of copper; each molecule binds six copper atoms.
- Acute-phase proteins are those where their circulating levels alter in response to inflammation, infection, and trauma.
- Urine strip tests for albumin and protein will often not detect excess light chains.
- Monoclonality type prevalence is often IgG (around 60%), less commonly IgA (around 25%), and rarely IgD, M, or E.
- Multiple myeloma patients receiving antiCD38 humanized monoclonal antibody (daratumumab) may exhibit an IgG kappa band on the electrophoretic gels.
- The glomerular is impermeable to large molecular weight proteins and thus their presence in urine is indicative of glomerular damage.
- Pathological proteinuria is a reflection of a spectrum spanning from impaired filtration restriction sieving effect at the glomerular levels to that of impaired tubular reabsorption.
- Biochemical analysis for CSF includes those for investigation of infection, hemorrhage, malignancy, neurological dysfunctions, multiple sclerosis, and biomarkers of traumatic brain injury.
- β-2-transferrin is relatively specific for CSF and is used to detect CSF rhinorrhea and otorrhea.
- Analysis of ascetic fluid post paracentesis is of diagnostic value in patients with new onset ascites. Causes of interest are those of suspected infection (bacterial peritonitis) and of suspected malignancy.

References

1. de Serres F, Blanco I. Role of alpha-1 antitrypsin in human health and disease. *J Intern Med.* 2014;276(4):311–335.
2. McElvaney NG. Diagnosing alpha1-antitrypsin deficiency: how to improve the current algorithm. *Eur Respir Rev.* 2015;24(135):52–57.
3. Shih AW, McFarlane A, Verhovsek M. Haptoglobin testing in hemolysis: measurement and interpretation. *Am J Hematol.* 2014;89(4):443–447.
4. Raj S, Guha B, Rodriguez C, Krishnaswamy G. Paraproteinemia and serum protein electrophoresis interpretation. *Ann Allergy Asthma Immunol.* 2019;122(1):11–16.
5. Desbois AC, Cacoub P, Saadoun D. Cryoglobulinemia: an update in 2019. *Joint Bone Spine.* 2019;86(6):707–713.
6. Bokenkamp A. Proteinuria-take a closer look! *Pediatr Nephrol.* 2020;35(4):533–541.
7. Porcel JM, Light RW. Pleural fluid analysis: are light's criteria still relevant after half a century? *Clin Chest Med.* 2021;42(4):599–609.

Suggested reading

Marson BA, Deshmukh SR, Grindlay DJC, Scammell BE. Alpha-defensin and the Synovasure lateral flow device for the diagnosis of prosthetic joint infection: a systematic review and meta-analysis. *Bone and Joint Journal.* 2018;100-B(6):703–711.

Lo Sasso B, Agnello L, Bivona G, Bellia C, Ciaccio M. Cerebrospinal fluid analysis in multiple sclerosis diagnosis: an update. *Medicina (Kaunas).* 2019;55(6).

Delanghe JR, Langlois MR. Hemopexin: a review of biological aspects and the role in laboratory medicine. *Clin Chim Acta.* 2001;312(1-2):13–23.

Chapter 11

Gastrointestinal disorders and nutritional assessment

Introduction

The role of the clinical chemistry laboratory in the investigation and management of patients with gastrointestinal disorders has been declining despite the increase in the prevalence of both irritable bowel syndromes and reflux esophageal disturbances. This is due in part to the increased utility of radiological examinations such as ultrasound, MRI, and CT imaging studies as well as endoscopies and tissue biopsy. In contrast, the role of the laboratory in the assessment and management of nutritional status is increasing.

This chapter describes the laboratory investigation of gastrointestinal dysfunction including malabsorption, gastric and pancreatic insufficiency, as well as biomarkers in the assessment of nutritional status.

Digestion

The gastrointestinal tract comprises the mouth (teeth and salivary glands), esophagus and stomach, pancreas (pancreatic fluids and enzymes), and small and large intestines. Digestion of food begins in the mouth where mechanical grinding and enzymatic degradation of food beings.

Salivary functions

Saliva is produced by the parotid, sublingual, and submandibular glands. The parotid gland is the major source. In addition to saliva fluid, the salivary glands secrete hormones and proteins (including enzymes and peptide hormones). Some originate from the serum and diffuse into the saliva (free hormones (nonprotein bound)) following passage from the blood through capillary and glandular epithelia, diffusing down a concentration gradient.

Saliva is a clear and slightly acidic (pH 6 to 7) secretion of the salivary glands. It is not an ultrafiltrate of blood. The average daily production is about 1 to 1.5 L. Predominantly (99%) water, it contains the electrolytes sodium, potassium, calcium, phosphate, magnesium, and bicarbonate. The protein content includes enzymes (e.g., amylase) and immunoglobulins. Mucins content affords protection against microorganisms. The functions of saliva are taste and digestion, buffering and clearance, protection, antibacterial activity, and maintenance of tooth integrity.

Salivary amylases initiate the breakdown of starch and carbohydrates before passage through the esophagus to the stomach. Salivary lipase initiates the breakdown of dietary fat, however, most (~85%) reaches the duodenum undigested.

Disorders of saliva production and flow leading to dry mouth (xerostomia) include infection (bacterial or viral (mumps)), obstruction, cancer, Sjogren's syndrome, and rheumatoid arthritis. Inflammation and stones (sialolithiasis) cause blockade of the salivary ducts and the resultant xerostomia leads to dental and gum disease.

Saliva contains important biomarkers such as glucose, vitamin D, calcium, nitrates, nitrites, fluoride, and a number of peptide and steroid hormones (e.g., cortisol). Salivary and blood glucose and calcium exhibit a poor correlation while vitamin D exhibits a positive correlation with circulating levels. Salivary fluoride and nitrate showed elevated levels in patients receiving respective supplementation.

The above markers are used to assess the body's nutritional status as well as antioxidant capacity.

Nonprotein bound and lipophilic unconjugated steroids such as free cortisol diffuse into the saliva which is in contrast to conjugated dehydroepiandrosterone sulfate (DHEA-S) which cannot diffuse passively and is actively transported into the saliva.

In addition to the above diffusion of steroids which correlates with blood levels, actively secreted peptides include insulin, and this active energy-dependent transport mechanism impairs the correlation with their respective circulating peptides with some (e.g., epidermal growth factors) reported higher in saliva compared to circulating levels.

Salivary glands secrete 11-β-hydroxysteroid dehydrogenase (11β-HSD) which converts most of the free cortisol to cortisone. Androstenedione is converted to testosterone by glandular tissue 17-hydroxysteroid-oxidoreductase activity. Likewise, the high salivary aldosterone level is thought to originate from glandular tissue conversion of 11-deoxycorticosterone by aldosterone synthase.

Peptide hormones in saliva include epidermal growth factor and transforming growth factor-alpha involved in cell

Tutorials in Clinical Chemistry. https://doi.org/10.1016/B978-0-12-822949-1.00003-6

proliferation and the regulation of the inflammatory reactions contributing to local wound healing. Saliva androgens act as pheromones. The use of salivary hormone measurements is now widely accepted, for instance, the use of cortisol in screening for Cushing syndrome, and profiling of salivary steroid hormones have been used as tumor markers.

Saliva provides an easily accessible and abundant sample, however, the lack of standardization of saliva-based assays and the lack of correlation with blood-based markers renders salivary biomarkers not reliable as stand-alone, and often measurement of blood biomarkers is required for confirmation.

Pancreatic function

The pancreas secretes about 1.5 L daily of alkaline enzyme-rich fluid. Increased water and bicarbonate flow after a meal neutralizes gastric chyme for optimal digestion. The secretion is controlled by the actions of secretin and cholecystokinin. Impaired pancreatic enzyme release leads to impaired digestion of fats. Common causes of pancreatic insufficiency include pancreatitis, cystic fibrosis, and pancreatic duct obstruction. Congenital and inborn errors leading to pancreatic insufficiency include trypsinogen deficiency; intestinal enterokinase deficiency causes defective activation of pancreatic proenzymes.

Digestion is facilitated by pancreatic enzymes produced by the pancreatic acinar cells, pancreatic fluid (rich in bicarbonate), and the presence of an intact pancreatic duct system. The presence of food (fatty acids and amino acids) and gastric acid in the duodenum as it passes along the digestive tract, stimulates duodenal mucosa to release cholecystokinin which stimulates the secretion of pancreatic enzymes by the acinar cells and secretin which stimulates bicarbonate secretion by the ductal ducts.

Pancreatic exocrine insufficiency, a complication of chronic pancreatitis is a common cause of maldigestion leading to weight loss and steatorrhea. The pancreatic exocrine function is assessed by measuring pancreatic fluid following stimulation using cholecystokinin and pancreatin hormones.

In the direct pancreatic function tests, the concentration of pancreatic enzymes and bicarbonate in pancreatic fluid is measured. An inserted tube placed in the duodenum, following stimulation by secretin and/or cholecystokinin, collects the pancreatic fluid.

A bicarbonate level of less than 80 mmol/L is a sensitive indicator for chromic pancreatitis. Those invasive diagnostic procedures have been superseded by advances in imaging techniques and are rarely performed.

The gold standard, although not routinely performed, is the 3-day fecal fat quantification in the investigation of pancreatic insufficiency. The patient is required to keep a strict diet of 100 g of dietary fat for 5 days, and fecal samples are collected for 3 days.

Stomach

The stomach is considered a mixing pot reservoir for ingested food with acid and pepsin before being released into the duodenum in a controlled process. Acid is secreted by the parietal cells lining the stomach and pepsinogen by the secreting chief cells. Pepsinogen is converted to active pepsin in the presence of acids. The hydrochloric acid produced kills ingested bacteria. The mucus produced by stomach lining cells protects the stomach from the acidic environment. The intrinsic factor (see later) is produced by the parietal cells of the stomach.

Most of the fat reaches the stomach undigested, however, the peristalsis and churning action of the stomach mixed with pancreatic enzymes including lipase and colipase helps in fat digestion. Each triglyceride is degraded to mono-acyl glyceride and two fatty acids.

In the stomach, protein digestion is achieved by the action of gastric pepsin released as pepsinogen 1 and 2 and activated by the low stomach pH.

In the duodenum, proteases digest proteins into amino acids. Amino acids cause the release of cholecystokinin from the duodenal and jejunal endocrine epithelial cells. Enterokinases released from the duodenal cells by the action of bile salts convert pepsinogen to trypsin, which catalyzes the conversion of all pancreatic proteases to their active forms.

Contrary to earlier understanding, *Helicobacter pylori* infection is now accepted as the main cause of gastric and duodenal ulcers. *H. pylori* elicits an asymptomatic inflammatory response that develops into chronic gastritis and acute inflammatory infiltration with about 10% of patients developing ulcers. Prolonged inflammation leads to dysfunction of gastrin-producing G-cells that become hyperactive with marked increased gastrin production. Gastrin increases the number and activity of parietal cells producing more gastric acid, leading to duodenal ulceration.

Atrophy of the gastric mucosa due to either autoimmune antibody-mediated loss of parietal cells or infection by *H. pylori* leads to impaired acid production. Circulating anti-*H. pylori* IgG and IgA have 92% and 83% sensitivity and specificity, respectively. In the autoimmune form, loss of parietal cells results in achlorhydria as well as loss of intrinsic factor causing pernicious anemia.

Small intestine

The small intestine is the major site of absorption of many nutrients. It is the site for the absorption of amino acids following protein digestion. It is 3–5 m in length and divided into the duodenum (20–25 cm long), the proximal end surrounding the pancreas in a "C" shaped format receiving chyme from the stomach, pancreatic enzymes, and hepatic bile, and where absorption starts; it is followed by the jejunum (2.5 m long) containing villi and muscular flaps, and where most of the carbohydrates, amino acids, and fatty acids are absorbed, followed by the final portion, the ileum (about 3 m) where absorption of B12 and bile acids, as well as final unabsorbed nutrients, takes place, before ending in the cecum.

The layers of the small intestine are made up of the mucosa; the innermost layer contains villi increasing the absorption surface area; the submucosa contains connective tissue, blood vessels, lymphatics, and nerves; and the muscularis comprising smooth muscle facilitating constriction and elongation propagating food distally along the intestine. The serosa layer is made up of mesothelium and epithelium.

Most of the dietary lipids (>94%) are absorbed in the proximal two-thirds of the jejunum, thus in a daily diet of 100 g fat, the presence of >6 g in fecal matter indicates fat malabsorption.

Duodenal ulceration, Crohn's disease (chronic inflammation), primarily the ileum, and ischemic injury (Wilke's syndrome-SMA syndrome) compression of the duodenum between the superior mesenteric artery (SMA) and abdominal aorta (seen in patients with cancer or anorexia nervosa) (due to lack of intraabdominal fat) cause destruction and shortening (short bowel syndrome) with decreased absorption of nutrients and essential vitamins.

Large intestine

In adults, the large intestine length ranges from 1100 to 2100 mm with its development continuing up to 4–5 years of age. It extends from the distal ileum to the anus. The longest parts are the transverse (30%) and the sigmoid colon (27%) followed by the cecum (3%), ascending colon (12%), descending (14%), and rectum (14%).

The large intestine has three main functions: absorption of water (90% had already been absorbed by the small intestine) and electrolytes from unabsorbed digested food, production and absorption of vitamins, and forming and propelling feces towards the rectum for elimination.

Dysfunctions of the large intestine include irritable bowel syndrome where the motility is disrupted by factors primarily psychological cause. Diverticulosis, which are pockets in the colonic mucosa, develops due to weakness of the colon muscle layer and is common with 1 in 10 over the age of 40 having diverticulosis, and if infected, the patient develops diverticulitis.

Inflammatory bowel disease includes Crohn's disease and ulcerative colitis. Whereas ulcerative colitis is confined to the large intestine, Crohn's disease can be anywhere in the gastrointestinal tract (see small intestine). Decreased blood flow in the intestine leads to ischemia commonly seen among the elderly. Infections and inflammation due to infections impair absorption of water and electrolytes leading to diarrhea with water and electrolytes loss. Infectious

agents are viral, bacterial, and/or parasitic. Commonly encountered agents are *Escherichia coli*, *Campylobacter*, *Shigella*, *Salmonella*, and *Clostridium difficile* (part of the flora but can be problematic when there is overgrowth due to long-term antibiotic use).

Enterohepatic circulation

This section is described in detail in Chapter 4, on liver disorders. Bile acids are required for the absorption of lipids and fat-soluble vitamins (K, A, D, and E). They are formed in the liver and excreted into the bile following conjugation with glycine and taurine. Bile is released as bile salts into the intestine where it solubilizes dietary fats. They are actively reabsorbed in the terminal ileum, transported to the liver, and re-excreted into the bile (Fig. 1). Manifestations of abnormalities with bile and thus the enterohepatic cycle are steatorrhea and vitamin deficiency.

Gastrointestinal dysfunction

Malabsorption

Food malabsorption is defined as a decrease in gut absorptive function but not requiring intravenous supplementation for health or for growth maintenance. Adequate gastrointestinal absorption requires adequate luminal digestion and brush border function, effective absorption into the intestinal mucosa, and transportation into circulation.

Nutritional deficiencies can be a combination of both malabsorption and maldigestion. Conditions leading to malabsorption include Crohn's disease, celiac disease, lactose

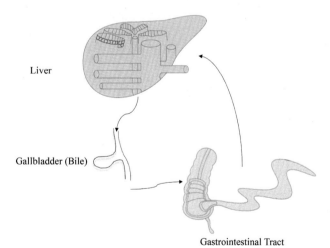

FIG. 1 Enterohepatic circulation: Circulation of bile acids (salt), bilirubin, and other metabolites from the liver to the bile, small intestine, absorbed by enterocytes and returned back to the liver. *Modified from Barkun AN, Love J, Gould M, Pluta H, Steinhart H. Bile acid malabsorption in chronic diarrhea: pathophysiology and treatment. Can J Gastroenterol. 2013;27(11):653-9. https://doi.org/10.1155/2013/485631. PMID: 24199211; PMCID: PMC3816948.*

intolerance, small intestine resection, small intestine bacterial overgrowth, Whipple's disease, radiation in tritest, and pernicious anemia.

Maldigestion occurs when there is pancreatic insufficiency, gastric resection, bile acid deficiency, and liver cirrhosis.

Malabsorption is secondary to either reduced absorptive surface due to either short bowel syndrome (less than 200 cm in adults), or less than 25% of that expected for age. The most common causes of short bowel syndrome in adults are Crohn's disease, ischemia, and postoperative complications. In children, malformations and necrotizing enterocolitis are common. In addition to the above, structural limitations and reduction in the absorptive size by bacterial overgrowth impeach digestion and absorption. More than 90% of the three nutrients are absorbed in the duodenum. The ileum compensates but there are permanent changes in enzyme secretion, which may lead to rapid gastric emptying.

The ileum secretes proteases and carbohydrate enzymes, which are responsible for the breakdown of proteins and carbohydrates. It is also the site for reabsorbing most of the daily secretions such as fatty acids and glycerol. It is also responsible for vitamin B12, bile acids, and magnesium absorption. Resection of the ileum results in diarrhea with sodium chloride and water loss, fat malabsorption, leading to fat-soluble vitamin deficiency and B12 deficiency. Blockage of the lymphatic system leads to fat malabsorption, steatorrhea, and protein losing enteropathy.

Fat malabsorption and steatorrhea

Absorption and metabolism of dietary fat requires bile acids, digestive enzymes, and intact functioning of intestinal mucosa. Dietary fat (primarily triacylglycerols) is emulsified by bile acids and hydrolyzed by pancreatic lipase and colipase into free fatty acids and monoglycerides. Fatty acids are absorbed in the form of chylomicrons and transported to the liver.

Disorders of the pancreas lead to fat malabsorption; they include chronic pancreatitis, pancreatic duct obstruction (as in cystic fibrosis), and pancreatic tumor. Similarly, bile acid disorders (cholestasis due to primary biliary cholangitis, primary sclerosing cholangitis), ileal resection, Crohn's disease of the ileum, as well as intestinal disorders include celiac disease, tropical sprue, lymphoma, amyloidosis, Whipple's disease, and infections (giardiasis, HIV enteropathy, etc.).

Increased excretion of fat in stools is termed steatorrhea. Patients may experience weight loss, poor nutritional status, and deficiency of fat-soluble vitamins (vitamins K, A, D, and E). Causes include insufficient exocrine pancreatic activity, celiac disease, and tropical sprue. The diagnosis is confirmed by quantitative estimation of fecal fat where excretion of more than 7 g of fecal fat per 24 h is diagnostic of steatorrhea.

The coefficient of fat absorption (CFA) is calculated which is the percentage of dietary fat that is absorbed using a standard quantity of fat ingestion. Patients follow a strict diet for 5 days containing 100 g of fats daily. The stool is collected in the last 72 h of the 5 days. CFA above 92% is considered normal. The test is cumbersome and unpleasant for most patients. However, a more acceptable test is a single sample for fecal elastase estimation for pancreatic insufficiency. Fecal elastase levels >200 μg/g stool are considered normal, levels 100–200 μg/g are considered indeterminant, and levels <100 μg/g are considered abnormal and supports a diagnosis of exocrine pancreatic insufficiency as the cause of fat malabsorption.

Celiac disease with a prevalence of 1.4% is investigated by measuring serum tissue transglutaminase IgA antibodies with total serum IgA, which is the recommended screening test. IgA endomysial antibodies have higher sensitivity compared to the transglutaminase IgA test. Of note is that patients with IgA deficiency will exhibit falsely low test results, hence the need for the combined measurement of IgA levels. Positive serological tests are confirmed by a follow-up biopsy confirmation.

Elevated antimitochondrial antibodies are seen in 90%–95% of patients with primary biliary cholangitis. Primary biliary cholangitis prevalence is 40 per 100,000 population.

Carbohydrate malabsorption

Carbohydrate provides most of the calories in a typical western diet. Individuals in the developed world consume about 200 to 300 g per day accounting for only 22% of total daily calories. Digestion of carbohydrates occurs in two stages; in the initial luminal stage, large branched chain starch is broken down to smaller polysaccharides and monosaccharides, that is, glucose, galactose, and fructose, amylase playing a central role, including sucrase-isomaltase, lactase-phlorizin hydrolase, maltase-glucoamylase, and the second stage in the mucosa where products of carbohydrate digestion are further reduced by brush border enzymes to monosaccharides that are then actively absorbed across the intestinal epithelium.

Malabsorption of carbohydrates leads to loss of calories as well as complications due to the metabolism of absorbed carbohydrates within the gastrointestinal tract. Carbohydrates are fermented by bacterial metabolism. The metabolic products have been implicated in the pathogenesis of various functional abdominal symptoms. Clinical symptoms of carbohydrates malabsorption are abdominal pain, flatulence, bloating, and alteration in bowel habits. The symptoms are secondary to the metabolism and fermentation of unabsorbed carbohydrates by colonic bacteria and the production of hydrogen, methane, and carbon dioxide gases, causing bloating, flatulence, and distension, or to increased osmotic load leading to diarrhea. Similarly, the accumulation of short-chain fatty acids results in cramps and diarrhea.

Causes of carbohydrate maldigestion and malabsorption may be either primary due to congenital lactase deficiency, sucrose-isomaltase deficiency, maltase-glucoamylase deficiency, trehalase deficiency, as well as SGLT1 sodium-glucose cotransporter deficiency, or secondary due to pancreatic insufficiency or secretion, age-related decrease in lactase activity, celiac disease, Crohn's disease, surgical intestinal resection or bypass, small intestinal bacterial overgrowth, use of drugs and toxins such as antineoplastic agents and antibiotics, and radiation injury.

Lactose intolerance related to an age-related decreasing lactase activity is common worldwide with increasing prevalence.

A hydrogen breath test is helpful in the diagnosis of carbohydrate malabsorption disorder, and many common gastrointestinal disorders including small intestine bacterial overgrowth and irritable bowel syndrome. Several substrates at various dosages are used in the breath test, such as glucose, lactulose, fructose, sorbitol, sucrose, and inulin (see later).

Amino acids malabsorption

Free amino acids make up only approximately 2% of the total amino acid content of the body and their respective concentrations are regulated by the modulation of their respective catabolic pathways, the rest being present as protein.

They are transported between tissues in the plasma and transported into cells by a variety of transport mechanisms that are relatively specific for particular groups of amino acids (see Table 1).

Digestion and absorption of dietary proteins require proteases, peptidases, and amino acid and peptide transporters. The transporters are essential for intestinal and renal absorption and intracellular, between cellular compartments, and between organs uptake. Defects in transport occur leading to impaired intestinal absorption and impaired renal reabsorption evidenced by aminoaciduria.

Protein synthesis and degradation

Protein degradation is suppressed following a protein meal and the rate of protein synthesis increased which is the net storage of amino acids as proteins. In the postabsorptive states, protein synthesis and degradation are reversed with a net release of amino acids. In the nongrowing adult, there is a net change in body protein content over a 24 h period.

Inherited amino acid absorption disorders may be classified as three types of transport defects. Brush border membrane of epithelial cells of the small intestine and kidney tubules defects (Hartnup disease, blue diaper syndrome, cystinuria, iminoglycinuria, and lysine malabsorption syndrome), basolateral membrane transport defect (lysinuric protein intolerance), and membrane of intracellular

TABLE 1 Amino acid transporters, their characteristics (i.e., sodium (Na⁺) dependent), and respective amino acid targets.

Transporter	Sodium dependence	Amino acids
A	Yes	Alanine, serine, glycine, methionine, proline
L	No	Leucine, isoleucine, valine, methionine, phenylalanine, tyrosine, tryptophan, histidine
ASCP	Yes	Alanine, serine, cysteine, proline
Ly	Yes	Lysine, histidine, arginine, ornithine
x^-_A	Yes	Aspartate
x^-_G	Yes	Glutamate
x^-_C	No	Aspartate, glutamate, cystine
y^+	Yes	Lysine, arginine, histidine
β	Yes	β-Alanine, taurine
$b^{0,+}$	No	Lysine, leucine
Gly	Yes	Glycine, sarcosine
N	Yes	Histidine, glutamine, asparagine
Imino	Yes	Proline

Modified from Emery PW. Encyclopedia of Human Nutrition; 2013; vol. 1. https://doi.org/10.1016/B978-0-12-375083-9.00009-X. AMINO ACIDS Chemistry and Classification.

organelles defect (cystinosis, hyperornithinemia-hyperammonemia-homocitrullinuria syndrome).

The handling (reabsorption and metabolism) of certain amino acids may be affected by deficiency in gastrointestinal handling, for instance, in Hartnup disease, a rare inherited disorder due to mutations in the SLC6A19 gene encoding amino acid transporter (B^0AT1) resulting in defective neutral amino acids transport in the kidney and small intestine leading to neutral aminoaciduria and thus deficiency. Patients develop various neurological and psychiatric symptoms.

Transporters and thus their defects causing Hartnup disease, cystinuria, iminoglycinuria, and dicarboxylic aminoaciduria are located in the apical membrane in the jejunum. Transport defects causing lysinuric protein intolerance and blue diaper syndrome are present in the basolateral membrane of the intestinal epithelium.

Cystinuria is the most common primary inherited aminoaciduria and because of compensation by alternative transporters, the patient does not experience nutritional deficiency symptoms except for risk for urinal cysteine stones due to excessive urine levels and accosts for 6%–8% of all urinary tract stones in children. Lysinuric protein intolerance (LPI) is the second most common disorder of amino acid transport defects. It is caused by the y^+LAT-1 (SLC7A7) carrier at the basolateral membrane of the intestinal and renal epithelium and the failure to deliver cytosolic dibasic cationic amino acids into the paracellular space.

The disorder is characterized by low plasma concentrations of dibasic amino acids (in contrast to high levels of citrulline, glutamine, and alanine) and massive excretion of lysine (as well as orotic acid, ornithine, and arginine in moderate excess) in the urine.

Gastric dysfunction

Common gastric disorders are upper and lower duodenal ulcers. It is now known that *H. pylori* infection is the cause. Syndromes of increased gastrin production lead to increased gastric acid secretion.

Zollinger-Ellison syndrome

Gastrin is a polypeptide (molecular weight 2.1 kDa) produced by the G cells of the gastric antrum and duodenum. It stimulates gastric cell hypertrophy and thus increases the secretion of gastric acid. Less than 0.5% of patients with gastroduodenal ulcers are attributable to increased production of gastric acid.

In patients with gastrinoma with elevated gastrin and thus gastric acid, it will lead to the Zollinger-Ellison syndrome. Gastrin could be from pancreatic or gastrin-producing cells. They could also be part of the MEN1 syndrome where about 60% are malignant.

Gastroesophageal reflux disease (GERD), peptic ulcer, and fat malabsorption (steatorrhea) all constitute an acid environment that inhibits pancreatic lipase. High levels of gastrin in the presence of symptoms of peptic ulcers and GERD are diagnostic of gastrinoma. It is recommended that H proton pump blockers (PPIs) are discontinued before testing. In cases of equivocal gastrin levels or where gastrin is normal but still, with high clinical suspicion, gastrin stimulation by injection (intravenous) of secretin produces a twofold increase in gastrin levels and is diagnostic of gastrinoma (10% of patients require stimulation testing to achieve diagnosis).

Intrinsic factor

Intrinsic factor is a glycoprotein synthesized by the parietal cells of the stomach. It is required for the absorption of vitamin B12. The most common cause of intrinsic factor deficiency is the autoimmune destruction of parietal cells by antibodies or by intrinsic factor antibodies neutralizing the intrinsic factor activity. The detection of autoantibodies to parietal cells and/or to intrinsic factors in the presence of vitamin B12 deficiency and macrocytic anemia indicates the presence of pernicious anemia. Low intrinsic factor levels are seen post gastrectomy, in patients with achlorhydria, and congenital deficiency of intrinsic factor.

Pancreatic dysfunction

The pancreas has two main functions, endocrine function where the islet cells of Langerhans secrete insulin and glucagon, and exocrine function, where the acinar cells secrete digestive enzymes (amylase and lipase) for food digestion in the small intestine, and also secretes bicarbonate which neutralizes gastric acid to facilitate the optimal function of the digestive enzymes. Those are produced in response to food entry (secretin and cholecystokinin respectively by the small intestine).

Metabolic causes of acute pancreatitis include hypertriglyceridemia, hypercalcemia, and alcohol. Causes of chronic pancreatic insufficiency are chronic alcohol intake. Pancreas has a large excretion reserve capacity and symptoms of insufficiency are present when less than 5% of its normal function remains.

Pancreatic insufficiency

Pancreatic insufficiency is caused by the progressive depletion of pancreatic acinar cells.

It is defined as an insufficient amount of pancreatic enzymes resulting in steatorrhea and fat malabsorption. The pancreas has a large reserve capacity and fat malabsorption does not occur until enzyme secretion is reduced by more than 90%. Pancreatic insufficiency can either be acute or chronic. The prevalence of pancreatic insufficiency varies between 6.1% and 15%.

Investigation of exocrine pancreatic insufficiency includes measurement of bicarbonate secretion as well as pancreatic enzymes amylase and lipase. Measurement of pancreatic bicarbonate levels is an invasive procedure following intravenous administration of secretin or cholecystokinin and periodic collection of pancreatic secretions from the duodenum via inserted Dreiling tube.

Noninvasive pancreatic function test includes fecal chymotrypsin or elastase measurement. Seventy-two-hour fecal fat estimation is considered the gold standard among noninvasive function tests.

Acute pancreatitis

Acute pancreatitis is one of the most common causes of acute abdomen presentation to the emergency department with annual visits ranging from 13 to 45 per 100,000 persons. The average hospital length of stay is 8 days. The mortality rate remains high at 5% associated with multiorgan failure.

The diagnosis of acute pancreatitis is established and characterized into early or late phases of the disease according to the revised Atlanta Classification. Acute mild pancreatitis is the most common form without organ failure or local or systemic complications. Transient (<48 h) organ failure with or without systemic complications is characteristic of moderately severe acute pancreatitis, whereas the severe form is characterized by persistent single or multiple organ failure lasting >48 h.

In general, the classification requires the finding of two out of three. The presence of abdominal pain and elevated lipase or amylase at least 3 times the upper limit of normal and/or a characteristic radiological finding (contrast CT, or MRI, transabdominal ultrasound) supports the diagnosis of acute pancreatitis.

Amylase increases up to 3 times the upper limit of normal reaching a peak at 3–6 h following onset of symptoms and with a half-life of 10–12 h, the elevation persists for 3–5 days.

Common causes include gallstones causing biliary tract obstruction (40% of cases) and alcohol abuse (35% of cases); less common causes include postendoscopic retrograde cholangiopancreatography (ERCP), hypercalcemia (calcium >10.4 mg/dL (2.6 mmol/L)), hypertriglyceridemia (>10 mmol/L), infection, drugs, tumors, trauma, and obstruction in cystic fibrosis.

Amylase is secreted by the acinar cells of the pancreas and by the salivary glands, and to a smaller degree by the intestinal tract, adipose tissue, fallopian tubes, and gonads. Circulating amylase is filtered through the glomerulus, reabsorbed by proximal renal tubules, and degraded by hepatocytes. Little appears in the urine except in patients with acute pancreatitis where the rapid increase (see later) overwhelms renal reabsorption and high levels detected in urine and thus of diagnostic value in late presentations. In patients with acute pancreatitis, pancreatic amylase lasts for 3–4 days in circulation with high levels lasting up to 7–10 days in urine.

Although an immunoassay-based assay specific to pancreatic amylase isoform is available, total amylase activity is relatively cheaper and is in general routine use.

In addition to the markedly elevated circulating salivary gland amylase (inflammation of the salivary glands (e.g., mumps)), elevated amylase is encountered in pancreatic obstruction (e.g., cystic fibrosis), pancreatic cancer, breast cancer, colon, lung, ovarian cancers, hepatitis, cirrhosis, peritonitis, head injury, acute aortic dissection, drugs, and pregnancy. Furthermore, reduced renal clearance results in high sustained amylase levels in those conditions.

Circulating amylase levels >5 times the upper limit of normal is encountered in 50% of patients presenting with either acute abdomen, drugs (e.g., morphine-causing spams of the sphincter of Oddi), diabetic ketoacidosis, and without evidence of acute pancreatitis.

Few patients exhibit macroamylasemia (amylase-antiamylase immunoglobulin (often IgA) complex or molecular aggregates). This molecular aggregate increases its half-life in the circulation and it is not filtered into the urine due to its large molecular size, thus low or normal urinary amylase levels are found.

The lack of tissue specificity of amylase where elevated levels are seen in patients without acute pancreatitis favors the measurement of lipase. Lipase affords a higher degree of pancreatic specificity compared to amylase, which is also elevated in nonpancreatic conditions. Recently, the use of lipase in place of amylase is recommended.

Similar to amylase, lipase is produced by pancreatic acinar cells. It is also produced to a much lesser degree (to the 100th) by hepatocytes, endothelial cells, and lipoprotein lipase activity. It has increased permeability compared to amylase. This leads to lipase levels rapidly increasing by 3–6 h following the onset of symptoms reaching a peak by 24 h and remaining elevated up to 2 weeks. It has a much wider diagnostic window compared to amylase. Lipase now has improved and automated assays. Additionally, it has improved diagnostic sensitivity (ranging from 64% to 100%) compared to amylase with reported 45% to 87% sensitivity.

Normal amylase and lipase levels may be observed in patients with clinical and radiological evidence of acute pancreatitis. This has been attributed to the time frame the patient presents. A very early (<4–5 h from onset of symptoms) or late (days later) presentation might produce normal level results.

Chronic pancreatitis

Chronic pancreatitis is a chronic and repetitive inflammation of the pancreas with variable intensity and duration. This complex inflammatory condition leads eventually to pancreatic fibrosis and calcification and ultimately to exocrine and endocrine pancreatic insufficiency.

The prevalence is variable with a possibility of about 25.4 to 98.7 per 100,000 people with an annual incidence of about 5 new cases per 100,000 persons. Approximately, 3%–35% of patients with a first episode of acute pancreatitis will progress to chronic pancreatitis over 3–8 years.

Risk factors and their prevalence include alcohol (40%–70%), frequent nicotine use (60%), genetic mutations predisposition, pancreatic duct obstruction (2%–9%), hypertriglyceridemia (3%–1%), chronic kidney disease (2%–5%), and autoimmune pancreatitis—IgG4 (1%–2%).

Cystic fibrosis, with a prevalence for the common type up to 7%, is an autosomal recessive mutation in the cystic fibrosis transmembrane conductance regulator (CFTR) gene with 80% of patients developing progressive damage secondary to blockade and obstruction of the pancreatic duct.

Pancreatic insufficiency leads to malabsorption, diabetes, and an increased risk for pancreatic cancer. Patients' quality of life and life expectancy are reduced.

Although diagnosis is based on clinical features and imaging evidence as well as the presence of known risk factors, abnormal serum or urine pancreatic enzymes (amylase or lipase) activities that are 3 times the upper limit of normal may be encountered. Similarly, abnormal exocrine functions with stool elastase <200 μ/g (see later) are encountered.

Intestinal (bowel) dysfunction

Diarrhea

Diarrhea is defined as a watery stool formation; it can be either secretory or osmotic in nature. The clinical chemistry laboratory plays an important role in its distinction.

Diarrhea represents an alteration of bowel function where stool water content is high secondary to reduced absorption by the intestine. Although acute diarrhea is self-limiting and is often associated with infection or ingestion of drugs and toxins, chronic diarrhea lasting more than 4 weeks often requires extensive investigation.

Eight liters of intestinal secretions are produced daily. The secretions are primarily reabsorbed in the jejunum and ileum and colon. Significant and life-threatening losses in K and other electrolytes can occur following dysfunction in reabsorption, due to either infection (dysfunction in sodium reabsorption in jejunum) or to osmotic substance presence or to anatomical factors such as postsurgical resection and thus reduced surface of absorption.

Disordered gut mobility may also contribute to diarrhea. This is often seen in patients with diabetic autonomic neuropathy and in patients post vagotomy.

Essential laboratory investigation includes complete blood count, metabolic profile, IgA antitissue transglutaminase and total IgA levels, and C-reactive protein. Investigation of stool electrolytes and osmolar gap is also performed. The following investigations are also carried out: fecal occult blood testing, stool culture, fecal calmodulin and/or lactoferrin activity, ova and parasite assessment, *clostridium difícile* toxin, and fecal fat by microscopy.

Imaging studies often followed in patients with abnormal laboratory findings include cross-sectional abdominal imaging MRI, barium fluoroscopic test, as well as colonoscopy and endoscopic procedures in patients with steatorrhea.

The fecal osmolar gap is calculated by (serum osmolality) − (2× fecal sodium-Fecal K). A gap of more than 100 mOsmol/L suggests osmotic diarrhea possibly due to ingestion of a poorly absorbed substance such as magnesium salts or lactose in a patient with lactase deficiency, or polyethylene glycol, whereas a large negative osmotic gap suggests ingestion of sulfate or phosphate salts, an osmolar gap <100 mOsmol/L indicates secretory diarrhea.

Carbohydrate malabsorption is associated with stool pH <6 due to fermentations of malabsorbed carbohydrates to short-chain fatty acids. Diarrhea with a small osmotic gap suggests secretory diarrhea, which may be due to one of the many conditions described above.

Laboratory findings for blood fecal leukocytes and fat content in diarrhea can be characterized as being watery, inflammatory, and fatty. This will help direct further evaluation and investigation.

Watery diarrhea can be either osmotic or secretory. Osmotic diarrhea is secondary to medication such as the use of osmotic laxatives containing magnesium, sulfate, or phosphate. Poorly absorbed and unmetabolized sugar such as lactose as in lactose intolerance due to enzymes dysfunction (lactase or sucrase), diet and foods containing sorbitol and mannitol, among others also lead to osmotic diarrhea. Secretory diarrhea is often seen in small intestinal bacterial overgrowth, colitis, and in medications such as stimulant laxative antibiotics. Diarrhea is also encountered in patients with carcinoid syndrome, gastrinoma, medullary thyroid carcinoma, and VIPoma, adrenal insufficiency, and hyperthyroidism.

Fatty diarrhea is associated with malabsorption and maldigestion syndromes. Digestion is decreased due to lack of bile salt seen in cirrhosis, bile duct obstruction, ileal resection, and cholecystectomy as well as in pancreatic dysfunction, cystic fibrosis, chronic pancreatitis, and pancreatic duct obstruction, and malabsorption in patients was due to short bowel syndrome, small intestinal bacterial overgrowth, and lymphatic obstruction.

Chronic diarrhea[1] is a common clinical problem annually affecting about 5% of the population.

The differential diagnosis is extensive, and many patients will have structural problems such as inflammatory bowel disease or celiac disease, or irritable bowel syndrome. Causes of irritable bowel syndrome associated with diarrhea range from bacterial overgrowth, bile acid malabsorption, food intolerance, and motility disorders.

The frequency of celiac disease in patients with chronic diarrhea is less well documented and maybe as much as 5% and all patients with chronic diarrhea should be screened for celiac disease with anti-IgA antitissue transglutaminase and total IgA levels.

Food intolerance may be the cause of diarrhea particularly when it is fluctuating in intensity from day to day. Carbohydrate malabsorption with carbohydrates accumulating due to malabsorption are converted to short-chain fatty acids contributing to the low fecal pH and the observed osmotic diarrhea.

Diarrhea related to nonallergic food intolerance may account for symptoms in at least 20% of patients with irritable bowel syndrome.

Food allergy in addition to diarrhea is often associated with other acute allergic symptoms such as swelling of the mucus of the membranes of the mouth or the skin rash.

TABLE 2 Types of gastrointestinal disorders associated with bile acids malabsorption.

Type 1	Ileal resection/dysfunction
Type 2	Idiopathic Mutations in hepatic bile acid transporter
Type 3	Gastrointestinal disorders Small bowel bacterial overgrowth Cholecystectomy Celiac disease

Modified from Barkun AN, Love J, Gould M, Pluta H, Steinhart H. Bile acid malabsorption in chronic diarrhea: pathophysiology and treatment. Can J Gastroenterol. 2013;27(11):653-9. https://doi.org/10.1155/2013/485631. PMID: 24199211; PMCID: PMC3816948.

Microscopic colitis, lymphocytic or collagenous, is a common cause of chronic secretory diarrhea; it might be identified in up to 5% to 10% of irritable bowel syndrome patients. Inflammatory markers such as C-reactive protein and fecal calprotectin are not reliable and endoscopic investigation coupled with anatomical pathological investigations of biopsies is often required.

Bile acid malabsorption can lead to secretory diarrhea. Excess conjugated bile acids secretion into the colon reaches a concentration of 3 to 5 mM, which reduces mucosal sodium absorption and stimulates chloride secretion producing water and secretory diarrhea.

Excess fecal bile acid excretion in a timed stool collection confirms the presence of bile acid malabsorption. There are three different types of gastrointestinal disorders (ileum, idiopathic, intestinal) that are common causes of secondary bile malabsorption. They are classified according to etiology and gastrointestinal defect site (Table 2).

Inflammatory bowel disease

Inflammatory bowel disease (IBD) represents a group of chronic and incurable disorders characterized by relapsing-remitting inflammation of the gastrointestinal tract with 0.3% prevalence in the developed world. There are primarily two main types, Crohn's disease affecting any segment of the upper or lower gastrointestinal tract, and ulcerative colitis which the name implies is limited to the colon. Although suggested to be secondary to an inflammatory response to intestinal microbes, the etiology remains poorly understood.

Crohn's disease

Crohn's disease is characterized by inflammation of the small intestine. It causes damage to the mucosa lining leading to malabsorption and can affect any part of the gastrointestinal tract, but the small bowel is mostly affected, and in an estimated 70% of patients, and indeed 33% of patients, who have this, it is confined to the small bowel. Malabsorption depends on the portion of the bowel that is affected. In terminal ileum involvement, bile salt and B12 malabsorption occur. Jejunum involvement can lead to protein-energy malnutrition because protein and carbohydrates and fats are absorbed there. Malabsorption in general and the constituents and the nutrients that are malabsorbed or affected depend on the site of the gastrointestinal tract that is involved.

Irritable bowel syndrome

A variable noninflammatory gastrointestinal condition leads to what is commonly termed irritable bowel syndrome (IBS). This is distinct from inflammatory bowel disease (IBD). Most patients complaining of chronic diarrhea are given a diagnosis of irritable bowel syndrome with diarrhea.

New serological markers for irritable bowel syndrome include anticytolethal distending toxin B (CdtB)b antibodies. The toxin is commonly produced by bacteria that cause gastroenteritis. The antibodies cross-react with vinculin when the protein is present in the gastrointestinal mucosa and enteric nervous system. High titers of antiantibodies are associated with lower probabilities of being normal, having inflammatory bowel disease, or celiac disease. The test has a high cut-off value leading to low sensitivity with fewer than 50% of all irritable bowel syndrome patients with diarrhea having a positive test.

Inherited disorders of the gastrointestinal tract

Lactose intolerance

Lactase deficiency can either be primary or secondary. Primary lactase deficiency is the most common and consists of three types of genetic mutations in the lactase enzyme activity gene. It is an autosomal recessive disorder. Secondary causes of lactase deficiency are underlying intestinal disease, small intestinal bacterial overgrowth infections, or inflammation as in Crohn's disease and celiac disease. Infections causing inflammation and damage to the epithelium result in lactose malabsorption.

Autoimmune disorders

Celiac disease

Celiac disease is an autoimmune disorder directed against gastrointestinal gliadin. The disease presents with symptoms that could be mild or atypical and thus a high index of suspicion is required, often by the general practitioner. Celiac disease affects 1% of the population, making it one of the most common gastrointestinal disorders. The disease has a strong genetic component, the most important genetic risk factor being HLA-DQ2 (encoded by alleles A1*05 and B1*02) and HLA-DQ8 (encoded by alleles A1*03 and

B1*0302) heterodimers. Almost all patients will have one of these HLA types (HLA-DQ2 among about 95%, and HLA-DQ8 among 5%) and that absence of mutations has a high negative predictive value (>99%) essentially excluding the Celiac disease as a diagnosis. However, HLA typing is not performed routinely because about 30% of the white population carries HLA-DQ2 or HLA-DQ8 with only 4% developing Celiac disease.

However, serological tests, antigliadin, anti-tissue transglutaminase (anti-TTG), and anti-endomysium and anti-deamidated gliadin peptides antibodies are commonly ordered, with antigliadin and antitissue transglutaminase antibodies being the most common in patients suspected with gastrointestinal disorders. IgA antibodies to tissue transglutaminase have high diagnostic sensitivity and specificity with biopsy confirming the diagnosis.

A typical algorithm for the investigation of Celiac disease is to initially measure IgA levels. If the levels are within the normal range, then measure anti-TTG IgA. If the latter is weakly positive, endomysial antibodies IgA and anti-deaminated gliadin IgA are measured.

If the initial IgA levels were low, measure anti-TTG IgA and IgG, and anti-deaminated gliadin IgA and IgG. However, if the initial IgA levels were undetectable, this indicates the presence of selective IgA deficiency and requires measurement of anti-TTG IgG, and anti-deaminated gliadin IgG.

IgA deficiency

General use IgA assay does not have the required sensitivity to detect IgA deficiency and assays with high sensitivity need to be used. Selective IgA deficiency occurs in 1:500 in the population and 2%–3% of patients with celiac disease.

Inflammation

Activated neutrophils, following inflammation, produce calprotectin (calcium-binding protein). Thus, elevated fecal levels indicate gastrointestinal infection but it is also elevated in colorectal carcinoma, polyps, and diverticulosis. A negative calprotectin rules out the need for a colonoscopy.

Gastrointestinal malignancy

There are a number of gastrointestinal malignancies. Common laboratory investigations are described in the following section.

Colorectal carcinoma

Adenocarcinoma is the most common cause of cancer-related mortality in the developed world with survival correlating with the stage of cancer at the time of presentation. Therefore, early detection is essential where screening an asymptomatic population reduced associated mortality by 15% to 33%.

Fecal occult blood testing

Although the utility of fecal occult blood testing is occasionally questioned, it continues to be widely used in a number of settings including as part of the physical examination at hospital admission and during annual health screens. The assays are designed to detect hemoglobin molecules in fecal samples as an indication of gastrointestinal (GI) bleeding that can be due to various pathologies including GI inflammation and colorectal carcinoma (CRC). Guaiac-based fecal occult blood tests (FOBTs) utilize the peroxidase-like activity of the heme molecule in hemoglobin. An upper GI bleed is only detected by heme-based assays. Newer, more sensitive, and specific antibody-based assays, such as fecal immunochemical testing, do not detect an upper GI bleed because the antigen (hemoglobin) will be digested and epitopes lost during GI passage.

The role of FOBTs in screening for CRC is well documented and multisociety guidelines for early detection of CRC include their use. However, there is little evidence for the appropriate use of guaiac-based FOBTs among hospitalized patients. In the era of evidence-based medicine, continued usage of guaiac-based FOBTs must be assessed in terms of outcomes. Ideally, test results should impact further management. In the case of a positive FOBT result, standard protocols recommend that a clinical assessment and a GI investigation, such as an endoscopy should follow.

Carcinoid syndrome

Carcinoid tumors arise in the gut, terminal ileum, and the ileocecal region or the lungs. Tumors produced vasoactive intestinal peptides (VIPs) such as 5-hydroxytryptamine and serotonin, metabolized to 5-hydroxyindole acetic acid (5-HIAA). Some tumors will produce 5-hydroxytryptophan. Elevated 24-h urinary 5-HIAA levels are indicative of carcinoid syndrome. Dietary bananas and tomatoes contain large amounts of 5-hydroxytryptophan and should be avoided for at least 48 h before the beginning of sample collection. Sample collection during the attack provides the best diagnostic sensitivity.

VIPs released by tumors are metabolized by the liver and thus symptoms appear when there is metastasis to the liver. Symptoms include abdominal colic and diarrhea, flushing, and may include asthmatic attack.

Edema and hyponatremia are present. Some carcinoid tumors produce ACTH or ACTH-like peptides leading to apparent Cushing's syndrome.

Verner-Morrison syndrome

In addition to gastrin, secretin, and cholecystokinin, as mentioned above, other gastrointestinal peptides (vasoactive peptides (VIP), pancreatic polypeptides, and gastric inhibitory polypeptide (GIP)) are produced by various gastrointestinal tumors. Excessive VIP causes excessive potassium loss and watery diarrhea, a clinical presentation known as the Verner-Morrison syndrome.

Insulinoma

Insulinomas are common pancreatic neuroendocrine tumors with the incidence being 4 per million person-years. 5% to 10% of cases are associated with MEN type 1.

Intraoperative localization of insulinomas is difficult in 9%–23% of cases and imaging studies are successful in small tumors, which can also occur at different sites.

Selective hepatic venous sampling following calcium stimulation helps with localization of the tumor and leads to successful surgical resection with 5-year survival in successful cases being at 100%. Arterial branches supplying each portion of the pancreas are selected and injected with calcium sequentially. Blood from hepatic veins is sampled at a time from 10 to 180 min post calcium injection in each artery. Calcium stimulates the release of insulin from hyperfunctioning insulinoma beta cells but not from normally functioning beta cells. When an artery supplying the functioning insulinoma is stimulated, the corresponding venous sample will secrete high insulin levels relative to other nontumor-containing areas. The accuracy of the procedure in identifying insulinomas ranges from 67% to 100% mostly ≥90%. Of note, the pancreatic body and tail are the most valuable as those site areas are difficult to visualize radiologically. Proximal or distal splenic stimulation with increased insulin in hepatic venous suggests pancreatic tail insulinoma, whereas hepatic insulin response following proper hepatic or gastroduodenal arteries suggests pancreatic head insulinoma.

Insulin produced by the insulinomas results in Whipple's triad of (1) symptomatic fasting post exercise hypoglycemia, (2) glucose levels less than 40 mg/dL (2.2 mmol/L), and (3) experiencing symptomatic relief following glucose administration.

The finding of sustained hypoglycemia in the presence of hyperinsulinemia confirms the diagnosis. C-peptide and proinsulin are often measured in addition, and they afford higher sensitivity compared to insulin. A comparison of the different imaging procedures with calcium-stimulated hepatic venous sampling is shown in the following Table 3.

Somatostatinoma

Somatostatinoma is a rare neuroendocrine tumor (NET) with an incidence of 1 in 40 million individuals and accounts for less than 5% of pancreatic NETs (pNETs). The tumor originates from the delta cells of the pancreas and predominantly contains somatostatin with trace quantities of other pancreatic hormones such as insulin, glucagon, gastrin, and vasoactive intestinal polypeptide. It remains

TABLE 3 Insulinomas detection rate by the different radiological and imaging studies and by selective arterial calcium stimulation.

Procedure	Detection rate
Operative exploration	77%–91%
Transabdominal Ultrasound	9%–63%
Contrasts enhanced CT	63%–94
Contrast enhanced MRI	60%–90%
Endoscopic ultrasound	40%–93%
Somatostatin—enhanced MIRI	60%–90%
SACST	67%–100%

The clinical laboratory participates in the localization studies by measuring insulin, C-peptide, and proinsulin in the samples collected following calcium stimulation. Insulin (C-peptide and proinsulin) results provide "a biochemical hot spot" and aids with the localization of the tumor for a successful surgical resection.
Modified from Zhao K, Patel N, Kulkarni K, Gross JS, Taslakian B. Essentials of insulinoma localization with selective arterial calcium stimulation and hepatic venous sampling. J Clin Med 2020;9(10):3091. https://doi.org/10.3390/jcm9103091. PMID: 32992761; PMCID: PMC7601191.

localized in the pancreas in 56% to 70% of the cases, out of which 36% occur in the head, 14% in the pancreatic body, and 32% in the tail. Other common sites include duodenum (19%), ampulla of Vater (3%), and small bowel (3%). Functional somatostatinomas release excessive amounts of somatostatin suppressing gallbladder motility and inhibiting the secretory activity of various endocrine and exocrine cell types. Nonfunctional somatostatinomas tend either to be asymptomatic or to present with obstructive symptoms. Diagnosis is mostly by imaging studies and histopathological examination and staining of the tissue. Some studies employed the detection of high levels of circulating somatostatin induced by the calcium-pentagastrin test as a supportive biochemical test. However, somatostatin measurement is not widely available.

Biomarkers of gastrointestinal dysfunction

Essential aspects of biomarkers frequently used in the assessment of gastrointestinal dysfunction (irritable bowel syndrome, irritable bowel disease, and pancreatic insufficiency) are discussed in the following section.

Fecal alpha-1-antitrypsin (AAT)

Fecal clearance of alpha-1-antitrypsin (AAT) is used as a marker of gastrointestinal protein losses. Immunonephelometric methods are used to measure the alpha-1-antitrypsin (AAT) in the stool. As a protease inhibitor, it resists gastrointestinal degradation and appears in feces. In inflammatory bowel disease, a high AAT fecal clearance of 200 mg/day is suggestive of 6 g of albumin. Many commercially available kits are available. Bloody stool causes false positive results. The analysis usually includes both AAT and hemoccult tests.

AAT is deactivated by gastric acid, thus its fecal detection represents gastrointestinal stricture beyond the pylorus. Elevated levels are indicative of chronic pancreatitis.

Fecal lactoferrin

Fecal lactoferrin is produced by neutrophils. It is an iron-binding protein. The amount of lactoferrin produced correlates with the severity of inflammation. It is used to differentiate between inflammatory bowel syndrome and irritable bowel disease; it correlates with severity and with endoscopic findings. Fecal lactoferrin level < 7.25 µg/g suggests no intestinal inflammation in patients with gastrointestinal symptoms. It is stable for a few days at room temperature and for longer if stored refrigerated or frozen. Human breast milk contains 8 to 10 mg of lactoferrin and thus testing is limited in infants undergoing breast-feeding. Lactoferrin testing is valuable in pregnant patients with gastrointestinal symptoms, this is because colonoscopies are often contraindicated, and circulating marker of inflammation such as erythrocytes sedimentation rate (ESR) is elevated in pregnancy and relatively nonspecific. C-reactive protein measurement has been suggested but it is similarly nonspecific to inflammatory bowel syndrome.

Resolution of inflammation can be followed by serial measurement of lactoferrin, which helps avoid repeat endoscopic colonoscopies.

Fecal elastase-1[2,3]

Elastase-1 is produced by acinar cells of the pancreas. It has a protease activity. It passes through the small intestine without being degraded and thus elevated levels are detected in the stool. Fecal elastase-1 levels are 3 to 4 times those found in duodenal fluid. Thus, decreased fecal levels are suggestive of exocrine pancreatin insufficiency. The stability of the test and the lack of need to stop pancreatic replacement therapy makes it a favorite first-line test. However, the test has a high false positivity rate.

The assay is ELISA based with two monoclonal antibodies directed against human elastase 1. The degree of specificity allows its measurement to assess pancreatic function in the presence of therapeutic enzyme supplementation. It is stable and unaffected by exogenous pancreatic enzyme treatment and correlates very well with stimulated exocrine pancreatic function test. It is sensitive and specific and correlates well with endoscopic retrograde cholangiopancreatography.

Levels < 200 µg/g are suggestive of pancreatic insufficiency. The test diagnostic sensitivity is 77% and the specificity is 88%.

A normal fecal elastase 1 level in low pre-test probability can be used to rule out pancreatic insufficiency, whereas, in patients with high pre-test probability, abnormal levels confirm pancreatic insufficiency. Similarly, false positive and negative levels are observed in low and high-risk patients (suspected irritable bowel syndrome with diarrhea and in patients with chronic pancreatitis, respectively).

The assay requires less than 1 g of fecal sample and levels are not influenced by prandial status or diet. Samples are stable for up to 14 days if stored refrigerated at 4°C. Watery and diluted samples are not suitable.

Fecal calprotectin[4]

Calprotectin is a cytosolic protein derived primarily from neutrophils. It is found in body fluids including the stool. Normally it is present at six times higher than circulating levels with concentrations proportional to the degree of inflammation. Thus, reflecting the degree of bowel inflammation. Many assays for calprotectin measurement, including point-of-care lateral flow assays and laboratory-based ELISA's are commercially available.

It is a 36-kDa protein and represents about 60% of the cytosolic protein in neutrophils, which thus constitute the primary source of calprotectin with smaller amounts in monocytes and macrophages.

Calprotectin is measured in symptomatic patients to screen for inflammatory bowel disease (IBD). In patients with known IBD, it is used to monitor mucosal healing in both Crohn's disease and ulcerative colitis, monitor disease recurrence following intestinal resection in Crohn's disease, and in predicting clinical relapse in both Crohn's disease and ulcerative colitis.

A threshold of 50 µg/g is considered the upper limit of normal in patients greater than 4 years old. High levels in normal infants and levels are 112 µg/g for >65 years old.

Relative change value ranges from 118% to 131% depending on the assay platform, thus changes beyond at least 100% are required to be of clinical relevance.

Fecal calprotectin has a sensitivity of 99% and specificity of 65% detection of inflammatory bowel syndrome. Fecal calprotectin levels less than or equal to 40 µg/g were associated with less than 1% probability of having inflammatory bowel disease and a negative predictive value of 99% for levels ≤ 100 µg/g. In addition to its role as a screening tool, fecal calprotectin is used to monitor disease activity in patients with levels < 100 µg/g suggesting that active IBD is unlikely. Similarly, it is also used for predicting clinical relapse.

Gastrointestinal dynamic test (breath) tests

Biochemical tests of bacterial overgrowth/colonization

Small intestine bacterial overgrowth with malabsorption is associated with greater than 10^5 colony forming units/mL on the quantitative culture of proximal jejunal aspirate and positive breath hydrogen test in greater than 80% of patients. Diagnosis is made by lactulose breath hydrogen test.

Hydrogen breath test[5]

The breath test is helpful in the diagnosis of carbohydrate malabsorption disorder and many common gastrointestinal disorders including small intestine bacterial overgrowth and irritable bowel syndrome. Several substrates at various dosages are used in the breath test, such as glucose, lactulose, fructose, sorbitol, sucrose, and inulin. The test measures gases (hydrogen (H_2) and methane (CH_4), the main gases of the tests, and carbon dioxide (CO_2)) produced in the intestine following carbohydrate metabolism (by intestinal bacteria). The gases diffuse into the circulation and are exhaled in the lung where they are captured into a breathing bag, followed by measuring bag gases content in expired air every 30 min for up to 3 h.

The principle behind the breath test in carbohydrate malabsorption is the fermentation of unabsorbed substrate by bacterial flora of the colon, thus time must allow for both passage and metabolism. This is suggested to range from 30 to 180 min (peak gas concentration at 77 min) for fructose and up to 3 h for glucose and lactulose. Thus, a 2-h test would be appropriate for the assessment of carbohydrate malabsorption.

Although the breath test is increasingly being used, lack of standardization with respect to indication, patient preparation, test performance, and interpretation has led to considerable heterogeneity in reported results and interpretation.

Among healthy individuals, intestinal gas volume ranging from 30 to 200 mL predominantly includes hydrogen, carbon dioxide, and methane, with fewer amounts of oxygen, nitrogen, hydrogen sulfide, indole, skatole, and ammonia.

Fructose either in the form of sucrose or as a monosaccharide increasingly is found in sweeteners and other food additives. Fructose ingested at an excess rate of 30 to 50 g per hour will not be absorbed. Foods containing factors and excessive glucose promote the incomplete absorption of fructose and sorbitol can aggravate fructose malabsorption.

To improve the diagnosis, utility of the various variables must be limited. In preparing the patient for the test, antibiotics are avoided for 4 weeks before the test, laxatives and promotility medication stopped for at least 1 week, fermentable food (complex carbohydrate) be avoided 24 h before testing, overnight fasting (or 8–12 h) before the test, smoking avoided on the day of the test, and that physical activity limited to that during the breath test.

The test relies on the metabolism of carbohydrates by intestinal bacteria. Levels $\leq 10^3$ colony-forming units (cfu) are shown in normal subjects, whereas levels $> 10^3$ cfu are generally considered overgrowth and thus significant.

Glucose is absorbed in the proximal small intestine. Exhaled hydrogen is indicative of metabolism. The test has a sensitivity ranging from 20% to 93% and a specificity ranging from 30% to 86%.

The lactulose breath test is used to diagnose lactose intolerance and maldigestion secondary to lactase deficiency. Lactulose breath test sensitivity ranges from 31% to 68% and specificity ranges from 44% to 100%.

The fructose breath test is used to diagnose fructose intolerance and maldigestion. A dose of 25 g of fructose has been recommended.

Interpretation of breath test results

All breath testing should incorporate measurement of carbon dioxide (CO_2) or oxygen (O_2) to adjust the breath sample for nonalveolar dilution of exhaled air. Methane (CH_4) is also measured to assess intestinal motility and constipation. The methane-producing bacteria utilized hydrogen (H_2) in the generation of CH_4 thus impacting H_2 levels (4 mol of H_2 and 1 mol of CO_2 to produce 1 mol of CH_4).

A rise of ≥ 20 ppm from baseline in H_2 is indicative of fructose and lactose malabsorption.

Similarly, a rise in H_2 by ≥ 20 ppm by 90 min is considered positive for small intestine bacterial overgrowth. Methane levels ≥ 10 ppm are indicative of constipation and reduced motility.

Both hydrogen and methane should be measured, as 20%–30% of patients may not excrete hydrogen producing a false negative result if methane was not measured.

The recommended dosage for the various carbohydrates is shown in Table 4.

The test is limited by the presence of intestinal bacterial overgrowth which produces excessive hydrogen and methane and thus interferes with test interpretation.

Methane is known to reduce gut motility and detection of methane in breath is indicative of constipation, and that levels correlate with the extent of constipation. Methane levels are higher than hydrogen. It also directs antibiotic therapy where *Methanobrevibacter smithii* is resistant to many antibiotics.

There is lack of "gold standard" although, couture of collected biopsies and bacterial isolation and identification are often referenced as the gold standard, limitations due to poor and unsuccessful sample collection, contaminations, invasive nature of the tests limit its routine use.

TABLE 4 Recommended dosages in the breath test for glucose, lactulose, lactose, and fructose.

Carbohydrate	Dosage (recommended)	Ideal Test duration	Absorption mediator	Interpretation ≥rise from baseline
Glucose	75 g			
Lactulose	10 g	90 min		
Lactose	25 g	180 min	Lactase	≥20 ppm
Fructose	25 g		Facilitative diffusion GLUT-5	≥20 ppm

(GLUT-5) Glucose transporter member 5 is the main transporter of fructose by passive diffusion, has a low saturable uptake capacity, and is stimulated by glucose and inhibited by sorbitol.
Modified from Rezaie A, Buresi M, Lembo A, Lin H, McCallum R, Rao S, Schmulson M, Valdovinos M, Zakko S, Pimentel M. Hydrogen and methane-based breath testing in gastrointestinal disorders: the North American consensus. Am J Gastroenterol. 2017;112(5):775-784. https://doi.org/10.1038/ajg.2017.46. Epub 2017 Mar 21. PMID: 28323273; PMCID: PMC5418558.

Urea breath test

The presence of *H. pylori* is detected following ingestion of C13 or C14 labeled urea. The presence of *H. pylori* urease (which hydrolyzes urea into ammonia and bicarbonate) (protective role against the acidity of the stomach) is the test principle. The released now labeled CO_2 into the breath is trapped (the patient breathes into a bag) and the isotopic CO_2 is measured. Detectable levels suggest active infection.

An alternative to the breath test is PCR molecular testing of fecal samples. Additionally, *H. pylori* antigen may be measured in the stool. Circulating anti-*H. pylori* antibodies can also be used to indicate exposure, but they cannot discriminate between current and recent exposure.

D-Xylose absorption test

This test is not widely used and only a few laboratories offer xylose absorption tests in the assessment of suspected carbohydrate malabsorption. Following an overnight fast, the patient is encouraged to drink water freely in the early morning of the test. The patient empties the bladder and urine is discarded before a D-xylose dose of 0.5 g/kg (maximum 5 g) is administered orally with plenty of water (250 mL). Venous blood samples are collected at 2 h (at 1 h for children) and urine is collected for the next 5 h into a dark urine bottle. Xylose levels are measured in both blood and urine. Urinary excretion of 16%–33% of ingested doses in children is considered a normal response. The accuracy of the procedure depends not only on the rate of absorption but also on the rate of excretion of xylose by the kidneys. Thus, patients with renal insufficiency will excrete a decreased amount of xylose. To eliminate misinterpretations as a result of renal retention, a blood determination of xylose is carried out, along with the determination of xylose in urine. A high blood xylose level in the presence of decreased urine xylose excretion would suggest renal retention. False positive (low) results may also occur in the presence of

TABLE 5 Normal blood and urinary xylose levels post intake in use by the author's laboratory.

	Urine (5 h collection)	Blood
Child	16%–33% of the ingested dose	30 mg/dL (>2.0 mmol/L) (at 1 h post dose)
Adult	>1.2 g (>8.0 mmol)/5 h urine	>20 mg/dL (>1.33 mmol/L) at 2 h post dose

vomiting, gastric stasis, dehydration, myxedema, massive ascites, edema, or bacterial gastrointestinal overgrowth. Low urine volumes, especially if below 100 mL may lead to unreliable results. Side effects of D-xylose ingestion include nausea, vomiting, and diarrhea. If vomiting occurs, the test is invalid and must be repeated. Expected values are shown in the following Table 5.

The acute abdomen

The etiology of patients presenting with the acute abdomen is varied and often requires clinical biochemistry testing. The term "acute abdomen" encompasses a spectrum of medical and surgical conditions ranging from trivial to life threatening that require hospital admission, investigation, and treatment. The following are common examples and their associated laboratory investigations.

Acute pancreatitis

A common presentation of acute abdomen is due to acute inflammation of the pancreas. This is precipitated by either gallstone or alcohol (both accounting for >80% of cases).

Markedly increased amylase and lipase are observed. Amylase often elevated within 2–12 h of the onset of symptoms and returned to normal within 35 days. Lipase is elevated in parallel to that of amylase with the exception that it decayed much slower than amylase, thus remaining elevated in circulation longer and thus having an improved sensitivity. Lipase is more specific to the pancreas although present in other tissues, amylase is elevated in nonacute pancreatitis, e.g., salivary glands infection.

Acute cholestasis

Acute cholestasis occurs due to biliary stones, obstruction, cholecystitis, etc. Laboratory investigation includes liver enzymes, γ-glutamyl transferase, alkaline phosphatase, AST, and ALT as well as total and direct bilirubin.

Markedly elevated cholestatic enzymes (γ-GT and alkaline phosphatase) in proportion to the cytosolic liver enzymes (AST and ALT) support clinical suspicion of cholestasis. Additionally, biliary obstruction is evident by the finding of elevated total bilirubin and the majority being direct conjugated bilirubin.

In acute hepatitis, pain occurs in the right upper quadrant and epigastrium, radiating up to the shoulder or to the back along the rib cage. In this case, hepatic cytosolic enzymes (AST and ALT) are very high compared to the cholestatic enzymes, which continue to increase following presentation.

Ectopic pregnancy

Ectopic pregnancy is not a common cause of acute abdomen. It is where a fertilized ovum implants outside the uterus (most commonly the fallopian tube). This is detected by a markedly elevated serum β-HCG that is less than the doubled (every 2–3 days) response encountered in normal pregnancy.

Acute porphyria

Acute porphyrias are rare but important to recognize and to identify the cause of acute abdomen presentation. The attacks almost never occur before puberty and affect a minority of porphyria patients (10%–20%). In adolescence and childbearing age, it is often triggered by the initial intake of contraceptive therapy. Drugs, alcohol, infection, reduced calorie intake, and stress are recognized factors in precipitating acute attacks.

Acute neurovisceral attacks are a common presentation in patients with acute intermittent porphyria (AIP), hereditary coproporphyrin (HCP), variegate porphyria (VP), and aminolevulinic acid dehydratase porphyria (ADP). AIP, VP, and HCP are autosomal dominant disorders whereas ADP is a rare autosomal recessive disorder.

Laboratory detection is by measurement of urinary porphobilinogen (PBG) and total urine porphyrin (TUP) on a random urine sample ideally collected during the attack at presentation. The sample is immediately sent to the laboratory protected from light.

PBG is the primary and initial test in the investigation of suspected acute porphyria. PBG levels are always markedly elevated and a normal PBG level excludes an acute porphyria.

Presentation of active acute porphyria in children is very rare, and testing should include measurement of urinary aminolevulinic acid (ALA) excretion to exclude the rare ALA dehydratase deficiency porphyria as well as possible lead poisoning, which inhibits ALA dehydratase activity and leads to a similar clinical presentation.

Biochemical assessment of nutritional status

Adequate intake of nutrients is essential for normal growth and development and maintenance of health.

Nutrients include proteins to supply amino acids, energy substrates (carbohydrates and fats), inorganic salts, vitamins, essential fatty acids, and trace elements. Nutrients are easily defined into two categories as macronutrients and micronutrients.

Daily requirements are influenced by age, gender, the degree of physical activity, and the presence of disease. Individuals are at risk of developing symptoms when requirements are not met, on the other hand, excessive intake of nutrients is harmful leading to metabolic derangements, obesity, coronary heart disease, hypertension, some types of cancer, and clinical symptoms of toxicity.

The clinical biochemistry laboratory plays a role in monitoring nutrients and in the diagnosis and management of patients with nutritional disorders.

Vitamins and their deficiencies

Vitamins are essential for body function and metabolism. They are not produced in the body (except for vitamin D). They are required in trace amounts.

Vitamin deficiencies arise as a result of inadequate intake, impaired absorption, impaired metabolism, increased requirements, and increased loss. It is important to note that vitamin functions are mainly intracellular and indicate that plasma level does not often reflects status (time of sample post diet, etc.). Clinical presentations are often specific to and indicative of the specific vitamin deficiency such as osteomalacia in vitamin D deficiency. In generalized malnutrition, deficiency is often of multiple vitamins.

Water soluble vitamins

Water-soluble vitamins include vitamin B complex (B1, B6, B12), vitamin C, vitamin H, and niacin.

Vitamin B1 (thiamine)

Thiamine pyrophosphate is a cofactor in the metabolism of pyruvate to acetyl CoA and succinyl CoA to 2-oxoglutarate. The body contains adequate amounts at 30 folds daily requirements.

Deficiency causes beriberi (Wernicke's encephalopathy) characterized by memory loss and nystagmus, peripheral neuropathy, muscle weakness, dementia, and cardiac failure.

Clinical response is rapid following thiamine supplementation and this rapid therapeutic response confirms the suspected deficiency.

Contributors to thiamine deficiency include: low vitamin B diet (e.g., white rice), excessive alcohol consumption, chronic diarrhea, dialysis, malabsorption (celiac disease), postoperative bariatric surgery, parenteral nutrition, and administration of high dose diuretics.

Laboratory tests are seldom required. However, thiamine status is assessed by measuring transketolase in RBC hemolysate. Transketolase activity is measured both with and without the addition of thiamine pyrophosphate. A whole blood sample is preferred for measurement. False results are observed in nonfasting samples associated with recent thiamine supplementation. Direct exposure to light of blood samples as well as nutritional supplementation should be minimized as it causes loss of vitamin activity.

Niacin

Niacin includes nicotinamide and nicotinic acid. Nicotinamide (in NAD and NADP) acts as a coenzyme for many dehydrogenases. In addition to dietary input, a larger component comes from tryptophan metabolism. Therefore, abnormality in tryptophan metabolism as in the carcinoid syndrome leads to niacin deficiency.

Nicotinic acid

Nicotinic acid is a precursor of nicotinamide, which is a constituent of coenzyme NAD and NADP (essential for glycolysis and oxidative phosphorylation). It is an essential water-soluble vitamin mainly found in protein-rich diets. Tryptophan in the diet is converted by the liver to niacin (60 mg of tryptophan yields 1 mg of niacin). The recommended daily allowance for niacin is 2 to 4 mg for infants, 6 to 8 mg for children, 12 mg for teenagers, 16 mg for men, 14 mg for women, and 17 and 18 mg for lactating and pregnant women, respectively.

Deficiency causes pellagra (dermatitis, diarrhea, dementia, and death). It is a clinical diagnosis and biochemical testing is rarely used.

Folic acid

Folate, a derivative of folic acid, is required for purine and pyrimidine, and hence nucleic acid synthesis. Deficiency results in macrocytic anemia.

Folate fortification of food has reduced the incidence of folate deficiency (from 16% to 0.5%) and has questioned the need for continued measurement of its levels. Depending on the population served, there remains a need to measure folate levels and assess both deficiency and risk for toxicity among those receiving supplementation.

Assessment of folate status is achieved by measuring either red blood cell or serum folate levels. RBC folate is considered a better sample type for assessment of folate status compared to serum; however, historically, it has been cumbersome to perform due to the need for sample preparation and the need for extra washing cycles on the automated analyzers. Serum, however, provides an adequate assessment and is widely used by many laboratories.

Vitamin B12

Vitamin B12 comprises many closely related substances called cobalamins. It is essential to nucleic acid synthesis, myelin synthesis, and to amino acids and fatty acids metabolism. Patients exhibit abnormal complete blood counts showing macrocytosis and anemia. The clinical presentation is similar to that of folate deficiency.

Deficiency causes megaloblastic anemia and in severe cases, leads to subacute combined degeneration of the spinal cord. Dietary deficiency is rare except in strict vegetarians. It is commonly seen in pernicious anemia, an autoimmune disease due to the lack of intrinsic factors essential for the absorption of the vitamin from the gut. Vitamin B12 is measured using immunoassays and the presence of circulating intrinsic factor autoantibodies interferes with the B12 assay producing falsely elevated results. Functionally, elevated methylmalonic acid is a more specific marker of B12 deficiency.

Vitamin C

Ascorbic acid is essential for the hydroxylation of proline residues in collagen, thus for the normal structure and function of this protein. Deficiency leads to scurvy. It acts by maintaining iron in hydroxylating enzyme in reduced form (antioxidant). It also facilitates the absorption of nonheme iron. Serum concentration is a poor indicator of tissue status.

Biotin (vitamin H)

Biotin is a cofactor for five carboxylases in the amino acids and fatty acids metabolism and in gluconeogenesis. Biotin also participates in the expression of oncogenes. Deficiency is associated with growth retardation, neurological and dermatological abnormalities, as well as fetal congenital anomalies.

Levels are reduced due to decreased absorption, increased utility, and/or metabolism, in patients on long-term anticonvulsant therapy, patients on total parenteral nutrition, chronic alcoholism, pregnancy, and inflammatory conditions.

Inborn errors in biotin metabolism are due to either biotinidase deficiency or to holocarboxylase synthase deficiency disorders presenting during infancy. In the latter, binding to carboxylases is impaired whereas in the biotinidase deficiency form, biotin is deficient due to impaired reutilization of biotin and of utilization from the diet. Carboxylases are essential in the catabolism of several amino acids, in gluconeogenesis, and in fatty acid synthesis, and that lack of biotin causes deficiency in their activity leading to multiple, life-threatening metabolic derangements, eliciting characteristic organic aciduria and neurological symptoms. Characteristic symptoms include metabolic acidosis, hypotonia, seizures, ataxia, impaired consciousness, and cutaneous symptoms, such as skin rash and alopecia.

Fat-soluble vitamins

Fat-soluble vitamins are vitamins K, A, D, and E. They are obtained from dietary sources except for vitamin D (see later). Their absorption is influenced by conditions leading to fat malabsorption. They are discussed separately below.

Vitamin A

Vitamin A is a constituent of the retinal pigment rhodopsin. It is essential for the normal synthesis of mucopolysaccharides and the growth of epithelial tissues. Mild deficiency causes night blindness. Severe deficiency leads to permanent retinal damage and loss of vision. It is stored in the liver and deficiency is rare in the developed world. It is present in the diet and can also be synthesized from dietary carotenes. It is bound to prealbumin and to retinol-binding protein. Low-binding proteins lead to low vitamin A delivery to tissues.

Vitamin D

Vitamin D3 (cholecalciferol) is derived from endogenous synthesis by the action of sunlight (ultraviolet beam, UV: 280–320 nm) on 7-dehydrocholesterol in the skin to form precholecalciferol which isomerizes to vitamin D3 in a thermosensitive process. Vitamin D2 (ergocalciferol) is obtained from the diet. It is derived from the UV conversion of plant (and fungi) ergosterol to ergocalciferol (vitamin D2). Structurally, it differs from D3 in that D2 has a double bond between C22 and C23 and a methyl group at the C24 side chain. This chemical change renders vitamin D2 with a lower affinity to binding proteins and faster clearance from the circulation.

Vitamin D3 and D2 are initially hydroxylated to 25-hydroxy vitamin D3, and D2 by cytochrome P450 mixed function oxidases (CYPs) which have 25-hydroxylase activity in hepatocytes. The CYPs are located either in the endoplasmic reticulum or in the mitochondria.

Unlike 25-hydroxylation, there is only one enzyme (1,α-hydroxylase (CYP27B1)) that converts 25-OH vitamin D (25-OH vitamin D) to 1,25-$(OH)_2$ vitamin D. The kidney is the main site for this hydroxylation activity. The enzyme is tightly regulated by PTH, FGF23, and by 1,25-$(OH)_2$ Vitamin D itself. PTH stimulates, whereas FGF23 and 1,25-$(OH)_2$ Vitamin D inhibit CYP28B1. Hypercalcemia suppresses CYP27B1 through suppression of PTH. Hyperphosphatemia suppresses CYP27B1 by stimulating FGF23, although both calcium and phosphate may have a direct effect on renal CYP28B1 activity.

Further hydroxylation of the active 1,25-$(OH)_2$ vitamin D form to the inactive 24- and 23-hydroxy vitamin D is effected via CYP24A1, which is the only established 24-hydroxylase involved with vitamin D metabolism. This enzyme has both 24-hydroxylase and 23-hydroxylase activity.

The 24-hydroxylase pathway results in the biologically inactive calcitroic acid, whereas the 23-hydroxylase pathway produces the biologically active 25-OH vitamin D-26, 23-lactone and 1,25-$(OH)_2$ Vitamin D-26,23 lactone.

Inactivating mutations in CYP24A1 have been found in children with idiopathic infantile hypercalcemia and more recently in adults who present with severe hypercalcemia, hypercalciuria, and nephrocalcinosis with decreased PTH, low 24,25-1,25-$(OH)_2$ Vitamin D, and inappropriately normal to high 1,25-$(OH)_2$ Vitamin D. Measuring the ratio of 24,25$(OH)_2$:25-OH vitamin D has proven useful in diagnosing these cases.

The 3-epimerase activity was first identified in the keratinocyte, which produces large amounts of the C-3-epi form of 1,25-$(OH)_2$ vitamin D. The C-3 beta epimer of 25-OH vitamin D has reduced binding to DBP relative to 25-OH vitamin D, and the C-3 beta epimer of 1,25-$(OH)_2$ Vitamin D has reduced affinity for the VDR relative to 1,25-$(OH)_2$ Vitamin D, thus reducing its transcriptional activity and most biologic effects. Surprisingly, however, it is equipotent to 1,25-$(OH)_2$ Vitamin D with respect to PTH suppression.

Clinically, interest in the C-3 epimerase arises because the C-3 beta epimer of the vitamin D metabolites is not readily distinguished from their more biologically active alpha epimers by liquid chromatography-mass spectrometry unless special chromatographic methods to separate the epimers before mass spectrometry are employed. Thus, the measurement of these metabolites using standard LCMS procedures results in a value increased above true levels of the C-3 alpha epimers to the extent that the sample contains the C-3 beta epimer. Immunoassays by in large do not recognize the C-3 beta epimer and so are not affected. This issue is particularly important in assessing 25-OH Vitamin D levels in infants where levels of the C-3 beta epimer of

25-OH Vitamin D can equal or exceed that of the C-3 alpha epimer of 25-OH vitamin D.

Vitamin D3 is present in meat and fatty fish whereas vitamin D2 is present in vegetables and/or supplantation. Not all immunoassays detect D2 and D3 equally, although assays continue to improve.

Breast milk contains relatively little vitamin D. If the mother is vitamin D deficient or if the baby is premature, vitamin D supplementation is needed, however, cholecalciferol has little biological activity. It is converted in the liver to 25(OH)D and then by the kidney to the active form 1,25-(OH)$_2$ Vitamin D.

Vitamin K

Vitamin K is required for gamma-carboxylation of glutamate residue in coagulation factors II, VII, IX, and X. It permits the binding of calcium to proteins. Deficiency leads to increased prothrombin time.

Vitamin E

Tocopherol (vitamin E) is an important antioxidant. It protects unsaturated fatty acids that reside in the cell membrane from free radical attack; clinical deficiency occurs in severe malabsorption. Clinical manifestations include hemolytic anemia and neurological dysfunction.

Trace elements

Trace elements are required for the maintenance of normal health. By definition, they are present in concentrations of less than 100 ppm. None is required in more than 1 mg per day. Deficiency occurs for the same reasons as for vitamins. FE is a common deficiency (particularly in reproduction age). Iodine deficiency causes goiter and, if severe, hypothyroidism.

Deficiency of trace metals is uncommon except under special circumstances such as severe malnutrition, prolonged parenteral nutrition, and in states of recessive utility and loss such as chronic inflammation, skin, and gastrointestinal dysfunction. Trace elements, their roles and function, and associated disorders are summarized in Table 7 below.

Zinc

Zinc is essential for the activity of many enzymes, including those involved in nucleic acid synthesis. Clinical presentation includes dermatitis, and delayed wound healing occurs in patients on prolonged TPN. Zinc deficiency is observed in catabolic patients following trauma. Plasma zinc levels fall in acute-phase response and in chronic liver diseases. In patients with acrodermatitis enteropathica, severe zinc deficiency occurs due to a defect in intestinal zinc absorption. For the assessment of zinc status, blood sample is collected in fasting states as levels drop by 20% following a meal. Zinc is extensively bound to albumin (albumin-corrected measurements are required).

Copper

Copper is essential for the activity of cytochrome oxidase and superoxide dismutase. In blood, 80%–90% of copper is present in ceruloplasmin. Copper deficiency is uncommon. Manifestation includes anemia and leucopenia. Wilson disease is characterized by excess tissue deposition of copper.

Selenium

Selenium is required as a prosthetic group for the enzyme glutathione peroxidase. With vitamin E, it is part of the antioxidant system protecting membranes and other vulnerable structures from free radicals. Selenium deficiency is only seen in areas of low intake. It is endemic in some parts of China, which have low selenium soil content, and can also be seen in patients on long-term total parenteral nutrition.

Clinical features of deficiency include myopathy and cardiomyopathy. It is measured either in plasma or in red blood cell (RBC) glutathione peroxidase activity which provides a measure of tissue levels.

Iodine

Sources of dietary iodine are sea fish, seafood, dairy products, eggs, broccoli, and peas. Ninety percent of dietary iodine is absorbed in the stomach and small intestine. Adequate iodine intake is 150 mg/day (adults) and 120 mg/day (children), and 250 mg/day (during pregnancy).

In addition to being central to the synthesis of thyroid hormones, its antioxidative property plays a role in inflammation protection.

Iodine deficiency leads to hypothyroidism, goiter, mental retardation, and congenital anomalies, whereas iodine excess leads to hyperthyroidism.

In 1993, the World Health Organization and the United Nations ICEF recommended the iodination of salt as a carrier. Iodized salt is accessible to over 70% of households worldwide. However, limited consumption of salt is recommended for patients with hypertension and cancer, the prevalence of which is increasing with incidents of iodine deficiency.

Iodine deficiency is prevalent in the eastern Mediterranean, Asia, Eastern Europe, and Africa. Mild deficiencies are observed in Australia, the United Kingdom, and New Zealand, and among vegans, vegetarians, and pregnant women. It is the most common cause of childhood mental retardation.

Iodine deficiency is identified when a 24-h urine concentration is less than 100 μg/day.

Iodine measurement

Iodine levels are measured in urine in the assessment of suspected iodine toxicity and in monitoring excretion rate as an index of replacement therapy. Concentration below 100 µg/L is indicative of iodine deficiency. Levels are monitored following thyrotoxic treatment before initiation of therapy or interventions.

The WHO criteria for assessing both intake and deficiency status are shown in the following table (Table 6).

Albumin

Albumin, a 67-kDa protein and predominant in circulation with a half-life of 21 days, is often considered a marker of nutritional status where reduced levels are assumed to reflect long-standing malnutrition. However, this concept is clearly problematic as changes in albumin levels are influenced largely by its volume of distribution and by hepatic and renal function. Chronic liver disease and nephrotic syndrome are associated with hypoalbuminemia.

Concentration can be affected by a change in hydration status, and redistribution to the extravascular space with a decrease by about 5 g/L following a change to prolonged recumbent posture. Increased intravascular osmotic pressure causes the movement of water from extravascular to intravascular space.

Albumin is a negative acute-phase reactant with levels decreasing as part of the body's acute-phase response to infection and inflammation due to the inhibition of albumin synthesis by cytokines, namely, IL-6.

Therefore, its measurement is not useful for nutritional assessment. However, markedly decreased levels are indicative of poor prognosis in critically ill and cachectic patients as well as correlate with disease severity, morbidity, and mortality.

Transthyretin (Prealbumin)

Prealbumin is a 55-kDa protein with four identical subunits. It has several functions where it binds to retinol-binding protein and transports thyroxine.

It has a short half-life in plasma of about 2.5 days, which makes it a useful indicator of short-term response to parenteral nutritional support. Concentration can increase by 10 mg/L/24 h with adequate support. Concentrations of prealbumin may decrease and hence of limited value in some disorders such as end-stage renal disease and in significant inflammation.

Retinol-binding protein

Retinol (vitamin A) binding protein, a 21-kDa protein, binds and transports retinol from the liver to target tissues. It is filtered through the glomerular membrane and degraded by the proximal tubules.

The protein has a very short half-life of 12 h, which makes it an ideal marker for responding to short-term changes in energy intake. However, measurement to assess nutritional status is not valid in states of vitamin A deficiency. Concentrations may decrease in liver disease, it is a negative acute-phase reactant, and its concentration is also influenced by renal disease. Furthermore, circulating levels vary by both age and gender and thus appropriate reference intervals are required respectively.

TABLE 6 Urinary iodine levels and associated degree of iodine status.

Urinary iodine (ug/L)	Iodine intake	Iodine status
<20	Insufficient	Deficiency (severe)
20–49	Insufficient	Deficiency (moderate)
50–99	Insufficient	Deficiency (mild)
100–199	Adequate	Adequate
200–299	Above requirements	Risk of excess
≥300	Excessive	Risk of adverse effects

Modified from Berger MM, Shenkin A, Schweinlin A, Amrein K, Augsburger M, Biesalski HK, Bischoff SC, Casaer MP, Gundogan K, Lepp HL, de Man AME, Muscogiuri G, Pietka M, Pironi L, Rezzi S, Cuerda C. ESPEN micronutrient guideline. Clin Nutr. 2022;41(6):1357-1424. https://doi.org/10.1016/j.clnu.2022.02.015. Epub 2022 Feb 26. PMID: 35365361.

TABLE 7 Trace elements, roles and functions, and associated disorders.

Element	Function/Role
Chromium	Deficiency causes glucose intolerance
Cobalt	Component of B12
Copper	Cofactor for cytochrome oxidase
Fluorine	Present in bone and teeth
Iodine	Component of thyroid hormones
Manganese	Cofactor for several enzymes
Molybdenum	Cofactor for xanthine oxidase
Selenium	Cofactor for glutathione peroxidase
Silicon	Present in cartilage
Tin	Essential for growth in animal studies
Zinc	Cofactor for many enzymes
Iron	Component of heme

Modified from Berger MM, Shenkin A, Schweinlin A, Amrein K, Augsburger M, Biesalski HK, Bischoff SC, Casaer MP, Gundogan K, Lepp HL, de Man AME, Muscogiuri G, Pietka M, Pironi L, Rezzi S, Cuerda C. ESPEN micronutrient guideline. Clin Nutr. 2022;41(6):1357-1424. https://doi.org/10.1016/j.clnu.2022.02.015. Epub 2022 Feb 26. PMID: 35365361.

C-reactive protein

C-reactive protein (CRP) is a 120-kDa large protein synthesized by the liver in response to proinflammatory cytokine IL-6. It is a positive acute-phase protein with levels rapidly and markedly increased in response to injury (levels often increased 4–6h post insult).

However, CRP concentrations reflect catabolic status and since catabolism and nitrogen balance are closely linked, it can thus be used in nutritional assessment.

Relationship between inflammation and nutritional parameters lead to the development of the Prognostic Inflammatory and Nutritional Index (PINI) calculated as follows: $PINI = (AGP \times CRP)/(ALB \times PA)$, with AGP = acid glycoprotein (mg/L), CRP = C-reactive protein (mg/L), ALB = albumin (g/L), and PA = prealbumin (mg/L). PINI level > 30 correlates with the risk of death and the index has been used as a screening tool for assessment of risk for malnutrition, as well as risk for mortality and morbidity even in the absence of overt malnutrition.

Alpha-1 acid glycoprotein and sometimes prealbumin are not routinely measured and thus limit the routine use of the indicator.

Insulin-like growth factor I (IGF-I)

IGF-1 is produced predominantly in the liver. Its concentration is regulated by growth hormone and by nutritional status. It has a very short half-life of 2–4h and thus is considered a sensitive marker of acute changes in nutritional status.

It is a strong predictor of life-threatening complications. Circulating levels are wide and are influenced by age and gender. Thus, appropriate respective reference intervals are required. This as well as the wide circulating range limits its routine application in nutritional assessment.

Fibronectin

Fibronectin is a 220-kDa glycoprotein synthesized in the liver and by fibroblasts, macrophages, and endothelial cells. It has a central role in wound healing, opsonization, and phagocytosis.

Fibronectin has a short half-life of about 25h (20 to 30h) making it a marker of recent changes in nutritional status. Concentration declines after 2days of starvation and is markedly increased by the fifth day of refeeding. However, it is not used routinely as a predictor of clinical outcomes.

Transferrin

Transferrin is a 76-kDa protein with two homologous iron-binding domains. It has a half-life of 8–10days. It binds and transports ferric iron to cell membranes, limits the availability of free ionized iron necessary for bacterial growth, and thus restricts bacterial infection.

Transferrin concentration reflects protein status but not energy intake. It is a negative acute-phase reactant, which limits its usefulness in nutritional assessment. Furthermore, its levels increase in states of iron deficiency. Therefore, it is no longer considered useful in assessing nutritional status.

Other markers

Other candidate makers in the assessment of nutritional status are amino acids and leptin levels. Circulating essential amino acids concentration declines in instances of protein deficiency, whereas nonessential amino acids remain normal or increased in plasma. This results in decreased ratio of essential to nonessential amino acids with the ratio being a marker of the degree of malnutrition. However, the ratio exhibits poor sensitivity and is affected by recent food intake. Furthermore, it requires complex measurement methods.

Leptin is a 16-kDa molecular weight peptide hormone secreted by adipose tissue. In a steady state, it acts as a marker for fat stores. It may have a role in nutritional assessment in the future but is not currently used in routine clinical care.

Nitrogen balance

Assessment of the body's nitrogen balance would in theory provide an accurate assessment of the body's nutritional status. It should indicate both negative and excess nitrogen and thus protein energy metabolism. It requires the calculation of the difference between nitrogen intake and nitrogen losses. Nitrogen input is gauged from dietary assessment or calculated directly in patients receiving support, whereas nitrogen output is assessed by measuring urinary nitrogen (traditionally) using the Kjeldahl method or chemiluminometric techniques.

Although losses are preliminary in the urine in the form of urea, determination of urine urea excretion is helpful but nonurinary losses of up to 4g/24h lost in hair, skin, and feces lead to underestimation of the nitrogen excretion rate.

Increased nitrogen losses occur in inflammatory conditions; additionally, significant protein loss can occur in burns, fistulae, and gastrointestinal disorders. There is considerable interindividual and intraindividual variation in the amount of nitrogen excreted as urea. Given the above limitations with potential summative errors, inaccuracy with timed urine collections, and contribution from nonurinary nitrogen has reduced its application in routine practice.

Creatinine-height index

The creatinine-height index is used to assess muscle mass, considered the largest protein reserve in the body, and thus as a nutritional assessment aid. It was formulated for use in children but later adapted for adults. Creatinine is the end product of the metabolism of creatine and creatine phosphate in skeletal muscle. In normal renal function, the creatinine excretion rate is an index of creatinine production.

The creatinine height index (CHI) is expressed as a percentage of measured 24-h urinary creatinine excretion/expected 24-h urinary creatinine excretion (for age and gender) × 100.

It represents the amount of skeletal muscle in the body. Assessment of muscle mass can be made from urine creatinine excretion: Assuming 24h excretion of 1 g (9 mmol) this represents about 17–20 kg of skeletal muscle. It is influenced by dietary and ethnic considerations. Values >80% suggest normal protein status whereas values 60% to <80% or 40%–60% indicate mild and moderate protein depletion, respectively.

It compares the 24-h urinary creatinine excretion with normal values for height and gender, however, the estimation can be obtained by measuring serum creatinine alone (see below).

Collection of 24-h urine samples is difficult and has inaccuracies. In a patient with normal kidney function (BUN<20 mg/dL), and thus assuming a normal creatinine clearance of 80 ml/min, urinary creatinine can be estimated from the creatinine clearance formula (U (Urine creatinine) × V (Urine volume)/P (plasma creatinine)); this helps avoid the collection of a 24-h urine sample. That is urine creatinine multipled by volume (UV) equals creatinine clearance multiplied by plasma creatinine value.

The presence of metabolic stress influences the rate of nitrogen metabolism, and estimation of the creatinine index requires adjustment for the severity of metabolic stress. It is assumed that about one-half of dietary nitrogen would increase urinary nitrogen beyond that due to metabolic stress. There is also an obligatory urinary urea loss of about 3 g per 24h. The catabolic index may then be estimated as (24-h urinary nitrogen excretion) − (1/2 dietary nitrogen intake +3). Values >5 represent moderate stress and > 10 represent severe stress. Correcting the catabolic index (CI) for body muscle mass (as determined by creatinine height index CHI) (CI divided by CHI) improves the prediction of the nutritional status and thus the need for intervention.

Patients on total parenteral and enteral nutrition (TPN)

Artificial nutrition support has evolved into a primary therapeutic intervention to prevent metabolic deterioration and therefore loss of lean body mass. It is also aimed to improve the outcomes of critically ill patients. The clinical biochemistry laboratory is an integral member of the hospital nutrition team providing testing and advice on frequency, sample requirements, test methodologies, and results interpretation.

The timing of initiation of therapy, the contents of macronutrients and the targeted amount of macronutrients, and the route of delivery are important determinants of the effect of the nutritional intervention.

Parenteral nutrition (PN) is preferred for rapid initiation and delivery of nutritional support but it carries a risk of infection and complications most likely due to hyperalimentation and hyperglycemia. Using the enteral route is considered to be more physiologic, providing nutritional and various nonnutritional benefits including maintenance of structural and functional gut integrity.

Management of patients receiving total parenteral nutrition requires periodic monitoring of electrolytes, metabolites, and markers of liver and renal function integrity (Table 8).

Enteral nutrition

In contrast to the above-described parenteral nutrition support, using the enteral route is considered to be more physiologic, where in addition to providing nutrition it facilitates the maintenance of structural and functional gut integrity. However, the disadvantages are related to a potential lower nutritional adequacy, particularly in the acute disease phase and in patients with gastrointestinal dysfunction.

There appears to be no difference in overall mortality among critically ill patients between enteral nutrition compared to the parenteral route for nutritional support. However, the enteral route of nutritional support was associated with decreased infection-related complications and reduced intensive care units length of stay which may be explained by the benefit of reduced macronutrient intake rather than the enteral route itself.

The placement of nasogastric enteral feeding tubes can be problematic, particularly in children and the pediatric population. Insertion of enteral feeding tubes is at risk of misplacement, injury, and exposure of the operator to body fluids.

The aspiration of a small sample aliquot from the location of the inserted tube is important to ascertain placement. The detection of gastric fluid (acidic environment) helps confirm the correct placement spot. A pH of ≤4.5 indicates gastric environment acidity and thus correct gastric tube placement. The use of a commercially available pH indicator such as (RightSpot) is widely used. The gastric sample is stable for a short time (2 min) at room temperature and blood contamination interferes with pH measurement.

Food and inhalants allergy

IgE-mediated allergic response

IgE is produced by B cells in response to T-cell activation following allergen exposure and uptake by dendritic cells. Stimulated T-helper cell produces cytokines IL-4, IL-5, and IL-13. Produced and released IgE binds to its receptors on mast cells leading to stimulation of the mast cells and production of allergic response in the form of histamine and vasoactive metabolites.

TABLE 8 Biomarkers, the frequency, rationale, and interpretation of their biochemical measurements in the assessment and management of patients with nutritional deficiency and those receiving enteral and parenteral nutritional support.

Parameter	Frequency	Rationale	Interpretation
Sodium, potassium, urea, creatinine	Baseline. Daily until stable. 1–2 times weekly	Assessment of renal function, fluid status, and Na and K status	Interpret with knowledge of fluid balance and medication. Urine Na may be helpful in complex cases with gastrointestinal fluid loss
Glucose	Baseline. 1–2 times daily (or more if required) until stable. Then weekly	Glucose intolerance is common	Good glycemic control is necessary to prevent metabolic complications and sepsis
Magnesium, phosphate	Baseline. Daily if risk of refeeding syndrome. Three times weekly until stable Then weekly	Depletion is common and under-recognized	Low concentrations indicate poor status
Liver testing (including INR)	Baseline. Twice weekly until stable, then weekly	Abnormalities common during PN	Complex. May be due to sepsis, other disease, or nutritional intake
Calcium, albumin[a]	Baseline Then 1–2 times weekly	Hypocalcemia or hypercalcemia may occur	Hypocalcemia may be secondary to Mg deficiency. Low albumin reflects disease, not protein status
C-reactive protein	Baseline Then 2–3 times weekly until stable	Assists interpretation of protein, trace element, and vitamin results	To assess the presence of an acute-phase reaction (APR). The trend of results is important
Zinc, copper	Baseline Then 2–4 weeks depending on the results	Deficiency is common, especially when increased losses	Patients are most at risk when anabolic APR causes ZN ↓ and Cu ↑
Selenium[b]	Baseline if risk of depletion Repeat test depends on baseline	Se deficiency likely in severe illness and sepsis, or long-term nutrition support	APR causes Se ↓ Long-term status is better assessed by glutathione peroxidase
Complete Blood Count and MCV	Baseline 1 or 2 times weekly until stable Then weekly	Anemia due to iron or folate deficiency is common	Effects of sepsis may be important
Iron, ferritin	Baseline Then every 3–6 months	Iron deficiency common in long-term PN	Iron status is difficult if ongoing APR (Fe ↓, ferritin ↑)
Folate B12	Baseline Then every 2–4 weeks	Folate deficiency is common	Serum folate/B12 sufficient, with complete blood count
Manganese[c]	Every 3–6 months if on home parenteral nutrition	Excess provision to be avoided—more likely if liver disease	Red blood cells or whole blood better measure of excess than plasma
25-OH Vit D[c]	6 monthly, if on long-term support	Excess provision to be avoided—more likely if liver disease	Requires normal kidney function for effect
Bone densitometry[c]	On starting PN Then every 2 years	Metabolic bone disease diagnosis	Together with lab tests for metabolic bone disease

[a]Although some experts recommend the measurement of the transthyretin (prealbumin) as a marker of protein-energy status, it is also affected by the acute-phase response (see above). It may also be of value in monitoring response to treatment.
[b]These tests are needed primarily for patients receiving parenteral nutrition (PN) in the community (also required in those in hospitals with prolonged serious illness); however, the evidence is still weak for when to supplement, and how much selenium.
[c]These tests are rarely needed in patients having enteral nutrition (in the hospital or the community) unless there is cause for concern.
Modified from Shenkin A. Biochemical monitoring of nutrition support. Ann Clin Biochem. 2006;43(Pt 4):269-72. https://doi.org/10.1258/000456306777695609. PMID: 16824276.

Patient history and clinical presentation direct immunological testing to identify the allergen. Skin prick testing is common for the determination of IgE sensitization. In this "bioassay," the skin response reaction is graded and recorded. The test requires medical supervision as the host may produce a severe anaphylactic response requiring immediate medical attention.

Measurement of circulating total IgE levels and allergen-specific IgE is often performed and has become the mainstay of allergy testing. However, allergen-specific serum tests, often performed in immunology or clinical biochemistry laboratories, involve the use of an array of target allergens (food and environmental (inhalants)) that are covalently coupled to a solid phase. Aliquots of patient's serum are incubated with the allergens and circulating allergen-specific antibodies bind to their respective antigens. Nonreactants are washed away and a detection signal is measured. Results are typically reported in allergen-specific kilounits (kU_A) per liter.

The degree of elevation of serum IgE levels correlates with an increased risk of clinical allergy, but the level of serum IgE does not accurately predict the severity of allergic reactions that can be triggered by the allergen.

A positive test indicates sensitization to the allergen (food or inhalants); however, the results themselves are not diagnostic of clinical allergy. In addition, serum IgE levels may be low and undetectable to an allergen that triggers clinical allergy, so a compelling history and negative serum IgE results warrant further evaluation. Serum IgE levels are influenced by ongoing symptoms such as eczema or urticaria.

As part of the normal inflammatory immune response, IgG levels are elevated. High levels of IgG4 are however associated with immunological tolerance linked to the activity of the regulatory T-cells to the food substance, but do not indicate imminent food allergy or intolerance. Testing for IgG4 is thus irrelevant for laboratory workup of food allergy or intolerance and its application in this setting is discouraged.

Summary

- The role of the clinical chemistry laboratory in the investigation and management of patients with gastrointestinal disorders has been declining due in part to the increased utility of radiological examinations.
- Saliva contains important biomarkers such as glucose, vitamin D, calcium, nitrates, nitrites, fluoride, and many peptide and steroid hormones (e.g., cortisol).
- Impaired pancreatic enzyme release leads to impaired digestion of fats. Common causes of pancreatic insufficiency include pancreatitis, cystic fibrosis, and pancreatic duct obstruction.

- Pancreatic exocrine insufficiency, a complication of chronic pancreatitis is a common cause of maldigestion leading to weight loss and steatorrhea.
- Acid is secreted by the parietal cells lining the stomach and pepsinogen by the secreting chief cells.
- Atrophy of the gastric mucosa due to either autoimmune antibody-mediated loss of parietal cells or infection by *H. pylori* leads to impaired acid production.
- Most of the dietary lipids (>94%) are absorbed in the proximal two-thirds of the jejunum, thus in a daily diet of 100 g fat, the presence of >6 g in fecal indicates fat malabsorption.
- Inflammatory bowel disease includes Crohn's disease and ulcerative colitis.
- Food malabsorption is defined as a decrease in gut absorptive function but not requiring intravenous supplementation for health or growth maintenance.
- Increased excretion of fat in stools is termed steatorrhea.
- Disorders of the pancreas lead to fat malabsorption, they include chronic pancreatitis, pancreatic duct obstruction (as in cystic fibrosis), pancreatic tumor.
- Causes of carbohydrate maldigestion and malabsorption are either primarily due to congenital enzymes deficiencies or secondary to pancreatic insufficiency celiac disease, Crohn's disease, surgical intestinal resection or bypass, small intestinal bacterial overgrowth, use of drugs and toxins such as anti-neoplastic agents, and antibiotics and radiation injury.
- Digestion and absorption of dietary proteins require proteases, peptidases, and amino acid and peptide transporters.
- Inherited amino acid absorption disorders may be classified as three types of transport defects. Those affecting intestinal and renal absorption and intracellular, between cellular compartments, and between organs uptake.
- Pancreatic insufficiency is caused by the progressive depletion of pancreatic acinar cells.
- Pancreatic insufficiency leads to malabsorption, diabetes, and increased risk for pancreatic cancer.
- Diarrhea defined as watery stool formation can either be secretory or osmotic in nature.
- There are two main types of inflammatory bowel disease, Crohn's disease affecting any segment of the upper or lower gastrointestinal tract, and uncreative colitis and the name implies is limited to the colon.
- Celiac disease is an autoimmune disorder directed against gastrointestinal gliadin.
- Carcinoid tumors arise in the gut, terminal ileum, and the ileocecal region or the lungs. They produced vasoactive intestinal peptides (VIPs) such as 5-hydroxytryptamine, and serotonin, metabolized to 5-hydroxyindole acetic acid (5-HIAA).
- Fecal clearance of alpha-1 antitrypsin is used as a marker of gastrointestinal protein losses.

- Markers of pancreatic insufficiency include fecal elastase and lactoferrin, as well as calprotectin.
- The etiology of patients presenting with the acute abdomen is varied and often requires clinical biochemistry testing. Differential diagnosis includes cholestasis, ectopic pregnancy, and porphyria among other gastrointestinal malignancy and ischemia.
- Parenteral nutrition (PN) is preferred for rapid initiation and delivery of nutritional support but it carries a risk of infection and complications most likely due to hyperalimentation and hyperglycemia. Using the enteral route is considered to be more physiologic.
- Detection of gastric fluid (acidic environment (pH $\leq$ 4.5)) helps confirm the correct placement of the enteral feeding tube.
- IgE is produced by B cells in response to T-cell activation following allergen exposure and uptake by dendritic cells.
- Measurement of circulating total IgE levels and allergen-specific IgEs are often performed and have become the mainstay of allergy testing.

References

1. Schiller LR. Evaluation of chronic diarrhea and irritable bowel syndrome with diarrhea in adults in the era of precision medicine. *Am J Gastroenterol.* 2018;113(5):660–669.
2. Vanga RR, Tansel A, Sidiq S, El-Serag HB, Othman MO. Diagnostic performance of measurement of fecal elastase-1 in detection of exocrine pancreatic insufficiency: systematic review and meta-analysis. *Clin Gastroenterol Hepatol.* 2018;16(8):1220–1228 e1224.
3. Dominici R, Franzini C. Fecal elastase-1 as a test for pancreatic function: a review. *Clin Chem Lab Med.* 2002;40(4):325–332.
4. Ricciuto A, Griffiths AM. Clinical value of fecal calprotectin. *Crit Rev Clin Lab Sci.* 2019;56(5):307–320.
5. Rezaie A, Buresi M, Lembo A, et al. Hydrogen and methane-based breath testing in gastrointestinal disorders: the North American consensus. *Am J Gastroenterol.* 2017;112(5):775–784.

Further reading

Clark R, Johnson R. Malabsorption syndromes. *Nurs Clin North Am.* 2018;53(3):361–374.

Elke G, van Zanten AR, Lemieux M, et al. Enteral versus parenteral nutrition in critically ill patients: an updated systematic review and meta-analysis of randomized controlled trials. *Crit Care.* 2016;20(1):117.

Guerrero RB, Kloke KM, Salazar D. Inborn errors of metabolism and the gastrointestinal tract. *Gastroenterol Clin N Am.* 2019;48(2):183–198.

Ismail OZ, Bhayana V. Lipase or amylase for the diagnosis of acute pancreatitis? *Clin Biochem.* 2017;50(18):1275–1280.

Omer A, Quigley EMM. Carbohydrate maldigestion and malabsorption. *Clin Gastroenterol Hepatol.* 2018;16(8):1197–1199.

Patterson JW, Kashyap S, Dominique E. Acute Abdomen. Treasure Island (FL): StatPearls; 2022.

Singh P, Arora A, Strand TA, et al. Global prevalence of celiac disease: systematic review and meta-analysis. *Clin Gastroenterol Hepatol.* 2018;16(6):823–836.e822.

Stellaard F, Lutjohann D. Dynamics of the enterohepatic circulation of bile acids in healthy humans. *Am J Physiol Gastrointest Liver Physiol.* 2021;321(1):G55–G66.

Woolf J, Marsden JT, Degg T, et al. Best practice guidelines on first-line laboratory testing for porphyria. *Ann Clin Biochem.* 2017;54(2):188–198.

Chapter 12

Common and rare metabolic disorders

Introduction

This chapter describes the metabolic disorders of iron homeostasis, cobalamin (vitamin B12) and folate metabolism, porphyria, uric acid, and purine and pyrimidine metabolism, as well as inherited metabolic disorders of the newborn. Pathophysiology and the role of the clinical biochemistry laboratory in their diagnosis and management are discussed.

Iron metabolism and associated anemia

Iron is an essential component of hemoglobin, myoglobin, cytochromes, catalases, and oxidase enzymes. It is also a cofactor of ribonucleotide reductase.

Iron is present in two stable oxidized forms, ferrous (Fe^{2+}) which is soluble, and ferric (Fe^{3+}) which is insoluble. Its presence in soluble and insoluble forms renders it a valuable metabolic element in redox potential reactions. Dietary sources, with meat being the richest, are mostly in the form of Fe^{3+}. Absorption, transport, and storage of iron are illustrated in Fig. 1.

Body iron content is 3–5 g with 60% being in hemoglobin, 10% in myoglobin, and the remainder in iron-containing enzymes and in reticuloendothelial cells. It is stored in hepatocytes and reticuloendothelial macrophages where iron is recycled. A normal daily loss of 1 mg must be replenished form dietary sources (Table 1). While there is no identified mechanism of iron excretion, the extent of its absorption is tightly regulated and is influenced by the body's iron content.

Absorption of organic iron present in food occurs in the acidic environment of the proximal duodenum and in the presence of ascorbate (reducing substance) which maintains it in its soluble Fe^{2+} ferrous state. Absorption seems to be dependent on iron storage levels. Iron sequestered in ferritin in enterocytes is lost days later via sloughing of intestinal epithelial cells. There is no iron excretion mechanism; deficiency is thus predominantly a consequence of loss and poor dietary intake. The prevalence of iron deficiency is about 1% in men and 11% in women.

Absorbed cytosolic iron is released through basolateral ferroportin-I following the oxidation of Fe^{2+} to Fe^{3+} (Fig. 1). Ferroportin-1 is a universal iron exporter from the intracellular pool. It is present in intestinal epithelial cells, hepatocytes, and macrophages. Expelled cytoplasmic iron binds to circulating transferrin, which has two iron binding sites. Transferrin is the major circulating iron carrier (transporter). It is present in three forms (apo-transferrin, mono-ferric, and di-ferric species). Iron binding to transferrin maintains it in a soluble form (Fe^{3+} alone being insoluble compared to Fe^{2+}). About 33% of transferrin is saturated and virtually all of the circulating iron is bound to transferrin.

The amount of iron in transferrin is represented as the percentage of transferrin iron saturation, calculated as a ratio of serum iron to total iron binding capacity (TIBC). TIBC is a measure of circulating iron plus transferrin unoccupied iron binding sites (UIBC).

Hepcidin, a 25 amino acid low molecular weight protein, is produced by hepatocytes in response to high iron levels and to interleukin-6 during inflammation (hence anemia of chronic disease). Hepcidin regulates iron influx by binding the iron exporter ferroportin-I triggering its internalization and degradation by lysosomes. When ferroportin-I is degraded, iron cannot be absorbed thus available circulating iron is markedly reduced.

During iron deficiency, there is decreased hepcidin production at the transcription level. Acquired hepcidin deficiency is seen in, erythropoiesis, conditions leading to increased RBC turnover, liver disorders, alcohol intake, iron deficiency, and in hypoxia. It is also deficient in hemochromatosis (see later).

Polymorphism in the iron metabolism protein (TMRPSS6) (type II transmembrane serine protease) causes elevated hepcidin and thus reduced iron absorption (see above). There is genetic polymorphism and variability among individuals with protective polymorphism against iron loss expressed in menstruating women.

Most of the available iron to the erythroid bone marrow arises from cellular recycling by tissue macrophages. Such recycled iron is temporarily stored in intracellular ferritin before being transferred to transferrin for deployment to bone marrow for immediate use in red blood cell synthesis or to hepatocytes for storage. Transferrin and transferrin receptors are recycled back to the cell surface. Iron-containing transferrin is recognized by two hepatocytes transferrin receptors. Transferrin-bound circulating iron is taken up via transferrin receptors expressed on cell membranes and is internalized through receptor-mediated endocytosis.

Tutorials in Clinical Chemistry. https://doi.org/10.1016/B978-0-12-822949-1.00018-8

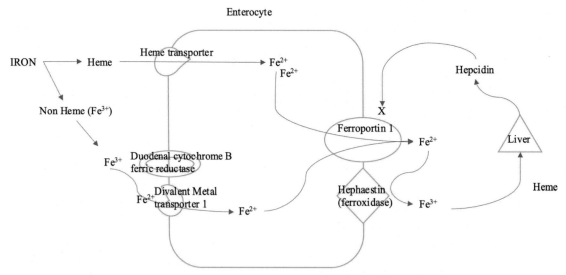

FIG. 1 Iron metabolism. Organic and nonorganic iron enters the enterocytes via either a heme transporter or divalent metal transporter, respectively. Fe^{2+} is oxidized to Fe^{3+} and is taken up by hepatocytes. Hepcidin produced by hepatocytes in response to iron content inhibits ferroportin-I transmembrane protein leading to the release of iron into the circulation. *Modified from Gattermann N, Muckenthaler MU, Kulozik AE, Metzgeroth G, Hastka J. The Evaluation of Iron Deficiency and Iron Overload. Dtsch Arztebl Int. 2021;118(49):847–856. https://doi.org/10.3238/arztebl.m2021.0290. PMID: 34755596; PMCID: PMC8941656, and Chifman J, Laubenbacher R, Torti SV. A systems biology approach to iron metabolism. Adv Exp Med Biol. 2014;844:201–25. https://doi.org/10.1007/978-1-4939-2095-2_10. PMID: 25480643; PMCID: PMC4464783.*

TABLE 1 Iron distribution in the body, losses, and daily requirements.

Source/content	Iron
Total body content	3–4 g
Hem-iron (Hemoglobin, myoglobin)	1.8–2.4 g (hemoglobin) 0.3–0.4 g (myoglobin)
Non-heme iron	Variable (enzymes)
Losses	1 mg/day (+0.5 mg (menstrual) (16 mg in 35 mL blood loss))
Daily requirements	18 mg (adult men) 27 mg (pre-menopausal) 30 mg (New RBC hemoglobin) Increased requirements during growth
Dietary sources	15 mg (mostly insoluble Fe^{3+}) 0.8–1.5 mg absorbed

Modified from Chifman J, Laubenbacher R, Torti SV. A systems biology approach to iron metabolism. Adv Exp Med Biol. 2014;844:201–25. https://doi.org/10.1007/978-1-4939-2095-2_10. PMID: 25480643; PMCID: PMC4464783 and Bothwell TH, Baynes RD, MacFarlane BJ, MacPhail AP. Nutritional iron requirements and food iron absorption. J Intern Med. 1989;226(5):357–65. https://doi.org/10.1111/j.1365-2796.1989.tb01409.x. PMID: 2681512.

Ferritin is the iron-storage protein synthesized by the liver. Iron bound ferritin is the main storage format and accumulates in macrophages and hepatocytes. It is made up of 24 subunits surrounding up to 4500 iron molecules. In general, serum ferritin levels are proportional to the amount of iron stored in macrophages and thus a measure of the total body iron levels. Ferritin is an acute-phase protein, thus elevated in infection, and is markedly elevated in macrophage activation syndromes of primary and secondary hemophagocytosis. Measurement of inflammatory markers (such as C-reactive protein) often indicates the inflammatory cause of elevated ferritin levels.

Hemosiderin, similar to ferritin, is an iron-storage protein. Most of the nonheme iron content of hemosiderin is thought to originate from degraded ferritin. It is not present in circulation and accumulates in macrophages in the liver, spleen, kidneys, lymph nodes, and in bone marrow. It is detected by immunohistochemical staining of the tissue.

Increased tissue deposition of protein bound iron as well as nonprotein bound iron increases the risk for free radical formation and tissue damage.

The red blood cell

Red blood cells (RBCs) are produced in the bone marrow with a typical 100 to 120 days lifespan in circulation. RBC morphology associated with various anemia types as well as biochemical findings is summarized in the following Table 2. Less than 5% of body iron content is contained in red blood cells.

Microcytic anemia is seen in iron deficiency anemia, anemia of chronic disease, thalassemia, lead poisoning, and congenital sideroblastic anemia. Normocytic anemia is indicative of blood loss, hemolysis, and of suppressed RBC production.

Macrocytic anemia is seen in patients with B12 and folate deficiency. Morphology, although performed by hematology laboratories, is essential in the assessment of

TABLE 2 RBC morphology associated with various anemia types as well as biochemical findings.

Cause of anemia	RBC morphology	Biomarkers
Blood loss, acute	Normochromic-normocytic, with polychromatophilia	If severe, possible nucleated RBCs and left shift of the WBCs, leukocytosis, thrombocytosis
Blood loss, chronic	Microcytic, with anisocytosis and poikilocytosis. Reticulocytopenia	Low serum iron. Increased total iron-binding capacity. Low serum ferritin
Folate deficiency	Oval macrocytes. Anisocytosis Reticulocytopenia. Hypersegmented WBCs	Serum folate <5 ng/mL (<11 nmol/L). RBC folate <225 ng/mL RBCs (<510 nmol/L). Nutritional deficiency and malabsorption (in sprue, pregnancy, infancy, or alcohol use disorder)
B12 deficiency	Oval macrocytes. Anisocytosis. Reticulocytopenia. Hypersegmented WBCs	Serum B12 <200 pg/mL (<145 pmol/L). Increased LDH, antibodies to intrinsic factor in serum (pernicious anemia), and sometimes the absence of gastric intrinsic factor secretion
Hemolysis	Normochromic-normocytic. Reticulocytosis.	Increased serum indirect bilirubin and LDH, increased stool and urine urobilinogen, hemoglobinuria in fulminating cases, hemosiderinuria
Infection, cancer, or chronic inflammation	Normochromic-normocytic early, then microcytic. Normal or increased iron stores	Decreased serum iron. Decreased total iron-binding capacity, normal serum ferritin, normal or increased marrow iron content
Sickle cell anemia	Anisocytosis and poikilocytosis. Some sickle cells in peripheral smear. Sickling of all RBCs in preparation with hypoxia or hyperosmolar exposure. Reticulocytosis	Largely limited to people of African ancestry in the United States, urinary hyposthenuria, Hb S detected during electrophoresis
Thalassemia	Microcytic. Target cells. Basophilic stippling. Anisocytosis and poikilocytosis. Nucleated RBCs in homozygotes. Reticulocytosis	Elevated Hb A2 and Hb F (in beta-thalassemia). Mediterranean ancestry (common), In homozygotes, anemia from infancy

Modified from Gattermann N, Muckenthaler MU, Kulozik AE, Metzgeroth G, Hastka J. The Evaluation of Iron Deficiency and Iron Overload. Dtsch Arztebl Int. 2021;118(49):847–856. https://doi.org/10.3238/arztebl.m2021.0290. PMID: 34755596; PMCID: PMC8941656, and Ford J. Red blood cell morphology. Int J Lab Hematol. 2013;35(3):351–7. https://doi.org/10.1111/ijlh.12082. Epub 2013 Mar 9. PMID: 23480230 and from Chifman J, Laubenbacher R, Torti SV. A systems biology approach to iron metabolism. Adv Exp Med Biol. 2014;844:201–25. https://doi.org/10.1007/978-1-4939-2095-2_10. PMID: 25480643; PMCID: PMC4464783., and from Characteristics of common anemias. https://www.merckmanuals.com/professional/hematology-and-oncology/approach-to-the-patient-with-anemia/evaluation-of-anemia. Accessed 9th March 2023.

anemia in directing laboratory investigations. The biochemical investigation of iron, B12, and folate deficiency is discussed in detail (see later).

Anemia

Anemia describes a decrease in the number of red blood cells (RBCs) as measured by red cell counts, measurement of hematocrit or of the red cell hemoglobin content.

There is gender deference in the definition of anemia. In men, anemia is defined as any of the following: hemoglobin <14 g/dL (140 g/L), hematocrit <42% (<0.42), and/or RBC <4.5 million/µL (<4.5 × 10^{12}/L). Whereas in women, anemia is defined as any of the following: (hemoglobin <12 g/dL (120 g/L), hematocrit <37% (<0.37), and/or RBC <4 million/µL (<4 × 10^{12}/L)). Among menstruating women, iron deficiency anemia prevalence is about 10%, whereas iron deficiency without anemia is about 20% to 40%. The

difference is due to cyclical blood loss. Hemoglobin levels <11 g/dL (110 g/L) define anemia among the elderly and during pregnancy.

Causes of iron loss contributing to anemia are heterogenous. In addition to hematuria (blood loss in the urine), pathological gastrointestinal losses are associated with malignancy (10% of patients), gastritis, ulcers, and postsurgical procedures as in bariatric surgery (23%). Malignancy-associated gastrointestinal losses are often gradual over a long period of time and often symptoms are not recognized until hemoglobin levels are critically low (≤5 g/dL). Iron deficiency in male patients (>50 years old) and a hemoglobin of less than 9 g/dL directs investigation for possible malignancy.

Iron deficiency in patients with celiac disease is thought to be due to inflammation-induced hepcidin levels and blood loss as well as to reduced absorption via the atrophied villus.

Achlorhydria impairs the conversion of dietary iron from ferric to ferrous form thus limiting its absorption. Similarly, gastric ulcers secondary to *Helicobacter pylori* infection are common pathways for iron deficiency.

Drugs, such as aspirin and nonsteroidal anti-inflammatory, lead to iron deficiency secondary to gastrointestinal bleeding. For aspirin, 0.8–5 mL of daily blood loss has been reported. Daily losses of 5 mL of blood can lead to iron deficiency anemia. Of important consideration is iatrogenic anemia following serial blood collections for repeated and standing laboratory test orders in patients. A daily CBC and complete metabolic panel could add up to about 7–10 mL blood loss per day. Several laboratories attempt to reduce blood volume collections using small blood tubes (manufacturers specify the minimum blood volume required when using tubes containing anticoagulant additives). Similarly, the need for repeated and serial laboratory testing is questioned from a test utilization point. Recommendations on the frequency of tests and their clinical utilities have been reported (see the section on laboratory tests utilization—Chapter 16 on aspects of laboratory management).

Biochemical markers of iron deficiency anemia include hemoglobin, transferrin, transferrin saturation (total iron binding capacity), and ferritin. The common difficulty with their interpretation is in patients with ongoing inflammatory conditions where some of those biomarkers are also acute-phase reactants and therefore their levels change irrespective of iron status.

Anemia is where hemoglobin concentration is below normal levels (see above). Regardless of its cause, the impact is the same, that is reduced oxygen delivery to tissue, and thus clinical symptoms and sequelae are similar. It arises either due to decreased production of hemoglobin (red blood cells) and/or increased losses of hemoglobin (red blood cells).

Iron deficiency causes reduced hemoglobin (red blood cells) production. Sixty-eight percent of patients with iron deficiency anemia will have a mean red blood cell volume (MCV) of <75 fL whereas MCVs >95 fL have a low probability of iron deficiency as a cause.

Biochemically, ferritin measurement is preferred to iron, transferrin, and to total iron binding capacity (TIBC) where a serum ferritin <15 ng/mL supports the diagnosis of iron deficiency and that levels >100 ng/mL rule iron as a cause of the anemia. In patients with chronic inflammation, ferritin increases as part of the acute-phase response, and levels between 15 and 40 ng/mL and up to 70 ng/mL can be seen in patients with chronic iron deficiency anemia.

Increasing hemoglobin levels following iron replacement therapy confirm the diagnosis and adequate response when hemoglobin rises by about 2 g/dL every 3 weeks. Repeated measurement at 9 weeks confirms recovery. There is no need to repeat ferritin measurement to assess iron status; the hemoglobin measured being the desired endpoint.

The investigation of the cause of iron deficiency is variable depending on clinical presentation and could vary from nutritional (reduced intake) to increased losses (GI bleeding) or to ineffective erythropoiesis.

Gastrointestinal (GI) blood loss contributes to iron deficiency anemia. Fecal occult blood tests are used to screen for GI hemoglobin loss. Fecal occult blood test (FOBT) assays are designed to detect hemoglobin molecules in fecal samples as an indication of GI bleeding that can be due to various pathologies including GI inflammation and colorectal carcinoma (CRC). Guaiac-based fecal occult blood tests (FOBTs) utilize the peroxidase-like activity of the heme molecule in hemoglobin, in the presence of hydrogen peroxide to catalyze the oxidation of alpha-guaiaconic acid to a blue-colored quinone compound. An upper GI bleed is only detected by heme-based assays. HemoQuant which measures fluorescent porphyrin (obtained following degradation of hemoglobin) is more sensitive to upper GI tract bleeding than HemoOccult guaiac-based tests. Positive tests are obtained when GI blood loss exceeds 10 mL remembering that anemia can arise following 5 mL losses. Newer, more sensitive, and specific antibody-based assays such as fecal immunochemical testing (FIT) do not detect an upper GI bleed because the antigen (hemoglobin) will be digested and epitopes lost during GI passage. The role of FOBTs in screening for CRC is well documented and multisociety guidelines for early detection of CRC include their use. Testing for fecal occult blood should be limited to screening for colon cancer using the most sensitive, specific, and easy-to-use methodology. Lack of visual melena (black stool) is misleading as pale stool may be seen in patients with up to 100 mL of gastrointestinal blood loss.

Hemolytic anemia

Hemolytic anemia may be either acquired or hereditary. It is characterized by an increased red blood cell destruction.

Causes of hemolytic anemia include RBC membrane abnormalities, hereditary spherocytosis, hemoglobinopathies, and red blood cell enzyme deficiencies (glucose-6 phosphate dehydrogenase deficiency, pyruvate kinase deficiency, and adenylate kinase). The latter catalyzes the conversion of adenosine triphosphate (ATP) and adenosine monophosphate (AMP) to two molecules of adenosine diphosphate (ADP). The deficiency of the enzyme leads to spherocytic hemolytic anemia. The deficiency is rare and is autosomal recessive with hemoglobin levels in the 8–9 g/dL range. The RBC enzyme activity is less than 30% of normal. Heterozygotes are asymptomatic with the normal phenotype (normal RBC and no anemia).

Laboratory investigation includes blood cell count and morphology. Biochemically, there are increased serum bilirubin levels (due to the increased heme metabolism load), elevated LDH, decreased haptoglobin (often below assay detection limit), and increased urinary-free hemoglobin.

Biochemical investigation of iron deficiency anemia and iron excess status

The finding of reduced iron staining in bone marrow samples is the definitive diagnostic test for iron deficiency anemia; however, it is invasive, labor intensive, and not amenable to routine measurement and assessment of iron status. Hematological indices show low MCV in patients with severe iron deficiency and those with anemia of chronic inflammatory disease. Patients with hepatic dysfunction ameliorate the magnitude of decrease in MCV. However, the rate of change in hemoglobin levels is helpful. For instance, a rapid decline indicates loss via bleeding whereas a slow decline in a male, >50 years old, to levels below 9 g/dL is suspicious for malignancy.

Serum iron levels itself is markedly variable throughout the day and are influenced by dietary intake and undergo significant biological variation. However, the presence of very high iron levels is indicative of iron overload. It is therefore helpful in identifying iron overload but not in the investigation of iron-deficiency states.

Measurement of circulating transferrin is preferred as part of the initial screen. It is expressed as a percentage of iron content. Levels <20% indicate iron deficiency; normal levels range from 20% to 50% in males and 15% to 50% among females. Elevated levels are indicative of iron overload. Levels >45% identify 97.9% to 100% of C282Y homozygous cases of iron overload hemochromatosis.

Transferrin receptors are shed into the circulation in iron deficiency and are not influenced by inflammation. Soluble transferrin levels depend on cellular volume and are elevated in patients with hemolytic anemia, and chronic lymphocytic leukemia, and thus mimic overt iron deficiency anemia.

UIBC test performance is equivalent to that of transferrin when screening for hereditary hemochromatosis. UIBC levels <26 μmol/L affords high degree of sensitivity and specificity (both at 90%) for detecting homozygous hemochromatosis.

In iron deficiency, TIBC is increased (the ability of transferrin to bind exogenous iron, i.e., a measure of transferrin saturation). TIBC is reduced in inflammation and in malnutrition.

Ferritin stores intracellular iron and reflects the body's iron store but although highly sensitive, it lacks the specificity of a screening test, as being a positive acute-phase protein, falsely high ferritin levels are seen in inflammation, and liver disorders (alcoholic disease, hepatitis, nonalcoholic fatty liver disease (NAFLD), malignancy).

A combination of ferritin levels <200 ng/mL in premenopausal women, <300 ng/mL in men and postmenopausal women, and transferrin <45% in all, have a high (97%) negative predictive value excluding iron overload. Ferritin remains the most preferred test for iron deficiency compared with iron, transferrin, and total iron binding capacity, where low levels supports the diagnosis.

Gene mutation analysis of patients suspected of hemochromatosis is routinely performed to confirm the high clinical suspicion. Genetic mutation of C282Y is part of the evaluation of suspected hemochromatosis (based on clinical or elevated iron studies) and detects 83% of cases. Analysis for H63D and S65C mutations are often reported with C282Y.

H36D mutation is more common and is found in most ethnic groups (20% carrier among whites (heterozygous)). S65C mutation is the least common (<2% among whites (heterozygous)).

Circulating zinc-protoporphyrin (formed due to lack of iron) is released into circulation. It is also elevated in lead poisoning (as lead substitutes iron binding) leading to the formation of free zinc-protoporphyrin. In inflammation, there is decreased incorporation of iron into hemoglobin leading to the formation of zinc-protoporphyrin.

Iron excess

The human body lacks functional excretion of excess iron. Iron is stored in the form of ferritin and hemosiderin to minimize iron toxicity. Symptoms of iron overload are seen when ferritin levels are >1000 ng/mL. Elevated levels are predictors of poor prognosis in patients with ferritin >1000 ng/mL, high AST, and ALT, and low platelet count predicts cirrhosis in >80% of patients. Many hereditary conditions result in uncontrolled iron absorption and thus increased total body iron including hemochromatosis (mutations in the HFE1, HFE2 genes). Inherited deficiencies in hepcidin cause the iron overload seen in genetic hereditary hemochromatosis (see later).

The amount of ferritin iron compared to hemosiderin is slightly larger in the lower range of iron deficiency to normal, whereas the opposite is true in the iron overload range. The ratio of hemosiderin iron content to that of ferritin correlates with the rate of iron tissue deposition.

Serum ferritin is a marker of iron stores and is used in the diagnosis and management of iron levels; however, overestimation occurs in patients with inflammation and malignancy.

Iron overload is decreased by either phlebotomy (in hereditary hemochromatosis) and by the use of iron-chelating agents such as deferoxamine in anemic patients with iron overload (repeated transfusion).

Hemochromatosis

Hemochromatosis is an autosomal recessive disorder leading to body iron overload. Genetic mutations affecting the hepcidin-ferroportin interaction lead to increased absorption and deposition in tissues and organs (commonly liver, pancreas, heart, pituitary, skin, and joints) causing damage. Free radical production leads to an increased risk of hepatocellular carcinoma.

In most types of hereditary hemochromatosis, mutations lead to either deficiency in hepcidin or to hepcidin resistance. It is common among northern Europeans. Diagnosis is made in the 4th and 5th decade with typically asymptomatic mild elevation in liver enzymes and high ferritin (>200–300 ng/mL) and transferrin saturation (>45%). There are four types of hemochromatosis genotypes-phenotypes described: 1A, 1B, 1C, 2A, 2B, 3, 4A, and 4B (Table 3).

General population screening is not recommended due to the variable prevalence of the C282Y gene among different ethnic groups. However, testing in patients with strong family history is warranted.

Secondarily acquired iron overload

Acquired iron overload is either due to frequent blood transfusions or to ineffective erythropoiesis seen in patients with thalassemia, myelodysplasia, and in hematopoietic stem cell transplant. In addition to therapeutic transfusions, there is excessive gastrointestinal absorption in beta-thalassemia.

In multiple transfusions as a cause, each blood unit contains about 200–250 mg of iron. The iron load initially accumulates in the reticuloendothelial macrophages and is subsequently deposited in the hepatic parenchyma, pancreas, and in endocrine tissue. Patients receiving a median of 21 units of red blood cells increased ferritin levels to about 1000 μg/mL.

Dietary-related intake is seen in some parts of the world where the use of nongalvanized steel utensils leads to increased iron intake. Excessive iron supplementation in parenteral nutrition may also be the cause of acquired iron overload.

In patients with nonalcoholic fatty liver disease (NAFLD), about a third of them show signs of iron overload. There are elevated ferritin levels and normal or mildly elevated transferrin saturation, a syndrome now termed dysmetabolic iron overload syndrome (DIOS). It is mainly due to impaired iron mobilization from hepatocytes and Kupffer cells. Additionally, associated inflammation impacts iron regulatory proteins such as hepcidin, ferroportin-I, transferrin receptor, ferritin, and/or copper.

Elevated ferritin levels are seen in patients with chronic inflammation and in those with hematological malignancies and hepatocellular and breast carcinoma, and in patients with chronic liver disease (viral hepatitis), and in porphyria cutanea tarda (PCT).

Alcohol use downregulates hepcidin expression transcription factor and thus increases iron transport into the cytoplasmic compartment. Additionally, insulin resistance causes downregulation of the hepcidin transcription factor.

Porphyria

Porphyria is a group of eight metabolic disorders of heme biosynthesis. They are either inherited or acquired. Clinical features are neurovisceral (abdominal pain) and/or cutaneous dermatological (blisters) characteristic of the pathway precursors accumulating upstream of the blockade in the metabolic pathway (Fig. 2). Acute neurological presentations are associated with precursors 5-aminolevulinic acid and porphobilinogen. Skin lesions are mostly seen following the accumulation of precursors further down in the pathway.

Heme is synthesized (80%) in the bone marrow (for hemoglobin), 15% in the liver, and 5% in other cell types for other cytochromes and hemoproteins. Differences are due to the different rates of 5-ALA synthases I and II. 5-Amino levulinic acid synthase II being erythroid-specific and is induced during active heme synthesis rate is not inhibited by heme but is limited by iron availability. Intracellular heme negatively controls the nonerythroid 5-ALAS I isoform. Heme-containing proteins are predominantly hemoglobin and myoglobin, and enzymes of the cytochromes P450, catalases, tryptophan pyrrolase, nitric oxide synthase, cyclo-oxygenase, prostaglandin-endoperoxide synthase, among others. Porphyria is classified as either hepatic or erythropoietic reflecting the site of precursor accumulation. The synthetic pathway begins and ends in the mitochondria with three enzymatic steps: porphobilinogen deaminase,

TABLE 3 Different mutations and presentations characterized as four types of hemochromatosis.

Type		Mutation
1	A	C282Y (homozygote)
	B	C282Y and H63D (compound heterozygote)
	C	S56C
2	A (Juvenile)	Hemojuvelin gene (HJV)
	B (Juvenile)	Hepcidin (HAMP) on 19q13
3		Transferrin receptor-2 (TFR2) on 7q22
4	A	SLC04A1 (Loss of function for ferroportin-I secretion)
	B	SLC40A1 (Gain of function ferroportin-hepcidin complex not internalized)

Modified from Kowdley KV, Brown KE, Ahn J, Sundaram V. ACG Clinical Guideline: Hereditary Hemochromatosis. Am J Gastroenterol. 2019;114(8):1202–1218. https://doi.org/10.14309/ajg.0000000000000315. Erratum in: Am J Gastroenterol. 2019;114(12):1927. PMID: 31335359.

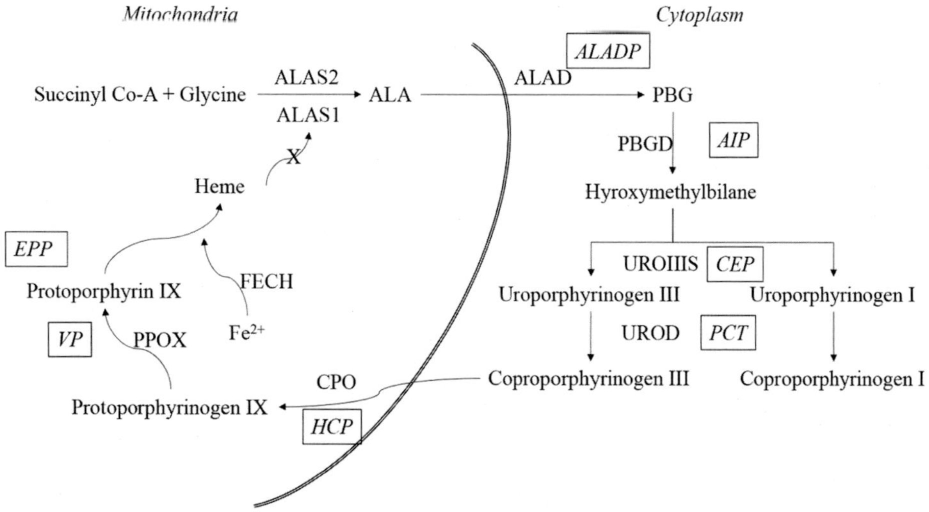

FIG. 2 Porphyria metabolism. *ALA*, 5-aminolevulinic acid; *ALAS*, ALA synthase; *PBG*, porphobilinogen; *PBGD*, PBG deaminase; *UROIII*, uroporphyrinogen III synthase; *UROD*, uroporphyrinogen decarboxylase; *CPO*, coproporphyrinogen oxidase; *PPOX*, protoporphyrinogen oxidase; *FECH*, ferrochelatase; *AIP*, acute intermittent porphyria; *HCP*, hereditary coproporphyria; *VP*, variegate porphyria; *PCT*, porphyria cutanea tarda; *EP*, erythropoietic protoporphyria; *CEP*, congenital erythropoietic porphyria; *HEP*, hepatoerthropoietic porphyria; *ALADP*, 5-aminolevulinic acid dehydratase porphyria. *Modified from Puy H, Gouya L, Deybach JC. Porphyrias. Lancet. 2010;375(9718):924–37. https://doi.org/10.1016/S0140-6736(09)61925-5. PMID: 20226990.*

uroporphyrinogen synthase, and uroporphyrinogen decarboxylase, leading to the formation of hydroxymethylbilane, uroporphyrinogen, and coproporphyrinogens, respectively.

The disorders are autosomal dominant with low penetrance in acute intermittent porphyria, variegate porphyria, and coproporphyria. Skin lesions (due to photosensitivity) are absent in intermittent porphyria (early step in the pathway with predominant 5-ALA and PBG accumulation). Further down the pathway, 60% of patients with the acute variegate porphyria developed skin lesions (due to accumulation of the photosensitive porphyrin precursors), and rarely 5% in patients with coproporphyria (due to accumulation of porphobilinogen precursors).

Acute intermittent porphyria (AIP)

The prevalence of AIP is variable, for instance, ranging from 1:75,000 to 1:1000 in northern Sweden among women of productive age. It is rare in men and women before puberty and after menopause.

Clinical manifestations are nonspecific and thus biochemical assessment is vital for both diagnosis and identification of the type of porphyria. About 10% of patients develop recurrent attacks. Hyponatremia is present in 40% and is due to SIADH. Severe AIP presentation is associated with seizures as well as hypomagnesemia.

Attacks last for 1–2 weeks and are life threatening due to severe neurological complications and muscle weakness leading to tetraplegia, bulbar and respiratory failure and eventually death. Psychological manifestations present in 20%–30% of patients and include: anxiety, disorientation, depression, confusion, paranoia, and hallucination. The

acute neurological symptoms are due to the accumulation of the neurotoxic 5-aminolevulinic acid (5-ALA) and porphobilinogen (PBG) metabolites.

Factors stimulating 5-ALAS I include menstrual cycle hormonal changes, fasting, smoking, inflammation, infection (upregulation of the acute-phase protein hemoxygenase I, which catabolizes heme), and certain drugs. The drugs are those stimulating cytochrome P450 (leading to increased heme metabolism).

The tetrapyrrolic nucleus of porphyrins makes them photosensitive whereby absorbing at 400 nm, they become excited, and energy is transferred promoting peroxidation of biomolecules in membranes and lipids, nucleic acids, and polypeptides.

Porphyria cutanea tarda (PCT)

PCT is diagnosed by the finding of fluorescence plasma emission at 618–620 nm. Precipitating factors include alcohol abuse, viral hepatitis, estrogens use, HIV infection, and hemochromatosis.

Erythropoietic porphyria (EP)

EP is due to partial deficiency of the mitochondrial ferrochelatase, the final enzyme in the heme synthesis pathway (Fig. 2). Accumulation of protoporphyrin in tissues and skin leads to photosensitivity. Protoporphyrin is lipophilic and therefore, it is not detected in urine. It is present in bile and feces. Diagnosis of EP is based on the finding of high levels of free protoporphyrin in RBCs using fluorescence excitation-emission is at 634 nm. Biochemically, a reduction in ferrochelatase activity by 10%–35% of normal is seen in symptomatic patients. Whereas up to 50% reduction in ferrochelatase activity is seen in asymptomatic patients. In otherwords, determining ferrochelatase residual activity helps identify both the proband and carrier status respectively.

Liver dysfunction occurs in about 10%–20% of patients and that porphyrin-containing gallstones are seen in patienst with PE and leads to cholelithiasis.

Congenital erythropoietic porphyria (CEP)

CEP is an autosomal recessive disorder due to a deficiency of uroporphyrinogen III synthase activity. It is characterized by the accumulation of uroporphyrin and coproporphyrin. Patients exhibit severe photosensitivity. In children, the presentation is severe ranging from erythrodontia, osteodystrophis, and hypercellular bone marrow (in all patients); red fluorescent urine in nappies provides an early diagnosis. Mild to severe hemolysis is suggestive of impaired hematopoietic heme synthesis. Adult late onset is often confined to skin photosensitivity presentation.

Hepatoerythropoietic porphyria (HEP)

Biochemical findings in HEP resemble those of PCT caused by a deficiency of uroporphyrinogen decarboxylase (homogenous or compound heterogenous deficiency).

There is rare recessive acute genetic porphyria of the AIP, 5-ALA dehydratase porphyria, VP, and HC. Those rare variants manifest in early infancy and childhood. Patients exhibit severe developmental delay, neurological deficit, psychomotor retardation, ataxia, convulsions, short stature, and cataract. Biochemical abnormalities indicative of hepatic dysfunction are seen. However, genetic mutation studies often reveal the disorder.

Laboratory diagnosis: Porphyria

The ideal urine sample is obtained during a suspected porphyria attack (Table 4). Testing for porphobilinogen is an essential first-line investigation. Dark coloration of the urine on standing (due to photo-oxidation) directs towards porphyria investigation. Biochemical analysis is central to the diagnosis of porphyria.

Measurement of 5-aminolevulinic acid (5-ALA) is elevated in the much rarer porphyria of the first enzyme in the pathway, 5-aminolevulinic acid dehydratase deficiency. The three acute porphyrias (AIP, variegate porphyria, and coproporphyrin) deficiency leads to the accumulation of 5-ALA and PBG, and thus their measurement (PBG mostly) is diagnostic of the acute presentation. PBG levels are much higher >10 ULN, in AIP, compared to VP and HCP. Patients with lead poisoning may present with acute abdominal pain, and 5-ALA levels but not PBG will be

TABLE 4 Summary of porphyria, their clinical presentation, and biochemical findings in urine, feces, and red blood cells.

Disorder	Presentation	Test: (Urine)	(Feces)	Red blood cells
AIP	Acute attack (100%)	PBG, ALA, Porphyrins		
HCP	Acute (80%) or cutaneous (5%), or both (15%)	PBG, ALA, porphyrins	Coproporphyrin III, ratio III: *I* > 2.0	
VP	Acute (20%), cutaneous (60%), or both (20%)	PBG, ALA, coproporphyrins	Protoporphyrin IX > coproporphyrin III	
PCT	Cutaneous (skin fragility and blisters) (100%)	Urobilinogen I/III, heptacarboxyl porphyrin I or III	Isocoproporphyrin, hepatcarboxyl porphyrin I or III	
EP	Burning feeling following sun exposure (100%)	Fecal: Protoporphyrin IX	Isocoproporphyrin, hepatcarboxyl porphyrin I or III	
CEP	Severe photosensitivity (100%)	Uroporphyrin I, coproporphyrin I	Protoporphyrin IX	Zinc protoporphyrin IX
HEP	Severe photosensitivity (100%)	Uroporphrin II, heptacrboxyl porphyrin I or III	Isocoproporphyrin, hepatcarboxyl porphyrin I or III	Zinc protoporphyrin IX
ALA	Acute-chronic neuropathy (100%)	Urine ALA, coproporphyrin III		

AIP, Acute intermittent porphyria; *HCP,* hereditary coproporphyria; *VP,* variegate porphyria; *PCT,* porphyria cutanea tarda; *EP,* erythropoietic protoporphyria; *CEP,* congenital erythropoietic porphyria; *HEP,* hepatoerthropoietic porphyria; *ALA,* 5-aminolevulinic acid dehydratase porphyria.
Modified from Puy H, Gouya L, Deybach JC. Porphyrias. Lancet. 2010;375(9718):924–37. https://doi.org/10.1016/S0140-6736(09)61925-5. PMID: 20226990.

elevated. Lead competes with iron binding to heme and causes an elevation in 5-ALA.

Coproporphyria is common in many disorders and thus measurement of total porphyrins rather than specifically PBG is unhelpful and can be misleading.

Elucidating the different porphyria in the proband requires assessment of plasma for fluorescence emission 624–628 nm to confirm VP as the presenting cause of the acute attack. The fluorescence test is also helpful during the asymptomatic period. Fecal protoporphyrin level is higher compared to fecal coproporphyrin and is indicative of VP. Fecal coproporphyrin is elevated in hereditary coproporphyria, with a ratio of isomer III to I being greater than twofold (Table 4).

Fecal coproporphyrin isomers III and I are diagnostic for coproporphyria (isomer III to isomer I ratio being >2) indicative of HCP.

Once the disorder is identified in the proband, family screening is essential to identify latent disease. With genetic mutation analysis being the gold standard, enzyme studies are also conducted for those where a mutation cannot be identified.

Clinical features of porphyria range from solely acute attacks of neuropathy, mixed acute attacks and bullous dermatosis, erosive photodermatitis, and acute photosensitivity.

Acute visceral, dermatological manifestations range from bullous to erosive, to acute photosensitivity. The autosomal dominant erythropoietic protoporphyria and the x-linked dominant erythropoietic porphyria mainly exhibit acute photosensitivity; porphyria cutanea tarda, hepatoerythropoietic porphyria, and congenital erythropoietic porphyria present with predominant erosive photodermatitis; and variegate porphyria and hereditary coproporphyria present with all mixed acute neurologic attacks and dermatological photosensitivity with variegate mostly presenting with erosive dermatitis, and hereditary coproporphyria predominantly presenting with acute neurological presentation. Acute intermittent porphyria and the rare 5-aminolevulinic acid dehydrate porphyria exhibit acute neurological attacks (Fig. 2).

When porphobilinogen (a tetrapyrrole) reacts with dimethyl amino benzaldehyde in acidic circumstances, a red-colored complex is formed. Urobilinogen reacts similarly but is extractable into amyl alcohol, whereas porphobilinogen is not. The presence of porphyrins is determined by acidification of urine and the extraction of porphyrins (colorless) into an amyl alcohol solvent phase, and subsequent detection of fluorescence in ultraviolet light. Freshly collected random urinary sample, approximately 10–20 mL, in a sterile urine container, is wrapped in foil after collection to prevent ultraviolet denaturation of the sample. Analysis should be performed as soon as possible and should be stored at 2–4°C if there is any delay in processing.

Urine porphobilinogen (PBG) screen

Chemical assays are commercially available for the detection of PBG in urine. They use Ehrlich's reagent and partition it into amyl alcohol. The presence of red color in the upper organic phase (amyl alcohol) denotes the presence of urobilinogen, indicating that the sample is negative for porphobilinogen. However, the presence of a pink or red color in the lower aqueous phase denotes the presence of porphobilinogen, that is, positive for PBG.

Limitations of the procedure are that in "concentrated" urine samples, urobilinogen in trace amounts may be observed in the organic phase, this is a normal phenomenon. Samples taken for diagnosis of acute intermittent porphyria must be taken during the suspected attack as PBG may be negative during transient periods.

The activity of the enzyme porphobilinogen deaminase should be measured in red cells in these cases. Liver disease may increase urinary coproporphyrin due to decreased biliary excretion, this is the most common cause of porphyrinuria.

In addition to identifying and treating the causative agents, treatment with opioids, saline, dextrose, chlorpromazine, and intravenous hemin is used to inhibit 5-ALAS I (nonerythroid enzymes in the first committed step). Decreasing urinary levels of PBG indicates a response to therapy.

Folic acid (folate)

In contrast to the microcytic anemia seen in pure iron deficiency anemia, megaloblastic macrocytic and hypersegmented neutrophils characterize anemia associated with folate and cobalamin (vitamin B12) deficiency.

Pteroylglutamic acid is folic acid, however, the term folate encompasses related compounds of similar nutritional activity. It is available in fruits and plants and fortified dietary sources (e.g., bread) and an average daily intake of 0.2–0.3 mg is close to the requirement. Body stores are 5 to 10 mg (about 4 months' supply); this suggests that deficiency can occur fairly rapidly compared to the relatively high body stores of B12.

Dietary folate is absorbed in the upper small intestine, converted to 5-methyl-tetrahydrofolate (THF) bound to a carrier protein, and it is transported into circulation. The majority of circulating 5-methyl THF is free with 30% being bound to albumin.

Folates act as coenzymes in the synthesis of purines and pyrimidines (DNA and RNA) and as methyl donors in the synthesis of methionine.

Both serum and red blood cell folate levels are measured to assess the body's folate status. However, red blood cell folate is considered a better indicator of body store compared to serum levels that are influenced by recent dietary intake. B12 deficiency causes a reduction in the enzymatic conversion of the major circulating 5-methyl-THF to THF and thus falsely elevated folate levels may be observed.

Although folate fortification of diet has reduced the incidence of folate deficiency, and that the Chose Wisely campaign of the American Society for Clinical Pathology recommends cessation of laboratory assessment of folate levels supported by a decrease in the incidence of folate deficiency from 16% to 0.5%. However, a significant number of certain populations suffer from folate deficiency, including those in pregnancy, and assessment of folate status is required.

Folate deficiency has been reported during pregnancy, in pediatric and geriatric patients where there is increased demand for folate, and in conditions such as hemolysis, leukemia, and exfoliative dermatitis that are associated with rapid cellular proliferation. Jejunum disease and short-bowel syndrome cause malabsorption, and bacterial overgrowth as well as drugs such as alcohol, anticonvulsant, and oral contraceptives have been shown to cause folate deficiency.

Cobalamin (vitamin B12)

Cobalamin is a synthesized metabolite that is present in dietary products of animal sources. Vegetable sources are much lower. Liver and milk are good dietary sources. The dietary daily requirement is relatively low at 1 microgram compared to a body storage of about 2–3 mg. Therefore, deficiency can take several years to develop. Dietary B12 is liberated from protein binding by gastric acid and protected from proteolysis by binding to the intrinsic factor secreted by the stomach parietal cells.

B12 is a large complex nonpolymeric molecule with a molecular weight of 1.3 kDa. Cyanocobalamin is the most stable form of B12.

The B12-intrinsic factor (IF) complex is taken up by terminal ileal enterocytes, released from the IF, and becomes bound to transcobalamin-II before being released into circulation. Congenital deficiency in transcobalamin II causes infantile megaloblastic anemia.

The B12 molecule is made up of four pyrrole units with a cobalt atom center. Variations in two subunits above and below the ring give rise to the various forms of the vitamin.

It plays a role in the conversion of methyl malonyl-CoA to succinyl-CoA and a circulating form converting homocysteine to methionine (Fig. 3).

Laboratory assessment of B12 status includes measurement of transcobalamin II, which provides a better marker than measuring B12 itself. The latter has a wide normal range of 160–1000 ng/L. With this range, a low B12 level is not specific and low levels occur in in a third of normal pregnancies and those with folate deficiency.

Surrogate markers of B12 deficiency include elevated homocysteine (B12 cofactor in the conversion of homocysteine to methionine). However, levels may be elevated in renal dysfunction and among 30% of normal subjects.

Autoantibodies to both parietal cells and intrinsic factor lead to B12 deficiency and pernicious anemia. Intrinsic factor antibodies are more specific than antiparietal cells antibodies, which are positive in 15% of normal elderly subjects. Anti-IF antibodies are positive in 50% of patients with pernicious anemia.

Uric acid metabolism

Uric acid (ionized, urate anion, at physiological pH) is a product of purine metabolism where the end product of hypoxanthine and xanthine is converted to uric acid by xanthine oxidase (Fig. 4). Deficiency in the purine salvage pathway (hypoxanthine-guanine phosphoribosyl transferase (HPRT)) known as Lesch-Nyhan syndrome leads to hyperuricemia and gout characterized by high plasma uric acid and high urine-urate creatinine ratio.

Circulating levels of uric acid represent a balance between production following the metabolism of purines and

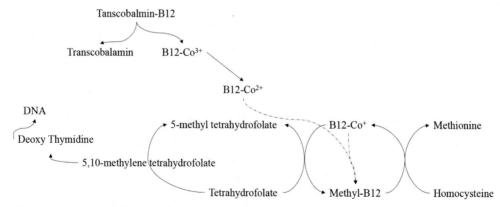

FIG. 3 B12 metabolism and conversion of homocysteine to methionine. *Modified from Rush EC, Katre P, Yajnik CS. Vitamin B12: one carbon metabolism, fetal growth and programming for chronic disease. Eur J Clin Nutr. 2014;68(1):2–7. https://doi.org/10.1038/ejcn.2013.232. Epub 2013 Nov 13. PMID: 24219896*

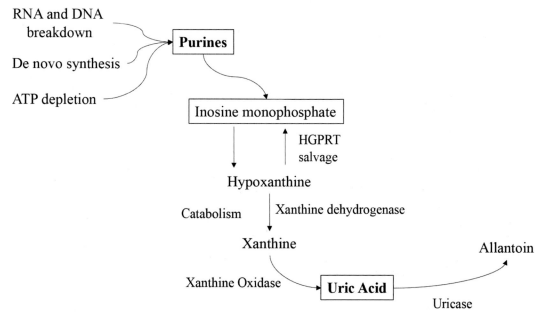

FIG. 4 Uric acid metabolism. Purines obtained from either nucleic acid breakdown or de novo synthesis are metabolized to inosine monophosphate (IMP), which is converted to hypoxanthine and xanthine. The latter is oxidized by xanthine oxidase to uric acid. *HGPRT*, hypoxanthine-guanine phosphoribosyl-transferase. *Modified from Gherghina ME, Peride I, Tiglis M, Neagu TP, Niculae A, Checherita IA. Uric Acid and Oxidative Stress-Relationship with Cardiovascular, Metabolic, and Renal Impairment. Int J Mol Sci. 2022;23(6):3188. https://doi.org/10.3390/ijms23063188. PMID: 35328614; PMCID: PMC8949471.*

kidney clearance. The kidney clears about 70% with some excretion by the intestine.

Males have higher urate levels compared to females; furthermore, obesity, high protein diet, and alcohol consumption are associated with higher circulating urate.

Hyperuricemia, secondary to increased cellular breakdown is seen in patients with tumor lysis syndrome. Hyperuricemia causes gout (precipitation of uric acid crystals in joints) leading to arthritic comorbidities and associated hypertension. It is also associated with the metabolic syndrome of obesity, glucose intolerance, dyslipidemia, and hypertension. Deposition in the renal tract leads to uric acid nephrolithiasis.

It is important to note that in patients presenting with an acute gout attack, circulating urate levels are likely to be within normal limits as it has precipitated into crystals in the joints, leading to inflammation and associated severe arthritic pain. In contrast, its antioxidative properties are thought to afford a protective role in neurodegenerative disorders such as multiple sclerosis.

Uric acid is both secreted and reabsorbed by the renal tubules and by the intestine. Renal handling of uric acid is complex, where it is completely filtered through the glomerulus, reabsorbed by proximal tubules, and actively both secreted and reabsorbed in the distal tubules.

Distal tubular secretion is inhibited by lactic acid, 3-betahydroxybutyrate, and thiazide diuretics which compete with urate for excretion. There is also distal tubular reabsorption of urate with a net 10% of filtered loads being finally excreted. Uricosuric drugs inhibit distal tubular reabsorption of uric acid. Salicylates have a dose-specific effect where a high dosage inhibits reabsorption and a low dose reduces tubular secretion.

Urinary uric acid concentration exceeding its solubility leads to the formation of uric acid stones.

Hypouricemia is seen when using xanthine oxidase inhibitors (allopurinol) and in loss of renal reabsorption as a result of loss of function mutation. Similarly, loss of renal tubular secretory mechanism is either due to reduced glomerular filtration rate or to a mutation in the secretory mechanism.

Hypouricemia is seen in dilutional hypervolemic states (SIADH) and in pregnancy, liver dysfunction, deficiency of xanthine oxidase (xanthinuria), Fanconi syndrome (defective renal reabsorption), and use of urate oxidase in tumor lysis syndrome (it converts uric acid to water-soluble allantoin).

It is recommended to bring uric acid levels to less than 6.0 mg/dL to resolve urate deposition.

Purine and pyrimidine disorders

Xanthine oxidase is required for the synthesis of purines and pyrimidines, which are the basic building blocks of DNA and RNA. Xanthine oxidase deficiency (Lesch-Nyhan syndrome) as well as sulfite oxidase deficiency (molybdenum cofactor deficiency) present with intractable seizures. The disorders are characterized by low plasma uric acid levels (impaired synthesis) and low urinary urate/creatinine ratio.

Inborn errors of metabolism

It was A. Garrod (1908) who coined the term inborn errors of metabolism (IEM) describing alkaptonuria, benign pentosuria, albinism, and cystinuria. The main cause is a genetic mutation or deficiency of a protein central to a metabolic pathway. A metabolic process may be involved in either synthesis, degradation, or transportation of molecules. The consequences are thus either accumulation of the substrate of a defective enzyme, diversion into a secondary pathway, or accumulation of molecules normally degraded as in storage disorders. The clinical presentations are variable and secondary to the above metabolic abnormalities.

There are currently over 400 disorders described, mostly (85%) present with neurological disorders in addition to hematological, cardiac, and hepatic dysfunctions. The neurological presentations are varied from lethargy, weakness, and loss of suck and swallow reflexes to convulsions and myotonia. The neurological deficit may be due to the accumulation of neurotoxic metabolite (e.g., phenylalanine in phenylketonuria), hypoglycemia (e.g., glycogen storage disorders), or to accumulation of elements such as copper (Wilson's disease) or iron (hemochromatosis).

Patients may exhibit specific clinical presentation later in life or nonspecific in the newborn. In addition to the earlier neurological symptoms, the affected patient my present with failure to thrive, persistent vomiting, abnormal odor or staining of dippers, hypoglycemia, metabolic acidosis and ketosis, prolonged jaundice, hepatomegaly, acute hepatic failure, renal impairment, renal calculi early in life, abnormal hair and pigmentation, resistant rickets, early cataract (galactosemia), and abnormal hematological indices (neutropenia, thrombocytopenia), and biochemical abnormalities such as hyponatremia and hyperkalemia among others.

The majority of IEMs involve dysfunctional enzymatic processes or transport proteins. The incidences are invariably rare ranging from 1: 10,000 to 1: 25,000 for phenylketonuria, cystinuria, Hartnup disease, and congenital adrenal hyperplasia, 1:50,000 to 1:100,000 in galactosemia, and 1:200,000 to 1:400,000 in tyrosinemia and maple syrup urine disease.

The disorders present in a wide variety of ways and although they are individually rare, collectively form significant proportions of illness. They are characterized by the accumulation of substrates (often diagnostic). Recognized disorders affect amino acids and organic acids metabolism, and lipids metabolism, among others.

Although most inborn errors of metabolism will exhibit some form of neuropathy, the fact that there remains about 3% of pediatric patients with unexplained isolated developmental delay and or intellectual disability makes obvious the need to search for an inborn error.

Newborn screening (NBS) for inborn errors of metabolism

Screening for metabolic disorders is performed during the neonatal period dictated by various local, national, and nation-wide programs. Examples of recognized and mandated screening programs and disorders tested for are shown in the following Tables 5 and 6.

Advancements in technologies such as tandem mass spectrometry and next-generation sequencing (NGS) employing a massively parallel sequencing strategy have facilitated the expansion of the disorders being tested for as well as an expanded understanding of the disorders and development of therapies.

Inborn errors of metabolism can in general be described in two groups. The first includes mutations that affect energy production and the other affects the synthesis and/or degradation of specific biomolecules.

Clinical presentation is variable. Patients with small molecule disorders often associated with either degradation pathways and those to generate energy or building blocks (amino acids, organic acids, urea cycle defects, glycogen storage disorders) often present with acute illness. Whereas patients with organelle metabolism present with neurological, neuromuscular, and hepatic dysfunction. Disorders of synthetic processes (porphyria, glycosylation), and those transporters and channel proteins present in both (e.g., iron metabolism).

When an inborn error of metabolism is suspected, initial biochemistry tests should include the determination of anion gap, lactate, glucose, ammonia, liver, and renal function test as well as liver enzymes, glucose, and blood gases if possible.

Primary testing is performed in patients (often neonates) undergoing screening for a set of inborn errors of metabolism. The inherited disorders being screened for vary between countries and various health and regional variation within the same country. Examples of those mandated by certain regions (for example the state of Texas) are shown in Table 6.

Disorders screened for are very variable worldwide, for instance, in Sub-Saharan Africa, there is limited screening for glucose-6-phosphate dehydrogenase deficiency and sickle cell-related programs (with only two countries participating in the CDC NBS quality assurance program). In Brazil, six conditions (cystic fibrosis, biotinidase deficiency, congenital adrenal hyperplasia, congenital hypothyroid, phenylketonuria, and severe combined immunodeficiency) are screened for. Among Asian countries, there is significant geographical variation in screening coverage and about 50% of the population coverage includes glucose-6-phosphate dehydrogenase deficiency and phenylketonuria screening.

TABLE 5 Inborn errors of metabolism.

Program	Disorders routinely tested	Additional tests (Mostly in North America and Europe)
	Amino acid disorders (PKU, HCY, MSUD, CIT, ASA, TYR-I)	Argininemia, Citrullinemia II, Hypermethioninemia, benign hyperphenylalaninemia, biopterin defects, tyrosinemia II, III
Organic acid disorders	PA, MUT, GA-I, 3-MCC, HMG, MCD, BKT, IVA	Malonic acidemia, isobutylglycinuria, 2-methylbutyrylglyciuria,3-methylglutaconic acidurias, 2-methyl-3-hydroxybytyruic acidurias
Fatty acid oxidation defects	MCAD, VLCAD, LCHAD, TFP, CTD, CPT-I,II, CACT, GA-II,	Short-chain acyl-CoA dehydrogenase deficiency, medium/short-chain L-3 hydroxy acyl-CoA dehydrogenase deficiency, medium-chain ketoacyl-CoA thiolase deficiency, 2,4-dienoyl-CoA reductase deficiency
Other disorders	BIOT, GALT, GSD-II, MPS-I, X-ALD	Galactoepimerase deficiency, galactokinase deficiency, T-cell-related lymphocyte deficiencies, glucose-6-phosphate dehydrogenase deficiency, and other lysosomal diseases

Neonatal screening program contents and additional tests are often in certain geographical locations.
PKU, Phenylketonuria; *HCY*, homocystinuria; *MSUD*, maple syrup urine disease; *CIT-I*, Citrullinemia type I; *ASA*, Argininosuccinic aciduria; *TYR I*, tyrosinemia type I; *PA*, propionic acidemia; *GA-I*, glutaric acidemia type I; *3-MCC*, 3-methylcrotonyl glycinuria; *HMG*, 3-hydroxy-3-methylglutaruic aciduria; *MCD*, holocaboxylae synthase deficiency; *BKT*, B-ketothiolase deficiency; *IVA*, isovaleric acidemia; *MCAD*, medium chain acyl CoA dehydrogenase deficiency; *VLCD*, very long chain acyl-CoA dehydrogenase deficiency; *LCHAD*, long chain 3-hydroxyacyl-CoA dehydrogenase deficiency; *TFP*, trifunctional protein deficiency; *CTD*, carnitine transport defect; *CPT-I, II*, carnitine palmitoyl transferase I (II) deficiency; *CACTY*, carnitine acylcarnitine translocase deficiency; *GA II*, glutaric acidemia type II; *BIOT*, biotinidase deficiency; *GALT*, classic galactosemia; *GSD-II*, glycogen storage disease type II (Pompes); *MPS-I*, mucopolysaccharidosis type I; *X-ALD*, X-linked adrenoleukodystrophy.
Modified from Keskinkılıç B. Neonatal screening programs. Clin Biochem. 2014;47(9):692. https://doi.org/10.1016/j.clinbiochem.2014.05.009. Epub 2014 May 18. PMID: 24845716, and Villoria JG, Pajares S, López RM, Marin JL, Ribes A. Neonatal Screening for Inherited Metabolic Diseases in 2016. Semin Pediatr Neurol. 2016;23(4):257–272. https://doi.org/10.1016/j.spen.2016.11.001. Epub 2016 Nov 16. PMID: 28284388, and Mak CM, Lee HC, Chan AY, Lam CW. Inborn errors of metabolism and expanded newborn screening: review and update. Crit Rev. Clin Lab Sci. 2013;50(6):142–62. https://doi.org/10.3109/1040836 3.2013.847896. PMID: 24295058, and Ombrone D, Giocaliere E, Forni G, Malvagia S, la Marca G. Expanded newborn screening by mass spectrometry: New tests, future perspectives. Mass Spectrom Rev. 2016;35(1):71–84. https://doi.org/10.1002/mas.21463. Epub 2015 May 7. PMID: 25952022.

TABLE 6 Examples of disorders in use in Texas.

Amino acid disorders	
Core conditions	**Secondary**
Argininosuccinic aciduria (ASA) Citrullinemia, Type I (CIT) Homocystinuria (HCY) Maple syrup urine disease (MSUD) Classic phenylketonuria (PKU) Tyrosinemia, Type I (TYR I)	Argininemia (ARG) Benign hyperphenylalaninemia (H-PHE) Biopterin defect in cofactor biosynthesis (BIOPT BS) Biopterin defect in cofactor regeneration (BIOPT REG) Citrullinemia, Type II (CIT II) Hypermethioninemia (MET) Tyrosinemia, Type II (TYR II) Tyrosinemia, Type III (TYR III)
Fatty acid disorders	
Core conditions	**Secondary**
Carnitine uptake defect (CUD) Long-chain L-3-hydroxyacyl-CoA dehydrogenase deficiency (LCHAD) Medium-chain Acyl-CoA dehydrogenase deficiency (MCAD) Trifunctional protein deficiency (TFP) Very long-chain Acyl-CoA dehydrogenase deficiency (VLCAD)	2,4 Dienoyl-CoA reductase deficiency (DE RED) Carnitine acylcarnitine translocase deficiency (CACT) Carnitine palmitoyltransferase Type I deficiency (CPT I) Carnitine palmitoyltransferase Type II deficiency (CPT II) Glutaric acidemia Type II (GA2) Medium-chain ketoacyl-CoA thiolase deficiency (MCKAT) Medium/short chain L-3-hydroxyacyl-CoA Dehydrogenase deficiency (M/SCHAD) Short-chain Acyl-CoA dehydrogenase deficiency (SCAD)

Continued

TABLE 6 Examples of disorders in use in Texas—cont'd

Organic acid disorders

Core conditions	Secondary
3-Methylcrotonyl-CoA carboxylase deficiency (3-MCC) 3-Hydroxy-3-methylglutaric aciduria (HMG) Beta-ketothiolase deficiency (BKT) Glutaric acidemia Type I (GA1) Isovaleric acidemia (IVA) Methylmalonic acidemia (Cobalamin disorders-Cbl A, B) Methylmalonic acidemia (Methylmalonic-CoA mutase) Holocarboxylase synthase Deficiency (multiple carboxylase deficiency-MCD) Propionic acidemia (PROP)	2 Methylbutyrylglycinuria (2MBG) 2-Methyl-3-hydroxybutyric aciduria (2M3HBA) 3-Methylglutaconic aciduria (3MGA) Isobutyrylglycinuria (IBG) Methylmalonic acidemia with homocystinuria (Cbl C, D) Malonic acidemia (MAL)

Endocrine disorders

Primary	Secondary
Congenital adrenal hyperplasia (CAH) Primary congenital hypothyroidism (CH)	N/A

Hemoglobin disorders

Primary	Secondary
S, S (Sickle Cell Anemia) S, C disease S Beta-Thalassemia	Various other hemoglobinopathies

Other disorders

Core conditions	Secondary
Severe combined immunodeficiencies (SCID) Biotinidase deficiency (BIOT) Classic galactosemia (GALT) Cystic fibrosis (CF) X-linked adrenoleukodystrophy (X-ALD) Spinal muscular atrophy due to homozygous deletion of exon 7 in SMN1 (SMA)	T-cell-related lymphocyte deficiencies

Secondary conditions may be detected following screening for the cord conditions.
Modified from Texas Newborn Screening Program. https://www.dshs.texas.gov/newborn-screening-program. Accessed 9th March 2023.

Amino acid disorders

Phenylketonuria

This is a disorder characterized by the accumulation of phenylketonuria and its detection in the urine. It was identified in 1934 by Folling when he detected phenylketone bodies in the urine of patients, and the development of a screening test by Guthrie in 1960 facilitated its population-wide screening and thus became the first inhered disorder to benefit from newborn screening. It is an autosomal recessive disorder caused by a deficiency of the phenylalanine hydroxylase that converts phenylalanine to tyrosine (Fig. 5). Deficiency of the enzyme leads to accumulation and appearance in the urine of phenyl ketone bodies (phenylalanine, phenylpyruvate, phenylacetate) and accumulation of phenylalanine in the blood and brain tissue. The enzyme requires cofactor tetrahydrobiopterin (B4), molecular oxygen, and iron.

The patient presents with vomiting and irritability (first few weeks of life), mental retardation (4–6 months later if not treated), and a fair complexion (secondary to deficient melanin).

Accumulation of phenylalanine in the brain is associated with irreversible mental retardation, disability, and motor deficits with the blood phenylalanine levels correlating with a degree of neurocognitive outcome and hence reduction in blood phenylalanine levels is essential.

A strict diet of phenylalanine is the mainstay treatment. The goal of therapy is three folds, first, prevent accumulation of excessive dietary phenylalanine in the body; second, substitute with amino acid mixture low in phenylamine, and

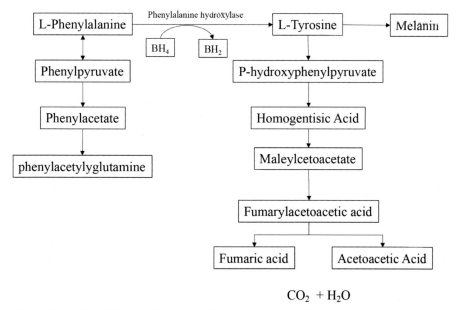

FIG. 5 Metabolism of phenylalanine. Phenylalanine hydroxylase catalyzes the conversion of phenylalanine to tyrosine and requires BH_4 as a cofactor. Deficiency in the enzyme of its cofactor leads to the accumulation of phenylalanine and phenylketones appearing in the urine, and thus the term phenyl-ketonuria. *BH_4*, tetrahydrobiopterin as a cofactor; *BH_2*, dihydrobiopterin. *Modified from Matthews DE. An overview of phenylalanine and tyrosine kinetics in humans. J Nutr. 2007;137(6 Suppl 1):1549S–1555S; discussion 1573S]1575S. https://doi.org/10.1093/jn/137.6.1549S. PMID: 17513423; PMCID: PMC2268015, and Elhawary NA, AlJahdali IA, Abumansour IS, Elhawary EN, Gaboon N, Dandini M, Madkhali A, Alosaimi W, Alzahrani A, Aljohani F, Melibary EM, Kensara OA. Genetic etiology and clinical challenges of phenylketonuria. Hum Genomics. 2022;16(1):22. https://doi.org/10.1186/s40246-022-00398-9. PMID: 35854334; PMCID: PMC9295449.*

promote and attain normal growth and nutritional status. This is achieved by ensuring that the diet contains a balanced intake of all nutrients and energy. Vitamins and minerals supplements are either added to the protein substitute or given as a separate supplement.

A commonly used cutoff is blood phenylalanine levels >120–130 μmol/L are considered abnormal, with a phenylalanine: tyrosine ratio > 2.

However, other causes of hyperphenylalaninemia need to be excluded. Hyperphenylalaninemia is seen in tetrahydrobiopterin defects, high protein diet, and liver dysfunction. Defects in BH_4 leading to high phenylamine levels can be treated by supplementation with BH_4.

Tyrosinemia

Tyrosinemia is a disorder characterized by hypoglycemia secondary to acute and severe liver disease and failure. This occurs due to a deficiency in the enzyme fumarylacetoacetase, which catalyzes the metabolism of fumarylacetoacetic acid to fumaric acid and acetoacetic acid. The deficiency leads to the accumulation of succinyl acetoacetic acid and succinyl acetone and increased tyrosine, p-hydroxyphenyl pyruvate, and p-hydroxyphenyl lactate due to inhibition of p-hydroxyphenylpyruvate oxidase. Diagnosis is suspected by the finding of increased plasma tyrosine levels, associated with increased methionine and phenylalanine as

well as urinary succinyl acetone. Alkaline phosphatase is often markedly elevated in tyrosinemia patients (>2000 IU/L).

The disorder is confirmed by the finding of decreased fumarylacetoacetase levels in leukocytes. It is known as tyrosinemia type I. NMTBC (2,2, nitro-4-trifluoromethyl benzoyl-1,3-cyclohexanedione) inhibits p-hydroxyphenylpyruvate oxidase and is used to manage patients with tyrosinemia type I and may help reduce the need for a liver transplant. Therapy is immediate dietary restriction followed by a liver transplant (Fig. 6).

Urea cycle defects

Disorders of the urea cycle (Fig. 7) onset are often early in life and present with neonatal hyperammonemia (often exceeding 800 μmol/L in the first 1–3 days). There are six possible urea cycle inherited defects.

Ammonia formed from amino acid deamination is converted in the urea cycle to urea and excreted into the urine. Urea cycle defects lead to hyperammonemia. Ammonia is a respiratory stimulus, and the patient often has respiratory alkalosis. The enzymes involved in the conversion of ammonia to urea (in the urea cycle, Fig. 7) are; carbamoyl phosphate synthase I (encoded for by CPS1 gene) the initial enzymatic step is the detoxification of ammonia. It catalyzes the condensation of ammonia with bicarbonate and requires *N*-acetyl glutamate. Ornithine transcarbamylase binds

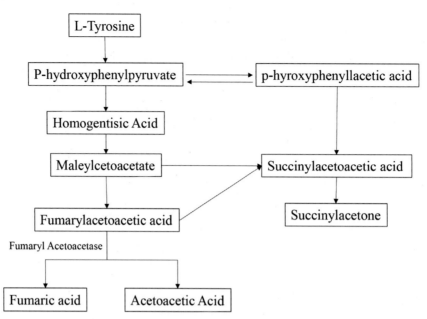

FIG. 6 Tyrosine metabolism: Tyrosinemia due to the accumulation of tyrosine and its metabolite fumarylacetoacetic acid and the succinylacetoacetic acid and succinyl acetone due to the deficiency of the enzyme fumaryl acetoacetates. The deficiency is termed tyrosinemia type 1. *Modified from Chinsky JM, Singh R, Ficicioglu C, van Karnebeek CDM, Grompe M, Mitchell G, Waisbren SE, Gucsavas-Calikoglu M, Wasserstein MP, Coakley K, Scott CR. Diagnosis and treatment of tyrosinemia type I: a US and Canadian consensus group review and recommendations. Genet Med. 2017;19(12). https://doi. org/10.1038/gim.2017.101. Epub 2017 Aug 3. PMID: 28771246; PMCID: PMC5729346.*

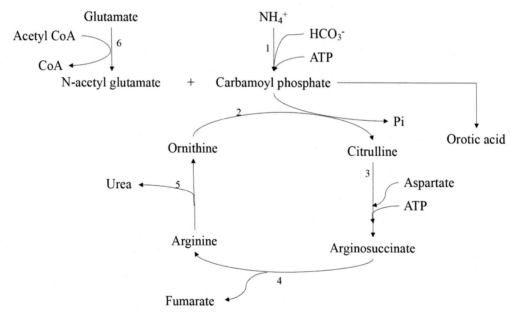

FIG. 7 Urea cycle. Enzymatic steps (1–6) have been identified as possible deficiencies in the metabolism of ammonia and the synthesis of urea. 1: carbamoyl phosphate synthetase, 2: ornithine carbamoyl transferase, 3: argininosuccinate synthetase, 4: arginosuccinate lyase, 5: arginase, 6: N-acetylglutamate synthetase. *Modified from Summar ML, Mew NA. Inborn Errors of Metabolism with Hyperammonemia: Urea Cycle Defects and Related Disorders. Pediatr Clin North Am. 2018;65(2):231–246. https://doi.org/10.1016/j.pcl.2017.11.004. Epub 2018 Feb 2. PMID: 29502911.*

carbamoyl phosphate to ornithine producing citrulline. Formed citrulline is transported out of the mitochondrion and attached to aspartate by arginosuccinate synthase. The formed argininosuccinate is converted into fumarate and arginine by arginosuccinate lyase. Arginine is hydrolyzed

by arginase to ornithine and urea. Thus, urea carrying two nitrogen residues is excreted into the urine (Fig. 7).

Dietary protein restrictions (0.8–1.5 g/kg/24 h) are required to reduce hyperammonemia, in addition to therapeutics such as benzoates which conjugate with glycine forming hippurate, which is excreted and thus diverts nitrogen away from the urea cycle. Patients with urea cycle defects exhibit lethargy, seizures, tachypnea, and vomiting.

Ornithine carbamoyl transferase (ornithine transcarbamylase (OTC))

OTC combines carbamyl phosphate with ornithine to produce citrulline (Fig. 7).

The deficiency of the enzyme ornithine carbamoyl transferase is X-linked with the incidence of 1:14,000. As such, it is the most common urea cycle defect and the majority of the severely affected are males. Carrier females may rarely be affected. Patients with partial OTC deficiency present anytime following a triggering event, such as infection.

The SLC25A15 gene encodes the mitochondrial ornithine translocator and its deficiency is associated with hyperornithinemia, hyperammonemia, and homocitrullinuria syndrome.

Arginosuccinate synthetase (ASS)

ASS conjugates citrulline and aspartate forming arginosuccinate (Fig. 7).

The deficiency of the enzyme arginosuccinate synthase leads to citrullinemia type I, with levels of citrulline >100 times the upper limit of normal. The patients exhibit severe hyperammonemia during the newborn period.

An adult form, citrullinemia II, results from the deficiency of a mitochondrial membrane glutamate-aspartate transporter. The reduced availability of aspartate for arginosuccinate synthetase results in citrullinemia and hyperammonemia.

Arginosuccinate lyase (ASL)

ASL gene encodes for arginosuccinate lyase. The enzyme converts argininosuccinate to arginine and fumarate (Fig. 7). Since the substrate arginosuccinate is freely excreted into the urine, hyperammonemia is less severe. In addition to hepatomegaly and elevated liver enzymes (AST and ALT), patients develop trichorrhexis nodosa (nodelike appearance of hair) which responds to arginine supplementation.

Arginase

Arginase is the final step in the urea cycle (Fig. 7). It cleaves arginine into ornithine and urea. Patients with arginase deficiency present with developmental delay, progressive spasticity, and gradual loss of cognitive abilities. It is encoded by the RG1 gene. Deficiency is often missed and it is wrongly misdiagnosed as cerebral palsy.

N-Acetyl glutamate synthetase (NAGS)

NAGS gene codes for N-acetyl glutamate synthase 1. The enzyme catalyzes the conversion of glutamate and acetyl-CoA to N-acetyl glutamate (NAG) (Fig. 7). The latter is a cofactor of carbamyl phosphate synthase-1 and thus in its absence, CPS-1 is not active. Patients exhibit significant and repeated bouts of hyperammonemia.

Organic acids disorders

Organic acids are low molecular weight intermediate metabolites of amino acids, carbohydrates, and fatty acids. Disorders in the metabolism of amino acids, carbohydrates, or fatty acids are often associated with the buildup of upstream metabolites (organic acids) leading to clinical presentation and often a high degree of morbidity and mortality if not diagnosed and managed appropriately.

The most common inborn errors of metabolism leading to organic acidurias are branched-chain amino acids disorders leading to maple serum urine disease (see later).

Although patients with organic acid disorders such as in methylmalonic and propionic acidemia may present with hyperammonemia, the levels of ammonia are relatively much lower (400–800 μmol/L (680–1362 μg/dL)) than those observed in patients with urea cycle defects. Blood and urinary amino acid measurements are required in the differential diagnosis.

Branched chain amino acids defects

Branched-chain amino acids (valine, leucine, and isoleucine) metabolism defects are also termed maple serum urine disease (MSUD). It is characterized by the sweet odor of urine and sweat. There is defective decarboxylation of the branched-chain amino acids (Fig. 8). Valine, leucine, and isoleucine accumulate in the circulation and their corresponding oxoacids in the urine.

MSUD is an autosomal recessive disorder with reduced/deficient branched-chain alpha-ketoacid dehydrogenase enzyme (BCKDH) complex.

It is characterized by failure to thrive, developmental and neurological delay, encephalopathy, branched-chain ketoacids in urine, and branched-chain amino acids in plasma.

Testing for MSUD is part of the newborn screening program, and that early treatment is effective with good clinical outcomes.

The initial step (branched chain aminotransferase) takes place in skeletal muscle; the majority is in skeletal muscle and not in hepatic in contrast to other amino acids metabolism. The amino acids are essential for protein synthesis, function, cellular signaling, and glucose metabolism.

In the second step of the metabolic pathway, branched chain α-ketoacid dehydrogenase (BCKDH) complex initiates oxidative decarboxylation of alpha-ketoacids

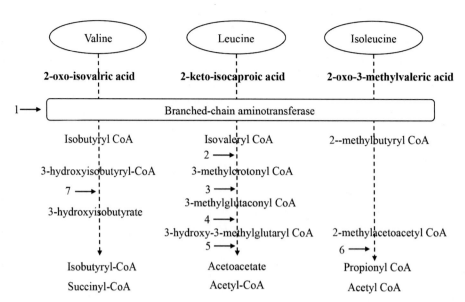

FIG. 8 Diagram showing branched-chain amino acids metabolism pathway. Enzyme deficiencies leading to specific disorders are, 1: classical branched-chain amino acid transferase (MSUD), 2: isovaleryl-CoA dehydrogenase (isovaleric acidemia), 3: 3-methylcrontonyl-CoA carboxylase deficiency (3-methytlcrotonylglycinuria), 4: 3-methylglutaconyl-CoA-hydratase (3-methylglutaconic acidemia) 5: 3-hydroxyl-3-methytlglutaryl-CoA-lyase (3-hydroxy-3-methytl glutaric aciduria), 6: acetoacetyl-CoA thiolase (2-methylacetoacetic aciduria), 7: 3-hydroxisobyutyryl CoA decarboxylase (valine catabolism). *Modified from Blackburn PR, Gass JM, Vairo FPE, Farnham KM, Atwal HK, Macklin S, Klee EW, Atwal PS. Maple syrup urine disease: mechanisms and management. Appl Clin Genet. 2017;10:57–66. https://doi.org/10.2147/TACG.S125962. PMID: 28919799; PMCID: PMC5593394.*

which converts them into acetoacetate, acetyl-CoA, and succinyl CoA. The BCKDH complex is made up of subunits E1-alpha, E-1Beta, E2, and E3. The dihydro-lipoamide branched chain transacylase (E2) gene provides instructions for synthesis of the BCKDH enzyme complex.

There are five clinical phenotypes identified by their presentations and biochemical profile, age at onset, and response to thiamine supplementation. Variants occur due

to different mutations in the genes encoding the BCKDH complex (Table 7).

Patients will also have elevated lactate, alanine, and alpha-ketoglutarate, which are related to mitochondrial dysfunction.

Other disorders (Fig. 8) of the branched-chain amino acids include the following: isovaleric acidemia is due to deficiency of isovaleryl-CoA-dehydrogenase, 3-methylcrotonylglycinuria due to deficiency of

TABLE 7 Type and genetics of MSUD.

Type	Genes	Enzyme subunits	Comments
Classic	BCKDH(A), BCKDH(B), DBT (E2)	E1alpha, E1beta, E2	BCAA and alloisoleucine in plasma, elevated BCAA in urine
Intermediate	BCKDH(A), BCKDH(B), DBT (E2)	E1alpha, E1beta, E2	As above but less severe
Intermittent			Normal BCAA
Thiamine responsive			Improved BCAA levels when on thiamine
E3-deficient			Elevated BCAA, alloisoleucine, lactate, pyruvate, and alanine in plasma. Elevated branched-chain ketoacids and alpha-ketoglutarate in urine

BCKDH, Branched chain α-ketoacid dehydrogenase; *BCKDH(A)*, branched chain α-ketoacid dehydrogenase-alpha; *BCKDH(B)*, branched chain α-ketoacid dehydrogenase-beta; *DBT*, dihydrolipoamide branched chain transacylase (E2); *BCAA*, branched chain amino acids.
Modified from Blackburn PR, Gass JM, Vairo FPE, Farnham KM, Atwal HK, Macklin S, Klee EW, Atwal PS. Maple syrup urine disease: mechanisms and management. Appl Clin Genet. 2017;10:57–66. https://doi.org/10.2147/TACG.S125962. PMID: 28919799; PMCID: PMC5593394.

3-methylcrotonyl-CoA-carboxylase, 3-methylglutanonic aciduria due to deficiency of 3-methylglutaconyl-CoA-hydratase, 3-hydroxy-3-methyl glutaric aciduria due to deficiency of 3-hydroxyl-3-methytlglutaryl-CoA-lyase, 2-methylacetoacetic aciduria due to deficiency in the enzyme acetoacetyl-CoA thiolase, and 3-hydroxyisobutyryl CoA decarboxylase deficiency involved in valine catabolism.

Other amino acid disorders

Homocysteine metabolism defect

Several enzymes and cofactors are involved in the conversion of the essential amino acid methionine to other amino acids (e.g., cysteine) (Fig. 9). Homocystinuria is a rare autosomal metabolic disorder secondary to the deficiency of the enzyme cystathionine beta-synthase. The enzyme requires the cofactor vitamin B6 (pyridoxine). Mutations in the methylenetetrahydrofolate reductase (MTHFR) genes result in deficient 5, methyl-TFH required in the conversion of methionine to homocysteine (Fig. 9) leading to homocystinuria.

Cystinuria

This disorder is characterized by failure of the renal tubules to reabsorb cystine and is often part of a collective inability to reabsorb basic amino acids (ornithine, arginine, and lysine) (COAL). High levels of cystine appear in urine with the risk of cystine renal stone formation, and that adequate hydration reduces the risk.

Carbohydrate disorders

Galactose metabolism disorder

Galactosemia is caused by the impairment of one of the three galactose metabolizing enzymes (Galactokinase, galactose-1-phosphate uridyltransferase, and UDP-galactose 4-epimerase). Classical glucosemia is the most severe form and a consequence of galactose-1-phosphate uridylphosphate transferase deficiency (Fig. 10). The classical form has a prevalence of 1:40,000-60,000. Galactose-1-phosphate accumulates in circulation and appears in the urine producing a positive reducing substance test. Neonate on lactose-free formula will not exhibit urine-reducing substances. Galactitol and galactonate accumulate in tissue and patients present with cataracts due to deposition of galactitol over 2–3 years if not diagnosed and managed appropriately with galactose-free diet.

Diagnosis is established by finding reduced erythrocyte galactose-1-phosphate uridyltransferase (Gal-PUT) enzyme activity and/or by Gal-PUT gene analysis. Genetic analysis per se is sufficient if the detected variations were consistent with those disease-causing genes and each of the biological parents carries one of the identified variations. In the neonatal period, the patient presents with failure to thrive, jaundice, and hepatomegaly. In severe cases, the patient develops septicemia. Patients will later develop neurological impairment leading to functional and cognitive deficits.

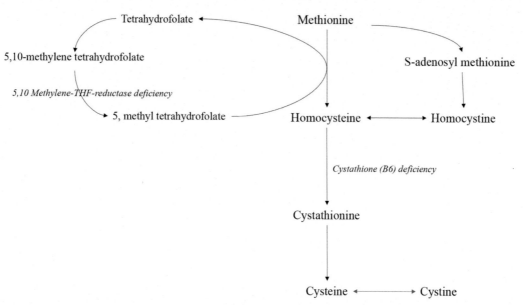

FIG. 9 Homocysteine metabolism: Classical form is a deficiency of cystathione (B6). The tetrahydrofolate (THF) is required for the metabolism of methionine to homocysteine. Deficiency in the enzyme 5,10 methylene THF reductase causes homocystinuria. *Modified from Huemer M, Diodato D, Schwahn B, Schiff M, Bandeira A, Benoist JF, Burlina A, Cerone R, Couce ML, Garcia-Cazorla A, la Marca G, Pasquini E, Vilarinho L, Weisfeld-Adams JD, Kožich V, Blom H, Baumgartner MR, Dionisi-Vici C. Guidelines for diagnosis and management of the cobalamin-related remethylation disorders cblC, cblD, cblE, cblF, cblG, cblJ and MTHFR deficiency. J Inherit Metab Dis. 2017;40(1):21–48. https://doi.org/10.1007/s10545-016-9991-4. Epub 2016 Nov 30. PMID: 27905001; PMCID: PMC5203859.*

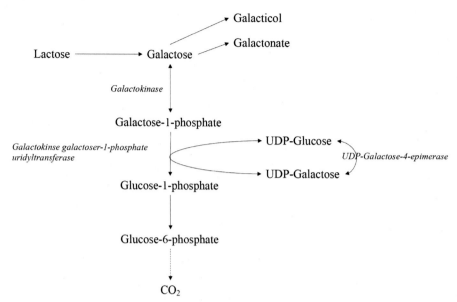

FIG. 10 Galactose metabolism: Galactose is phosphorylated to galactose-1-phosphate by galactokinase, which is converted to glucose-1-phosphate by galactose-1-phosphate uridyltransferase. Epimerase converts glucose-1- phosphate to UDP-galactose. *Modified from Demirbas D, Coelho AI, Rubio-Gozalbo ME, Berry GT. Hereditary galactosemia. Metabolism. 2018;83:188–196. https://doi.org/10.1016/j.metabol.2018.01.025. Epub 2018 Jan 31. PMID: 29409891.*

Treatment for patients is with a lifelong galactose-restricted diet. RBC Gal-1-P levels should be measured at diagnosis, at 3 and 9 months following initiation of therapy, and at 1 year until the patient baseline has been established. Gal-1-P accumulation is associated with reduced cellular phosphate and ATP levels.

Laboratory findings in the classical form show a circulating galactose level of >10 mg/dL. With >120 mg/dL in the classical form, levels decline to <1 mg/dL on successful restricted diet therapy.

Patients with the biochemical variants are asymptomatic and the biochemical variants have been identified in an abnormal newborn screening showing moderately elevated total blood galactose and decreased galactose-1-phosphate uridyltransferase activity. A recent guideline does not recommend treating the Duarte variant (partial deficiency of erythrocyte galactose-1-phosphate uridyltransferase).

Hereditary fructose intolerance

The disorder is discovered following exposure to fructose or sucrose (fructose plus glucose). Patients present with hypoglycemia, lactic acidosis, and hypophosphatemia.

The disorder is autosomal recessive and is due to the deficiency of the enzyme fructose-1.6-diphosphate aldolase. The enzyme converts fructose-1-phosphate to glyceraldehyde and dihydroxyacetone phosphate. The prevalence of the disorder is estimated to range from 1 in 20,000 to 1 in 60,000. The accumulation of fructose-1-phosphate inhibits phosphomannose iosomerase enzyme responsible for N-glycosylation and thus to impaired N-glycosylation of proteins. Hepatic fibrosis and renal dysfunction are seen among untreated patients. Patients may exhibit Fanconi syndrome as well as nephrocalcinosis.

Fatty acids oxidation defects

Fatty acids are essential nutrients stored in adipose tissue as triglycerides and are metabolized releasing energy. This allows the body to withstand extended periods of fasting and reduced energy intakes as well as produce energy at times of need as in increased metabolism in illness and activity.

Beta-oxidation of fatty acids takes place in the mitochondria with three different acyl-CoA dehydrogenases having been identified.

It is characterized by fasting-induced hypoglycemia secondary to defects in beta-oxidation of fatty acids and thus inability to be metabolized into ketone bodies. Patients present with episodes of nonketotic hypoglycemia that may progress to Reye-like syndrome.

The first fatty acids oxidation defect was described in the 1970s. Several defects are known; they are based on the fatty acids chain length that is affected. The most common is medium chain length acetyl CoA dehydrogenase deficiency (MCAD) affecting fatty acids with carbon length C6–C10.

The disorders become apparent during periods of fasting, stress, infection, and sepsis.

TABLE 8 Glycogen storage disease types, associated genes, liver histology, and biochemical tests.

GSD type	Enzyme deficiency	Glycogen storage in the liver (histology)	Genes involved	Other biochemical findings
0	Glycogen synthase	−ve	GYS1 (cardiac/skeletal) GYS2 (liver)	Hyperglycemia
1	Glucose-6-phosphatase alpha	+ve hepatomegaly	GSDIa,b	Hypoglycemia, hypertriglyceridemia, hyperuricemia
II	Acid-alpha-glucosidase deficiency (Pompe Disease)	Lysosomal accumulation of glycogen	GAA activity in leukocytes or fibroblasts. Muscle biopsy shows vacuolated myopathy and excessive lysosomal glycogen accumulation	High CK, LDH
III	Glycogen debranching enzyme deficiency (Cori/Forbes disease)	Accumulation of abnormal glycogen (very short outer chain)	Type IIIa: liver and muscle, IIIb muscle, IIIc (loss of glucosidase), IIId (loss of transferase)	High ALT, AST, hypoglycemia, hyperlipidemia, fasting ketosis, there is no high lactate level
IV	Glycogen branching enzyme deficiency (Andersen's disease)	Accumulation of abnormal glycogen with fewer branch points (polyglucans)		
V	Muscle glycogen phosphorylase deficiency (McArdle disease)	Two isoforms of glycogen phosphorylase encoded by two separate genes	PYGM	Impaired glycogenolysis. Markedly elevated CK and half of patients show myoglobinuria
VI	Liver glycogen phosphorylase deficiency (Hers' disease)			Ketotic hypoglycemia. Hyperlipidemia Normal CK and uric acid levels

GAA, Acid-alpha-glucosidase; *GYS*, glycogen synthase; *PYGM*, muscle associated glycogen phosphorylase.
Modified from Ellingwood SS, Cheng A. Biochemical and clinical aspects of glycogen storage diseases. J Endocrinol. 2018;238(3):R131-R141. https://doi.org/10.1530/JOE-18-0120. Epub 2018 Jun 6. PMID: 29875163; PMCID: PMC6050127.

Glycogen storage diseases

Many glycogen storage disorders have been identified (Table 8). The disorders are characterized by the deficiency of or reduced enzymatic activity of glucose-6-phosphatase (G6P) (in type I), the most common with over 80% of cases attributed to the enzyme deficiency resulting in the lack of degradation and accumulation of glycogen.

The patients often present with hypoglycemia, hepatomegaly (glycogen storage) and increased hepatic enzymes due to liver cells damage, ketosis and lactic acidosis, and hypertriglyceridemia and hyperuricemia (secondary to increased production and to reduced excretion).

Glucose 6 phosphatase is not expressed in fibroblast or red blood cells and that liver biopsy is often required to confirm the diagnosis. Histological examination shows the accumulation of glycogen. A variant type Ib is identified via enzymatic activity measurement in fresh (not frozen) liver tissue.

GSD 0

Inability to store glycogen due to deficiency in the enzyme glycogen synthase. The patients exhibit hyperglycemia rather than hypoglycemia due to the inability to convert to glycogen.

GSD II

A small amount of glycogen is degraded by acid alpha-glucosidase. Deficiency results in intralysosomal accumulation of glycogen leading to lysosomal dysfunction and rupture.

Manifestation can be either as congenital at birth or at a later onset. Hypoglycemia is often not present as the lysosomal contribution to glycogenolysis is minimal. Patients develop progressive muscle weakness with or without cardiac involvement. The congenital form of the enzyme activity is less than 1% and neonates present with cardiac and hepatic enlargement.

In the last onset form, the enzyme activity is often in the 1%–30% activity and rarely there is cardiac involvement. There is, however, motor delay, clumsiness, myopathic gate, obstructive sleep apnea, and exercise difficulty. Later on, the involvement of the diaphragm muscle leads to respiratory failure.

GSD III

This variant is characterized by the accumulation of abnormal glycogen with a very short outer chain. Glycogen debranching enzyme is deficient and glycogenolysis stops when the enzyme glycogen phosphorylase encounters a branch point that is four glucose residues away. Four subtypes have been described based on the tissue affected and the type of activity that is deficient. Type IIIa is the most common and affects the liver and muscle, type IIIb affects only the liver. In type IIIc, glucosidase is deficient, and in IIId, transferase activity is deficient.

Clinical presentation is variable depending on the tissue affected. Patients do not exhibit fasting high lactate levels since gluconeogenesis is present. Fasting ketosis is common and liver enzymes are markedly elevated. Hypoglycemia and hyperlipidemia are also encountered. There is hepatomegaly, and end-stage liver disease leading to hepatic carcinoma. In type IIIa, due to the involvement of muscle, creatine kinase is markedly elevated. In addition to genetic testing, a biopsy of liver, muscle, and fibroblast tissue confirms the disorder. Potential cardiac and muscle involvement helps to discriminate between GSD I and GSD III. Glucose levels are maintained (avoid hypoglycemia) by frequent consumption of carbohydrate-rich meals. A high-protein diet is also an option.

GSD IV

Glycogen branching enzyme deficiency (Andersen's disease):

Glycogen branching enzyme deficiency causes the accumulation of abnormal glycogen with fewer branch points (polyglucosans). Accumulation of the material leads to cell dysfunction and death.

Disease presentation is variable from intrauterine hydrops and perinatal death due to hypotonia and severe cardiomyopathy, failure to thrive, hepatosplenomegaly, and progressive hepatic cirrhosis leading to death by 5 years of age. In contrast, the adult form is mild presenting as isolated myopathy or as a multisystem disorder with upper and lower motor neuron involvement, bladder incontinence, gait disturbance, and lower limb paresthesia.

Diagnosis is via biopsy showing abnormal glycogen histology staining. Confirmation is by demonstration of the absence of the branching chain enzymatic activity in the liver, muscle, fibroblast, leukocytes, or erythrocytes.

GSD V

Muscle glycogen phosphorylase deficiency (McArdle disease):

The enzyme affected is glycogen phosphorylase. Two isoforms encoded for by two separate genes are described: a muscle isoform is encoded for by muscle associated glycogen phosphorylase (PYGM) and results in impaired glycogenolysis. Patients exhibit muscle weakness and exercise intolerance and cramping. Baseline creatine kinase is elevated (~5000 U/L) increasing to 1,000,000 U/L during rhabdomyolysis. Levels up to 400 U/L are considered normal. Myoglobinuria is encountered in about 50% of patients with GSD V.

GSD VI

Liver glycogen phosphorylase deficiency (Hers' disease):

This form is caused by a deficiency in the liver isoform of glycogen phosphorylase. Hepatic glycogenolysis is impaired and thus the patients exhibit ketotic hypoglycemia and hyperlipidemia. This form is characterized by normal creatine kinase and uric acid levels. Patients present with growth retardation and hepatomegaly.

Mucopolysaccharidosis

Mucopolysaccharidosis is a group of metabolic disorders of the degradation and metabolism of glycosaminoglycans. The overall incidence is about 1:25,000 and varies according to the type of mucopolysaccharidosis with geographical variation.

There are seven disorders characterized by the deficiency of respective enzymes involved in the degradation and metabolism (Table 9). Biochemical tests in addition to enzymatic activity involve the detection of the type of mucopolysaccharidosis excreted into the urine (e.g., heparan sulfate, keratan sulfate, dermatan sulfate, chondroitin 4- and 6-sulfate) (Table 9).

The disorders are often subtle and present a diagnostic challenge. Bone and joint involvements (erosive bone lesion without evidence of inflammation, claw hand, spinal deformities, or dysostosis multiplex) at a young age often trigger screening for MPS.

Cystic fibrosis

Cystic fibrosis was first described in 1935 as a fatal disorder in early childhood. With the advent of diagnostic and therapeutic measures, most patients survive into adulthood, to that effect, newborn screening is now included in most screening programs in high-income countries. Immunoreactive trypsin is measured as part of the screening program. The screen has a low positive predictive value and 10% of patients are

TABLE 9 Mucopolysaccharidosis (MPS), types, enzymes involved, and glycosaminoglycan compound appearing in the urine.

MPS type	Enzyme deficiency	Glycosaminoglycan metabolite
MPS-I (Hurler) MPS-I (Hurler-Scheie) MPS-I Scheie	α-L-iduronidase	HS, DS
MPS-II (Hunter)	Iduronate-2-sulfatase	HS, DS
MPS-IIIA Sanfilippo A	Heparan-N-sulfatase	HS
MPS-IIIB Sanfilippo B	α-N-acetylglucosaminidase	HS
MPS-IIIC Sanfilippo C	α-glucosaminide acyltransferase	HS
MPS-IIID Sanfilippo D	N-acetylglucosamine-6sulfatase	HS
MPS-IVA Morquio A	N-acetylgalactosmaine-6-sulfatase	KS, C6S
MPS-IVB Morquio B	β-galactosidase	KS
MPS-VI- Maroteaux Lamy	N-acetyl galactosamine-4-sulfatase	DS, C4S
MPS-VI Sly	β-glucuronidase	DS, HS, C6S, C4S
MPS-IX Natowicz	Hyaluronidase	Hyaluronan

HS, heparan sulfate; *DS*, dermatan sulfate; *KS*, keratan sulfate; *C6S*, chondroitin-6-sulfate; *C4S*, chondroitin-4-sulfate.
Modified from Nagpal R, Goyal RB, Priyadarshini K, Kashyap S, Sharma M, Sinha R, Sharma N. Mucopolysaccharidosis: A broad review. Indian J Ophthalmol. 2022;70(7):2249–2261. https://doi.org/10.4103/ijo.IJO_425_22. PMID: 35791104; PMCID: PMC9426054.

subjected to additional testing. The addition of CFTR gene mutation significantly improved positive predictive value. A positive screen is followed up by confirmatory sweat chloride testing (sweat chloride >60 mmol/L) or by the presence of two CF-associated mutations.

CF has a wide spectrum with some patients initially presenting in adulthood with mild symptomatic bronchiectasis.

Older publications suggested that it was a predominantly Caucasian disorder; however, cases are increasingly being reported from Africa, South America, Asia, Turkey, and the Middle East.

Several mutations in the cystic fibrosis (CF) transmembrane conductance regulator (CFTR) gene have been identified, in addition to the well-known F508 deletion. Seven classes have been reported for CF and vary from near absence of the CFTR protein (class 1) to lack of the CFTR mRNA (class VII) (Table 10).

The mutations are generally divided into two groups. One is decreased CFTRP protein synthesis and the other is related to the protein function and/or stability.

Class I mutations lead to the near absence of the CFTR proteins (stop codon and frameshift mutations), and class II mutations lead to defective intracellular protein processing resulting in the degradation of the protein. Although class II mutations end in synthesized CFTR protein reaching the cell membrane, it has a defective channel opening, similarly, in class IV, fewer chloride ions pass due to impaired conductance; class V mutations reduce the amount of normal

TABLE 10 CFTR gene mutations and associated abnormalities.

CF Class	Mutation	Defect
Class I	Gly542X, Trp128X	No conductance protein
II	Phe508del, Asn1303Lys, Ala561Glu	No traffic
III	Gly551Asp, Ser549Lys, Ala561Glu	Impaired channel gating
IV	Arg117His, Arg334Trp, Ala455Glu	Decreased conductance
V	Ala445Glu, 3272-26A to G, 3849+10kg to T	Reduced protein
VI	C120del23, rPhe508del	Less stable protein. Recycled and degraded
VII	Dele2,3(21 kb), 1717-1G to A	No mRNA

Modified from Chen Q, Shen Y, Zheng J. A review of cystic fibrosis: Basic and clinical aspects. Animal Model Exp Med. 2021;4(3):220–232. https://doi.org/10.1002/ame2.12180. PMID: 34557648; PMCID: PMC8446696, and from De Boeck K. Cystic fibrosis in the year 2020: A disease with a new face. Acta Paediatr. 2020;109(5):893–899. https://doi.org/10.1111/apa.15155. Epub 2020 Jan 22. PMID: 31899933.

CFRT protein. Unstable CFTR protein that is recycled and degraded in lysosomes is observed in class VI mutation. The CFTR protein in class VII is added to describe those patients unamenable to treatment.

There are significant advancements in therapeutic options from early treating and managing symptoms to modulating CFTR action and deficiency.

IEM biochemical investigations

Biochemical investigation of inborn errors of metabolism is best handled systematically. Initial screening, followed by confirmation testing may include genetic analysis and family studies. The range of screening tests is determined by the regional prevalence of the disorders, the availability of confirmatory tests, and the availability of therapeutic interventions, such as special diets, supplements, and transplant programs. Initial and confirmatory tests as well as clinical presentations are shown in Tables 11 and 12.

The presence of a high anion gap metabolic acidosis is seen in lactic acidosis, ketones, and organic acid accumulation. Organic acidemias (methylmalonic, propionic, and isovaleric) present with marked metabolic acidosis. When ketone bodies are negative and there is hypoglycemia, this indicates fatty acid oxidation defects.

Hypoglycemia is observed in patients with glycogen storage disorders (impaired conversion of stored hepatic glycogen to circulating glucose). Fasting hypoglycemia observed within 4h is suggestive of insulin-related disorders, hypoglycemia within 4 to 8h suggests impaired glycogenolysis and/or gluconeogenesis, whereas hyperglycosemia onset at >8h of fasting suggests fatty acid oxidation defects.

Ammonia is an intermediary metabolite that accumulates in severe liver dysfunction, urea cycle defects, and drug interaction (valproate). Ammonia is neurotoxic and elevated levels are associated with neurological dysfunction. In addition to urea cycle defects, the accumulation of organic acids in organic acidurias inhibits the urea cycle enzyme N-acetylglutamate synthase leading to hyperammonemia.

In patients with fatty acids oxidation defects, there is reduced production of the end product acetyl-CoA which is required for N-acetyl glutamate synthesis which in turn activates the urea cycle enzyme carbamoyl phosphate synthase-1. Accumulation of ketone bodies (3-hydroxybutyric acid, acetoacetic acid, and acetone) in fasting hypoglycemia or postprandial hyperglycemia and elevated lactate are suggestive of certain glycogenesis disorders.

Secondary and tertiary level tests include mass spectrometric analysis; tertiary level tests may include genetic and mutation analysis for confirmation and family and hereditary studies.

Postnatal testing (screening) for genetic disorders includes Wilson's disease and dyslipidemia.

The details of molecular genetic tests are beyond the scope of this chapter.

Sample requirements

Sample timings and type are essential in the investigation of inborn errors of metabolism (IEM). In patients suspected of IEM, urine samples (without preservative, and centrifuged to remove blood cells before analysis), plasma samples (lithium heparin or fluoride oxalate as anticoagulant and preservative), whole blood samples (collected in EDTA preservative tubes), or tissue biopsies are used in both enzymatic and genetic testing processed as per specific test requirements.

Capillary samples obtained by heel prick in neonates are used for neonatal screens (preferably 24 to 48h of age). The excessive squeezing of the heel and scrapping blood collection tube across the skin are likely to cause contamination as well as sample hemolysis and not be suitable for analysis. Peripheral circulation is improved by warming the heel to about 40°C using a warm pad , area cleaned with antiseptic, and allowed to air dray. The heel is then squeezed and skin punctured, not to exceed 2.4mm deep and 1.6mm wide. The heel area distant from the previous puncture is preferred and not on the posterior curvature of the heel where the bone is closest to the skin. A full-term neonate has a total blood volume of about 275mL (premature <1kg has about 80mL). Due to the high hematocrit in neonates, the plasma volume obtained from an older child is approximately 30-fold lower than in neonates. The high hematocrit in neonates interferes with many point-of-care devices due to reduced plasma water content, increased sample viscosity, and thus impaired fluidics.

Laboratory investigation

Tests no longer in use but of historical relevance include: ferric chloride test for aromatic hydroxyl/keto-groups (phenylketonuria). False positive results obtained in the presence of bilirubin and various drugs. Carbohydrate disorders were investigated using reducing substances (Benedict's), glucose oxidase, or qualitative thin-layer chromatography. Dinitrophenylhydrazine test for organic keto-acids in the detection of phenylketonuria (PKU), maple syrup urine disease (MSUD), Tyrosinemia, Isovaleric acidemia, and Methylmalonic aciduria, the test is falsely positive in early days of life and is subject to interference by various drugs. Toluidine blue-metachromatic spot test for glycosaminoglycans (for mucopolysaccharidoses). Cyanide-Nitroprusside test for cystinuria and homocystinuria. Amino acid disorders were investigated using urine/serum applied to thin-layer chromatography. Use of HPLC quantitative methods were considered significant improvements over the thin layer chromatography. Organic acids are investigated by gas chromatography.

TABLE 11 Clinical and initial biochemical findings suggestive of a metabolic disorder and may require further laboratory assessment.

Presentation	Possible metabolic disorder	Suggested investigations
Unexplained hypoglycemia	Organic acid disorders Amino acid disorders Glycogen storage disorders (types I) Disorders of gluconeogenesis Congenital adrenal hyperplasia Congenital lactic acidosis Galactosemia	Organic acids (U) Amino acids (U, P) 3-hydroxybutyrate (P) Free fatty acids (P) Lactate (P) Insulin (P) Cortisol (P) 17-hydroxyprogesterone (P) Galactose 1-phosphate uridyl transferase (B)
Acid-base imbalance: • Metabolic acidosis (exclude primary cardiac and respiratory disorders) • Respiratory alkalosis	Organic acid disorders Congenital lactic acidosis Urea cycle disorders	Organic acids (U) Lactate (P) Amino acids (U, P) Ammonia (P) Orotic acid (U) Amino acids (U, P)
Liver dysfunction (often associated with hypoglycemia and galactosuria)	Galactosemia Fructose 1,6 diphosphatase deficiency Hereditary fructose intolerance Tyrosinemia (type I) Glycogen storage disorders (type I) Disorders of Gluconeogenesis Alpha-1-antitrypsin deficiency	Galactose 1-phosphate-uridyl transferase (B) Sugars (U) Amino acids (U, P) Succinyl Acetone (U) Alpha-fetoprotein (P) Lactate (P) Oligosaccharides (U) Organic acids (U) Alpha-q-antitrypsin (P)
Neurological dysfunction: • Seizures • Depressed consciousness • Hypotonia with Zellweger's syndrome Organic acid disorders	Non-ketotic hyperglycinemia Urea cycle disorders Xanthine/sulfite oxidase deficiency Homocystinuria (remethylation defect) Congenital lactic acidosis	Amino acids (U, P, C) Orotic acid (U) Ammonia (P) Urate (P, U) Sulfite (U) Lactate (P) Organic acids (U) Very long-chain fatty acids (P)
Cardiomyopathy	Glycogen storage type II (Pompe's) Fatty acid oxidation disorders Tyrosinemia (type I)	Lactate (P) 3-hydroxybutyrate (P) Free fatty acids (P) Oligosaccharides (U) Organic acids (U) Carnitine (P) Amino acids (U, P)

B, blood; *P*, plasma; *U*, urine; *C*, cerebrospinal fluid sample type.
Modified from Saudubray JM, Garcia-Cazorla À. Inborn Errors of Metabolism Overview: Pathophysiology, Manifestations, Evaluation, and Management. Pediatr Clin North Am. 2018;65(2):179–208. https://doi.org/10.1016/j.pcl.2017.11.002. PMID: 29502909, and from Balakrishnan U. Inborn Errors of Metabolism-Approach to Diagnosis and Management in Neonates. Indian J Pediatr. 2021;88(7):679–689. https://doi.org/10.1007/s12098-021-03759-9. Epub 2021 Jun 7. PMID: 34097229, and from Ferreira CR, van Karnebeek CDM. Inborn errors of metabolism. Handb Clin Neurol. 2019;162:449–481. https://doi.org/10.1016/B978-0-444-64,029-1.00022-9. PMID: 31324325, and from Kruszka P, Regier D. Inborn Errors of Metabolism: From Preconception to Adulthood. Am Fam Physician. 2019;99(1):25–32. PMID: 30600976.

Summary

- Iron is an essential component of hemoglobin, myoglobin, cytochromes, catalases, and oxidase enzymes. It is also a cofactor of ribonucleotide reductase.
- Body iron content is 3–5 g with 60% being in hemoglobin, 10% in myoglobin, and the remainder in iron-containing enzymes and in reticuloendothelial cells.
- Hepcidin regulates iron influx by binding the iron exporter ferroportin-I triggering its internalization and degradation by lysosomes.
- Ferritin is the iron-storage protein synthesized by the liver. It is made up of 24 subunits surrounding up to 4500 iron molecules.
- Ferritin is an acute-phase protein and is thus elevated in infection.

TABLE 12 Initial and additional follow up biochemical tests, findings, and associated metabolic disorders.

	Further investigations	Diagnoses
Metabolic acidosis	Plasma lactate Plasma 3-hydroxybutyrate Plasma-free fatty acids Urine organic acids	Glycogen storage types I Congenital lactic acidosis Disorders of gluconeogenesis Fatty acid oxidation defects
Liver dysfunction	Plasma and urine amino acids Galactose-1-phosphate uridyl transferase Urine sugars Urine organic acids	Tyrosinemia type I Galactosemia Hereditary fructose intolerance Fatty acid oxidation effects
Absence of acidosis and liver dysfunction	Plasma cortisol Plasma 17-hydroxyprogesterone Plasma insulin (when hypoglycemic) Plasma growth hormone and TSH	Adrenal insufficiency Adrenal hyperplasia Nesidioblastosis Hypopituitarism
Hyponatremia	Plasma 17-hydroxyprogesterone Plasma cortisol Plasma growth hormone and TSH	Adrenal hyperplasia Adrenal insufficiency Hypopituitarism

Modified from Saudubray JM, Garcia-Cazorla À. Inborn Errors of Metabolism Overview: Pathophysiology, Manifestations, Evaluation, and Management. Pediatr Clin North Am. 2018;65(2):179–208. https://doi.org/10.1016/j.pcl.2017.11.002. PMID: 29502909, and from Balakrishnan U. Inborn Errors of Metabolism-Approach to Diagnosis and Management in Neonates. Indian J Pediatr. 2021;88(7):679–689. https://doi.org/10.1007/s12098-021-03759-9. Epub 2021 Jun 7. PMID: 34097229, and from Ferreira CR, van Karnebeek CDM. Inborn errors of metabolism. Handb Clin Neurol. 2019;162:449–481. https://doi.org/10.1016/B978-0-444-64,029-1.00022-9. PMID: 31324325, and from Kruszka P, Regier D. Inborn Errors of Metabolism: From Preconception to Adulthood. Am Fam Physician. 2019;99(1):25–32. PMID: 30600976

- In men, anemia is defined as any of the following: (hemoglobin <14 g/dL (140 g/L), hematocrit <42% (<0.42), and/or RBC <4.5 million/μL (<4.5×10^{12}/L)).
- In women, anemia is defined as any of the following: (hemoglobin <12 g/dL (120 g/L), hematocrit <37% (<0.37), and/or RBC <4 million/μL (<4×10^{12}/L)).
- Biochemical markers of iron deficiency anemia include hemoglobin, transferrin, transferrin saturation (total iron binding capacity), and ferritin. TIBC is a measure of circulating iron plus transferrin unoccupied iron binding sites (UIBC).
- Gastrointestinal (GI) blood loss contributes to iron deficiency anemia. Fecal occult blood tests are used to screen for GI hemoglobin loss.
- The presence of very high iron levels is indicative of iron overload. It is therefore helpful in identifying iron overload but not in the investigation of iron-deficiency states.
- Hemochromatosis is an autosomal recessive disorder leading to body iron overload.
- Porphyria is a group of eight metabolic disorders of heme biosynthesis.
- Clinical features distribution of porphyria ranges from solely acute attacks of neuropathy, mixed acute attacks and bullous dermatosis, erosive photodermatitis, and acute photosensitivity.
- The ideal urine sample is obtained during a suspected porphyria attack.
- The three acute porphyrias (AIP, variegate porphyria, and coproporphyrin) deficiency leads to the accumulation of 5-ALA and PBG, and thus their measurement (PBG mostly) is diagnostic in the acute presentation.
- Megaloblastic macrocytic and hypersegmented neutrophils characterize anemia associated with folate and cobalamin (vitamin B12) deficiency.
- Folates act as coenzymes in the synthesis of purines and pyrimidines (DNA and RNA) and as methyl donors in the synthesis of methionine.
- Laboratory assessment of B12 status includes measurement of transcobalamin II, which provides a better marker than measuring B12 itself.
- It is important to note that in patients presenting with acute gout attacks, circulating urate levels are likely to be within normal limits.
- Uric acid a product of purine metabolism where the end product of hypoxanthine, xanthine is converted to uric acid by xanthine oxidase.
- The majority of inborn errors of metabolism involve dysfunctional enzymatic processes or transport proteins.
- Screening for metabolic disorders is performed during the neonatal period dictated by various local, national, and nation-wide programs.
- Inborn errors of metabolism include amino acid disorders, carbohydrate disorders, urea cycle defects, glycogen storage disorders, and of mucopolysaccharide disorders, among others.

Further reading

DeLoughery TG. Iron deficiency anemia. *Med Clin North Am.* 2017;101(2):319–332.

Blackburn PR, Gass JM, Vairo FPE, et al. Maple syrup urine disease: mechanisms and management. *Appl Clin Genet.* 2017;10:57–66.

Villoria JG, Pajares S, Lopez RM, Marin JL, Ribes A. Neonatal screening for inherited metabolic diseases in 2016. *Semin Pediatr Neurol.* 2016;23(4):257–272.

Guerrero RB, Salazar D, Tanpaiboon P. Laboratory diagnostic approaches in metabolic disorders. *Ann Transl Med.* 2018;6(24):470.

Saudubray JM, Garcia-Cazorla A. Inborn errors of metabolism overview: pathophysiology, manifestations, evaluation, and management. *Pediatr Clin N Am.* 2018;65(2):179–208.

Ferreira CR, van Karnebeek CDM. Inborn errors of metabolism. *Handb Clin Neurol.* 2019;162:449–481.

Sobczynska-Malefora A, Delvin E, McCaddon A, Ahmadi KR, Harrington DJ. Vitamin B12 status in health and disease: a critical review. Diagnosis of deficiency and insufficiency—clinical and laboratory pitfalls. *Crit Rev Clin Lab Sci.* 2021;58(6):399–429.

Ellingwood SS, Cheng A. Biochemical and clinical aspects of glycogen storage diseases. *J Endocrinol.* 2018;238(3):R131–R141.

Ramsay J, Morton J, Norris M, Kanungo S. Organic acid disorders. *Ann Transl Med.* 2018;6(24):472.

Green R, Miller JW. Vitamin B12 deficiency. *Vitam Horm.* 2022;119:405–439.

Lehman TJ, Miller N, Norquist B, Underhill L, Keutzer J. Diagnosis of the mucopolysaccharidoses. *Rheumatology (Oxford).* 2011;50(Suppl 5):v41–v48.

Gattermann N, Muckenthaler MU, Kulozik AE, Metzgeroth G, Hastka J. The evaluation of iron deficiency and iron overload. *Dtsch Arztebl Int.* 2021;118(49):847–856.

Chapter 13

Biomarkers of malignancy

Introduction

This chapter describes tumor biomarkers and their utility in clinical practice. Several biochemical markers are utilized in screening, diagnosis, establishing prognosis, monitoring progress, and follow-up post-therapeutic interventions of various malignancies. The biomarkers, termed tumor markers, are either produced by the tumor and secreted (into blood, serous fluids, urine, or cerebrospinal) or expressed (at the cell surface) in larger quantities by malignant cell or their environment than by their normal counterparts. In addition, the biomarkers may also be tumor associated that are produced in response to or impacted by the presence of the tumor.

Types of tumor markers

Tumor markers are either those produced by the tumor or produced in response to the presence of the tumor. That is, they can be tumor specific or tumor associated. They are either peptide proteins, carbohydrate antigens, or metabolites. Chromosomal abnormalities, gene rearrangement, and mutations are often tested for to establish diagnosis and to assess prognosis.

Ideal tumor marker

An ideal tumor marker will be sensitive (detects small tumors at an early stage) and specific (not present in health—benign) and characteristic of the type of cancer. Most tumor markers are individually neither specific nor sensitive. Low diagnostic sensitivity and specificity coupled with low prevalence among asymptomatic individuals (that is low positive predictive values) puts their utility in screening into question.

Several attempts to improve both diagnostic sensitivity and specificity include a combination of markers or other investigational procedures such as colonoscopy in patients with positive fecal occult blood with significant improvement in diagnostic utility (see later).

For a marker to be of value, it has to offer at least one or more of the following roles; screening, diagnosis, prognosis, monitoring response to therapy, and follow-up for reoccurrence. Although few markers (see later) may offer any one of the utilities mentioned, none provide adequate support for all.

Tumor markers classification

Tumor biomarkers are classified as either tumor specific or tumor associated. Furthermore, tumor-specific biomarkers are produced either exclusively by the tumor or in relative abundance to their normal tissue counterpart. They are tumor derived (for example, oncofetal antigens). Those markers often afford a higher degree of specificity. On the other hand, biomarkers may be tumor associated, that is, produced as a result of the tumor presence or the extent of its involvement. Examples are cholestatic enzymes gamma-glutamyl transferase (γGT) and alkaline phosphate (indicating hepatic infiltration and metastasis), calcium (hypercalcemia associated with either bone resorption due to bone metastasis, or the production of parathyroid hormone-related peptide (PTH-rp) by the tumors), glucose (hypoglycemia, secondary to increased metabolic rates and/or to the production of insulin-like growth factor-1 (IGF-1) by the tumors), and to changes in acute phase proteins, among others.

Oncofetal antigens derived

Proteins and antigens are normally produced during fetal development; however, following genetic mutations they are expressed in post-fetal life and are characteristics of the developing malignancy. An example is AFP (the predominant circulating fetal protein that declines after birth and albumin becomes the major circulator protein), transformed hepatocytes re-expresses AFP, are produced in large amount, and thus become a biomarker of hepatic cancer (hepatoma). Similarly, carcinoembryonic antigen (CEA) is produced by many cell types and thus lacks the tissue specificity seen with AFP. However, βhCG, an oncoprotein, offers better sensitivity and specificity and has been used in patients with germ cell tumors (see later).

Protooncogenes derived

Proto-oncogenes are a group of genes that encode proteins responsible for cell division and growth. Examples are epidermal growth factor receptor (EGFR) (in nonsmall cell lung cancer, head and neck, colon, and pancreas); RAS gene expresses a family of proteins with GTPases

Tutorials in Clinical Chemistry. https://doi.org/10.1016/B978-0-12-822949-1.00007-3

activities and acts as an oncogene. Point mutations in codons 12 and 13 of the RAS gene increase its affinity for GTP and those in codon 61 inactivate its autocatalytic GTPase function, resulting in permanent RAS activation and stimulation of its downstream targets with mutations resulting in H and K-RAS, among others. HRAS (in 10%–20% of papillary, 40%–50% in follicular, and 10% in medullary thyroid cancer) and KRAS (in pancreatic, colorectal, and nonsmall cell lung carcinoma) proteins, and tumor suppressor genes. The encoded proteins also inhibit cell differentiation and apoptosis. Mutations in proto-oncogenes (typically dominant in nature) promote tumorigenesis of normal cells to become cancerous. The transformation into oncogenes leads to abnormal expression of proteins associated with cell growth leading to cancer. The detection of oncogenes is often performed in molecular and hematological laboratories and is beyond the scope of this book; examples are summarized in Table 1. Biomarkers detected are the product of those oncogenes and they are either different in quantity and/or in a structure that can be used as markers of the presence of those transformed cells.

Structural molecules (epitopes on structural molecules) and mucins

A number of large molecular weight proteins that are highly glycosylated (termed mucins) and expressed on cell surfaces are expressed and released in larger amounts and are associated with certain cancers. They are identified by numbers following a designation CA (carbohydrate antigens). Examples are CA 125, CA 19-9, CA 15-3, etc. The terminal carbohydrates are highly immunogenic and form the basis for the development of the humanized anticancer monoclonal therapy.

Mucins (glycoproteins) on the cell surface (consist of protein core plus carbohydrates) examples are carcinoembryonic antigen (CEA), β-2-microglobulin (light chain of class I major histocompatibility antigen) present on the surface of all nucleated cells (hence used in monitoring B cell tumors (in multiple myeloma—see later), cytokeratins (intermediate filaments of the cytoskeleton), CYFRA 21 (soluble fragment of cytokeratin-19), among other tissue-polypeptide-specific antigen).

Secretion products and enzymes

Tumor-specific proteins produced in excess and are indicative of tumor presence include alpha-fetoprotein (AFP), human chorionic gonadotrophin hormone (βhCG), prostate-specific antigen (PSA), neuron-specific enolase (NSE), alkaline phosphatase (placental-like Regan isoenzyme), thyroglobulin, Bence Jones protein (BJP), and catecholamines.

TABLE 1 Proto-oncogenes and mutations associated with tumors.

Proto-oncogene	Detection	Tumor
EGFR	EGFR gene mutations (G719A/C/S) and exon 19 deletion	Nonsmall cell lung cancer, head and neck, colon, pancreas
HER-2 (ERBB2)	Quantitative circulating HER-2 levels	Breast (overexpression associated with sensitivity to anti-HER2 agents) (Trastuzumab)
KRAS	Mutations in codons 12, 13, 61, and 146	Colon, small intestine, pancreas
HRAS	Mutation at codons 12 and 13 of the RAS gene (coding for GTPases). A rare mutation in codon 61	Thyroid (10%–20% of papillary carcinomas, 40%–50% of follicular carcinomas, 10% of medullary carcinomas, and 20%–40% of poorly differentiated and anaplastic carcinomas) Kidney, bladder
BCR/ABL	(Chromosome 9,12 translocation)	Chronic myeloid leukemia
BRAF	Mutations at codon 600 (V600E/K)	Melanoma, hairy cell leukemia, papillary thyroid cancer
Cyclin D1	Translocation cyclin-D1 and IgH (t(11:a4))	Low-grade B cell lymphoma

Adapted from Chial H. Proto-oncogenes to oncogenes to cancer. Nature Educ 1(1);2008:33.

Nonspecific markers of cell turnover

Neopterin (a breakdown product of pteridine) is released from active macrophages, interferon-gamma production from activated T-lymphocytes, thymidine kinase (reflects DNA proliferation activity), and tumor-associated trypsin inhibitor (in renal and gastric carcinoma).

Measurement and detection of tumor markers

Soluble and circulating tumor markers are routinely measured by immunoassay-based methodologies. Markers exhibiting enzymatic activity are measured utilizing their activity through monitoring reaction components, and by molecular genetics applications (PCR) in tumor genes detection. Body fluids include blood, cerebrospinal fluid, urine, and cavity fluids (peritoneal, pleural, and drainage fluids). Although some immunoassays are not validated or approved for body fluids other than blood, several literature sources support their use in other body fluid types, they offer value in detecting tumor spread (metastasis).

The presence of tumor makers on the cell surface in paraffin sections, smears, or fresh biopsy tissue is also performed; however, those are often carried out in histopathological laboratories.

Immunoassays in the measurement of tumor markers although offer rapid and reliable measurements, there are a number of limitations that need to be released; (1) analytical measurement range; tumor makers are likely to be at very high concentrations, often beyond the assay analytical measurement range. This may lead to antigen excess (known as the hook effect), resulting in unreliable and often falsely low results. Samples are performed in dilution to overcome this limitation. Appropriately diluent, as recommended, should be used to minimize matrix effect as often the dilution factor is high, and (2) the often presence of circulating antibodies (human anti-mouse antibodies) or those used during therapy (humanized antibodies) or radiological imaging investigation and therapeutics. For example, the use of Daratumumab (anti-CD38) in the management of patients with multiple myeloma causes an apparent IgG kappa (the nature of the Daratumumab) band in the electrophoretic gel. This may lead to either overestimation of a patient monoclonal IgG kappa or reporting its presence as a newly observed monoclonal component.

Reproducibility (defined by precision) is required and is favored since the assays are utilized for serial monitoring and often in periodic screens and to assess recurrence. Most of the available assays offer acceptable imprecision performance assessed against the marked biological variations of the biomarkers (see chapter on laboratory management). Therefore, serial monitoring should be performed by the same assay. Furthermore, due to differences between the assays and lack of standardization of some assays between manufacturers, the laboratory reports must indicate the specific assay used in reporting the tumor value.

Tumor markers in routine clinical practice

Human chorionic gonadotropin (hCG)

HCG member of the glycoprotein hormone family (includes LH, FSH, TSH) is produced by the normal placenta and reaches a maximum concentration in the plasma during the 8th week of gestation. The hormone consists of an alpha (α) and beta (β) and subunits. The β subunit is encoded for by genes cluster on chromosome 19q13.3, whereas the α subunit is encoded for by a single gene on chromosome 12q21.1-23.

The α subunit is common to the other glycoprotein hormones, and it is the β units that confer specificity. The α subunit contains 92 amino acids. The hCG β subunit contains 145 amino acids with a 24 amino acid extension, comprising the C-terminal peptide.

Although the hCG β unit confers specificity for hCG, it exhibits 80% homology with the LH β unit which caused interference in the earlier polyclonal antibody immunoassays.

Antibody-based immunoassays in routine use have been directed at the β chain which is specific for hCG. However, some commercially available assays detect both β and intact hCGαβ molecule (see later).

Carbohydrates constitute about 30% of the hCG molecular weight. In total, there are eight carbohydrate moieties (N-linked to asparagine (Asn) 13, 30, 52, and 78) and four O-linked to serine (Ser) 121, 127, 132) with an additional O-linked on serine 138 in the C-terminal peptide of βhCG. Thus, there are six carbohydrate moieties attached to the βhCG subunit and two to the αhCG subunit (Fig. 1).

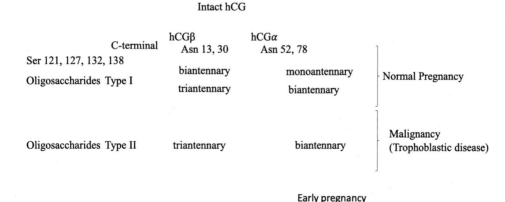

FIG. 1   hCG variants (carbohydrate contents) in normal and early pregnancy and in patients with gestational trophoblastic disease. A total of six carbohydrate moiety complexes are attached to asparagine amino acids (N-linked) or to serine amino acids (O-linked) at the positions indicated. The moieties are either monoantennary, biantennary, or tri-antennary. (*Modified from Cole LA. HCG variants, the growth factors which drive human malignancies. Am J Cancer Res 2012;2(1):22–35. Epub 2011 Nov 20. PMID: 22206043; PMCID: PMC3236569.*)

Importantly and of diagnostic relevance is the extent of glycosylation of hCG when produced by malignant tissue. Termed "hyperglycosylated" hCG denotes an hCG molecule with additional carbohydrate moieties. This form is produced both early in normal pregnancy by cytotrophoblasts and is the major circulating form in patients with the gestational trophoblastic disease and by various germ cell tumors (Fig. 1). Normally glycosylated hCG is produced by the syncytiotrophoblasts later on in pregnancy.

Additionally, a terminal sialic acid demonstrates heterogeneity and causes charge differences in the degree of acidity with isoelectric focusing (pI) ranging from 3 to 7 with βhCG being more acidic (pI: 3–5) and the α subunit being more basic (pI: 5–8). In patients with the trophoblastic disease, produced hCG exhibits reduced sialic acid content (that is more basic with high pI), whoever, few patients have high sialic acid content (that is more acidic with low pI).

The number of antennary increases for both β and α subunits in hCG produced by gestational trophoblastic diseases and germ cell malignancy. The extent of glycosylation is also high early in pregnancy. Additionally, a difference at the C-terminal of the β unit is the change in oligosaccharide types from I to II in normal pregnancy to that of malignancy, respectively.

Isoforms of hCG in clinical practice

In addition to the carbohydrate differences highlighted above, the hCG molecule exhibits amino acid chain lengths and structural differences. Identified and approved hCG structural variants nomenclatures are shown in Table 2.

In addition to the α and β subunits discussed above, isoforms (structural variants) of the βhCG exist (Table 2) and

TABLE 2 Recognized hCG isoforms and their associated structural differences.

hCG variant	Structural differences
Intact hCG	hCG devoid of nicked forms and free subunits
Nicked hCG	Partially degraded hCG, missing peptide bonds in the βhCG-40–50 region
α-subunit hCG	αhCG, dissociated from intact hCG
β-subunit hCG	βhCG, dissociated from intact hCG
nicked β-subunit βhCGn	Partially degraded βhCG, missing peptide bonds in the βhCG-40–50 region
β-core fragment βhCGcf	Residues βhCG-6–40, joined by disulfide bonds to βhCG-55–92

Adapted from Stenman UH, Tiitinen A, Alfthan H, Valmu L. The classification, functions and clinical use of different isoforms of HCG. Hum Reprod Update 2006;12(6):769–84. https://doi.org/10.1093/humupd/dml029. Epub 2006 Jul 28. PMID: 16877746.

their respective determinations aid in the investigation and management of gestational trophoblastic tumors, testicular tumors, as well as nongestational trophoblastic disease.

The majority of the circulating hCG is metabolized by the liver with 20% appearing in the urine. The major form in urine in both normal pregnancy and in patients with the trophoblastic disease is the core fragment βhCGcf and a minor component of nicked hCG (βhCGn) (Fig. 3). The nicked isoform is also detected in serum from patients with trophoblastic disease.

The hCG β subunit is cleared from the circulation relatively slowly compared to intact hCG and determining the relative proportion of βhCG to the total intact hCG prior to and during therapy in patients being investigated for germ tumors and gestational trophoblastic diseases is helpful (see later). Core βhCG fragment is detected in the urine (Fig. 3).

Structural isoforms include nicked β subunit (βhCGn) where peptide bonds in the 40–50 amino acids region are missing (degraded). β subunit fragments 6–40 are joined by disulfide bridges with 55–92 fragment, forming what is termed β core fragment (βhCGcf), and the carbohydrate moieties on Asn 13 and 30 are smaller compared with βhCG. Nicked hCG (βhCGn) and core β fragment (βhCGcf) are present in the urine of both normal pregnancy and form cancer patients.

Routinely availably laboratory assays measure the combined intact hCGαβ and βhCG subunit. However, differential measurement of the βhCG subunit and its circulating proportion is important for the following diagnostic utility; in patients with molar disease, the relative proportion of circulating βhCG is higher in patients with molar disease compared to those with normal pregnancy and the relative proportion is even higher when in patients with choriocarcinoma when compared to relative proportion during pregnancy. Overall, a relative circulation βhCG >5% is suggestive of gestational trophoblastic disease and requires further follow-up and investigations. Furthermore, the higher the relative proportion of βhCG, the more likely is aggressive. βhCG levels that continue to rise during therapy indicate possible resistance to therapy.

Patients with trophoblastic disease are very sensitive since it is produced by about 100,000 cells and recurrence following the failure of therapy is detected by elevated and increasing hCG before the tumor is large enough to be detected by other means. Therefore, hCG measurement in patients with trophoblastic disease exhibits almost 100% sensitivity and specificity.

The frequency of hCG production and its detection among the various trophoblastic, germ cell tumors, and nontrophoblastic diseases is shown in Fig. 2.

In patients with germ cell tumors, about 50% of nonseminomatous testicular tumors exhibit elevated circulating hCG levels compared with only 10% and 15% of seminomatous tumors. The finding of elevated AFP supports the

Trophoblastic disease:	↑ hCG in about 100%		
Placental site trophoblast:	Rare tumor. <25% produce hCG		
Germ cell tumors	Testicular:	Seminomatous	↑ hCG in about 10 - 15%
		Nonseminomatous	↑ hCG in about 50%
	Ovarian:	Rarely hCG detected (when contains trophoblastic tissue)	

Non-trophoblastic hCG:

Pituitary (ectopic) hCG:	Stimulated by GnRH. Values values <20 IU/L
Non-trophoblastic tumors:	↑ hCG in about 30-70% of patients
Cervical, endometrial ovarian, and vulvovaginal cancers	

FIG. 2 The frequency of hCG production among the various trophoblastic, germ cell tumors, and nontrophoblastic diseases. *(Modified from Stenman UH, Tiitinen A, Alfthan H, Valmu L. The classification, functions and clinical use of different isoforms of HCG. Hum Reprod Update 2006;12(6):769–84. https://doi.org/10.1093/humupd/dml029. Epub 2006 Jul 28. PMID: 16877746.)*

presence of nonseminomatous tumors. In patients with ovarian germ cell tumors, the presence of hCG is rare and is only when trophoblastic tissue is present.

Placental site trophoblasts are rare tumors that arise in remnant placental tissue, they produce little hCG, and that 25% of the tumors do not produce hCG.

Patients with cervical, ovarian cancers, and vulvovaginal cancers exhibit circulation and urinary core beat hCG isoform (βhCGcf). Similarly elevated levels are associated with poor outcomes.

About 30%–70% of patients with nontrophoblastic tumors show isolated elevation of βhCG values and indicate poor prognosis,

Ectopic hCG

Nontrophoblastic hCG is produced by the pituitary often seen secondary to ovarian failure (ovariectomy, iatrogenic following treatment of gynecological malignancy, or following testicular tumor removal). About 30%–70% of patients with nontrophoblastic tumors produce βhCG.

A positive hCG in postmenopausal women or rarely in men (typically with levels ≥14 IU/L, and FSH <40 IU/L) should be repeated and preferably by a different immunoassay, if the results were different by more than 10%. It is likely a false positive result; if the results were concordant (<10% variance), βhCG is specifically measured. If the relative proportion is >30%, suggests a possible underlying malignancy or an ectopic source; however, if <30%, GnRH antagonist (e.g., following high dose estrogen dosage). A nondetectable hCG suggests underlining malignancy, whereas a suppressed hCG suggests nonmalignancy and possible ectopic pituitary source (Fig. 3).

False isolated positive isolated hCG results in the absence of pregnancy may be misinterpreted for the presence of occult malignancy. Proper investigation in consultation with the clinical laboratory for the assay characteristic and possible causes of interference. Repeat analysis, serial dilutions, and blocking for the presence of heterophile and human anti-mouse antibodies (HAMA) (see the chapter on analytical method) often reveal the cause of interference.

Accurate measurement of hCG is important for effective management of gestational trophoblastic disease. An assay with a wide analytical measurement range and sample dilution protocols provide high hCG levels and also avoid false negative and low results secondary to antigen excess (hook effect).

The use of appropriate reference intervals (normal ranges) is important to avoid misclassification. For instant postmenopausal hCG (secondary to gonadal failure) can be as high as 7 to 25 IU/L.

In patients receiving chemotherapy and those with ovariectomy, detectable hCG is derived from the pituitary.

Trophoblastic tumors

Germ cell tumors include trophoblastic tumors, choriocarcinoma, epithelioid tumors, and testicular tumors.

The gestational trophoblastic disease has a wide spectrum from molar hydatidiform to choriocarcinoma.

Choriocarcinoma

Gestational choriocarcinoma is the most common among trophoblastic tumors and mainly occurs during the reproductive years with a mean age of 30 years. Half of the

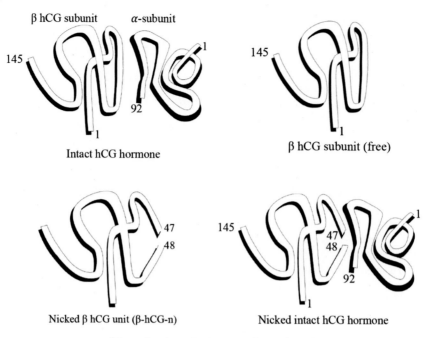

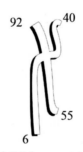

β core hCG fragment (urine)

Urinary hCG molecular form

FIG. 3 Molecular isoforms of hCG in circulation and in urine. *(Modified from Cole LA. hCG, five independent molecules. Clin Chim Acta 2012;413(1-2):48–65.)*

tumors (50%) arise after pregnancy, 25% after molar gestation, and 25% following any other type of gestational event.

Uterine and extra-uterine (lung, liver, gastrointestinal tract, and central nervous system) are common spread sites. It is often present with uterine mass and extensive bleeding. Histologically, the tumor stains were positive for hCG, HSD3B1, Mel-CAM, HLA-G, MUC-4, and cytokeratin AE1/AE3. Biochemically, high circulating hCG levels are often seen.

Although this form is associated with a prior gestational event, nongestational tumors occur in children and patients below the fourth decade. Patients present with abdominal pain and elevated hCG levels. In children, the markedly elevated hCG causes presentations of precautious puberty.

Raised serum concentrations of βhCG correlate well with choriocarcinoma tumor mass and the assay is sensitive enough to detect a tumor bulk of approximately 1 mg. Serum levels are used to judge the progress and necessary duration of chemotherapy and for the early detection of metastases. Elevation in normal pregnancy is characterized by near doubling of levels every 48 h, this is often lost in patients with hydatidiform or a demised pregnancy. HCG is measured routinely in all cases of hydatidiform mole after the evacuation of the uterine mass. Persistent trophoblastic disease: characterized by plateaued or rising hCG concentration.

Testicular teratoma

Elevated serum βhCG (above 5 IU/L (1–2 ng/mL)) is found in about half (40%–60%) of patients presenting with testicular teratoma and in a few with apparently pure seminoma. Serum βhCG in teratoma is routinely assayed simultaneously with AFP.

Pineal tumors

Germinomas secrete low levels of βhCG. This is helpful when discriminating between mixed malignant germ cell tumors often requiring intensive therapy and are the more common type. Making up 65% of central nervous system tumors. Elevated AFP levels in the serum or the CSF correlate with the diagnosis of mixed ger cell tumors. In contrast, patients with germinomas will only exhibit elevated βhCG and no AFP. However, about 60% of germinomas will have normal βhCG. Thus, it cannot be used for diagnosis but may have a role in monitoring response to therapy in the remaining 40% of cases.

Human placental lactogen (HPL)

Placental lactogen is encoded by the growth hormone-placental lactogen genes. It is a 191 amino acid peptide with two disulfide bonds. Molecular weight is 22 kDa and is normally produced by the placenta.

Placental site trophoblastic tumors where the placenta remains attached to the uterus following a normal delivery. Measuring placental lactogen is helpful in following response to therapy. The tumors respond well to chemotherapy as well as to surgical excision.

Epithelioid trophoblastic tumor

The epithelioid trophoblastic tumor is a rare usual variant of the trophoblastic tumor, closely related to choriocarcinoma but with a monomorphic growth rather than the dimorphic pattern of choriocarcinoma. The tumor occurs in women aged 15 to 48 years (mean 36.1 years) with a significant percentage in pre- and postmenopausal women.

In addition to staining for human gonadotrophin, the tumor stains for human placental lactogen, as well as for placental alkaline phosphatase. Circulating human placental lactogen (HPL) in patients with epithelioid trophoblastic malignancy is measured to monitor post-treatment for recurrence, initially every 3 months for 2 years, then every 6 months for three more years.

Alpha-fetoprotein (AFP)

AFP is synthesized by the fetal yolk sac, liver, and gastrointestinal tract. It is the major serum protein during fetal life declining to <10 ng/mL at 12–18 months. It is a 70-kDa glycoprotein with carbohydrates constituting 4% of its molecular weight. Multiple glycoforms are present evident by affinity chromatography and have been utilized to improve diagnosis (see later).

Circulating AFP levels are elevated in hepatocellular carcinoma (HCC) (in 50%–70% of patients), normal pregnancy, hepatitis (elevated levels in 25% of patients), liver cirrhosis, gonadal, and gastrointestinal tumors. Patients with hepatitis B and C are at higher risk of developing cirrhosis, fibrosis, and hepatoma and that screening asymptomatic hepatitis patients leads to early and effective treatment.

Normal AFP reference intervals appear to be assays dependent with an upper limit of normal being 10–25 ng/mL. At an AFP cutoff of 20 ng/mL, sensitivity ranges between 41% and 65%, and specificity between 80% and 94%. In patients with hepatitis and liver cirrhosis, AFP is often <500 ng/mL, and patients with AFP > 500 ng/mL are at high risk of hCC. The diagnostic specificity of AFP is improved when combined with ultrasound.

The AFP glycoform L3 may help identify the aggressive form of the tumor and the AFP-L3 proportion of <10% identifies patients at risk of small tumors <2 cm. However, it is not useful in the early detection of HCC where elevated AFP levels are required.

AFP in measurement in conjunction with βhCG is used to identify patients with testicular teratoma. About 75% to 95% of all patients presenting with testicular teratoma will have abnormalities in one or both AFP and βhCG.

AFP levels that are raised before orchidectomy and that fall to normal levels after surgical excision suggest that the disease was limited to the testis. Circulating AFP has a half-life of 3.5 to 4 days. Serial measurements showing slow decline indicate residual AFP-producing tumor.

Combined AFP levels below <60 ng/mL and hCG <50,000 IU/L are associated with a 10% mortality rate, whereas AFP levels >1200 ng/mL and hCG levels >100,000 IU/L carry a mortality rate over 40%.

In patients suspected of testicular cancer: Alpha-fetoprotein, hCG, and LDH measurements are helpful in diagnosis, staging prognosis, recurrence, and therapy monitoring. Alpha-fetoprotein is recommended for differential diagnosis of nonseminomatous and seminomatous germ cell tumor where it is detected in nonseminomatous germ cell tumors that contain embryonal carcinoma, yolk sac tumor, or teratoma. AFP is not elevated in patients with seminomatous or choriocarcinoma.

Germ cell tumors

Germ cell tumors are a histologically diverse group of neoplasms. They are in the gonadal tissue of the testis and ovaries.

Nearly all testicular tumors are gems cell tumors where 40% are classified as seminomas and 40% as nonseminomatous germ cell tumors and 20% are mixed.

Alpha-fetoprotein (AFP) is not secreted by pure seminoma tumor similar to pure choriocarcinoma. It is markedly elevated in nonseminomatous tumor and the level correlates with tumor burden.

Human chorionic gonadotropin (hCG) is produced choriocarcinoma and 60% to 80% of nonseminomatous germ cell tumors in men. Levels are usually greater than 1000 mIU/mL compared with <500 mIU/mL seen in the 10%–20% seminoma germ cell tumors having the same prognosis as those that do not produce hCG.

LDH may be elevated in 40% to 60% of patients with testicular germ cell tumors and levels correlate with tumor burden.

In females, less than 5% of malignant ovarian tumors are germ cell tumors with the majority (70%) of new ovarian tumors in the young 10–30 years old.

Elevated AFP levels in the serum or the CSF correlate with the diagnosis of mixed ger cell tumors.

Hepatocellular carcinoma

Hepatocellular carcinoma (HCC) is the fifth most common cancer and the second most common cause of death worldwide. Wide geographical variation (possibly due to variable hepatitis B and/or C risk for exposure). Similarly, high-risk primary biliary and alcoholic cirrhosis and hemochromatosis.

The liver has a large reserve capacity, and most patients are asymptomatic at the early stages of the disease. The late presentation contributes to the poor prognosis of less than 5% 5-year survival.

The normal range for AFP which is the most commonly used tumor marker for hepatocellular carcinoma is 10 to 20 ng/mL with sensitivity and specificity of 41% to 65% and 80% to 94%, respectively, at 20 ng/mL (positive predictive value at 3.3%), where about 80% of patients with small HCC show no increase in AFP levels.

Due to its low sensitivity, the use of AFP in screening for HCC is not recommended. Its sensitivity for HCC is 25% when the lesion is <3 cm and about 52% when the lesion is >3 cm. Well-differentiated tumors express lower levels of AFP.

A number of professional bodies (laboratory and hepatology) recommend the use of AFP in high-risk subjects coupled with abdominal ultrasound particularly where AFP levels >20 ng/mL, and for areas where ultrasound is not available.

AFP levels are elevated in cirrhosis, and AFP cutoffs for HCC above 400 ng/mL are recommended. In practice and due to late presentation, AFP levels are often in the 1000s ng/mL with higher levels suggestive of vascular invasion in 61% of cases. Additionally, increasing AFP levels indicate recurrence, metastasis, and poor prognosis. High pretreatment AFP levels are associated with a 3.3-fold increase in the probability of HCC recurrence following transplantation. Furthermore, increasing AFP levels over time predicts the risk for nontransplant.

AFP half-life is 3.5–4 days and serial measurements for a follow-up every 3 months for the first 2 years and then every 6 months up to 5 years are performed to monitor response to therapy. AFP is combined with liver ultrasound examination in the surveillance of high-risk patients.

Elevated AFP levels are seen in non-HCC conditions such as acute and chronic hepatitis, and in pregnancy. It is elevated in gastric cancer and in biliary and pancreatic malignancy.

A glycosylated form of AFP known as *Lens culinaris* agglutinin-reactive fraction (AFP-L3) is primarily produced by cancer cells and thus offers improved specificity for HCC. Elevated AFP-L3 is correlated with tumor poor differentiation, aggressiveness, vascular invasion, intrahepatic metastasis, and thus poor prognosis.

Des-gamma-carboxy prothrombin (DCP) is an abnormal prothrombin induced by vitamin K2 absence/antagonist II. It is increased in patients with HCC and its combined use with AFP significantly improves sensitivity for HCC to >85% and that combined use of AFP, AFP-L3, and DCP improves sensitivity and specificity of diagnosing and monitoring HCC to >88%.

Carcinoembryonic antigen (CEA)

CEA is a complex family of glycoproteins, synthesized by tumor cells and also by normal colonic epithelium. It is carried on the surface membrane of these cells and shed into the surrounding medium (thus detectable in serum and serous fluids) in cancer patients and into the intestinal lumen and feces in normal subjects. It is a glycoprotein 150.3 kDa, with a 45%–55% carbohydrate. It is part of the immunoglobulin gene "superfamily" and is elevated in patients with; colorectal cancer (70%), lung (45%), gastric (50%), breast (40%), pancreatic (55%), uterine (40%), and ovarian (25%). It is present in benign disease; however, levels that are 5–10 times the upper limit suggest colorectal carcinoma (CRC). It is most widely used tumor marker for CRC. Circulating CEA levels are normally <2.5 ng/mL and <5.0 ng/mL in nonsmokers and smokers, respectively.

CEA has a half-life of 5 days and measurement is recommended for follow-up of CRC patient post-resection with 80% sensitivity and 70% specificity for detection of recurrence. Baseline CEA levels should be obtained before elective surgical intervention to establish baseline values.

Serial measurements (three times per year for 2 years) provide a median lead time of ~5 months. Furthermore, the rate of rise can be used to predict localized recurrence or metastatic spread noting that 20%–30% of localized recurrence will have normal CEA levels and that 80%–90% will likely be hepatic metastasis. The rise in levels postoperatively is used to trigger an investigation for recurrence.

Additionally, intensive follow using CEA results in a 20%–30% reduction in mortality by facilitating early therapeutic interventions.

Raised serum concentration in patients without tumors: Circulating CEA is largely cleared by the liver. Raised levels are found in patients without tumors who have cirrhosis, cholelithiasis (particularly involving the common bile duct), cholangitis, liver abscess, biliary obstruction due to various causes, diverticulosis, and pancreatitis. It is also found elevated in heavy smokers necessitating separate reference intervals/cutoff for those. It is also elevated in patients with inflammatory bowel disease.

The role of CEA in the management of colorectal cancer is still unclear. Serum concentration is raised in about 60% of all cases of colorectal cancer. The circulating levels depend on the following; the stage of the tumor—the serum concentration is raised in 90% (range 80%–100%) of patients with hepatic metastasis, the site of the tumor—left colonic tumors, particularly of the sigmoid colon, produce the highest levels while lower or absent circulating CEA levels occur in the right colonic and rectal tumors; and the degree of differentiation of the tumor—although even tumors that are apparent nonproducers of CEA are positive for CEA by immunohistochemistry, and tumors that are well encapsulated may be secreting CEA into the gut lumen without raising the serum concentration, and a functional hepatic status.

CEA has no role in detecting cancer among the normal population (i.e., in screening). As a prognostic indicator: Very high preoperative levels suggest a poor prognosis, but may provide no more information than through clinical evaluation of tumor node metastasis by histopathological staging. CEA is an adjunct to these tests. As an indicator for "second-look" surgery: Some studies showed CEA concentrations rising 9 months or so before the recurrence of the tumor was detected by other means. Some patients (possibly 20%–30%) do not show an elevated CEA level despite biopsy-proven recurrence, while others show unaccountable transient rises. Even with the most careful monitoring, CEA is not a sufficiently reliable indicator of early and curable recurrence. In monitoring therapy: Falling CEA levels suggest, but are not diagnostic of, response to chemotherapy or radiotherapy. Rising CEA levels during therapy are incompatible with tumor regression, but CEA levels do not relate directly to tumor bulk.

For colorectal cancer; CEA can be used for prognosis, postoperative surveillance, and therapy monitoring in advanced disease. Fecal occult blood testing (FOB) is used for screening asymptomatic adults 50 years and older.

Fecal occult blood testing (FOBT)

Colorectal carcinoma (CRC) is the third most common malignancy worldwide. Each year 1 million new cases and 0.5 million deaths. The lifetime risk for developing CRC is 6% and 50% of developing colorectal adenoma.

Early detection (stage I) affords 90% and only 5%–15% at (stage IV) five-year survival. Screening and early detection are therefore important. Screening reduces mortality significantly with a 25% reduction in overall mortality.

There are two stool-based assays in use for the detection of fecal hemoglobin. The principle is the detection of blood or occult blood component contaminating stool as it passes over a friable bleeding cancerous tissue. However, by design the assays will detect hemoglobin due to gastrointestinal bleeding, the etiology is varied from inflammation, peptic ulcers, anemias, and secondary to the use of various drugs. Positive fecal occult blood tests as well as clinical symptoms alone or combined guide patient management directs additional endoscopic investigations.

The earlier assay (guaiac) utilized the peroxidase-like activity of hemoglobin, where in the presence of hydrogen peroxide, it catalyzes the oxidation of alpha-guaiaconic acid to a blue-colored quinone compound. This sassy detects both upper and lower gastrointestinal bleeding as it detects peroxidase activity rather than intact hemoglobin molecule or its antigenic determinants. The assay is affected by dietary peroxidases as well as meat content. Manufacturers recommend storage of the test card with the sample, unprocessed, for 3 days to allow for deterioration of dietary peroxidases. This practice is often adhered which may result in false positive results.

Adequate performance is obtained when three separate collections are made, which is often a compliance challenge.

The second assay formulation in current use is antibody based often termed fecal immune testing (FIT). The antibody detects hemoglobin in the stool. It does not detect upper gastrointestinal bleeding because the antigen (hemoglobin) is digested, and epitopes are degraded during the gastrointestinal passage. FIT has a sensitivity of 80%. A single test is adequate with improved patient compliance compared to the minimum of three required with the guaiac-based test.

Most protocols in place require three sequential FOBTs when screening for CRC. However, single test is adequate when using FIT-based assays.

Recent development in screening for colorectal carcinoma is a measurement of fecal DNA-based makers. Mutations in the KRAS, APC, and P53 genes as well as a marker of microsatellite instability BAT-25 and L-DNA (a marker of DNA integrity) have all been recommended for screening but the relative cost at this time is prohibitive.

FIT-DNA testing is performed every 3 years compared to the annual fit of FOBT testing. It offers increased sensitivity for cancers, advanced adenomas, and serrated polyps compared with FIT alone.

Fecal occult blood tests are designed to detect hemoglobin molecules and fecal samples. The presence of hemoglobin in stool is considered an indication of gastrointestinal bleeding that could be due to various pathologies including gastrointestinal malignancy and inflammation.

Although the utility of fecal occult blood testing is sometimes questioned, it continues to be widely used in practice as part of the periodic physical examination and in inpatient and outpatient settings. Its use in screening for colorectal carcinoma is on several protocols and guidelines.

Prostate specific (sensitive) antigen (PSA)

PSA is a 237 amino acid glycoprotein with serine protease activity encoded by the KLK3 gene. It is produced by liminal epithelial cells of prostate glandular tissue. It is also produced by the breast and is detectable in breast milk with no identified clinical significance. Normal ranges for total PSA (protein-bound and free) are often reported as ≤4.0 ng/mL with a sensitivity of 21%. However, levels ≤2.5 ng/mL are recommended for men aged <50 years old.

It is present in free (5%–45%) and in complex forms bound to antichymotrypsin (ACT), α-2-macroglobulin. With available assays for total, free, and complex forms, the sensitivity of detection is increased by measuring free PSA and reporting it as a percentage of the total. The sensitivity for cancer detection is improved when using %free PSA particularly in the gray zone of 4.0 to 10.0 ng/mL. The lower the percentage of free PSA, the higher the probability of cancer.

The assays exhibit variable calibrant and antibody specificity. However, traceability efforts using the WHO (96/670) reference material containing 90% PSA-ACT plus 10% Free PSA, and the WHO (96/668) reference material containing free PSA only has reduced discrepancies among assays. Historically, the reference methodology was the Hybritech (Beckman Coulter) assay with the clinical decision point being at 3–4 ng/mL. The assays had variable abilities to detect free and PSA-ACT complexes.

Equimolar assays detect free and ACT-complexed forms equally, whereas in nonequimolar assays, changes in free/ACT complexed relative proportions result in overestimating increasing free PSA and overestimating total PSA.

Traceability and standardization efforts have reduced variations among assays considerably from about 62% to 10% over time.

The use of PSA for prostate screening has been controversial with discrepancies among different randomized controlled studies. Although screening diagnosed more prostate cancer, early detection of those cancers did not reduce the risk of dying 7–10 years of follow-up, where some studies suggested screening reduced mortality by 20% but was associated with a high risk of overdiagnosis.

Although PSA mass screening is not recommended, high-risk individuals (positive family history, African descent) with 10 to 15 years of life expectancy should be offered screening with an explanation of test limitations and utility.

Increasing PSA levels in patients with urinary tract symptoms is an indication for biopsy and may be suggestive of metastatic prostate cancer.

Although there is no defined PSA level below which risk for prostate cancer can be eliminated, and many conditions other than prostate cancer may cause an elevation in PSA levels, elevated levels per se are not diagnostic but can be used to stratify risk.

Three categories are defined based on total PSA levels. Low risk when a total PSA is <=4.0 ng/mL with cancer risk being at 2.7% (3.1–4.0), moderate risk for PSA between 4.0 and 10.0 ng/mL with cancer risk being 25%–35%, and high risk for PSA >10 ng/mL with risk for cancer being 40%–50%.

Continued elevation in PSA levels is an indication of re-biopsy. The prostate cancer antigen 3 (PCA3) score determines whether a repeat biopsy is needed after an initial negative biopsy. PCA3 score is the ratio of PCA3 mRNA (noncoding segment from chromosome 9q21-22) overexpressed (60–100-fold) in >95% of prostate cancer. Urinary PCA3 mRNA to PSA mRNA is more cancer specific than PSA. PCA3 requires the collection of 20–30 mLs of urine voided after a digital rectal examination (DRE) (accuracy is lower at 80% without DRE and increases to 98% for samples collected following DRE).

mRNA is very labile (disappears in 20 minu in the absence of ribonuclease inhibitors (to be added to about 2 mLs of collected urine)). mRNA counts ≥7500/mL are considered an adequate sample for testing. The PSA mRNA corrects for the number of prostatic epithelial cells and thus controls for valid PCA3 mRNA results. The sensitivity and specificity of PCA3 at different cutoff ratios are shown in Fig. 4.

Clinical staging and risk stratification are required, for instance, preoperatively in patients with PSA >10 ng/mL. Radiological CT and bone scan are performed.

Patients at risk but with PSA < 10 ng/mL require active surveillance at 3–6-month intervals with the determination of PSA doubling time. Postoperatively (radical prostatic resection) PSA is measured 4–12 weeks post-surgery, where

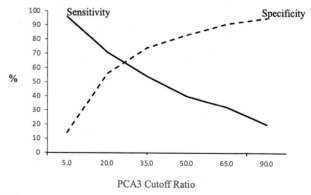

FIG. 4 PCA3 ratio sensitivity and specificity at different cutoffs. *(Modified from Marks LS, Bostwick DG. Prostate cancer specificity of PCA3 gene testing: examples from clinical practice. Rev Urol 2008 Summer;10(3):175–81. PMID: 18836536; PMCID: PMC2556484.)*

PSA should be undetectable (current assay detection limits are about 0.1 ng/mL). That is <0.1 ng/mL. However, in patients receiving radiotherapy only, it takes a long time for the PSA to reach its nadir and plateau. This could take 6 to 12 months and in some cases up to 3 years.

Periodic PSA measurement is required to detect disease recurrence, where two consecutive PSA levels >0.2 after radical prostatectomy suggest recurrence. However, post-radiotherapy recurrence is suspected when PSA is ≥2.0 ng/mL above the lowest values (nadir) attained.

Bone and tissue organs surveillance for metastasis is initiated when postsurgical PSA is >10 ng/mL and/or PSA velocity is >0.5 ng/mL/per month or PSA doubling time is <6 months.

In patients with advanced disease and those on hormonal therapy, both PSA and testosterone levels are monitored every 6–8 months.

In patients with PSA < 50 ng/mL and with three consecutive rising PSA levels that are less than 1 week apart, or >50% increase in PSA levels over the lowest nadir value (with PSA >2 ng/mL) is suggestive of hormone (testicular removal)-resistant prostate cancer.

Although PSA is clinically prostate specific, it is not prostate specific. It is produced to a smaller degree by other tissue such as the breast (present in breast milk). However, its specificity for prostate tissue malignancy can be improved by measuring free PSA, complexed PSA, free PSA isoforms, PSA density, PSA velocity, and age-specific PSA cutoffs.

Free PSA is often measured in a reflex format when total PSA is 4–10 ng/mL and is expressed as both absolute and percentage format ((Free PSA/total PSA) X100). Free PSA at >25% indicates low risk (probability 8%), and free PSA < 10% indicates high risk (probability 56%). A cutoff of 25% detected 95% of cancers and reduced the biopsy rate by 20%.

There is method dependent analytical variability with lack of comparability between assays (College of American Pathologist (CAP) proficiency testing participants summaries indicate a 20% to33% analytical variability among the different PSA assays in routine use). However, using the same manufacturer for total and free PSA measurement improves performance.

There is a lack of standardized pre-analytical protocols/ sample handling. For example, sample storage for >7 days at 4°C decreases free PSA%, and if the sample was to be kept for >24h, stability is maintained if stored frozen at −70°C. Avoid sample collection within 48–72 h of prostatic manipulation as this leads to transient falsely elevated PSA levels.

The increased total prostate volume reduces the difference in free PSA between normal and cancer patients. In prostate volume <35 cc, a cutoff of 14% is applied and a >35 cc cut off of 25% is used.

PSA Velocity: represents a change in total PSA over time (PSA velocity = 0.5 × (PSA$_2$ − PSA$_1$)/(Time$_1$) + 0.5

(PSA$_3$ − PSA$_2$)/(Time$_2$)), offers improved discrimination between cancer and BPH, and identifies those with the curable disease, useful in identifying those for biopsy in patients with total PSA <10 ng/mL and unremarkable DRE. It is helpful in early cancer detection where patients with a PSA velocity >3.5 ng/mL/year are recommended to have a prostate biopsy to investigate the cause.

Test Limitations: There are wide biological variability (20%–46%) changes in total PSA due to biological and assay variation. PSA elevation due to inflammation affects velocity calculation performed over short periods. The same PSA assay should be used for velocity calculations.

PSA Density: PSA density is defined as; (total PSA/ prostate volume) determined by transrectal ultrasound. It is based on the positive relation between PSA levels in blood and prostate volume. Volume determined by TRUS is operator dependent. The ratio of stroma and epithelial tissues is different in individual prostates. It is not helpful in the early detection of cancer.

The use of age-specific reference intervals improved the utility of PSA. As the prostate increase in size with age, younger men have lower normal levels than older men and a cutoff value of 2.5 ng/mL has been proposed instead of 4.0 ng/mL.

Prostate cancer influences the proportion of the PSA-ACT complex in blood and its measurement may improve cancer specificity of complexed PSA over total PSA, but not over free PSA measurement.

In untreated patients, total PSA levels correlate with the disease stage, and levels >20 ng/mL are suggestive of bone metastasis.

Following total prostatectomy, PSA levels are below the detection of the assay <0.1 ng/mL, and although low detectable levels do not indicate the presence of malignancy, rising levels do. In the authors laboratory, the detection limit was lowered to 0.05 ng/mL allowing for early detection of recurrence with levels rising >0.2 ng/mL indicating relapse after total prostatectomy.

Debate on the utility of PSA screening given the natural history of early prostate lesions suggests that routine PSA measurement may lead to unnecessary biopsies, detection of indolent tumors, and overtreatment. This led the US preventative services task force in May 2012 to recommend the removal of PSA screening from primary care for old men. However, professional urological and cancer societies support that PSA measurement continues to be performed in men aged between 55 and 69 years old or for all above 50 years old with a minimum of 10-year life expectancy.

CA125

CA 125 is a glycoprotein expressed in epithelial tissue. It is thus common in tubular, endometrial, endocervical, peritoneum, pericardium, and pleura tissue.

This is a heavily glycosylated mucin. First-generation assay antibody directed against OC125 epitope for capture and detection. Second-generation assay OCT125 and M-11 epitopes sandwich assay with improved specificity and linearity. The cutoff for most assays is 35 U/mL; however, results are not interchangeable.

There is a low prevalence of epithelial ovarian cancer (1 in 2500), and therefore, effective screening must have sensitivity >75% and specificity >99.6% for a positive predictive value (PPV) of 10%. Thus, not recommended alone to screen asymptomatic women for ovarian cancer.

CA 125 is neither sensitive nor specific. Among premenopausal women, it is elevated in pregnancy, endometriosis, ovarian cysts, pelvic inflammation, and carcinoma of breast and lungs.

Elevated levels of CA 125 in patients without gynecological malignancy are common. It is elevated in patients with lung and pancreatic cancer. Mildly elevated levels are seen in patients with hepatitis, cirrhosis, hepatitis, pelvic inflammatory disease, endometriosis, and in pregnancy.

Measurement of CA 125 alone has a low positive predictive value (3.7%), which increases to 23.5% when combined with pelvic ultrasound. Several attempts have been utilized to improve CA 125 utility and algorithms developed for instance, stable levels suggest benign disease, and progressively rising level suggests ovarian cancer. An arbitrary cutoff of 30 U/mL showed 62% sensitivity.

In ovarian cancer, CA 125 measurement is recommended with transvaginal ultrasound (TVUS) for early detection of ovarian cancer in women with high risk. It is recommended for differential diagnosis of a suspicious pelvic mass in postmenopausal women as well as for detection of recurrence, monitoring therapy, and determination of prognosis in women with ovarian cancer.

Ovarian cancer

Ovarian cancer is the second most common gynecological malignancy and the 4th most common cause of tumor-related death among women. Unfortunately, the most patient presents late stage III and IV with poor prognosis, and therefore, early detection is important. Most patients (80%) will exhibit CA 125 greater than 35 U/mL. with 50%–60% in stage I, 80%–90% in stage II, and >90% in stages III and IV.

CA 125 has low sensitivity for cancer detection at an early stage and is thus not used for screening for asymptomatic patients as it will provide significant false negative results. It can be elevated in nonovarian malignancies as well as in benign (endometriosis, uterine fibroids, and in liver cirrhosis) and in physiological (pregnancy) causes.

Despite combined CA 125 and transvaginal ultrasound (TVUS) screening as well as serial measurements of CA 125, there is little evidence that screening improved

outcomes and/or reduced mortality. Its use alone or in combination with ultrasound is not recommended.

In patients with hereditary ovarian cancer syndrome, Lynch syndrome, and in BRCA-positive patients, annual screening for ovarian cancer using CA 125 is recommended.

In patients with pelvic mass CA 125 > 95 U/mL discriminates between benign and malignant tissue in postmenopausal women.

Serial measurement of CA 125 is more informative where increasing levels or more are associated with malignant pathology. Similarly, serial measurements are useful when assessing response to therapy, where declining levels indicate a favorable response.

The possibility of germ cell tumors in patients >40 years old with complex ovarian mass requires the measurement of AFP, hCGβ, and LDH to aid in the differential diagnosis of possible germ cell tumor. Additionally, their measurement is recommended for routine follow-up in patients with nonepithelial ovarian cancer.

AFP, βhCG, and LDH are used to assess prognosis in epithelial ovarian cancer, whereas the same in addition to inhibin are helpful in the routine follow-up of patients with nonepithelial ovarian cancer.

In the presence of elevated CA 125, preoperative imaging is recommended to rule out metastasis.

Various risk scores have been developed to improve on the 84% sensitivity and 66.3% specificity for CA 125. The risk score, in addition to CA125 values, includes menopausal status and radiological findings. For example, the risk of malignant index (RMI) where a total score of greater than 200 has a high specificity for malignancy. An algorithm of risk of ovarian malignancy algorithm (ROMA) uses both CA 125 and human epididymis protein-4 (HE4) (see below) to improve the sensitivity of diagnosing ovarian malignancy. ROMA values >13.1% and >27.7% are indicative of high risk for ovarian cancer among pre- and postmenopausal patients, respectively.

Another algorithm utilizes five markers, namely, CA 125, β-2-microglibulin, prealbumin, transferrin, and apolipoprotein A1. In a multivariate score scale of 0 to 10, scores ≥5 and ≥4.4 are considered high risk in pre- and postmenopausal patients, respectively, with respective sensitivity of 85% and 96%, and specificity of 40% and 28%.

CA 125 has a half-life of 2 weeks; therefore, a decline in levels following surgical resection and/or the initiation of therapy indicates a good response. A decrease of 50% after the second cycle of therapy predicts that a good response is likely. Similarly, increasing CA 125 levels indicate recurrence and treatment failure with 95% accuracy and guides radiological examination and/or changes in cytotoxic regimens. Serial CA 125 measurement is important as it often detects recurrence 3–5 months prior to clinical symptoms. Additionally, 40-day doubling time predicts median survival of 10.6 months compared to 22.1 months for doubling times greater than 40 days.

Human epididymis protein-4 (HE4) is a glycoprotein produced by epithelial cells. It is detected in ovarian, endometrial, breast, and lung carcinomas. Although its performance compared to CA 125 remains under investigation, about 50% of ovarian cancer patients with low CA 125 have elevated HE4 levels.

Elevated CA 125 in patients with endometrial cancer indicates the need for preparative imaging studies to rule out metastasis.

CA 15-3

CA 15-3 is a large glycoprotein of 300–450 kDa. It is elevated in breast cancer (69%), pancreatic cancer (80%), lung cancer (71%), ovarian cancer (64%), colorectal cancer (63%), and liver cancer (28%). It is thus not useful in screening; however, it is useful in monitoring response to therapy in patients with breast cancer where a change >25% correlates with progression, and no change indicates stability in 60% of patients. There is a temporary paradoxical increase following therapy which may be associated with tumor lysis. Similarly, a carcinoembryonic antigen (CEA) tumor marker may also be used to monitor response to therapy in advanced disease.

For patients with breast cancer; estrogen and progesterone receptors are mandatory for predicting response to hormone therapy. Human epidermal growth factor receptor-2 is mandatory for predicting response to trastuzumab. Urokinase plasminogen activator/plasminogen activator inhibitor 1 may be used for determining prognosis in lymph node-negative patients.

CA 27.29 is equivalent to CA 15-3 in the management of patients with breast cancer. The respective assays target epitopes on the same glycoprotein-mucin 1 (MUC1). Although various studies have shown concordance (90%) between the two assays, significant differences between the results of the two assays exist, and the two biomarkers (CA 15-3 and CA 27.29) should not be used interchangeably. Furthermore, since not all breast cancer cells express CA 27.29, its utility has declined in favor of CA 15-3.

CA 19-9

CA 19-9 is a glycoprotein expressed on the surface of cancer cells. It is elevated in patients with colorectal carcinoma and pancreatic carcinoma. It is useful in monitoring patients with pancreatic carcinoma where levels >37 U/mL discriminate between pancreatic cancer and mild pancreatic disease. Elevated preoperative values are suggestive of poor prognosis.

Patients with pancreatic cancer present at an advanced stage of the disease due to the lack of tests for early detection.

Five-year survival is very low at 20%. CA 19-9 has low positive predictive value and thus has no role in screening asymptomatic patients. However, it is used to distinguish benign from malignant pancreatic disorders. To this effect, it has prognostic where levels >100 U/mL are indicative of poor prognosis (normal values <37 U/mL). Serial measurements are important to assess response to therapy. Levels declining >20% at 8 weeks post-chemotherapy indicate a longer median survival compared to patients with slower CA 19-9 levels decline.

Elevated CA 19-9 levels are seen in patients with cholangiocarcinoma, stomach, colon, gallbladder, bile duct, and lung cancers. It must also be noted that CA 19-9 is elevated in patients with pancreatitis, obstructive jaundice, cholangitis, rheumatoid arthritis, rheumatoid arthritis, diverticulitis, and liver disease in the absence of pancreatic carcinoma.

Lactate dehydrogenase (LDH)

A family of at least six NAD^+-dependent isoenzymes (LD1-5 and LD6, among others) are observed. They all catalyze the conversion of pyruvate to lactate and the oxidation of NADH to NAD^+.

Under normal circumstances, NADH is oxidized by oxygen to NAD+ which is required for ATP generation, essential for glycolysis. However, in cases of hypoxia, the conversion of pyruvate to lactate provides the required NAD^+.

In cancer cells, despite the presence of adequate oxygen, anaerobic conversion of pyruvate to lactate by LDH occurs with lactate being an end product, accumulating and exhibiting lactic acidosis.

Reflects increased glycolysis in rapidly growing cells.

Normally circulation LDH levels are from cell turnover (cell damage). Thus, a measure of cell injury.

Increased urinary LDH activity is a candidate for bladder and kidney neoplasm markers, it is also elevated in urinary tract infection and inflammation.

In addition to increased total LDH activity in malignancy, changes in the relative ratio of the isoenzymes have been observed. The A subunit isoform is the most predominant. Low LDH activity may be suggestive of remission or improved prognosis.

Due to a lack of both sensitivity and specificity, it is not used in diagnosis but is of value in monitoring the course of the disease, response to therapy, and prognosis in certain cancers (Table 3).

LDH reflects tumor burden and is helpful in monitoring response to therapy and the early detection of selective tumors. It is helpful in the early detection of the recurrence of renal carcinoma. It is also of prognostic value in renal cancer patients receiving system therapy and with advanced metastatic disease.

LDH is helpful in combination with AFP and βhCG (intact plus free beta assay) in the differential diagnosis

TABLE 3 LDH isoforms predominately elevated in selected malignancies.

Tumor	Isoform
Bladder cancer	Urine LD5
Breast cancer	LD1
Testicular (germ cell)	LD1
Colorectal carcinoma, Gastric, pancreatic, hepatocellular, and squamous cell carcinoma	LD5
Lung cancer (both small and nonsmall)	LD5

Modified from Forkasiewicz A, Dorociak M, Stach K, Szelachowski P, Tabola R, Augoff K. The usefulness of lactate dehydrogenase measurements in current oncological practice. Cell Mol Biol Lett 2020;25:35. https://doi.org/10.1186/s11658-020-00228-7. PMID: 32528540; PMCID: PMC7285607.

of testicular cancer. It is also helpful in the testicular postoperative and prognosis assessment when measured pre-orchiectomy with AFP and βhCG. The marker measurements are then repeated after surgical removal, and then weekly until values are normalized or become stable. Continually increasing levels indicate the presence of recurrence and metastatic disease. In patients with nonseminomatous germ cell tumors (NSGCTs), combined LDH, AFP, and βhCG are monitored for at least 10 years and at least 5 years in patients with seminomas, with more frequency during the initial 2 years.

In patients with advanced NSGCT disease and receiving chemotherapy, LDH, AFP, and βhCG measurements are at the beginning of each chemotherapy cycle when the cycle is complete. This helps classify patients with metastatic disease into good, intermediate, or high-risk groups according to the classification of the international germ cell consensus classification (IGCCC).

Paraproteins

Paraproteins are monoclonal immunoglobulins. If light chains are produced in excess, these appear in the urine as Bence Jones protein which is almost always an indication of malignancy. Bence Jones protein is also catabolized by the renal tubule so that in advanced renal failure urinary levels rise. Additionally, it is filtered by the year by the kidney and is detected in circulation in patients with reduced GFR.

Serum paraprotein concentrations correlate with tumor bulk. Remission in myelomatosis is defined in terms of the percentage reduction of initial paraprotein levels. The paraprotein concentration at presentation does not correlate with long-term survival nor does the rate of fall of paraprotein level during chemotherapy.

Multiple myeloma

Serum total protein may be significantly increased and there may be associated pseudohyponatremia.

The most commonly encountered monoclonal immunoglobulin is IgG (~60% of patients), less commonly IgA (~25%), less commonly IgM, and rarely IgD or IgE.

In only 80% of myeloma cases, is a serum paraprotein detected and approximately 20% have light-chain (Bence Jones protein) excess only. The presence of a paraprotein is usually accompanied by suppression of the other immunoglobulins.

In 70% of myeloma, light chains are made in excess over heavy chains component and because of their low molecular weight (20,000 Dalton), they are excreted in urine. They may form amyloid deposits in the kidney.

A discrete band follows the electrophoretic separation of serum proteins (Fig. 5) and the presence of a monoclonal (M) band indicative of clonality of plasma cells (Fig. 5). Bands suspected of clonality are further characterized by immunostaining (immunofixation) (Fig. 6). In the latter, separated serum proteins are incubated with anti-heavy chains (G, M, A as well as D and E) and anti-free light chains (kappa and lambda) antibodies (Fig. 6). Cross-reactivity with the heavy and light chain antibodies identifies the monoclonality. 5–20% of patients will exhibit no M band and often in the presence of hypogammaglobulinemia. Difficulties in the detection of an M band when levels are either low or when the band is comigrating within an elevated gamma or beta globulin region. This is often encountered when there is IgA or IgD paraproteinemia as those often migrate within the beta region. False positive M band detection is seen in patients being infused with therapeutic monoclonal antibodies, often within 2 days of infusion. For instance, Daratumumab was reported as IgG kappa detected within the gamma region (Fig. 7).

Of concern is the difficulty in detecting low levels of monoclonal component comigrating within normal proteins of the respective electrophoretic region. An SPEP will indicate a negative result that shows a positive monoclonal band present when subjected to immunofixation. The latter should be performed in the presence of an apparently normal electrophoretic pattern but when there is a high index of clinical suspicion.

In patients classified as having monoclonal gammopathy of undetermined significance (MGUS), 1% of IgM will develop into multiple myeloma and 0.5% per year for progression to malignancy. The risk of progression to multiple myeloma is determined by the level of the immunoglobulin, the abnormality in the free kappa/lambda, and the degree of bone marrow involvement.

CRAB criteria (calcium >11 mg/dL), renal dysfunction with creatinine >2 mg/dL, anemia with hemoglobin <10 g/dL (or >2 g/dL decline from baseline) and the presence of

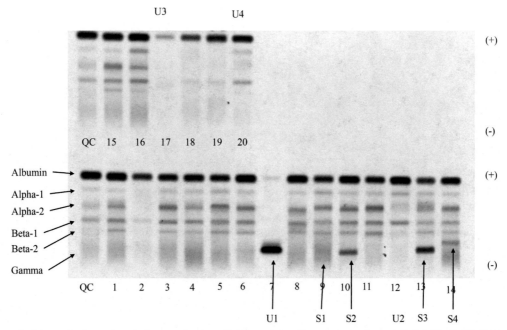

FIG. 5 Serum and urine protein electrophoresis for several patients (1–20) are shown. Serum samples (lanes; 1, 3–6, 8–11, 13–16). Urine samples (lanes; 2, 7, 12, 17–20). QC; quality control samples (serum; showing albumin band and alpha-1, alpha2, beta-1, beta-2 and gamma globulins regions of electrophoretic separation). Pattern suspected of M-component is indicated by arrows (samples U1, S1–4). Samples exhibiting abnormal patterns are subjected immunofixation to confirm and identify the abnormal band (see Fig. 6). Patterns that are abnormal (increased or decreased band intensity, beta-gamma bridging, split alpha-2 band, etc.) but without a clear M-component band are commonly seen and may reflect ongoing pathology (e.g., renal and hepatic dysfunction, acute phase reaction, and chronic inflammation, etc.). Detection of other than a very faint albumin in urine is abnormal. The degree of abnormality ranges from selective (<3 bands) to nonselective proteinuria (>3 bands), to marked proteinuria, and nephrotic syndrome. The pattern may suggest predominantly glomerular (e.g., sample 17, 18) or mixed glomerular and tubular proteinuria (samples 12, 20). *(Courtesy of the author's laboratory.)*

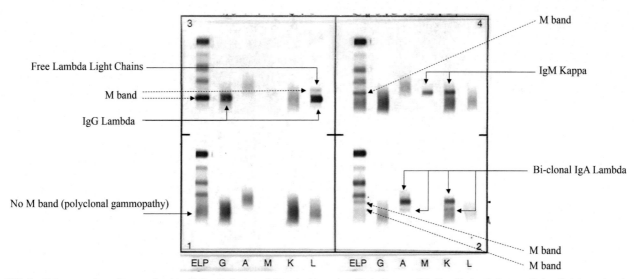

FIG. 6 Gel pattern shows immunofixation. Patient 1 shows no M band with nonspecific background binding. Patient 2 shows a distinct IgA kappa bands. Patient 3 shows IgG lambda and free lambda light chains, whereas patient 4 shows IgM kappa band. *(Courtesy of the author's laboratory.)*

A

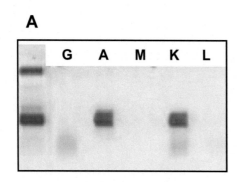

B

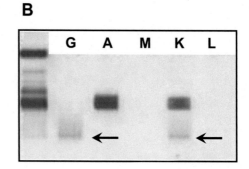

A: IFE of multiple myeloma patient serum from Parkland Hospital with Iga Kappa M-protein prior to daratumumab treatment.

B: 5 months after the start of daratumumab, both Iga Kapa and IgG Kappa (indicated with arrows) are seen on IFE which can be interpreted as presence of biclonal multiple myeloma since there is no certainty if there is a switch in clonality post-daratumumab treatment.

FIG. 7 Daratumumab detected as IgG kappa in a patient with IgA kappa monoclonal bands. *(Courtesy of the author's laboratory and from Vakili H, Koorse Germans S, Dong X, Kansagra A, Patel H, Muthukumar A, Hashim IA. Complete Depletion of Daratumumab Interference in Serum Samples from Plasma Cell Myeloma Patients Improves the Detection of Endogenous M-Proteins in a Preliminary Study. Diagnostics (Basel). 2020;10(4):219. https://doi.org/10.3390/diagnostics10040219. PMID: 32295157; PMCID: PMC7235820.)*

bone disease with ≥1 lytic lesion distinguish multiple myeloma from MGUS. The finding of <10% plasma cells in bone marrow, an M band less than 3 g/dL and the absence of CRAB, and serum-free light chains ratio less than 100, suggest MGUS.

Measurement of light chains (kappa and lambda) often quantitatively by nephelometry and determining the ratio of kappa and lambda is helpful in detecting unbalanced ratio and the presence of light chain disorders. Mean normal kappa/lambda ratio is 0.9 (ranging from 0.25 to 1.65). Free light chain measurement is helpful in detecting light chain multiple myeloma, light chain deposition disease, light chain amyloidosis, and nonsecretory multiple myeloma.

Daratumumab

Approved for newly diagnosed patients with refractory remission of multiple myeloma. It is the first fully humanized monoclonal antibody against CD38 IgG1-K used in the treatment of newly diagnosed refractory remission either as a single agent or in combination.

By binding to CD38, it induces cell death (Fc dependent, complement dependent, and antibody-dependent cell-mediated cytotoxicity).

CD38: glycoprotein present on the surface of hematopoietic and nonhematopoietic cell lines. It is a transmembrane protein acting as both a cell antigen receptor (interacting with its ligand CD31 on T cells stimulating cytokine cascade) and as a channel receptor (Fig. 7).

Hormones

Hormones produced by tumors are termed eutopic if they are appropriate to the tissue of origin. Examples include some of the most useful endocrine markers in malignancy (Prolactinoma, Insulinoma, Glucagonoma).

Hormone receptors

Some breast cancers go into remission during periods of hormonal manipulation. Estrogen receptors (ER) are found in approximately 60% of cases presenting with breast cancer with a higher percentage in postmenopausal than in premenopausal patients. Progesterone receptors (PR) may also be present.

Assessing prognosis: Patients whose tumors are rich in ER (ER+) have a longer disease-free interval than patients with tumors that have little or no ER (ER−), even when stratified according to lymph node status.

Selection of therapy: Patients with ER+ tumors have a 50%–60% chance of responding to some form of endocrine therapy, but for ER- tumors the figure is less than 5%. The antiestrogen tamoxifen is effective only in those postmenopausal patients with ER+ tumors. Tumors that are ER + PR+ have a 70% response to endocrine therapy while those that are ER + PR− have a 20%–30% response.

Alkaline phosphatase (Regan isoenzyme)

Alkaline phosphatase is an enzyme present in all tissues. Five isoforms have been identified and confer some degree of organ specificity. The liver and bone isoforms are the most represented in the circulation. A kidney and an intestinal isoform. A placental-like isoenzyme (Regan isoenzyme) has been identified in association with various tumors such as renal cell carcinoma and bronchial carcinomas.

The liver isoform is a microsomal enzyme and is elevated in the presence of intrahepatic filtration and cholestasis by the secondaries to the liver.

Prostatic acid phosphatase

Prostatic acid phosphatase (PAP) is the traditional marker of prostatic cancer. However, it has a low sensitivity and is elevated in about one-third of patients with stage I prostatic cancer (intracapsular lesion) and in 92% of patients with stage IV disease (distant metastases).

In patients with benign prostatic hypertrophy, PSA is elevated in >40% of cases, whereas PAP is elevated in <5%. Taken overall, in patients with the clinically apparent prostatic disease, PSA correctly classifies about 75%, and PAP correctly classifies about 60%. PSA is generally a more sensitive marker of tumor progression or regression. Neither test is of value in screening for prostatic cancer.

Organ-specific tumors

Medullary carcinoma of the thyroid

Rare comprising about 3% of all thyroid cancers. It arises from neuroendocrine parafollicular C cells of the thyroid. The most common mutation leading to MTC is RET mutation characterized by overexpression of tyrosine kinase receptors (VEGFR, EGFR, and MET).

Diagnosed cytologically following ultrasound-guided fine-needle aspiration biopsy of the suspect thyroid nodule.

RNA sequencing for indeterminate FNA cytology provides 100% sensitivity and specificity in identifying MTC.

Following confirmed diagnosis, preoperative calcitonin levels are often obtained to provide a baseline level to follow the response to therapeutic intervention. CEA, as well as CA 19-9 biomarkers, provides prognosis. Positive CA 19-9 post-therapy less than 1 year predict mortality.

It has a familial incidence and serum calcitonin levels are useful as markers of established disease, and in the screening of asymptomatic members of an affected family. Calcitonin is a single-chain polypeptide 32 amino acids.

Secreted by the parafollicular or C cells of the thyroid in response to an increase in calcium level. It inhibits osteoclastic activity and thus bone resorption. At the kidney, calcitonin reduces calcium reabsorption. It lowers blood calcium levels

Neuroendocrine tumors

Neuroendocrine tumors account for about 2% of all cancers. They arise from the cells of the endocrine and nervous system. Commonly involved organs are the gastrointestinal tract, pancreas, lung, and thymus.

Chromogranin A (CgA) is a glycoprotein stored in the secretory granules of neuroendocrine cells. High circulating levels are seen in 50%–100% of patients with neuroendocrine tumors (with or without hormone secretion) with diagnostic sensitivity ranging from 27% to 63% according to the stage of disease and grade of differentiation. Serial measurement is used for monitoring therapeutic response to therapy and for evaluating progression of the disease, and tumor recurrence.

Chromogranin A lacks specificity where elevated levels are seen in other nonneuroendocrine tumors, such as hepatocellular carcinoma, ovarian cancer, colorectal cancer, small cell lung cancer, neuroblastoma, prostate carcinoma, and breast cancer, and in nonmalignancy inflammatory bowel disease, gastritis, rheumatoid arthritis, and in patients using proton pump inhibitors.

Pheochromocytoma

Tumors of the adrenal medulla are termed pheochromocytomas (brown-black colored cells when react with dichromate). They are chromaffin cell tumors derived from the neural crest.

Epinephrine and norepinephrine are converted to metanephrine and normetanephrine and by catecholamine-o-methyltransferase (COMT).

Incidence 2.0–9.1 per million persons. Many of the tumors are benign, clinically silent, and detected at autopsy. Genetical, pheochromocytomas arise sporadically or in the familial MEN type 2 syndrome associated with RET mutation, neurofibromatosis type 1, and the VHL gene mutation syndrome (Hippel-Lindau).

First-line investigation in patients suspected of pheochromocytoma is plasma or urine-fractioned metanephrines. Elevated levels confirm the diagnosis. Dopamine is usually part of the test profile, but if not, few patients with dopamine-only tumors as well as those with small tumors (<1 cm) secreting low metanephrines will be missed as hormone levels correlate with the size of the tumor. Discussed in detail in the chapter on neurology. Plasma metanephrines have a diagnostic sensitivity ranging from 89.5% to 100% and specificity ranging from 79.4% to 97.6%. This is compared with 85.7% to 97.1%, and from 68.6% to 95.1% when measured in urine, respectively.

Periodic postsurgical follow-up is required. Plasma and urinary fractionated metanephrines should be performed within the first month postoperatively, at 6 months, at 1 year, and yearly.

Other neuroectodermal tumors

Malignancies of the more primitive neural crest cells include neuroblastoma in which serum levels of adrenaline and noradrenaline are often normal while the urinary homovanillic acid level is almost always raised.

Carcinoid syndrome

Carcinoid syndrome is the most frequent of the neuroendocrine tumor ectopic hormonal syndrome. Neuroendocrine neoplasms per se are relatively rare and humorous. They are heterogeneous and arise from the neuroendocrine cells commonly in the gastrointestinal and bronchopulmonary systems.

Patients present with diarrhea, cutaneous flushing, wheezing, and asthma-like symptoms, and pellagra-like skin lesions with hyperkeratosis and pigmentation. Fibrosis of the heart secondary to neuroendocrine tumors gives rise to carcinoid heart disease which is associated with poor prognosis. The neoplasm-associated fibrosis may occur at local or distant sites.

Carcinoid syndrome symptoms occur when a sufficient amount of tumor-related biomarker reaches the systemic circulation as they are inactivated if reaches portal circulation.

Biomarkers mediators of the clinical syndrome include serotonin (98%–100% in most cases) identified by its metabolite 5-hydroxyindole acetic acid (5-HIAA), serotonin precursor (5-hydroxytryptophan (5-HTP)), prostaglandins, substance-P, neurokinin A, GI peptides, bradykinin, and histamine. Some investigators add chromogranin A measurement (see later) for neuroendocrine tumors as part of the initial investigation.

5-HIAA is a metabolite of serotonin measured in urine in 24-h samples or plasma and provides a measure of the functionality of the tumor. In patients with carcinoid heart disease (CHD), levels range from 226 to 1381 μmol/24 h compared to 67.5 to 575 μmol/24 h in non-CHD involvement. Values >300 μmol/24 h are associated with a two- to threefold increased risk of developing CHD.

Cardiac biomarker for CHD includes NT-proBNP where levels >260 pg/mL has a sensitivity of 92% and specificity of 91%. Furthermore, NT-proBNP levels correlate with disease progression and survival. Activin A is a member of the TGF family, and those levels ≥0.34 ng/mL are found to have 87% sensitivity and 57% specificity for the detection of carcinoid heart disease.

Initial investigation of the clinical syndrome includes measurement of 24-h urinary 5-HIAA. The sensitivity is 73%–91% (similar to blood) and the specificity of 100%. Although blood levels were not influenced by meals and the time of day, they are affected by renal function.

Limitations with urinary 5-HIAA testing include dietary sources of 5-HIAA, diurnal changes,

A small number of argentaffin cells are normally found in tissues derived from the embryonic gut. The carcinoid syndrome is usually associated with an excess of circulating 5HT. Ileal and appendiceal tumors do not produce the clinical syndrome until they have metastasized, usually to the liver. The clinical syndrome includes flushing, bronchospasm, and diarrhea which may be so severe as to cause malabsorption syndrome. Urinary 5-HIAA secretion is usually greatly increased. Excretion of more than 130 umol (25 mg) in 24 h is diagnostic.

Gastrinomas

May cause Zollinger-Ellison syndrome. G cells, usually in the pancreatic islets (most commonly in the form of tumors), produce large amounts of gastrin. About 60% are malignant; of the remaining 40% two-thirds are multiple and only one-third (13% of the total) are single, resectable adenomas. Acid secretion by the stomach is very high.

Associated benign adenomas may be found in other endocrine glands, such as the parathyroid, pituitary, thyroid, and adrenal (multiple endocrine adenopathy): these are rarely functional.

Fasting plasma gastrin concentrations in the Zollinger-Ellison syndrome is from 5 to 30 times the upper limit of normal. Gastrin concentration may be high in many other conditions, e.g., renal failure and achlorhydria. A very low gastric juice pH and a very high plasma gastrin level indicate autonomous hormone secretion not under normal feedback control and is therefore diagnostic. Ectopic hormones are involved in many tumors. Syndromes of ectopic ACTH and ADH secretion are well recognized in oat cell carcinoma. Peptides secreted react with antibodies to the hormones, but they may not be identical to the true hormone molecule produced in the appropriate tissue.

Bladder cancer

Bladder cancer is the 8th most common worldwide. The majority (80%) of patients present with nonmuscle invasive bladder cancer. The remaining 20% exhibit muscle invasive form. The tumor has a high recurrence with nearly half of the noninvasive form recurring despite radical therapy. Therefore, periodic surveillance is recommended, for instance, every 3 months on high-grade tumors.

Urinary nuclear matrix protein-22 (NMP22) is expressed in urothelial tumors and released into the urine following cell death. It is one of a family of proteins involved in DNA replication and gene expression. The marker has 52%–69% sensitivity and about 77% to 89% specificity for bladder cancer. NMP22 is the most characterized marker and several assays, including point-of-care tests, are available for its measurement.

Human complement factor H-related protein is detected in the urine of patients with bladder cancer. Commercially available assays are known as bladder tumor antigen assays (BTA). However, the assays reportedly have higher sensitivity for bladder cancer when compared with urine cytology

(67% to 95% compared to 43%–95%), respectively. This marker compared to NMP22 is falsely elevated in patients with the inflammatory urinary tract.

Several assays are FDA approved and are commercially available for urinary NMP22 and MCM5 tumor makers. The markers are ideally used in conjunction with cystoscopy to detect invisible tumors. None of the liquid-based markers are unhelpful in screening, follow-up or assessing response to therapy.

There are commercially available urinary-based genetic tests. They include; DNA methylation analysis, mutations (telomerase reverse transcriptase (TERT) promotor), DNA microsatellites, RNA-microsatellites (used in cancer detection and surveillance), and mRNA tests. They reflect increased cellular metabolism, for instance, mRNAs of GTAse-activating proteins. This is found to be elevated in patients with bladder cancer (Table 4).

Currently, available biomarkers lack sensitivity (low positive predictive values) influenced by nonmalignancy inflammation and that cytology analysis remains the mainstay for the detection of bladder cancer. However, a multi-marker approach may provide improved sensitivity and specificity (Tables 5 and 6).

Multiple endocrine neoplasia syndromes

Multiple endocrine neoplasia (MEN) syndrome is a group of heterogeneous disorders characterized by a predisposition for tumors involving two more endocrine glands. Four syndromes are recognized (MEN 1–4). They are autosomal dominant syndromes involving two or more endocrine glands or that a single key gland tumor in a patient with a first-degree relative with a diagnosis of the MEN type.

TABLE 4 Bladder cancer soluble biomarkers, mRNA, and DNA-based available assays.

Test	Biomarker	Sensitivity (%)	Specificity (%)	Comment
NMP22		53.4	77.4	Grade 1/Grade 3 malignancy
BTA	Bladder tumor antigens (complement factor H-related protein)	57–82	68–93	Higher sensitivity than cytology but false positive in patients with urinary tract infection and inflammation
CYFRA-21-1	Soluble fragments of cytokeratin 19	55.7	91.0	
K17	Keratin 17	100	96	Elevated in low and grade high-grade tumor and urothelial cancer
Cellular-based markers				
ImmunioCyst (use of three fluorescently labeled antibodies)	CEA, sulfated mucin glycoproteins	60–100	75–84	Antigens are expressed on the cell surface Influenced by the presence of UTI
UroVysion In situ hybridization assay	For positive results, at least one of the following is found: ≥4 cells (of 25) with gains of ≥2 chromosomes in the same cell ≥10 cells with a gain of a single chromosome. ≥10 cells with tetrasomic signal patterns Homozygous deletion of the 9p21 locus in 20% or more cells	69–87	89–96	Detects chromosome 3,7, 17 aneuploidy or loss of the 9p21 locus Used for both diagnosis and surveillance
Genes-based tests	IGFBPS, HOXA13, MDK, CDKI, CXCR2	82	90	mRNA based
		46.2	77	mRNA based
	FGFR3, TERT, HRAS, methylation of (OTX1, ONECUT2, TWIST1)	97	83	DNA based

Modified from Ng K, Stenzl A, Sharma A, Vasdev N. Urinary biomarkers in bladder cancer: a review of the current landscape and future directions. Urol Oncol 2021;39(1):41–51. https://doi.org/10.1016/j.urolonc.2020.08.016. Epub 2020 Sep 9. PMID: 32919875.

TABLE 5 Tumor markers and their utility as recommended by various professional bodies.

Cancer type	NCCN	ASCO	ACS	EGTM
Breast	ER and PR on all cancers CA 15-3/CA 27.29 for monitoring advanced disease	Routine use of CA 15-3 or CA 27.29 alone not recommended Increasing levels suggest Rx failure	None	ER/PR CEA and one MUC-1-gene-related protein for prognosis and monitoring Rx
Ovarian	CA125 monitoring RX	None	None	CA125 in Dx and monitoring Rx
Prostate	PSA + DRE %PSA when total PSA 4-10 ng/mL	–	PSA + DRE	PSA + DRE %PSA when total PSA 4-10 ng/mL
Germ cell	AFP, hCG, and LDH for detecting and monitoring testicular tumors AFP is Dx for NSGCT	None	None	AFP, hCG, and PLAP (in nonsmokers) for case finding, staging, prognosis, follow-up, and monitoring response to therapy AFP diagnostic for NSGCT
Colon	CEA for monitoring response to therapy	CEA for prognosis, detection recurrence & monitoring response to therapy	None	CEA for case finding, prognosis, follow-up, and monitoring response to therapy
Neuro-endocrine	Ur CATS Calcitonin (thyroid carcinoma)	None	None	None
Myeloma	SPEP IGGs BJP, B2M	None	None	None
Lung	None	None	None	NSE in differential diagnosis, CEA, and/or NSE for follow-up & response to therapy.

NCCN, National clinical practice guidelines in oncology; *ASCO*, American Society of Clinical Oncology; *ACS*, American Cancer Society; *EGTM*, European Group on Tumor Markers.
Modified from Febbo PG, Ladanyi M, Aldape KD, De Marzo AM, Hammond ME, Hayes DF, Iafrate AJ, Kelley RK, Marcucci G, Ogino S, Pao W, Sgroi DC, Birkeland ML. NCCN Task Force report: Evaluating the clinical utility of tumor markers in oncology. J Natl Compr Canc Netw 2011;9 Suppl 5:S1–32; quiz S33. https://doi.org/10.6004/jnccn.2011.0137. PMID: 22138009, Sturgeon CM, Duffy MJ, Stenman UH, Lilja H, Brünner N, Chan DW, Babaian R, Bast RC Jr., Dowell B, Esteva FJ, Haglund C, Harbeck N, Hayes DF, Holten-Andersen M, Klee GG, Lamerz R, Looijenga LH, Molina R, Nielsen HJ, Rittenhouse H, Semjonow A, Shih IeM, Sibley P, Sölétormos G, Stephan C, Sokoll L, Hoffman BR, Diamandis EP; National Academy of Clinical Biochemistry. National Academy of Clinical Biochemistry laboratory medicine practice guidelines for use of tumor markers in testicular, prostate, colorectal, breast, and ovarian cancers. Clin Chem. 2008;54(12):e11–79. https://doi.org/10.1373/clinchem.2008.105601. PMID: 19042984, and Harris L, Fritsche H, Mennel R, Norton L, Ravdin P, Taube S, Somerfield MR, Hayes DF, Bast RC Jr.; American Society of Clinical Oncology. American Society of Clinical Oncology 2007 update of recommendations for the use of tumor markers in breast cancer. J Clin Oncol. 2007;25(33):5287–312. https://doi.org/10.1200/JCO.2007.14.2364. Epub 2007 Oct 22. PMID: 17954709.

Different multiple endocrine neoplasia syndromes have been identified: MEN type 1: the tumor at pancreatic islet cells, parathyroid gland, and anterior pituitary (3P's). MEN-2: medullary thyroid carcinoma, pheochromocytoma, hyperparathyroidism. MEN-3: predominantly aggressive and early onset medullary carcinoma of the thyroid. MEN-4 is similar to the MEN-1 where the pituitary adenoma is smaller and less aggressive. The tumors are associated with adrenal, kidney, and reproductive organ tumors.

Multiple endocrine neoplasia MEN type 1 (MEN-1)

Tumors in the pancreatic islet cells, parathyroid gland, and anterior pituitary (the 3 Ps) are a cluster of tumors in MEN-1. The prevalence is estimated at 1:30,000 in the general population, but higher and often missed in the subpopulation with one of the key tumors. In addition to the three key glands, patients with MEN may also develop adrenocortical tumors, meningiomas, facial angiofibroma, collagenomas, lipomas, and carcinoid tumors of the thymus and small intestine.

However, the most common (95%) tumor is parathyroid adenoma (primary hyperparathyroidism), with biochemical characteristics of hypercalcemia and inappropriately elevated parathyroid hormone (see Chapter 1). Pancreatic islet cell insulinomas represent about 4% of MEN-1 patients. Pituitary tumors are seen in 15%–50% of patients with MEN-1 with the majority 60% being prolactinomas, 25% growth hormone tumors, and 5% ACTH tumors with the remainder being nonfunctional. Pancreatic islet cell

TABLE 6 Various tumors and their associated biomarkers. The indicated biomarkers are usually performed in the investigation and monitoring of patients.

Tumor	Biomarker
Teratoma	AFP, hCG
Seminoma	hCG, AFP, LDH, placental alkaline phosphatase
Choriocarcinoma	HCG, HPL
Prostate cancer	PSA, prostatic acid phosphatase
Hepatoma	AFP
Small cell lung cancer	NSE
Myeloma	Immunoglobins, Bence Jones protein, beta 2-microglobulin
Gastrointestinal/pancreatic tumors	Gut hormones pancreatic polypeptide, vasoactive intestinal peptide, glucagon, gastrin, somatostatin, neurotensin, insulin.
Ovarian tumor	CA 125
Granulosa cell of the ovary	Estradiol
Medullary carcinoma of the thyroid	Calcitonin
Carcinoid tumor	5-hydroxyindole acetic acid (urine)
Pheochromocytoma	Catecholamine (fractionated metanephrines) (urine/blood)
Adrenal cortex tumors	Androgen

Modified from Febbo PG, Ladanyi M, Aldape KD, De Marzo AM, Hammond ME, Hayes DF, Iafrate AJ, Kelley RK, Marcucci G, Ogino S, Pao W, Sgroi DC, Birkeland ML. NCCN Task Force report: Evaluating the clinical utility of tumor markers in oncology. J Natl Compr Canc Netw 2011;9 Suppl 5:S1–32; quiz S33. https://doi.org/10.6004/jnccn.2011.0137. PMID: 22138009, Sturgeon CM, Duffy MJ, Stenman UH, Lilja H, Brünner N, Chan DW, Babaian R, Bast RC Jr., Dowell B, Esteva FJ, Haglund C, Harbeck N, Hayes DF, Holten-Andersen M, Klee GG, Lamerz R, Looijenga LH, Molina R, Nielsen HJ, Rittenhouse H, Semjonow A, Shih IeM, Sibley P, Sölétormos G, Stephan C, Sokoll L, Hoffman BR, Diamandis EP; National Academy of Clinical Biochemistry. National Academy of Clinical Biochemistry laboratory medicine practice guidelines for use of tumor markers in testicular, prostate, colorectal, breast, and ovarian cancers. Clin Chem. 2008;54(12):e11–79. https://doi.org/10.1373/clinchem.2008.105601. PMID: 19042984, and Harris L, Fritsche H, Mennel R, Norton L, Ravdin P, Taube S, Somerfield MR, Hayes DF, Bast RC Jr.; American Society of Clinical Oncology. American Society of Clinical Oncology 2007 update of recommendations for the use of tumor markers in breast cancer. J Clin Oncol. 2007;25(33):5287–312. https://doi.org/10.1200/JCO.2007.14.2364. Epub 2007 Oct 22. PMID: 17954709.

tumors or neuroendocrine tumors are seen in 30%–80% of MEN-1 patients. In addition to insulinoma, they include gastrin-secreting gastrinoma (Zollinger-Ellison syndrome), glucagonomas, and vasoactive intestinal peptide (VIP)-omas.

The gene, coding for a tumor suppressor protein, is located on chromosome 11 (11q13). Pituitary adenoma, commonly prolactinoma, and parathyroid chief sell hypertrophy progress to adenoma.

Multiple endocrine neoplasia type 2 (MEN-2)

The MEN-2 syndrome comprises medullary thyroid carcinoma (MTC) in 95% of patients, pheochromocytoma in 50% of patients, and hyperparathyroidism in 20%–30% of patients. It has a prevalence of 1:25,000. It is caused by mutations in the RET (rearranged during transfection) proto-oncogene. A 21-exon gene located on chromosome 10q11.2 encodes a membrane-bound tyrosine kinase cell surface receptors.

Biomarkers are those of calcitonin for medullar thyroid carcinoma, catecholamines for pheochromocytoma, and PTH and calcium for hyperparathyroidism.

MEN-2 A

MEN-2 A syndrome comprises; parathyroid adenoma/hyperplasia, medullary carcinoma of the thyroid, pheochromocytoma. All patients will have medullary carcinoma of the thyroid. Pheochromocytoma is present in half of the patients, about 30% of patients will develop hyperparathyroidism. c-ret proto-oncogenes coding for tyrosine kinase receptor gene located on chromosome 10 (10q11.2).

Men-2 B

MEN-2 B comprises; medullary carcinoma of the thyroid, pheochromocytoma, and ganglioneuroma with point mutations on exon 16.

Multiple endocrine neoplasia type 3 (MEN-3)

Aggressive early onset medullary thyroid carcinoma (MTC) is the initial manifestation followed by pheochromocytoma in 50% of patients. It has a low prevalence of 0.2 per 100,000. Similar to the MEN-2, it is caused by mutations in the RET. The majority (98%) of patients will have RET mutation (about 50% de novo germline mutation) with about 95% harboring highly specific M918T mutation which confers a high risk for early MTC metastasis.

Biochemical monitoring is by measuring calcitonin for MTC (basal levels or following pentagastrin stimulation), and periodic measurement of fractionated serum or 24-h urinary metanephrines and normetanephrines for pheochromocytoma.

Multiple endocrine neoplasia type 4 (MEN-4)

The most common phenotype is similar to that of MEN-1 with predominant (80%) parathyroid neoplasm; with pituitary adenoma (smaller and less aggressive than in MEN-1) and pancreatic neuroendocrine tumors (gastrinomas with decreased penetrance compared to MEN-1), the tumors are associated with kidney, adrenals, and reproductive organs tumors. It is associated with eight heterozygous mutations in the CDNK1B gene.

Biochemical markers are similar to those in MEN-1 in addition to adrenal adenoma (aldosterone) biomarker.

Neuroendocrine tumors

Neuroendocrine tumors are heterogeneous and rare (incidence of about 7 per 100,000), mostly of gastrointestinal and bronchopulmonary origin.

Nontumor organ involvement

Tissue fibrosis is a common finding and complication in patients with neuroendocrine tumors. The formation of fibrosis is thought to be mediated by the combined effects of serotonin, growth factors, and several peptides (Table 7).

The heart is the most affected organ leading to congestive heart failure and to increased morbidity and mortality.

5HIAA

5 Hydroxyindole acetic acid (5HIAA) is a metabolite of serotonin. Blood or 24-h urinary level reflects tumor activity. Higher levels are observed in patients with congestive heart disease.

NT-proBNP

Screening patients with carcinoid syndrome for congestive heart disease where levels >260 ng/mL had a sensitivity of 92% and specificity of 91% for congestive heart disease.

Chromogranin A

Glycoprotein produced by neuroendocrine tumors was measured to monitor response to therapy but not to screen for congestive heart disease in patients with carcinoid syndrome.

TABLE 7 Neuroendocrine modulators associated with tissue fibrosis.

Growth factors	Peptides
TGF-alpha, beta, TGFR, FGF, VEGF, IGF, CTGF, and PDGF	Kinins, Tachykinins GRP FAO-alpha Tenascin C
Serotonin	5HIAA

Modified from Laskaratos FM, Rombouts K, Caplin M, Toumpanakis C, Thirlwell C, Mandair D. Neuroendocrine tumors and fibrosis: an unsolved mystery? Cancer 2017;123(24):4770–4790. https://doi.org/10.1002/cncr.31079. Epub 2017 Nov 7. PMID: 29112233.

Activin A is a member of the TGF family elevated in patients with congestive heart disease where levels ≥0.34 ng/mL had an 87% and 57% sensitivity and specificity for congestive heart disease in carcinoid patients, respectively.

Metabolic impact of malignancy

Cachexia, hypercalcemia, hypoglycemia, and metastatic liver involvement lead to cholestatic hyperbilirubinemia and cholestatic enzymes (alkaline phosphatase and gamma-glutamyl transferase (γGT)).

Cachexia

As many as 80% of patients with advanced cancer disease exhibit wasting states known as cachexia. It is mainly seen in patients with solid tumors and accounts for more than 20% of cancer-related mortality. Although there is no effective therapy, nutritional support is shown to have a positive impact. Cachexia is characterized by a state of enhanced catabolism and several biomarkers may be used to assess the severity and progression of the cachexia. Muscle wasting is a prominent condition and is thought to be secondary to increased protein degradation and decreased synthesis. A state of insulin resistance among patients with advanced cancer. Although not currently available, the degradation products (e.g., β-dystroglycan, glycerol, free fatty acids, hexosyl-ceramides, and lactosyl-ceramides) may offer a way to monitor muscle wasting in cancer cachexia.

Transforming growth factor beta family proteins (activin A, myostatin, and growth differentiation factor 15) induces muscle wasting and fat loss. Zinc-alpha-2-glycoprotein is a lipid mobilizing factor where it promotes the browning of white adipose tissue and thus increased metabolism and energy-associated wasting. Parathyroid hormone-related peptide (PTHrp) promotes the browning of fat and expression of thermogenesis genes in fat cells and thus lipolysis. Angiotensin II stimulates the expression of IL-6, TNF-α, and glucocorticoids and acts on the hypothalamus to reduce appetite. Reducing food intake is a component of cachexia.

Circulating levels of inflammatory cytokines such as IL-6, TNF-α, IL-1β, IL-8, monocyte chemoattractant protein-1 (MCP-1), and C-reactive protein (CRP) are possible biomarkers of cancer cachexia, where levels correlate with survival and lean body mass, tumor staging, and weight loss. It is worth noting that the biomarkers are also elevated in infections and other conditions and that the majority are produced by both the tumor and the normal cells in response alike.

MicroRNAs have been suggested as possible biomarkers of cancer cachexia. They are 17-22 nucleotides long noncoding RNA. They regulate gene expression in skeletal muscle and adipose tissue. Circulating levels of MicroRNA-21, −203, and 130a have been proposed as possible biomarkers for cachexia.

Therefore, cachexia biomarkers are those of inflammation, muscle, and fat-wasting products, and PTHrp and microRNA products. They are either host or tumor derived. However, there are no clear clinical biomarkers for cancer cachexia. It is possible that the measurement of more than one biomarker in profiles may improve the diagnostic utility of the various markers in the detection and monitoring of cancer cachexia.

Hypercalcemia

Ten percent of patients with advanced cancer have hypercalcemia which indicates a poor prognosis. Symptoms of hypercalcemia (>14 mg/dL (>3.5 mmol/L)) include nausea, vomiting, lethargy, renal failure, and coma. The degree of hypercalcemia as well as the duration of onset dictates the severity of symptoms. Termed humoral hypercalcemia of malignancy, 80% of the hypercalcemia is due to secretion of parathyroid hormone-related peptide by tumor cells. PTHrp increases calcium resorption from bone and renal reabsorption with resultant hypercalcemia, most common in patients with squamous cell tumors. The remaining 20% of hypercalcemia is from bone secondary to metastatic resorption and increased osteolytic activity seen is often seen in patients with multiple myeloma, lymphomas, and breast cancer.

The finding of hypercalcemia must be confirmed by repeat measurement and by measuring ionized calcium, if available, or correcting total calcium for albumin levels applying the formula (albumin corrected calcium=measured calcium (mg/dL)+0.8 (4.0-albumin (mg/dL))). This is followed by measuring PTH which is inappropriately high in patients with primary hyperparathyroidism, and either inappropriately low or near the lower end of the normal reference interval, when measuring PTHrp and the finding of elevated levels confirms humoral hypercalcemia of malignancy.

Humeral hypercalcemia is of malignancy secondary to bone metastasis and increased resorption, due to parathyroid hormone-related peptide (PTH-rp) production by tumors.

PTHrp was identified in 1987. It is larger than PTH with strong homology at N-terminal. Thus, it binds to PTH receptors in bone and renal tubules. It is, however, not tumor specific since mRNA is found in most fetal tissues (paracrine, autocrine function in growth and development of the embryo). In normal adult tissue, it is expressed in the epidermis and lactating breast.

Syndrome of inappropriate anti diuretic hormone secretion (SIADH)

SIADH syndrome secondary to ADH section occurs in 1%–2% of all cancer patients. It is characterized by hyponatremia and low serum osmolality. 10%–45% of small cell lung cancer develop SIADH.

Cushing's syndrome

Ectopic production of ACTH commonly (50%–60%) by small cell lung tumors and bronchial carcinoid results in Cushing's paraneoplastic syndrome. Patients often present with hypertension, hypokalemia, muscle weakness, and generalized edema. Weight gain and centripetal fat distribution are more common in nonparaneoplastic Cushing's. Biochemical findings of ACTH-dependent Cushing's are elevated serum cortisol >29 μg/dL urinary free cortisol >47 μg/24 h and a midnight ACTH >100 ng/L. An inferior petrosal sinus sampling (IPSS) procedure may be required to confirm ectopic Cushing's (see Chapter 1). Failure to suppress cortisol following a high-dose dexamethasone suppression supports the presence of ectopic ACTH.

Hypoglycemia

Nonpancreatic cause of hypoglycemia (resulting in paraneoplastic syndrome) represents recurrent episodes of glucose <20 mg/dL (<1.1 mmol/L). The hypoglycemia is secondary to IGF-2 production by tumors (more rarely tumor cell insulin). Insulin and C-peptide are low (<1.44–3.6 uIU/mL) and <0.3 ng/mL, respectively. Reduced growth hormone and IGF-1 levels and normal or elevated IGF-2 and a high IGF-2/IGF-1 ratio support tumor-associated hypoglycemia.

Paraneoplastic neurology syndromes

This syndrome is present in 7%–15% of patients with malignancy. Patients with small cell carcinoma of the lung, melanoma, gastrointestinal and endocrine tumors, and prostatic carcinoma.

The causative biomolecules are either tumor-derived such as hormones, neurotransmitters, and cytokines. They can also be host derived such as antibodies.

Antibody-mediated paraneoplastic syndromes affect less than 1% of patients with cancer.

In response to cancer, patients produce tumor-directed antibodies known as onconeural antibodies. The antigen is either neuroendocrine proteins produced by small cell lung cancer and neuroblastoma, or contain neural components (teratomas), immunoregulatory (thymomas), and immunoglobin production regulators (lymphoma and myeloma).

The antibodies are detected before cancer is diagnosed in 80% of cases. Because of antigenic similarity, both the antibodies and antigen-specific T-lymphocytes inadvertently attack the components of the nervous system as well as the tumors.

The syndrome is developed in 5% of patients with small-cell lung cancer and 10% of patients with multiple myeloma and lymphoma.

Malignancy and associated antibodies are described (Tables 8 and 10). The onconeural antibodies fall into three

TABLE 8 Antibodies and their associated cancers and paraneoplastic syndrome.

Associated cancer	Antibodies	Paraneoplastic syndrome
Small cell lung cancer (SCLC)	Anti-Hu	Limbic encephalitis (LE)
Testicular	Anti-Ma2	
	Anti-CRMP5 (anti-CV2)	
	Anti-amphiphysin	
SCLC, gynecologic, breast, Hodgkin lymphoma	Anti-You	Paraneoplastic cerebellar degeneration
	Anti-Hu	
	AntiCRMP5 (ant-CV2)	
	Anti-Ma	
	Anti-Tr	
	Anti-Ri	
	Anti-VGCC	
	Anti-mGluRI	
SCLC, prostate, cervical, lymphomas, adenocarcinoma	Anti-VGCC (P/Q type)	Lambert-Eaton myasthenia syndrome (LEMS)
Thymoma	Anti-AchR	Myasthenia gravis (MG)
	Anti-Hu	Autonomic neuropathy
	Anti-CRMP5 (anti-CV2)	
	Anti-nAchR	
	Anti-amphiphysin	
Lung (70%–80% SCLC) Breast Ovarian Sarcoma Hodgkin lymphoma	Anti-Hu	Subacute (peripheral) sensory neuropathy
	Anti-CRMP5 (anti-CV2)	
	Anti-amphiphysin	

Antibodies are mostly detected in serum and rarely in cerebrospinal fluid samples.
Modified from Binks S, Uy C, Honnorat J, Irani SR. Paraneoplastic neurological syndromes: a practical approach to diagnosis and management. Pract Neurol 2022;22(1):19–31. https://doi.org/10.1136/practneurol-2021-003073. Epub 2021 Sep 11. PMID: 34510016.

TABLE 9 Antibodies and the extent of their association with malignancy.

Association categories	Antibodies
Strong cancer association	Anti-amphiphysin, anti-CRMP5 (CV2), anti-Hun (ANNA-1), anti-Ma2, anti-recoverin, anti-Ri (ANNA-2), anti-Yo (PCA-1)
Partially associated	ANNA-3, anti—mGluR1, anti-Tr, Anti-Zic4, PCA-2
Cancer and noncancer associated	Anti-AchR, anti-nicotinic AchR, anti-VGCC, anti-VGKC

Modified from Pelosof LC, Gerber DE. Paraneoplastic syndromes: an approach to diagnosis and treatment. Mayo Clin Proc 2010;85(9):838–54. https://doi.org/10.4065/mcp.2010.0099. Erratum in: Mayo Clin Proc. 2011;86(4):364. Dosage error in article text. PMID: 20810794; PMCID: PMC2931619.

unlikely and that may be T cell-mediated immunity plays a role in the pathogenesis in this case. Some of the antibodies are directed against structural neuronal sites such as the anti-acetylcholine receptor antibodies, and the anti-voltage gated calcium channel antibodies which suggest a putative functional role in the paraneoplastic syndrome. The pathogenesis and mechanism for most of the antibodies remain unclear, some offer prognostic value; for example, patients with small cell lung cancer and positive for anti-Hu are more likely to achieve remission after treatment compared with patients negative for anti-Hu (Table 10).

Miscellaneous conditions associated with paraneoplastic syndromes

A number of dermatological syndromes are described that are present either alone or in combination with paraneoplastic syndrome. Few have clinical biochemistry laboratory involvement. Those include dermatomyositis, where patients present with skin changes followed by proximal muscle changes. Patients present with upper eyelid rash, scaly papules on bony surfaces, and erythematous rash on face, neck, chest or back, or shoulders. Rash may be photosensitive, proximal muscle weakness, difficult swallowing, respiratory difficulty, and muscle pain. Laboratory findings are those of elevated muscle serum creatinine kinase, aspartate transaminase, alanine transaminase, lactate dehydrogenase, and aldolase. Diagnosis is obtained using skin biopsy.

Hematological manifestation in paraneoplastic syndrome

Hematologic disorders associated with paraneoplastic syndromes are rarely symptomatic. They are typically seen in

categories. (1) Those with strong cancer association, (2) partially cancer-associated, or (3) occurring in both cancer and then cancer-associated syndromes (Table 9).

Many antineuronal antibodies are directed against intracellular antigens which suggest that in vivo binding is

TABLE 10 List of common names of antibody targets and respective codes abbreviations in use.

Code	Name	Code	Name	Code	Name
AchR	Acetylcholine receptor	G-CSF	Granulocyte colony-stimulating factor	VGCC	Voltage-gated calcium channel
ANP	Antineuronal nuclear antibody	$mGluR_1$	Metabotropic glutamate receptor-subtype-I	VGKC	Voltage-gated potassium channel
CRMP	Collapsing response mediator protein	PCA	Purkinje cell cytoplasmic autoantibody	GM-CSF	Granulocyte-macrophage-colony stimulating factor
$FGFR_1$	Fibroblast growth factor receptor I	PDGFR	Platelet-derived growth factor receptor	JAK_2	Janus kinase 2

Modified from Pelosof LC, Gerber DE. Paraneoplastic syndromes: an approach to diagnosis and treatment. Mayo Clin Proc 2010;85(9):838–54. https://doi.org/10.4065/mcp.2010.0099. Erratum in: Mayo Clin Proc. 2011;86(4):364. Dosage error in article text. PMID: 20810794; PMCID: PMC2931619.

advanced stages of associated malignancy. Laboratory findings are most those of hematological abnormalities, and there are little clinical biochemistry laboratory findings with the exception of elevated cytokines, namely, IL-5, IL-3, IL-2, and GM-CSF in eosinophilia syndrome, and IL-6 in thrombocytosis associated syndrome.

Summary

The field of tumor markers in detection, diagnosis, and prognosis is rapidly expanding with advancements in technologies, namely, liquid chromatography-mass spectrometric (LCMSMS) methodologies and those of molecular next-gene sequencing as well as expansion of application or artificial intelligence.

- Tumor markers are either produced by the tumor and secreted or expressed (at the cell surface).
- Tumor biomarkers are classified as either tumor-specific or tumor-associated.
- Soluble and circulating tumor markers are measured by immunoassay-based methodologies, markers exhibiting enzymatic activity are measured utilizing their activity, and molecular genetics applications in tumor genes detection.
- Tumor markers are often oncofetal, protooncogene products, structurally modified proteins, and as well as abnormally (often excessively) expressed normal proteins.
- Tumor markers in clinical practice include hCG, AFP, PSA, CEA, CA 19-9, CA 125, CA 15-3, PTH-rp, calcitonin, LDH, and glands hormones (e.g., prolactin in prolactinoma)
- Structural heterogeneity in hCG and its β subunit is utilized to improve diagnostic utility (specificity and sensitivity) for gestational trophoblastic disease and germ cell tumors.
- Gestational choriocarcinoma is the most common among trophoblastic tumors and raised serum

concentrations of βhCG correlate well with choriocarcinoma tumor mass.
- AFP is synthesized by the fetal yolk sac, liver, and gastrointestinal tract. Circulating AFP levels are elevated in hepatocellular carcinoma.
- AFP in measurement in conjunction with βhCG is used to identify patients with testicular teratoma.
- AFP is not elevated in patients with seminomatous or choriocarcinoma.
- CEA measurement is recommended for follow-up of patients with colorectal carcinoma post-resection with 80% sensitivity and 70% specificity for detection of recurrence.
- Fecal occult blood tests are designed to detect hemoglobin molecules and fecal samples.
- The presence of hemoglobin in stool is considered an indication of gastrointestinal bleeding that could be due to various pathologies including gastrointestinal malignancy and inflammation.
- The use of PSA for prostate screening has been controversial with discrepancies among different randomized controlled studies.
- High-risk individuals (positive family history, African descent) with 10 to 15 years of life expectancy should be offered screening with an explanation of test limitations and utility.
- In ovarian cancer, CA 125 measurement is recommended with transvaginal ultrasound (TVUS) for early detection of ovarian cancer in women with high risk.
- CA 15-3 is a large glycoprotein of 300–450 kDa. It is elevated in breast cancer (69%), pancreatic cancer (80%), lung cancer (71%), ovarian cancer (64%), colorectal cancer (63%), and liver cancer (28%).
- CA 19-9 is a glycoprotein. It is elevated in patients with colorectal carcinoma and pancreatic carcinoma.
- Paraproteins are monoclonal immunoglobulins. If light chains are produced in excess, these appear in the urine as Bence Jones protein which is almost always an indication of malignancy.

- Multiple endocrine neoplasia (MEN) syndrome is a group of heterogeneous disorders characterized by a predisposition for tumors involving two more endocrine glands. Four syndromes are recognized (MEN 1–4).
- About 15% of patients with malignancy exhibit paraneoplastic neurology syndrome.
- Ten percent of patients with advanced cancer have hypercalcemia which indicates poor prognosis.

Further reading

Faria SC, Sagebiel T, Patnana M, et al. Tumor markers: myths and facts unfolded. *Abdom Radiol (NY)*. 2019;44(4):1575–1600.

Johnson PJ, Pirrie SJ, Cox TF, et al. The detection of hepatocellular carcinoma using a prospectively developed and validated model based on serological biomarkers. *Cancer Epidemiol Biomarkers Prev.* 2014;23(1):144–153.

Montminy EM, Jang A, Conner M, Karlitz JJ. Screening for colorectal cancer. *Med Clin North Am.* 2020;104(6):1023–1036.

Laskaratos FM, Davar J, Toumpanakis C. Carcinoid heart disease: a review. *Curr Oncol Rep.* 2021;23(4):48.

Pelosof LC, Gerber DE. Paraneoplastic syndromes: an approach to diagnosis and treatment. *Mayo Clin Proc.* 2010;85(9):838–854.

McDonnell JE, Gild ML, Clifton-Bligh RJ, Robinson BG. Multiple endocrine neoplasia: an update. *Intern Med J.* 2019;49(8):954–961.

Ng K, Stenzl A, Sharma A, Vasdev N. Urinary biomarkers in bladder cancer: a review of the current landscape and future directions. *Urol Oncol.* 2021;39(1):41–51.

Forkasiewicz A, Dorociak M, Stach K, Szelachowski P, Tabola R, Augoff K. The usefulness of lactate dehydrogenase measurements in current oncological practice. *Cell Mol Biol Lett.* 2020;25:35.

El Hage L, Hatipoglu B. Elevated hCG can be a benign finding in perimenopausal and postmenopausal women. *Cleve Clin J Med.* 2021;88(11):635–639.

Cole LA. hCG, five independent molecules. *Clin Chim Acta.* 2012;413(1-2):48–65.

Chapter 14

Therapeutic drugs and toxicology testing

Introduction

Drugs (therapeutic and abused) testing in clinical laboratories is performed for the following reasons: (1) assessment of adequacy and safe dosing of therapeutic drugs with narrow therapeutic window, (2) detection of drugs of abuse, (3) in the clinical investigation of the unconscious patient and patients suspected of poison ingestion in the emergency department and in critical care, and (4) in support of pain management and rehabilitation programs in monitoring compliance and in detecting deviation.

Provision of personalized therapeutic drug monitoring by measuring direct or surrogate biomarkers of the drug pharmacology effect in addition to its circulating concentration is essential for many and expanding list and an area of increasing interest.

This chapter describes the pharmacokinetics and pharmacodynamics of the various drugs that are routinely measured in the clinical laboratory including drugs of abuse and selected poisons. The classes of drugs, preferred sample type, and relevant methodology aspects of detection, cross-reactivity, and reporting are discussed.

Pharmacokinetics

Pharmacokinetics (PK) is a mathematical representation of what the body does to the drug, that is absorption, distribution, metabolism, and excretion. The two most important parameters of the pharmacokinetics of drugs are the volume of distribution (V_d) and clearance (CL).

The volume of distribution is defined as a proportionality constant that links the amount of the drug administered and the dosage to the measured plasma concentration, whereas clearance is a measure of the drug elimination and represents the volume of the blood or plasma from which given drugs are completely removed per unit of time. That is metabolism and excretion.

The elimination half-life is a combination of the volume of distribution and clearance. That is a prolonged half-life can be due to either reduced clearance or an increased volume of distribution, or both.[1]

Most drugs encountered in the clinical laboratory are administered either orally or intravenously. Oral administration is subject to the drug characteristics as well as to physiological parameters such as gastric pH, intestinal transit time, drug metabolizing enzymes and drug transporters, and by food intake and its constituents such as milk. For example, milk causes an alkaline stomach pH reducing the absorption of weak acids such as phenytoin due to increased ionization and to decreased absorption of weak bases such as ketoconazole due to reduced solubility.

The type of food is also thought to influence gastric emptying. Prolonged gastric emptying results in reduced drug absorption and that increased gastric emptying increases the rate of drug absorption. This is not the case for all drugs where for digoxin increased gastric emptying causes a decrease in its rate of absorption.

A number of metabolizing enzymes and transporter receptor proteins are present in the intestine and play an important role in the metabolism, absorption, and tissue uptake of the drugs. Enzymes include cytochrome P450 complex, glutathione S transferase, and carboxylesterase-2. Transporters include ATP-binding P-glycoprotein, and multidrug resistance-associated protein, among others. Respective transporters and metabolizing enzymes will be stated for the specific drugs later as relevant.

Upon absorption into the systemic circulation, the drugs will distribute in different tissues and organs and the distribution pattern will depend on the physical and chemical properties of the drug such as its solubility, the degree of ionization, and protein binding. This will be influenced by systemic blood flow and by the permeability of the blood-brain and placental barrier.

Protein binding influences drug distribution. The most relevant plasma proteins are albumin, alpha-1 acid glycoprotein, and globulins. The concentrations of those proteins vary due to various physiological conditions, such as pregnancy, and pathological states such as renal and or hepatic dysfunction.

Reduce protein binding secondary to reduction in the protein concentration or to changes in pH and or to interference by other drugs or free fatty acids lead to an increase in the free fraction of the drugs. Free drugs diffuse more easily resulting in a higher volume of distribution and may lead to increased levels in tissue and organs and therefore to possible toxicity. The influence of protein binding on free plasma drug concentration is limited to drugs that are known to have moderate-to-high degrees of protein binding and narrow therapeutic index, examples being phenytoin. Minor differences in protein binding will result in a significant difference in the free concentration of the drug.

Tutorials in Clinical Chemistry. https://doi.org/10.1016/B978-0-12-822949-1.00020-6

Hepatocytes are the major site of drug metabolism although first-pass effect takes place in the intestine for orally administered drugs. Other organs such as the kidney, lungs, blood cells, the placenta, and brain may also contribute to respective drug metabolism.

Two major pathways are involved in drug metabolism. They are divided into either phase 1 or phase 2 reactions. Phase 1 results in structural changes of the drug such as oxidation, reduction, and hydroxylation, whereas phase II reactions are synthetic such as conjugation with molecules leading to increased water solubility.

Elimination of the drugs is mostly by the kidney which involves filtration, tubular excretion, and reabsorption. Filtration by the glomerulus is very rapid and depends on the glomerular filtration rate, whereas tubular reabsorption/excretion is a slow process.

Pharmacodynamics

Pharmacodynamics (PD) describes the relationship between a given concentration of a drug and the extent of a specific response and shows what the drug does to the human body. That is the action of the drug in terms of the end effect. The actions of drugs relevant to the clinical laboratory are described separately for each of the drugs.

Timing of sample collection

Central to the correct interpretation of the drug levels is the relationship between the dosing time and blood sample collection. The drug level should be measured when at a steady state.

The therapeutic window is governed by a concentration level below which the drug is not effective and above which the drug is toxic (Fig. 1). The spectrum is a continuum that takes 5–7 half-life's ($T_{1/2}$) for a particular drug to reach its therapeutic window. Few drugs meet those criteria and are thus high candidates for therapeutic drug monitoring and are discussed in this chapter.

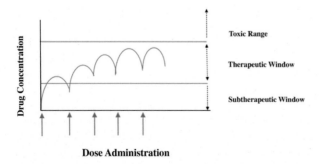

FIG. 1 Drug circulating concentration in relation to dosage regimens and to the therapeutic window. *Modified from Kang JS, Lee MH. Overview of therapeutic drug monitoring. Korean J Intern Med. 2009;24(1):1-10. https://doi.org/10.3904/kjim.2009.24.1.1. PMID: 19270474; PMCID: PMC2687654.*

Factors influencing the relationship between dosage and drug concentration reaching its action site describe the pharmacokinetics of the drug are; absorption, liberation quantified as bioavailability (F), and distribution (volume of distribution (V_d)) governed by its relative solubility in fat and in water.

The amount of the drug reaching the target ($S \times F \times V_d$) depends on the volume of distribution, the bioavailability (F), and the salt factor (S) (the fraction of the drug present in the administered material).

Drug metabolism, protein binding, elimination, and physiological or pathological factors causing changes in those will alter the drug's desired concentration levels, for instance, changes in renal function and hepatic function for drugs where those are the predominant metabolism sites. Changes in albumin (predominant binding protein), e.g., in pregnancy as well as in patients with renal and hepatic dysfunction. Coadministration of other drugs may influence metabolism. For example, coadministration of phenytoin and lamotrigine where hepatic metabolism of the latter is enhanced by the phenytoin induction of microsomal enzymes. Additionally, the use of herbal supplements (often not mentioned and overlooked during patient clinical assessment) may explain the observed discordance, examples that include St John's Wort on cyclosporine metabolism. Pharmacogenetics factor's contribution to pharmacodynamics (metabolism, etc.) has been identified and shown to be of value when assessing TDM in some drugs.

Clinical samples used routinely are blood (plasma/serum), urine samples, saliva, and meconium. However, hair, nails, and vitreous humor are often used in specialized testing supporting forensic and legal cases.

Sample (blood) is taken prior to the next dose when there is no contribution to levels due to continued absorption and that elimination predominates and levels represent trough concentration. In practice, a lack of correlation between dosage and observed clinical outcomes is often attributed to inappropriate sample collection time in relation to dosage. Another contributing factor is not waiting for the drug to reach equilibrium (5–7 its respective half-live), i.e., for digoxin which has a 36h $T_{1/2}$, drug levels should be assessed for adequacy after 8 days from initiation of therapy.

Therapeutic drug monitoring

Laboratory monitoring for certain therapeutic drugs is essential and with appropriate interpretation and assessment influences drug administration and prescription.

Therapeutic drug monitoring (TDM) is relevant and of value for very few drugs particularly those with a narrow therapeutic window (Fig. 1), the blood concentration of the drug correlates with its action, but the dosage does not correlate with the blood concentration. The spectrum of response is a continuum from ineffective, through effective to toxic. The ultimate goal is to individualize drug dosage by maintaining drug concentration within its therapeutic window (Fig. 1). This goal has been extended to include assessing for compliance, confirmation of intake and cessation, as well as for drug-drug interaction. A target range of desirable concentrations is often quoted. This infers that there is a concentration-effect relationship. If this is similar to the dose-effect relationship, this suggests that there is no need to measure the drug concentration. However, if a relationship has been established; the drug (and, if of proven value, its active metabolite) should be measured.

For the purpose of therapeutic drug monitoring, the sample is usually taken just prior to the next dose, i.e., when elimination predominates, i.e., there is no contribution from continuing absorption nor continuing distribution. Analytical considerations are discussed separately (see later).

While measuring the concentration of the drug is important, it is limited by the fact that it does not reflect the pharmacodynamics of the drug and its interactions. To provide personalized drug therapy monitoring, the following parameters must be known.

(1) The drug's pharmacokinetics (its absorption rate, distribution, clearance, and half-life).
(2) The dose of the drug given.
(3) The frequency and duration of dosing.
(4) The patient's weight (and height if ideal body weight is important).
(5) The time of sampling relative to the last dose.
(6) Is the patient in steady state?
(7) Is there an underlying disease state likely to affect the drug kinetics or dynamics?
(8) Is there a drug interaction?

Drug monitoring is of value when the therapeutic effect correlates with plasma levels better than does the prescribed dose. This is important when considering the interactions in multiple drug therapy, when compliance is questioned, and when metabolite formation may produce pharmacologically active substances.

The finding of high drug levels is suggestive of one or a combination of the following (Table 1); Excessive dosage, enhanced absorption, decreased distribution, decreased clearance, drug-drug interaction, sample drawn at the wrong time, i.e., during absorption phase, or analytical error.

The finding of an unexpectedly low drug concentration level may be due to any of the following (Table 2), inadequate dose, diminished absorption, increased distribution, increased clearance, drug interaction, and analytical error.

Dose increments are dictated by the range of doses available. Often the only change is in the dose and hence the plasma concentration will change proportionately (first-order kinetics). However, target ranges are just that, targets. If a patient responds adequately to a "low" con-

TABLE 1 Causes and examples leading to high drug levels.

Cause	Comment
Excessive dosage	Inappropriate dosing regimen and frequency. Lack of compliance with dosage
Enhanced absorption	Rapid gastric emptying
Decreased distribution	Hypovolemia, circulatory failure, protein binding
Decreased clearance	Renal and/or hepatic dysfunction
Drug-drug interaction	Coadministered drug-reducing clearance and metabolism
Inappropriate sample collection time	Sample collected in relation to dosage. Ideal is just before the next dosage. That is the nadir (highest clearance rate)
Analytical error	Wrong result obtained due to either interference or sample contamination

Modified from Kang JS, Lee MH. Overview of therapeutic drug monitoring. Korean J Intern Med. 2009;24(1):1-10. https://doi.org/10.3904/kjim.2009.24.1.1. PMID: 19270474; PMCID: PMC2687654.

TABLE 2 Causes and examples leading to unexpectedly low drug concentration level.

Cause	Comment
Inadequate dosage	Inappropriate dosage regimen. Lack of compliance
Diminished absorption	Delayed gastric emptying. Dietary content interfering with absorption. Fat contents, etc.
Increased distribution	Volume overload, ascites
Increased clearance	Coadministered drug enhances metabolism and clearance
Drug-drug interaction	Coadministered drug enhances metabolism and clearance
Analytical error	Wrong result obtained due to either interference or sample contamination

Modified from Kang JS, Lee MH. Overview of therapeutic drug monitoring. Korean J Intern Med. 2009;24(1):1-10. https://doi.org/10.3904/kjim.2009.24.1.1. PMID: 19270474; PMCID: PMC2687654.

centration of the drug, then it is the right concentration for that patient. Thus, therapeutic drug monitoring is adjunct to clinical judgment. It takes roughly five half-lives—regardless of dose—to reach a new steady state following a dose change. Thus, for a drug with a half-life of 48 h, it will be at least 10 days before a steady state is reached. It is not impossible to interpret drug levels taken before this time, but it is certainly more difficult.

Most drugs (orally taken) show a first-order kinetics. The dosage interval of a drug is influenced by its half-life where the interval is usually half of the drug's half-life.

The selection of drugs to be monitored is dictated by the criteria described above. That is the drug has a narrow therapeutic window, there is marked interindividual variability in its pharmacodynamics and kinetics, coadministration of other drugs, and changes in the patient's condition. Established benefit for therapeutic drug monitoring has been established for several drugs (Tables 1 and 2).

Therapeutic drugs

Antiepileptics

There are about 30 antiepileptic drugs in use for the treatment of patients with epilepsy, some are also used in the management of pain and bipolar disorders (Table 3). The group constitutes the larger components of the therapeutic drug monitoring workload.

The drugs satisfy the requirements for TDM, the serum concentration correlates better with clinical symptoms than dosage, and since the drugs are given prophylactically and seizures occur sporadically clinical assessment alone is problematic and that is often difficult to recognize clinical signs of toxicity which may be confused with that of subtherapeutic levels (toxic levels often exacerbate seizure). Furthermore, there are interindividual variabilities in pharmacokinetics.

Pediatric dosages are much higher (2–3 times higher weight for weight) compared to adults given the high volume of distribution volume.

Antiepileptic drugs continue to be used in pregnancy to control seizures despite their known teratogenic effect. Frequent monitoring is required to maintain seizure-free terms. In general, pregnancy causes plasma concentration of antiepileptics to decline throughout gestation. Pregnancy-associated changes in pharmacokinetics due increased body total volume (decreasing total drug levels while the free biologically active form level to increase). Decreased intestinal motility (marked during the third trimester), renal hepatic blood flow, and cardiac function all influence drug metabolism and elimination. Increased estrogens and progesterone alter hepatic enzymes metabolizing capacity. Metabolism by the placenta and redistribution of the drugs also alters their levels.

In general, antiepileptics with high protein binding are affected by physiological and pathological conditions affecting albumin levels and thus measurement of the free active form of the drug might be more appropriate in those conditions.

The characteristics and utility of the first-generation and newer antiepileptics are shown in Table 3. The indications for monitoring the presence of pharmacologically active metabolites are shown in Table 3.

Several patients (about 30%) are receiving multiple antiepileptics (2 or more), and thus, the likelihood of drug-drug interactions is high. The interaction leads to either increased or decreased circulating levels due to either inhibition or enhanced metabolism by the cytochrome P450 system, respectively. Therapeutic drug monitoring helps monitor and adjusts therapy to compensate for the interaction. It also helps to determine deviation from the median half-life of the drug and identify if the patient is a slow or fast metabolizer and thus allows rapid adjustment of dosage and target concentrations.

Phenytoin

Phenytoin has been in clinical use since 1938. It is used in the treatment and management of tonic-clonic and partial seizures.

It is considered a voltage-gated sodium channel blocker. It binds to the sodium channel in its inactivated state and in doing so prolongs the inactivated states causing a reduction in the high-frequency firing that occurs during seizure. It is also thought to stabilize the brain cell membranes by increasing the levels of neuroinhibitory 5-hydroxtryptamine (serotonin) and gamma-aminobutyric acid (GABA) in the brain.

It is available as either oral, parenteral, or as a sodium-salt intravenous formula. The drug has nonlinear kinetics and a narrow therapeutic window and thus is a candidate for measurement and therapeutic monitoring with a target circulating concentration of 10 to 20 mg/L.

Toxic effects of phenytoin are cerebellar dysfunction (ataxia, diplopia, nystagmus, and tremor), dyskinesia, and peripheral neuropathy. Tremors occur at about 20 mg/L and ataxia at 30 mg/L, and coma at 40 mg/L.

Side effects include allergic reactions, gastrointestinal irritations, gingival hyperplasia (not favored by some patients due to this cosmetic effect), and lymphomas.

Phenytoin is highly protein bound (90%–95%). Total phenytoin measurement accounts for both protein-bound and free fractions. The free fraction (1–2 mg/L target range) diffuses into the blood-brain barrier and thus is considered the pharmacologically active moiety and the development of side effects correlates better with free phenytoin levels compared to total phenytoin.

Patients with hypoalbuminemia and normal total phenytoin levels may exhibit signs of toxicity due to high free phenytoin levels. This is identified by measuring free phenytoin levels.

Factors reducing protein binding include physiological and pathological states of hypoalbuminemia,

TABLE 3 Antiepileptic drugs (year introduced) and their respective pharmacologically active forms (free and their respective percentage) and active metabolites and indications for their respective therapeutic drug monitoring. The free drug species are either of clinical significance and measured (Y) or not (N) measured. N/A (not applicable) where the metabolites are either inactive or their specific measurements add no value.

Antiepileptic drug (year introduced)	Free fraction measured (% Free)	Active metabolites (measured)	TDM indication
Phenobarbital (1912)	Y (52%)	N/A	Predictable pharmacokinetics
Phenytoin (1938)	Y (8%)	N/A	Nonlinear pharmacokinetics. Interindividual variability makes it impossible to predict blood concentration and therapeutic response. Significant drug-drug interactions. TDM invaluable in guiding treatment
Fosphenytoin (1996)	Y (<10%)	Free phenytoin	Phenytoin prodrug. Free phenytoin levels are helpful to guide reloading dosages
Primidone (1952)	Y (≥67%)	Phenobarbital	Not for primidone. Metabolite phenobarbital was measured except when needed to assess compliance. Dosage adjustment is required in liver disease
Ethosuximide (1960)	N (>95%)	N/A	Not indicated. Adjustment based on clinical response. Except in multidrug use to identify drugs causing toxicity
Carbamazepine (1963)	Y (25%)	Carbamazepine epoxide (≤2.3 mg/L)	Interindividual variability with the narrow therapeutic range. Coadministered drugs influence metabolism
Valproate (1974)	Y (7%–26%) concentration dependent	N/A	Interindividual variability with the narrow therapeutic range. Coadministered drugs influence metabolism. Hepatic and polycystic ovary disease side effects
Clobazam (1982)	Y (10%–20%) parent 30% metabolite	N-Desmethylclobazam (0.3–3.0 mg/L)	Dosage adjustment needed in hepatic impairment
Vigabatrin (1989)	N (100%)	N/A	Linear pharmacokinetics. Routine monitoring is not recommended except in patients with renal impairment. Levels 0.8–36 mg/L
Lamotrigine (1991)	Y (34%)	N/A	Monitoring is valuable due to interindividual differences between dose and concentration. Drug-drug interactions. Therapeutic levels at 2.5–15 mg/L. Severe toxicity present with cutaneous rash
Gabapentin (1993)	Y (75%)	N/A	Monitoring is helpful due to nonlinear pharmacokinetics. Interindividual variation in dosage to concentration. Therapeutic levels at 2–20 mg/L.
Felbamate (1993)	N (75%)	N/A 50% unchanged	Not indicated levels do not predict rare adverse effects
Topiramate (1995)	N (83%–91%)	N/A. Inactive metabolites	Linear pharmacokinetics. Routine monitoring is not recommended. Need to monitor bicarbonate levels. Assess hyperchloremic metabolic acidosis
Phenobarbital (1912)	N (45%)	N/A. Inactive metabolites	Monitoring is helpful due to interindividual variability in clearance. Large dose concentration differences
Piracetam (1997)	N (100%)	N/A	Routine monitoring not required except when assessing compliance and signs of toxicity

Continued

TABLE 3 Antiepileptic drugs (year introduced) and their respective pharmacologically active forms (free and their respective percentage) and active metabolites and indications for their respective therapeutic drug monitoring. The free drug species are either of clinical significance and measured (Y) or not (N) measured. N/A (not applicable) where the metabolites are either inactive or their specific measurements add no value—cont'd

Antiepileptic drug (year introduced)	Free fraction measured (% Free)	Active metabolites (measured)	TDM indication
Tiagabine (1998)	N (5%)	N/A	Monitoring is not required. Clinical assessment for side effects and toxicity is required
Oxcarbazepine (2000)	Y (55%)	10-Hydroxycarbazepine	Monitoring helpful. Measure metabolite. Interindividual differences in dose/concentration relationship
Levetiracetam (2000)	N (>90%)	N/A Minor inactive metabolite	Monitoring is not helpful except in suspected drug-drug interaction and compliance. Therapeutic range is 20–40 mg/L
Pregabalin (2004)	N (>95%)	N/A	Little information on target values. Not helpful routine application variable concentration with dose
Zonisamide (2005)	N (50%)	N/A	Monitoring helpful. Levels do not correlate with dosage and drug-drug interaction occurs. Dosage adjustment in renal and hepatic dysfunction is required
Rufinamide (2007)	N (35%)	N/A	Monitoring is valuable due to nonlinear pharmacokinetics. Therapeutic values about 30–40 mg/L or lower in non-Lennox-Gastaut syndrome-associated seizures
Stiripentol (2007)	Y (4%)	Children with severe myoclonic seizures (Dravet syndrome)	Monitoring helpful, nonlinear pharmacokinetics. It is used as an adjunct to other antiepileptics with drug-drug interaction leading to interindividual differences
Lacosamide (2008)	No (>85%)		Dosage adjustment required in renal and hepatic dysfunction
Eslicarbazepine acetate (2009)	N (>60%)	Eslicarbazepine	Dosage adjustment in renal disease
Perampanel (2012)	Y (2%)	N/A	Routine monitoring is not required due to the wide range, except to assess compliance, toxicity, and drug-drug interactions
Brivaracetam (2018)	N (>80%)	N/A	Dosage adjustment in hepatic disease. Inhibits epoxide hydrolase causing an increase in active carbamazepine epoxide metabolite

Modified from Patsalos PN, Spencer EP, Berry DJ. Therapeutic Drug Monitoring of Antiepileptic Drugs in Epilepsy: A 2018 Update. Ther Drug Monit. 2018;40(5):526-548. https://doi.org/10.1097/FTD.0000000000000546. PMID: 29957667.

coadministration of drugs displacing phenytoin from binding, and renal impairment where the accumulation of 3-carboxy-4-methyl-5-propyl-2-furanpropanoic acid impairs phenytoin binding to albumin. Additionally, renal impairment is often accompanied with hypoalbuminemia. Calcium and antacids reduce the bioavailability of phenytoin when administered together.

Phenytoin is metabolized by hepatic cytochrome P450 (CYP-2C9) and to a lesser extent by (CYP 2C19). It is also a potent inducer of the cytochrome P450 enzymes. Phenytoin is metabolized to 5-(p-hydroxyphenyl)-5-phenylhydantoin with further possible metabolism to catechol and quinone and semiquinone.

Phenytoin has zero-order or saturation kinetics that is a slight increase in dose will result in a marked increase in plasma concentration. Most other drugs have first-order kinetics. That is there is a dose/concentration relationship within individuals.

The metabolism of phenytoin is reduced by amiodarone, fluoxetine, fluvoxamine, isoniazid, and azole antifungal agent.[2] Prolonged administration interferes with vitamin D metabolism, leading to an increased risk for osteomalacia. Additionally, prolonged administration may lead to folate deficiency.

In addition to its antiepileptic usage, phenytoin is often used in wound healing, dizziness, migraine, hiccups, myocardial infarction, and in burns patients.

Patients on phenytoin exhibit elevated hepatic gamma-glutamyl transferase (γGT) and alkaline phosphatase metabolizing enzymes as well as increase HDL-cholesterol levels.

Carbamazepine

Carbamazepine is the first-line drug for the treatment of partial and generalized primary tonic-clonic seizures. It is also used in the treatment of epilepsy and bipolar disorder refractory to lithium. It has been in use since the early 1970s.

Carbamazepine, a member of the anticonvulsant drugs, inhibits voltage-gated sodium channels and thus stabilizes membrane excitability. Used for generalized tonic-clonic and partial focal seizures. It is not indicated for the absence of seizures. Its pharmacokinetics are shown in Table 3. With a therapeutic range between 4 and 12 mg/L. The relationship between the carbamazepine concentration and the clinical response is complex. In some patients, the relationship is linear, once a stable level is reached. However, the presence of the active metabolite and individual variability results in a lack of dosage/concentration relationship making therapeutic drug monitoring necessary when seizure control is difficult.

Carbamazepine has fewer side effects than phenytoin or phenobarbital. Toxic effects include blurred vision, ataxia, and dizziness, syndrome of inappropriate antidiuretic hormone (SIADH) may also be present.

It is metabolized by the liver and levels are not influenced by renal function. It stimulates the upregulation and is metabolized by the cytochrome P450 (CYP3A4 and CYP2CB) to carbamezapine-10,11-epoxide with circulating levels at 15%–55% and 5%–81% of total carbamazepine among adults and children, respectively, representing significant interindividual variability with similar activity to the parent drug and a much reduced half-life of the parent drug which is 50% protein bound. Chronic administration enhances clearance.

It is further metabolized to the inactive metabolite carbamazepine-10,11-trans-dihydrdiol by microsomal epoxide hydrolase. About 15% of carbamazepine undergoes glucuronidation by UDP-glucuronosyltransferase.

Similar to other antiepileptics, its metabolism is induced by phenobarbital and phenytoin; however, it is inhibited by valproate and lamotrigine resulting in doubling of the metabolite circulating concentration. It stimulates its

elimination by up to threefold and thus exhibits nonlinear pharmacokinetics.

Clobazam, stiripentol, cimetidine, ciprofloxacin, erythromycin, fluconazole, and ketoconazole among many others inhibit metabolism of carbamazepine leading to increased concentration, whereas coadministration of phenobarbital, phenytoin, primidone, rifampicin, St John's Wort, theophylline, probenecid, among others, induce carbamazepine metabolism and thus decrease its circulating concentration.

Therapy is associated with hyponatremia (<135 mmol/L) as carbamazepine stimulates ADH secretion causing water retention and leading to the observed hyponatremia among 50% of patients beaning treated for epilepsy. Other side effects include cognitive deficits (attention and language), hypersensitivity skin reactions (DRESS; drug rash with eosinophilia and systemic symptoms) in 16% of patients, hepatotoxicity (ALT ≥3 upper limit of normal), cholestasis (alkaline phosphatase ≥2 upper limit of normal), hematological disorders associated with carbamazepine including aplastic anemia, pancytopenia, and decreased RBC granulocytes (neutrophil count $<0.5 \times 10^9$/L).

Bone disorders with a prevalence of 80% low bone density, 48.2% osteopenia, and 31.8% osteoporosis are observed among adults with epilepsy receive carbamazepine. It is possible that carbamazepine induces increased metabolism leading to hypocalcemia, hypophosphatemia, and reduced vitamin D levels associated with increased parathyroid hormone levels. The patients are at increased risk for bone fracture.

Valproate (valproic acid)

Valproic acid is effective in the treatment of myoclonic seizures, generalized absence seizures, and in general and partial epilepsy. It has been in use since the late 1970s with an injectable formulation since the 1990s. It increases gamma-aminobutyric acid (GABA)ergic and glutamatergic neurotransmission.

It exhibits saturable protein binding and thus its pharmacokinetics are nonlinear. It is strongly bound to albumin (≥90%) and thus during pregnancy and in patients with renal disease protein binding is reduced and clearances increased. The free fraction is the pharmacologically active moiety and represents 5%–10%. The total valproate therapeutic range is 50 to 100 mg/L.

Among critically ill patients with marked changes in albumin levels, free valproate levels may be significantly elevated beyond the therapeutic target of 20 mg/L, in the presence of low total valproate measurement. In such patients, measuring total valproate levels cannot predict the free fraction thought to be at 5%–10%. The free fractions are very variable making an estimate based on total concentration highly inaccurate. Therefore, in critical ill patients and in those with low albumin, measuring free valproate levels is preferred. Although formulas are available that predict the amount of free valproate from total measurements, however those appear to be unreliable in critically ill patients. In addition to the low albumin, the presence of uremia may alter albumin binding. Free fatty acids displace valproate from its binding to albumin thought to contribute to the variability seen between fasting and postprandial states.

Valproate causes hyperammonemia and hepatic encephalopathy with little other evidence of hepatic injury. The mechanism of hyperammonemia is that valproate inhibits carbamoyl phosphate synthetase I, the first enzyme in the urea cycle where ammonia, a product of amino acids breakdown and deamination, is converted to urea and as a consequence ammonia levels rise in the absence of other biochemical evidence of liver injury such as elevated transaminases.

The drug pharmacokinetics is shown in Table 3. The drug is metabolized by the cytochrome P450 system. Its clearance is increased by coadministration of phenytoin and phenobarbital as they also stimulate the cytochrome P450. The half-life of the active metabolite (2-N-propyl-3-oxo pentatonic acid) is relatively short compared to the parent drug. Toxic levels are associated with ataxia, nystagmus, unsteady gait, and vomiting.

Common side effects are weight gain, nausea, tremer and vomiting. Hyperammonemia may also occur and the drug is teratogenic.

The development of rare hepatotoxicity is thought to be due to the accumulation of the principal metabolite 4-en-vaproic acid.

Although routine measurement and monitoring of valproic acid are not recommended due to the poor relationship between pharmacokinetics and pharmacodynamics of the drug, measurements may be helpful in the presence of therapeutic failure despite an apparently adequate dosing and that monitoring is less frequent once therapy is established.

Phenobarbital

Phenobarbital, initially used as a sedative and sleep aid, binds to the gamma-aminobutyric acid (GABA)-A-receptor prolonging the opening of the associated chloride channel. It is effective against focal seizures and generalized tonic-clonic seizures but it is not effective against generalized absence seizures. It is the first-line anti-seizure drug in neonatal seizures.

Adverse side effects include sedation, decreased concentration, and mood changes, particularly depression, and in pediatric patients it can cause hyperactivity. Prolonged use is associated with decreased bone density. It has a teratogenic activity and thus it is not recommended for use in pregnancy. Similar to most antiepileptics, it is a potent activator of the hepatic cytochrome P450 enzymes (CYP2C19) and thus enhances the metabolism and clearance of drugs metabolized by CytP450.

It has a long half-life of 80 to 100 h, and although it is mostly metabolized in the liver a quarter of the dose is eliminated unchanged in the urine. For the drug pharmacokinetics, see Table 3. Its predictable pharmacokinetics and long half-life support its therapeutic monitoring. The therapeutic range is 10 to 30 μg/mL with levels >40 μg/mL associated with toxicity.

Clonazepam

It is used for the treatment of absence, tonic and myoclonic seizures. It is also used in the management of status epilepticus and in the treatment of Lennox-Gastaut syndrome as well as off-label use in neonatal seizures.

It exhibits linear pharmacokinetics with rapid absorption and >80% bioavailability. It is metabolized by the CYP3A4 system. Coadministration of carbamazepine, phenobarbital, primidone, and phenobarbital enhances clonazepam metabolism and thus reduces its circulating concentration, whereas felbamate inhibits its metabolism and thus increases its circulating concentration. The therapeutic range is from 0.2 to 0.08 μg/mL with levels >0.08 μg/mL being associated with toxicity.

Gabapentin

It is used in the treatment of partial seizures and in the management of peripheral neuropathic pain. It is rapidly absorbed, not metabolized, and is cleared by the kidney. Its absorption by the L-amino acid transporter is saturable and thus exhibits nonlinear pharmacokinetics. Although gabapentin exhibits little drug-drug interaction and is not metabolized, the variability in absorption between individuals supports its therapeutic level monitoring. The therapeutic range is from 2.0 to 20.0 μg/mL and levels >25.0 μg/mL are associated with toxicity.

Lamotrigine

It is used for monotherapy of partial seizures and primary generalized tonic-clonic seizures in adults and children greater than 12 years old. It exhibits linear pharmacokinetics and rapidly absorbed with >95% bioavailability with 66% protein binding. It is metabolized in the liver primarily by UGT1A4, and to less extent by UGT1A1 and UGT2B7.

Valproic acid inhibits UGT1A4 and thus increases lamotrigine circulating levels, whereas carbamazepine, methsuximide, phenobarbital, phenytoin, primidone, and rufinamide induces the UGT1A4 and thus decreases lamotrigine circulating levels.

There are significant interindividual differences in dose/plasma drug relationship as well as susceptibility to drug-drug pharmacokinetics interactions. This in addition to toxicity causing life-threatening cutaneous rush makes lamotrigine therapeutic monitoring very valuable. The therapeutic range is wide from 2.5 to 15 μg/mL with levels >15 μg/mL associated with toxicity.

Vigabatrin

It is used for the treatment of partial seizures with and without secondary generalization. It is also used for the treatment of infantile spasms. It is rapidly absorbed with a bioavailability of 60% to 80%, not metabolized, and is excreted into the urine. Therefore, its pharmacokinetics are linear, and its routine therapeutic monitoring is not recommended except in patients with impaired renal function to ascertain compliance. Therapeutic range is wide from 0.8 mg/mL to 36 mg/mL.

Primidone

It is used as mono- and polytherapy for focal seizures and generalized tonic-clonic seizures. It is also effective in controlling essential tremors. It exhibits nonlinear pharmacokinetics. It is rapidly absorbed with >90% bioavailability and <33% protein binding. Therapeutic range is narrow from 5 to 10 mg/L.

It is metalized by hepatocytes into two major active metabolites; phenobarbital (25% of oral dose) and phenylethylmalonamide. Its metabolism is enhanced by the coadministration of carbamazepine, and phenytoin, and inhibited by clobazam, ethosuximide, and stiripentol.

Side effects include acute toxic reactions, drowsiness, dizziness, ataxia, nausea and vertigo, and vomiting. Since it is the least tolerated compared with other anticonvulsant drugs, it is the least used in clinical practice.

Rufinamide

It is used for in patients 4 years and older with Lennox-Gastaut syndrome seizures. It is also used off-label in the treatment of partial seizures, myoclonic-astatic epilepsy, and status epilepsy. Mode of action likely delayed sodium channel action potential.

Its pharmacokinetics are concentration dependant being linear up to 1600 mg/dL. It is metabolized by hepatocytes by hydrolysis into carboxylic acid derivative which is excreted into the urine following glucuronidation. Coadministration with carbamazepine, phenobarbital, phenytoin, primidone, and vigabatrin enhances rufinamide metabolism, whereas valproic acid inhibits its elimination and thus increases its circulating levels. It has exhibited significant interindividual variability in the dosage/concentration relationship due to its nonlinear pharmacokinetics. Therefore, therapeutic drug monitoring of rufinamide is valuable. The therapeutic target is 5.0 to 30.0 μg/mL.

Levetiracetam

Used in patients with focal epilepsy (monotherapy) and patients with myoclonic and tonic-clonic seizures. In contrast to other antiepileptics, it is not metabolized by CYP450, and about 75% are exceeded into the urine unchanged. About a third is enzymatically hydrolyzed and excreted as inactive metabolite into the urine. Similar to other antiepileptics, its metabolism is stimulated by coadministered carbamazepine, phenytoin, and phenobarbital increasing clearance by 25% to 37%. Therapeutic levels range from 20 to 40 mg/L; however, routine therapeutic monitoring is not recommended except when drug-drug interactions are suspected.

Cardioactive drugs

A number of cardioactive in use and those with interest in clinical laboratory and are candidates for therapeutic monitoring are discussed.

Digoxin

Digoxin, a cardiac glycoside, and a member of the digitalis group. It binds and inhibits the sodium-potassium ATPase (Na/K ATPase pump) resulting in a primary increase in intracellular sodium content and a secondary increase in intracellular calcium. This causes an increase in the force of myocardial contraction. It also reduces the conductivity of AV nodes (antiarrhythmic) and slows the heart rate. It is used in the management of chronic cardiac failure due to systolic dysfunction. Used in the management of supraventricular arrhythmias and chronic atrial fibrillation.

Following oral administration, 70% is absorbed. Twenty-five percent of digoxin is bound to albumin. The volume of distribution is very large due to the extensive binding to muscle and tissue.

The therapeutic range for digoxin is 0.5 to 2 ng/mL. There is a large interindividual variability. Digoxin is excreted virtually unchanged in the kidney, with 30% to 50% of the daily dose appearing in the urine. Enterohepatic circulation is insignificant. The elimination half-life of the drug is 1.5 to 2 days and in renal patient it is prolonged for 4 to 6 days.

Absorption is decreased by antacids, cholestyramine, and dietary fiber and by drugs such as phenytoin and tacrolimus, which enhances its clearance by inducting the hepatic cytochrome P45 (3A4). St John's Wort reduces plasma digoxin by about 25% which might be due to a combined effect of induction of metabolic clearance by cytochrome P450 and by inhibition of binding to P-glycoprotein in the intestine.

Although food causes a delay in the absorption of digoxin, it will not affect its total absorption and bioavailability. Green tea is shown to significantly reduce digoxin bioavailability.

Patients with severe digoxin toxicity have a mortality rate of 20%. Digoxin cannot be removed from plasma by dialysis; hence, the use of anti-digoxin therapy in the form of "DigiBind" fab fragments binding to circulating digoxin levels and inhibiting its biological activity. DigiBind interferes with immunoassay measurements and once the patient is on DigiBind, digoxin levels cannot be reliably measured where high false values will be obtained.

Hypokalemia and hypermagnesemia potentiate digoxin activity and lead to toxicity. Thus, coadministration of corticosteroids and diuretics (thiazide, furosemide) requires monitoring and appropriate adjustments.

Quinidine, amiodarone, propafenone, and spironolactone increase the concentration of digoxin levels.

Digoxin-like immune reactive substances have been reported in samples from neonates, the elderly, and pregnant patients. Those substances, including adrenocortical hormone and biologically active inhibitors of the sodium/potassium ATPas, variably interfere with commercially available assays, causing falsely high or less frequently falsely low digoxin results, although the interference is less reported with newer assays.

Hypercalcemia potentiates digoxin activity and thus toxicity may occur at an apparent within therapeutic levels of digoxin. Toxicity is also potentiated by hypermagnesemia and hypokalemia.

In summary, circulating digoxin levels directed by therapeutic drug monitoring, may not reflect digoxin tissue concentration in patients on amiodarone, similarly for calcium, potassium, and magnesium levels where abnormal values potentiate digoxin toxicity. Clinical symptoms and signs of toxicity need to be assessed.

Antiarrhythmic drugs

Antiarrhythmic drugs verapamil, diltiazem, and quinidine have an important role in the management of atrial and ventricular arrhythmia. They have a narrow therapeutic window that overlaps with their proarrhythmic effect. They are classified into four different classes depending on their mode of action.

Class I drugs are relatively toxic and their mode of action is the blockade of fast-inward sodium channel in the myocardium (Sodium channel blockers). Therapeutic monitoring is required to avoid toxic levels. They include quinidine, an alkaloid *D*-isomer of the antimalarial drug quinine. It is considered a membrane-stabilizing antiarrhythmic agent with complex cellular effects. It blocks the rapid sodium channel (decreasing the phase of the rapid depolarization of the action potential). It is metabolized by the hepatic cytochrome P450 enzymes with 60% to 80% converted into active metabolites. The volume of distribution of the drug increases with cirrhosis and decreases with congestive heart failure.

Class II agents are antisympathetic, beta-adrenoreceptor blockers are safe and do not require

therapeutic measurement monitoring. Class III are potassium channel blocker antiarrhythmic drugs including sotalol and amiodarone with therapeutic monitoring useful for amiodarone to monitor compliance and toxicity. Class IV are calcium channel blockers and include verapamil and diltiazem. Therapeutic monitoring is often required, and their efficacy is by monitoring their hemodynamic effects.

Bronchodilators

Bronchodilator drugs are used in the treatment of airway disorders such as asthma and chronic obstructive airway disease (COPD). A number of drugs are in routine clinical use and have a narrow therapeutic window and require therapeutic monitoring to minimize toxicity and assure compliance.

Theophylline

Theophylline, a bronchodilator, is used for asthma and stable chronic obstructive pulmonary disease. More effective and less toxic drugs such as anticholinergics bronchodilators are available and theophylline is becoming less widely used.

Theophylline is metabolized in the liver by hydroxylation to 1,3 dimethyl uric acid and by demethylation to 1-methyluric acid.

There is poor relation between dosage and plasma concentration which makes it a candidate for therapeutic drug monitoring. Therapeutic target values are from 10 to 20 mg/L.

Overdosage is commonly associated with hypotension and cardiac arrhythmia. Patients frequently develop hypokalemia and serum potassium levels need to be monitored as levels decrease in patients with theophylline overdosage. Patients develop metabolic acidosis. In patients taking erythromycin, circulating theophylline levels may not reflect tissue concentration.

Caffeine, (in neonates)

Caffeine is the preferred methylxanthine for the treatment of apnea of prematurity. In addition to its long half-life and broad therapeutic profile, it has a number of effects on multiple organs including the lung the brain and the cardiovascular system.

Psychoactive drugs

Antidepressants drugs include lithium, serotonin selective reuptake inhibitors (SSRIs), and tricyclic antidepressants, and although effective they suffer from side effects, and therapeutic monitoring of levels is required.

Lithium

It is used for bipolar disorders, however, the exact mechanism of action is still not clear. There is a poor correlation between dosage and serum concentration as well as significant interindividual variation. Therefore, monitoring is required to aid individualized therapy.

There is no protein binding. It is excreted by the kidney and accumulates at toxic levels in patients with renal impairment.

Lithium distribution exhibits two-compartment model, it is distributed throughout the body and accumulates in brain, thyroid, and kidney. Long-term use is associated with an increased incidence of hypothyroidism (about 20% of patients) and up to 40% develop goiter. Hyperthyroidism due to either thyroiditis or Graves' disease has been reported. Monitoring thyroid function in patients with long-term lithium therapy is required. Additionally, the interfering role of lithium has been utilized in the management of severe hyperthyroidism. Lithium accumulates in the thyroid gland at 3–4 times its circulating concentration. It inhibits colloid formation, and by altering the tertiary structure of thyroglobulin, it reduces tyrosine iodination and thus thyroid hormone formation. Lithium reduces the clearance of free thyroxine and hepatic deiodination.

Lithium interferes with sodium reabsorption in renal tubules. It causes nephrogenic diabetes insipidus secondary to accumulation in renal tubules. Lithium reduces distal tubule response to ADH and thus the ability to concentrate the urine.

Therapeutic targets are variable depending on the disorder, however, typically in the range of 0.5 to 2.8 mmol/L, whereas bipolar disorder may require concentration up to 1.2 mmol/L. Relapse is more likely for concentrations that are lower than 0.5 mmol/L.

It interferes with thyroid function leading to primary hypothyroidism. Measurement of TSH and assessment of eGFR are required every 4–6 months.

Therapeutic monitoring is helpful as plasma concentration is a good guide to effective therapy. Toxic levels are managed via saline infusion or by hemodialysis in severe cases.

The serum lithium levels vary in parallel with the patient's serum urea and creatinine concentrations and alterations in renal function can account for its variation.

Patients on lithium and thiazide diuretics exhibit drug-drug interaction and that measurement of lithium levels to adjust dosage accordingly to maintain therapeutic levels is required.

Amitriptyline (nortriptyline)

Amitriptyline is a tricyclic antidepressant; it blocks serotonin and noradrenaline reuptake in the brain. Its metabolite nortriptyline is more active than the parent drug.

The drug is metabolized by the cytochrome P450 system, and that metabolism is influenced by CYP 2D6 genotyping. It stimulates its own metabolism as well as by other coadministered drugs.

The therapeutic target range is 50 to 150 μg/L with nortriptyline metabolite being more active; it should be measured and that the target range is 80 to 250 μg/L.

Long-acting antipsychotic drugs

A number of new long-acting antipsychotic drugs are available for clinical use. The clinical laboratory plays a role in their therapeutic monitoring. Injectable and oral formulations are in current use. The drugs exhibit significant interindividual variation and therapeutic monitoring assists with dosage selection and with the transition from oral to the injectable formulation.

Therapeutic drug monitoring is recommended for the following drugs, Haloperidol, Fluphenazine, clozapine, Olanzapine, Perazine, Perphenazine, Aripiprazole, Chlorpromazine, Flupentixol, Paliperidone, Quetiapine, N-desalkylquetiapine, Risperidone and metabolite 9-hydroxyrisperidone, Sertindole, and Ziprasidone. Furthermore, therapeutic monitoring is recommended in developing a transition formula for the following antidepressant drugs. Haloperidol, Fluphenazine, and Risperidone.

The pharmacokinetics of long-acting injectable antipsychotic medications are different from their oral formulations. When using the injectable formulations, appropriate sampling is that immediately before the next injection. Peak concentrations are often reached within 1 to 14 days after the initiation of therapy.

Imipramine (and desipramine)

Imipramine and its active metabolite desipramine are used in the treatment of depressive affective disorders. They have narrow therapeutic ranges of 180 to 350 ng/mL, and 115 to 250 ng/mL, respectively, with toxicity at 500 ng/mL for both. Half-life is 12 to 28 and 6 to 28 h for imipramine and desipramine, respectively. There is significant interindividual pharmacokinetics variability for imipramine and desipramine and that therapeutic drug monitoring is helpful in quickly achieving the optimal dosage and in confirming the suspicion of overdose or noncompliance. Furthermore, hydroxylated metabolites exhibit cardiotoxicity, and the levels follow the parent compound concentration.

Antibiotics

Aminoglycosides

Aminoglycosides are broad-spectrum antibacterial antibiotics for gram-negative organisms. They include gentamicin, amikacin, tobramycin, neomycin, and streptomycin. Aminoglycosides interfere with protein synthesis in susceptible microorganisms. The aminoglycosides have poor oral bioavailability and are therefore given parenterally. They are not metabolized, not protein bound, and are excreted by the kidney. Therapeutic drug monitoring is important since the relationship between dosage and concentration is very poor. There is significant intraindividual variation in the rate of absorption distribution and plasma half-life which is dependent on renal function. They have a little therapeutic index where toxicity might occur just above the plasma concentration required for bactericidal activity. Therefore, monitoring the antibiotic levels as well as monitoring for adverse reactions are required. Aminoglycosides can lead to nephrotoxicity, ototoxicity, and rarely to neuromuscular blockade.

In patients with adequate renal function measurement of the trough level of the drug taken within an hour before the second dose is recommended. If the renal function is stable and the trough level is low less than 1 mg/L, no adjustment is necessary, whereas if the level is greater than 1 mg/L the dosing interval may be extended. For patients with renal impairment, dosage adjustment is required.

For patients with extended dosing intervals, the use of established nomograms is helpful. Two nomograms are widely used (Fig. 2). Gentamicin levels at 6 to 14 h after the first dose are measured and the results are plotted on the nomograms to predict the time of the next dose. If the levels are above the Q 48 line, drug administration is stopped and levels are monitored until the time of trough of less than 1 mg/L is ascertained.

The area-under-the-curve measurements have also been used in the management of aminoglycoside dosing regimens. At least two measurements are required for the calculations of the area under the curve. Manual and statistical methods are available for the calculation.

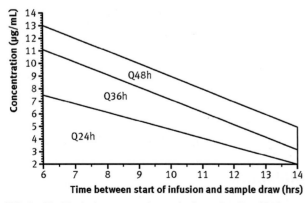

FIG. 2 The Hartford nomogram for monitoring aminoglycoside therapy. *Modified from Banerjee S, Narayanan M, Gould K. Monitoring aminoglycoside level. BMJ. 2012;345:e6354. https://doi.org/10.1136/bmj.e6354. PMID: 23044986.*

The frequency of monitoring aminoglycoside levels depends on the patient's situation. The levels should be monitored at the start of therapy and whenever there are dose adjustments or changes in renal function, the clinical condition of the patient is unstable when frequent monitoring is required.

A number of aminoglycosides have been synthetically modified to overcome resistance due to acetyltransferases, phosphotransferases, and nucleotidyltransferases.

Amikacin is semisynthetically acylated to afford stability against acetyltransferases. Its optimal antibacterial effect occurs when the maximum concentration in serum is 8 to 10 times higher than the minimal inhibitory concentration.

Vancomycin

Active against aerobic and anaerobic gram-positive bacteria.

One of the few available antibiotics to treat methicillin-resistant staphylococcus aureus and methicillin-resistant coagulase-negative staphylococcus species.

It is a 1.45-kDa glycopeptide, unmetabolized where the majority (80%–90%) appear in the urine within 24 h post-dosage. It is given intravenously and distributed throughout body compartments, albeit to varying degree. There is a risk for nephrotoxicity and ototoxicity that increases several folds (three- to fourfold when administered in combination with other aminoglycosides). However, recommended peak and trough therapeutic levels are 30–40 mg/L and 5–10 mg/L, respectively. There is little evidence to support the relationship between serum levels and efficacy or toxicity; additionally, the multicompartment distribution of vancomycin and the fact it is a time-dependent and not a concentration-dependent antibiotic, interpretation of peak values is troublesome and most measurements are now performed on trough levels. Since there is a risk of developing resistance when concentrations are kept prolonged near the minimum inhibitory concentration (MIC), maintaining adequate circulating levels is important and more so in patients with changing renal clearance. Poor penetration to the lungs and the central nervous system may require high circulating concentration to achieve efficacy. It has been recommended that patients with ventilator-associated pneumonia have trough levels in the 15 to 20 mg/L range, hence the need for therapeutic monitoring.

Amikacin

First described in 1972, a broad-spectrum aminoglycoside antibiotic, semisynthetic derivative of kanamycin is typically used in severe gram-negative infections and gram-negative bacteria such as Acinetobacter baumannii and *Pseudomonas aeruginosa*. It is also used in the treatment of neonatal sepsis. It exhibits low protein binding (<12%) and has a half-life of 2–3 h.

Although associated with a risk for nephrotoxicity, there is insufficient evidence to support therapeutic drug monitoring for amikacin. Published target levels are 15–25 μg/mL at peak and <5 μg/mL at trough. Levels >35 and >5 μg/mL at peak and trough, respectively, are associated with toxicity.

Gentamycin

Initially discovered in 1963, it is effective against gram-negative and limited gram-positive organisms; it is not metabolized and excreted in the kidney. Although patients exhibit a slight increase in serum creatinine, persistent renal impairment is relatively rare. It exhibits low protein binding (<10%) and has a half-life of 2–3 h. Published target levels are 4–10 μg/mL at the peak, and <2 μg/mL at the trough with toxicity associated with levels >12 μg/mL and >2 μg/mL for peak and trough, respectively.

Tobramycin

A broad-spectrum aminoglycoside antibiotic appears to have no advantage over commonly used gentamycin. It is used for severe infection, bacteremia, and pneumonia. Organisms include pseudomonas, Enterobacter, Klebsiella, Acinetobacter, Proteus, and Serratias. Its action is via irreversible inhibition of protein synthesis. Similar to the other aminoglycosides, it is not metabolized and excreted into the urine unchanged. It exhibits low protein binding (<10%) with a 2–3-h half-life. Target levels are 5–10 μg/mL at the peak and <2 μg/mL at the trough. Levels >12 μg/mL and >2 μg/mL at peak and at trough, respectively, are associated with toxicity.

Antifungal drugs

Triazole antifungal agents (voriconazole, posaconazole, and itraconazole (hydroxyitraconazole)) are used to treat and prevent systemic fungal infection. They are used as prophylactic in patients receiving immunosuppressants following organ transplant. Monitoring blood concentrations of antifungal agents is important for several reasons; first, there is interindividual variability in the pharmacokinetics of the drug (absorption, metabolism, and clearance), the drugs also have a narrow therapeutic index. The drugs are metabolized by the liver and in patients with liver transplant metabolism may be varied.

The drugs are often given in combination; thus, their simultaneous determinations are helpful. LC-MSMS based methods provide both sensitivity and identification of all coadministered drugs as well as their active metabolite. The availability of rapid, sensitive, and specific assays with a quick turnaround time is important. Trough levels are measured after reaching the steady state which is between 5 and 7 days of therapy.

Fluconazole is used in prophylaxis, empirical therapy, and treatment of superficial and systemic fungal infections. Voriconazole is effective in pulmonary invasive aspergillosis. Posaconazole is used in patients with invasive aspergillosis and prophylaxis for patients with neutropenia and hematopoietic stem-cell transplant, itraconazole, is used in dermatological and those caused by dematiaceous fungus.

Fluconazole and voriconazole exhibit high oral bioavailability compared with itraconazole and posaconazole which are much lower and more variable.

Fluconazole has a wide therapeutic index and thus its routine TDM is not required. Itraconazole, voriconazole, and fluconazole are available as both oral and intravenous preparations, whereas posaconazole is only available orally.

Fluconazole is highly water soluble with low protein binding (11%–12%) and volume of distribution approximating that of total body water achieving 50%–60% of its levels in CSF compared to that in serum.

Fluconazole is excreted unchanged (80%) into the urine with minimal hepatic metabolism, thus requiring dosage adjustment in patients with renal failure with half-life increasing from 30 to 100 h in patients with eGFR <20 mL/min.

Triazoles (itra- and voriconazole) are metabolized in the liver by the cytochrome P450.

Therapeutic target levels are voriconazole and itraconazole is >1 μg/L and posaconazole >1.5 μg/mL. The steady state reached 5–7 days.

Itraconazole, posaconazole, and voriconazole have moderate water solubility and thus volume of distribution ranging from 5 to 25 L/Kg following oral intake. Itraconazole and posaconazole are highly protein bound (>98%), whereas voriconazole is moderately protein bound (58%).

Itraconazole is predominantly metabolized by hepatic CYP3A4 to an active metabolite hydroxyitraconazole. Forty percent of inactive metabolites are excreted into the urine and 3%–18% in stool. It is a strong inhibitor of CYP3A4 and thus extends its half-life. Additionally, the coadministration of drugs metabolized by the CYP3A4 may interact with its metabolism. Thus dosage requires adjustment in patients with hepatic and renal dysfunction.

Voriconazole is predominantly metabolized by hepatic CYP2C19 and to a limited extent by CYP2C9 and CYP3A4, the metabolites are inactive and less than 2% are excreted unchanged in the urine. Genetic variability in the CYP2C19 is the cause of the interindividual variability in circulating levels among patients. Similarly, CYP3A4 plays a role when there is drugs coadministration. Patients with liver dysfunction will have toxic levels of voriconazole and dosages are halved in patients with mild to moderate cirrhosis. Some formulation (e.g., cyclodextrin) is accumulated in patients with renal failure.

Posaconazole is primarily metabolized by UGTs in the liver and is not a substrate for CYP3A4, CYP2C9, or

CYP2C19. Fourteen percent of the conjugated metabolite is excreted into the urine with 66% in the stool. Dosage adjustments are not required in patients with renal or hepatic dysfunction.

Triazole antifungals inhibit fungal cell membrane synthesis by inhibiting the synthesis of ergosterol from lanosterol (inhibits 14-alpha-demthylase enzyme (converts lanosterol to ergosterol)). The differences in the activities of the different antifungals are a reflection of their varied affinities for the 14-alpha-demthylase enzyme.

Although posaconazole has a broader antifungal activity, the combination therapy is important as itraconazole has limited activity against zygomycetes, and voriconazole is effective against some candida (*Candida krusei*) but not all of the fluconazole-resistant species (Candida glabrata and Fusarium).

Immunosuppressants

Patient and graft survival were markedly increased following the introduction and use of immunosuppressants. However, they often have narrow therapeutic window and cause significant toxicity putting the transplanted organ at risk, and their pharmacokinetics are influenced by the coadministration of other drugs.

Mechanism of action is different. They either act as, (1) calcineurin inhibitors (cyclosporin-A, tacrolimus), (2) antimetabolites (mycophenolate mofetil, azathioprine), and (3) mammalian targets of rapamycin inhibitors (mTOR) (sirolimus, everolimus). Commonly used immunosuppressants, cyclosporin, tacrolimus, sirolimus, everolimus, and the antimetabolite mycophenolic acid and azathioprine are individually discussed.

Cyclosporin

An 11 amino acid cyclic polypeptide (molecular weight 12 kDa) is observed. One of the first immunosuppressants was derived from the fungus *Tolypocladium inflatum* in 1972. Its immunosuppressive activity is due to specific and reversible inhibition of immunocompetent lymphocytes in the G0 or G1 phase of the cell cycle where it inhibits calcineurin enzyme (calcium-dependent phosphatase).

It binds to cyclophilin and inhibits calcineurin. Cyclosporin-cyclophilin-immunophilin binds to and inhibits calcineurin.

Cyclosporin dephosphorylates several transcription factors including the nuclear factor of activated T cells (NF-AT) which is present at the promotor regions of regulatory cytokines IL-2, IL-3, Il-4, GMCSF (granulocyte-macrophage colony-stimulating factor), INF-gamma (interferon gamma), and TNF-alpha. This inhibits cytokines production and limits T cell activation.

The increase in TGF-alpha and TGF-beta due to cyclosporin is thought to be responsible for the development of fibrosis in transplanted organs (liver).

Lymphocyte activation and co-stimulation are termed signal 2 pathway where several ligands on the antigen-presenting cells bind to various T cell receptors (CD28, CD154, CD2, CD11a, and CD54). This activates the calcium-calcineurin and the mitogen-activated protein, and the nuclear factor-kB (NF-kB). Cyclosporin and tacrolimus are both calcineurin inhibitors and thus inhibit the signal 2 immune response activation pathway.

The activated T cell nuclear factors do not translocate to the nucleolus in the absence of calcineurin and IL-2 production is inhibited. There is also a decrease in the T cell response to both class I and class II antigens. The outcome is a marked reduction in organ rejection.

It is metabolized by the CYP3A enzyme system in the liver and the gut. Monitoring of circulating levels is required particularly during the first 6 months.

It is highly lipophilic, and is present at higher concentrations in tissue (adipose, renal, hepatic, pancreatic, and adrenal tissue). In blood, cyclosporin is mostly intracellular (41%–58% in erythrocytes, 5%–12% in granulocytes, and 4%–9% in lymphocytes). The intracellular blood levels are approximately threefold higher compared with plasma and the relative distribution between plasma and red blood cells appears to be influenced by temperature.

Circulating levels in plasma are highly bound to protein (greater than 98%), mostly to lipoproteins HDL and LDL and VLDL lipoproteins, and to a lesser extent binding to albumin. Rifampin, nafcillin, rifabutin, and octeriod, among others, increase the CYP450 metabolism of cyclosporin. In contrast, protease inhibitors (indinavir and nelfinavir) inhibit CYP450 and thus lead to increased cyclosporin concentration. Similarly, grapefruit and grapefruit juice increase cyclosporin concentrations.

Side effects are nephrotoxicity, neurotoxicity, hypertension, and dyslipidemia leading to cardiovascular complications. Other side effects include gingival hyperplasia and hirsutism.

Tacrolimus

Tacrolimus inhibits calcineurin but is approximately 100 times more potent than cyclosporin, increasingly replacing the use of cyclosporin. It binds to intracellular FK506 binding protein inhibiting IL-2 mRNA transcription, it inhibits calcineurin phosphatase, and thus inhibits T lymphocyte activation.

Its absorption following oral administration is very variable (5%–67%) influenced by the presence of a high-fat diet decreasing the rate of absorption.

It is present in red blood cells 20- to 30-fold higher compared with plasma. In plasma, it has a high protein binding greater than 98% mostly to albumin and alpha-1 acid glycoprotein. It has a half-life of about 32–48 h. It is extensively metabolized by the CYP3A4 and that 13-dimethyl tacrolimus is the major metabolite. Less than 1% is excreted unchanged in the urine.

Side effects are nephrotoxicity, neurotoxicity, hypertension, diabetes, and dyslipidemia leading to cardiovascular complications.

Drug interactions are mainly related to those stimulating the CYP450 system, they include anticonvulsants, herbal supplements. St John's Wort causes a marked reduction in blood concentration leading to subtherapeutic levels and risk of rejection of the transplanted organ.

Other drugs inhibiting CYP450 and thus increasing the immunosuppressants examples are calcium channel blockers (diltiazem, verapamil, nicardipine), antibiotics (e.g., azithromycin,), antifungals, as well as amiodarone, allopurinol, bromocriptine, colchicine, and metoclopramide.

Sirolimus

A macrolide, although originally isolated as an antifungal agent as rapamycin (from Rapa Nui—Eastern Island), was subsequently shown to have antitumor and immunosuppressive activity. It is a potent inhibitor of antigen-induced proliferation of T and B cells and of antibody production.

Sirolimus forms in an immunosuppressive complex with the intracellular protein FKBP12. The complex blocks the activation of the cell cycle-specific kinase TOR.

The correlation between steady-state trough levels and the area under the curve favors its therapeutic drug monitoring given the narrow therapeutic window. Target trough concentration ranges from 5 to 15 µg/L when coadministered with cyclosporin (trough levels at 75–15 µg/L). Weekly monitoring is recommended for the first month and then biweekly for the next month and then after only measured when its clinically indicated.

Marked interindividual variability in P-glycoprotein and Cyt P450 (8.5- to 9.4-fold variability) supports its therapeutic measurement.

It is distributed among red blood cells (94.5%), plasma (3.1%), lymphocytes (1%), and granulocytes (1%); this is in contrast to tacrolimus and cyclosporine where the distribution is not temperature dependent. Their sequestration inside red blood cells may be partially related to binding to immunophilin. Blood samples are collected in EDTA whole blood tubes.

Tacrolimus as well as cyclosporin forms a complex with calcineurin, calcium calmodulin-dependent serine/threonine phosphatase causing its inactivation. This inhibits calcineurin ability to phosphorylate the cytoplasmic subunit of the nuclear factor of activation of T cells, blocking its translocation to the nucleus which is required for the transcription of the cytokine genes.

Everolimus

A macrolide immunosuppressant with a molecular weight of 957.6 Da. It has a 2-hydroxyethyl chain substitution at position 40 on the sirolimus structure producing everolimus with a higher degree of polarity improving its bioavailability when taken orally. Its bioavailability is 16% when taken orally compared to sirolimus 10%. Its absorption is affected by the variability of the P-glycoprotein.

Similar to the other macrolide immunosuppressants (cyclosporin, tacrolimus, and sirolimus), more than 75% of everolimus is bound to erythrocytes; thus, whole blood sample collected in EDTA blood tubes is the specimen of choice.

It blocks the T cell response to alloantigen which is at a later stage compared to that of cyclosporin and tacrolimus calcineurin inhibition.

Similar to sirolimus, it inhibits cell proliferation by blocking cell cycle progression from the G1 phase to the S phase-mediated binding to immunophilin FK506-binding protein 12 (FKBP12). The everolimus/FKBP12 complex inhibits protein kinase TOR (target of rapamycin) leading to the arrest of the G1 cell cycle. Its binding to the FKBP12 protein affinity is twofold lower than that for sirolimus.

Although at steady state trough concentration is a reliable index of everolimus dosage, variable oral bioavailability and narrow therapeutic index support its routine measurement of its blood concentration. Target levels are in the range of 3 to 15 µg/L when coadministered with cyclosporin, and trough levels at 100–300 µg/L when given with prednisolone.

This difference in mechanism provides a synergistic effect and thus allows for the administration of cyclosporine and everolimus at much lower doses reducing side effects.

It is rapidly absorbed reaching a peak concentration at 1.3 to 1.8 h and steady state is reached within 7 days. It has lower nephrotoxicity compared with cyclosporine and tacrolimus. Side effects of the drug include hypertriglyceridemia, hypercholesterolemia, opportunistic infections, thrombocytopenia, and leukocytopenia.

The drug is metabolized by the cytochrome P450 (3A4, 3A5, and 2C8). Hepatic impairment and coadministration of drugs metabolized by this cytochrome system leads to differences between individuals. The clearance of the drug is significantly reduced in patients with liver impairment requiring a reduction in the dosage of the drug (reduced by half).

Mycophenolate

Mycophenolate mofetil (MMF) is the first-line drug in use for solid organ transplantation and has been widely used for years. Mycophenolic acid is an inhibitor of the inosine monophosphate dehydrogenase enzyme required for the de novo synthesis of purines. Thus deleting guanosine nucleotides, this action blocks both T and B lymphocyte proliferation. It is a fivefold more potent inhibitor of the type II isoform expressed in activated lymphocytes, whereas type I is expressed in most other cell types.

MPA induces apoptosis of activated T-lymphocytes (eliminating antigenic targeted clones). It suppresses glycosylation and thus the expression of adhesion molecules, decreasing the recruitment of lymphocytes to rejection and inflammation sites. By depleting guanosine nucleotides, it depletes tetrahydrobiopterin a cofactor for an inducible form of nitric oxide synthase.

It is coadministered with cyclosporine, tacrolimus, sirolimus, everolimus, and corticosteroids as an immunosuppressant in kidney, heart, and liver transplants.

The two widely used formulations are enterically coated to reduce gastrointestinal side effects such as bleeding.

The principal metabolite phenolic glucuronide formed following conjugation in the liver is subject to enterohepatic recycling when de-glucuronidation in the intestine followed by reabsorption of mycophenolic acid exhibits a second serum peak 6–8 h following ingestion.

Factors affecting mycophenolate concentrations include coadministration with cyclosporin which inhibits the enzyme transporter multidrug resistance-associated protein-2 found in the bile canalicular membrane. This leads to a reduction in mycophenolate glucuronide entering the gut and thus a reduction of the enterohepatic recirculation.

Changes in albumin concentration and renal function following renal transplantation lead to reduced clearance of mycophenolic acid.

The drug has a relatively wide therapeutic index; however, significant interindividual variation between the drug dose and concentration (area under the curve) supports the need for therapeutic drug monitoring initially and during coadministration with other immunosuppressants and in changing kidney and hepatic function.

Drugs in oncology

Methotrexate

Initially, it is used in the treatment of choriocarcinoma and is considered as the first chemotherapeutic agent. Methotrexate is effective in the treatment of childhood leukemias. Lower doses are used to treat rheumatoid arthritis and psoriasis. It inhibits dihydrofolate reductase leading to a reduction in folate levels required for the synthesis of purines.

It does not cross the blood-brain barrier and intrathecal introduction is required when used for the treatment of central nervous system tumors.

Methotrexate exhibits a triphasic elimination profile with the initial phase reflecting distribution, the second phase reflecting renal elimination, and the final phase reflecting elimination from the intracellular distribution. Its elimination may be reduced in the presence of renal failure. It is excreted 90% unchanged in the urine, and if given in high dosage, it carries a risk for renal toxicity.

Cisplatin (Carboplatin)

Cisplatin, the first metal-based chemotherapeutic agent, it is used in a number of solid malignancies such as testicular, ovarian, and lung, including head and neck squamous cell carcinoma, among others. It results in apoptosis following a sequence of events. It interacts with DNA purine bases, followed by the activation of several signal transduction pathways. Cisplatin has significant side effects by accumulating inside cells. Additionally, DNA repair and inactivation of cisplatin by glutathione and metallothionein lead to drug resistance. To minimize the side effects and resistance, combination therapies are often used.

Cisplatin undergoes irreversible protein binding and accumulates within cells leading to a risk of toxicity and thus a major risk for nephrotoxicity. Therapeutic drug monitoring by determining the area under the curve and the clearance rate following initiation of therapy is shown to be helpful particularly in pediatrics and in reducing toxicity and side effects. Patients who are not candidates for cisplatin may be treated with carboplatin. Carboplatin has less nephrotoxicity and neurological sequelae compared to cisplatin.

Thiopurine methyl transferase (TPMT)

Thiopurine drugs (mercaptopurine, azathioprine, and 6-thiouguanine) are used as antimetabolites in the treatment of acute lymphoblastic leukemia, as immunosuppressants in organ transplant, and in the management of patients with inflammatory bowel disease.

The drugs are metabolized by intestinal and hepatic enzymes (thiopurine methyltransferase (TPMT), hypoxanthine phosphoribosyl transferase (HPRT), xanthine oxidase (XO), and inosine monophosphate dehydrogenase (IMPDH)) with a number of metabolites detected. Those metabolites actively mediate the pharmacological effect of thiopurines (6-thioguaniner nucleotides (6TGN) and 6-methylmercaptopurine ribonucleotides (6MMPR) and inactive the metabolites 6-thiouruic acid (6RU) and 6-mercaptopurine (6MMR)).

6MMPR is produced by TPMT and levels >5700 pmol/$8 \times 10^*8$ red blood cells are associated with hepatotoxicity. 6TGN is catalyzed by IMPDH and concentrations ≥ 235 pmol/$8 \times 10^*8$ RBCs and ≥ 450 pmol/$8 \times 10^*8$ RBCs are associated with clinical remission and hematological toxicity, respectively, although the values remain controversial.

Hepatotoxicity is classified into: hypersensitivity, idiosyncratic cholestatic reaction, and nodular regenerative hyperplasia.

There is interindividual variability partially due to pharmacogenetics variation in drug metabolism and thus therapeutic drug monitoring is essential to maintain efficacy. Monitoring of 6MMPR helps identify patients at risk of hepatotoxicity.

A deficiency of TPMT activity leads to the accumulation of thiopurine and myelosuppression.

Red blood cell thiopurine methyl transferase enzyme activity is measured to assess the risk of myelotoxicity.

Although there is good correlation between genotyping and phenotyping of the enzyme in most patients, it is reported to be poor in patients treated for acute lymphoblastic leukemia and that genotyping assessment is preferred.

Patients should be assessed for TPMT activity before initiation of thiopurine therapy.

Red blood cell 6TGN and 6MMPR levels are measured 4 to 8 weeks after initiation of thiopurine therapy where levels above 230–260 pmol/$8 \times 10*8$ RBC are more likely to be in clinical remission. Therapeutic drug monitoring of red blood cells TGN and MMPR levels guides dosage adjustments to maintain efficacy and reduce toxicity.

Patients considered to be hyper-methylators of thiopurine will have a subtherapeutic TGN levels and a ratio of red blood cells MMPR to TGN of >11 and thus poor response to therapy.

Thiopurine metabolites monitoring in children with inflammatory bowel disease

Thiopurine therapy in children is widely used (>70% of children with inflammatory bowel disease). Mercaptopurine and azathioprine are commonly used in children.

Thiopurine methyltransferase red blood cell activity and genotype as well as thiopurine metabolites are measured as part of therapeutic drug monitoring and adjustments are largely based on white blood cell count to minimize the risk for myelosuppression.

Azathioprine

Azathioprine (Imran) is used as an immunosuppressant in the prevention of kidney transplant rejection among other indications such as rheumatoid arthritis, systemic lupus erythematosus, and ulcerative colitis. Patients homozygous or heterozygous for thiopurine methyltransferase deficiency are at risk of developing myelosuppression. Red blood cell thiopurine methyltransferase activity is measured to assess the adequacy of enzymatic activity prior to initiation of therapy.

6-Mercaptopurine

6-Mecraptopurine is a metabolite of azathioprine. Its measurement reflects azathioprine therapy, whereas therapeutic target levels have not been established, circulating 6-mercaptopurine levels below 1000 ng/mL is indicative of usual dosage regimens. It is also available as standalone therapy (Purinethol).

Busulfan/Melphalan

Busulfan is an alkylating agent used to obliterate bone marrow cells in preparation for hemopoietic stem cell transplantation.

Cytotoxic DNA alkylating agents are used in conditioning regimen for hematopoietic stem cell transplantation.

Busulfan is used as a component of the chemotherapy regimen prior to hematopoietic stem cell transplantation. It is used to ablate bone marrow cells prior to stem cell transplantation. Therapeutic monitoring of busulfan is helpful in avoiding veno-occlusive disorders, disease relapse, and engraftment failure.

The drug is administered intravenously, and its pharmacokinetics are monitored to avoid toxicity while ensuring delivery of adequate dosage to achieve complete bone marrow ablation. The area under the curve is determined and the clearance rate is calculated following the administration of the initial dose. The usual dosage regimen is 0.8 mg/Kg body weight (or ideal body weight—whichever is lower) every 6 h for a total of 16 doses. Time blood collection samples (at end infusion, a minimum of four samples with the initial sample collected immediately after the infusion is stopped, followed by samples at 1, 2, and 4–2 h after infusion stop) are used to calculate the area under the curve and the drug clearance rate. The ideal area under the curve (cumulative dose) is 1100 μmol/L/min with values above 1500 μmol/L/min associated with toxicity, whereas values lower than 900 μmol/L/min are seen in incomplete bone marrow suppression. Normal clearance rate is 2.1 to 3.5 mL/min/Kg.

Melphalan is used to treat malignant disease especially prior to the stem cell transplant for multiple myeloma and amyloidosis. The two drugs are often given together shortening patient length of stay (Table 4).

Biomarkers in immunotherapy

Several humanized monoclonal antibodies-based therapeutics are available. They are often measured to assess compliance to optimize and individualize therapy. Commonly used drugs are discussed here.

Ustekinumab and vedolizumab antibodies levels

Immunotherapy is increasingly being used to individualize therapy and manage the disease. For example, anti-TNF-alpha,

TABLE 4 Drugs commonly measured in therapeutic monitoring. Protein binding (PB), volume of distribution (V_d), and half-life ($T_{1/2}$).

Drugs		PB (%)	V_d (L/Kg)	$T_{1/2}$ (h)	Therapeutic target range
Antiepileptics	Phenytoin	90	0.65	6–24	5–20 mg/L
	Phenobarbital	50	0.6	80–120	10–40 mg/L
	Carbamazepine	75	1.0–1.8	10–20	4–12 mg/L
	Valproate	95	0.15–0.3	11–17	50–100 mg/L
	Primidone	≤35		4–22	5–15 mg/L
Cardioactive	Digoxin	25	7	36	1.0–1.2 µg/L
	Quinidine	80–90		6–9	2–5 mg/L
	Amiodarone	>98	70	50	0.5–2.5 mg/L
Bronchodilators	Theophylline	60	0.4–0.6	3–9	10–20 mg/L
	Caffeine	35	0.9	40–230	5–20 mg/L
Psychoactive	Lithium	0	0.5–0.8	10–35	0.5–0.8 mmol/L
	Amitriptyline	95	15	20	50–150 µg/L (nortriptyline metabolite 80–250 µg/L)
	Imipramine	63–96		6–28	150–250 µg/L
Oncology	Methotrexate	50%–60%		2–4 (initial), 8–15 (terminal)	≥5 µmol/L (24 h), ≥ 0.5 µmol/L (48 h), ≥0.05 µmol/L (72 h)
Aminoglycosides antibiotics	Gentamicin	<0.1%	0.18–0.52	2–3 h	5–10 mg/L (peak), <2 mg/L (trough)
	Amikacin	<0.1%	0.14–0.36	2–3 h	20–30 mg/L (peak), < 5 mg/L (trough)
	Vancomycin	10%–50%	0.4–1	6–12 h	20–40 mg/L (peak), 5–10 mg/L (trough)
	Tobramycin	<0.1%	0.1–0.3	2–3 h	5–10 mg/L (peak), < 2 mg/L (trough)
Antifungals antibiotics	Voriconazole	58%	4.6	6–24	1.0–6.0 µg/mL
	Posaconazole	99%	7–25	15–35	0.5–0.7 µg/mL
	Itraconazole	99%	11	35–64	1–2 µg/mL
	Fluconazole	12%	0.7–0.8	22–81	15–35 mg/mL
Immunosuppressants	Cyclosporin	98%	6.4	11.6	150–350 µg/L
	Tacrolimus	98%	0.5–1.4	10–20	5–20 ng/mL
	Sirolimus	92%	5.6–16.7	62	5–15 ng/mL
	Everolimus		1.3–1.8		3–8 ng/mL
	Mycophenolic acid	98%	1.6	17	1–3.5 µg/mL

Modified from respective drug leaflet and British Pharmacopeia (2018): The Stationery Office; 2019th edition. ISBN-10: 0113230702. ISBN-13: 978-011323070.

IL-12/23p40 antibodies are widely used in the treatment of moderate-to-severe active inflammatory bowel disorders such as ulcerative colitis and Crohn's disease.

Ustekinumab

A fully human IgG1 monoclonal antibody targeting the p40 subunit of IL-12 and IL-23. Initially approved for use in psoriatic arthritis and psoriasis, it is used in patients with Crohn's disease. There is considerably interindividual variability in the pharmacokinetics. The median clearance in patients with weight >100 kg is 55% higher compared with the patients with lower weight; furthermore, clearance is also affected by albumin, C-reactive protein, gender, and race. This interindividual variability in clearance supports therapeutic drug monitoring at dosing troughs.

Vedolizumab

Vedolizumab antibody is an IgG1 fully humanized antibody directed toward α4-β7 integrin expressed on a subset of leukocytes and thus modulates lymphocyte trafficking in the intestine without introducing systemic immunosuppression. The antibody does not bind to the majority of memory CD4 T-lymphocytes (60%), neutrophils, and monocytes. The predominant binding is to 25% of peripheral blood memory CD4 T-lymphocytes including IL-17 T-helper lymphocytes. The pharmacological properties of the drug limit its action to the gastrointestinal system and thus avoid systemic effects.

There is a concentration-dependent clearance of the antibody with a slow linear elimination at a concentration of about 10 μg/mL and a more rapid nonlinear elimination at lower concentration. Increased clearance is seen in patients with low albumin (<3.2 g/dL) and high body weight (>120 kg). This interindividual variation supports its therapeutic drug monitoring.

Other drugs of clinical interest

Nicotine and metabolites

This is used to identify patients using tobacco and to monitor patients on nicotine replacement therapy. It is often measured in candidates for and those undergoing plastic surgery. It influences the operative plan and surgical outcomes; it interferes with wound healing in patients with elective cosmetic surgery. The success of plastic surgery judged by patients by symmetry, contour, and minimal scarring. Each area is adversely affected by cigarette smoke.

Nicotine stimulates alpha receptors causing vasoconstriction and poor oxygen delivery to the tissue. This particularly affects large flaps of skin and cutaneous tissue operation where survival and attachment are determined solely by a random pattern of blood supply. Those effects are seen in abdominoplasty, rhytidectomy (face lifting), and breast surgery.

Nicotine present in tobacco is metabolized by hepatocytes to cotinine which is excreted into the urine. The amount of urinary cotinine is proportional to the amount of tobacco dosage and to hepatic metabolism which appears to be genetically predetermined. Nicotine and cotinine levels in urine range from 1000 to 5000 ng/mL and from 1000 to 8000 ng/mL, respectively.

In addition to nicotine, tobacco products include anabasine and nornicotine. The finding of those alkaloids in urine indicates the recent use of tobacco. Nornicotine is present in nicotine replacement products and its detection in the absence of anabasine indicates that tobacco is not the source, and the patient is compliant with replacement therapy.

Anabasine >10 ng/mL and/or nornicotine >30 ng/mL indicates tobacco use. Passive exposure to tobacco shows contine levels up to 20 ng/mL with nornicotine and anabasine undetectable.

Rivaroxaban

An anticoagulant is used in the treatment of vein thrombosis and prophylactically in atrial fibrillation and post-knee replacement. It is a competitive inhibitor of free and clot-based factor Xa. It is administered orally at 20 mg daily with mean and range circulating blood concentration 270 ng/mL (189–419) reached 2–4 h post-dosage and median trough 26 ng/mL (range 6 to 87 ng/mL). It is cleared by the kidney (36%), and thus, its measurement is of value in patients with impaired renal function, in the elderly and in obese patients, in the assessment of compliance and of suspected overdosage, and in suspected drug-drug reactions. Routine monitoring of levels is not indicated.

Leflunomide levels

Leflunomide is used in the management of rheumatoid arthritis. Therapeutic monitoring is required due to marked pharmacokinetics interindividual variability. Measurement performed to confirm compliance and clearance. Levels above 40 mg/L are associated with improved clinical outcomes. Drug levels should be <0.02 mg/L if wanting to start a pregnancy. Lower levels are needed when the hepatic function is decreased. Cholestyramine helps with clearance.

Dexamethasone

Dexamethasone levels are measured to confirm therapeutic compliance. Its measurement is particularly helpful in patients receiving long term low dose and exhibiting dexamethasone suppression test failure.

Urine screening for other synthetic steroids (see below) is performed in patients suspected of taking nonprescribed steroids, or to confirm therapeutic compliance.

Urine levels <0.1 μg/dL is considered negative for the following synthetic steriods (Betamethasone, dexamethasone, fludrocortisone, fluticasone propionate, megestrol acetate, methylprednisolone, prednisolone, prednisone, and triamcinolone acetonide. Levels <0.2 μg/dL cutoff for budesonide is considered negative.

Drugs-associated biomarkers

Ammonia

Sodium valproate causes a significant elevation of blood ammonia levels. Patients may present with significant hyperammonemia. Lipids (hypertriglyceridemia and hypocholesteremia) are seen in patients receiving macrolides immunosuppressants (sirolimus, everolimus, and tacrolimus). Urea and creatinine are measured in the assessment of renal function in patients on aminoglycosides.

Renal and haptic dysfunction markers

Drugs undergo hepatic and/or renal metabolism and clearance. Hepatic and renal functions are often assessed prior to and during drug therapeutic drug administration. The glomerular filtration rate is assessed using the Cockcroft formula and/or the newly adopted CKD-Epi refit formula. Although the latter is widely used in clinical practice, the Cockcroft formula is preferred in therapeutics as it incorporates body weight in the calculation often required for dosage assignment.

Drugs, by nature of the need for their therapeutic monitoring, require continued assessment for hepatic and/or nephrotoxicity from the drug, its metabolites, or to unrelated changing hepatic and renal functions.

Hepatic function is monitored by measuring its synthesis and clearance for bilirubin and ammonia, respectively. Liver enzymes (ALT and AST) are measured as indicators for liver injury and/or hepatitis.

Herbal supplements and interference

Thousands of herbal supplements are commercially available, and their consumption is rapidly increasing with about 80% of the world population having used or attempted herbal supplements. About 12% of herbal supplements have reported safety concerns and approximately 2000 patients a month visit the emergency department with complaints related to herbal supplements. The most commonly used are echinacea, ginseng, St John's Wort, chamomile, and kava among many others. Herbal supplements may interfere with laboratory biomarkers either in vivo or in vitro testing. For instance, St John's Worts, as herbal antidepressant, (hypericin, hyperforin, and quercetin stimulates CYP3A4) stimulates metabolism of cyclosporin and is reported to

reduce blood concentration by as much as 50% leading to subtherapeutic levels and putting the transplanted organ at risk for rejection. Similar reduction in the anticonvulsant drugs, phenytoin and phenobarbital, is observed.

In vitro interference examples include; bufalin present in Chan Su and Lu-Shen-Wan Chinese herbal medicine, and oleandrin present in oleander-containing herbs are structurally similar to digoxin and interfere with digoxin immunoassays.

Furanocoumarins present in grapefruit juice inhibit intestinal CYP3A4 but not hepatic. This leads to an increase in the affected drugs' bioavailability, an effect lasting up to 12 h. It also has P-glycoprotein. It significantly increased bioavailability of many drugs (immunosuppressants, amiodarone, statins, carbamazepine, methadone, oxycodone, benzodiazepines, and antiplatelet agents, among many). Drugs administered in their prodrug form and require to be metabolized to the active form will exhibit reduced bioavailability.

Clinical toxicology

Poisoning accounts for around 10% of acute medical admissions. Clinical toxicology investigations account for <1% of biochemistry tests. This is mainly because, often the history and circumstances indicate the agent, symptoms of some important poisonings allow a clinical diagnosis, and many poisonings require conservative management, i.e., symptomatically.

The decision to test for suspected abuse or poisoning and the reason for the request depends on if knowing the drug's identity or concentration will provide no change in therapy or have no diagnostic or prognostic significance.

About 8.8% of adolescence age 12 to 17 admitted to using any illicit drugs including marijuana, prescription medication, cocaine, hallucinogens, methamphetamine, inhalants, and heroin. The range of drugs encountered is often influenced by what is trending and what is readily and affordably available on the street or as over-the-counter items. The frequency and types are dynamic, and the clinical toxicology laboratory must keep track of trends. Presentations at the emergency department, media, drug enforcement agencies reports, and seizures often guide the laboratory to ensure the availability of appropriate tests. The following drugs are often encountered.

Although qualitative determination is necessary, quantitative measurements are of value in limited poisoning and toxicology scenarios.

Toxicology testing is valuable in the differential diagnosis between poisoning and other causes of symptoms, e.g., coma. When an antidote is available, and that therapy will be changed if the drug can be identified. Toxicology testing is performed as part of employment screening, licensing, organ donation, and surgical management, e.g., nicotine in plastic surgery, among others.

Misinterpretation can have significant consequences for the patient. (Interference positive or negative results).

Point-of-care testing is widely and increasingly being used at pain management psychiatric clinics allowing for the clinician to discuss with the patient in real time and make necessary adjustments to prescriptions. Awareness of the limitation of the different assays (false positives as well as more importantly negative) results. The POCT devices often include adulterant checks in the form of specific gravity (indication of how to dilute the urine sample). A highly dilute sample (excessive intentional water drinking) dilutes the concentration of the substances to below the assay cutoff values, and oxidative measures (presence of oxidizing agents interfering with color formation and with assay reaction).

Testing for possible sample adulteration. Check urine temperature (should be 90–100 F) within 4 min of collection. Specific gravity should be between 1.002 and 1.030, and urine pH variable between 4.5 and 8.0, and urine creatinine is >20 mg/dL.

Adulterants commonly used include household bleach, table salt, vinegar, lemon juice, ammonia, and eye drops all those with the exception of the latter may be inferred by using the adulterants checks mentioned earlier.

Cutoffs are designed to avoid false-positive results particularly in the workplace (poppy seeds ingestion causing false-positive opiates, and passive inhalation of marijuana cause positive cannabinoid test).

Alcohols and metabolites

Alcohols of clinical interest are ethanol, methanol, ethylene glycol, isopropanol, and their respective metabolites. They are detectable in blood, urine, and saliva. In forensics postmortem settings, samples such as vitreous humor and skeletal muscle are alternate samples. Methods for alcohol measurements are either enzymatically based spectrophotometric analysis or gas chromatographic and mass spectrophotometric methods.

Ethanol

It is widely abused with characteristic clinical signs. Plasma concentration is poorly guided except at high levels of severity. Serum osmolar gap provides a rough guide to concentration/.

It is metabolized by hepatic ADH to acetaldehyde which is oxidized by aldehyde dehydrogenase to acetic acid. Its elimination rate is about 15 mg/dL/hr. which is prolonged, nearly doubled at about 30 mg/dL/hr. in chronic alcoholics.

Alcohol is measured to assess intake either in an acute setting presentation in the emergency department or as part

of the rehabilitation programs. Alcohol can be measured either in blood or in urine and its measurement indicate a very recent consumption. It is cleared from the blood and thus cannot assess the extent of chronic consumption where measurement of its metabolites is more helpful.

The metabolites are fatty acid ethyl esters, ethyl glucuronide (EtG), ethyl sulfate (EtS), and phosphatidyl ethanol (PEth).

Fatty acid ethyl esters (FAEE) are formed by enzymatic esterification of ethanol with free endogenous fatty acids, triglycerides, lipoproteins, and phospholipids by FAEE synthase and acyl-CoA ethanol O-acyl transferase.

FAEE does not cross the placenta, whereas ethanol does; therefore, FAEE in meconium is an indicator of fetal exposure to alcohol. Detection of alcohol metabolites (EtG, FAEE, and PEth) confirms chronic consumption. The detection cutoff for meconium EtG is recommended to be 2 nmol/g.

EtG is a minor metabolite of ethanol formed after conjugation with glucuronic acid by UDP-glucuronyl transferases. It is thus very sensitive and specific to alcohol consumption.

0.02% to 0.06% of consumed alcohol is eliminated in the urine and EtG can be detected in urine 3–5 days after alcohol is negative in blood. It can be detected in blood up to 18 h after alcohol is negative.

Several diagnostic cutoffs have been used for the detection and classification of alcohol consumption. The difficulties are in considering variation in social and occasional consumption. Detection times for alcohol metabolites are EtG (up to 80 h in urine), 18 h in blood, and 8 h in plasma. PEth is detectable up to 7 days in blood following alcohol ingestion and up to 29 days in the chronic abuser. The following are widely used (Table 5).

Phosphatidyl ethanol (PEth)

Phosphatidyl ethanol is formed by when ethanol reacts with phosphatidylcholine, present in cell membranes, catalyzed by phospholipase D.

PEth exists in a number of species with a common nonpolar head group with two attached double-bond fatty acid moieties are attached. The chain lengths are varied depending on alcohol consumption history, with the body disorders, diet, and genetic variability, the different species and their predominance are shown in Table 6.

Gamma glutamyl transferase (gGT)

Microsomal hepatic enzyme is stimulated by alcohol and is elevated in chronic alcohol intake. It is elevated in cholestatic liver disease and is also stimulated by anticonvulsants such as phenytoin and carbamazepine alone and without the

TABLE 5 Biomarkers of alcohol intake (amount and chronicity) and observed test sensitivity and specificity.

Analyte	Amount	Sample levels	Sensitivity	Specificity
Ethanol		>14 ng/mL		
Ethanol glucuronide (EtG) (Urine)	Blood alcohol level 1.2 g/L after 24 h	Urine: ≥100 ng/mL	100	
	Blood alcohol level 0.2 g/L after 24 h		50% after 24 h 100% after 12 h	
	Abstinence monitoring		89%	99%
Phosphatidyl ethanol (PEth)	Moderate intake Heavy or chronic intake	Blood: ≥20 ng/mL >200 ng/mL	88%–100%	48%–89%
CDT	Chronic and excessive drinking	Blood: ≥1.7% (2–3 weeks)	46%–90%	70%–100%
gGT	Chronic and excessive intake	Blood: >54 IU/L	37%–95%	18%–93%
MCV	Chronic and excessive intake		40%–50%	80%–90%
Combined (CDT, MCV, and gGT)	Chronic and excessive intake		88%	95%

EtG, Ethyl glucuronide; EtS, Ethyl sulfate; PEth, Phosphatidyl ethanol; CDT, Carbohydrate deficient transferrin; MCV, Mean corpuscular volume.
Modified from Andresen-Streichert H, Muller A, Glahn A, Skopp G, Sterneck M. Alcohol biomarkers in clinical and forensic contexts. Dtsch Arztebl Int 2018;115(18):309–315.

TABLE 6 Phosphatidyl ethanol metabolites ratios as indicators of chronic alcohol abuse.

Consumption	PEth species	Percentage of blood total PEth
Abusive drinkers	16:0/18:1, 16:0/18:1	46%, 26%–28%
	16:0/20:4, or 18:1/18:1 and 18:0/18:2	8%–13%, 11%–12%
	16:0/16:0, 16:0/20:3, 18:0/18:1, and 18:1/18:2	1%–5%

Modified from Nathalie Hill-Kapturczak, Donald M. Dougherty, John D. Roache, Tara E. Karns-Wright, Marisa Lopez-Cruzan, Martin A. Javors, Chapter 58. Phosphatidylethanol Homologs in Blood as Biomarkers for the Time Frame and Amount of Recent Alcohol Consumption, Editor(s): Victor R. Preedy, Neuroscience of Alcohol, Academic Press, 2019, Pages 567-576, ISBN 9780128131251.

presence of alcohol intake. Patients without the above and chronic heavy alcohol use is usually below 54 IU/L.

Carbohydrate-deficient transferrin (CDC)

Levels increased in patients with heavy alcohol use. Value >1.6% indicative of heavy alcohol consumption. Excessive alcohol intake >50–80 g per day over a period of 1–2 weeks leads to loss of transferrin carbohydrate side chains. Levels within the normal range in patients with intermittent or moderate alcohol consumption are observed.

Mean corpuscular volume (CV)

Hematological indices are indicative of red blood cell volume. It increased in patients with alcohol abuse due to alcohol toxicity rather than due to possible associated vitamin deficiency.

Fatty acid ethyl esters (FAEE)

Produced in the presence of ethanol reacting with free fatty acids and triglycerides by FAEE synthases. Detected in blood, tissue, and in hair. The metabolite measured is ethyl palmitate with cutoff for abstinence being less than 0.12 ng/mg per 3 cm of hair.

Cocaethylene

The combined use of alcohol and cocaine is common among drug abusers. The combination has more than additive (due to each one separately) effects. They affect heat rate, the formation of cocaethylene potentiates cardiotoxicity, or alcohol or cocaine alone. They also may potentiate a tendency toward violent thoughts and threats, and to an increase in violent behaviors. Most commercially available urine cocaine assays do not detect cocaethylene which may be misleading when investigating patients with clinically extreme behaviors seen in cocaine or ethanol alone. In the author's laboratory, the immunoassay cross-reactivity for cocaethylene is 0.4% at the 300 ng/mL detection cutoff.

Methanol

Often used as a contaminant or substitute for ethanol. Presenting symptoms confused with those for ethanol.

Patient is present with severe acidosis with little methanol contribution to the serum osmolar gap.

Ethanol is administered as effective therapy diverting metabolism from toxic formaldehyde to alcohol. Formic acid causes marked acidosis and optic neuritis leading to blindness.

Methanol is oxidized by hepatic alcohol dehydrogenase (ADH) at 1/10th the rate of ethanol to formaldehyde. Formaldehyde is rapidly oxidized to formic acid by aldehyde dehydrogenase. Formic acid correlates better than methanol with clinical symptoms.

Isopropanol

Often a contaminant or accidental intake. It is rapidly metabolized to acetone by ADH.

Ethylene glycol

Accidental intake. Clinical presentation is confused with that of ethanol. There is little contribution, in presenting cases, to the serum osmolar gap. Patients present with severe acidosis and oxalate metabolite cause hypocalcemia.

Historically, ethanol was an effective therapy (diverting metabolism); however, fomepizole is a competitive inhibitor of alcohol dehydrogenase and is the preferred antidote. Rapid ethylene glycol measurement is required to guide therapy.

Ethylene glycol levels (0.06–4.3 g/L) are associated with mortality. Toxic metabolites are oxalic and glycolic acids.

Glycolic acid levels correlate better than ethylene glycol with clinical symptoms and mortality. Levels >10 mmol/L are associated with a 33% mortality rate. Levels ≥10 mmol/L predict acute renal failure (90% of survivors develop acute renal failure) and require hemolysis (particularly when pH <7.25), whereas antimetabolic (Fomepizole) therapy is applied when levels are 1 < 10 mmol/L.

Glycolic acid interferes with the measurement of lactate by blood gas analyzers where it falsely elevated values (often in the 20's mmol/L). However, it does not interfere with laboratory-based enzymatic lactate measurement. This observed "lactate gap" provides a high index in patients suspected of ethylene glycol poisoning. Measurement of ethylene glycol takes time and often the sample is referred to a reference laboratory for measurement with delay in results. The finding of "lactate gap" in suspected patients may help institute early therapy until results of the ethylene glycol and its metabolites become available. Interference is seen with most of the cassette-based lactate measurements that are sensitive to glycolate; however, it is important to note that some blood gas analyzers, e.g., Siemens RL1265, may not interfere.

Osmolar gap

Alcohols are osmotically active and the presence of an osmotic gap indicates the presence of alcohol. The amount of alcohol can also be estimated. The osmolar concentration of ethanol is equal to the serum concentration divided by 4.6 given that its molecular weight is 46 g/mol.

The relationship between osmolar gap and ethanol concentration is given by the formula:

$$Osmolar\ gap = 0.23 \times ethanol\ concentration\ (mg / dL) - 1.43.$$

Alcohol molecular weight is 46 g/mol. An osmolar gap of 26 mOsmol/L is indicative of 120 mg/dL ethanol.

Acetaminophen

Acetaminophen (N-acetyl-p-aminophenol (APAP)) is also known as paracetamol: common and widely used analgesic. It is available as a counter item in different preparations. It is also available in prescription combined with an opioid such as codeine and oxycodone.

Early symptoms and clinical findings of toxicity are nonspecific and patients are sometimes identified following retrospective measurement of acetaminophen levels in samples 2 days earlier upon admission, when symptoms and biochemical findings for liver toxicity become apparent (elevated transaminases (ALT, AST)).

Pharmacokinetics

It has analgesic and antipyretic activity. However, it is anti-inflammatory activity and is much lower. It exhibits minimal anti-inflammatory activity compared to NSAIDs. It has a half-life of 2–3 h. Therapeutic levels are maintained at 10 to 20 μg/mL for approximately 6–8 h.

Ninety percent is metabolized by the liver to glucuronide and sulfate conjugates excreted by the kidney. About 4% is excreted unchanged into the urine (Fig. 3).

A small fraction is metabolized by the cytochrome P450 system to N-acetyl-p-benzoquinone imine (NAPQI) which has a short half-life and conjugates with hepatic glutathione to produce APAP-cysteine and APAP-mercapturate metabolites excreted in the urine.

Toxicity occurs at a dosage of greater than 250 mg/kg (all patients taking greater than 350 mg/kg will develop toxicity) or greater than 12 g over a 24-h period; furthermore, it occurs during the 8 h post-ingestion. Toxicity is due to overload of the glutathione and thus detoxification by glucuronide and sulfate conjugation. The increased glucuronide rapidly deletes any glutathione. Unconjugated (bound) NAPQI binds to hepatocytes leading to hepatic necrosis with marked elevated transaminases. ALT and AST levels above 1000 IU/L are indicative of hepatic toxicity. Hyperbilirubinemia and prolonged prothrombin time become apparent 24 to 72 h post-ingestion. Within the first 24 h post-ingestion, the mild nonspecific symptoms (nausea, malaise, lethargy, anorexia, diaphoresis, and vomiting) are accompanied by normal laboratory findings.

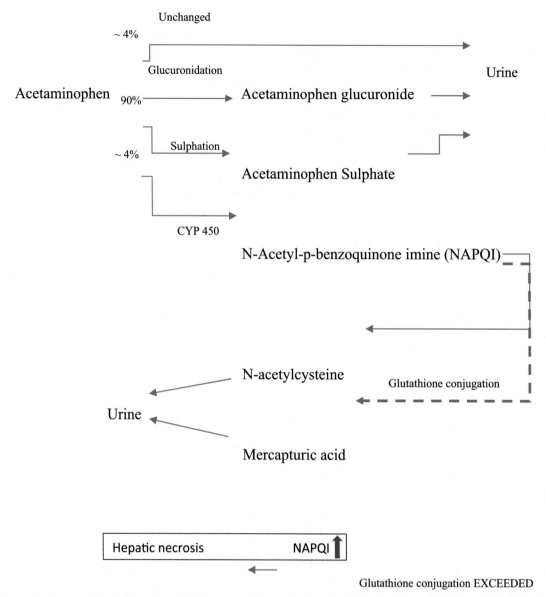

FIG. 3 Acetaminophen metabolism. The majority (90%) undergoes glucuronidation and sulfation to yield water-soluble acetaminophen glucuronides and subplate metabolites. A small amount (~4%) of acetaminophen is excreted unchanged into the urine. A small amount (~4%) is metabolized by the hepatic cytochrome P450 into toxic metabolite *N*-acetyl-p-benzoquinone imine (NAPQI) which is conjugated by hepatic glutathione to inactive *N*-acetylcysteine and mercapturic acid which are excreted into the urine. Excessive amounts of NAPOQI in acetaminophen overdose (~150 mg/kg) exceed the glutathione capacity and accumulate in the liver leading to hepatic necrosis. *Modified from Forrest JA, Clements JA, Prescott LF. Clinical pharmacokinetics of paracetamol. Clin Pharmacokinet. 1982;7(2):93-107. https://doi.org/10.2165/00003088-198207020-00001. PMID: 7039926.*

Toxicity is responsible for at least 500 deaths a year in the USA, 50,000 emergency room visits, and 10,000 hospitalizations per year.

The Rumack-Matthew nomogram (Fig. 4) describes the relationship between plasm acetaminophen level, time from ingestion, and risk for hepatic toxicity and thus provides a window for intervention. The nomogram is to be used after a single acute acetaminophen ingestion. Therefore, acetaminophen levels are used as an indication for treatment. The antidote is *N*-acetylcysteine (NAC) which acts as a substitute for glutathione and is a precursor for sulfate.

It also reduced the toxic metabolite NAPQI to acetaminophen. Additionally, NAC exhibits anti-inflammatory and antioxidant activities as well as acting as a vasodilator thus improving both anti-inflammatory mechanism and improved circulation. Its use is recommended during the 8–10-h window. However, due to its vasodilatory and anti-inflammatory effects, its use beyond that window for up to 36 h post-acetaminophen ingestion reduces morbidity and mortality.

Levels below the line indicate unlikely or no risk for hepatic toxicity, whereas levels above the line indicate

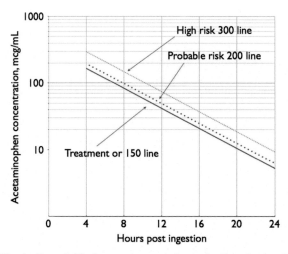

FIG. 4 Rumack-Matthew nomogram. Acetaminophen levels plotted versus time post-ingestion to assess potential toxicity and decision on administering antidote *N*-acetyl cysteine. *Modified from Hodgman MJ, Garrard AR. A review of acetaminophen poisoning. Crit Care Clin 2012;28(4):499-516.*

levels leading to probable hepatic toxicity. It is important that acetaminophen levels are measured 4 or more hours after injection. If the exact time is not known, repeat measurements 2 h apart will help identify if the levels are increasing that is absorption is still occurring, may be associated with extended-release preparation, or a decreasing level will indicate the half-life and thus help estimate the time since ingestion and thus the point on the nomogram. The nomogram cannot be used for ingestions of more than 24 h prior to acetaminophen sample collection and measurement.

Conditions potentiating toxicity include Gilbert's syndrome, alcohol abuse, and use of medications metabolized by CYP 450 (anticonvulsants competing with metabolism).

Salicylate

Acetylsalicylic acid (aspirin) is over 120 years old and the most extensively prescribed analgesic, anti-inflammatory, and antipyretic drug. It is rapidly absorbed from the stomach with a half-life of 2–4 h when given in therapeutic doses and prolonged up to 20 h in overdosage due to saturation of the metabolic pathway. It has also been prescribed at low dosage as prophylactic to improve hemodynamics and coagulation, in risk reduction of myocardial infarction, and colon cancer, and in the prophylaxis and treatment of preeclampsia.

It is a reversible inhibitor of cyclooxygenase enzymes (prostaglandin—endoperoxide synthase).

It is metabolized in the liver by conjugation to glycine and glucuronides and is eliminated in the kidney.

Although prophylactic dosages are low, circulating levels are not routinely measured. However, plasma concentration is a good guide to severity during overdoses. Acute

poisoning is a common medical emergency and carries still a high mortality.

Present presenting symptoms of toxicity include nausea, vomiting, tinnitus, dizziness, and sweating. Acid-base disturbances are those of respiratory alkalosis secondary to hyperventilation stimulated by the respiratory center, and metabolic acidosis due to the accumulation of lactic acid secondary to the uncoupling of oxidative phosphorylation.

Biochemical abnormalities include hypokalemia, hyponatremia, hypoglycemia, or hyperglycemia. Toxicity is observed for values above 350 mg/L. Serial 2–3-h measurements are required to assess the presence of delayed-release/absorption and thus possibly increasing levels.

Treatment is directed at correcting the dehydration in metabolic disturbances. Effective therapy (hemodialysis) or urinary alkalinization is available.

In situations where the time of dosage is unknown, collecting two timed measurements aids in determining whether the drug is still being absorbed (increasing levels), and its elimination rate, giving an indication of the peak dosage for risk assessment, and elimination rate (K_d) in response to intervention, $K_d\,(h^{-1}) = \ln\,(C_1/C_2)/(t_1 - t_2)$.

Salicylates act as an uncoupling agent in oxidative phosphorylation, resulting in the accumulation of lactic acid and subsequently metabolic acidosis.

Respiratory alkalosis in children is rare under the age of 4 years. Metabolic acidosis is more common in comparison with adults where there is an initial respiratory alkalosis due to a direct effect on the respiratory center.

Respiratory alkalosis is shown by a raised pH and a decreased pCO_2. This is an early abnormality in salicylate overdose and is usually followed by metabolic acidosis.

Salicylate uncouples oxidative phosphorylation and may lead to hyperpyrexia.

Carbon monoxide

Carbon monoxide poisoning is a common presentation to the emergency department following inhalation of car exhaust fumes, gases from defective heating systems during winter, or fire victims. Presenting symptoms range from headache and dizziness to coma and death with a mortality rate from one to 3%. Effective treatment is normo- and hyperbaric oxygen.

Laboratory measurement is performed on arterial or venous blood samples and analyzed on laboratory-based or point-of-blood gases devices with co-oximetry. Levels higher than 25% carboxyhemoglobin require admission to critical care units with poor >50% of patients at risk for prognosis.

Smokers will have a background (COHb levels up to 10%–15%). It is also worth noting that oxygen therapy (given in ambulance) can markedly affect COHb levels.

Heavy elements toxicity

Heavy metals are inorganic elements with a density higher than $5 \, g/cm^3$. They are classified as either essential or nonessential heavy metals. Essential metals are relatively harmless and are often present at low concentrations. They include lead, copper, zinc, iron, cobalt, and manganese. Nonessential metals are often highly toxic even at low concentrations they include arsenic, mercury, cadmium, and chromium. Metals differ from other toxic substances in that they are neither created nor destroyed. Essential heavy metals are cofactors in various metabolic pathways (Table 7). Metal-metal interactions are common, for instance, iron, copper, and zinc metabolism are influenced by levels of lead, arsenic, cadmium, and mercury.

Heavy elements toxicity is secondary to Inhibiting cell signaling leading to impaired cell metabolism and function, inhibiting proteins and enzymes function, inhibiting DNA replication leading to mutagenesis, impaired gene transcription, and thus leading to abnormal protein function.

They also induce oxidative stress, leading to protein and membrane damage and protein dysfunction.

Iron

Iron body content is very well regulated via restricted intestinal absorption.

Excessive iron intake (overdose) of vitamins and over-the-counter supplements, repeated blood transfusions as well as a genetic abnormality of hemochromatosis and thalassemia. However, excessive iron exposure is due to environmental factors such as water supply (corrosive pipes), mining, industrial manufacturing, and industrial waste contamination. Symptoms of iron toxicity include vomiting, diarrhea, nausea, abdominal pain, dehydration, and lethargy.

Therapy includes the use of iron chelating agents such as deferoxamine with plasma concentration of $>90 \, \mu mol/L$ in children and $>145 \, m\mu ol/L$ in adults helps guide therapy.

Some toxicology centers require the collection and storage of urine, blood, and gastric content (not lavage) on the admission of patients suspected of overdose for further investigation should be required.

Some poisonings cause metabolic changes and the diagnostic and therapeutic significance of these should not be neglected.

Lead

Sources of lead toxicity among adult population is chronic and occupational exposure such as in lead-related industries (automotive and battery manufacturing), refining, and smelting. Whereas sources among children include ingestion by chewing on surfaces painted with old lead-containing paint. Other usual sources of lead exposure are the use of ceramic vessels, and cosmetics containing lead.

Lead is readily absorbed by inhalation whereas, only 10%–15% of ingested lead is absorbed. Most of the lead in blood is in red blood cells inhibiting heme synthesis. The majority (95%) of absorbed lead is deposited in bones and teeth.

Symptoms of electricity or headache, anemia, abdominal pain, convulsions, and severe cases need to be calmer and death.

Blood lead levels $>100 \, \mu g/L$ ($0.49 \, \mu mol/L$) are associated with illness in children and levels in adults $>700 \, \mu g/L$ ($3.4 \, \mu mol/L$) suggest occupational exposure and workers are removed from further immediate exposure. Urine lead concentration $>159 \, \mu g/L$ ($0.73 \, \mu mol/L$ indicates excess exposure while working with organic lead compounds).

Endogenous elimination of lead is extremely low. Succimer and CaNa2EDTA are used for the therapeutic chelation of lead.

Several methods are available for the measurement of lead, they include point-of-care methods, used in community screening programs for children at high risk, and utilize capillary blood samples. Laboratory-based methodology includes atomic absorption.

Copper

Toxic exposure to copper is mainly through environmental exposure and manufacturing operations, mining, farming, and industrial wastewater operations. Symptoms of Copper Texas City include vomiting, hypertension, jaundice, and abdominal pain with gastrointestinal pain. Chronic exposure and delayed therapeutic intervention result in hepatic,

TABLE 7 Metals and their biological activities.

Element	Metabolic activity
Cu, Zn, Fe, Co	Oxygen utilization, cell growth, immunity, enzymatic reactions, and biosynthesis
Fe	Hemoglobin, myoglobin, cytochromes (a,b,c), catalase, aconitase, succinate dehydrogenase, aldehyde oxidase, peroxidases, 2,3-dioxygenase
Cu	Tyrosinase, superoxide dismutase, cytochrome *c* oxidase, ceruloplasmin, dopamine-B-hydroxylase
Zn	Protein folding, conformational changes, DNA synthesis, male fertility, and growth hormone
Co	B12 synthesis

Modified from Jomova K, Makova M, Alomar SY, Alwasel SH, Nepovimova E, Kuca K, Rhodes CJ, Valko M. Essential metals in health and disease. Chem Biol Interact. 2022;367:110173. https://doi.org/10.1016/j.cbi.2022.110173. Epub 2022 Sep 22. PMID: 36152810.

kidney, and brain damage. Penicillamine and tetrathiomolybdate are used in therapy for copper toxicity.

Arsenic

Exposure to high levels of arsenic is from food and drinking water. Chronic exposure leads to peripheral neuropathy and peripheral vascular disease as well as the risk of lung, skin, and other cancers.

Therapeutic chelation using 3-dimercaptopropanesulfonate (DMPS), dimercaptosuccinic acid (DMPS), and penicillamine.

Other elements (cadmium (Cd), aluminum (Al), and mercury (Hg))

Aluminum: Most 95% of the aluminum in the body comes from food with a minor contribution from environmental air inhalation, and topical skin applications. AL is in bone, liver, lungs, and nervous system. In circulation, 90% of AL is bound to transferrin and 8% is complexed with citrate. AL is cleared into the urine and thus accumulates in bone in patients with CKD and the brain leading to encephalopathy in patients with long-term CKD. In normal renal function, circulating AL has a half-life of 8 h, whereas AL bound to tissue, e.g., bone, has a much longer half-life of several weeks that may extend to years in cases of prolonged exposure and accumulation in trabecular and cortical bone.

Organophosphate insecticides

Most but not all organophosphorus compounds inhibit cholinesterase activity, allowing naturally formed acetylcholine to accumulate in nerve endings and the walls of blood vessels. The inhibition of cholinesterase is irreversible, and recovery depends on the synthesis of new enzymes, which may take weeks. It is readily absorbed through the gut, respiratory tract, and skin. It is thought to be responsible for much chronic ill health, nonfatal poisoning, and death in the developing world.

Diagnosis of poisoning can be confirmed by finding reduced serum or preferably RBC cholinesterase activity. Among asymptomatic subjects, 50%–70% of normal cholinesterase activity is found, 10%–20% of activity in moderate poisoning, and <10% activity in severe poisoning.

The most sensitive indicator is a marked reduction in red cell cholinesterase, but as this assay is not available routinely, the analysis of serum cholinesterase activity is used.

Drugs of abuse

Testing for drugs of abuse is for support of a clinical toxidrome. Test selection for cholinergic syndrome (associated with increased acetylcholine levels), anticholinergic (acetylcholine antagonism), sympathomimetic, opiates, sedative-hypnotic, and opiates is observed. In support of pain management programs, urine is screened for both evidence for compliance with prescribed medication (positive for prescribed drug and its metabolites) and/or detection of other nonprescribed drugs as evidence for diversion and thus noncompliance with the program and evidence for dismissal from the program.

Initial screening using immunoassay-based methods which is followed by confirmatory LC-MSMS methodologies (Table 8). False-positive immunoassays are observed due to inferences from similar compounds (cross-reactivity), whereas some assays produce false-negative results. Common examples are immunoassays for opiates that do not detect commonly used oxycodone. This has in many cases resulted in the erroneous dismissal of patients from pain management programs.

Drugs of abuse detection are of clinical value in differential diagnosis of symptoms and patient management and support of rehabilitation programs. Drugs commonly encountered in abuse/misuse include opiates, opioids (fentanyl), amphetamines (methylamphetamine), cocaine, benzodiazepines, cannabinoids, barbiturates, phencyclidine, and alcohols.

The drug test menu offered by the clinical laboratory must reflect the changing seen often positivity rates are in the 20% and low positivity rates may reflect inappropriate utilization. Consultation with emergency departments, toxicology (poison center), psychiatry, and pain management healthcare personnel as well as drug seizure records on the local law enforcement data are helpful guides in selecting a test menu. Other variable frequencies depend on geographical location.

The medicolegal implications of positive or negative results require a circumspect use of such tests unless absolutely necessary, usually as part of a drug rehabilitation program.

In addition to confirmation of intake compliance, the drugs exhibit interindividual variation in their pharmacokinetics and pharmacodynamics as well as their narrow therapeutic index. Drugs in this category include methadone, for opioid addiction, buprenorphine for opiate dependency, amphetamine for amphetamines dependency, heroin, and cocaine for controlled rehabilitation withdrawal programs.

Amphetamines

Amphetamines are central nervous stimulants. They are anorexiant. Toxic values lead to hallucinations, psychosis, dysphoria, and depression on withdrawal. Rapidly absorbed from the small intestine and is detected in urine within 20 min. An oral dose of 10–30 mg is associated with an elevation of mood, increased self-confidence, increased alertness, and improved physical performance. Chronic abuse leads to tolerance for values as high as 2000 mg/daily.

TABLE 8 Initial drug of abuse screen and cutoff levels for positivity. Respective test confirmatory test and associated cutoff value.

Initial test	Initial test cutoff concentration (ng/mL)	Confirmatory test	Confirmatory test cutoff concentration (ng/mL)
Marijuana metabolites	50	THC	15
Cocaine metabolites	150	Benzoylecgonine	100
Opiate metabolites (Codeine/Morphine)	2000	Codeine Morphine	2000 2000
6-Acetylmorphine	10	6-Acetylmorphine	10
Phencyclidine	25	Phencyclidine	25
Amphetamines (AMP/MAMP)	500	Amphetamine Methamphetamine	250 250
MDMA[3]	500	MDMA MDA[4] MDEA[5]	250 250 250

THC, Delta-9-tetrahydrocannabinol-9-carboxylic acid; *MDMA*, Methylenedioxymethamphetamine; *MDA*, Methylenedioxyamphetamine. Morphine is the target analyte for codeine/morphine testing. Methamphetamine is the target analyte for amphetamine/methamphetamine testing. To be reported positive for methamphetamine, a specimen must also contain amphetamine at a concentration equal to or greater than 100 ng/mL. Either a single initial test kit or multiple initial test kits may be used provided the single test kit detects each target analyte independently at the specified cutoff.
Modified from DOT Rule 49 CFR Part 40 Section 40.87. Subpart F—Drug Testing Laboratories. https://www.transportation.gov/odapc/part40/40-87. Accessed March 9th, 2023.

There are a number of designer drugs, methyl-amphetamines (Ecstasy (MDMA) 3,4-methylenedioxmethyl-amphetamine) with high potency causing hallucinogenic activity at 100–200 mg doses, and lead to hyperthermia, severe dehydration, convulsions, rhabdomyolysis, acute renal failure, and death (Fig. 5).

Amphetamines metabolism

Amphetamine (parent drug) 30%–74% may be seen in acidic urine. Norephedrine (Active) is about 2% of dose.

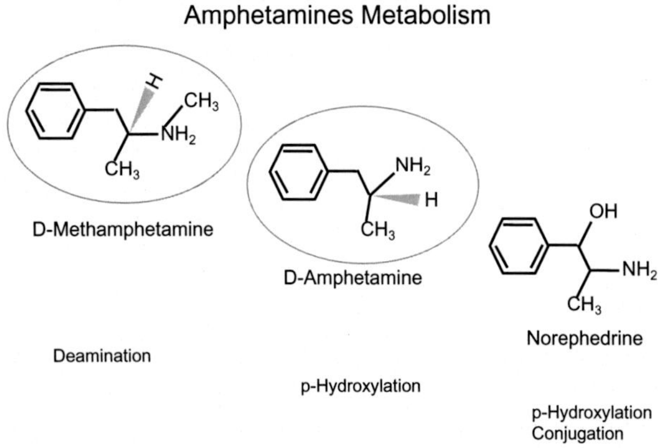

Amphetamines Metabolism

FIG. 5 Amphetamines and metabolites. *Modified from Heal DJ, Smith SL, Gosden J, Nutt DJ. Amphetamine, past and present—a pharmacological and clinical perspective. J Psychopharmacol 2013;27(6):479-96. https://doi.org/10.1177/0269881113482532. Epub 2013 Mar 28. PMID: 23539642; PMCID: PMC3666194.*

p-hydroxynorephedrine (active) 2%–4% of dose. p-hydroxyamphetamine (active) 0.3% of dose. Phenylacetone (inactive) 0.9% of dose. (Fig. 6). Urinary excretion of amphetamines is pH dependent (Table 10).

Methods

Most assays utilize antibodies detecting the parent drug and the main metabolites (amphetamine, methamphetamine, (MDMA, MDA, MDEA)) (Tables 9 and 10).

Cocaine

The third most commonly used drug of abuse after cannabis and tobacco. Some preparations are contaminated with methamphetamine and heroin.

The clearance of cocaine is variable with half-life ($T_{1/2}$) ranging from 16 to 90 min (Fig. 7). Urinary excretion is pH dependent and about 1.9% of cocaine appears in urine unchanged.

Benzoylecgonine is the major metabolite of cocaine, and it is against which the assays (antibodies) are developed.

Cocaine detection time depends on the size of the dose, mode of administration, urine volume, and pH.

It is detected 2–4 h after an intranasal dose of 1.5 mg/kg and up to 40 h following a 20 mg intravenous injection (Table 11).

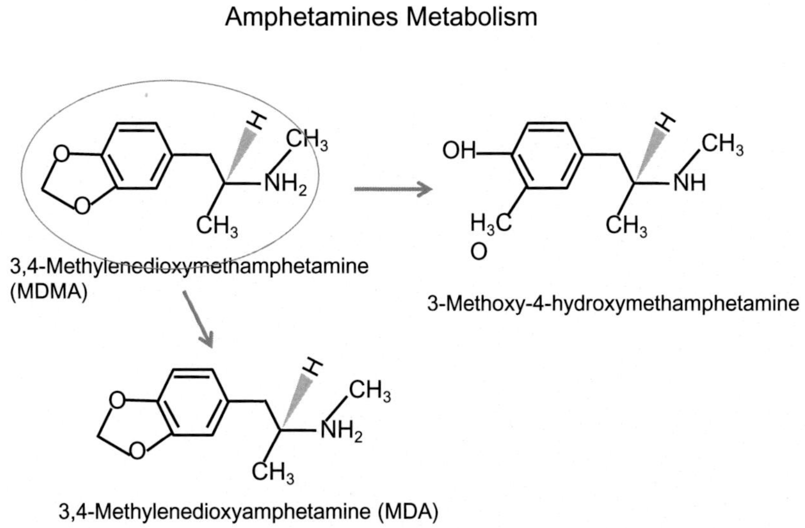

Amphetamines Metabolism

FIG. 6 Metabolism of synthetic amphetamines. *Modified from Heal DJ, Smith SL, Gosden J, Nutt DJ. Amphetamine, past and present—a pharmacological and clinical perspective. J Psychopharmacol 2013;27(6):479-96. https://doi.org/10.1177/0269881113482532. Epub 2013 Mar 28. PMID: 23539642; PMCID: PMC3666194.*

Cannabinoids

Cannabinoids are lipophilic, have instant absorption, and slow release into circulation with a marked half-life ($T_{1/2}$) of 20–30 h. It accumulates in chronic use—detectable 72 days after smoking the last cigarette. Over a period of 72 h, 40% is eliminated in feces and 30% of dose is eliminated in urine.

Cannabinoids commonly known as Marijuana *grass* texturally are dried finely chopped leaves, stems, and seeds. It contains between 1% and 2% of the main metabolite tetrahydrocannabinol (THC).

In other preparations, "Hashish" is a mixture of dried and pressed flowers with/resin and contains higher up to 6% THC. Cannabinol oil from crushed seeds has a much higher THC content at 15%–40%.

Hemp seed oil consumption produces positive cannabinoids. The assay does not distinguish between synthetic drug dronabinol metabolites and marijuana metabolites. It depends on the quality of marijuana, body metabolism, and body fat content.

The assays are designed to detect the major carbonylated metabolites of THC (9-tetrahydrocanabinol) which is 11-nor-delta-9-tetrahydrocanabinol-9-carboxylic acid. (Table 12).

False-positive results are obtained by nonsteroidal anti-inflammatory drugs (NSAIDs) such as ibuprofen and naproxen. False-positive results are obtained in patients receiving antiretroviral (efavirenz). Recent reports also showed false-positive results by select baby soap which is troublesome and must be realized to void unwarranted child protection actions.

Cannabinoids (passive smoking)

Common defense claim. Studies ($n=2$) exposed volunteers to an intense atmosphere of cannabis smoke in a small unventilated space for ~1 h on consecutive days. Urine is positive within the first 5 h. Studies ($n=5$) exposed volunteers to less extreme conditions. Most urine samples were negative with only a few positives for a few hours post-exposure. Although this is often used as a defense claim, harsh exposure conditions are required for a claim of passive smoking to test positive in urine.

High potency marijuana about 12% may produce positive cannabinoids in the setting of passive smoking in unventilated room exposure for at least 1 h and samples tested within a day at the recommended detection limit of 50 ng/mL. Lower cutoffs (e.g., 20 ng/mL likely to identify more subjects with passive smoking).

Recommendations to identify positivity due to passive smoking include measuring carboxyl metabolites which would be higher compared to those seen in active smoking, false-positive oral saliva test (within 30 min in the car) may be observed.

Synthetic cannabinoids

Examples are synthetic cannabinoids which are chemically synthesized analogues of natural cannabinoids they are not cannabis products. They are cannabinoid receptor agonists with similar or increased potency compared with natural cannabinoids.

Several generations of synthetic cannabinoids are increasingly available, with over 175 synthetic cannabinoids

TABLE 9 Cross-reactivity of the amphetamine assays (in use by the author's laboratory) for amphetamines and its metabolites in urine. The cross-reactivity for over-the-counter items and various drugs such as nasal decongestants (ephedrine and pseudoephedrine) are shown.

Amphetamine	Cutoff 1000 (ng/mL) Cross-reactivity (%)	Plasma $T_{1/2}$ (h)	Detection time (days)
d-Amphetamine	101	7–24	2–4 (9)
l-Amphetamine	3.0		
d,l-Amphetamine	58		
l-Ephedrine	0.4		
d-Methamphetamine	100	6–15	2–4 (6)
d,l-Methamphetamine	65	6–15	1.5–3
l-Methamphetamine	12		
3,4-Methylenedioxyamphetamine (MDA)	1.9		1–2
3,4-Methylenedioxymethamphetamine (MDMA)	69	6–9	1–2
Phentermine	1.9		
d,l-Phenylpropanolamine	0.3		
d-Pseudoephedrine	0.6		
Selegiline (metabolized to amphetamine)			

Modified from Moeller KE, Kissack JC, Atayee RS, Lee KC. Clinical Interpretation of Urine Drug Tests: What Clinicians Need to Know About Urine Drug Screens. Mayo Clin Proc 2017;92(5):774–796. https://doi.org/10.1016/j.mayocp.2016.12.007. Epub 2017 Mar 18. PMID: 28325505. from DOT Rule 49 CFR Part 40 Section 40.87. Subpart F, and SAMHSA. 2022-06886 Mandatory Guidelines for Federal Workplace Drug Testing Programs using Urine. file:///Users/ihashim/Downloads/SAMHSA-2022-0002-0001_content.pdf. Accessed 9th March 2023, and from test reagents information sheets.

TABLE 10 Amphetamines excretion is pH dependent.

Urine pH	<5.0	6–7	> 7
Amphetamine (A)	74%	30%	1.0%
Methyl-amphetamine (MA)	76% MA 7% A	43% MA 4.7% A	<2% MA <0.1% A

Modified from Heal DJ, Smith SL, Gosden J, Nutt DJ. Amphetamine, past and present—a pharmacological and clinical perspective. J Psychopharmacol 2013;27(6):479-96. https://doi.org/10.1177/0269881113482532. Epub 2013 Mar 28. PMID: 23539642; PMCID: PMC3666194.

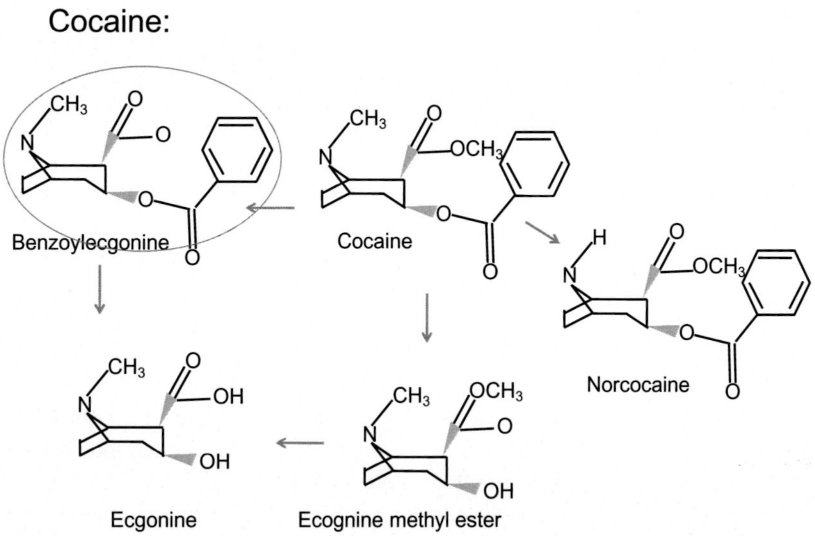

Cocaine:

FIG. 7 Cocaine metabolism. *Modified from Cone, Edward J.; Tsadik, Abraham; Oyler, Jonathan; Darwin, William D.. Cocaine metabolism and urinary excretion after different routes of administration. Therapeutic Drug Monitoring 20(5):pp. 556-560, October 1998.*

TABLE 11 Cross-reactivity and detection of cocaine and its metabolites. The assays are designed to detect the main metabolite benzoylecgonine and it does not detect the parent drug with an antibody cross-reactive of <2% for the assays in use by the author's laboratory.

Cocaine	Cutoff 300 ng/mL Cross-reactivity (%)	Plasma $T_{1/2}$ (h)	Detection time
Benzoylecgonine	100	0.7–1.5	17–72 h (2–4 days single dose) (11–22 days chronic abuse)
Cocaine	1.7	–	–
Cocaethylene	0.4	–	–
Ecgonine	<0.05	–	–
Norcocaine	<0.05	–	–
Ecgonine Methyl ester	<0.05	–	–

Modified from Moeller KE, Kissack JC, Atayee RS, Lee KC. Clinical interpretation of urine drug tests: what clinicians need to know about urine drug screens. Mayo Clin Proc 2017;92(5):774-796. https://doi.org/10.1016/j.mayocp.2016.12.007. Epub 2017 Mar 18. PMID: 28325505, from DOT Rule 49 CFR Part 40 Section 40.87. Subpart F, and SAMHSA. 2022-06886 Mandatory Guidelines for Federal Workplace Drug Testing Programs using Urine. file:///Users/ihashim/Downloads/SAMHSA-2022-0002-0001_content.pdf. Accessed 9th March 2023, and from test reagents information sheets.

TABLE 12 Cannabinoids metabolites and cross-reactivities (assay detection) in use by the author's laboratory. The cutoff for detection is 50 ng/mL. LC-MSMS methodologies offer a lower cutoff at 15 ng/mL.

Cannabinoids (Marijuana)	Cutoff 50 ng/mL Approx. Cross-reactivity (%)	Plasma $T_{1/2}$ (h)	Detection time
9-Carboxy-11-nor-8-THC	69	20–57	Casual use: 2–7 days Chronic use: Up to 30 days (95)
9-Carboxy-11-nor-9-THC Glucuronide	54	5–6 days (>1 week in heavy users)	
8-β-11-dihydroxy-9-THC	30.9		
Cannabinol	0.6		

Modified from Moeller KE, Kissack JC, Atayee RS, Lee KC. Clinical interpretation of urine drug tests: what clinicians need to know about urine drug screens. Mayo Clin Proc. 2017;92(5):774-796. https://doi.org/10.1016/j.mayocp.2016.12.007. Epub 2017 Mar 18. PMID: 28325505, from DOT Rule 49 CFR Part 40 Section 40.87. Subpart F, and SAMHSA. 2022-06886 Mandatory Guidelines for Federal Workplace Drug Testing Programs using Urine. file:///Users/ihashim/Downloads/SAMHSA-2022-0002-0001_content.pdf. Accessed 9th March 2023, and from test reagents information sheets.

recognized. In addition to posing a health risk, they are not detected by currently available clinical assays, and continued assay development and validation are required to keep pace.

The most prevalent synthetic cannabinoid, at least in the United States, is 5F-MDMB-PICA, 4-cyano CUMYL-BUTINACA, and 5F-EDMB-PINACA. LC-MSMS based methodologies are the methods of choice due to their sensitivity and ability to detect metabolites and identify previously unknown compounds.

Synthetic cannabinoids and their metabolites often tested for include 4-carboxy-AMB-PINACA a metabolite of the synthetic cannabinoid AMB-PINACA(AB-PINACA) and may also be a metabolite of other synthetic cannabinoids with similar structures. 5-fluoro-PIC-ACID (5-fluoro-PB-22 3-carboxyindole) is known to interfere with this measurement.

5-fluoro-PICA 3,3-dimethylbutanoic acid is a metabolite of the synthetic cannabinoid 5-fluoro-MDMB-PICA and may also be a metabolite of other synthetic cannabinoids with similar structures.

FUBICA 3,3-dimethylbutanoic acid is a metabolite of the following synthetic cannabinoid(s): ADMB-FUBICA (ADB-FUBICA); MDMB-FUBICA (5-fluoro AMB) and may be a metabolite of other synthetic cannabinoids with similar structures.

5-fluoro-PINAC-ACID a metabolite of the following synthetic cannabinoid(s): 5-fluoro-EDMB-PINACA; 5-fluoro-MDMB-PINACA (5F-ADB); 5-fluoro-EMB-PINACA (5F-AEB); 5-fluoro-MMB-PINACA (5-fluoro AMB); 5-fluoro-QU-PINAC (5F-NPB-22) and may also be a metabolite of other synthetic cannabinoids with similar structures.

Opioids

Opioids are either natural (codeine, morphine, opium, thebaine), synthetic (fentanyl, methadone, tramadol, and meperidine), whereas semisynthetic includes (buprenorphine, dihydrocodeine, hydrocodone, hydromorphone, oxymorphone, levorphanol, and heroin). Importantly, most commercial screening assays may not detect oxycodone, methadone, fentanyl, or tramadol in their "opiates" assays screen, and specific assays for those substances are needed (Figs. 8–10).

Most important is that opioid metabolism often converges at several common metabolites. That is codeine, heroin, and morphine will exhibit a positive urine morphine.

Codeine (present in many over-the-counter medications) is metabolized to morphine and hydrocodone, and subsequently to hydromorphone (Figs. 8–10).

Free codeine (inactive) 5%–17%. Norcodeine (active) 10%–21%. Morphine (active) 5%–13% of dose. Codeine conjugates 32%–46% (inactive) of the dose.

The relative proportion of the parent drug and metabolites are; dihydrocodeine parent drug (active) 31% of dose, dihydrocodeine conjugates (inactive) 28% of dose, dihydrocodeine (active) 16% of dose, dihydromorphine (active) 0.5% free and 8.4% conjugates of dose, dihydromorphine (active) 1.8% of dose, and hydrocodone (active) 0.2% of dose.

Oxycodone has opioid activity and represents 13%–19% of dose. It is converted to oxycodone conjugates which are inactive and represent 7%–29% of dose. Oxycodone is metabolized to noroxycodone which is inactive. The metabolite oxymorphone is active and represents 1.9% of the dose. Oxymorphone conjugates are inactive and represent 44% of dose (Fig. 10).

Codeine excretion

Time-dependent appearance of codeine and metabolites in urine. Primarily, codeine conjugates predominate during the early phase of intake, whereas morphine conjugates predominate 20 to 40h (late phase) following intake. That is

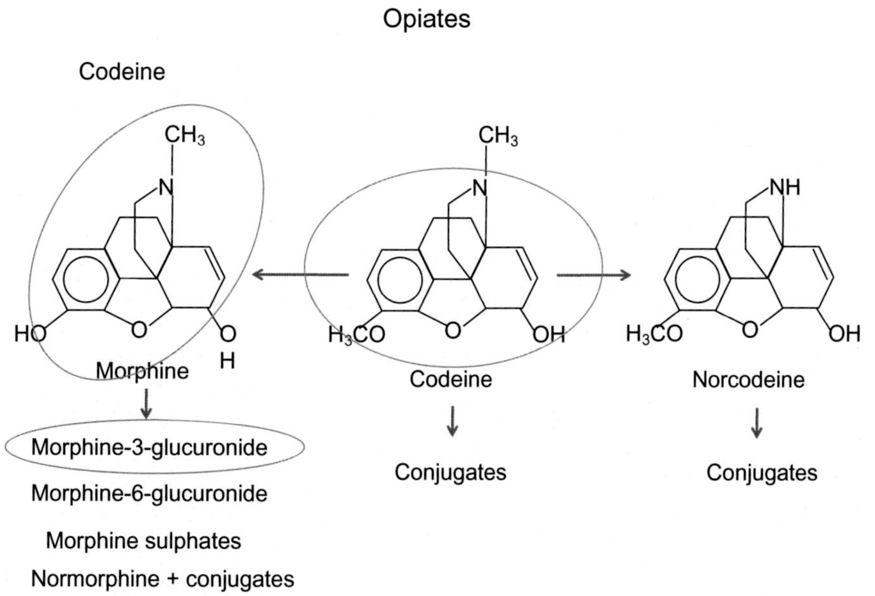

Opiates

Codeine

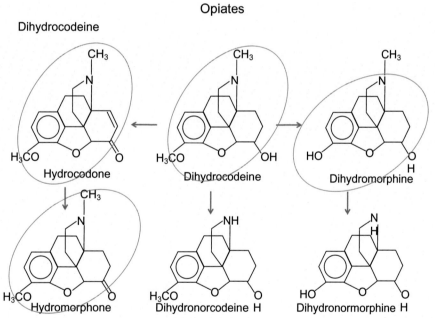

FIG. 8 Opiates metabolism (codeine). *Modified from Milone MC. Laboratory testing for prescription opioids. J Med Toxicol 2012;8(4):408-16. https://doi.org/10.1007/s13181-012-0274-7. PMID: 23180358; PMCID: PMC3550258.*

Opiates

Dihydrocodeine

FIG. 9 Opiates metabolism (dihydrocodeine). *Modified from Milone MC. Laboratory testing for prescription opioids. J Med Toxicol 2012;8(4):408-16. https://doi.org/10.1007/s13181-012-0274-7. PMID: 23180358; PMCID: PMC3550258.*

the sample collected 2–3 days after codeine ingestion may appear to contain only morphine which may be erroneously interpreted as representing morphine intake following the diversion of prescribed codeine. However, dihydrocodeine is not metabolized into morphine.

Opiate measurements are detected by immunoassays as a group. However, differences exist in the cross-reactivity and thus detection among the various opiates and their metabolites (Table 13). The clinical laboratory should be aware

and should indicate what opiates are detected. For instance, some assays may not detect oxycodone and negative results for an opiate screen may incorrectly indicate patient non-compliance in a drug rehabilitation program,

Methadone

Methadone an opiate similar to morphine and binds to the *u* receptor. It exhibits significant protein binding (>90%)

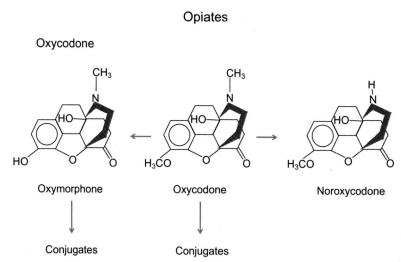

FIG. 10 Opiates metabolism-oxycodone. *Modified from Milone MC. Laboratory testing for prescription opioids. J Med Toxicol 2012;8(4):408-16. https://doi.org/10.1007/s13181-012-0274-7. PMID: 23180358; PMCID: PMC3550258.*

TABLE 13 Opiates assays cross-reactivity with various metabolites. The detection limit in use is 300 ng/mL in the author's laboratory.

Opiates	Cutoff (300 ng/mL) Cross-reactivity	Plasma $T_{1/2}$ (h)	Detection time (days)
Codeine	134	1.9–3.9	2–4
Ethyl morphine	101		
Diacetylmorphine	82		2–4
6-Acetyl morphine (Heroin metabolite)	78	1.3–6.7	2–4 h (2–4 days as morphine)
Dihydrocodeine	59		
Morphine-3-glucuronide	54		
Hydrocodone	28	4	2–4
Thebaine	25		
Hydromorphone	21	1.5–3.8	2–4
n-Norcodeine	2		
Oxycodone	<0.4	4–6	2–4

Modified from Moeller KE, Kissack JC, Atayee RS, Lee KC. Clinical interpretation of urine drug tests: what clinicians need to know about urine drug screens. Mayo Clin Proc 2017;92(5):774-796. https://doi.org/10.1016/j.mayocp.2016.12.007. Epub 2017 Mar 18. PMID: 28325505, from DOT Rule 49 CFR Part 40 Section 40.87. Subpart F, and SAMHSA. 2022-06886 Mandatory Guidelines for Federal Workplace Drug Testing Programs using Urine. file:///Users/ihashim/Downloads/SAMHSA-2022-0002-0001_content.pdf. Accessed 9th March 2023, and from test reagents information sheets.

and has a long half-life. Patients on long-term methodone maintenance develop tolerance requiring the application of increasing dosage. Its metabolism is induced by phenytoin and rifampicin. The main metabolite is 2-thylidende-1,5-dimethyl-3,3-diphenyl-pyrrolidine (EDDP).

Target therapeutic values between 150 and 250 µg/L with levels less than 50 µg/L are associated with withdrawal symptoms.

Fentanyl

Fentanyl is a short-acting synthetic opioid agonist that is about 100 times more potent than morphine. There is a significant increase in fentanyl seizure by law enforcement agencies with almost an increase of 400% in 1 year. Synthetic formulations such as carfentanil are 10,000 times more potent than morphine. Similar to other synthetic illicit drugs, fentanyl analogues will not be detected by standard fentanyl assays.

The patient will present with the typical opioid toxidrome that is CNS depression, meiosis, and respiratory depression. Treatment includes the use of naloxone and respiratory support.

Buprenorphine

Synthetic opioids are used for pain management and treatment of opioid abuse disorders. It is a *mu*-opioid partial agonist. The major metabolite is norbuprenorphine which is measured as well as the parent drug. It is more potent than morphine by a factor of 20-fold. The main metabolite is norbuprenorphine and its parent drug exhibits a dose-related concentration. Urine is the sample of choice.

Tramadol

Synthetic codeine analog is used in the treatment of moderate-to-severe pain. It is metabolized by hepatic CYP2B6, 2D6, 2C19, and 3A4 to the more active metabolite *O*-desmethyl-tramadol. Tramadol's half-life is approximately 8 h which is dose dependent in overdose and is prolonged in patients with renal impairment.

Benzodiazepines

Large family of drugs. They exhibit different activities with different half-lives ($T_{1/2}$ for Temazepam is 7–8 h, Diazepam 20–40 h, and for Nordiazepam 50–100 h).

Widely available on the illicit drugs market. Detection in urine is variable, long-term abuse → detectable in urine weeks-months after stopping, 10 mg/day for 5 days → positive urine 2–7 days afterward (Table 14). Major benzodiazepines and their common metabolites are shown in Fig. 11.

Barbiturates

Barbiturates have a sedative effect through their action of binding and inhibiting central nervous system (CNS) gamma amino-butyric acid-A (GABAA) receptors causing and potentiating the opening of neural chloride ion channels. In addition to its sedative action, it has gained use in a number of clinical conditions such as traumatic brain injury and brain ischemia, among others.

Common barbiturates detection time, metabolites, and their cross-reactivities in the assays in use by the author's laboratory are shown (Table 15).

Phencyclidine

Phencyclidine (PCP), historically used as an anesthetic agent, is abused as a hallucinogenic drug. Effects include acute psychosis, aggressive and violent behaviors, status epilepticus, hyperthermia, rhabdomyolysis, and respiratory and hepatic failure.

PCP, ketamine, and their novel analogues antagonize *N*-methyl-D-aspartate receptors. Illicit forms include methoxetamine, and 3- and 4-methoxy phencyclidine.

Ketamine has only 10% of the receptor binding affinity compared to PCP. Symptoms include tachycardia, nystagmus, hypertension, euphoria, nausea, and vomiting. Life-threatening complications include coma, hyperventilation, apnea, seizures delirium, hallucinations, and agitation.

Common PCP drug detection time, metabolites, and their cross-reactivities in the assays in use by the author's laboratory are shown (Table 16).

Other drugs of increasing clinical interest

It is important to note that the drug scene is dynamic and changes due to various factors including economic. The clinical laboratories must be aware of what is available on the street and in use and be able to provide the appropriate tests and detection methods. Examples of drugs of interest are shown in Table 17 .

Cathinone

Khat (*Catha edulis*) is a plant commonly used as a stimulant in the Middle East and Africa. It is chewed and the active ingredient cathinone is degraded to cathine which has about 1/10th of the stimulant effect of D-amphetamine. The drug causes agitation, increased alertness, insomnia, euphoria, anxiety, and hyperactivity; it is also associated with cardiac and gastrointestinal complications, and acuter kidney injury. Some patients may exhibit hyponatremia. Cathinones are not detected using standard amphetamine assays. Supportive care includes sedation to prevent significant acidosis.

Gamma-aminobutyric acid (GABA) and its analogues

Nonopioid central nervous system depressant. It is developed as an anticonvulsant and is used in the treatment of partial seizures in adults and children. Its application has been extended to moderate-to-severe restless legs syndrome, neuralgia.

Sample types

Several body fluid types are used in therapeutic and toxicological testing, and some have been validated as acceptable sample samples. They include blood (whole blood), plasma (anticoagulated blood), serum (clotted sample), urine (random), saliva, meconium, hair, and nails.

TABLE 14 Benzodiazepine metabolites cross-reactivity in the assay at a cut of 200 ng/mL in use by the author's laboratory.

Benzodiazepines	Cutoff 200 (ng/mL) Cross-reactivity (%)	Plasma $T_{1/2}$ (h)	Detection time (days)
Diazepam	93	21–37	2–7 (up to 30)
Demoxepam	99	–	–
Alprazolam (α-OH-, 4-OH-, α-OH-Glucuronide)	91 (88,81,54)	6–27	1–5
Estazolam	92	10–24	1.5–5
Bromazepam	83	–	–
Nitrazepam (7-amino-, 7 aceto-)	81 (84, 0.2)	–	–
Triazolam (α-OH-, 4-OH-)	85 (82,80)	1.8–3.9	0.5–1
Oxazepam	77	4–11	1–2
Clobazam	84	–	–
Clorazepate	85	–	–
Flunitrazepam (7-amino, desmethyl, 3-OH-)	71 (94, 73, 56)	–	4–12.5
Temazepam (glucuronide)	78 (0.7),	3–13	1–3
Chlordiazepoxide, (desmethyl chlordiazepoxide)	65 (70)	6–27	1.5–5.5
Clonazepam (7-aminoclonazepam)	68 (69)	19–60	4–12.5
Lorazepam (glucuronide)	59 (1.0)	9–16	2–3.5
Flurazepam (OH-, desalkyl-, didesethyl-)	57 (88, 88, 73)	1–3	10–21
Midazolam (α-OH-)	65 (75)	1–4	0.5–1
Pinazepam	69	–	–
Halazepam	57	–	–
Medazepam (desmethyl-)	51 (33)	–	–

Modified from Moeller KE, Kissack JC, Atayee RS, Lee KC. Clinical Interpretation of Urine Drug Tests: What Clinicians Need to Know About Urine Drug Screens. Mayo Clin Proc 2017;92(5):774-796. https://doi.org/10.1016/j.mayocp.2016.12.007. Epub 2017 Mar 18. PMID: 28325505, from DOT Rule 49 CFR Part 40 Section 40.87. Subpart F, and SAMHSA. 2022-06886 Mandatory Guidelines for Federal Workplace Drug Testing Programs using Urine. file:///Users/ihashim/Downloads/SAMHSA-2022-0002-0001_content.pdf. Accessed 9th March 2023, and from test reagents information sheets.

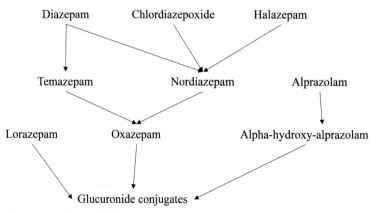

FIG. 11 Common benzodiazepines and outlines of their metabolites. *Modified from Moeller KE, Kissack JC, Atayee RS, Lee KC. Clinical interpretation of urine drug tests: what clinicians need to know about urine drug screens. Mayo Clin Proc 2017;92(5):774-796. https://doi.org/10.1016/j.mayocp.2016.12.007. Epub 2017 Mar 18. PMID: 28325505.*

TABLE 15 Barbiturates metabolites cross-reactivity at 200 ng/mL cutoff in use by the author's laboratory.

Barbiturates	Cutoff 200 (ng/mL) Cross-reactivity (%)	Detection time (days) (at 300 ng/mL)	Plasma $T_{1/2}$ (h)
Amobarbital	29	2–4 (3–8)	15–40
Butalbital	71	2–4 (7–18)	35–88
Pentobarbital	36	2–4 (4–6)	20–30
Phenobarbital	22	Up to 30 (10–30)	48–144
Secobarbital	n/a	2–4 (4.5–6.)	22–29
Cyclopentobarbital	101	–	–
Aprobarbital	93	–	–
Allobarbital	71	–	–
p-Hydroxyphenobarbital	19	–	–
Barbital	11	–	–
1,3-Dimethylbabituric acid	0	–	–
Mephobarbital	<0.1	–	–
Barbituric acid	<0.01	–	–
Hexobarbital	<0.01	–	–
Diphenylhydantoin	<0.02	–	–
Glutethimide	<0.04	–	–

Modified from Moeller KE, Kissack JC, Atayee RS, Lee KC. Clinical interpretation of urine drug tests: what clinicians need to know about urine drug screens. Mayo Clin Proc 2017;92(5):774-796. https://doi.org/10.1016/j.mayocp.2016.12.007. Epub 2017 Mar 18. PMID: 28325505, from DOT Rule 49 CFR Part 40 Section 40.87. Subpart F, and SAMHSA. 2022-06886 Mandatory Guidelines for Federal Workplace Drug Testing Programs using Urine. file:///Users/ihashim/Downloads/SAMHSA-2022-0002-0001_content.pdf. Accessed 9th March 2023, and from test reagents information sheets.

TABLE 16 Phencyclidine metabolites cross-reactivity at 25 ng/mL cutoff in use by the author's laboratory.

Drug	Cutoff 25 (ng/mL) Approx. Cross-reactivity (%)
Phenylcyclohexylpiperidine	51
Dextromethorphan	0
Ketamine	0

Modified from Moeller KE, Kissack JC, Atayee RS, Lee KC. Clinical interpretation of urine drug tests: what clinicians need to know about urine drug screens. Mayo Clin Proc 2017;92(5):774-796. https://doi.org/10.1016/j.mayocp.2016.12.007. Epub 2017 Mar 18. PMID: 28325505, from DOT Rule 49 CFR Part 40 Section 40.87. Subpart F, and SAMHSA. 2022-06886 Mandatory Guidelines for Federal Workplace Drug Testing Programs using Urine. file:///Users/ihashim/Downloads/SAMHSA-2022-0002-0001_content.pdf. Accessed 9th March 2023, and from test reagents information sheets.

The nature of sample is often dictated by the clinical needs. Requests received; Clinical; Diagnostic, Therapeutic. Legal/Law enforcement; Workplace, Insurance, Forensic Science, Prisons, anti-doping programs in sports. Hair/nails sweat not in clinical setting, often criminal and forensic settings. Testing for Olympics sports competition requirements are different from those in use for clinical testing with different accreditation systems and requirements.

Blood

Blood is the sample of choice in therapeutic drug monitoring. Whereas few therapeutic drugs such as the immunosuppressants cyclosporine, tacrolimus, and sirolimus are measured using whole blood samples due to their sequestration in red blood cells, most other drugs are measured in either plasma or serum following separation from red blood cells by centrifugation. Blood sample is ideal for pharmacokinetic studies, where samples are often collected at trough levels (just prior to the next dose) to determine levels within the therapeutic window (Fig. 1), or during the drug peak levels, 2 h Postoral administration to define maximum concentration and the derivation of the drug distribution are under the curve. Blood is also used to establish clearance studies in patients with renal and/or hepatic dysfunction.

Total drug concentration does not reflect any changes in the relative proportion between the free and bound drug.

TABLE 17 The above drugs are of increasing clinical interest and requests for laboratory testing are rapidly increasing.

Drug	Plasma $T_{1/2}$ (h)	Detection time (days)
Meperidine	2–5	0.5–1
Methadone	15–55	3–11
Tramadol	4.3–6.7	0.5–1.5
Propoxyphene	8–24	2–7 (casual use) <30 (chronic use)
Dextropropoxyphene	24–50	<9
Fentanyl	3–12	<1

Modified from Moeller KE, Kissack JC, Atayee RS, Lee KC. Clinical interpretation of urine drug tests: what clinicians need to know about urine drug screens. Mayo Clin Proc 2017;92(5):774-796. https://doi.org/10.1016/j.mayocp.2016.12.007. Epub 2017 Mar 18. PMID: 28325505.

This is significant in situations where significant protein binding changes.

Changes in protein levels and protein binding, drug-drug interaction, and renal and hepatic functions. Some drugs have significant protein binding (mainly acidic drugs to albumin) and to alpha-1-acidglycoprotein (mainly basic drugs) and changes in protein levels as in kidney and/or liver disorders will affect the relative proportion of the free drug (nonprotein bound fraction), which is often the pharmacologically active fraction.

Blood sample facilitates the measurement of protein-bound and free drug routinely measured and reported as total drugs concentration.

For drugs that are highly protein bound and that have a relatively smaller free fraction (<10%), significant changes in protein levels, such as in renal loss and decreased hepatic synthesis or in changes due to acute inflammatory response, the relative proportion of the free drug component, often the biologically active form, is markedly altered sometimes by as must as 50%. In patients with marked changes in protein levels, the drug being administered exhibits high protein binding (e.g., phenytoin) (Table 4) measurement of the free form indicated in pediatrics and during pregnancy where albumin levels are physiologically low and that the free drug levels better reflect the drug pharmacodynamics. Patients with renal and/or hepatic dysfunction and those with acute inflammatory response will exhibit significant changes in protein levels. Technical challenges are those of the assay sensitivity for the low free drug concentration and for the need to remove protein-bound drug component.

Coadministration of drugs that either inhibit or stimulate the cytochrome P450 system might significantly change the elimination and half-life of the drug and its circulating level.

Urine

Urine is a preferred sample in drugs of abuse and toxicological testing. It is readily available in large volumes, and

contains both parent drug and metabolites, the latter often in high concentrations.

The appearance of drugs and metabolites in urine depends on the dose and drug pK_a, urine pH, and the lag time between drug administration and urine void.

Metabolites detected in the urine are conjugated and may not be detectable by immunoassays or mass spectrometry. Sample pretreatment by hydrolysis of conjugation and sulfation although improves detection, it may lead to deterioration of metabolite as well as interconversions. For instance, acid hydrolysis leads to the conversion of hydrocodone to hydromorphone and oxycodone to oxymorphone. More significant is the conversion of 6-monoactlylmoprohine (6-MAM) (heroin) to morphine which may thus lead to false heroin reporting.

In general, clinical practice is random and consensual, without the need for chain of custody, nor the need for observed collection. Chain of custody is required for legal requests and if the patient is known/suspected to adulterate the specimen.

Limitations of toxicology and drug tests include differences in renal and hepatic function (i.e., clearance and metabolism). Other factors influencing laboratory analysis include urine sample concentration, volume (minimum volume required for point-of-care testing cups), and the presence of interfering substance.

While, urine drug testing indicates the presence or absence of the drug, it does not provide information as to how much drug was taken, when it was taken, and for how long after use will the drug screen give positive results. Although some of this information may be available in scientific literature and the laboratory procedure, they rarely accompany the toxicology report.

Hair and nails

Hair and nail have been used as a sample for drug analysis. Hair grows at approximately 1 cm per month, and finger nail grows by 0.35 cm per month and provide a historical picture of the drug use in the previous weeks or months. It is often used in forensic toxicology testing. Limitations include environmental contamination and lack of standardization in the preanalytical protocol for sample instruction and handling. It is not used in routine clinical practice.

Cord blood

Drugs administered during pregnancy have the potential to cross the placenta and reach the fetus. Drugs and their metabolites may be detected in cord blood samples obtained immediately after birth.

Meconium

Meconium is formed by the fetus as early as the 12th week of gestation and thus serves as an indicator of substance exposure by the fetus for the last 2 to 3 months prior to birth. It comprises epithelial cells, mucus, amniotic fluid, bile, and water that are ingested by the fetus during the entire pregnancy. Therefore, drugs administered during pregnancy may accumulate in the meconium throughout pregnancy compared to urine and blood that only reflect acute exposure. Meconium is the first stool passed by the newborn within 72 h of birth. It is dark viscous and contains 60%–80% water.

Limitations for the use of meconium as a sample include a small sample volume, the possibility of missing collections, need for repeat collections as it might be expelled in stages. The sample is often heterogeneous, sticky, and contaminated with stool. Extensive sample preanalytical preparation is required from mixing to solvent extraction and thus analysis is limited to specialized toxicology laboratories. Immediate refrigeration of the sample is required to minimize the deterioration of drug contents.

Saliva

Saliva is an ultrafiltrate of plasma and has been used for drug measurement. The drugs are in their free (nonprotein bound) form and are present at relatively low concentrations. Assays with a high degree of sensitivity are thus required.

Salvia is mostly water (99%) with 0.3% protein composition. The proteins are salivary proteases and enzymes. Its pH is acidic (6 to 7.5) and is maintained by bicarbonate, phosphate, and protein buffering.

Drugs appear in saliva within minutes of its administration. The diffusion of the drug into saliva is dependent on the drug pK_a and for drugs that have pK_a values around 8.5, their diffusion is unaffected by saliva pH. The appearance of methadone in saliva is hindered by binding to P-glycoprotein, transport protein present in salivary glands.

Sweat as a sample

The majority of sweat is produced by eccrine glands, in the transdermal layer, and apocrine glands present in the axilla, pubic region, and around nipples.

Sweat glands are developed in close association with hair follicles and sometimes empty directly into the hair follicle. The volume of sweat produced depends on the anatomical location, 50% by the trunk, 25% by the legs, and 25% by the head and upper extremities. The amount of sweat highly variable depends on daily activity, emotional state, and environment temperature.

The sweat is a clear hypotonic solution with approximately 99% water. It contains electrolytes: Na, Cl, K, urea, pyruvate, lactate, peptides, antibodies, cytokines, and xenobiotics (drugs, cosmetics, ethanol, etc.) with partial reabsorption of Na and CL. The sweat is slightly acidic (pH: 4.0–6.8) (average 5.8) and is influenced by a flow rate with pH of 6.8 when the flow rate is high. Disease states alter sweat composition by altering the concentration of common components or the presence of a disease-specific biomarker. Sweat is stored in the eccrine and apocrine glands before secretion into sweat and transported through sweat pores to the epidermal surface.

The mechanism of drug presence in sweat is not clear, plausible mechanism being positive diffusion (from blood to sweat glands), and transdermal migration across the skin, and the stratum corneum acts as a temporary reservoir.

Sweat patches

Sweat patches are adsorbent occlusive/nonocclusive, waterproof, contains NaCl crystals, resistant to tampering, and allows the skin to breathe with O_2, CO_2, and water vapor allowed to escape. It facilitates the monitoring of drug intake over several weeks using a single patch. Drug concentrations are much lower than in urine (sensitive assay required) (repeat testing limited). False-positive and false-negative results may be obtained and be due to changes in pH, infection, and hydration status. Body areas with a high rate of sweat production are the shoulders, upper dorsal, and anterior parts of the body.

Sweat patches offer continuous drug monitoring over a long period (up to 7–14 days) compared to urine and saliva. They are less invasive sample collection compared to urine. Patch application easy little training required for both patient and healthcare personnel.

False-positive and false-negative results may be obtained. Contributing factors include variable sweat production (precludes quantitative analysis). Environmental contamination before application and following application. Removal of the collection patch (unintentional or intentional) during the monitoring period. The most notable and nonobvious contributor to results variability is changes in lifestyle (often a component of adjustments and rehabilitation efforts) such as vigorous and prolonged exercise that may lead to false-positive results (evidence of outward transdermal migration of some accumulated drugs) assumed to be new drug usage. Possibility of time-dependent drug loss from the patch by drug degradation on the skin and possible re-absorption into the skin, and that lipophilic drugs (stored in adipose tissue) may reach episodically, or over an extended timespan and may erroneously suggest a false new episode of drug intake.

Sweat testing considerations when testing selected drugs

Amphetamines: Both parent drug and its metabolites are present and the metabolite concentrations are variable. Furthermore, in contrast to the urine, the parent compound is present in higher concentration than metabolites.

Cannabinoids: Cannabinoids are lipophilic and accumulate in fat with positive results obtained for up to 28 days after cessation of smoking. Only parent compound is detectable in sweat compared to urine.

Cocaine: Both parent and metabolites are detected (compared to urine where the majority detection is for the metabolite benzoylecgonine). This is limited by the fact that the urine immunoassays are targeted toward benzoylecgonine. Detection variable depends on patch location (the back is 8× higher than the shoulder). Sweat patch testing for cocaine has a sensitivity of 68.6%, specificity of 86.1%, and diagnostic efficiency of 78.6%. There were 13.5% false-negative and 7.9% false-positive sweat results as compared to urine tests. The percentage of false-negative results in their study indicates that weekly sweat testing may be less sensitive than thrice weekly urine testing in detecting opiate use.

Sample adulteration efforts

Several approaches are attempted by those wishing to interfere with toxicology results. The attempts, which include sample adulteration, are for either obtaining negative or positive results depending on the need.

For a negative result, the sample may be adulterated as follows; dilute with water (in vitro), drink large volumes of fluid before providing a sample (in vivo), use of diuretics, substitute urine sample from drug-free associate, add bleach, salt, liquid soap, oxidizing agents, vitamin B drinks (dilution/fluorescence) which interferes with immunoassay antibody-antigen binding and/or with signal production. The patient may refrain from taking illicit drugs for several days or wear devices (containing drug-free urine) (e.g., Urinator).

For obtaining a positive, the patient may add drugs directly to urine (only parent compound would be detected without the presence of metabolites) or substitute a urine sample from a drug-positive colleague.

Sample collection protocols to detect possible adulteration

A number of protocols (precautions) may be followed to detect and to minimize the possibility of sample adulteration.

At the preanalytical phase: For a urine sample, direct observation (if possible), patient washes hand before sample cup is provided (this removes possible hand contamination with detergents or oxidizing agents), patient is given a marked urine container, immediate recording of sample appearance, temperature (32–38°C within 4 min), pH, specific gravity (>1.003), and creatinine (>0.45 g/L (4 mmol/L)).

At the analytical phase, use of metabolites-specific assays; use of automated adulteration detection (measurement of oxidizing agents, creatinine, specific gravity).

There are several challenges, they include a well-informed drug user with extensive literature available on adulteration, dedicated websites, and web-based information.

Assay methodologies

Assays for the measurement of therapeutic drugs and detection of drugs of abuse are in two categories. The first category employs immunoassay-based technology. Immunoassays are either homogeneous or heterogeneous in composition. The second category is chromatographic techniques (confirmation/quantification); LC-MS/GC MS, Tandem MS.

Detection thresholds are those for clinical, pain management, and employment and are defined by various agencies such as NIDA (National Institute on Drug Abuse). Detection "cutoff values" and positivity may vary for different point-of-care devices and comparison and validation studies with clinical laboratory-based screen methods may be required to avoid discrepancy in results.

Screening usually by immunoassay, class "group" specific and often detects parent compound and metabolites. Confirmation and quantification are by chromatographic methods (identifies drugs and metabolites). Rules-out interference and claims for passive and accidental ingestion (e.g., Cannabis).

The characteristics of laboratory-based and point-of-care (near-patient) testing are summarized in Table 18.

Immuno-based assays

Antibody-based immunoassays are used in both therapeutic drug monitoring and drugs of abuse screening. They are available either as laboratory-based assays on automated chemistry analyzers or as reagents in point-of-care urine testing cups. Both setups allow for rapid testing with point-of-care providing the opportunity for real-time discussion with patient at the point of care.

TABLE 18 Characteristics and differences between laboratory-based and point-of-care (near-patient) testing modality. Several assay configurations are in use for therapeutic drugs and toxicology testing. They are either immunoassay-based, chromatography-based assays, or a combination of both.

	Laboratory-based	Point-of-care testing
Nature of the assay	Qualitative/ quantitative	Qualitative
Assay time	30 to 60 min	Rapid 5–10 min
Performance	High-performance characteristics Controlled and high level of accuracy	Performance limitations Compliance and regulatory concerns
Cost	Relatively low cost	Relatively high cost

In the automated laboratory based assays, the antibody binding to drugs either causes a decrease or increase in turbidity that is proportional to the amount of drugs. Examples of assay formations include KIMS (kinetic immunoassay), where in the absence of the drugs, the reagent antibodies bind to a latex-attached reagent antigen. This causes aggregation and an increase in turbidity, whereas in the presence of drug, the binding of the antibody preferentially to the free drug (in patients' sample) and not to the latex-bound reagent drug forms no aggregates and thus no turbidity, degree of which is related to the level of the drug in the patient sample.

Similarly, the use of enzyme multiplied immunoassay assay (EMIT), where the reagent drug is conjugated to an enzyme often (alkaline phosphates, etc.). This reagent drug-enzyme conjugate competes with drug in the patient's sample with reagent antibody, the binding of the enzyme labeled antigen inhibits enzymatic activity and thus reduces the significant color of the enzymatic reaction following addition of substrate, and is inversely proportional to the amount of the drug in patient samples. Manufacturers list the degree of antibody cross-reactivity with parent drugs and metabolites, and they vary from one manufacture and is reflective of the antibody specificity and the assay formulation.

The use of antibodies directed against either the groups of drugs, for example, amphetamines where the antibody detects the parent compounds as well as metabolites is common. Not all metabolites are detected and not all synthetic materials are detected. Such assays are designed for screening purposes, and they are whether available as point-of-care testing devices or in reagents for automated laboratory-based instrumentation. As screening assays, confirmation may be required to avoid false positives due to interferences, often

by chromatographically based assays (see later). Some immunoassays are directed toward specific drugs such as those for methadone, or oxycodone, that may not be recognized by the general group-targeted antibodies.

Chromatography-based assays

Liquid chromatography coupled with mass spectrometry detections (LC-MSMS) is becoming widely available in routine clinical laboratories. They are applicable to both therapeutic drugs monitoring and toxicological testing.

They afford both a higher degree of sensitivity and specificity and are often used to confirm initial immunoassay-based laboratory findings. See the chapter on analytical methods for more details.

Assays characteristics

Commonly tested for toxicology drugs, their half-life, time remaining positive post dosage, their respective assays detection limits, cross-reactivities as well as recommended cutoffs for workplace and clinical application are shown in Tables 19–21.

Cutoffs for positivity

The above tables show urine and sweat cutoffs for positivity as recommended by statutory agencies, assay performance and utility (clinical, workplace, forensic, etc..) (Tables 20 and 21).

Limiting interference

Interference in toxicology testing is common and both clinical correlation and confirmatory testing are often required. The screening assays, as the name implies, are often designed to be group or class specific to allow for detection of both parent compound and/or its metabolites as well as possible synthetic or adulterated compound. Clinical correlation (toxidromes, drug history, review of assay kit instructions for manufacturer documented interferent/cross-reactant) often resolves the suspicion of interference in an urgent setting. However, laboratory confirmation is often warranted. This is achieved using a higher specificity and sensitivity methodology such as liquid chromatography coupled to tandem mass spectrometry, or even the use of analyte-specific immunoassay such as those specifically for 6-monoacetylmorphine (heroin), methadone, oxycodone. Pretreatment and technical manipulation of the patient sample may improve detection and specificity such as in hydrolysis of glucuronides conjugates of benzodiazepines prior to testing by immunoassays. The following interferences have been reported for some of the commercially available assays (Table 22).

TABLE 19 Half-life of various toxicology drugs and their detection window. *MDMA*, 3,4-methyenedioxy-methamphetamine; *6-AM*, 6-acetylmorphine (heroin); *PCP*, phencyclidine; *TCA*, tricyclic antidepressants.

Drug/metabolite	Half-life (T½) (h)	Initial detection on intake (h)	Time remaining positive post-dose
Amphetamines	7–24	4–6	2–4 (up to 9) days
Methamphetamine	6–15	4–6	2–4 (up to 6) days
Barbiturates	Variable: 15–144	2–4	2–30 days
Benzodiazepines	Variable: 1–37	2–7	1–4 days (Diazepam: 2–7 (up to 30) days)
Cannabinoids	20–57	1–3	1–7 days casual use 1–30 (up to 95) days chronic use
Cocaine	0.7–1.5	2–6	1–4 days single use 11–22 days chronic use
Ecstasy (MDMA)	6–9	2–7	1–4 days
Fentanyl	3–12	24–72	<1 day
Hydrocodone	4	6–11	2–4 days
Hydromorphone	1.5–3.8		2–4 days
Methadone	15–55	3–8	1–3 (up to 11) days
Opiates (codeine)	1.9–3.9	2–6	1–4 days
Opiates (heroin-6 AM)	1.3–6.7	2–6	2–4 h 2–4 days as morphine
Oxycodone	4–6	1–3	1–4 days
PCP	7–46	4–6	2–7 days casual use 71–30 days chronic use
TCA	15–30	8–12	2–7 days
Tramadol	4.3–6.7		0.5–1.5 days

Modified from Moeller KE, Kissack JC, Atayee RS, Lee KC. Clinical interpretation of urine drug tests: what clinicians need to know about urine drug screens. Mayo Clin Proc 2017;92(5):774-796. https://doi.org/10.1016/j.mayocp.2016.12.007. Epub 2017 Mar 18. PMID: 28325505.

TABLE 20 SAMHSA: Substance abuse and mental health services.

Screening test	Screening test Cutoff	Confirmatory test	Confirmatory test Cutoff
Marijuana metabolites	50 ng/mL	THCA	15 ng/mL
Cocaine metabolites	150 ng/mL	BE	100 ng/mL
Opiate metabolites Codeine/morphine	2000 ng/mL	Codeine/morphine	2000 ng/mL 2000 ng/mL
6-AM	10 ng/mL	6-AM	10 ng/mL
PCP	25 ng/mL	PCP	25 ng/mL
Amphetamine/ methamphetamine	500 ng/mL	Amphetamine/ methamphetamine	250 ng/mL 250 ng/mL
MDMA	500 ng/mL	MDMA MDA MDEA	250 ng/mL 250 ng/mL 250 ng/mL

NIDA, National Institute on Drug Abuse; *THCA*, tetrahydrocannabinolic acid; *BE*, benzoylecgonine; *6-AM*, 6-acetylmorphine (heroin); *PCP*, phencyclidine; *MDMA*, 3,4-methyenedioxy-methamphetamine; *MDA*, 3,4-methylenedioxyamphetamine, 3,4-methylenedioxy-N-ethylamphentamine.
Modified from SAMHSA. 2022-06886 Mandatory Guidelines for Federal Workplace Drug Testing Programs using Urine. file:///Users/ihashim/Downloads/SAMHSA-2022-0002-0001_content.pdf. Accessed 9th March 2023.

TABLE 21 Cutoffs in use by different agencies and for different purposes. Note those of the workplace are much higher compared to those of clinical needs.

Drug assay Cutoff (ng/mL)	Federal workplace	Clinical laboratories	Pain management	Confirmation GC-MS/ LC-MSMS	Sweat (skin patch PharmCheK)
Opiates	2000	300	300	100	10
Amphetamines	1000	1000	500	75–250	10
Oxycodone	–	–	100	50–100	10
Oxymorphone	–	–	100	50	10
Methadone	–	–	100	100	–
Barbiturates	–	200	200	100	–
Benzodiazepines	–	200	200	100	–
Cannabinoids	50	50	20	5–15	0.5
Cocaine (Benzoylecgonine)	300	300	300	100–150	10
Phencyclidine	25	25	25	25	7.5
Propoxyphene (norpropoxyphene)	–	–	300	200	–
Ethyl alcohol (ethyl glucuronide)	–	100	100	100	–
Adulteration Check	✓	✓	✓		

Modified from Moeller KE, Kissack JC, Atayee RS, Lee KC. Clinical interpretation of urine drug tests: what clinicians need to know about urine drug screens. Mayo Clin Proc 2017;92(5):774-796. https://doi.org/10.1016/j.mayocp.2016.12.007. Epub 2017 Mar 18. PMID: 28325505, from DOT Rule 49 CFR Part 40 Section 40.87. Subpart F, and SAMHSA. 2022-06886 Mandatory Guidelines for Federal Workplace Drug Testing Programs using Urine. file:///Users/ihashim/Downloads/SAMHSA-2022-0002-0001_content.pdf. Accessed 9th March 2023, and from test reagents information sheets.

TABLE 22 Test drug group and reported interferences by different commercial assays and different cutoff values.

Test drug group	Drugs with observed interference
Amphetamines	Bupropion, chlorpromazine, 1,3-dimethylamylamine (DMAA), Labetalol, Metformin, Ofloxacin, Promethazine, Trazodone
Tricyclic antidepressants	Quetiapine
Benzodiazepines	Efavirenz, Sertraline
Cannabinoids	Efavirenz, Ibuprofen, Naproxen, Niflumn acid
Opiates	Amisulpride, Sulpiride, Codeine, Morphine, Methadone, Morphine-3-glucuronide, Dihydrocodeine, Diphenhydramine, Levofloxacin, Ofloxacin, Pefloxacin, Enoxacine, Gemifloxacin, Lomefloxacin, Moxifloxacin, Ciprofloxacin, Norfloxacine, Morphine, Naloxone, Pentazocine, Quetiapine, Rifampicin, Tapentadol, Tramadol, Verapamil
PCP	Lamotrigine, methylenedioxypyrovalerone (MDPV), Tramadol, Venlafaxine
LSD	Ambroxol, Fentanyl, Sertraline, Amitriptyline, Benzphetamine, Bupropion, Buspirone, Cephradine, Chlorpromazine, Desipramine, Diltiazem, Doxepin, Fluoxetine, Haloperidol, Imipramine, Labetalol, Metoclopramide, Prochlorperazine, Risperidone, Thioridazine, Trazodone, Verapamil, Ergonovine, Lysergol, Brompheniramine maleate, Imipramine HCl, and Methylphenidate HC
Barbiturates	Ibuprofen, Naproxen

Modified from Saitman A, Park HD, Fitzgerald RL. False-positive interferences of common urine drug screen immunoassays: a review. J Anal Toxicol 2014;38(7):387-396.

Novel drugs of abuse

Novel illicit drugs either newly synthetic or analogues of known drugs are continuously being produced commonly known as designer drugs. They are continuously evolving and thus the prevalence remains unknown. Illicit drugs may also be contaminants of traditional drugs of abuse, for example, the addition of fentanyl to heroin.

The new or modified drugs are likely to have either enhanced physiological response or heterogenous symptoms. Standard laboratory assays, although being by design are group specific, are often unlikely to detect designer drugs. Surrogate markers such as anion gap, biochemical abnormalities, osmolar gap as well as clinical symptoms may suggest a particular group of drugs. Testing often requires specialized laboratory but the results take a long time to come back and not in a timely manner to influence clinical management. Clinical management is often conservative by correcting for dehydration, acid-base status, and sedation to limit any accompanied agitation and central nervous system excitation.

Summary

- The clinical laboratory is central to; (1) support therapeutic drug monitoring, and (2) the toxicological investigations and support of drug dependency rehabilitation programs.
- Some clinical laboratories may extend their activities to support forensic, law, and workplace testing. The latter in addition to the provision of chain of custody requires the availability of both screening and confirmatory testing.
- Drugs are characterized by their pharmacokinetics and pharmacodynamic characteristics. Pharmacokinetics describes the drug absorption, bioavailability, metabolism, and excretion (handling by the body), whereas pharmacodynamics describes the action of the drug and the relationship between dosage and effect (drug actions).
- Candidate drugs for therapeutic drug monitoring are those with narrow therapeutic window, high risk of toxicity, difficult to ascertain toxicity and/or subtherapeutic levels, and when needed to confirm patient compliance.
- Therapeutic drug monitoring should be performed once the drug has reached steady state which is typically at five to seven times the half-life of the drug.
- Immunoassay-based methods detect both parent and drug metabolites. They are rapid but often suffer from variable degree of cross-reactivity with metabolites and possibly other drugs as well as a lack of sensitivity for some.

- Chromatography-based assays (LC-MSMS) are used for both screening and confirmation. They afford higher levels of sensitivity and specificity when compared with immunoassays. However, they are considered laboratory-developed tests, cumbersome to develop, and are not amenable to rapid and STAT analysis.

References

1. van den Anker J, Reed MD, Allegaert K, Kearns GL. Developmental changes in pharmacokinetics and pharmacodynamics. *J Clin Pharmacol.* 2018;58(Suppl 10):S10–S25.
2. Abou-Khalil BW. Update on antiepileptic drugs 2019. *Continuum (Minneap Minn).* 2019;25(2):508–536.
3. Lass-Florl C. Triazole antifungal agents in invasive fungal infections: a comparative review. *Drugs.* 2011;71(18):2405–2419.
4. Jenkins N, Black M, Schneider HG. Simultaneous determination of voriconazole, posaconazole, itraconazole and hydroxy-itraconazole in human plasma using LC-MSMS. *Clin Biochem.* 2018;53:110–115.
5. Restellini S, Khanna R, Afif W. Therapeutic drug monitoring with Ustekinumab and vedolizumab in inflammatory bowel disease. *Inflamm Bowel Dis.* 2018;24(10):2165–2172.

Further reading

Shipkova M, Christians U. Improving therapeutic decisions: pharmacodynamic monitoring as an integral part of therapeutic drug monitoring. *Ther Drug Monit.* 2019;41(2):111–114.

Garcia-Bournissen F, Rokach B, Karaskov T, Gareri J, Koren G. Detection of stimulant drugs of abuse in maternal and neonatal hair. *Forensic Sci Med Pathol.* 2007;3(2):115–118.

Patsalos PN, Spencer EP, Berry DJ. Therapeutic drug monitoring of antiepileptic drugs in epilepsy: a 2018 update. *Ther Drug Monit.* 2018;40(5):526–548.

Sandilands E, Bateman DN. Analgesics. *Clin Med (Lond).* 2008;8(1):96–99.

Kim JJ, Kim YS, Kumar V. Heavy metal toxicity: an update of chelating therapeutic strategies. *J Trace Elem Med Biol.* 2019;54:226–231.

Wang GS, Hoyte C. Novel drugs of abuse. *Pediatr Rev.* 2019;40(2):71–78.

Banerjee S, Narayanan M, Gould K. Monitoring aminoglycoside level. *BMJ.* 2012;345, e6354.

Konidari A, Anagnostopoulos A, Bonnett LJ, Pirmohamed M, El-Matary W. Thiopurine monitoring in children with inflammatory bowel disease: a systematic review. *Br J Clin Pharmacol.* 2014;78(3):467–476.

Hodgman MJ, Garrard AR. A review of acetaminophen poisoning. *Crit Care Clin.* 2012;28(4):499–516.

Saitman A, Park HD, Fitzgerald RL. False-positive interferences of common urine drug screen immunoassays: a review. *J Anal Toxicol.* 2014;38(7):387–396.

Andresen-Streichert H, Muller A, Glahn A, Skopp G, Sterneck M. Alcohol biomarkers in clinical and forensic contexts. *Dtsch Arztebl Int.* 2018;115(18):309–315.

Chapter 15

Blood gases and acid-base homeostasis

Introduction

Assessment of blood acid-base status is vital in the diagnosis and management of patients in critical care settings.

Responsibility for the availability of blood gases testing often belongs to clinical chemistry laboratories as well as to point-of-care testing sections and that testing is either performed by the clinical laboratory, by respiratory therapists, or by emergency room and critical care, and surgical clinical personnel. This chapter describes acid-base homeostasis, disorders, and their investigation, where accurate and timely measurement and interpretation are critical and lifesaving.

Acid-base homeostasis and buffering systems

Maintaining an optimal hydrogen ion (H^+) concentration is essential for optimum cellular function and metabolic activities. Several organs including the lungs, kidney, brain, liver, and blood play a major role in maintaining the acid-base status of the body.

Normal hydrogen ion concentration is very low at 0.00004 mmol/L expressed as (pH 7.4). It is best that the very low [H^+] concentrations are presented as pH derived using the negative logarithmic of H^+ concentration ($-\log_{10}$ [H^+]); hence, its reported value is not linear and changes *inversely* to [H^+]. For instance, a of 40 nmoL/L is a pH of 7.4 and a [H^+] of 80 nmoL/L is a pH of 7.10 (Fig. 1). Therefore, pH is an index of the blood degree of acidity or alkalinity and represents the net effect of simple or mixed acid-base disorders and any compensatory component.

The body is able to tolerate large changes in H^+ concentrations, as much as fourfold, for instance, a change from 40 to 175 mmol/L which may not be apparently obvious when described in pH terms, that is a change from pH 7.40 to 6.7 (Fig. 1).

The pH is affected by body temperature with a 0.015 units decrease for every 1°C increase, and in some clinical practice, blood gases results are reported corrected for the patient body temperature at the time of sample collection.

Hydrogen ion regulation

The body is constantly producing hydrogen ions (H^+) from metabolic processes at about 40–80 mmol of hydrogen ions per day. Metabolism and oxidation of sulfur-containing amino acids contribute the most. A high protein diet typically produces 1 mEq/Kg body weight per day (70 mEq per day for a 70 kg person). Phosphoric and sulfuric acids are major products of the metabolism of dietary proteins and phospholipids. Pathological acids are ketoacids and lactic acids. The rate of production of ketoacid and lactic acids is self-regulated where, for instance, their production is decreased in the presence of low pH. This accumulation of acid (or loss of HCO_3^{-}) if not corrected or if it exceeds the kidney's ability results in metabolic acidosis. A vegetarian diet high in fruits and vegetables is not acid-producing and produces a net alkali load.

Homeostatic mechanism is very efficient in maintaining blood pH at the normal range of 7.35 to 7.45. Both the kidneys and the lungs play an important role in the process of regulating nonvolatile and volatile acid-base components, respectively. The imbalance between the production and elimination of acid-base components and failure of homeostatic mechanism results in states of acidosis or alkalosis with either a primary sole component or an often mixed status.

Under normal circumstances, the control mechanisms work hard to maintain hydrogen ion homeostasis and adequate oxygenation, and prevent hypercapnia. This is achieved mainly through buffering mechanisms, lung function, and renal function. All three are interlinked and work together in health and in disease.

The kidney is the major regulator of acid-base status through reclaiming and generating bicarbonate, the metabolic component of acid-base balance, and in the process excreting excess acid (H^+) (see later).

At the lungs, the cycle of blood oxygenation and exchange of gases begins with oxygen and carbon dioxide is exchanged at the alveolar-capillary membrane levels by a process of diffusion down a concentration gradient. Oxygen bound to hemoglobin is delivered to the tissue and exchanged with carbon dioxide. Adequate blood supply is required for this process. Furthermore, decreased blood flow and reduced oxygen levels lead to tissue hypoxia and injury.

The movement of gases exerts pressure which is directly proportional to its concentration and directs the rate of diffusion across the tissue. Thus, the partial pressure of oxygen is high in the alveoli (high O_2 concentration) and that CO_2 is high in the blood reaching the lungs, the gases are exchanged down their partial pressure (concentration

Tutorials in Clinical Chemistry. https://doi.org/10.1016/B978-0-12-822949-1.00004-8

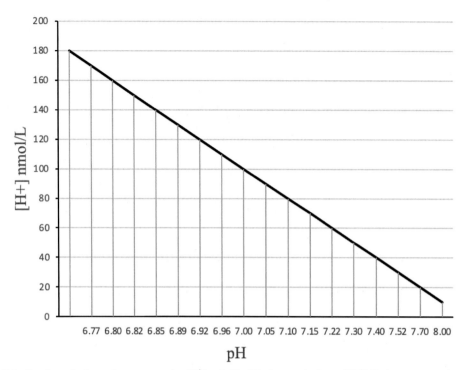

FIG. 1 Range of clinically relevant hydrogen ion concentration [H⁺] and pH. pH is the negative Log of [H⁺]. It changes *inversely* to [H⁺]. Note logarithmic change is not linear (for example, [H⁺] 40 mmoL/L = 7.4, and 80 mmoL/L = 7.10).

gradient), similarly at the tissue levels where O_2 diffuses into the tissue and CO_2 into the blood. The partial pressure of the gases is measured as an indication of its concentration and is denoted by pO_2 and pCO_2. The measurement of the O_2 and CO_2 partial pressures is indicative of the pressure (concertation) of the gases at the time of sample collection. Normal pO_2 and pCO_2 levels are 12–24 kPa (80 mmHg) and 4.6–6.0 kPa (35 mmHg), respectively.

Buffer systems and their capacity

Buffer systems resist changes in pH when acid or base components are added. Composed of a weak acid (easily dissociates) and a conjugate base. The buffering capacity is concentration dependent and works best with nearly equal amounts of each (acid/base) present and within one pH unit of the buffer system pK_a.

An acid donates a proton (H^+), whereas a base accepts a proton. Therefore, maintenance of acid-base status requires acid-base pairs. In this setting, examples are carbonic acid-bicarbonate base, monobasic and dibasic phosphate, ammonia and ammonium ion, and lactic acid lactate.

Therefore, in functional terms, buffering is the capacity of a weak acid and its associated base, for example, to resist ensuing change in pH.

As hydrogen ions are produced, they are buffered by a number of buffer systems within the body; bicarbonate buffer, proteins (mostly albumin and is mostly due to histidine imidazole group with a pK_a of 7.4), hemoglobin (binding H^+ and transporting it to the lung where it is exchanged

with O_2), tissue mostly bone, and phosphate and ammonia buffering exchange systems in urine (Figs. 2 and 3).

It is important to note that buffering of hydrogen ions is only a temporary measure as the hydrogen ion is still in the body. Buffering power will eventually be depleted if H^+ is not eliminated from the body. Hydrogen ions can only be lost from the body through the kidney and intestine. It cannot be excreted alone and is associated with a carrier cation (see later).

Bicarbonate buffer

The bicarbonate buffer is the most abundant and most important. About 12,000 mmol of carbonic acid (CO_2) is produced per day. In the presence of carbonic anhydrase, dissolved CO_2 (carbonic acid) dissociates into H_2O and HCO_3^-.

$$\left[CO_2 + H_2O \leftrightarrow H_2CO_3 \leftrightarrow H^+ + HCO_3^- \right]$$

The reaction is reversible, and hydrogen ions combine with HCO_3^- to form CO_2 and water ($H^+ + HCO_3^- \leftrightarrow H_2CO_3$). This is a reversible reaction catalyzed by carbonic anhydrase and H^+ will only continue to be neutralized (restricted) if CO_2 is removed (by the lung).

Approximately 15,000 mmol of carbon dioxide is generated each day by tissue metabolism and can be removed from the body in expired air. This results in the depletion of the buffer.

Regeneration of the buffer can take place by excreting the H^+ bound to another buffer, e.g., HPO_4^{2-} or NH_3 systems

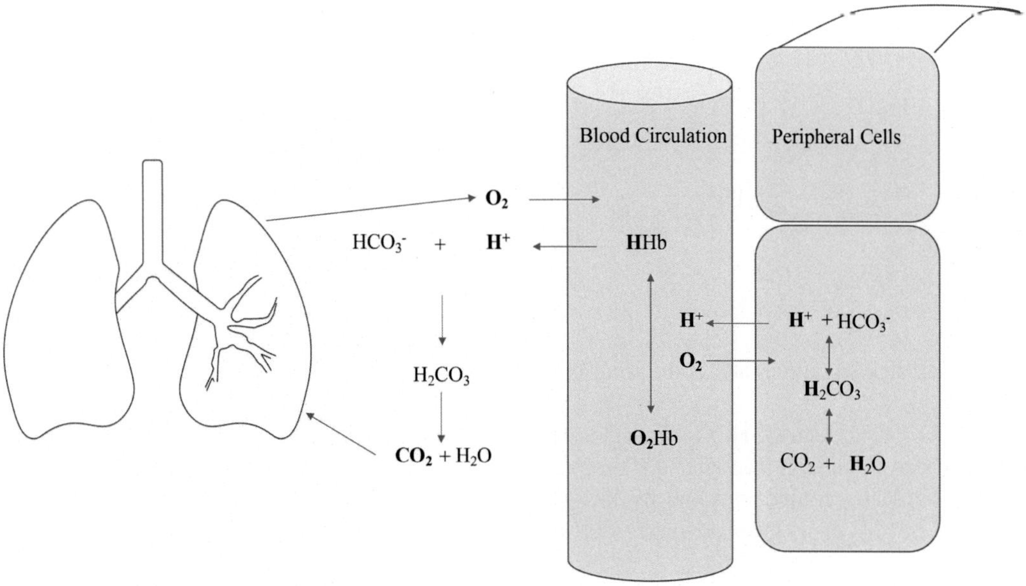

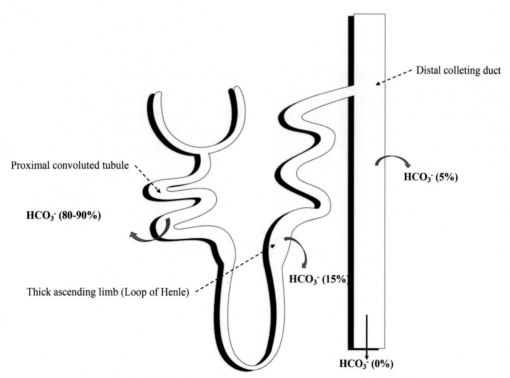

FIG. 2 Lung homeostatic role: Hydrogen ion is exchanged with O_2 in the lungs, where inhaled O_2 enters the blood circulation and CO_2 is exhaled. *Modified from Hamm LL, Nakhoul N, Hering-Smith KS. Acid-base homeostasis. Clin J Am Soc Nephrol. 2015;10(12):2232–42. doi: 10.2215/CJN.07400715. Epub 2015 Nov 23. PMID: 26597304; PMCID: PMC4670772.*

FIG. 3 Most of the filtered bicarbonate (HCO_3^-) is reabsorbed at the proximal convoluted tubule (80%–90%), some at the thick ascending limb of Henle, and at the distal collecting duct. Very little to nonbicarbonate is lost in the urine. *Modified from Hamm LL, Nakhoul N, Hering-Smith KS. Acid-base homeostasis. Clin J Am Soc Nephrol. 2015;10(12):2232–42. doi: 10.2215/CJN.07400715. Epub 2015 Nov 23. PMID: 26597304; PMCID: PMC4670772.*

in the kidney. The lung and the kidney work in tandem to regulate hydrogen ion concentration. The relatively rapid respiratory response acting initially followed by a slower renal response.

The above bicarbonate buffer reaction equation can be rearranged to provide what is known as the *Henderson-Hasselbalch* equation and is used to provide a mathematical relationship as derived below:

$$H^+ + HCO_3^- \leftrightarrow H_2CO_3$$

$$\left[H^+\right] = k \times \left[H_2CO_3\right] / \left[HCO_3^-\right]$$

$$\left[H^+\right] = k \times \left[pCO_2\right] / \left[HCO_3^-\right]$$

$$pH = pK_a - \log\left[H_2CO_3\right] / \left[HCO_3^-\right]$$

$$pH = pK_a + \log\left[HCO_3^-\right] / \left[pCO_2\right]$$

$$pH = 6.1 + \log\left[HCO_3^-\right] / \left(0.03 \times pCO_2\right)$$

(Henderson-Hasselbalch equation, 0.03 is the solubility coefficient)

Since pH and pCO_2 are measured, HCO_3^- can then be calculated using the above equation (see later). Therefore, pH is defined by pCO_2 (lung component) and by HCO_3^- (kidney component), not by their absolute values but by their relative ratio.

At the lungs (respiratory component), carbon dioxide is exhaled, and oxygen is inhaled in exchange for H^+ (Fig. 2). Inhaled oxygen is exchanged at the hemoglobin level with H^+ (Figs. 2 and 4).

The lungs in acid-base homeostasis

Breathing control and respiratory rate

Breathing is largely involuntary and produced by semi-autonomous neural networks known as central pattern generators (CPGs) (Fig. 5). It represents a control network of peripheral sensor neurons and central control termed and drives the activity of spinal motor neurons innervating respiratory pump muscles.

It comprises central chemoreceptors sensitive to H^+, CO_2, and pO_2. Therefore, respiratory rate is influenced by

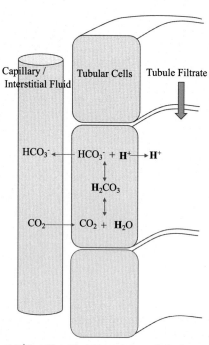

FIG. 4   Renal H^+ handling. The kidney plays a role in the excretion of H^+. Renal interstitial cells containing carbonic anhydrase catalyze the bicornate reaction described above. This regenerates bicarbonate diffusing into the blood and excretes hydrogen ions. However, hydrogen ions cannot be excreted into the urine alone and are accompanied by associated cations. *Modified from Hamm LL, Nakhoul N, Hering-Smith KS. Acid-base homeostasis. Clin J Am Soc Nephrol. 2015;10(12):2232–42. doi: 10.2215/CJN.07400715. Epub 2015 Nov 23. PMID: 26597304; PMCID: PMC4670772.*

acid-base status as well as alveolar and arterial blood gases (O_2 and CO_2). Several control mechanisms have been postulated; however, the endpoint is the central and neurological adjustment to maintain gases and acid-base balance. For instance, the response to hypercapnia (high CO_2).

In cases of increased O_2 need, as in exercise, and need to remove generated CO_2 and adjustment of the pH (acid-base

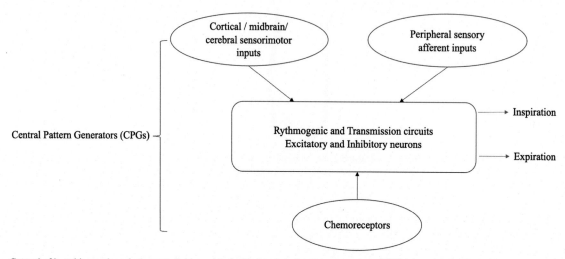

FIG. 5   Control of breathing and respiratory rate is hierarchical with the central pattern generators (CPGs) (a network of central and peripheral neuronal receptors) driving the respiratory process and its rate. The respiratory center is stimulated by and helps maintain pO_2, pCO_2, and acid-base status. *Modified from Smith JC, Abdala AP, Borgmann A, Rybak IA, Paton JF. Brainstem respiratory networks: building blocks and microcircuits. Trends Neurosci 2013;36(3):152–62. doi: 10.1016/j.tins.2012.11.004. Epub 2012 Dec 17. PMID: 23254296; PMCID: PMC4080795.*

status) due to increased metabolism and/or lactic acidosis, in severe exercise.

In patients with respiratory disorders such as chronic obstructive airway disease (COPD), the stimulus to hypercapnia is impaired and hence the rapid respiratory correction for the acid-base abnormalities (respiratory acidosis) due to hypercapnia.

The kidney in acid-base homeostasis

The kidney plays an important role in acid-base status through the excretion of excess acid (H^+) and reclaiming of filtered bicarbonate. Hydrogen ions cannot be excreted alone but are associated with a carrier base such as ammonia and phosphatase (see later). Additionally, central to the buffering system is carbonic anhydrase in renal tubular cells. Bicarbonate is regenerated and reclaimed while hydrogen ions are generated and excreted coupled to other anions primarily phosphate and ammonia.

Most (about 90%) of filtered bicarbonate is reabsorbed at the renal proximal tubules (Fig. 3). Filtered bicarbonate combines with hydrogen ions to form carbonic acid. Carbonic anhydrase present in the brush borders of the renal tubules converts carbonic acid to carbon dioxide and water. CO_2 passively diffuses into renal tubular cells, wherein the presence of water is converted back into bicarbonate and hydrogen ions catalyzed again by the reversible action of carbonic anhydrase ($[CO_2 + H_2O \leftrightarrow H_2CO_3 \leftrightarrow H^+ + HCO_3^-]$).

Hydrogen excretion in the kidney is coupled with the excretion of phosphate (HPO_4^{2-}), ammonia (NH_3), and bicarbonate (Figs. 4, 6, and 7). Therefore, the excretion of H^+ depends on the presence of urinary phosphate and ammonia.

The kidney excretes about 50–100 mEq/day of nonvolatile acids compared with about 15,000 to 25,000 mmol/day by the lungs. Compensatory mechanisms in acid-base homeostasis are, however, slower in the kidney compared to that of the rapid lung respiratory process.

Phosphate as buffering system

It has been stated that hydrogen ions cannot be excreted alone. It is associated with phosphate cations. To maintain neutrality, sodium ions are exchanged (see Fig. 6), and this results in the reabsorption of filtered sodium. Phosphate is predominately intracellular. Circulating concentration is maintained at about 0.97 to 1.3 mmol/L. At physiological pH 7.4, the major (75%) inorganic phosphate form is HPO_4^{2-} and a minor (25%) H_2PO^{4-}.

Homeostatic mechanisms include extracellular shifts, bone resorption (bone contains 80% of the body's phosphate content as hydroxyapatite), and renal and gastrointestinal absorption stimulated by vitamin D. Most >90% of filtered phosphate is reabsorbed and is inhibited by parathyroid hormone.

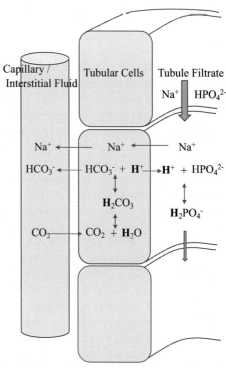

FIG. 6 Phosphate as a buffer system: Phosphate is coupled to H^+ facilitating its excretion. Active reabsorption of sodium maintains electrical neutrality. *Modified from Hamm LL, Nakhoul N, Hering-Smith KS. Acid-base homeostasis. Clin J Am Soc Nephrol. 2015;10(12):2232–42. doi: 10.2215/CJN.07400715. Epub 2015 Nov 23. PMID: 26597304; PMCID: PMC4670772.*

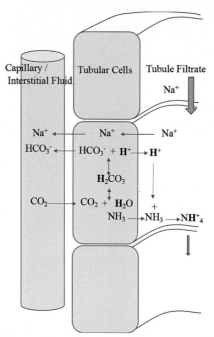

FIG. 7 Ammonia as a buffer: Ammonia generated in the deamination of proteins diffuses into the lumen down a concentration gradient where it is coupled to H^+ ions and thus facilitates both its excretion and removal of ammonia. Electroneutrality is maintained following active reabsorption and thus reclamation of filtered sodium. *Modified from Hamm LL, Nakhoul N, Hering-Smith KS. Acid-base homeostasis. Clin J Am Soc Nephrol. 2015;10(12):2232–42. doi: 10.2215/CJN.07400715. Epub 2015 Nov 23. PMID: 26597304; PMCID: PMC4670772.*

Ammonia as a buffering system

Ammonia is generated by haptic and gastrointestinal deamidation of proteins. The main precursor is glutamine in the renal tissue. It is produced as NH_4^+ by mitochondrial phosphate-dependent glutaminase deaminates glutamine to glutamate and NH_4^+. A second NH_4^+ is generated following the conversion of glutamate to alpha-ketoglutarate by glutamate dehydrogenase. Alpha-ketoglutarate is then converted to glucose or metabolized yielding HCO_3^-.

Ammonium ion (NH_4^+) is the other major buffer system for the excretion of H^+ ions accounting for 50 to 75% of the next acid excretion (and bicarbonate generation) of about 40–50 mmol/day.

The ammonia buffer system ($H^+ + NH_3 \leftrightarrow NH_4^+$) has a pK_a of 9.2 (too high), i.e., at physiological pH most of the ammonia is in the NH_4^+ form which renders it not as effective as bicarbonate.

Renal production of ammonia is enhanced in states of chronic metabolic acidosis. Hyperkalemia suppresses ammonia production and handling by the proximal and thick limb, whereas hypokalemia increases ammonia production by the kidneys (Fig. 7).

Most of the renal NH_4^+ is excreted into the urine and not via blood circulation.

Hemoglobin as a buffering system

Hemoglobin inside red blood cells also provides a buffer system for H^+ where it binds to negatively charged Hb^- (Fig. 8). HCO_3^- is exchanged for chloride (known as the chloride shift Bohr effect).

Acid-base disorders

Acid is produced as a result of body metabolism and strict maintenance of normal acid-base status, that is a blood pH within 7.35 to 7.45 is essential for metabolic activities (enzymatic action, electrolytes neutrality balance, bone health, and kidney function, etc.) where, for instance, chronic acidosis results in decreased bone density, skeletal muscle wasting, progression of chronic kidney disease (stages 1 to3), and formation of kidney stones. The intracellular pH is about 7.2. At the extreme ends, hydrogen ions that are compatible were life ranges from 0.126 mmol/L (pH 6.9) to 0.025 mmol/L (pH 7.6).

About 1.5 mmol of acid (H^+) is produced per kilogram body weight per day (70 to 100 mmol H^+). The lung removes about 15,000 to 25,000 mmol of volatile acid in the form of CO_2 per day, whereas the kidney removes about 70 mEq H^+ per day.

As mentioned above, the lung and kidney play a central role in acid-base metabolism and homeostasis. Acid-base disorders are classified as either respiratory (lung) or metabolic (kidney) in nature and either exhibiting acidosis (low pH – high H^+ concentration) or alkalosis (low pH – low H^+ concentration). Normalization of blood pH in the presence of pCO_2 and HCO^{3-} abnormalities is considered a saucerful compensatory mechanism in either the lung (rapid in minutes) or the kidney (slow—days) or both (see later). Compensation could be either complete, partial (pH slightly outside normal limits), or unsuccessful (uncompensated).

Interpretation of blood gas measurements as a standalone, although often possible, can sometimes be difficult and clinical integration is often required for accurate

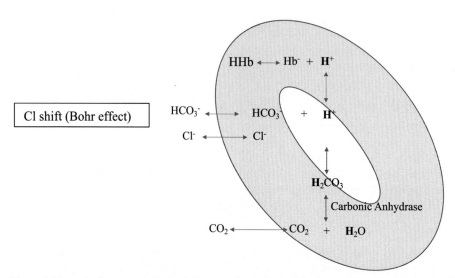

FIG. 8 Red blood cell hemoglobin as a buffer system buffering hydrogen and regenerating bicarbonate. Neutrality is maintained by exchange for chloride ions a process known as the Bohr effect. *Modified from Jensen FB. Red blood cell pH, the Bohr effect, and other oxygenation-linked phenomena in blood O_2 and CO_2 transport. Acta Physiol Scand 2004;182(3):215–27. doi: 10.1111/j.1365-201X.2004.01361.x. [PMID: 15491402].*

diagnosis. Patient history and cause of disease often provide a clue as to the origin of the acid-base disorder.

Laboratory assessment of acid-base disorders includes the measurement of arterial blood gases, co-oximetry, as well as electrolytes, lactate, osmolality, and urine results.

Blood gases and relevant components and applied terminologies

In addition to pH, several blood gas components measured as well as derived, their diagnostic utility, as well as normal limits are shown in Table 1.

Acid-base disorders are termed either being metabolic in nature. This refers to a primary change in HCO_3^- and/or H^+. Respiratory classification refers to a primary change in pCO_2 excretion by the lungs. In general, respiratory acidosis and alkalosis cannot exist simultaneously.

Compensatory mechanisms

In intact homeostatic mechanisms, adaptive response to return pH toward normal by restoring the normal ratio of pCO_2 to HCO_3^- is termed a compensatory process. Driven directly by abnormal pH only (not directly affected by pCO_2 or HCO_3^-). However, the degree of compensation depends on the extent of change in pH, diminishes as pH returns to normal, and disappears when primary acid-base disorder resolves. In most disorders to maintain charge Cl^- changes in the opposite direction to HCO_3^- but by the same amount, respiratory disorders alter the renal excretion of HCO_3^-. Metabolic disorders alter respiratory rate to change pCO_2 (Table 2).

In metabolic compensation: Renal HCO_3^- excretion alters slowly (reaching maximum compenstation at 48–72h). In patients with acute respiratory disorders, bicarbonate changes by 1–2 mmoL/L per 10 mmHg. Whereas, in chronic

TABLE 1 Measured and calculated parameters in the assessment of acid-base status. Partial pressure of oxygen (pO_2), partial pressure of carbon dioxide (pCO_2), bicarbonate (HCO_3^-).

Component	Utility	Analysis	Reference intervals SI units/(conational)
pH (−Log [H$^+$])	Index of acidity/alkalinity of blood	Measured pH electrode	pH: 7.35–7.45 H$^+$: 35–45 mmol/L
pO$_2$	Tension/pressure of dissolved O$_2$	Measured Clark electrode	Arterial: Adult: <60yrs.: 11.3–13.3 kPa (85–100 mmHg), >60yrs.: 8.7–10.6 kPa (65–80 mmHg)
pCO$_2$	Tension/pressure of dissolved CO$_2$	Measured	Arterial: 4.7–5.8 kPa (35–44 mmHg)
HCO$_3^-$	Indicator of the buffering capacity of blood	Calculated $(0.0307 \times pCO_2 \times 10^{(pH-6.105)})$	mmol/L
Actual bicarbonate:	Reflects both respiratory and metabolic effects on HCO$_3^-$ of limited use in critically ill patients.	Calculated using pH and pCO$_2$	21–25 mmol/L
Standard bicarbonate	Eliminates the contribution of the respiratory component to blood HCO$_3^-$ estimation. Measures metabolic nonrespiratory contribution to HCO$_3^-$. Used with pCO$_2$ to interpret respiratory and metabolic components.	Calculated using pH and substituting a normal pCO$_2$ (5.3 kPa)	21–25 mmol/L
Base excess	Describes the amount of bicarbonate in mmol added to a liter of blood under standard condition (37°C and pCO$_2$ 5.3 kPa to return pH to 7.4)	Calculated $[HCO_3^-] - 24.8 + 16.2 \times (pH - 7.4)$	+ 2 mmol/L to −2 mmol/L
FO$_2$Hb	Percentage of total Hb that is saturated with O$_2$	(O$_2$Hb/(O$_2$Hb + HHb + COHb + MetHb))	90%–98%
Oxygen Saturation. (SaO$_2$)	Percentage of functional Hb that is saturated with O$_2$ (a fraction of 1)	(O$_2$Hb/(O$_2$Hb + HHb))	>95% (~92% on room air)
FiO2	Fraction of inspired oxygen		

Continued

TABLE 1 Measured and calculated parameters in the assessment of acid-base status. Partial pressure of oxygen (pO_2), partial pressure of carbon dioxide (pCO_2), bicarbonate (HCO_3^-)—cont'd

Component	Utility	Analysis	Reference intervals SI units/(conational)
Co-oximetry			
Hemoglobin		Measured. Spectrophotometrically	Male:13.2 to 16.6 g/dL Female: 116 to 15.0 g/dL
Carboxy Hemoglobin	Carbon monoxide poisoning/exposure	Measured. Spectrophotometrically	<2.5%
Methemoglobin		Measured. Spectrophotometrically	<1.5%
Other biomarkers			
Sodium	Electrolytes disorders	Measured (ISE) Nernst equation	135–145 mmol/L
Potassium	Electrolytes disorders (secondary to acid-base status)	Measured (ISE.) Nernst equation	3.7–4.7 mmol/L
Calcium (ionized)	Measured using a blood gas sample (maintain the acid-base status of the specimen)	Measured (ISE.) Nernst equation	1.15–1.30 mmol/L
Magnesium (ionized)	Measured using a blood gas sample (maintain the acid-base status of the specimen)	Measured Nernst equation	0.4–0.6 mmol/L 1.5–2.5 mg/dL
Glucose	Glucose status (i.e., diabetic ketoacidosis)	Measured (glucose dehydrogenase/Oxidase)	3.5–4.5 mmol/L 63–81 (mg/dL)
Lactate	Lactic acidosis	Measured (lactate oxidase)	<2.0 mmol/L

ISE, ion selective electrode.

TABLE 2 Primary and secondary acid-base disorders and associated biomarkers.

	Primary	Compensatory
Metabolic acidosis	Low HCO_3^-	Lung expels CO_2 (hyperventilation)
	(low) pH ~ (Low) HCO_3^-/pCO_2	pH ~ (low) HCO_3^-/(low) pCO_2
Respiratory acidosis	High pCO_2	Kidney increase HCO_3^- reabsorption
	(low) pH ~ HCO_3^-/(High) pCO_2	pH ~ (Inc) HCO_3^-/(Inc.) pCO_2
Metabolic alkalosis	High HCO_3^-	Lung reduces the elimination of CO_2 (hypoventilation)
	High pH ~ (Inc.) HCO_3^-/pCO_2	pH ~ (Inc.) HCO_3^-/(Inc.) pCO_2
Respiratory alkalosis	Low pCO_2	Kidney increases the excretion of HCO_3^-
	(high) pH ~ HCO_3^-/(low) pCO_2	pH ~ (low) HCO_3^-/(low) pCO_2

respiratory disorders bicarbonate changes by 3–5 mmoL/L per 10 mmHg.

In respiratory compensation: Pulmonary PCO_2 excretions alter rapidly reaching maximum by 12 h. A rule of thumb in respiratory acidosis; PCO_2 often equates to the 2 digits after decimal in pH (e.g., 25 if pH is 7.25). In respiratory alkalosis compensation: pCO_2 changes by 3–5 mmHg per 10 mmoL/L HCO_3^-.

Disorders of hydrogen ion metabolism

Acidosis is an accumulation of H^+, whereas alkalosis is a deficit of H^+. Metabolic refers to factors that govern the formation and excretion of acid. Because HCO_3^- regulation is important in this respect, it is referred to as the metabolic component. The respiratory component refers to the status of CO_2 production (represented by pCO_2 measurement).

Although four primary disorders can exist (Tables 2 and 3), they are often mixed and will have a compensatory component.

Physiological compensation

Under normal circumstances, a specific acid-base primary disturbance will evoke a compensatory response that

TABLE 3 Four primary disorders exist: Biochemical findings and their primary compensatory mechanism are shown.

	pH	H$^+$	HCO$_3^-$	pCO$_2$	Compensation
Metabolic acidosis	↓	↑	1°↓		↓ pCO$_2$
Respiratory acidosis	↓	↑		1°↑	↑ HCO$_3^-$
Metabolic alkalosis	↑	↓	1°↑		↑ pCO$_2$
Respiratory alkalosis	↑	↓		1°↓	↓ HCO$_3^-$

opposes the primary disturbance (Tables 2 and 3). The mechanism (lung and kidney) in play to restore pH can be easily explained by the Henderson-Hasselbalch equation.

$$\text{Since pH} \propto \frac{\left[\text{HCO}_3^-\right]}{\text{pCO}_2}$$

Adaptive response to return pH toward normal by restoring normal ratio of pCO$_2$ to HCO$_3^-$. Driven directly by abnormal pH only (not directly affected by pCO$_2$ or HCO$_3^-$). The degree of compensation depends on the extent of change in pH, diminishes as pH returns to normal, and disappears when primary acid-base disorder resolves. Thus, respiratory disorders alter the renal excretion of HCO$_3^-$ and metabolic disorders alter the respiratory rate to change pCO$_2$. The extent of the various compensatory components are discussed above under compensatory mechanisms.

An absent or inadequate compensatory response or an excessive alteration in the compensating factor represents the existence of a second acid-base disorder.

Pure disturbances are very rarely seen and mixed disorders are clinically the most common derangements.

Differential Diagnosis of Metabolic Acidosis: (↓pH ↑[H$^+$] ↓ HCO$_3^-$, (compensatory: hyperventilation ↓pCO$_2$)).

Metabolic acidosis is characterized by reduced bicarbonate levels in the presence of arterial blood pH <7.35.

It results from increased production or decreased excretion of H$^+$ (both may exist). Increased H$^+$ formation is seen in ketoacidosis (diabetic), lactic acidosis (hypoxia), poisoning (ethanol, methanol, ethylene glycol), organic acidurias, acid ingestion (poisoning), and excessive total parenteral nutrition TPN (arginine, lysine, histidine).

If anion accumulation occurs due to either the generation or impaired excretion of fixed acid the anion gap is increased. Anion gap calculated as: (AG = Na$^+$ − (Cl$^-$ + HCO^{3-}). Elevated anion gap acidosis is secondary to bicarbonate loss. Normal anion gap acidosis indicates hyperchloremic acidosis. This is relevant clinically as the differential diagnosis and management are different (Table 4).

If decreased H$^+$ excretion or inability to reabsorb filtered bicarbonate (renal (RTA, generalized renal failure)) or to bicarbonate loss (gastrointestinal causes; diarrhea,

TABLE 4 Causes of increased and normal anion gap in patients with metabolic acidosis.

Elevated anion gap (AG) metabolic acidosis (Acid production consumes H$^+$)	Normal anion gap (AG) metabolic acidosis (Bicarbonate loss—impaired regeneration)
Ketoacids (diabetes, ethanol) Lactic acids (sepsis, hypovolemia, seizures, carbon monoxide poisoning, liver dysfunction) Drugs (metformin), methanol, ethylene glycol	Gastrointestinal loss: Diarrhea, fistula (pancreatic, small bowl) Renal cause: Hypokalemia: proximal renal tubular acidosis (RTA-II). Drug induced (acetazolamide, topiramate), Distal RTA-I: drug induced (amphotericin B, ifosfamide). Hyperkalemia: distal nephron dysfunction RTA-IV. Adrenal insufficiency (mineralocorticoid deficiency, hypoaldosteronism), intrinsic tubulointerstitial dysfunction Hyperkalemia plus renal insufficiency: Diuretics (K-sparing), ACE-inhibitors, NSAID, trimethoprim Exogenous: Acid intake, ammonium chloride, TPN

pancreatic, intestinal, and biliary fistulae or drainage), carbonate anhydrase inhibitors (lack of HCO$_3^-$ generation). The anion gap will be normal or low in the presence of high chloride levels.

Respiratory compensatory mechanism (hyperventilation) increases CO$_2$ excretion evident by the observed low pCO$_2$ levels. Successful compensation leads to the normalization of pH level.

Respiratory Acidosis: (↓pH ↑[H$^+$] ↑pCO$_2$, (compensatory ↑HCO$_3^-$)).

The primary defect is the retention of CO$_2$ usually due to generalized respiratory impairment either acute in nature or chronic. It is characterized by the findings of decreased pH (increased [H$^+$]), and increased pCO$_2$. The renal compensatory mechanism is by increased bicarbonate regeneration.

In acute respiratory acidosis as in asthma, bronchopneumonia, and acute pulmonary failure, serum bicarbonate is mildly elevated 1–2 mmol/L for every 10 mmHg (1.3 kPa) increase in pCO_2 and/or a base excess of 0 mmol/L. There is an acute rise in pCO_2 (7.5 mmHg associated with 1 mmoL/L HCO_3^- and 5.5 nmol H^+).

Chronic presentation as in chronic bronchitis, emphysema, and serum bicarbonate is increased by 4–5 mmol/L for every 10 mmHg (1.3 KPa) increased in pCO_2 and/or a base excess of $(0.4 \times (pCO_2-40)$ mmol/L).

There is chronic CO_2 retention, when renal compensation is maximal, the H^+ is increased by only 2.5 nmoL/L for each 7.5 mmHg rise in pCO_2.

In the short term, pCO_2 is restored to normal and that compensation occurs through increased renal H^+ excretion. Very often a low pO_2 is associated with respiratory dysfunction such as chronic obstructive pulmonary disease (COPD).

Associated conditions include decreased alveolar ventilation, depression of the respiratory center, use of anesthetics and sedatives, cerebral trauma, neuromuscular disease (poliomyelitis, Gillian-Barre syndrome, and motor neuron diseases), and tetanus infection.

Patients with pulmonary disease (fibrosis, severe pneumonia, respiratory distress), extra-pulmonary thoracic disease, flail chest, severe kyphoscoliosis, and in lung malignancy.

Metabolic Alkalosis: ($\uparrow$pH $\downarrow[H^+]$, $\uparrow HCO_3^-$, (compensatory: $\uparrow pCO_2$)).

Characterized by rise in pH (low H^+), increased bicarbonate ($\uparrow HCO_3^-$), and evidence of moderate respiratory compensation ($\uparrow pCO_2$).

Most commonly due to excessive loss of H^+ evident by a primary disorder, or that there is a primary increase in HCO_3^- accompanied by a loss of H^+. Causes are; gastrointestinal (gastric aspiration, vomiting with pyloric stenosis, loss of intravascular fluid and chloride secondary to diuretics use, congenital chloride-losing diarrhea). Patients receiving parenteral nutrition low in chloride and high in acetate will exhibit metabolic alkalosis.

Renal causes are mineralocorticoid excess, Cushing's syndrome, and Conn's syndrome. Other causes; diuretic therapy, potassium depletion, rapid correction of chronic rise in pCO_2, administration of alkali, and antacid abuse (very high urine sodium, negative urine anion gap). Inappropriate treatment of acidotic states, hypovolemia (evident by high BUN/creatinine ratio), and occasionally due to citrate after massive blood transfusion.

Urine chloride levels are low (<10 mmol/L) in patients likely to respond to volume replenishment (saline responsive) and represent >95% of cases. Patients with chloride levels >10 mmol/L are classified as saline-resistant metabolic alkalosis (often secondary to excessive glucocorticoids and mineralocorticoids, excessive potassium and

magnesium depletion, Bartter syndrome, Gitelman syndrome, renin-secreting tumors, and in renal artery stenosis).

Respiratory Alkalosis: ($\uparrow$pH $\downarrow[H^+]$ $\downarrow pCO_2$, (compensatory: $\downarrow HCO_3^-$)).

This is the most frequent acid-base disorder. It occurs in anxiety and hysterical breathing, normal pregnancy, and at high altitude (hypoxemia), and in patients with pulmonary disease and hypoxemia (see later).

A primary fall in arterial blood pCO_2 levels due to abnormally deep or rapid respiration. Respiratory alkalosis is characterized by the following findings, an increase in arterial blood pH (>7.45) (decreased $[H^+]$), and a decreased pCO_2 due to increased alveolar ventilation (excretion).

The above biochemical findings are observed in, acute, chronic, and mixed disorders. However, without appropriate clinical information and other laboratory tests, definite diagnosis can be difficult.

In acute respiratory alkalosis, H^+ concentration declines by 5.5 nmol/L for each 7.5 fall in pCO_2, or a decrease in serum bicarbonate by 1–2 mmol/L for every 10 mmHg (1.3 kPa) decline in pCO_2 and/or a base excess of 0 mmol/L is assumed. This is observed in patients with pneumonia, sepsis, and anxiety.

In chronic respiratory alkalosis, serum bicarbonate is significantly decreased by 4–5 mmol/L for every 10 mmHg (1.3 kPa) decrease in pCO_2 and/or a base excess of $(0.4 \times (pCO_2-40)$ nmol/L, a chronic respiratory alkalosis is assumed. This is seen in pregnancy, hyperthyroidism, hepatic cirrhosis, hypoxia, high altitude, and severe anemia.

Secondary to hyperventilation (usually due to anxiety, pain, or artificial ventilation). Chronic due to chronic hypoxia, high altitude, severe anemia, and fall in pCO_2 ($[H^+]$ fall by 5.5 nmoL/L for each 7.5 fall in pCO_2). Causes: Hypoxia, high altitude, severe anemia, pulmonary disease (hyperventilation), pulmonary edema, and pulmonary embolism.

Increased respiratory derive by respiratory stimulants (salicylates), cerebral disturbances (trauma, infection, tumors), hepatic failure, and gram-negative septicemia[1].

Mixed disorders

Mixed acid-base disorders are common and often suspected when the compensatory mechanism say for HCO_3^- is much higher than would be expected.

Respiratory compensation occurs within minutes compared with days for renal to achieve full compensation.

The degree of compensation thus depends on lung and kidney functions and also on whether the disorder is acute or chronic in nature.

In metabolic acidosis, pCO_2 correction (decrease) is about 1.2-fold the decrease in bicarbonate. However, if the rate of change is higher, this suggests the presence of nixed disorder with a respiratory alkalosis component.

The respiratory compensation in metabolic alkalosis (hypoventilation) increased pCO_2 levels. If the increase in pCO_2 is 0.6 times the increase in HCO_3^-, this is a compensatory mechanism; however, a higher degree of compensation suggests the presence of a mixed disorder in the form of respiratory acidosis.

The renal compensatory correction for respiratory disorders begins about 2h but takes up to 2–3 days to complete. Compensation occurs in two phases; in phase one, the change in HCO_3^- is 0.1 times the change in pCO_2, whereas in the second phase, the change in HCO_3^- is about 0.4 times the change in pCO_2. In general, a change >10% in the predicted correction of either pCO_2 or HCO_3^- in response to acid-base disturbance (alkalosis or acidosis) suggests the presence of a mixed acid-base disorder.

Patients may have more than one of the acid-base disorders, with both metabolic acidosis and alkalosis present. Similarly, patients receiving ventilation could change from respiratory alkalosis to respiratory acidosis. However, there are not often seen present in combination.

pO$_2$/FiO$_2$ ratio

For patients on ventilation, the pO_2/FiO_2 ratio provides a measure of oxygenation. A ratio between 300 and 500 mmHg is considered normal, with values below indicating abnormal gas exchange and values <200 mmHg indicating severe hypoxemia.

Interpretation of acid-base data

Interpretation of acid-base results should always be considered in the clinical context and a well-thought-out logical approach will overcome most difficulties (Fig. 9). Hydrogen ion (pH) indicates acid-base status, pCO_2 indicates the respiratory component, pO_2 confirms the respiratory component, whereas HCO_3^- indicates the metabolic component.

Considering the presence of mixed disorders, pCO_2 and HCO_3^- have changed in opposite directions, whereas if they move in the same direction this indicates the presence of a compensatory mechanism, the degree of which requires assessment. If the pH [H$^+$] were normalized, then this suggests complete compensation. Abnormal pH and [H$^+$] suggest inadequate and unsuccessful compensation.

When interpreting acid-base status, best understood using the Henderson eq. ($H = pCO_2/HCO_3^-$), in this order, first establish if the disorder is compensated for (pH is within normal range, successful compensation, e.g., by the metabolic (kidney) in respiratory disorder (lung component)). If pH is high uncompensated alkalosis; if pH is low uncompensated acidosis.

If H$^+$ is high (acidosis), consider pCO_2; if decreased, the patient has metabolic acidosis (hyperventilation removing pCO_2 to correct pCO_2/HCO_3^- ratio. If pCO_2 is normal, the patient has an uncompensated metabolic acidosis. The lack of pCO_2 response may be related to a lung pathology (i.e., mixed disorder present). If H$^+$ is high and the pCO_2 is

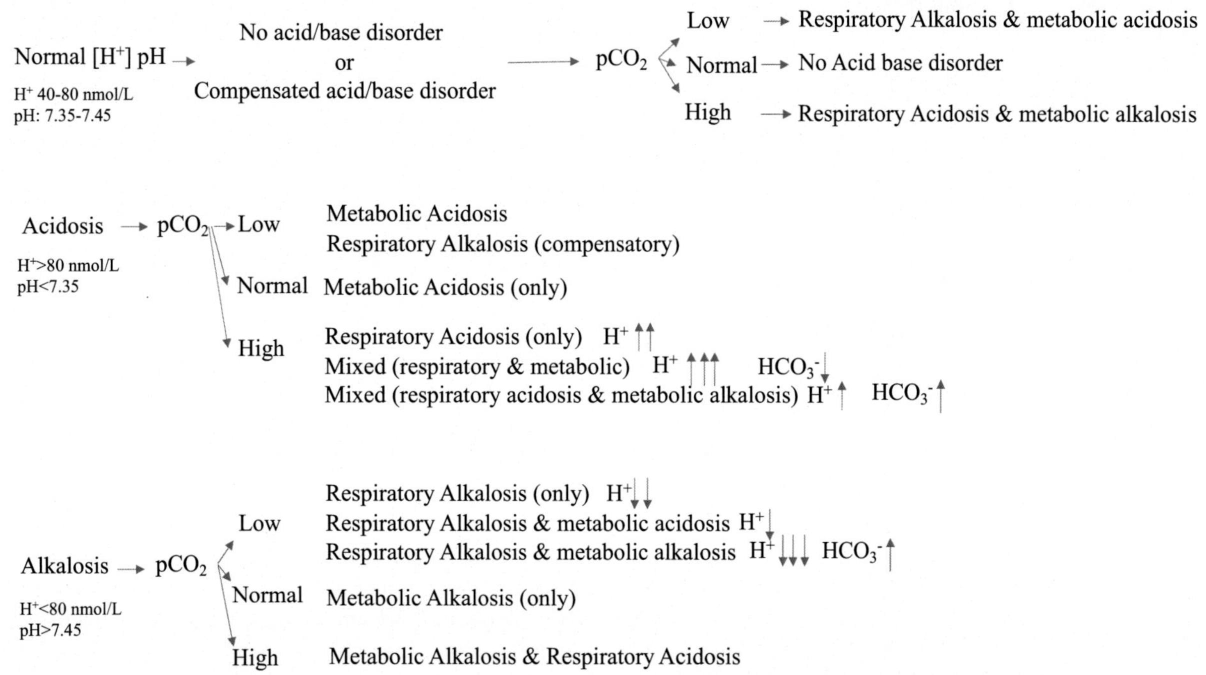

FIG. 9 Stepwise approach to the interpretation of acid-base disorders in the absence of clinical findings. *Modified from Rodríguez-Villar S, Do Vale BM, Fletcher HM. The arterial blood gas algorithm: proposal of a systematic approach to analysis of acid-base disorders. Rev Esp Anestesiol Reanim (Engl Ed). 2020;67(1):20–34. English, Spanish. doi: 10.1016/j.redar.2019.04.001. Epub 2019 Dec 9. PMID: 31826801.*

high, the patient has respiratory acidosis. Normal or slightly elevated HCO_3^- suggest acute (uncompensated), and high HCO_3^- suggests chronic.

If H^+ is low (alkalosis), pCO_2 is decreased. The patient has respiratory alkalosis (hyperventilation), and HCO_3^- may be slightly low (simple respiratory alkalosis). If pCO_2 is normal and H^+ is low, this is uncompensated metabolic alkalosis, HCO_3^- will be elevated. If pCO_2 is increased and H^+ is low (alkalosis), this is metabolic alkalosis with some respiratory compensation (hypoventilation is not a significant compensation to metabolic alkalosis). That is, some other mixed disorders must be present, such as mixed metabolic alkalosis and respiratory acidosis. HCO_3^- will also be increased. If H^+ is normal, the patient either has no acid-base disorder or that compensatory mechanisms are in play. If pCO_2 is decreased, then H is normal, suggesting respiratory alkalosis and metabolic acidosis (mixed). If pCO_2 is normal and H is normal, this suggests no acid-base disorder as HCO_3^- is also likely to be normal. If pCO_2 is increased and H^+ is normal, the patient has compensated respiratory alkalosis, or a mixed respiratory acidosis and metabolic alkalosis.

Anion gap calculations and diagnostic value

The difference between regularly measured cations (sodium, and potassium) and regularly measured anions (chloride and bicarbonate) is observed. Thus, the difference "the gap" represents unmeasured anions such as lactate, ketones, and albumin (predominant protein negatively charged).

$Na^+ + (K^+$ not always applied)$-Cl^- - HCO^{3-}$. Normal gaps are from 8 to 16 and from 12 to 20 when potassium is included in the calculation.

Evaluation of metabolic acidosis is difficult without knowing the unknown gap. The gap is a measure between the positive and negative anions and accounts for unmeasured anions.

The anion gap increases when HCO_3^- decreases relative to Na and Cl secondary to increase acids with lactic acid accounting for 50% of cases. Patients with lactic acid 5–9.9 may have normal AG and thus cannot replace lactate measurement (sensitivity/specificity about 80%). However, it can be used to follow the resolution of the lactic acidosis in response to therapeutic interventions (Tables 5–7).

Low or negative AG is seen when chloride levels are high (hyperchloremia seen in patients with lithium toxicity, high levels of calcium and magnesium in patients with IgG monoclonal gammopathy). Falsely, high chloride results may be seen in patients with salicylate intoxication.

Normal AG in metabolic acidosis suggests hyperchloremia, loss of bicarbonate is neutralized by increased absorption of chloride.

TABLE 5 MUDPILES mnemonic.

Anion gap acidosis	
M	Methanol
U	Uremia
D	Diabetic ketoacidosis (ketocidosis: alcoholic, starvation)
P	Paraldehyde, phenformin, paraldehyde
I	Iron; isoniazid, inborn errors of metabolism
L	Lactic acidosis
E	Ethylene glycol
S	Salicylate

Modified from Andrew L. Schwaderer and George J. Schwartz (2004) Back to basics: acidosis and alkalosis. Pediatr Rev 25, (10), 350–357.

TABLE 6 MUDPILECATS mnemonic.

Anion gap acidosis	
M	Methanol/metformin
U	Uremia
D	Diabetic ketoacidosis
P	Phenformin/paraldehyde
I	Iron-isoniazid/ibuprofen
L	Lactic acidosis
E	Ethanol/ethylene glycol
C	Cyanide
A	Acetylsalicylic acid
T	Toluene
S	Starvation/solvents

Modified from Klauer KM. Life beyond MUDPILES. Air Med J 2002;21(5):37-41. PMID: 12196739.

HCO_3^- loss via gastrointestinal, in diarrhea, renal loss in renal tubular acidosis, saline Na 0.9% overload (chloride content is high at 154 mmol/L compared to normal serum levels of 106 mmol/L. HCO_3^- is lost to maintain neutrality). The urine anion gap helps to indicate the chloride factor.

This provides an estimate of NH_4^+ (ammonium urinary excretion secondary to the increased reabsorption of chloride and potassium and in response to metabolic acidosis). The increased urinary ammonia increases urine pH to >5.5. The urine anion gap is often referred to as a cation gap (positive in normal states). It is calculated as follows;

$$UAG = Na^+ + K^+ - CL^-$$

TABLE 7 GOLD MARK mnemonic; Glycols (ethylene and propylene), oxoproline, L-lactate, D-lactate, methanol, aspirin, renal failure, and ketoacidosis.

Anion gap acidosis	
G	Glycols
O	5-Oxoproline
L	Lactic acidosis
D	D-Lactic acidosis
M	Methanol
A	Alcohols and acetylsalicylic acid
R	Renal failure and rhabdomyolysis (cell lysis)
K	Ketoacidosis (diabetic, alcoholic, or starvation)

Modified from Mehta AN, Emmett JB, Emmett M. GOLD MARK: an anion gap mnemonic for the 21st century. Lancet 2008;372(9642):892. doi: 10.1016/S0140-6736(08)61398-7. PMID: 18790311.

Normally, the urine anion gap is positive in the range of 20 and 80 mmol/L. In hyperchloremic metabolic acidosis, the urine gap is negative due to the increased chloride being much higher than the combined sodium and potassium levels. The urine anion gap is not reliable in patients with renal impairment and in those with diabetic ketoacidosis.

In theory, the anion gap should reflect the following shown below,

$$Na^+ + K^+ + 2 \times Ca^{++} \ 2 \times Mg^{++} + H^+ + \text{unmeasured cations} =$$

$$Cl^- + HCO_3^- + 2 \times CO_3^{2-} + OH^- + \text{albumin} + \text{phosphate}$$

$$+ \text{sauphate} + \text{lactate} + \text{unmeasured anions}$$

The most important contributors are those with significant large concentration, thus;

AG (mmol/L) = $Na^+ - Cl^- - HCO_3^-$ (considering a mean Na^+ of 140 mmol/L, Cl^- of 106 mmol/L, HCO_3^- of 24 mmol/L, a gap of 10 mmol/L is obtained which mainly represents albumin).

Although not widely adopted, correction for albumin may be applied. 0.23–0.25 × albumin in g/L. That is, each g/L albumin decreased AG by about 0.25 mmol/L. AG (mmol/L) = $Na^+ - Cl^- - HCO_3^- - 0.25$ (albumin in g/L).

An increase in AG in metabolic acidosis suggests the presence of organic acids (endogenous or exogenous). The normal range for an anion gap is considered to be 3 to 12 mmol/L.

A change of 20 g/L in albumin (correct anion gap by multiplying 20 × 0.25 = 5) that is the upper limit of AG being 12–5 = 7, that is levels above 7 are considered abnormal when corrected for the decreased albumin levels.

Because many substances and conditions can lead to an increased unknown gap in metabolic acidosis various

mnemonics are used. (GOLD MARK, MUDPLIES, MUDPILECATS) (Tables 5–7).

In patients with acidosis (low pH) and hypoxia (low pO_2), the finding of increased anion gap points toward lactate. The higher the anion gap, the greater likelihood of metabolic acidosis due to the increased anions such as lactate and acetoacetate.

Titratable acids in urine

Titratable acid (urine) is mostly phosphate (the major buffer system in the urine. It is more important than ammonia as it has a pK_a of 6.8); however, its capacity is limited due to a max filterable load of 20 to 50 mmol/day. Titratable acid is defined as the volume of sodium hydroxide (NaOH) that need to be added to normalize the urine pH. This test is not widely performed but can help investigate urinary anion gap using the formula; titratable acidity = volume of NaOH (mls) added × 0.75.

Osmolality and osmolal gap

Osmolality can either be measured or calculated and that the difference between the two values is known as the osmolal gap. It indicates the presence of an osmotically active substance (e.g., ethanol) that is not accounted for. It is helpful in patients with high and unexplained anion gap acidosis.

Osmolality is measured by freezing point depression and normal individuals having a smaller gap of less than 10 mOsmol/L (ranges from −14 to +10).

Calculated osmolality: 2 × [Na^+] + (Glucose in g/dL/18) + (BUN g/dL/2.8) + (ethanol in mg/dL/3.7).

In methanol and ethylene glycol, osmolal gap is high but symptoms must not be present due to the delayed metabolizing to the acidic metabolites. Co-ingestion of ethanol delays the metabolism due to competition for the metabolizing alcohol dehydrogenase.

Standard Base excess (SBE)

Standard base excess is calculated using the formula below. It is used to estimate the amount of base that is needed to correct acid-base disorders.

$$SBE(mmol/L) = \left[HCO_3^- \right] - 24.8 + 16.2 \times (pH - 7.4)$$

For practical purpose, normal SBE is considered 0 mmol/L, that is no base addition is required. This assumes a normal pH of 7.40, a normal pCO_2 at 40 mmHg, and a mean normal bicarbonate of 24 mmol/L.

Co-oximetry analysis

Hemoglobin, oxyhemoglobin, carboxyhemoglobin, and methemoglobin are measured spectrophotometrically. Light is passed through a hemolyzed sample. The absorption spectrum of at least two different wavelengths is recorded and used to measure the hemoglobin and its derivatives.

Hemoglobin

Hemoglobin and oxyhemoglobin are measured using either pulse oximetry or co-oximetry. Most of the oxygen (97%) dissolved in blood is bound to hemoglobin with 3% being in plasma. Oxygen saturation (SaO_2) is a measure of the percentage of oxygen that is bound to hemoglobin. However, the relationship between the oxygen saturation and partial pressure of oxygen is described by the oxyhemoglobin disassociation curve (Fig. 10). The dissociation curve is influenced by body temperature, pH, pCO_2, and concentration of 2,3 diphosphoglycerate.

Increase in temperature, H^+ (low pH), increase in pCO_2, and increase in 2,3 DPG shift the dissociation curve to the right, that is adequate saturation requires higher partial pressure of oxygen. In contrast, low temperature, low H^+ (high pH), low pCO_2, and low 2,3 DPG shift the curve to the left, that is high oxygen saturation is achieved at a lower partial pressure of oxygen. This increased affinity to hemoglobin reduces its diffusion intracellular at the tissue capillary interface, thus leading to relative tissue hypoxia compared to the reduced affinity at higher temperature.

Carboxy hemoglobin

Carbon monoxide is tightly bound to the oxygen hemoglobin binding site. Values more than 10% of hemoglobin in the carboxyhemoglobin form is considered a critical value and requires immediate notification.

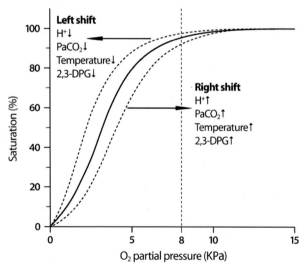

FIG. 10 Oxyhemoglobin dissociation curve. *Modified from Hall, J.E. (2015). Guyton and Hall Textbook of Medical Physiology (Guyton Physiology), 13th ed. Saunders. ISBN-10: 1455770051ISBN-13: 978-145577005.*

TABLE 8 Symptoms associated with carboxyhemoglobin levels.

Carboxyhemoglobin (%)	Symptoms
5%–20% (Mild)	Headache, nausea, vomiting, blurred vision, palpitation, dizziness
20%–50% (Moderate)	Moderate: Syncope, chest pain, shortness of breath, altered coordination, altered mental ability
>50% (Severe)	Life-threatening: Cardiac dysrhythmias, cardiac arrest, cerebral infarction, severe metabolic acidosis, seizures, pulmonary edema, coma, hemodynamic abnormalities

Modified from Chenoweth JA, Albertson TE, Greer MR. Carbon monoxide poisoning. Crit Care Clin 2021;37(3):657–672. doi: 10.1016/j.ccc.2021.03.010. PMID: 34053712.

One carbon monoxide molecule binding to one O_2 binding site causes a positive cooperativity with stronger binding to O_2 on the remaining three hemoglobin sites leading to hypoxia. Symptoms associated with various carboxyhemoglobin levels are shown below (see Table 8).

Normally carboxyhemoglobin is <2% among nonsmokers and <5% among smokers. Levels >9% indicate exogenous exposure. Carboxyhemoglobin levels do not always correlate with either symptoms nor outcomes and thus elevated levels are only indicative of exposure and associated risks and that levels guide therapeutic intervention.

Methemoglobin

Methemoglobin is formed when the hemoglobin ferrous iron (Fe^{2+}) is oxidized to its ferric form (Fe^{3+}). This transformation impairs hemoglobin ability to bind oxygen (ferric form unable to bind and transport oxygen). Oxidation of iron is caused by drugs. For example, in clinical practice, it is mostly due to use of local anesthetics, (benzocaine and procaine), antibiotics (dapsone,) and nitrites (nitroglycerine/nitric oxide), antimalarials (chloroquine, primaquine), and to industrial household products (aniline dyes, naphthalene, aminophenol). Symptoms depend on levels (see Table 9).

Hemoglobin by blood gas analyzers

In the blood gases instrument, hemoglobin is determined spectrophotometrically compared with chemical methodology on the automated hematology analyzers (cyanohemoglobin or cyanide-free sodium lauryl sulfate). There are often slight differences not considered significant, where

TABLE 9 symptoms associated with methemoglobin levels.

Methemoglobin concentration	% of Total hemoglobin	Symptoms
<1.5 g/dL	<10	None
1.5–3.0 g/dL	10–20	Cyanotic skin discoloration
3.0–4.5 g/dL	20–30	Anxiety, lightheadedness, headache, tachycardia
4.5–7.5 g/dL	30–50	Fatigue, confusion, dizziness, tachypnea, coma
7.5–10.5 g/dL	50–70	Seizures, arrhythmias, acidosis, tachycardia
>10.5 g/dL	>70	Death

Modified from Ludlow JT, Wilkerson RG, Nappe TM. Methemoglobinemia. [Updated 2022 Aug 29]. In: StatPearls [Internet]. Treasure Island (FL): StatPearls Publishing; 2022 Jan. Available from: https://www.ncbi.nlm.nih.gov/books/NBK537317/.

blood gas analyzers hemoglobin showed a slightly negative bias (about 0.4 g/dL) when compared with laboratory-based chemical assays. Although its uses in management were not endorsed by professional bodies, they offer rapid assessment and trending of patient hemoglobin status.

Calculated parameters

Blood gas parameters and other parameters provided by the instruments are either measured or derived following calculations utilizing some of the measured parameters (see Table 1).

Bicarbonate is a calculated parameter when determined by blood gas instruments. The calculation is based on the Henderson-Hasselbalch equation ($pH = pK_a + Log\,[HCO_3^-]/pCO_2$). Thus, calculating entered values for pH and pCO_2, bicarbonate was obtained (HCO_3^- ($0.0307 \times pCO_2 \times 10^{(pH-6.105)}$)).

This is in contrast to measured bicarbonate in automated chemistry analyzers which is enzymatic reaction rate methodology. Bicarbonate HCO_3^- reacts with phosphoenolpyruvate in the presence of phosphoenolpyruvate carboxylase to oxaloacetate and phosphate. Oxaloacetate is coupled with NADH in the presence of malate dehydrogenase to produce malate and NAD. A decrease in NAD is monitored at 340 nm and the rate of change is directly proportional to bicarbonate concentration.

Blood sample types in acid-base assessment

Whole blood sample is required, prefilled heparinized (anticoagulant) syringes are commercially available and are required when collecting samples for bold gases analysis (Arterial, venous, capillary, cord blood).

Sample collection precautions include avoiding tourniquet use (restrict blood flow leading to hypoxemia and lactic acidosis), avoid pull on the syringe plunger to minimize air bubbles and sample hemolysis, and that sample is analyzed immediately (within 15 min of collection).

Samples collection using syringes that contain heparin as an anticoagulant. Avoid the use of a tourniquet, avoid pull on the syringe plunger, avoid air bubbles, and analyze the sample immediately (within 15 min of collection).

Air bubbles lead to erroneous pO_2 and pH results. The ambient air contains 21% oxygen (pO_2 159 mmHg), (arterial blood being at 95–100 mmHg, and venous blood at 40–50 mmHg) dissolved air causes erroneous results. The air bubbles may not be visually apparent, and efforts (via training) are toward the expulsion of air bubbles from the syringe following collection and that the specimen is appropriately capped to prevent air. Samples are transported to the laboratory via a tube system, the tubes are subjected to g-force that can facilitate air bubble dissolution and thus produce high erroneous pO_2 results.

Similarly, to provide an accurate representation of the patient acid-base status at the time of sample collection, the sample may be kept on ice and analyzed immediately to avoid the impact of ongoing metabolic activity within the specimen.

Delayed sample analysis: Decreased pH due to metabolic activity, increased pCO_2 due to increased CO_2 production by glucose metabolism, and decreased pO_2 due to consumption of oxygen by leukocytes. Sample placement on the ice although preferred in some laboratories where samples are immediately processed, ice is avoided (some tube manufacturers suggest that ice promotes ambient gas diffusion through the plastic syringe material to the sample).

Rapid processing of blood samples is important. Gases diffuse through the wall of the collection tube. Oxygen diffuses through plastic more than glass containers. Available collection devices are plastic syringes of 1, 3, or 5 mLs self-filling plastic disposable syringes prefilled with a small amount of heparin anticoagulant. Additionally, continued metabolism in the blood can alter the blood gas values during the time between sampling and analysis. Leukocytes continue to consume oxygen at a rate that is dependent on temperature and time.

It is recommended that plastic syringes not be placed on ice but should be kept at room temperature as long as the blood is analyzed within 30 min of collection.

The presence of air bubbles, a common problem (in as much as 40% of blood gas specimens) (often small and invisible) affects pO_2 and pCO_2 results. A falsely high pO_2 and falsely low pCO_2.

Sample stored at 0°C for up to 1 h showed no change in pH, whereas a significant decrease is observed when stored at 22°C for 30 min.

Reference intervals for pH have not been established evident by the variation reported levels from a lower interval of 7.35 to 7.40 and an upper interval of 7.40 to 7.45. There is evidence of differences in acid-base reference intervals among gender, additionally, also during the menstrual cycle where a decrease of 3 mmHg in pCO_2 is observed during the luteal phase

Arterialized blood sample

When arterial collations are difficult to obtain, arterialized venous samples may be obtained following adequate warming of the site of collection (arm). This facilitates increased circulation and gas diffusion.

The well-perfused patient's venous pH is 0.03–0.04 lower and pCO_2 3–4 mmHg higher than arterial. May be used if evaluation of pO_2 is not needed.

Arterial samples assess oxygenation accurately. pCO_2 measurement is needed to evaluate respiratory component. Comparable samples are arterialized-venous and capillary blood samples.

Venous samples are inaccurate for pH and pCO_2. The well-perfused patient's venous pH is 0.03–0.04 lower and PCO_2 3–4 mmHg higher than arterial. May be used if evaluation of pO_2 is not needed.

Capillary blood samples

Capillary blood samples are often preferred due to its low pain. It is obtained by about 1 mm deep skin puncture delivery with a small sample volume of about 100–150 µL. Given the anatomy, capillary samples are expected to reflect blood gases midway between arterial and venous values; in practice, the blood collected is contaminated by both arterial and venous blood. Several studies showed no significant difference between arterialized (warmed) capillary samples' blood gases to those of arterial in the adult normal population. However, among patients only those of pH and pCO_2 were not clinically significant between capillary and atrial samples. pO_2 levels are significantly different and suggests that capillary pO_2 levels are of limited clinical utility.

Cord blood gases

During pregnancy, the fetus receives oxygen from the mother's arterial blood through the umbilical vein and by diffusion across the placenta. Deoxygenated fetal blood is transported back to the placenta via the umbilical arteries. The venous umbilical cord reflects the maternal placental acid-base status at birth. The venous umbilical cord reflects the maternal placental acid-base status at birth. It has a lower pH and a higher oxygen content than the arterial umbilical vein which has a higher carbon dioxide content than the venous umbilical veins. The composition of the venous umbilical cord veins resembles that of the adult arterial veins reflecting the new needle acid-base status.

Cord blood gases provide an indication of respiratory distress during fetal delivery. It provides a way to assess fetal metabolic status at birth and indicates possible fetal exposure to hypoxia and to associated metabolic acidosis that may potentially lead to encephalopathy and cerebral palsy.

Arterial umbilical cord blood gases are required at birth. It is often used to investigate a deteriorating neonate under the care of neonatology as to possible complication during delivery as the predisposing cause. Umbilical cord blood gas analysis assists with clinical management and excludes a diagnosis of birth asphyxia in approximately 80% of cases. Complete blood gas analysis provides information on the type in codes of acidemia and the arterial sample is preferred to venous. It is important to note that the blood circulation in the cord is reversed, i.e., what is considered arterial is venous and vice versa. Samples are often collected from cords up to 2 h following the dissection of the cord. Studies, however, have shown that results from cord samples collected several days later can be extrapolated back via calculations to represent acid-base status within 2 h of cord dissection.

Analytical and regulatory considerations

There are a number of commercially available blood gas machines ranging from handheld to benchtop instruments. Some offer an essential blood gases menu (pH, pCO_2, pO_2, and bicarbonate), some offer additional co-oximetry (carboxyhemoglobin, methemoglobin), and others add electrolytes such as sodium, potassium, chloride, ionized calcium, and ionized magnesium.

The instruments use ion-selective electrode technologies as well as electronic sensor-based technologies. The instruments are either located inside critical care laboratories, at nursing stations, and within the inpatient and operating room units.

Methods for the measurement of H^+ (pH) and blood gases (pO_2, pCO_2) are based on electrochemical (potentiometric and amperometric) selective electrode-based methods. Gases, electrolytes, and metabolites electrodes are often placed in-line. The application of a whole blood sample enters all the electrode chambers arranged in tandem. Some instruments may offer a diversion of flow to electrolytes/electrodes. Prior to analysis, the applied while blood sample is hemolyzed, to facilitate co-oximetry measurements (see analytical measurements chapter).

It is the development of accurate measurement of H^+ that has realized its physiological importance and the need for strict maintenance of its concentration within a very narrow limit. Blood samples (arterial, venous, cord, arterialized, capillary, and cord) are the samples that are often submitted for analysis.

Understanding measurements of the various parameters used in the assessment of acid-base status as well as gases (co-oximetry) is important. There are regulatory components (CLIA) that are different from those commonly applied to the automated clinical analyzer, for instance, in blood gas measurements, calibration (usually automated) is performed every 30 min, compared to the less frequent (as needed and as recommended by manufacturers of routine automated analyzers), and that at least one quality control sample is run every 8 h of instrument operation.

The laboratory is also expected to either have or contribute to a procedure on proper sample collection, the difference between arterial and venous collection, possible causes for preanalytical errors such as the presence of air bubbles, sample stability, and complication of arterial blood samples collection (see the section on sample quality).

Analytical interferences and limitations

The accuracy of blood gas results and their true representation of the patient acid-base status at the time of sample collection depends on the quality of the sample. Delayed processing results in falsely low pH, low bicarbonate, increased lactate, and potassium. The presence of air bubbles causes falsely elevated pO_2 (dissolved air), accelerated by G-force applied during transportation by pneumatic tube. A likely scenario is when invisible bubbles are present following the expulsion of visible air bubbles.

Ethylene glycol discrepancy

Patients presenting with ethylene glycol poisoning often exhibit metabolic acidosis due to its metabolites glycolate and glyoxylate. Conformation is by measurement of ethylene glycol levels which is often performed at a distant referral laboratory (by gas chromatography-mass spectrometry). However, a discrepancy in lactate levels (lactate gap) when determined by point-of-care devices (falsely elevated) compared with that performed in laboratory-based automated chemistry analyzers often gives a clue to the presence of ethylene glycol.

Hence, patients present to the emergency department and suspected of ethylene poisoning (abnormality in acid-base status) are likely to have blood gases and lactate (if available on the blood gas analyzer) performed for immediate management, subsequent samples for metabolic panels to assess renal function and electrolytes, are likely to have to follow up lactate measurements. The observed lactate gap between the two instruments is due to ethylene glycol metabolites interference. Ethylene glycol metabolites, glycolic acid, and glyoxylic acid cause a positive interference with the overestimation of blood lactate by blood gas instruments. The gap could be as high as 20 mmol/L when compared with that obtained by laboratory-based automated chemistry analyzers methodologies.

Blood gases instrument uses lactate oxidase-producing pyruvate and hydrogen peroxide, the latter is measured amperometrically following reaction with peroxidase and production of oxygen.

Poor specificity of the lactate oxidase enzyme used and possibly lack of sample separation (use of whole blood in blood gases analyzer). It is worth noting that not all blood gas machines exhibit such interference.

Oversight and management-related issues

The clinical chemistry laboratory and/or point-of-care testing are often responsible for the provision of blood gases measurement. The instruments may be located within the central clinical laboratory or more often in a rapid response laboratory serving critical care areas, or within patient care units under the auspices of point-of-care testing.

In addition to maintaining quality control procedures and accreditation requirements such as validation and comparison between multiple instruments (laboratory-based and POCT devices), the laboratory often provides training and competency assessment of clinical staff handling arterial blood gas samples and measuring blood gases on the instruments. In consultation with the critical care team, develop arterial and venous blood sample collection protocols.

Pulse oximetry devices

Transcutaneous monitors (being either transmissive or reflective) are used to monitor patient oxygenation status (pO_2). By recording absorbances at red region of the spectrum (650 nm) and the infrared region (910 nm), and oxygenated hemoglobin is estimated (Fig. 11). The noninvasive nature and ease of use helped avoid repeated arterial blood collections minimizing the risk of infection and iatrogenic anemia. The instrument does not provide accurate readings in the presence of carboxyhemoglobin, methemoglobin, and when there is strong vasoconstriction.

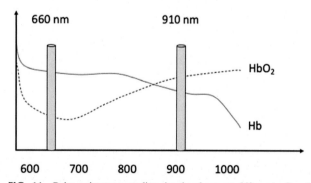

FIG. 11 Pulse oximeter recording the absorbance at 660 nm (*red*) and 910 nm (*infrared*) for estimation of oxygenated hemoglobin when using a pulse oximeter. *Modified from Jubran A. Pulse oximetry. Crit Care 2015;19(1):272. doi: 10.1186/s13054-015-0984-8. PMID: 26179876; PMCID: PMC4504215.*

Transcutaneous pCO_2 devices

Although $ptcCO_2$ (transcutaneous pCO_2) compares well with arterial pCO_2, in most cases, discrepancies arise and professional societies recommend against the use of transcutaneous devices when making appropriate treatment and ventilatory manipulations.

Differences between capillary and arterial. Capillary (as in NICU) may correlate better with transcutaneous. Transcutaneous pCO_2 was comparable to that of capillary blood gases; however, transcutaneous was higher when compared with arterial blood gases.

They are used for trending patient condition and not for guiding significant changes to management without the use of blood gas measurements.

Reporting of blood gases results

Critically ill patients are likely to exhibit changes in body temperature and the fact that the solubility of blood gases in the blood changes with temperature has led to the practice of adjusting blood gases for the body temperature (Fig. 6). Although the practice is not widely adopted, the evidence for its utility in hypothermia is convincing. Hyperthermia (body temperature > 38°C) is often seen in sepsis, infection, and brain tumors.

Mild hypothermia (body temperature 35 to 32°C), moderate (35–32°C) and severe <30°C were seen during sedative management, cardiopulmonary bypass, and following alcohol ingestion, drugs, and prolonged environmental exposure to low temperatures. Additionally, the beneficial outcome following induced hypothermia in patients with brain injuries and in those following cardiac arrest in the critical care environment.

Temperature correction of measured gases refers to applying mathematical adjustments to the measured 37°C values to obtain a more accurate reflection of the gas tensions as they existed in the artery (actual core temperature). Correction of pH and pCO_2 to body temperature in hyperthermia is not recommended. During hypothermia, arterial pH rises, and pCO_2 falls. This alkalotic change does not occur when measurements are made at 37°C.

At 40°C, correction for pH would be +0.045 and for pCO_2 would be +13%. pCO_2 correction is important for pulmonary gas exchange studies but not for clinical management of assisted ventilation. Available data support the practice that only uncorrected (37°C) blood gas values should be used and reported routinely. Temperature-corrected values should be calculated only when specifically requested.

The dissociation curve is influenced by body temperature, pH, pCO_2, and by concentration of 2,3 diphosphoglycerate.

Increase in temperature, H^+ (low pH), increase in pCO_2, and increase in 2,3 DPG shift the dissociation curve to the right, that is adequate saturation requires higher partial pressure of oxygen. In contrast, low temperature, low H^+ (high pH), low pCO_2, and low 2,3 DPG shift the curve to the left, that is high oxygen saturation is achieved at a lower partial pressure of oxygen. This increased affinity to hemoglobin reduces its diffusion intracellular at the tissue capillary interface, thus leading to relative tissue hypoxia compared to the reduced affinity at higher temperatures.

When blood gases results are corrected for body temperature, pCO_2 and H^+ decrease when corrected for low temperature (indicating respiratory alkalosis), whereas pCO_2 and H^+ increase (respiratory acidosis). It is thus clear that interchangeable use of temperature correction or not can lead to misinterpretation and unnecessary adjustment of ventilator settings.

Biomarkers in support of blood gases interpretation

It is not surprising that the availability of electrolytes, lactate, and glucose in a blood gas instrument is helpful in the interpretation of blood gas parameters. In the absence of the appropriate clinical information, the following biomarkers provide clues to the presence and type of disorder present (Tables 1–3 and 10). Serum sodium to assess volume status where hypovolemia is a common cause of metabolic alkalosis and, chloride levels where changes opposite to that of sodium indicate the presence of acid-base disorder. No change in chloride levels is suggestive of anion gap metabolic acidosis. Changes in serum potassium mirror that of pH where unchanged levels are suggestive of compensatory disorder. Changes in serum bicarbonate levels, in addition to being indicative of metabolic acidosis (low levels) or metabolic alkalosis (high levels), the degree of change reflects either, acute disorder (minimal change 1–2 mmol/L) versus chronic disorder (changes of 4–5 mmol/L). The availability of sodium, potassium, chloride, and bicarbonate allows the determination of the anion gap (see above). Glucose is also measured where high levels are indicative of diabetes and supportive of suspected metabolic acidosis secondary to diabetic ketoacidosis. It also allows the calculation of the osmotic gap and helps indicate the presence of osmotic substance such as methanol or ethanol in metabolic acidosis. Lactate provides an assessment of tissue perfusion and is elevated in metabolic acidosis.

Advantage of measuring sodium using whole blood sample and ISE on the blood gases instrumentation is that it is measured directly (i.e., no sample dilution), and hence not influenced by hyperlipidemia, and hyperproteinemia causing pseudohyponatremia seen in laboratory based-indirect ISE methodologies (due to sample dilution prior to measurement).

TABLE 10 Electrolytes (often available on blood gases instruments) are helpful in the interpretation of accompanied blood gases results in the absence of relevant clinical information.

Analyte	Indication
Sodium (serum/plasma)	Hypovolemia (common cause of metabolic alkalosis). Allows calculation of anion and osmotic gap
Chloride	Changes follow that of Sodium. Changes opposite to HCO_3^- (by the same amount) Exception is "anion gap" metabolic acidosis where Cl is unchanged if not the same as Na indicates acid-base disorder
Potassium	Abnormal if pH is abnormal Unchanged in compensated disorders Low in alkalosis High in most acidosis except in HCO_3^-—losing states
Bicarbonate	Evaluates metabolic component of acid-base disorders Required for anion gap calculation If increased = Metabolic alkalosis/respiratory acidosis If decreased = Metabolic acidosis/respiratory alkalosis
Anion gap	Detects additions of acid (usually organic acids) Increase equals the acid concentration in mmol/L Increased anion causes a decrease in HCO_3^-, if not then acid-base disorders are present
Glucose	Ketoacidosis common in diabetes mellitus Used in calculating osmolar gap (detecting added organic acids)
Osmotic gap	Calculated—Measured osmolality (2× Na + Glucose/18 + BUN/2.8) Osmotic gap concentration in mmol/L Indicates unmeasured substances usually alcohols/glycols
Lactate	High anion gap Product of anaerobic glycolysis Arterial and venous are similar unless perfusion is poor. The difference is a measure of tissue perfusion

Adapted from the author's laboratory.

Lactate

An intermediary metabolite, lactate, is a marker of tissue hypoxia and an indicator of anaerobic metabolism. It is elevated in cardiac and circulatory insufficiency as well as in sepsis, poisoning, among others.

Lactate assay, whether performed on a laboratory-based large automated analyzer, by a blood gas machine, or by a point-of-care handheld device, employs lactate oxidase. The assay is specific to L-lactate and shows very poor reactivity (<20% to D-Lactate). However, the difference is in the detection system utilized. L-Lactate is oxidized by lactate oxidase to pyruvate and hydrogen peroxide, the latter is metabolized to oxygen using peroxidase. The oxygen produced oxidizes a chromogen, the concentration of which is proportional to the sample lactate concentration. In the aerometric-based blood gas and point-of-care devices, oxygen produced oxidizes at the electrode surface generating an electric current that is proportional to the sample lactate concentration.

D-Lactate

D-lactate acidosis is due to excess production in the colon by yeast and lactobacillus microorganisms, it is facilitated by decreased colonic motility and by the presence of excessive carbohydrates. The latter are either due to ingestion of large carbohydrate amounts or to decreased malabsorption as in surgical short bowel syndrome. The acidosis is of short duration and is related to carbohydrate ingestion.

There is an apparent normal blood lactate level. This is because the routinely used lactate assay measures L-lactate and not D-lactate.

D-Lactate accumulates due to its slow metabolism (20% that of L-lactate) leading to a high anion gap metabolic acidosis in the absence of ketonuria and elevated L-lactate.

Summary

- H^+ and CO_2 are produced during metabolism
- H^+ homeostasis depends on:
  - Buffering in blood/tissue
  - Excretion of H^+ in urine
  - Excretion of CO_2 in expired air
- $[H^+]$ is:
  - Directly proportional to pCO_2
  - Inversely proportional to HCO_3^-
- Respiratory acidosis is result of CO_2 retention
- Respiratory alkalosis is due to excessive CO_2 loss
- Metabolic acidosis is due to either increased H^+ production or decreased excretion or both
- Metabolic alkalosis is due to excessive H^+ loss from the body
- Mixed disturbances are frequent
- Compensatory mechanisms help correct the acid/base disturbance. The correction may be complete or partial.
- Quality control for blood gases is performed every 8h (at least one quality control level).
- Umbilical cord blood gases predict fetal acid-base status at birth/delivery.

References

1 Berend K, Duits AJ. The role of the clinical laboratory in diagnosing acid-base disorders. *Crit Rev Clin Lab Sci.* 2019;56(3):147–169.

Further reading

Bisson J, Younker J. Correcting arterial blood gases for temperature: (when) is it clinically significant? *Nurs Crit Care.* 2006;11(5):232–238.

Hampson NB. Carboxyhemoglobin: a primer for clinicians. *Undersea Hyperb Med.* 2018;45(2):165–171.

Thorp JA, Rushing RS. Umbilical cord blood gas analysis. *Obstet Gynecol Clin North Am.* 1999;26(4):695–709.

Chenoweth JA, Albertson TE, Greer MR. Carbon monoxide poisoning. *Crit Care Clin.* 2021;37(3):657–672.

Ayers P, Dixon C, Mays A. Acid-base disorders: learning the basics. *Nutr Clin Pract.* 2015;30(1):14–20.

Hauvik LE, Varghese M, Nielsen EW. Lactate gap: a diagnostic support in severe metabolic acidosis of unknown origin. *Case Rep Med.* 2018;2018:5238240.

Jubran A. Pulse oximetry. *Crit Care.* 2015;19:272.

Smith JC, Abdala AP, Borgmann A, Rybak IA, Paton JF. Brainstem respiratory networks: building blocks and microcircuits. *Trends Neurosci.* 2013;36(3):152–162.

Chapter 16

Aspects of clinical laboratory management

Introduction

Before the appearance of the laboratory's result in a final patient report, there were many activities occurring behind the scenes; from day-to-day operational management to quality and regulatory essentials.

For example, when a clinician orders a glucose test on a patient with signs and symptoms suggestive of diabetes mellitus, the return of a glucose level of 300 mg/dL (16.7 mmol/L) confirms the clinician's suspicion. However, for the laboratory, that glucose test request is one of many hundreds, if not thousands, received daily by the laboratory and it is impossible for the laboratory staff to review every single patient chart to verify if the obtained glucose of 300 mg/dL was expected and consistent with a patient's symptoms. The laboratory, therefore, develops mechanisms and processes that ensure the very high likelihood of that result being correct.

This chapter describes the role of the medical director "consultant clinical chemist" (also called the chemical pathologist or the clinical biochemist); the organizational structure, accreditation, and regulatory aspects of the laboratory; requirements for quality control and proficiency testing; and quality indicators that are all components of the quality management program, as well as establishing reference intervals, the concepts of critical differences, and that of critical values. This chapter also discusses methods validation and factors to consider when selecting a reference laboratory, as well as the various financial aspects of determining the cost of a laboratory test. The chapter also describes the expanding field of laboratory informatics as well as the emerging new roles of the clinical laboratory central to patient care and patient outcome.

Medical directorship roles and responsibilities

As clinical chemist, you are likely to assume medical directorship and/or clinical consultant responsibilities as part of your professional duties. Your duties will often include clinical, teaching, and administrative components. You will provide interpretation and consultative advice to both healthcare practitioners and laboratory technical staff, and teach clinical chemistry to pathology residents, residents, and trainees from other medical specialties on laboratory aspects and disease pathophysiology. In addition to clinical, teaching, and administrative duties, you are likely to pursue basic or translational research in an area of your interest.

Upon completion of clinical chemistry training, you are expected to understand clinical needs in terms of laboratory tests and be able to translate those needs into analytical performance characteristics required to fulfill those needs. Users of the clinical laboratory—either the healthcare delivery team or patients cannot define the technical goals required to achieve the necessary analytical performance for their optimum care.

The clinical training of a clinical chemist covers methodologies, their performance characteristics and diagnostic efficiency, and balancing the business act of day-to-day operations such as test utilization and consultative activities. Furthermore, in addition to awareness of and compliance with regulatory requirements (accreditation standards), ethics of practice, and maintenance of competency and skills, a clinical chemist also requires credentialing and privileges as well as of maintenance of specialty board certification.

The medical director is responsible for ensuring that available clinical laboratory testing and services is of the highest quality in terms of the tests' repertoire appropriate to the population the laboratory serves, and that testing utilizes relevant and appropriate methodologies by providing instructions and advice on sample collection, patient preparation, test selection, as well as availability of laboratory results in an acceptable time frame, accompanied by appropriate reference intervals and interpretive comments. In addition, the medical director is responsible for ensuring laboratory compliance with local and accrediting agency's regulations.[1]

Although some of the day-to-day activities performed may be viewed as administrative in nature, they are essential to the provision of accurate and timely laboratory results. Administrative duties associated with regulatory aspects can account for about 50% (less than 20% of those activities can be delegated to a technical manager), followed by clinical activities (30%), and academic activities (20%). Those distributions are typical of a large academic medical center but can vary significantly depending on the institution and your expected role. In some practices, your clinical activities may require 95% of your duties, with the remaining time allocated to teaching, mentoring, and/or administrative roles.

Tutorials in Clinical Chemistry. https://doi.org/10.1016/B978-0-12-822949-1.00001-2

The administrative activities can be classified as those requiring clinical expertise, such as test utilization initiatives, diagnostic algorithms development, selecting methodologies based on clinical needs, and inclusion of appropriate reference intervals and relevant information in the report to aid accurate interpretation of the laboratory results. Activities requiring technical expertise focus on the analytical phase of the testing cycle, such as instrument and test selection and validation, establishing laboratory developed tests, establishing acceptable performance characteristics, and reviewing internal and external quality control. Administrative activities require administrative experience, and although few can be delegated to a nonclinically trained technical manager (about 20% of the activities), you remain responsible for many aspects such as oversight of operations, policy development and reviews, and approval and review of several documents. You will take part in periodic staff management meetings, conflict management sessions, and health and safety issues, and will ensure laboratory personnel's adherence to test procedures, instruments operating instruction, and staff competency assessments (i.e., reviewing and accepting corrective actions for technical errors), among other day-to-day operational activities.

The essence of directing determines the goals for your laboratory, by guiding and influencing staff to achieve those predetermined goals. You have the role of providing a vision as to what the laboratory will look like and how it will be run. Your manager colleagues will help ensure that activities are directed toward those goals and vision. In doing so, giving clear direction is pivotal to the success of your desired goals. Cornerstones for successful management of the required changes to achieve these desired goals is to exhibit a sense of urgency and to provide regular updates on progress.

The laboratory director also provides guidance, leadership, and a workspace and environment, for example, by helping to establish and maintain a productive work environment with adequate physical space, equipment, and supplies. You will also ensure the laboratory develops, implements, and maintains a quality systematic approach, as well as deliver accurate, reliable, and timely results. You will ensure that the laboratory has an overall quality management program with appropriate key indicators, and that corrective and preventative measures are implemented in a timely fashion. The laboratory director might also ensure that the laboratory provides a healthy and safe environment through compliance with federal, state, and local regulations.

Delegation of laboratory director activities

Although it is understood that the laboratory director holds the accreditation license and is responsible and accountable, there are too many activities that require specialized scientific, clinical, and administrative training. Therefore, the laboratory director may delegate some of those activities do others deemed qualified to do so. Some activities may be delegated by the laboratory director to other specialty laboratory area clinical consultants or medical, scientific, and technical staff that meet the required qualifications and experience as established by the laboratory accrediting agencies and local state regulations (see later section). Some of these specialized activities include selection of the appropriate testing methodology, define method performance verification (e.g., accuracy and precision), ensure appropriate utilization of quality control and proficiency testing programs and review their performance and advise on corrective measures as needed, ensure and provide supervision of the testing site, facilitate and ensure ease of access to approved testing and to operational procedures, and facilitate and ensure training and assessment of competency of testing personnel. However, there are many activities that may not be delegated by the laboratory director, which include taking responsibility for high-quality clinical laboratory services that meet the needs of the clinical department and those utilizing the laboratory service, ensuring the provision of safe laboratory environment, securing an adequate number of trained and appropriately certified staffing for provision of services, and approving all procedures and policies. Similarly, the director must ensure that all delegated activities are performed well, and that testing is performed within any licensure limitations or restrictions.

Accreditation and regulatory aspects

The operation of the clinical laboratory is governed by and subject to a number of legal acts and accreditation standards defined by Clinical Laboratory Improvement Act (CLIA) in the United States and administered with oversight by different agencies with deemed status. Historically, these were enacted to ensure safe practices and environment. In addition to promoting standardization of practice, accreditation facilitates a safe environment, attracts high-caliber staff, and assists with staff retention. Accreditation is also required for payments by some insurance and the government. Accredited laboratories often enjoy end-user trust and are favored over nonaccredited laboratories in countries where accreditation is not mandated.

In instances where different standards apply, that of the stricter ruling supersedes. For example, if the laboratory accrediting agency requires 5 years of data storage and the state where the laboratory practices mandates 10 years, the state rule is stricter and thus prevails.

The following are examples of regulatory agencies of clinical laboratories that you, as a clinical chemist and/or a medical director, must know.

Clinical Laboratories Improvement Act of 1988 (CLIA-88)

Following complaints about the quality and safety of laboratory tests (cytology), the Clinical Laboratory Improvement Act (CLIA) was passed in 1967 to cover independent and hospital-based laboratories. A second amendment was introduced in 1988 to cover all laboratory testing sites (physician offices, nursing homes, etc.). It mandated that any laboratory performing clinical testing for diagnosis, screening, or monitoring of illness and treatment monitoring is regulated. Administration of the act was given to the Centers for Disease Control and Prevention (CDC). The centers for medicare and medicaid services (CMS) regulates all clinical laboratory testing via CLIA and its amendments.

The license holder is the laboratory director who may delegate some of the responsibilities to one of the following personnel: clinical consultant, technical consultant, or technical supervisor. In the instance of high complexity testing, a general supervisor may also be assigned and delegated to.

The duties of the clinical consultant are to ensure appropriate testing; provide relevant interpretation; and be available for consultation with other healthcare practitioners, those duties extend to the technical consultant (for moderate complexity testing), and technical supervisor (for a high complexity testing). The clinical consultant will also oversee activities related to test performance such as appropriate test methodology and competent staffing, adequate methods verification, participation and review of proficiency testing, quality control, annual evaluation of high complexity testing staff competency, and review corrective actions and appropriate procedures are available to testing personnel, and that a general supervisor, who will provide onsite supervision, is available and responsible for the day-to-day supervision of all testing personnel.

The operation of the clinical laboratory is governed by and is subject to a number of acts administered by CMS (see later) with oversight by different agencies. Historically, those were enacted to ensure safe practices and environment to protect the health of both patients as well as laboratory personnel handling patient samples.

Operations and accreditation are based on standards that are classified into general aspects (termed Laboratory Common) that are common to all areas of the clinical laboratory such as quality, safety, competency of staffing, and informatics. Specialty standards that are specific to the clinical area of the laboratory completes the required accreditation standards.

The accreditation process mandates site visits and inspections every 2 years with self-inspection in the year in between. The findings of the latter are reviewed during the site inspection. Although site visit inspections are required, those were suspended during the COVID-19 pandemic, and in some instances, exclusively remote or a combination of remote and follow-up short onsite verification visits were performed.

United States Food and Drug Administration (FDA)

The FDA is responsible for ensuring the safety of medical devices and reagents used in clinical laboratories for the diagnosis and treatment of disease. It recently added oversight of laboratory-developed testing. It reviews items for safety and effectiveness before entering the market. The FDA clears moderate-risk devices for use if they have been demonstrated to be substantially equivalent to a legally marketed predicate device that did not require premarket approval. The FDA also categorizes testing based on complexity, which drives decisions on staffing and laboratory structure.

The FDA approval process can be lengthy and depends on the risk as well as complexity of the testing and its intended use. During the COVID-19 epidemic, the FDA issued emergency use authorization (EUA) to in vitro diagnostics tests for COVID-19. This is a restricted use and applies during a declared public health state of emergency. EUAs were either for individual molecular and serology tests, those of an umbrella EUA status for independently validated serology tests, or for molecular diagnostic tests for SARS-CoV-2 developed and performed by high complexity CLIA-accredited laboratories. Submission of completed templates were required for FDA EUA approvals. Information on assay characteristics such as limit of detection, reagents, and sample stability are required.

FDA Approval Process: The FDA reviews submissions for in vitro diagnostic tests and devices. The testing system is categorized as Class I, II, and III indicating low risk, moderate risk, and high risk, respectively. The length of time required for review is variable and is often about 3 weeks for Exempt, FDA-registered, or listed for Class I (low-risk) test systems; about 5 months for 510K, FDA-cleared (~5 months) Class II (moderate-risk) test systems; and about 18 months for Class III (high-risk or no predicate): Premarket Approval.

510K refers to the section of the FDA's Food, Drug, and Control Act in the Federal Register. When planning to provide an in vitro diagnostic test for commercial use, the manufacturer submits a 510K application; similarly, if the intended use of an approved IVD test has changed or the testing has been altered significantly in that it may affect safety and/or effectiveness of the previously approved test. A premarket approval follows submission to demonstrate to the FDA that the test system is safe, effective, and substantially equivalent to an approved test in the market. There is no specific form, but the format must include components described in 21CFR-807. It is worth noting that many analytes and specific reagents do not require 510K submission.

Alternative pathways exist for humanitarian, de novo, product development protocol, and custom device exception EUAs, in that the approval process takes about 5 weeks. One such example are COVID-19 serology (IgG, IgM) tests; these minimum validation studies recommended by the FDA include Cross-reactivity/analytical specificity, Class specificity, Clinical agreement study, and Sample type/matrix equivalency. The FDA recommends that clinical accuracy should be established on human specimens from patients with microbiologically confirmed COVID-19 infection.

For antigens, assessment for limit of detection/analytical sensitivity is required.

The FDA defines tests into three classes (I–III) based on their potential risk, with Class I being the lowest risk of causing harm. Additionally, FDA-cleared Class I and II means that the test performance is substantially equivalent to those already FDA-approved or cleared. Class III tests are those of either new technology or new medical use of an existing technology.

Centers for Medicare and Medicaid Services (CMS)

This is the US federal agency running programs of Medicaid, Medicare, and Heath Insurance Exchanges. Thus, it is responsible for payment for health services provided under those programs. Those health services include clinical laboratory testing, where a periodic fee schedule is published and updated with testing menus and payments. The CMS regulates all laboratory testing (except research) performed on humans in the United States through CLIA. The Center for Clinical Standards and Quality has the responsibility of implementing the CLIA program administered by the Division of Clinical Laboratory Improvement and Quality within the quality, safety, and oversight group. The objective of the CLIA program is to ensure quality laboratory testing. Laboratories must be CLIA-certified to receive Medicare or Medicare payments. It periodically publishes clinical laboratory fee schedules and caps for reduction in price, often in the range of 10%–15%.

The CMS is the single largest payer of healthcare, and thus its requirements tend to shape how clinical laboratory testing operates. For clinical laboratories to participate in CMS payment systems, they must be accredited by CLIA or by organizations with deemed status from CMS to provide laboratory accreditation. Those organizations developed accreditation standards that must meet minimum CLIA requirements and may exceed them. In some countries this is not required by payers for laboratory services; however, accredited laboratories are more likely to attract well-qualified and experienced staff and offer an environment of safety and high quality.

Accrediting agencies define personnel designations and qualification requirements based on testing complexity, and some accrediting organizations, e.g., College of American Pathologists (CAP) include testing volume as well (see Table 1). The laboratory director is designated as the license holder, and the term "medical director" often represents the subspecialty director in both clinical and technical aspects of the subspecialty.

Occupational Safety and Health Administration (OSHA)

OSHA was created following the Occupational Safety and Health Act of 1970 by the US Congress. The act covers both workers and their employers throughout the jurisdictions of the United States. The agency is tasked with developing required guidance and regulations to ensure safety of working men and women via enforcing standards and by providing training and education. It is part of the US Department of Labor.

Although state and local government workers are not covered by the Federal act, state-based health safety programs must exist and be at least as effective as the Federal program, as well as Federal agencies and their employees. In laboratory aspects, this covers health and safety documents and procedures within the clinical laboratory. Protective equipment, clothing, signs and placards, training, and education is required and be included in the accreditation program. In addition to provision of safety equipment and training, the employee is free from retaliation from their immediate supervisor or employer if they complain about safety, health, and safety-related issues to OSHA. Under the act, the employees may have a legal right to refuse work in an environment that poses hazards to their health and safety if there is a lack of protective measures. As the medical director, you are responsible for ensuring provision of a safe working environment.

Equal opportunity employment

Equal opportunity and employment legislation prohibits workforce discrimination. It is enforced by the Equal Opportunity Commission. The commission was established by the Civil Rights Act of 1964. The employment section of the act, Title VII, prohibits discrimination based on race, color, national origin, gender, and religion. The act also prohibits employer retaliation. The act was amended to give the commission the authority to conduct its own enforcement litigation. Furthermore, the commission strongly influences the judicial interpretation of civil rights legislation. A typical analytical framework would be that the plaintiff has the burden of proof to show that they were directly discriminated against in a hiring case by showing that (1) they are a member of a Title VII-protected group,[3] (2) had ap-

TABLE 1 Roles and qualification/credentials required as defined by CLIA-88.[2]

Role	Credentials/qualifications		
	High complexity	Moderate complexity	Waived testing
Laboratory Director	MD, DO (Certified CP/AP), DPM (Clin Lab training), PhD (Board Certified)	As in High Complexity or MD, DO, or DPM plus 1 year experience supervising nonwaived testing, or 20 CME credit hours in laboratory practice commensurate with director responsibilities, or equivalent laboratory training (20 CME) obtained during medical residency	As in High and Moderate Complexity or MD, DO, or DPM
Clinical Consultant	As in High Complexity	As in High Complexity	N/A
Technical Consultant	N/A	As above (with 20 CMEs), or Doctoral or Master's degree in a chemical, physical, biological, or clinical laboratory science with at least 1 year of training and/or experience in nonwaived testing, or Bachelor's degree in a chemical, physical, biological, or clinical laboratory science or medical technology with at least 2 years of experience in nonwaived testing	N/A
Technical Supervisor	MD or DO with a current medical license and board-certification in anatomic, cytopathology, and clinical pathology, or possess qualifications equivalent to those required for certification • Technical supervisors overseeing a clinical pathology specialty must have board-certification in clinical pathology or equivalent qualifications	N/A	N/A
General Supervisor	1. Qualified as a Director for high-complexity testing; OR 2. Qualified as a Technical Supervisor for high complexity testing; OR 3. Doctoral degree in clinical laboratory science or chemical, physical or biological science with 1 year training and experience in high complexity testing; OR 4. Master's degree in clinical laboratory science, medical technology or chemical, physical, or biological science and 1 year training and experience in high-complexity testing; OR 5. Bachelor's degree in clinical laboratory science, medical technology or chemical, physical, or biological science and 1 year training and experience in high-complexity testing; OR 6. Associate's degree in medical laboratory technology (or pulmonary function) and 2 years laboratory (or blood gas analysis) training or experience, or both, in high complexity testing Refer to the CLIA regulation 42CFR493.1461 for additional qualifications.	N/A	N/A

Continued

TABLE 1 Roles and qualification/credentials required as defined by CLIA-88.2—cont'd

Role	Credentials/qualifications		
	High complexity	Moderate complexity	Waived testing
Testing Personnel	MD or DO with a current medical license, or Doctoral degree in clinical laboratory science, chemical, physical, biological science, or Master's degree in medical technology, clinical laboratory, chemical, physical, or biological science, or Bachelor's degree in medical technology, clinical laboratory, chemical, physical, or biological, or Associate's degree in chemical, physical, or biological science or medical laboratory or equivalent education and training (refer to 42CFR493.1489(b) for details on required courses and training), or individuals performing high complexity testing on or before April 24, 1995, with a high school diploma or equivalent with documented training may continue to perform testing only on those tests for which training was documented prior to September 1, 1997 (refer to CLIA regulation 42CFR493.1489(b) for details on required training), or individual previously qualified or could have qualified as a technologist under CFR.493.1489 and CFR.493.1491 on or before February 28, 1992	1. MD or DO with a current medical license[1]; OR 2. Doctoral degree in clinical laboratory science, chemical, physical, or biological science; OR 3. Master's degree in medical technology, clinical laboratory, chemical, physical, or biological science; OR 4. Bachelor's degree in medical technology, clinical laboratory, chemical, physical, or biological science; OR 5. Associate's degree in chemical, physical, or biological science or medical laboratory technology; OR 6. High school graduate or equivalent and laboratory training/experience consisting of the following: a. Successfully completed military training of 50 or more weeks and served as a medical laboratory specialist; OR b. Appropriate training/experience as specified in 42CFR493.1423	Training/Competency records

Modified from Laboratory personnel qualifications and training requirements. Code of Federal Regulations. https://www.ecfr.gov/current/title-42/chapter-IV/subchapter-G/part-493/subpart-M. Accessed 28 February 2023.

plied and was qualified for the position sought, and (3) the employer rejected the plaintiff for the job and continued to seek applicants with similar qualifications after the rejection. Once the plaintiff succeeds in those points, the burden of proof shifts to the employer to provide a legitimate, nondiscriminatory reason for refusing to hire the plaintiff. Failing that, the employer is considered guilty of workplace discrimination. The workforce must be representative of the applicant pool and the interview pool. The following figure can be applied to monitor a representative workplace. The applicant, interview, and hire proportions of the workforce is representative of the applicant pool and the target qualified audience.

The goal is always to hire the best qualified applicant who possesses the required technical and clinical skills and desired behaviors. Review the application documents and curriculum vitae for meeting minimum job requirements and qualifications and if the work experience is consistent with your business model.

Tests classification

Tests are classified based on their degree of complexity in terms of performance, required handling steps, required knowledge, and if they are either waived, moderately complex, or highly complex. The classification is assigned by the FDA, which has the responsibility of ensuring safety and efficiency of the testing process. A scale of 1, 2, and 3 are assigned for low, medium, and high-risk, respectively, following seven testing criteria: (1) knowledge required to perform the test, (2) degree of training required at each of the three phases of the testing cycle of the testing personnel, (3) extent of reagent handling and preparation, including that of stability and storage requirements, (4) characteristics of the various operational steps such as the need for manual pipetting, the need for temperature monitoring, or for manual recording of reaction time, (5) stability of calibration, quality control, and proficiency material, (6) the extent of complexity of the test system maintenance and troubleshooting, the extent of technical knowledge required

to perform maintenance, and (7) extent of interpretation and judgment required at all three phases of the testing cycle, and the ability to resolve and perform interpretation independently.

Tests with less than 12 total points are classified as moderately complex, whereas tests with scores greater than 12 are considered highly complex.

The degree of complexity (waived, moderate, or high) mandates the level of personnel's qualification, and certification requirements are shown in Table 2. Personnel qualifications and certification are required and are recognized during privileging and credentialing by the employers. Some specialty certification boards expire and become inactive unless a maintenance program is completed such as completion and attainment of approved continuing medical education hours as required for recredentialling.

Quality management program

Clinical laboratories are one of the early clinical subspecialties adopting quality management programs in its routine practice. Quality processes are integral components of sample analysis and results reporting where the use of quality control samples of a known target value is assayed as part of the analytical run. If the expected value is obtained, it can be assumed that the analytical run is acceptable, and the unknown patient sample results are considered acceptable and are thus reported. Patient samples received into the laboratory are numerous, and although the indication for testing as well as differential diagnosis may be accessed, it is impractical for the laboratory to do so given a sample volume. This is in contrast where, for example, a physician order for a glucose test for a patient with polyuria, polydipsia, and weight loss who is suspected of having diabetes mellitus, a glucose result returned by the laboratory as 300 mg/dL and/or A1c of 8.9% confirms the clinical suspicion. The laboratory cannot review the clinical indications for every test request of the thousands of samples often received, hence the utility of quality control and the assumption for a valid laboratory result.

TABLE 2 Examples of high complexity, moderate complexity, and waived tests.

High complexity	Moderate complexity	Waived testing
All cytology, cytogenetics, histopathology, histocompatibility tests Nonautomated chemistry tests LCMSMS Bone marrow examination Abnormal cell identification on WBC differential Manual hematology procedures (WBC, RBC, Hb, Platelet count) Any modified FDA-cleared or approved tests, laboratory developed tests (LDTs)	Automated chemistry, hematology/coagulation Dipstick urinalysis Manual WBC differentials (identify normal cells only)	Glucose (point of care) hCG Pregnancy test Urine strip test

Modified from Test Complexity Classification. https://www.cdc.gov/clia/test-complexities.html. Accessed 9 March 2023.

Furthermore, quality management has evolved into all aspects of the three phases of the testing cycle. It has also become subject to various regulatory and accreditation standards for performance and is considered an integral component of good laboratory practices, for example, ISO 15189 guidelines for quality, CLSI quality management system, CAP, CLIA, Joint Commission, and CLOA, among others.

There are various definitions for quality, but all are centered around consumer requirements. The customer of the clinical laboratory is the patient, whereas the clinician/patient care provider is the consumer on behalf of the patient. This makes it clear that a relevant test menu must be available, and that the test results are accurate, reproducible, and available in a timely manner. Also, appropriate interpretation and information will accompany the result to aid timely and appropriate patient management.

The Institute of Medicine defined quality of care as "the degree to which healthcare services for individuals and populations increase the likelihood of desired health outcomes and are consistent with current professional practice." The six health domains identified are those related to patient safety, effectiveness, equity, patient-centeredness, timeliness, and efficiency. The clinical laboratory must have a written quality management program that covers all areas of the laboratory and specifically monitors all aspects of the testing cycle (preanalytical, analytical, and postanalytical). The monitoring is performed periodically to both identify trends and assess improvement (or lack of) following intervention. In essence, what is measured is then managed.

Selection of quality indicators is at risk of selection bias due to a case occurring. It should be a comprehensive program monitoring all aspects of the testing cycle with continuous review of all areas identifying potential problems and areas for improvement.

It is also important to note that quality assurance activities and associated documentation may be the subject of evidence in a patient-related legal case. The concept of negligent entrustment applies where an error was attributed to what could be a foreseen deficiency or risk for patient management and safety. Adequate documentation of quality measures and appropriate retention of those documents is important.

Samples and documents retention

The laboratory must have a policy to define and guide specimen and laboratory records, the period of retention, and the condition of retention and storage. Each laboratory defines its sample acceptance criteria guided by information gathered from manufacturers' instructions, published literature, clinical practice guidelines, and from actual practice and validation studies.

Requirements for retention are variable between agency and local government requirements as well as the nature of the test. Typically, samples for chemistry testing are held for 24 h and stored as per testing manufacturer recommendation. Laboratory reports are stored for a minimum of 2 years; however, for some areas of the laboratory such as histology and cytology tests, 10 years and cytogenetics for 25 years are mandated (CLSI, Quality Management, GP 26-A4) (see Table 3 for examples of retention periods).

A document may serve more than one purpose; hence, its retention is dictated by the purpose with the longest period of time. Bearing in mind, the nature of limitations varies from one local government to another and from one accrediting agency to another. Similarly, as to when the clock starts, some begin from the time of sample collection and others from the time the report becomes available. The time the event occurred versus when the time the patient complains or becomes aware of the issue may vary considerably. This then becomes a subject of risk management.

TABLE 3 Examples of retention times for documents.

Item/records	Retention period
Requisitions	2 years
Quality control	2 years
Instrument maintenance	2 years
Blood bank donor/recipient records	Indefinitely
Blood bank employee signature/initials	10 years
Blood bank QC	5 years
Reports	
Clinical pathology	2 years
Autopsy	Indefinitely
Surgical pathology	10 years
Cytogenetics	20 years
Specimen	
Serum/other body fluids	48 h
Blood smear routine	7 days
Pathology bone marrow slides	10 years
Pathology blocks	10 years
Microbiology smears	7 days
Blood bank donor/recipient specimens	7 days posttransfusion
Cytogenetics slides	3 years
Cytogenetics diagnostic images	20 years

Note: Considerations must be given to local rules and regulations that may require extended storage and availability beyond that deemed appropriate by the laboratory professional and accrediting agencies. Modified from CLSI GP26-A4. *Quality Management System: A Model for Laboratory Services; Approved Guideline.* 4th ed.

Quality and performance indicators

Performance indicators must cover all aspects of the laboratory testing cycle process, for example, patient and specimen identification, test accuracy orders, specimen suitability, critical values reporting, and corrected reports. The laboratory and medical director has responsibility for defining quality indicators and their respective acceptance criteria.

Total laboratory errors range from 0.33% to 0.61%. Clinical laboratories perform at about 3.5 sigma, therefore, a large laboratory reporting 20,000 tests per day would expect about 175 errors. The majority of the errors are likely to be in the preanalytical phase of the testing cycle often due to patient identification error, sample contamination, and/or to sample hemolysis.

Analytical errors occur at the analytical phase due to the advent of automation, autoverification, and quality control alerts. Manual analytical processes are often associated with manual entry errors (Table 4). Although the frequency of analytical errors is much reduced, the impact on patient care and outcomes is likely to be more significant in this phase.

Selected laboratory indicators are identified for each phase of the testing cycle. Examples are shown in Table 4. The frequency of data collection and monitoring of each indicator, as well as target goals for acceptable performance, are defined. Performance monitors are identified as meeting a threshold (goal); findings that exceed the goals will require increased monitoring frequency. Where goals are not met, corrective action should be implemented. Increased monitoring identifies the presence of random or systemic errors. Excessive outliers require that the process is stopped, investigated, and corrected. The goals are often selected based on guidelines and recommendations such as hemolysis rate of <2% or by establishing baseline data as a start and identifying corrective measures to reduce the baseline.

Quality control

When a clinician orders a glucose level on a patient with symptoms suggestive of diabetes mellitus, a fasting glucose results of 200 mg/dL (11.1 mmol/L) confirms clinical suspicion. For the clinical laboratory, the use of quality control samples provides timely assurance that the glucose result reported was within analytical goals. The large number of samples received into the laboratory makes it impractical to review the clinical indication for every test as a way of validating assays results. In using quality control samples, the clinical laboratory becomes one of the first clinical subspecialties that introduced quality performance integral to its operation. Although the findings of acceptable glucose quality control results assume acceptable analytical performance, it does not guarantee it. Random errors may still occur affecting samples between quality control runs, defined as the time or sample volume intervals between successive quality control samples review. In addition to the afore-mentioned quality control (internal), good laboratory practice and accreditation agencies require that the laboratory periodically assay unknown samples through participation in a proficiency testing program, as discussed later in this chapter.

When quality control failures are not promptly detected and assays performance corrected, patient results during a missed identification of a quality control failure requires repeat analysis of patient samples analyzed and reported since the last known acceptable quality control. This can be a very large number of samples for a busy high-volume laboratory. Samples spot-check may be selected at random from 10% of samples selected for rerun. If the repeated results ae similar to those reported earlier (within assay imprecision), the entire reported patient samples can be considered acceptable for some analytes. Otherwise, all patient samples since the last known acceptable quality control sample will have to be repeated. Some repeat analysis may not be feasible, such as blood gases governed by sample stability. Therefore, careful monitoring of assay performance is warranted.

Internal quality control samples

Samples of known values can be obtained commercially; they can be obtained from the same manufacturers of the

TABLE 4 Examples of selected performance (quality) monthly indicators in use by the author's laboratory.

Testing cycle phase	Indicator	Acceptable minimum	Failure
Preanalytical	Delayed sample	<3	>3
	Mislabeled	0	≥1
	Hemolyzed/clotted	<2%	≥2.1%
	Volume insufficient	0	≥1
Analytical phase	Failed quality control	<5	≥1
	Frequency of calibration	<2	≥3
	Manual entry errors	0	≥1
Postanalytical phase	Turnaround time	<30 min (95%)	≥30 min
	Critical values notification	<30 min (95%)	≥30 min
	Manual entry errors	<1	≥2

assay reagents or from a third party, which in the author's opinion would be good laboratory practice as it breaks the manufacturer's reagent calibrator's quality control circle and provides an independent assessment. The quality control material can also be purchased with values unassigned. In both cases (assigned and unassigned), the laboratory would analyze the samples in the same manner as they would for a patient sample, i.e., at least 20 measurements within and between assays, then calculate the mean and standard deviation. Another way of attaining quality control material is for the laboratory to develop its own. This can be prepared by either collecting pooled patient samples, patient samples spiked with known concentration of the analyte, or use of a material of similar matrix such as fetal calf serum or similar. Prepared quality control samples are often aliquoted and stored frozen to minimize repeated freeze-thaw cycles.

A minimum of two different quality control levels must be run every 24 h as per CLIA regulations; in practice quality controls are, however, often run much more frequently. They provide real-time assessment of analytical performance.

Analysis of the quality control and thus system performance for both random and systematic error is best assessed via a Levey-Jennings graphical chart (Figs. 1–3). It is a plot of serial quality control values at all different levels against their respective mean and standard deviations. The distribution of the data follows a Gaussian distribution with a percentage of random outliers being 31.7%, 4.6%, and 0.3%

at one standard deviation, two standard deviations, and three standard deviations, respectively. Therefore, 95% of the quality control data are expected to be within two standard deviations. The graphical presentation is reviewed for random error variation and systematic bias. Several rules apply; however, Westgard rules are the most popular and widely used. The rules define patterns for acceptance, rejection, and for warning and closer monitoring. The rules are shown in Table 5.

Interpretation of quality control performance

Sources of random error (imprecision) include incorrect reconstitution and mixing of control, inappropriate storage of control in frost-free freezers, incorrect pipetting of control samples, misplacement of control sample within the run, air bubbles, operator techniques, wrong quality control sample used, and use of nonreagent grade water in test system.

Sources of systemic errors (inaccuracy) represented by shifts and trends include improper alignment of sample or reagent pipettes; drift or shift in incubator chamber temperature; inappropriate temperature/humidity in testing area; failing light source; change in reagent or calibrator lot number; deterioration of reagent while in use, storage, or shipment; poor calibration or deterioration of calibrators while in use, storage, or shipment; and deterioration of control performance while in use, storage, or shipment. This is in addition to changes in operator-dependent handling and processing of any of the testing components.

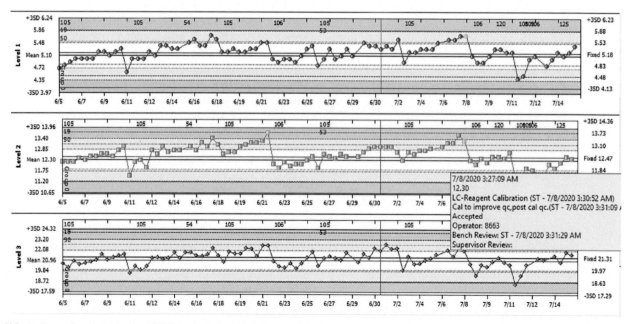

FIG. 1 Levey-Jenning's plot for TSH from the author's laboratory. All three quality control levels 1, 2, and 3 are within acceptable limits (2 standard deviation). A shift on 6/10 reflects performance following calibration. The drop on 7/13 for all three levels were due to the running of the wrong quality control material (did not contain TSH). Repeat run using the correct quality control bottles showed expected response. TSH is a stable and robust analyte compared with FT4 shown in Fig. 2. *(Courtesy of the author's laboratory.)*

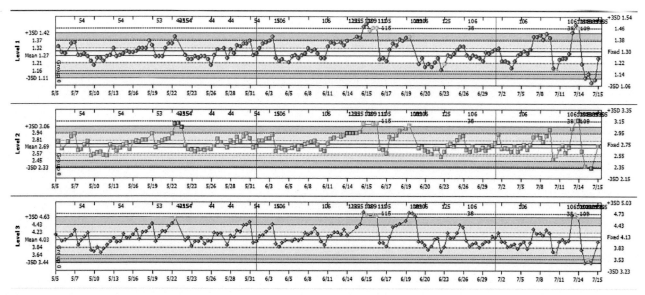

FIG. 2 Levey-Jenning's plot for FT4 from the author's laboratory. All three quality control levels 1, 2, and 3 are within acceptable limits (2 standard deviation). The assay results indicate periodic shifts that required frequent calibration to maintain within the acceptable 2 standard deviations. This is characteristic of the FT4 assay that required weekly calibration. The QC pattern thus dictates the frequency of calibration and often coincides with that recommended by the manufacturer. FT4 is a less stable and robust analyte compared with TSH shown in Fig. 1. *(Courtesy of the author's laboratory.)*

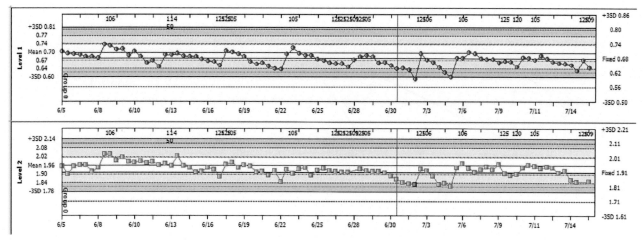

FIG. 3 Levey-Jenning's chart showing quality control pattern for lithium. The performance of the QC decays over time as shown, starts high and trends low. The assay is calibrated weekly. Calibration causes a reset and a higher QC value (all within the acceptable 2SD range). The performance of the quality control in this assay confirms the manufacturer and actual operational needs for weekly calibration.

Examples of quality control performance and interpretation are shown in Figs. 1-3. The troubleshooting algorithm in use by the author is shown in Fig. 4.

Desirable quality specification

The would-be acceptable and desirable performance of a test assay should be determined by its clinical utility and required performance characteristics. Of particular importance is the reproducibility (precision) of the assays, as most tests are used to monitor progression of a disease/disorder and a response to intervention. Thus, they are often used for determining trends. For this to be of value, the assay must be reproducible.

When compared to analytical variability (imprecision), which is characteristic of a particular test methodology, the biological variability (within the body) is of a much larger amplitude. The latter is influenced by diurnal rhythm, prandial status, physical activity, and environmental and genetic factors.

Assuming that preanalytical variables related to sample collection and handling (storage and transportation) are well controlled, the contribution to results variability (imprecision) is that of inherent assay imprecision and the within subject biological variability.

TABLE 5 Westgard's internal quality control samples acceptance criteria.[4]

Rule	Acceptance/failure	Action
1_{2s} One measurement > X ± 2SD:	*Warning* rule requires further assessment. Few laboratories consider this rule a failure rule. However, this is considered excessive since about 4.5% of acceptable performance is between 1_{2s} and 1_{3s} rules.	Consider performance of other controls in the run (and within the run) and in previous runs before accepting and reporting result.
1_{3s} One measurement > X ± 3SD:	Considered *out of control (Failure rule)*	The rule applies within the run only. Mainly detects random error but may also indicate the beginning of a large systematic error.
2_{2s} Two measurements > X ± 2SD:	Rejection rule *(Failure rule)*	Detects systematic error. It is applied within and between runs.
R_{4s} The difference in SD between 2 control values exceeds 4_s	Rejection rule *(Failure rule)*	Detects random error. Applied within run.
4_{1s} The last four QC values on the same exceed 1_s	Rejection rule *(Failure rule)*	Detects systematic bias. Within and between assays. Indicator of need for instrument maintenance or calibration.
10_x Ten consecutive control observations falling on one side of the mean	Rejection rule *(Failure rule)*	Sensitive to systematic error.

Modified from WESTGARD QC. https://www.westgard.com/mltirule.htm. Accessed 24 February 2022.

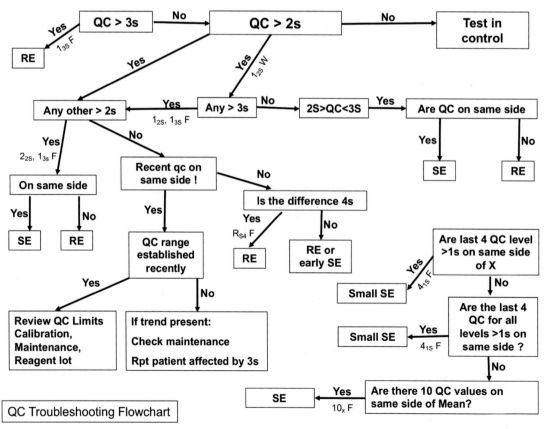

FIG. 4 Troubleshooting algorithm for internal quality control results. *(Courtesy of the author's laboratory.)*

If the analytical imprecision is CV_a (coefficient of variation-analytical) and the inherent biological variability is CV_i (coefficient of variation for an individual), the combined assay results variability is the sum of CV_a and CV_i. This is derived as shown here:

$$\text{Total } CV^2 = CV_a^2 + CV_i^2. \text{ That is combined}$$
$$CV = \sqrt{CV_a^2 + CV_i^2}$$

If the analytical precision equals that of the biological variability, the equation becomes:
$CV = \sqrt{2 \times CV_i^2}$ That is $1.414 \times CV_i$, which indicates an addition of about 40% to the total CV when the analytical CV is same as that of the biological variability.

If the analytical variability was half that of the biological variability, the contribution to the total CV would be 11.18%.

$$\text{Total } CV = \sqrt{(0.5 CV_a)^2 + CV_i^2} = \sqrt{5/4 CV_i^2} = 1.118 CV_i$$

The mathematical range of contributions to the total biological variability if the analytical variability was related is shown in Table 6. Therefore, for a contribution of about 10%, the analytical variability should be at least half of the biological variability.

Assuming variability of <0.5, biological variability adds about 10% to the test results obtained with no more than 12% variability added to the test result's variability. A desirable analytical variability (imprecision) should not exceed $0.5 CV_i$, which would add a maximum of 12%; an optimum $0.25 CV_i$ adds 3%, and minimum of $0.75 CV_i$ adds 20%.

TABLE 6 The would-be addition to the total result variability when the analytical variability is mathematically and hypothetical calculated as a fraction of the inherent biological variability of the test.

Magnitude of analytical imprecision compared to biological variability	Variability added to total result variability (CV_a plus CV_i)
0.25	3.1
0.50	11.18
0.745	25
1.0	41.4
1.5	80.3
1.73	100

A minimum addition of about 3% is seen when the analytical variability is 0.25 that of the biological variability. There is about a 10% contribution of the analytical variability to the total; variability observed with its inherent variability is half of the biological variability. This biological concept applies to define required assay performance (quality).
Modified from Fraser C. *Biological Variation: From Principles to Practice.* AACC Press; 2001. ISBN-10: 1890883492. ISBN-13: 978-189088349.

Analytical variability that is half the inherent biological activity ($CV_a < 0.5\ CV_i$) of a particular test is considered acceptable (desirable). However, in reality, the analytical variability for the majority of clinical chemistry tests are below their observed biological activity.

Mathematically, the total allowable errors (TEa) is a combination of both accuracy (bias) and variation (imprecision).

If bias is $<0.25\ \sqrt{(CV_a^2 + CV_i^2)}$ and imprecision is 1.65 ($0.5\ CV_i$), then the total allowable error (TEa) is given by the formula:

$$TEa < 0.25 \sqrt{(CV_a^2 + CV_i^2)} + 1.65(0.5 CV_i)$$

External quality samples (proficiency testing)

External quality control samples, also known as proficiency testing (PT), are analyzed in the same manner a patient sample would be. The PT samples are often purchased from supplies recognized by the laboratory's accrediting agency. Samples are often received two or three times a year (i.e., two or three challenges per year). Regulated analyte (see discussion later) requires three challenges annually. Results are reported to the program samples supplier who analyzes results for deviation from the expected value as determined by the manufacturer or by participating peer laboratories using the same measurement system (Table 8). Participation in a program such as CAP, American Standard Institute, etc., in addition to fulfilling quality requirements and accreditation standards, the data obtained include the number of participating laboratories using the participating laboratory's particular methods, the range of methods available, and the comparative results obtained. It provides information about the comparability of the test system, which in the end will aid in harmonization and thus commutability of laboratory results.

Participation in a PT program was enacted and became a requirement of accreditation of clinical laboratories following amendment of CLIA in 1988. To facilitate better assessment of analytical performance including imprecision, the frequency of testing was increased from two samples and four challenges annually to five samples and three challenges annually.

Tests are grouped into categories of specialties and subspecialties with respective analytes monitored (termed regulated analyte) in each group. Subspecialty groups with selected analyte in each group are shown in Table 7.

Total PT success is passing four of the five specimens for each analyte in that category with ≥8% successful performance in all of the three consecutive challenges. Performance was considered unacceptable (unsuccessful) when there are two or more successive failures in five specimens of an analyte or in two of the three successive challenges with an <80% overall success rate in the category. This is considered an indication of significant quality

TABLE 7 Tests for which proficiency testing is required.

Analyte	
ALT, AST, alkaline phosphatase, amylase, LDH	Urea nitrogen, creatinine, uric acid
Albumin, total protein	Iron, total
Bilirubin, total	Cortisol
Blood gases (pH, pCO_2, pO_2)	FT4, T3 uptake, T3, TSH, T4
Calcium, total	HCG
Sodium, potassium, chloride, magnesium	Blood alcohol
Cholesterol. Total, HDL-cholesterol, triglycerides	Blood lead
Creatine kinase	Carbamazepine, digoxin, ethosuximide, gentamicin, lithium
Glucose	Phenobarbital, phenytoin, primidone, procainamide and metabolite, quinidine, theophylline, tobramycin, valproic acid

Modified from CLIA approved proficiency testing programs. https://www.cms.gov/regulations-and-guidance/legislation/clia/downloads/ptlist.pdf. Accessed 8 March 2023. Tests for which proficiency testing is required. https://www.cms.gov/Regulations-and-Guidance/Legislation/CLIA/Downloads/List-of-Non-waived-Testing-Which-PT-Is-Required.pdf. Accessed 8 March 2023.

failure, and the laboratory is suspended from further testing in the affected specialty until it is reinstated following provision and assessment of corrective measures.

If the laboratory decides to voluntary stop testing for the analyte in question until corrective measures are implemented, the laboratory needs to inform CMS and the local CLIA office of their cessation to test that analyte prior to receiving a notification from CMS. If subsequent PT tests were acceptable, Medicare and Medicaid payments may not be impacted.

Remedial action includes determining the cause for the error, determining and implementing processes to eliminate them, and documenting the investigation, corrections, and outcomes. Corrective measures and documentation include review of patients' results and review of internal quality control performance at the time of PT analysis. Patient samples may not be available for rerun; however, performance of internal quality control at the time, instruments calibration, and maintenance records are reviewed as well as clinical correlation of results reported around the time of PT failure. Clinical correlations include assessment of serial laboratory results, if available, in concordance with other laboratory findings and clinical parameters. Documentation for corrective measures for patient results are also recorded. This may include notification to patient clinical care team (test requester), request

for repeat sample collection and analysis, and determination of extent of variance and whether it is of clinical significance and its contribution, if any, to patient harm.

Limitations of proficiency tests is that feedback on the laboratory assay performance is often obtained several weeks later when patient results have already been reported. This is in contrast to internal quality control results that are immediately available and provide the basis for timely assay acceptability.

Other options for blind assessment of assay performance include split sample analysis with another laboratory. Samples are split, often at a minimum of every 6 months, and results obtained are assessed for acceptance using defined criteria, often criteria published by CLIA is applied. Another form of proficiency testing is retrospective clinical correlation, where patient medical records are reviewed. Examples are tests that do not have proficiency testing or no comparator methodology available, so that a split sample may be sent is not viable. An example in clinical chemistry is the foam stability test of amniotic fluid in the assessment of fetal lung maturity. Retrospect review of the patient health records and delivery and baby outcomes for respiratory distress provides a clinical retrospective review of the performance of the test. Examples of interpretation and acceptance criteria for external quality control tests (proficiency testing) as defined by CLIA are shown in Table 8.

TABLE 8 Proficiency testing samples acceptance limits.

Analyte	Acceptance limits
AL, AST, alkaline phosphatase	TV ±15%
Albumin	TV ±8%
Bilirubin, total	TV ±20%
CA 125	20%
CEA	15%
Cortisol	20%
E2	30% or 1 ng/mL (whichever is greater)
FT4	15% or 0.3 ng/dL (whichever is greater)
HCG	18% or qualitative positive/negative
PTH	30%
Prolactin	20%
Testosterone	30% (20 ng/dL)
TSH	20% (2 mIU/L)
B12	25%

Those are regulated analytes for Clinical Chemistry. The target value (TV) (may also represent the mean derived using a minimum of 10 participants).
Modified from: https://www.westgard.com/2019-clia-changes.htm. Accessed 19 March 2021.

They vary depending on the analyte and the methodology. They range from ±10% to ±30% of the target value.

Calibration and verification assessment

Laboratory assays require frequent calibration to maintain accuracy and optimum performance. Some assays are calibrated on a weekly, biweekly, monthly, or longer interval as determined and recommend by the manufacturer. However, it is common that more frequent calibration intervals may be required. The need for calibration is judged by the performance of the quality control material as well as of a calibration verification material.

A constant bias, as well as proportional bias (decreasing or increasing), indicates calibration error and recalibration is often required. Improper sample handling, reconstitution, mixing, or storage results in proportional bias. Control samples and calibration verification samples outside the range may indicate sample handling errors such as sample degradation, pollution, reconstitution, mixing, and/or inappropriate sample storage. Results outside the range at the low or high end often indicate either sample degradation or dilution error.

Individualized quality control plan (IQCP)

We have learned that the minimum requirement for quality control should be two levels a day for internal QC and two challenges a year for proficiency testing. Although those are accrediting agencies' minimum requirements, and that the manufacturer may recommend less or more frequent quality control performance, those practices may be adequate to achieve CLIA compliance. However, depending on the laboratory testing cycle and individual laboratory process, additional quality control activities may be needed. An individualized quality control process can be tailored to the laboratory particular environment. To implement an individualized quality control plan (IQCP), all potential sources of error at the preanalytical, analytical, and postanalytical phases of the testing cycle are assessed. Once those are identified, appropriate quality control practices may be identified and established.

One major component of IQCP is to assess the chances of an error occurring. In other words, does the testing process include a step that could reduce or easily identify the error? If so, establish a process to minimize the likelihood of the error occurring.

There are three parts of a IQCP; they are (1) risk assessment, (2) developing a quality control plan, and (3) quality assessment of the three phases of the testing cycle.

Risk assessment identifies potential problems that can lead to errors in the testing system at all three phases of the testing cycle. Components that must be assessed are specimen, test system, reagents, environment, and testing personnel; other components may also be identified and must be included as the cycle is assessed.

Areas for risk assessment include, but are not limited to, accreditation agencies requirement; local and federal regulation; manufacturer kit inserts and instructions, with particular attention to the intended use of the assay, i.e., screening and or diagnosis; sample limitations and handling requirements; quality control frequency; interfering substances; instrument operator manual and troubleshooting guide; manufacturer technical bulletins and alerts; assays validation and performance verification outcomes; quality control and proficiency testing results; scientific literature; and testing personnel qualifications credentials and competency assessment records. Examples of potential sources of errors that could be identified during the risk assessment exercise are shown in Table 9.

It is the responsibility of the laboratory director to ensure that all aspects of the testing cycle are properly assessed for potential errors and that quality control processes are in place to capture and remedy errors. It is clear that most of

TABLE 9 The three steps and respective examples of risk assessment components to be considered when developing an individualized quality control program (IQCP).[5]

IQCP steps	Scope	Examples
Risk assessment	Evaluate potential failures and sources of errors	Specimen, test system, reagent, environment, testing personnel
Quality control plan	Written procedures of operations must ensure accuracy and reliability of test results and that they are relevant to patient care	Internal controls (including electronic), proficiency testing (external control), calibration, maintenance, training and competency of operators.
Quality assessment	Metrics of performance: All three phases of the testing cycle (preanalytical, analytical, and postanalytical)	Frequent reviews of quality control and proficiency testing results, chart reviews, specimen rejection logs, turnround time assessment, and complaint reports

IQCP-CMS. https://www.cms.gov/Regulations-and-Guidance/Legislation/CLIA/Downloads/IQCP-Workbook.pdf. Accessed 24 February 2022.

the data that is analyzed are data that already being gathered by the laboratory as part of a quality control assessment, instrument maintenance, proficiency testing participation, and staffing competency, among other routine examine processes, albeit they may be in isolation, such as patients' results reviews, specimen rejection records, turnaround time reports, critical values notification records, communication records, corrective actions record, compliant and incidents reports, etc.

Once a risk is identified, measures to reduce or eliminate it must be identified, controlled, and monitored regularly. There are no particular format or limits on what monitors to record and their numbers. It is at the discretion of the laboratory director to ensure that adequate monitors and reviews are in place and that an approach to assess risk and minimize errors, as deemed logical and plausible, is established and is in place. It must include the type, frequency, and criteria for acceptance of quality control measures. Although the number of quality control processes may be less than that required by an accrediting agency or CLIA, it must not be less stringent than the manufacturer's instructions for quality control testing. This is often encountered with point-of-care testing where the manufacturer may recommend a frequency of quality control and calibration that is less stringent than that required by CLIA. An IQCP should be developed for each testing system.

Sample acceptance criteria

It is obvious that the quality of the result depends on the quality of the sample. Sample quality indicators in clinical chemistry commonly include degree of sample hemolysis, icterus, and lipemia, in addition to sample volume, collection procedure (e.g., via intravenous line or direct stick for blood), sample transit time, and storage and handling conditions, among others.

The laboratory is responsible for providing guidance on sample acceptance and rejection criteria. Guidance includes information on the tube type, the tube additives acceptable, the volume of sample needed, the collection conditions as well as the transportation conditions, and that of patient preparation. Those instructions are likely to be available in electronic, online, or in paper handbook format. The laboratory is also required to perform periodic review of the sample requirements and update the handbooks accordingly.

Sample requirements and type of the assay characteristics and requirements as well as validation studies performed by the clinical laboratory are defined by the manufacturer. Guidance includes information on samples deemed precious, that is irreproducible, and deviation from criteria might be approved by the medical director. Precious samples include cerebrospinal fluid, knee joint fluid, pleural effusion, samples from premature neonates, timed samples, and samples that were collected premortem.

Common interferences in clinical biochemistry tests are those due to hemolysis, icterus, and/or lipemia (HIL). Quantitative assessment using multiple spectrophotometric measurement by automated analyzers, of sample hemolysis (H) (free hemoglobin), icterus (I) (bilirubin), and lipemia (L) (turbidity) are commonly known as HIL or serum indices.

Hemolysis index, icterus index, and lipemia index are often assessed by automated chemistry analyzers by recording absorbances of the sample aliquot diluted in saline (0.9% sodium chloride) and recording hemolysis at 570 nm (primary wavelength) and 600 nm (secondary wavelength), icterus at 480 nm (primary wavelength) and 505 nm (secondary wavelength), and lipemia at 660 nm (primary wavelength) and 700 nm (secondary wavelength).

Analyte-specific data on HIL interference levels are provided by manufacturers. However, few laboratories have validated the HIL levels for sample rejection, often extending the limits of acceptability (Table 10).

Sample hemolysis is a common preanalytical error affecting biochemistry results. Falsely elevated parameters such as potassium, AST, magnesium, phosphate, and LDH present at much higher concentrations compared to those in circulation. Additionally, free hemoglobin may interfere in a number of assays, such as colorimetric assays, with absorbance between 320 nm and 450 nm, and between 540 nm and 580 nm where oxygenated and deoxygenated hemoglobin absorbs, respectively. Example analytes are iron, lipase, albumin, and γGT. Additionally, free hemoglobin interferes with fluorescence-based assays. Released adenyl cyclase participates in the creatine kinase reaction and causes a falsely elevated result.[6] Sample collection techniques and sample handling are frequent contributors to in vitro hemolysis contributing up to 7% of potassium measurement rejections.

High bilirubin level, termed icterus due to the color of the sample, may also interfere in the measurement of analytes such as creatinine. Bilirubin absorbs between 400 and 540 nm of the creatinine in the Jaffe alkaline picrate method where reaction is measured at 500 nm. In addition to spectrophotometric interferences, bilirubin reacts with hydrogen peroxide due to its antioxidant properties that interferes with the measurements of urate, cholesterol, and triglycerides, as well as enzymatic creatinine assays. The extent and direction of interference varies between conjugated and unconjugated bilirubin, for example, unconjugated bilirubin causes a positive interference in some triglyceride assays, whereas conjugated bilirubin causes a negative interference.

The third component of the HIL indices assesses sample turbidity due to the presence of high lipoprotein particles. Those cause light scattering and thus interferes in assays that rely on light scattering such as turbidimetric and nephelometric-based assays. Lipemia causes scattering within the visual spectrum wavelength of 300–700 nm.

TABLE 10 Examples of hemolysis, icterus, and lipemia (HIL) serum indices in use by the author's laboratory.

Analyte	Hemolysis (H)	Icterus (I)	Lipemia (L)
Alpha-fetoprotein, PSA	2200	65	1500
Albumin	1000	60	1500
Alkaline phosphatase	200	60	2000
ALT	170	60	150
Ammonia	200	10	50
Amylase	500	60	1500
AST	100	60	150
Bilirubin, direct	30	N/A	100
Bilirubin, total	800	N/A	1000
BUN, calcium, CRP, glucose, LDL-cholesterol	1000	60	1000
C3 complement, chloride, IgA, IgG, IgM, lipase, sodium	1000	60	2000
CEA	2200	66	1500
Cholesterol	700	16	2000
Creatine kinase	200	60	1000
CO_2	600	60	1800
Cortisol	500	25	1500
Creatinine	800	15	2000
Ferritin	500	65	3300
Folate	100	29	1500
Free T3	1000	66	2000
Free T4	1000	41	2000
FSH	1000	64	1900
GGT	200	50	1500
Haptoglobin	10	60	200
hCG	1000	24	1400
HDL-cholesterol	1200	60	2000
Iron	200	60	1500
Lactate	1000	28	1500
Lactate dehydrogenase	15	60	900
LH	1000	66	1900
Magnesium	800	60	2000
NT-proBNP	1000	25	1500
Phosphorus	300	40	1250
Potassium	90	60	2000
Prealbumin	1000	60	100
Progesterone	1000	54	200
Prolactin	1500	30	1500

Continued

TABLE 10 Examples of hemolysis, icterus, and lipemia (HIL) serum indices in use by the author's laboratory—cont'd

Analyte	Hemolysis (H)	Icterus (I)	Lipemia (L)
Protein, total	500	20	2000
PTH	250	65	1500
Rheumatoid factor	300	40	2000
Testosterone	600	30	1000
Transferrin	1000	60	500
Triglycerides	700	10	N/A
Troponin T	100	25	1500
TSH	1000	41	1500
UIBC	40	60	300
Uric acid	1000	40	1500
Vitamin B-12	100	65	1500
25-OH vitamin D	600	66	300

Modified from the test manufacturer information.

Assays utilizing the NAD(P)H reactions are also subject to interference as its reaction is monitored at 340 nm. Interference can also be due to differential partitioning of analytes into the aqueous polar and nonpolar phases of the sample and to direct interactions with assay reagents. Partitioning is responsible for the observed pseudohyponatremia where sodium remains in the aqueous phase of the sample. If the sample is diluted prior to measurement, and the assumption is made for the aqueous partitioning, the assumption is not valid for lipemic samples and a falsely low result is reported. Potassium and chloride are similarly affected. Lipemia secondary to high fat diet and/or dyslipidemias contribute up to 7.4% of sample rejection.

A number of samples are commercially available to test serum indices. They can be used to assess the automated system operation for checking patient sample integrity via HIL measurements.

Method verification and validation (assessment of method error)

Method verification and validation shows that you comply with an accreditation requirement by providing a document that you can show at inspection, or to assess the total errors a method (total errors in the lab result) has that may or may not affect clinical decision and thus its utility.

Thus, method validation, in essence, determines the total errors of a method as performed in the clinical laboratory. Additionally, it determines whether the number of errors affects the interpretation of a result and thus influences patient care. Therefore, the assessment needs to take into context the clinical significance of the degree of error of the methodology. In other words, the degree of error must be smaller than the change in result imparting a change in interpretation or initiation of a clinical action. Understanding the clinical need and reasoning for the testing is thus important. Total errors includes random and systematic errors, with contributors to errors being accuracy (trueness) and reproducibility (imprecision).

The other characteristics of the assay such as detection limit, linearity, and reportable range do not contribute to total error. Trueness (accuracy) is assessed by determining bias from the expected target value. Target value includes comparison methods, samples with assigned values, reference material, those defined by reference methodologies, and those traceable to such material.

The extent of required validation depends on the complexity of the assay as defined by CLIA. Nonwaived test requires verification of manufacturers' claims for reportable range, precision, accuracy, and reference intervals. Laboratory-developed tests require verification of the detection limit (analytical sensitivity), analytical specificity (interference recovery), as well as extensive reference range studies.

Steps of method validation

The extent of method validation is dictated by the complexity of the methodology as well as its FDA approval and clearance status. Validation documents are kept for as long as the method is in use. A list of required samples and acceptance criteria (values) for each step of the method verifications steps is shown in Tables 8 and 11.

TABLE 11 Minimum and preferred number of test samples associated with a particular activity.

Activity (indication)	Sample numbers (minimum)	Frequency/findings
Quality control: Mean, standard deviation, and imprecision	20	Over a 2-week period (10 working days). Preferably 4 weeks (20 working days)
Method comparison	40	In parallel/subsequent
Reference intervals verification	20	Considered verified if no more than two outliers
Reference intervals estimation	40 (preferable 60)	Considered verified if no more than two outliers
Reference intervals derivation	120	Required when no published reference intervals available
Analytical reportable range	4 (preferably 5)	Using different levels of concentration spanning the analytical reportable range of the assay

Samples with known values may be used to verify accuracy, imprecision and measurements, and reportable ranges.
Modified from the author's laboratory and from CLSI document: EP28-A3c. *Defining, Establishing, and Verifying Reference Intervals in the Clinical Laboratory; Approved Guideline*. 3rd ed. 2010. CLSI document: EP09c. *Measurement Procedure Comparison and Bias Estimation Using Patient Samples*. 3rd ed. 2018. CLSI document: EP09-A3. *Measurement Procedure Comparison and Bias Estimation Using Patient Samples; Approved Guideline*. 3rd ed. 2013. From Linnet K. Necessary sample size for method comparison studies based on regression analysis. *Clin Chem.* 1999;45(6 Pt 1):882–894. PMID: 10351998.

Waived tests

Test that are FDA/CLIA waived have no testing requirement for method validation except that the operator is able and deemed competent to follow the manufacturer's instructions when performing the test.

FDA-approved assays

Experiments to verify the performance specifications as described by the manufacturer are required for FDA-cleared or approved tests. They include assessment for:

(a) Accuracy
Accuracy is the assessment of bias or the closeness of an obtained value to that of the true assigned value. The difference (bias) could be either negative or positive to that expected (assigned reference material) when calculated. It may be

constant along the entire measurement range, or it may be proportional (concentration dependent). The bias is often presented as an absolute value or as a percentage. The latter may exaggerate the bias when the values are low.

More often than not, the new methodology to be verified replaces a method that is either in existence in-house or being performed by the reference laboratory. In this case, accuracy of bias is determined via method comparison studies. It is preferred to use a minimum number of 20 different patient specimens (or 40 samples) with values spanning the measurement range and/or representative of points of relevant clinical decision points. It is also preferred that this is performed over several days to minimize systemic errors. A minimum of 5 days is recommended, although some laboratories may prefer to standardize the process using 20 days similar to the precision studies. Bland-Altman plot is used to visually express the degree of bias between the new method under verification and comparator methods (in current use) (Fig. 5).

Methods comparison is another way of assessing accuracy. Correlation and comparison studies are required when introducing a new methodology or when establishing the correlation of the in-house method with a comparator reference methodology. Plotting values obtained by both the comparator and the reference method identifies a number of assay characteristics. The slope of the line indicates the bias (systematic error) between the two methods; it can be either positive or negative and can either be constant or proportional (Fig. 6). Additionally, the range of data above and below the correlation line determines the intercept (line of best fit) and describes the inherent random error (imprecision).

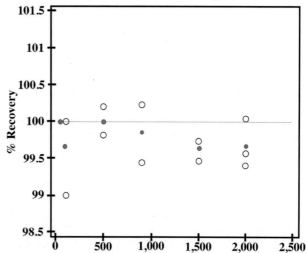

FIG. 5 Bland-Altman difference blot showing assigned (target) concentration and percentage recovery (deviation) from expected values. The plot shows data obtained using 6 points. *(Courtesy of the author's laboratory (Osmolality).)*

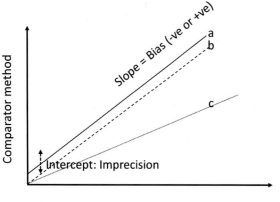

FIG. 6 Method correlation (comparison). Method (a) shows positive bias compared to the ideal response to the comparator method (b, ideal response). The positive bias in (a) is constant across the measurement range and shows a concentration-related proportional bias in (c). *(Modified from Westgard JO. Basic Method Validation and Verification. 3rd ed. Training in Statistical Quality Control for Medical Laboratories; 2008. ISBN1-886958-33-5. ISBN13: 978-1-886958-33-3.)*

(b) Imprecision (variability):

The reproducibility of the result is a reflection of the method's imprecision. This is clinically relevant since the majority of clinical laboratory testing is for trending purposes involving repeated measurements for monitoring progression of disease and/or response to therapy. This must be verified at critical clinical decision points.

Imprecision is a measure of the random error of the test system, and it has to be assessed over a long period of time to account for all possible and relevant testing variables. Typically, this is achieved by obtaining test results on 20 samples over a period of time to account for all of the experimental variables. The coefficient of variation (CV%) or imprecision is calculated by deriving the mean and the standard deviation (SD) and is expressed as a percentage ((SD/Mean) × 100). It is thus clear that imprecision is concentration-dependent (the mean of the 20 replicates). This is done at several concentrations spanning the analytical measurement range. A precision profile is thus obtained (Fig. 7).

(c) Reportable range:

The range of values, for example, from low to high that the test system can report both accurately and reliably (precisely) is known as the reportable range. It is also known as the analytical measurement range (AMR). When sample pretreatment such as dilution is performed, the AMR range is extended and is then known as the clinically reportable range (CRR). An example would be diluting a sample for the measurement of a tumor marker, the concentration of which falls far beyond the limit AMR of the assay, in other words, when sample pretreatment is applied to extend the AMR.

A minimum of four samples (preferably five or more) of known concentrations spanning the range are required. Three or four replicated measurements are often performed for each level. Commercially available sample type material with nonconcentrations, standards, dilutions of patients' specimens, or spiked specimens may be used to verify the measurement range.

When preparing serial dilutions to span the measurement range, it is important to maintain the sample matrix as close as possible to the test sample type. For example, if the test sample is serum or plasma, the diluent may be solutions of bovine or serum albumin or even serum/plasma samples containing low or negligible levels of the analyte to be measured. This is often essential for tests where changes

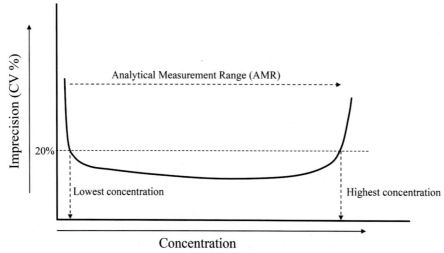

FIG. 7 Precision profile showing CV% as a concentration-dependent variable. Acceptable imprecision is often within 5% or 10% depending on the clinical needs. It is preferably at half of that of the biological variability of the analyte. The latter is obtained from the literature and published sources. *(Courtesy of the author's laboratory.)*

in matrix affect the performance of the assays. However, for some chemistry tests, distilled deionized water or saline may be used as a diluent.

Reportable range verification is very similar to calibration verification experiments, the difference being that, for calibration verification, each of the samples used must have assigned values, for example, commercially available calibrators used as patient samples, control samples with assigned values, proficiency testing samples of known values, and even patient samples with known values, whereas reportable range samples may include those but may also use serially diluted samples where only the starting high concentration is known and the serial samples have derived/calculated values.

Calibration verification

The process of verifying the calibration of the testing system is similar to that of measurement range verification. A minimum of three samples with concentrations spanning the measurement range are required and preferably at or close to clinical decision levels. They should include a low value, a midpoint value, and a high value. The verification of the calibration is repeated every 6 months at a minimum and every time there is a change of reagent lot numbers, major preventative maintenance, or replacement of what is considered a critical part of the test system such as measuring cells and washing stations of an automated analyzer, or more frequently when the performance of the control material indicates a systematic shift (bias).

Carryover studies

Although not specifically stated, the degree to which an automated pipetting and analytical system exibits carryover must be assessed. This is where a prior sample containing high concentration of an analyte results in contamination of the subsequent sample due to inefficient between-samples probe-washing. Samples (patient samples, calibrators, control material, commercial linearity material, e.g., CAP LNR) containing high and low analyte concentrations (four identical high (H) and four identical low (L)) are run in a particular sequence, for example, (HHHLLLHHLLHHLL). The percentage carryover is calculated using the formula:

$$Carryover\,(\%) = \frac{L1 - (L3 + L4)/2}{(L3 + L4)/2}$$

$$\times 100 \left(\begin{array}{l} \text{expressed as a percentage;} \\ \text{a carryover of not more than 2\%} \\ \text{is often considered acceptable} \end{array} \right)$$

Non-FDA-approved assays and laboratory-developed tests

For laboratory developed tests and for those that are non-FDA approved, in addition to the previous parameters, the following performance characteristics must be verified:

(1) Analytical sensitivity

Three terminologies are often used when analytical sensitivity is discussed: limit of blank, limit of detection, and limit of quantification. Some of these are used interchangeably, and some overlap is shown in Fig. 8.

Limit of blank is a theoretical and calculated parameter where the mean of analytical signal obtained (absorbance units, florescence, etc.) for a blank sample (i.e., 0 concentration), estimated as 95% one-side confidence limit, 1.65 times the standard deviation (LoB = Mean (signal) + 1.65 SD of the blank).

Limit of detection is the lowest amount of the analyte that can be detected. It is estimated as the 95% confidence interval to one side of the distribution, plus 1.65 times the standard deviation of the blank, plus 1.65 times the standard deviation of a low concentration of the sample (LoD = LoB + 1.65 SD of a spiked sample).

Limit of quantification is the lowest amount that can be reliably calculated. It takes into account the acceptable precision performance of the assay (Fig. 8).

(2) Analytical specificity to the test as well as impact of interfering substances

The specificity of the assay to the analyte and evaluation of possible interferences are needed. This could be done via spiking and recovery experiments of the possible interferents.

Common interferents are those of homolysis, icterus, and lipemia, which is interference from free hemoglobin when the sample is hemolyzed, interference from bilirubin,

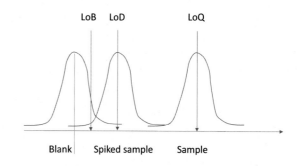

FIG. 8 The concepts of limits of blank (LoB), limits of detection (LoD), and limits of quantification (LoQ). *(Modified from NCCLS publication EP17-A2. Protocols for Determination of Limits of Detection and Limits of Quantitation; Approved Guideline. From Armbruster DA, Pry T. Limit of blank, limit of detection and limit of quantitation. Clin Biochem Rev. 2008;29(suppl 1):S49–S52. PMID: 18852857; PMCID: PMC2556583.)*

and interference from high triglycerides levels, respectively. These are also commonly known as serum indices (see earlier).

Possible interference substances must also be assessed, for example, assessing the effect of common drugs likely to be encountered when measuring a particular analyte; antitumor drugs for tumor marker assays; or interference by other vitamins (used in supplements) when validating a vitamin D assay for the degree of interference by metabolites such as 3-epimer. It is worth noting that metabolites may not be commercially available, and often the parent drug/compound is the only available alternative. Acceptable limits for interference are variable depending on the clinical need for the assay but often do not exceed 20%. An assay with low specificity (high degree of cross-reactivity) may be clinically favorable such as those for drug screening where the detection of drug group spectrum including metabolites and synthetic derivatives may be preferred.

(3) Reference intervals

Reference intervals provided by the assay manufacturer or in the literature may be transferred, adopted (verified), or established. This process is discussed in detail in "Reference intervals" section.

(4) Minimum and preferred number of test samples associated with a particular activity

The recommended minimum and preferred number of test samples associated with a particular validation activity are shown in Table 11. Although a larger number of samples is often desirable, those are usually difficult to obtain.

Emergency use authorization (EUA)

Following declaration of the health emergency status during the COVID-19 pandemic, the FDA allowed EUA approval of tests for its diagnosis. The categories allowed under the emergency provisions are (1) for diagnosis, i.e., PCR and (2) for confirmation of prior exposure to COVID-19, i.e., serology testing to identify current or past exposure but not for confirmation of presence of adaptive immunity. The application for EUA requires the following validation elements: (1) description of the test principles and steps, (2) the control material, and (3) interpretation of test results. Test performance evaluation must include assessment of analytical sensitivity and cross-reactivity (specificity) ($\geq$75 samples negative for COVID-19, i.e., from the US population prior to December 2019, before the first case of COVID-19 was recorded), which is the population with highest prevalence for infection or vaccination against flu, HCV, HBV, other corona viruses, HIV, positive for ANA, with the acceptance criteria being for specificity being >95%. A small number ($n=5$) of individuals from each of the previous patient populations may be acceptable. PCR data for COVID-19 is considered the reference for clinical correlation of the test results. Matrix equivalency, when

different sample types are to be used, is not available when collected in concordance. The positive presence of matrix effect is assessed by spiking the candidate alternate sample matrices with analyte at different concentrations to assess both the limit detection and analyte concentration of clinical relevance; 95% concordance with original sample type indicates matrix equivalency.

Acceptance criteria must be defined for all parameters tested. If the developed test under consideration offers advantages over existing tests, e.g., use of whole blood sample obtained by fingerstick, the performance claims must be assessed, i.e., 30 negative and 30 positive whole blood samples obtained by fingerstick must be included in the validation studies.

The FDA's EUA policy remains in effect as long as the public health emergency declared by the Secretary Of State For Health And Human Services (declared January 20, 2020, effective January 27, 2020) remains in effect, including any renewals made by HHS Secretary in accordance with the relevant part of the Public Health Service Act. It is worth noting that public comments for all the guidance documents was not sought; it was decided that prior public participation is not feasible or appropriate, and the guidance document was implemented immediately but remains subject to comments in accordance with the FDA's Good Guidance practice.

Reflex and reflective testing

Reflex testing

The clinical laboratory may automatically offer and perform additional testing to the initial request, a process known as reflex testing, on selected tests to improve the diagnostic value of the original test request. Once an assigned test result is exceeded the sample is subjected to additional testing as per agreed protocol, for example, a request for thyroid stimulating hormones (TSH), if within normal reference intervals (0.45–4.5 mIU/L for most laboratories), no additional testing is performed. However, if the TSH result is outside those reference interval limits, the sample is automatically forwarded for free thyroxine (FT4) measurement. A finding of elevated FT4 in the setting of low TSH indicates hyperthyroidism, and a fining of a low FT4 in the setting of an elevated TSH suggests hypothyroidism. Additionally, the finding of a normal FT4 in the setting of suppressed TSH may indicate nonthyroidal illness, similarly for a high TSH where it may suggest need for therapeutic dosage regimen review in a patient on thyroxine replacement therapy. This reflex action provides additional laboratory values that are of clinical value on a sample that is already in the laboratory without the need for additional laboratory samples, thus eliminating the need for additional phlebotomy and clinical visits before a final result is achieved. The measurement of only TSH in the initial phase is due to the inherent sensitivity of TSH in the detection of thyroid dysfunction, evident by the log-liner relationship between TSH and thyroid hormones.

The reflex test menu may contain few or many tests and are often specific for the clinical laboratory and clinical services provided. It is often developed in collaboration with clinical services that the laboratory supports, is reviewed periodically, and is approved by the medical executive committee of the institution. This is required to avoid inappropriate testing, self-referral, and possible fraud. Charging/billing for a reflex test performed without a provider's specific order can result in charges of false claims (billing fraud). The test ordering system must indicate that the test requested includes automatic reflexing to other tests such as TSH, serum protein electrophoresis, or drugs of abuse screening tests that are followed up with reflexing to confirmatory testing and species identification on liquid chromatography-mass spectrometry.

An example of the list in use by the author's laboratories is shown in Table 12. It is important to note that the list is not often foolproof. The selection of the primary index test or tests is important as levels not exceeding trigger values may provide a false sense of assurance. For example, TSH and

FT4 are ideal combined tests to avoid missing *sec*ondary hypothyroidism. The prevalence of the respective disorders must be considered.

Another example is that of reflexing serum protein electrophoresis to immunofixation (IFE) on the finding of suspected pattern abnormalities. Performing IFE on every sample is not practical due to the low incidence of abnormality as well as to the complexity and expense of IFE.

Similarly, for LCMSMS confirmation of drugs of abuse, a screening methodology provides a rapid answer (often at point-of-care in the clinic) for management. Unexpected findings are reflexed to laborious and time-consuming confirmatory testing.

Reflective testing

Reflective testing is a concept that is increasingly being used. It is when additional test(s) is added to an original request after reflection on the original result, taking into consideration other findings. They will often include interpretive commentaries and may or may not involve communication with the requester of the original test. They could be described as a case-finding scenario. An example would

TABLE 12 Examples of clinical chemistry reflex test protocols in use by the author's laboratory.

Original test	Reflexed test	Criteria for reflection
Total bilirubin	Direct bilirubin	For all patients >1 month of age if total bilirubin is 1.3 mg/dL then direct bilirubin will be performed. Direct bilirubin required for interpretation of all total bilirubin results 1.3 mg/dL to help distinguish between the need for surgical versus medical interventions.
Lipid panel (total cholesterol, HDL-cholesterol, LDL- cholesterol (calculated), triglycerides)	Direct (measured) LDL-cholesterol	The LDL calculation formula is not valid when negative results are obtained or when Triglycerides are >400 and <2000 mg/dL. Therefore, LDL must be directly measured. When Triglycerides are >2000, no LDL (calculated or direct) can be reported.
Opiate screen, urine	Opiate drug confirmation	If the result is positive (≥ to the cutoff of 300 ng/mL) and the order is from an outpatient location, a confirmatory Opiate LCMSMS will be performed. Morphine, codeine, hydromorphone, oxycodone, hydrocodone, 6-acetylmorphine, oxymorphone, noroxycodone, noroxymorphone, and norhydrocodone can be identified.
Protein electrophoresis (blood/urine)	Immunofixation-electrophoresis (serum/urine) and/or immunotyping (serum/urine)	Immunofixation electrophoresis (IFE) or immunotyping may be performed if any monoclonal component or irregular peak is present. IFE or immunotyping may be done to classify the M protein with respect to heavy and light chain type (e.g., IgG, Lambda, etc.). This is necessary for accurate diagnosis and patient management.
TSH (reflex)	Free T4 and/or free T3	If TSH value is abnormal based upon the age specific reference range, Free T4 will be performed. If free T4 is 0.8–1.8 ng/dL and the TSH <0.4 µIU/mL, free T3 will be performed. Free T4 will be performed to rule out hypo/hyperthyroidism. Free T3 will be done to rule out T3 thyrotoxicosis.

be adding PSA to an isolated alkaline phosphatase finding in a male patient or adding IgM and antimitochondrial antibodies when suspecting primary biliary cirrhosis.

Critical values

Laboratory test results may sometimes be at such variance that it indicates imminent risk to the patient and requires immediate intervention. There is no way for the laboratory to know if the patient care team is aware and/or expecting such a critical test value; it thus incumbent on the laboratory, as we are the first to identify and become aware of the test value, to notify the patient care team of the findings in a timely manner that facilitates immediate intervention and management.

Candidate tests as well as their values/findings are selected by the laboratory in collaboration with the clinical team and makes up what is often termed a Critical Values List.[7] It is understood that the laboratory cannot be a substitute for physician alertness on test results; however, the clinical laboratory is central to patient care. Similar to

the reflex testing protocol, it is good practice to have the list periodically reviewed and approved by the medical executive board.

The list has to be guarded as tests not meeting the definition of a critical values test may creep onto the list. This is often easy to do, since the laboratory would have a vehicle for identification of critical values test results and their notification, and such vehicle may prove convenient to address other issues due to operational difficulties or convenience, for example, notifying a pregnancy test result to an outpatient clinic afterhours. Although this may provide improved patient care team satisfaction, it is likely to take away resources from timely notification of a critical potassium result to the emergency department or in an unsuspecting inpatient unit. Examples from the author's laboratory are shown in Table 13.

Requirement for critical values notification carries the same weight as that of patient management litigation. Therefore, appropriate action and documentation of those actions according to approved policy is an essential component of patient management and safety.

TABLE 13 Examples of critical values in use by the author's laboratory.

Test	Low	High	Unit
Acetaminophen		>150	µg/mL
Ammonia		>110	µmol/L
Bilirubin, cord blood		>4.0	mg/dL
Bilirubin, total (neonate <30 days)		>14.0	mg/dL
Blood culture	Positive		–
Calcium, total	<6.0	>14.0	mg/dL
Calcium, total (neonate <30 days)	<7.0	>12.0	mg/dL
Calcium, ionized	<3.1	>6.3	mg/dL
Calcium, ionized (neonate <30 days)	<4.0	>6.0	mg/dL
Carbamazepine		>20.0	µg/mL
CO_2	<12		mmol/L
Digoxin		>2.5	ng/mL
Ethylene glycol		Detected (≥10 mg/dL)	mg/dL
Fibrinogen	<100		mg/dL
Glucose	<50	>500	mg/dL
Glucose (neonate <30 days)	<40	>300	mg/dL
Gram stain	Positive finding on normally sterile sites, e.g., CSF, synovial fluid, pleural fluid, surgically-collected tissue from normally sterile organs (brain, liver, heart, etc.)		

TABLE 13 Examples of critical values in use by the author's laboratory—cont'd

Hematocrit	<15	>60.0	%
Hematocrit (neonate <30 days)	<30	>70.0	%
Hemoglobin	<5.0	>20.0	g/dL
Hemoglobin (neonate <30 days)	<10.0	>23.0	g/dL
INR		>5.0	–
Iron		>500	mg/dL
Isopropanol		≥10	mg/dL
Lactate		>3.4	mmol/L
Lithium		>2.0	mmol/L
Magnesium	<1.2	>8.4	mg/dL
Methanol		Detected (≥10)	mg/dL
Methotrexate	All values ≥0.05 are called Critical Values and are time postdose-dependent 24 h postdose >5.00 48 h postdose >0.50 72 h postdose >0.05 Any time posttreatment: >20.0		µmol/L
Osmolality, serum	<250	>315	mOsmoL/L
pCO_2, arterial	<20	>70	mmHg
pH, arterial	<7.20	>7.59	–
pH, cord blood arterial and venous	<7.00		–
pH, cord blood arterial	<7.00		–
pO_2, arterial	<40		mmHg
Phenobarbital		>60.0	µg/mL
Phenytoin		>30.0	µg/mL
Phosphorus	<1.0		mg/dL
Platelet count	<20	>1000	×10⁹/L
Potassium	<2.9	>6.0	mmol/L
PTT		>100.0	seconds
Salicylate		>30	mg/dL
Sodium	<120	>160	mmol/L
Theophylline		>20.0	µg/mL
Troponin T—first instance		≥0.01	ng/mL
Valproic acid		>200.0	µg/mL
WBC	<0.50	>50.00	×10⁹/L
WBC, neutrophil absolute (first instance)	<0.50		×10⁹/L

Reference intervals

Test results are reported with appropriate reference intervals for normality to aid with identifying abnormality and with interpretation. Reference intervals may be adapted from published literature, including those provided by the assay manufacturers or previously established intervals.

The concept of reference intervals was realized in the late 1960s and explained in the landmark book by Galen and Gambino *Beyond Normality* in 1975. Years later, the concept was adopted by the International Federation For Clinical Chemistry, which defined a reference range serving as basis for a more-or-less intuitive assessment of biological information given by an observed value.

Although the concept of normality can be a subject of debate, for instance, is it the absence of sign of disease specifically related to the analyte? The term "normal" is discouraged as it assumes most suited for survival, follows a Gaussian distribution, is most representative of a class, and is statistically proven. Furthermore, the term "normal" implies that everything outside the range is abnormal. The interval encompasses 95% of the population, leaving 5% outside the range. This also implies that the probability of a result being outside the reference interval is governed by $1-0.95^n$, where n is the number of analytes. That is, for a group of 20 analytes in one sample ($1-0.95^{20}$), there is a 64% probability of being outside the range. Distribution of reference intervals is rarely clear-cut; it often overlaps those values seen in the patient population (Fig. 9).

In addition to its value in assessing the value of a laboratory analyte, it became a regulatory requirement for inclusion into a laboratory test report. The reference intervals, in addition to depending on the analytical method used, may also have gender and/or age stratification.

The laboratory may establish or verify reference ranges and periodically review their appropriateness to the patient population being tested. Therefore, changes in analytical methodology and patient population characteristics require re-evaluation of the reference intervals.

Validation of available reference intervals requires minimum testing, often at least 40 samples (Fig. 10). The intervals are considered verified if 95% of the data were within the intervals. However, establishing reference intervals is a more involved process and requires a much larger number of participants, often at least 120 subjects.

Reference intervals can be either verified or established. For both options, samples from normal volunteers are required. Normal volunteers should ideally be those representing the patient (reference) population. However, it is often derived from laboratory personnel, students, and staff volunteers. Volunteers complete a health questionnaire that defines inclusion and exclusion criteria. Information gathered include demographics (age, gender), recent or current illness, medications, and supplements intake. Samples are often collected in the morning with fasting status and information on the sample type and size (volume, tubes additives). Sample transportation and handling is standardized and controlled, and an analytical system must be in control and verified by quality control and system stability. Samples are analyzed in the same manner as patient samples. Results are collected and tabulated for statistical analysis.

The number of required samples in general should exceed 100/lower percentile limit required, that is, for a 95% percentile, the minimum number required is 40 to establish a reference interval. Clinical and Laboratory Standards Institute (CLSI) recommend 120 samples since confidence intervals improve as the number tested increases and imprecision decreases.

Parametric (for normally distributed analytes) and nonparametric (logarithmic transformation) statistical analysis is performed. Data is examined statistically for normality in preparation for analysis.

Reference intervals may exhibit stratification due to gender, age, or ethnicity. This requires separate reference

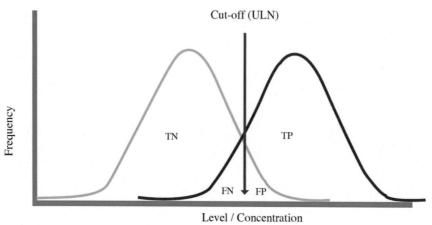

FIG. 9   Distribution of test values in normal *(green)* and disease *(red)* populations. There is often an overlap that leads to false positive (FP) and false negative (FN) results.

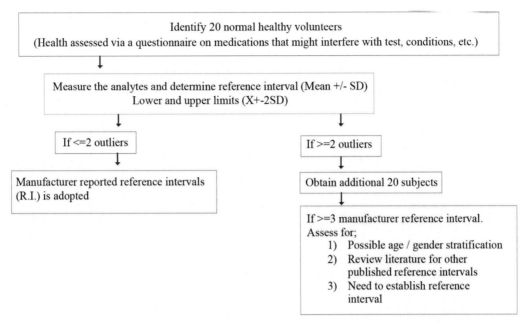

FIG. 10 Reference ranges verification schematic diagram. *R.I.*, reference intervals. *(Courtesy of the author's laboratory.)*

intervals for each of the different groups if the difference falls between respective subclasses distribution means >25% of that calculated from the combined distribution.

Transference of reference intervals

Alternative methods requiring either a smaller number of volunteers and samples collection, or no samples collection nor volunteers may also be applied. They involve transferring reference intervals, either from published literature or using those supplied by the assay manufacturer. This approach requires a small number of samples from normal volunteers. For example, 20 normal volunteers representing the reference population, samples are collected and analytes measured. For the published reference limits to be adopted, ≤2 of the measured values may fall outside the candidate reference interval.

Reference ranges may be estimated using 60 samples, this option may be used with fewer numbers but not less than 40. The mean and SD of the tested population and the published population are compared for agreement.

A calculation from comparative method is used to adjust or correct the reported reference interval on the basis of observed methodological bias. This approach is helpful when the reference intervals are previously established by the laboratory, and that a new methodology or analyzer is in use and reference intervals need to be verified. The formula $Y(lower) = a + bX$ (lower) and $Y(higher) = -a + bX(higher)$ can be used to derive the new reference intervals where "a" is the intercept and "b" is the slope of the correlation line. Typically, six or seven data points are used to calculate the line of correlation. This approach is sometimes used when bringing testing in-house from a reference laboratory. It can

only be performed once as frequent transferability may include and increase inherent errors.

Existing patients data can be used to establish reference intervals where there are thousands to millions of patients laboratory records already available in the laboratory database (electronic health system). Although it is inexpensive and relatively rapid, there are certain requirements and assumptions applied. First, the database must contain adequate clinical information; second, it is based on the assumption that the majority of laboratory results are normal; and third, statistical exclusion of outliers' "unhealthy" subjects are conducted using the frequency distribution. Limitations of this approach include; skewed distribution of the data (usually fail), little and no control over preanalytical variables (i.e., patient preparation), data may not be traceable to the testing methodology (historic data), the reference population is not defined beforehand, and that there is limited information about the subject. In this approach, reference intervals among patients (in-patients/out-patients) are established irrespective of health status.

Calculations include discarding top and bottom 10%–20% of data, extrapolating the central linear portion of the curve, and determining the 2.5th and 97.5th percentile for the data.

This approach is frequently used for pediatric and neonatal populations where collection of normal volunteers is not plausible. This approach is called Hoffman's approach. Example of reference intervals obtained by the author's laboratory using the Hoffman's approach for plasma sodium levels are shown in Fig. 11.

A less-popular and a last-resort method is a judgment decision by the medical director. The original data and protocols used to establish the reference intervals are required.

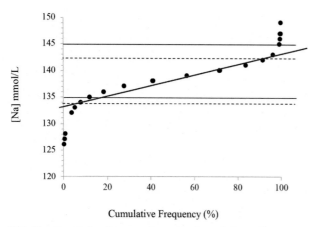

FIG. 11 Cumulative frequency for patients' population sodium ranges. *(Developed by the author.)*

The medical director would review and use their judgment as to the appropriateness of the ranges to be adopted. This approach only requires the medical directors' approval and signature.

The characteristics and differences between reference intervals and decision limits are shown in Table 14. Decision limits are determined using receiver operating characteristic (ROC) analysis as shown in Fig. 12.

Critical difference (relative change value) determination

Relative change value, also known as the critical difference, is a change in laboratory values that exceed that due to combined analytical and biological variability. When combining

TABLE 14 Characteristics and differences between reference intervals and decision limits determination.

	Reference intervals	Decision limits
Conditions influencing values	Type of population Age group Gender	Clinical question Patient category
Information gathered	Being or not being part of the reference population	Patient eligible for certain procedure
Data number	Two: Lower and upper limits	One or more according to the likelihood of clinical situation or different clinical questions
Statistics	95% central range of distribution	Receiver operating characteristic (ROC) curves and predictive values

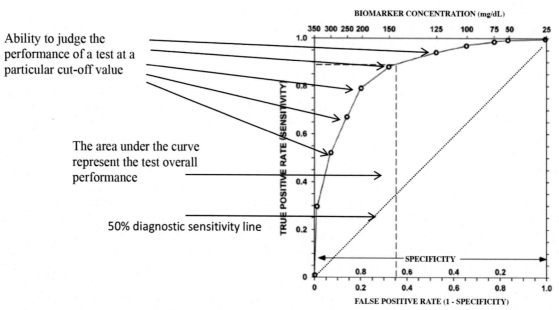

FIG. 12 ROC curve illustrating the process of construction of a receiver operating characteristic (ROC) curve. *Dashed vertical line* indicates 90% diagnostic sensitivity at about 40% false positive rate (60% specificity). *(Modified from Kampfrath T, Levinson SS. Brief critical review: statistical assessment of biomarker performance. Clin Chim Acta. 2013;419:102–107. ISSN 0009-8981.)*

variabilities, the square root of the combined squared analytical and biological variabilities is applied.

$$RCV = 2^{1/2} \times Z \times \sqrt{\left(CV_a^2 + CV_i^2\right)}$$

Where Z is the probability factor and equals 1.96 and 2.58 for probability factors of 95% and 99%, respectively.

Data for analytical variability is obtained from the clinical laboratory where the test is performed. As a rule of thumb, an acceptable analytical variability is <0.5 of the biological variability. Biological variabilities for the analyte of interest are obtained from the published literature. Examples of analytical and biological variabilities and relative change values in use by the author's laboratory are shown in Tables 15 and 16.

The concept of delta checks and its application

The concept of a delta check is widely practiced in clinical laboratories. It is the change in results in successive samples beyond that due to analytical and biological variability over a specific period of time. The value change in successive samples may be presented as absolute change, a percentage change, or as a rate change. The latter can also be presented as a percentage rate change as shown in Table 17.

The initial utility of delta check is to identify mismatched and mislabeled samples. However, the prevalence of sample label mismatch is variable and not often known. It ranges from <1.0% up to 6.3%. The sensitivity, specificity, and thus predictive value for utility of delta checks in identifying sample mismatch remains unknown. Furthermore, it is complicated by possible sample contamination with intravenous lines and therapeutics, as well as changing patient

TABLE 15 Examples of analytical and biological variabilities and relative change values in health and in disease in use by the author's laboratory.

Analyte	CV$_a$ (%)	CV$_i$ (%)
CA 125 antigen	6.2	24.7
CA 19.9 antigen	4.0	15.95
Carcinoembryonic antigen (CEA)	3.2	12.7
Cholesterol	1.5	5.95
Cortisol	3.8	15.2
Creatinine	2.8	6.4
Ferritin	3.6	14.2
Follicle stimulating hormone (FSH)	2.8	11.0
Iron	6.6	26.5
Parathyroid hormone (PTH)	6.5	25.9
Prolactin	5.8	23.0
Prostatic specific antigen (PSA)	4.5	18.1
Triglyceride	5.0	19.9
Thyroid stimulating hormone (TSH)	4.8	19.3

Analyte	CV$_i$ (%) healthy	CV$_i$ (%) disease	Disease
CA 19.9	15.95	24.5	Resected ovarian neoplasm
Calcium	1.9	1.3	Chronic renal failure
CEA	12.7	9.8	Radically resected breast cancer
Cholesterol	6.0	4.7	Mild hypercholesterolemia
Creatine kinase	23	43	Impaired renal function
Creatinine	6.4	2.5	Chronic renal failure

CV_a, analytical variability; CV_i, biological variability within an individual.
Modified from Desirable biological variation database specification. https://www.westgard.com/biodatabase1.htm. Accessed 8 March 2023.

TABLE 16 Calculated relative change values (critical differences) for selected analytes.

Analyte	Calculated relative change value (RCV) (critical difference)
Prolactin	55%
Follicle stimulating hormone	137%
Luteinizing hormone	76%
Thyrotrophin stimulating hormone	53%
Free thyroxine	82%
Testosterone	158%
Estradiol	47%
Cortisol	25%

A change in serial levels need to exceed the test respective percentage to indicate significant difference.

condition. A simulated sample mix-up study was performed where the prevalence was known, such that delta checks had low positive predictive value and high negative predictive value. This suggest that, in instances where the likelihood of sample mix up is very low—for example, following implementation of strict positive patient identification, sample labeling practices, and use of barcode labels as well as barcode reader technologies—the use of delta check offers very little value in detecting sample mismatches where the false positive rate is high. With a sensitivity of 82.8% and specificity of 99.4%, the changes in predictive value with simulated prevalence of specimen mix up is shown in Table 18.

Delta check values for analytes of interest are derived from either laboratory experience following retrospective review of data, literature review, or by calculating the relative change value, also known as the critical difference.

The time frame for change varies from hours for acute settings (e.g., glucose in emergency department and hospital setting), days and weeks for an outpatient clinic setting, and months (e.g., bilirubin and glycated hemoglobin,

TABLE 17 Examples of delta checks in use by the author's laboratory (a: numeric responses, b: alpha responses).

(a)

Test	Delta check	Time (min)	Absolute/% value
Na	%	360	15%
K	%	360	15%
Calcium, total	Absolute	360	1 mg/dL
Creatinine	Absolute	1440	0.4 mg/dL
Protein, total	%	1440	25%
Albumin	Absolute	1440	1 g/dL
Cortisol	%	2880	100%
Digoxin	%	1440	100%
Ferritin	%	2880	100%
FT4	%	10,080	50%
TSH	%	10,080	50%
Troponin T	%	2880	100%
hCG	%	2880	150%
Mean corpuscular volume (MCV)	Absolute	4320	4 fL
Hemoglobin	Absolute	360	4 g/dL

(b)

Test	Delta check	Time
Antinuclear antibody (ANA)	Alpha response	8 weeks
Hepatitis B core, total antibody	Alpha response	8 weeks
Hepatitis B surface antibody	Alpha response	8 weeks
Serum protein electrophoresis (SPEP) monoclonal component	Alpha response	8 weeks

TABLE 18 Relationship between prevalence and impact on predictive value (positive predictive value [PPV] and negative predictive value [NPP]).

Rate of specimen mix up (misidentification)	PPV	NPV
1% (1 in 100)	58.2%	99.8%
0.1% (1:1000)	12.1%	100%
0.01% (1:10,000)	1.4%	100%
0.001% (1:100,000)	0.1%	100%
0.0001% (1:1,000,000)	0%	100%

Modified from Ovens K, Naugler C. How useful are delta checks in the 21 century? A stochastic-dynamic model of specimen mix-up and detection. *J Pathol Inform.* 2012;3:5. https://doi.org/10.4103/2153-3539.93402. Epub 2012 Feb 29. PMID: 22439125; PMCID: PMC3307229.

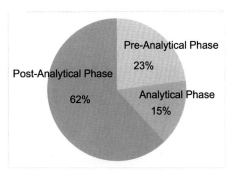

FIG. 13 The three phases of testing cycles and associated percentage of errors. The errors at the preanalytical phase range from incorrect patient identification, use of wrong tube additives, and incomplete tube filling; the analytical phase errors include unrecognized failed quality control, random errors and biases; whereas postanalytical errors include missed turnaround time targets, missed critical values notification, and incorrect reports and report entries such as reference intervals and interpretive comments, among others. (*Modified from Carraro P, Plebani M. Errors in a stat laboratory: types and frequencies 10 years later. Clin Chem. 2007;53(7):1338–1342. PMID 17525103.*)

respectively) or annually in cases of screening and monitoring (e.g., PSA, TSH). Examples of delta checks in use by the author's laboratory are shown in Table 17.

Mismatch can be reduced by implementing lean projects, staff training, positive patient identification, use of patient and specimen barcode labels, automated sample processing, and strict adherence to standardized sample collection and labeling practices. Minimizing analytical and biological variabilities are essential for delta check use, i.e., instrument maintenance, calibration, and use; standardized sample collection protocols (i.e., time of sample collection, patient prandial status, time of sample collection in relation to therapeutic drugs administration, etc.)

Errors within the different phases of the testing cycle

Errors occur at all phases of the testing cycle. However, their contribution to the total laboratory is varied. Most of the errors occur during the preanalytical phase followed by the postanalytical phase, whereas the analytical phase has a minimum number of errors (Fig. 13). This is probably due to implementation of quality measures and automation. Although a minimum number of errors occur at the analytical phase, they have the highest impact on patient outcomes. It is therefore important that errors at all phases of the testing cycle be identified and their reduction and elimination is sought.

Root cause analysis

These are tools to investigate patients' safety incidents. It is a requirement by various patient safety and accreditation agencies. Harmful events must undergo a thorough root cause analysis to determine why the event occurred and how similar events can be prevented from occurring in the future. Lessons learned and systems or cognitive

deficiencies addressed. It is important to note that failures are not linear, and they are often a consequence of more than one cause.

Fishbone diagram

A fishbone diagram is a structured approach for the investigation of complex problems such as diagnostic errors. It provides a systematic approach involving a cause-and-effect diagram to determine a root cause. It helps determine the major causes that might affect the outcomes but is not necessarily the end cause of the problem; it identifies root causes and generates ideas for potential solutions. Cause-and-effect diagrams are also known as fishbone diagrams because of their shape.

The horizontal arrow extending from left to right points toward the problem's potential causes that should be identified and grouped into major categories above and below the horizontal arrow. Common categories include equipment, personnel, materials, and environment. Offshoots corresponding to the identified category are causes or symptoms of that category. An example of a fishbone diagram is shown in Fig. 14.

Financial aspects

Budgetary elements

There are three separate budgets developed during the budgeting cycle:

(1) Operating budget, which is prepared at the level of the cost center, often by the area manager with consultation with the medical director on future developments and projections. The operational budget is comprised, in turn, of three different budgetary components: (a) statistical

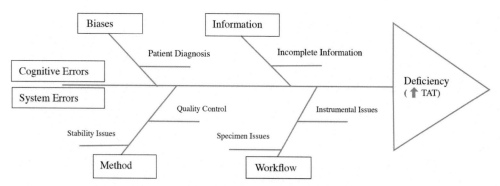

FIG. 14 Fishbone diagram showing categories and associated items leading to the error and interventions and possible remedies. Increased test result turnaround time (TAT) is an example of a deficiency under investigation. *(Modified from Harmening DM. Laboratory Management: Principles and Processes. 2nd ed. D.H. Publishing and Consulting, Inc.; 2007. ISBN:13: 978-0-9036-1599-1.)*

(volume) budget, which is a forecast for the activity of the unit; (b) revenue budget, which is the gross charges forecasted based on the projected volume; and (c) expense budget, which is projected expenditure and resources required to perform the projected volumes.

(2) Capital budget, which is prepared at the organizational level and is based on operational budgets and requests received from the departments within the organization. The capital budget is thus centrally arranged for priorities, needs, organizational goals, and available funds. The budget includes equipment needs for the upcoming year, property renew and or replacement costs, as well as needs by the physical plant.

(3) Cash budget, which is prepared by the organization's finance dept and is the most critical of all three budgets. This budget predicts cash flow in and out of the organization and calculates cash availability. Cash reserve must be managed carefully (timing of cash discernment, any borrowing or investment activities) to remain solvent and thus stay in business.

Competitor SWOT analysis

The marketplace and competition from other laboratories and organizations is a dynamic process that requires continuous assessment to remain successful. One way of assessing your laboratory position and predict the competitor's behavior is to perform an inward assessment of your laboratory's areas of strength, weakness, opportunities, and threats, known as SWOT analysis. Although the strategy and capabilities of the competitor's laboratory may limit your laboratory's ability and opportunities for growth in some areas, internal SWOT assessment may identify areas for growth.

Information about the cost of a test is essential for several decision-making processes such as whether the test is performed in-house or referred to a reference laboratory, profit loss and operating cost accounting, management and test utilization studies, and research studies costing.

It is also important because reimbursements are assigned by governmental agencies and by payers; furthermore, changes to the test fee schedule continues to occur, either capped or decreased, which will impact laboratory revenue and thus the cost-effectiveness to continue to perform the test. Knowing the cost is required when submitting a new test proposal.

However, it is difficult to determine cost with a high degree of specificity (what you really need is to capture major components) due to numerous factors being direct or indirect contributors to the cost. It is also good practice to examine the final figure for appropriateness. Once the cost and associated factors are known, they can be used to modify contributing factors to manage cost and preferably targets for cost reduction. Additionally, changes in staffing structure and workflow processes such as automation of manual steps or changes in methodology require redetermination of the test's cost.

As a medical director, some of your duties in accounting terms are considered nonproductive. Activities such as management meetings and conference attendance are activities not directly involved in test result production.

The cost of any test does not remain static; it is influenced by test volume, that is, the more tests we do, the lower the total cost and, usually, it does not require additional equipment or staffing. Factors contributing to the total cost of a test can be divided in general into two components, direct and indirect.

Direct components are those directly associated with performing the test in question, i.e., test reagents, calibrators, and quality control (labor involved in the testing and instrument depreciation, maintenance, and repairs), in addition to a portion of indirect costs, which include general laboratory supplies, labor cost associated with supervision, administration, informatics, accreditation, and other laboratory and hospital overheads.

Indirect costs are items that are required regardless of the test volume, even if the tests are performed or not. Examples are general laboratory supplies, labor costs associated with administration, training as well as hospital overhead, infrastructure utilities and buildings, administrative components of the laboratory such as accreditation and related activities, supplies and ordering, among other support activities. Nontesting and management staff expenses, office supplies, central receiving, and general and administrative support also fall under indirect costs.

Indirect costs also include the laboratory portion of hospital costs. Examples are patient services, patient registration and phlebotomy, human resources, management and finances, building utilities, and support services. Those are difficult to assess, and some laboratories add a 10% to the test cost toward those hospital activities. Additionally, the impact of the reimbursement rate must be considered as it will impact revenue regardless of test cost and volume. Some laboratories may assess a percentage to account for reimbursement rates which could be as high as 50%.

Share in the indirect expenses being fixed or variable could be assessed by determining the percentage of the test's volume out of all testing in the laboratory, i.e., the indirect cost both within the clinical laboratory and the associated hospital support services.

An example of cost associated with say pain management testing is when using both screening and confirmatory testing on LCMSMS, which is complex labor-intensive testing with significant lag time (development time) before revenue is generated. An example of costing analysis would be assessing correction factors (multipliers) and accounting for technical nonbillable components. Let's look at a $114 Medicare confirmatory pain management test. The cost to lab is $25.40. Now, allowing for 38% reimbursement rate and 10% hospital

indirect cost, this would be $45.26, which is an example of cost of introduction of a complexed new manual technology with significant lag time in development (laboratory developed test [LDT]) before results can be reported. Thus, revenue is generated as shown in Tables 22–25. An example of a relatively simple to introduce automated test such as procalcitonin is utility of an already existing equipment. For some assays, significant lead time is needed to reach a break even point.

Both direct and indirect costs will have associated fixed and variable components. Fixed costs are those present regardless of the test volume, whereas components are those changing with test volume, an example being point-of-care testing where, regardless of test volume, the instrument and associated peripherals are fixed, whereas the test cartridges used are variable depending on test volume. The cost of the instrument is often relatively cheap, whereas the cost of the variable number of cartridges is often relatively expensive compared with their laboratory-based counterparts. Therefore, the cost of the test in this case will vary with the test's volume. In this case, the more tests are performed, the higher the cost to the laboratory. Exceptions are batched tests such as in ELISA-based assays where batching and full use of a plate allows for the use of one set of calibrators and quality control material, which would otherwise be required for each run regardless of the number of tests or those subject to contractual arrangements where increased test volume attracts lower reagent costs.

Thus, the total cost of the test is the sum of direct costs and a proportion of indirect costs associated with the test, as well as fixed costs and those that are variable and a function of test volume (Fig. 15).

Fixed and Variable Cost

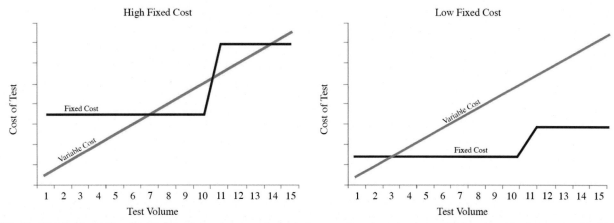

FIG. 15   Fixed and variable costs: Impact of changing test volume on the cost of test in environment of high and low fixed costs. *(Modified from Broughton PMG, Hogan TC. A new approach to the costing of clinical laboratory tests. Ann Clin Biochem. 1981;18(6):330–342. https://doi. org/10.1177/000456328101800603. Tarbit IF. Laboratory costing system based on number and type of test: its association with the Welcan workload measurement system. J Clin Pathol. 1990;43(2):92–97. https://doi.org/10.1136/jcp.43.2.92. PMID: 2318999; PMCID: PMC502286. Ma I, Lau CK, Ramdas Z, Jackson R, Naugler C. Estimated costs of 51 commonly ordered laboratory tests in Canada. Clin Biochem. 2019;65:58–60. https://doi.org/10.1016/j. clinbiochem.2018.12.013. Epub 2019 Jan 5. PMID: 30615855.)*

When considering the cost of a test, the focus is often on the analytical component of the testing cycle. Significant contributors to cost are present at both the pre- and postanalytical phases of the testing cycle, from sample collection and preparation, to generation of a report and notification of critical values. At the extreme end, a phlebotomy service may be provided for a test that is sent to another laboratory as required by a payer or by a patient, and the performing laboratory bills directly for the testing component, and the cost of the preanalytical component is not reimbursed. Components associated with cost are shown in Table 20.

Tests utilization initiatives

The clinical laboratory is central to optimal patient care and, in that regard, appropriate utilization of tests and resources is important. That is, the posttest probability for the disorder is significantly improved by performing the test. Several approaches have been tried to improve utilization of laboratory tests. They range from use of testing algorithms, review of sent-out referral tests (often those that are relatively expensive), and use of clinical decision support systems (see section on informatics below). This is preferred as being interactive and at the point of test requisition rather than after the sample was collected and received at the laboratory.

Many clinical laboratories have an established test utilization committee, similar to the formulary committee and pharmacy, that oversees the request for additional new tests, reviews of test utilization, and removal of tests considered obsolete. The committee includes physician representatives from major clinical specialties (high volume users of the laboratory) such as internal medicine, endocrinology, surgery, obstetrics, and emergency department, among others. Nursing representatives and those from support departments (i.e., informatics) are also included.

Central to test utilization initiatives is availability of evidence related to the appropriate test utility and impact on patient outcomes, which are not necessarily available at the time.

It is important to note that, although there will be attempts and ways of reducing laboratory test use, it is appropriate that utilization should be the target, i.e., it might also require the addition of new tests or replacement of current tests for ones that are more accurate or more informative, but may be more expensive. However, the impact of those interventions is on the overall system cost, i.e., avoidance of particular procedures such as diagnostic invasive procedures, changes to therapeutics or interventions, or changes to clinic visits and or reduction in hospital length of stay.

Knowledge of and reporting the cost of the test has been shown to impact test utilization. Some laboratories have elected to provide a range for the cost of the test (e.g., use of dollar signs; e.g., $: <$100, $$: $100–$300, $$$: >$300,

etc.) rather than the actual cost of the test. This approach allows for minor changes to test cost and to labor that is variable such as variability in direct and indirect costs, variability in overhead costs considered proprietary information from the vendor, and variability in service contract, other than operation of your activities such as the frequency of calibration and of quality control use.

Determining the cost of a laboratory test

In addition to operating profit and loss financial reporting, knowledge of the cost of the test is also important when deciding on introducing a new test or referring a test to an outside laboratory.

Two options can be used for determining the cost of a test. First is to estimate the direct and indirect costs, second is to measure and calculate all associated costs: direct, indirect, fixed, and variable. The definition for each item is described in Table 19.

Estimating cost of test (unit of service)

(1) Obtain cost of reagents (from vendor)
(2) Estimate cost of calibration and quality control (usually 10%–30%)
(3) Obtain monthly salary staff expenditure
(4) Obtain monthly test volume
(5) Obtain annual cost of instrument maintenance
(6) Obtain annual general supplies cost
(7) Calculate individual test portion of the previous expenditure
(8) Add to reagent cost
(9) Determine the relative percentage of volume of the test for which the cost is being estimated; for example, if complete "comprehensive" metabolic panel (CMP) represents 50% of the laboratory test volume, the cost of panel may be derived as shown in Table 20.

The advantages of this approach is that it's a fast determination and it considers hidden costs and allows for variation in staff and testing volume. The limitations are it is an approximation (actual equalization of effort and generalization), it is not applicable to laboratory developed tests (often associated with higher staff and equipment cost), it is not applicable to the addition of new instrumentation technology, and it must have limited esoteric (nonroutine) testing.

Measure and calculate all associated costs (direct and indirect, as well as fixed, variable, and semivariable)

This approach, in contrast to the estimate approach, requires identification of steps and gathering all pertinent information. This includes listing all components associ-

TABLE 19 Definitions of terminologies commonly used in cost and financial analysis.

Term	Definition
Operating budget	Personnel, consumables, reagents, instrument maintenance
Capital budget	Instruments (refrigerators, centrifuges, instruments), instruments interface, space, transport equipment. Typically has to be above a particular monitory value >$5000
Unit of service	Determined by dividing total cost (direct and indirect) by the volume of tests. Cost per unit of service allows for inclusion of variable costs
Break even point	Represents the volume of activity required for all fixed cost to be covered. Total Fixed cost divided by (selling price − variable cost)
Direct cost	Components that are directly associated with performing the test. Test reagents (standards, calibrators, quality controls), labor (personnel time), and equipment (cost, service, maintenance)
Indirect cost	Items that are required regardless of test volume/or test performance; share determined by apportioning expenditure and test volume
Fixed cost	Unaffected by test volume (even if the test is not performed)
Variable cost	Change with the specific test volume
Semivariable cost	Varies with test volume but in increments

Modified from Broughton PMG, Hogan TC. A new approach to the costing of clinical laboratory tests. *Ann Clin Biochem*. 1981;18(6):330–342. https://doi.org/10.1177/000456328101800603. Tarbit IF. Laboratory costing system based on number and type of test: its association with the Welcan workload measurement system. *J Clin Pathol*. 1990;43(2):92–97. https://doi.org/10.1136/jcp.43.2.92. PMID: 2318999; PMCID: PMC502286. Ma I, Lau CK, Ramdas Z, Jackson R, Naugler C. Estimated costs of 51 commonly ordered laboratory tests in Canada. *Clin Biochem*. 2019;65:58–60. https://doi.org/10.1016/j.clinbiochem.2018.12.013. Epub 2019 Jan 5. PMID: 30615855.

TABLE 20 Example of cost test (panel in this case) estimation using the generalized estimation approach.

	Monthly expenditure	CMP portion (50% lab volume)	Approx. cost per test
Test volume	5000	2500	
Personnel expenditure	$20,000	$10,000	
Supply expenditure	$8000	$4000	
Total ($)		$16,500	
Equipment purchases in the last 5 years	$150,000/60 = $2500		16,500/2500 = $6.60

An example cost analysis from the author's laboratory. *CMP*, complete "comprehensive" metabolic panel (i.e., sodium, potassium, chloride, bicarbonate, urea, creatinine, glucose, albumin, total protein, calcium, alkaline phosphatase, total bilirubin, ALT and AST).

ated with the test, determining the amount of time (labor) required for all associated activities, determining items contributing directly to the cost of the test, listing items contributing indirectly to the cost of the test, and identifying items that are fixed, variable, or semivariable. The direct and fixed cost items are those components directly associated with performing the test. Variable costs are those that change with test volume, which include reagents and consumables, test reagents, standards and calibrators, and internal quality control material. Fixed costs are the minimum number of staff required regardless of test volume, labor and personnel time associated with the test, and equipment cost and associated services and maintenance cost. Semivariable costs are those that vary

with test volume and include pay increases or reduction of staffing depending on test volume and peak times that include regular and overtime obviously, transportation costs, and need for additional equipment, for example, during excessive workload (Fig. 15).

You will need to determine the indirect costs, which are items not directly related to the production of a test but required for the testing environment and required regardless of test volume and/or test performance. The test share is determined by apportioning expenditure and include general laboratory supplies, labor costs associated with supervision and administration (overhead), building and utilities, regulatory expenses such as proficiency testing safety and support services, and expenditures related to the informatics.

Laboratory portion of hospital costs often levied at about 10% estimate.

Adjusting factors (multipliers) may be added to correct for nonbillable costs such as repeat testing (duplicates, triplicates, etc.), needed dilutions when the test exceeds the AMR of the assays, and proficiency testing. Overhead includes laboratory, hospital, and other support departments, often levied at 10%. Some institutions may factor in collection rates (variable 36%–38%) as well as expected or require profit margin, often at 15%.

The following example shows cost analysis carried out to assist with decision-making on implementing manual assay for Interleukin-6 measurement required during the COVID-19 pandemic. IL6 measurement was considered helpful in identifying patients at risk for cytokines storm.

The options were either to set it up in an ELISA format (automated ELISA processor available in-house and in use for autoimmune testing) or to send the test to a local reference laboratory with relatively longer turnaround time. Analysis for cost of material, reagents, and labor costs are shown in Tables 21–26. Example of activities from the author's laboratory and time spent on each activity and the level of personnel. Those parameters where applied when determining the cost of establishing an in-house LCMSMS-based measurement for antifungal drugs (Tables 22 and 23) and that of an ELISA-based interleukin-6 assay (Tables 24–26). Note the extent and cost of technical personnel activities between the LCMSMS-based antifungal assays and the ELISA-based IL-6 assays.

TABLE 22 Example of time expenditure by technical staff when measuring antifungal drugs by LCMSMS methodology.

Activity	Operator level	Time (min)
Sample retrieval	MLT	0.5
Sample allocating/dilution/internal standard/loading	MLT	3.5
Calibrators allocating/loading	MLT	1.0
Instrument start up and worksheet build	MLT	2
Run test	MLT	4
Integrate AUCs	MLT	5
Review integration and accept results	Supervisor	1.0
Manual entry into Epic	Supervisor	1.5
Total time (min)		18.5

LCMSMS, liquid chromatography-mass spectrometry (tandem); MLT, medical laboratory technologist.

TABLE 21 The various direct and indirect test components and their associated fixed and variable components at three phases of the testing cycle (preanalytical, analytical, and postanalytical).

Testing cycle phase	Activity
Preanalytical phase	Sample collection
	Sample handling and transportation
	Accessioning
	Centrifugation
Analytical phase	Instrument and reagent preparation (calibration, quality control, etc.)
	Testing process
	Calculations, etc.
Postanalytical phase	Reporting
	Interpretation
	Instrument shutdown

TABLE 23 Examples of labor costs for measuring antifungal drugs by LCMSMS.

Testing (hands on time)			
	Minutes	Rate/min	Labor cost/BT
Tech bench cost/BT	5	$0.60	$3.00
Supervisor cost/BT	2.5	$0.70	$1.75
Processing cost/BT	4	$0.30	$1.20
Verification cost/BT	5	$0.60	$3.00
Start up cost/BT	2	$0.60	$1.20
Total			$10.15
Non-BT factor (average specimen per run/average BT per run)			1.08
Labor cost/BT			$10.96

Samples tested in batches. BT, batched testing.

TABLE 24 Determination of materials and disposables cost for the measurement of interleukin-6 by ELISA-based assay.

Materials	Unit cost	Institution charge	# in Each set	Units	Cost/unit	Units/test	Cost/test	Cost/test
IL-6 kit	$236.00	$236.00	96	tests	$2.46	24	$59.00	$ 118.00
Reagent kit	$216.00	$210.00	96	tests	$2.19	24	$52.50	$ 105.00
10 μL tips	$43.65	$26.19	960	tips	$0.03	25	$0.68	$0.68
250 μL tips	$43.65	$26.19	960	tips	$0.03	75	$2.05	$3.71
1000 μL tips	$43.65	$26.19	960	tips	$0.03	5	$0.14	$0.14
96 well trays	$123.00	$125.68	50	trays	$2.51	1	$2.51	$2.51
Aluminum tray covers	$75.00	$75.00	100	covers	$0.75	8	$6.00	$6.00
Molecular grade water	$49.54	$49.54	6000	mL	$0.01	400	$3.30	$3.30
14 mL polystyrene round bottom tube	$125.00	$125.00	100	tube	$1.25	3	$3.75	$3.75
Reservoirs multipipetting	$0.70	$0.70	1	reservoir	$0.70	8	$5.60	$5.60
500 mL polypropylene	$36.00	$36.00	12	bottles	$3.00	1	$3.00	$3.00
125 mL polypropylene	$60.00	$60.00	24	bottles	$2.50	1	$2.50	$2.50
Sheath fluid	$25.00	$25.00	20,000	mL	$0.00	1000	$1.25	$1.25
				Total	$15.45	Regt cost	$142.28	$255.44
						#Test on batch	5	10
						Consumable cost/test	$28.46	$25.54

The cost for the measurement of IL-6 by the referral laboratory was $50 with a turnaround of less than 24 h. The ELISA assay was to be processed in a batch format once a day. It is apparent that referring the sample for IL-6 on what would have been a test on a critical patient was appropriate.

Reference laboratories and referred testing

Tests that are low in volume might not be either practical nor cost effective to perform in-house. They may also require additional instruments or expertise. The laboratory director in consultation with institution medical staff and physicians is responsible for selecting a referral laboratory to which the specimens may be sent. A number of reference commercial laboratories are available. However, when considering a referral laboratory, several aspects must be examined, such as quality of services, turnaround time, accreditation, test methodologies, sample requirement, and cost. Evidence of

performance and quality metrics as well as customer satisfaction reports should be examined, if available, as well as specimen type and collection requirements, availability of courier services and schedules and frequency of sample pick up, provisions of sample collection and packaging material, and mode of communication and reporting of results. The laboratory director should also consider the availability and cost of computer interfaces, scanning and paper reports, report contents, critical values notification, and availability of clinical consultation when needed. The latter is helpful when discussing appropriate tests to be performed and the availability of testing algorithms. Periodic meetings to review performance as well as quality metrics should be held, and reviews should also include reports on exceptions, canceled tests, unsuitable samples, and inability to perform testing. Feedback should be gathered on test utilization and recommendations on alternative testing as well as support in transferring the test in-house when volumes become cost effective and/or when turnaround times cannot meet clinical needs. Referral laboratories may support the main

TABLE 25 Determination of direct and indirect personnel cost for the measurement of interleukin-6 by ELISA-based assay.

Personnel time cost	Unit cost	Institution charge	# in each unit	Units	Cost/unit	Units/test	Cost/test	Cost/test
Test time	$36.00	$50.00	60	min	$0.83	260	$216.67	$216.67
Analysis of Results	$36.00	$50.00	60	min	$0.83	15	$12.50	$12.50
Computer entry	$36.00	$50.00	60	min	$0.83	30	$25.00	$25.00
Total technologist time	$50.00	$50.00	60	min	$0.83	305	$254.17	$254.17
Office personnel	$32.00	$50.00	60	min	$0.83	5	$4.17	$4.17
Computer system personnel	$50.00	$50.00	60	min	$0.83	5	$4.17	$4.17
Supervisor time	$42.00	$75.00	60	min	$1.25	5	$6.25	$6.25
Directors time	$127.00	$127.00	60	min	$2.12	5	$10.58	$10.58
						#Test on batch	5	10
						Subtotal personnel cost	$279.33	$279.33

laboratory during in-house method validation by provision of samples for comparison and validation studies.

Organizational structure

Organizational charts define the relationship between units and individual positions. An institution and/or hospital organizational chart indicates the reporting structure within the larger health and academic system.

The organizational structure models range from static and mechanistic models to an organic network model (Fig. 16). The static model promotes communication from the top-down with strict division of labor and centralized decision-making. The model insists on conformity to policy and procedures. This is in contrast to a network model that promotes decentralized decision-making with wide sharing of responsibilities. The network mode facilitates flexibility and adaptation to the changing environment. Most clinical laboratory models offer a static mechanistic model. It is considered to be a closed system with functional units. It tends to be hierarchical and bureaucratic in nature with a clear understanding of responsibility and authority. It provides a

stable controlled environment with repetitive efficient areas. The model creates areas of silos focused on their areas of responsibility where coordination between areas is often competitive and unresponsive. This model has become even more restrictive through efforts of cost-effectiveness resulting in flattening of the structure and eliminating some of the supervisory and management layers with fewer points in the decision process with top-down control remaining (Fig. 16).

Smaller laboratory units may offer more of a network model. Departments and many clinical laboratories have organizational charts that provide administrative and operational responsibilities and reporting structures at a glance (Fig. 19). The structure is hierarchical and defines how the work is divided depending on size and complexity. They indicate the levels of authority and lines of communication. It could be flat and simple, as in Fig. 17, or large and complex, as in Fig. 19. It is often divided along lines of specialties and subspecialties, also in lines of type of work provided, whether it is technical in nature with a degree of automation; a regulatory and financial administrative component such as billing, safety, and regulatory aspects; or informatics, which

TABLE 26 Determination of equipment and final (total) cost of the measurement of interleukin-6 by ELISA-based assay.

Equipment cost	Unit cost	Institution charge	# in each unit	Units	Cost/unit	Units/test	Cost/test	Cost/test
Computer equipment	$14.47	$14.47	1	per test	$14.47	0	$–	$–
Luminex (5 years)	$35,000.00	$35,000.00	6000	test	$5.83	0	$–	$–
Other equipment	$37.14	$37.14	1	per test	$37.14	0	$–	$–
						Subtotal equipment cost	$–	$–
						#Test on batch	5	10
						Total cost	$421.61	$534.78
						Costs per test	$84.32	$53.48
						Total cost+overhead (1.1158)	$892.05	$1131.48
						Cost per test (with overhead)	$178.41	$113.15
						Charge	$125.00	$125.00

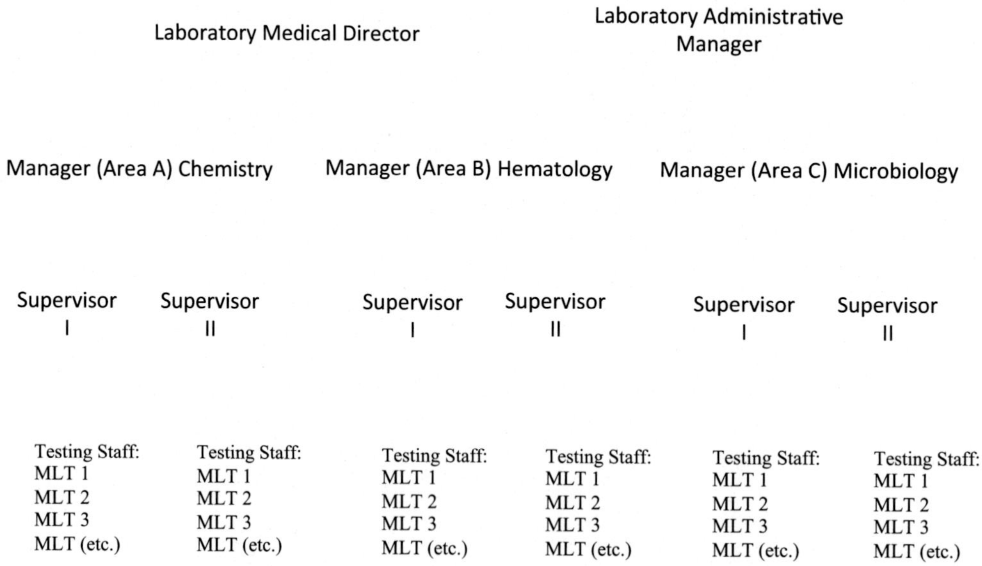

Laboratory Medical Director   Laboratory Administrative Manager

Manager (Area A) Chemistry Manager (Area B) Hematology Manager (Area C) Microbiology

Supervisor I Supervisor II Supervisor I Supervisor II Supervisor I Supervisor II

Testing Staff:	Testing Staff:	Testing Staff:	Testing Staff:	Testing Staff:	Testing Staff:
MLT 1	MLT 1	MLT 1	MLT 1	MLT 1	MLT 1
MLT 2	MLT 2	MLT 2	MLT 2	MLT 2	MLT 2
MLT 3	MLT 3	MLT 3	MLT 3	MLT 3	MLT 3
MLT (etc.)	MLT (etc.)	MLT (etc.)	MLT (etc.)	MLT (etc.)	MLT (etc.)

FIG. 16 Traditional multilayer organizational structure. *(Modified from the author's laboratory and from Harmening DM. Laboratory Management: Principles and Processes. 2nd ed. D.H. Publishing and Consulting, Inc.; 2007. ISBN:13: 978-0-9036-1599-1.)*

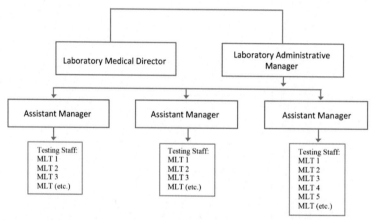

FIG. 17 Flattened design organizational model. *(Modified from the author's laboratory as well as from Harmening DM. Laboratory Management: Principles and Processes. 2nd ed. D.H. Publishing and Consulting, Inc.; 2007. ISBN:13: 978-0-9036-1599-1.)*

often have a separate line of accountabilities that touches every area of the laboratory. It is dynamic in nature in that it is updated and redesigned as changes in the environment or business model surface. This is evident with automation, as instrumentation and automation models evolve; the concept of core laboratory models with total automation results in mergers of clinical chemistry with hematology, coagulation, basic immunology, as well as urinalysis. Those are areas that, over time, evolved into unique areas of subspecialty and evolved into a hierarchy. However, the advances in automation has also led to evolvement of different organizational structure with multispecialty training of technologists, supervisory and management oversight, as well as medical directors' responsibility. The environment and expectations will be different. Its change is driven by goals and the strategy of the institution, technological advancement, as well as size of the laboratory. In addition to those factors, leadership style and patient care needs contribute to changes in structure. Although success depends on the capabilities of the individuals, talented individuals perform well in most structures but excel in well-organized structures (Fig. 18).

Availability of such charts are also required by accrediting agencies. There are different structural organizations within different laboratories, and there are no recommended or favored module as they depend on the organizational history, culture, financial structure, and affiliation, among others.

You can either be the laboratory director, holder of the accreditation license, or the medical director of your subspecialty, clinical chemistry, or point-of care testing. You would often have a dotted line of responsibility and

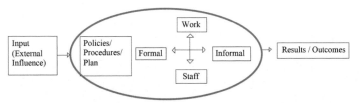

FIG. 18 Congruence model open structure. The four components involved are; tasks being performed, individuals skills required, policies and procedures, and culture and informal rules. *(Modified from Harmening DM. Laboratory Management: Principles and Processes. 2nd ed. D.H. Publishing and Consulting, Inc.; 2007. ISBN:13: 978-0-9036-1599-1.)*

reporting structure to a clinical laboratory staffing structure that is different from your academic institution (your direct employer). Medical technologists report to their respective section supervisor or team leader, and the latter reports to the laboratory manager. In a larger complex system, an assistant manager may be responsible for more than one section and report to a manager who would perform more of the larger administrative duties. The manager of the respective areas of responsibility may report to an administrative director on management and administrative issues and to a medical director on clinical, technical, as well as regulatory aspects.

The two models for open and closed organization systems contrast in their leadership styles where the latter is more collaborative and collegial compared with an independent superior-subordinate basis. The decision-making process is hierarchically determined in the closed system compared with an open system where the decision is made at the level of the problem and where the information resides. Authority and responsibility coexist together in the closed system whereas it is separate with multiple accountabilities. The closed system eliminates or suppresses conflict whereas the open system manages it. Performance

review and appraisal is hierarchal and external compared with self-review in the open system. The power base is hierarchical and within the system compared with control over certainty at the system boundary. Distribution of work is allocated in the closed system whereas it is negotiated among the groups.

The unit structure is often organized around a common cause, i.e., clinical chemistry specialty, location, technology, or customer group. The structure contains all of the relevant skills to operate and are responsible for their own outcomes. Each structure unit is grouped by function around centralized support and management services. Although team approach and good communication maximizes efficiency, there is duplication of work and thus required expertise as in specimen receiving required for each of the specialty units.

Matrix organization

This is an example of a core laboratory set-up. It is a move from the functional unit described previously toward a production core laboratory model (Fig. 19). The model requires interdependency on technical expertise and specialization. It promotes skill diversification and efficiency in sharing

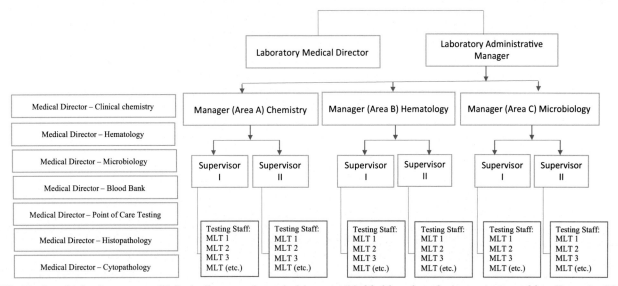

FIG. 19 Organizational structure model. Lacks direct reporting to the laboratory. *(Modified from the author's organization and from Harmening DM. Laboratory Management: Principles and Processes. 2nd ed. D.H. Publishing and Consulting, Inc.; 2007. ISBN:13: 978-0-9036-1599-1.)*

human resources. The drawback is that roles and reporting structures can be confusing as an individual may report to more than one supervisor/leader and may assume different roles. It takes time for the employees to adapt and to understand the structure and their access to resources.

Another model is the network structure model. This facilitates subspecialization and is often organized in frontline basic and specialized units with support backline facilities in a layer format (Fig. 20). Management here acts as a supporting role, and each functional unit has a high degree of autonomy.

It is a model of evolving network organizations as it allows access and distribution of data. Information technology models are customer-focused and information-sharing. Specialized units (internal or external) are linked together by informal or formal agreements. Network organizations have a center *not* a top. The role of management is to coordinate, facilitate, and serve from the customer/patient back and *not* from the top down by combining innovation and responsiveness of small entrepreneurial structures with the economies of scale of large organiza-tions. The frontline serves client needs and makes critical decisions (frontline, i.e., point of care testing [POCT] units, client services). The next layer represents less-urgent batched testing, and backline support includes specialized technical areas offering complex and esoteric tests, also serving as a resource (knowledge base) to the frontline on technical and clinical matters. Central management serves in a support function such as information technology, facilities, and personnel.

The healthcare system network model

This model consolidates testing at a centralized laboratory supporting several patient care facilities with regional laboratories reporting to the central laboratory and sending high complexity level testing (Fig. 21). Those regional units support more than one patient care facility, which consolidates and reduces duplication, expands revenue-generating services, and delivers high-quality, cost-effective results. They can also respond to dynamically changing environments but depends on strong collaborative leadership with radical changes in how we view working relationships and leadership/management roles.

Staff competency assessment

Employers at every field and level usually assess the performance of their employees for promotion and incentives as well as job-related merits. However, CLIA requires assessment of employees for their competency to perform laboratory testing. Competency is defined as the ability to perform correctly and safely and to recognize and solve minor problems without the need for assistance. It is a requirement by accrediting agencies that a competency program be in effect and that competency assessment is documented.

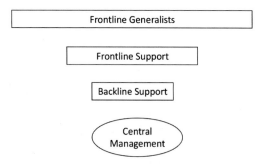

FIG. 20 Network structure model requires multilayers with frontline and support backline staffing. (*Modified from Harmening DM. Laboratory Management: Principles and Processes. 2nd ed. D.H. Publishing and Consulting, Inc.; 2007. ISBN:13: 978-0-9036-1599-1.*)

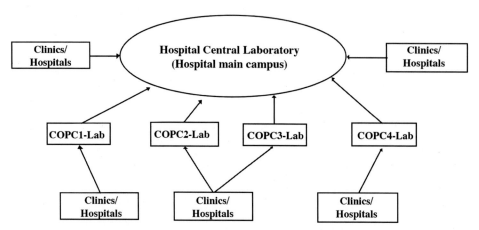

FIG. 21 Health system network model. Facilitates on-campus and remote testing facilities managed centrally (from the author's laboratory). *COPC,* Community Oriented Patient Clinics (*n* = 15) distributed across the Dallas, Texas metroplex. (*Modified from the author's hospital and from Harmening DM. Laboratory Management: Principles and Processes. 2nd ed. D.H. Publishing and Consulting, Inc.; 2007. ISBN:13: 978-0-9036-1599-1.*)

It is required that the technical consultant (moderate complexity laboratory) or a technical supervisor (high complexity laboratory) be responsible for evaluating and documenting competency of employees at least every 6 months during their first year of employment and then annually. The semiannual and annual cycle is repeated if test methodology or instrumentation changes took place. The employee has to be deemed competent before they begin testing patient samples.

Skills for which competency is assessed include sample collection, handling and processing, prior test methods, implementing laboratory standard procedures, instrument maintenance and operation, calibration, quality control, knowledge of test methodology and their limitations, interfering substances, reporting and information system entry, and verification of laboratory results.

Several methods can be used to assess employee competency: direct observation of all technical aspects stated for competency requirement in a blind fashion by testing previously tested samples and results compared for correctness and closeness (allowing for inherent analytical variability); proficiency testing sample analysis where results are known; using case-based studies or direct questions to assess problem-solving ability for instrumentation errors, sample quality issues, and presence of interferences such as lipemia and hemolysis on laboratory result; and ability to identify normal and abnormal results as well as those considered critical values and their notification.

Six elements used for assessment of competency

(1) Direct observation of routine patient test performance (whether its automated or manual chemistry, microscopic analysis, phlebotomy, sample handling, etc.).
(2) Monitor the recording and reporting of test results.
(3) Review intermediate test result worksheets, quality control (QC) records, proficiency testing results, and preventive maintenance records.
(4) Direct observation of performance of instrument maintenance and function checks.
(5) Assessment of previously analyzed specimens, i.e., internal patient samples (blind) or proficiency test (PT) samples (known values following evaluation).
(6) Assessment of problem-solving skills.

All likely performance variations must be included in the competency assessment, and competency assessment follows training and/orientation. The complexity, if waived assessment is performed annually; if nonwaived assessment is performed semiannually then annually. Similarly, qualification of those conducting the competency assessment depends on the complexity of the test to be performed.

If it's moderately complex, a technical consultant level is required, and if it's high complexity testing, a technical supervisor or general supervisor level is required.

This responsibility may be delegated, in writing, to a general supervisor meeting the required qualification for a high complexity testing.

Failing to demonstrate competency in any of the six elements, corrective action must be reviewed and documented as per established policy followed by re-education and training and retaking of the failed element. If the results remain unsatisfactory, the employee must repeat training, undergo a supervisor review, reassignment of duties, or other actions as deemed necessary.

Supervisors and consultants are required to undertake competency assessments; this will be at different levels and highlights what is important to the laboratory, i.e., compliance, communication, quality control review, TAT of reports signature, policy reviews, etc. Other laboratory system-specific facets could include corrected reports and error frequency, maintenance of board certification, participation in quality assurance activities, proficiency testing failure, attendance at faculty meetings, subordinate complaints, etc.

Laboratory informatics

Nearly all clinical laboratories employ a form of informatics from either simple software on a standalone computer to a fully integrated, large electronic information system that is interfaced to laboratory instruments and integrated into the clinical information systems of the hospital or the clinical entity in which the laboratory serves. The systems provide electronic or paper reporting of results, periodic instruments and quality reports, reference intervals, interpretive commentaries, and many other functionalities. The laboratory director and personnel, in collaboration with the informatics team, are responsible for selection and implementation of the appropriate information system that caters to the needs and services requirements, and complies with accreditation and regulatory rules. The laboratory is also responsible for validation and periodic assessment of the system for correctness of transmission of data, calculations, identification and flagging of abnormal and critical results, among many others.

Several interactive functions at the laboratory-clinical areas interface are available and have been utilized in test utilization activities. They include provision of electronic laboratory handbook, providing information of available tests menu (in-house and referrals), sample requirements (blood tube, container types, and any required preservatives), patient preparation (prandial status, time of day, pre- and posttherapeutic dosage), transportation and handling, test methodology, indications for the test, as well as reference intervals and commentaries on test results interpretation.

Clinical decision support systems in the form of best practice alerts (BPAs) are widely used to direct and advise users. For example, BPAs may be established to trigger when a duplicate test is being ordered. In addition to being timely and automated, it facilitates consistency and standardization. It can also be applied to both relatively low-cost tests and can be updated, modified, and changed as utilization changes. It can also be integrated within the health system including clinical information on the patient as well as therapeutics and procedural interventions, for example, the development of certain order sets for a particular indication precluding the use of tests that are not necessary or relevant for that particular procedure.

The laboratory director and clinical chemist participate in the periodic review and approval of how results appear in the electronic healthcare records, review of calculation formulas, associated electronic flags for abnormal, feasibility, and critical values, as well as incorporating interpretive comments.

Emerging roles of the clinical laboratory

Looking into the future of laboratory medicine, it is likely that there will be increased reliance on and expectation of a central role for the clinical laboratory for a patient-centered approach. There will likely be increased utility for point-of-care testing. There will also be increased demand for consultative roles for the clinical laboratory and increased emphasis on appropriate utilization of tests. This will be mainly driven by increased autonomy of nonphysician practitioners with limited training in clinical pathology. There may also be increased utility and dependence on informatics and on some degree of artificial intelligence such as results reporting in a user-friendly format that, at a glance, identifies if the test is within or outside the reference intervals, where the test exceeded relative change values, allowing for easily identify trends in laboratory test results, as shown in Fig. 22.

These futuristic needs and advancements depend on a well-trained clinical chemist and on additional training in informatics and test utilization management.

Summary

- As a clinical chemist and medical director of the laboratory, you are responsible for the day-to-day running of the laboratory, providing clinical consultative services, participating in teaching and in education activities, and possibly conducting research projects.
- The different roles within the clinical laboratory—from clinical consultant to technical supervisor, manager, general supervisor, and testing personnel—are all governed by accrediting agencies with respect to qualifications and required training and competency.
- Accreditation of the laboratory by CLIA-CMS or by agencies with deemed status is required by several payers and local and central governments.
- Based on their characteristics, laboratory tests are classified as either waived, moderated, or high complexity, and this classification in turn directs personnel experience and training reequipments.
- Quality management programs are designed to monitor each aspect of the testing cycle.
- Local and state rules on document and specimen retention supersedes those defined at the federal level.
- Quality and performance indicators are set by the laboratory and are best defined into preanalytical, analytical, and postanalytical phases of the testing cycle. They must be systematic, transparent, consistent, comprehensive, and cover all aspects of the testing cycle. They should focus on areas considered more likely to have an impact and undesired consequences on patient care and outcomes.
- Quality control procedures (internal and external) are essential for assurance of accurate and reproducible laboratory results. The integration and measurement of samples with unknown concentrations termed proficiency testing samples (external quality control samples), and obtained from a proficiency testing program.

Patient	Test	Results	
1234567	Creatinine	0.9	Failed delta
1223344	Creatinine	3.0	Actionable
2223334	Creatinine	0.6	
3344556	Glucose	95	
4455566	Glucose	137	Pre-Diabetic
1245567	Alk Phos	16	Normal Mg
5545678	TSH	4.5	Low FT4

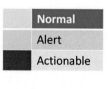

| Normal |
| Alert |
| Actionable |

FIG. 22 Abnormal results such as outside predefined limits, critical, or exceeded relative change values (critical differences) are identified at a glance *(color coded). (Modified from Cadamuro J, Hillarp A, Unger A, et al. Presentation and formatting of laboratory results: a narrative review on behalf of the European Federation of Clinical Chemistry and Laboratory Medicine (EFLM) Working Group "postanalytical phase" (WG-POST). Crit Rev Clin Lab Sci. 2021;58(5):329–353. https://doi.org/10.1080/10408363.2020.1867051. Epub 2021 Feb 4. PMID: 33538219.)*

- Serum indices describe spectrophotometric analysis of hemolysis, icterus, and lipemia for possible interference and testing the specific analyzed levels.
- Critical values are those at variance with health, critical for survival, and that corrective action is available. The laboratory in collaboration with physicians defines both the analytes to be included as well as the limits/values for notification.
- Reference intervals are either established for the population and the methodology in use or obtained from the manufacturer and published literature and verified as appropriate for the patient population.
- Relative change values (also known as critical difference values) represent percentage change in serial laboratory values that exceeds the combined inherent analytical and biological variation for a particular test.
- The laboratory testing cycle comprises three phases (preanalytical, analytical, and postanalytical). Errors occur most frequently in the preanalytical phase when compared to the other phases; however, it is those errors occurring in the analytical phase that often impart clinical significance.
- The cost of a test includes both direct and indirect elements. Direct cost items are essential components of a single test (i.e., reagents). Indirect costs are shared with other testing activities (e.g., facilities cost, etc.). Apportioned contributions by indirect elements must be accounted for.
- Various laboratory organizational models are in use, and they reflect the essentials and characteristics of each laboratory environment, its testing menu, and served population.
- Informatics are integral to clinical laboratory activities, and basic knowledge of data management systems is helpful for the clinical chemist.

- The role of the clinical laboratory continues to evolve into a more clear patient-centered role with direct involvement with patient outcomes assessment and various utilization and risk-reduction activities. The clinical chemist is central to all of those activities and should be prepared to participate at that clinical interface.

References

1. Friedberg RC, Rauch CA. The role of the medical laboratory director. *Clin Lab Med.* 2007;27(4):719–731. v.
2. Code of Federal Regulations. https://www.ecfr.gov/current/title-42/chapter-IV/subchapter-G/part-493/subpart-M. Accessed 24 February 2022.
3. Commission USEEO; 2022. https://www.eeoc.gov/employers/small-business/3-who-protected-employment-discrimination. Accessed 16 March 2022.
4. WESTGARD QC. https://www.westgard.com/mltirule.htm. Accessed 24 February 2022.
5. IQCP-CMS. https://www.cms.gov/Regulations-and-Guidance/Legislation/CLIA/Downloads/IQCP-Workbook.pdf. Accessed 24 February 2022.
6. Farrell CJ, Carter AC. Serum indices: managing assay interference. *Ann Clin Biochem.* 2016;53(Pt 5):527–538. https://doi.org/10.1177/0004563216643557. Epub 2016 May 3. PMID: 27147624.
7. Hashim IA, Cuthbert JA. Establishing, harmonizing and analyzing critical values in a large academic health center. *Clin Chem Lab Med.* 2014;52(8):1129–1135.

Further reading

Harmening DM. Laboratory Management Principles and Processes. D.H. Publishing & Consulting Inc.; 2007.
Ho CKM, Chen C, Setoh JWS, Yap WWT, Hawkins RCW. Optimization of hemolysis, icterus and lipemia interference thresholds for 35 clinical chemistry assays. *Pract Lab Med.* 2021;25:e00232. https://doi.org/10.1016/j.plabm.2021.e00232. PMID: 34095417; PMCID: PMC8145753.

Chapter 17

Analytical methods and special considerations

Introduction

This chapter describes the principles and characteristics of selected methods commonly used in clinical biochemistry laboratories, applicable sample types, precautions required in patient preparation, sample collections, and handling as well as methods limitations.

The chapter is divided into the testing cycle components of the preanalytical phase which includes patient preparation and sample collection, and handling, the analytical phase which describes the methodologies in use, their principle and characteristics, and the postanalytical phase which describes the reporting of test results.

Preanalytical considerations

Patient preparation

Many if not most of the biomarkers are influenced by physiological and environmental factors such as patient prandial status (i.e., fasting, or nonfasting), example tests affected include glucose and triglycerides, patient posture where a change from supine to upright posture causes fluid redistribution and increases the concentrations of many analytes. Several biomarkers, e.g., cortisol, exhibit significant circadian rhythm (e.g., circulating cortisol levels which are high in the morning and significantly lower in the evening). Patients may experience anxiety and stress (white coat syndrome) when attending a clinical environment for blood sample collection and certain biomarkers are influenced by stress (e.g., prolactin).

The above factors are discussed separately below; however, the clinical laboratory has a central role in assisting with patient and clinical staff avoidance of possible patient preparation errors and helping with adherence to recommended protocols by providing clear instructions to both patients and clinical teams on sample requirements and on patients' preparation. Those instructions are available in easy-to-find and follow format with appropriate languages (translations as needed) relevant to the patient population being served.

Prandial status

Although it is common that patients present fasting (overnight) for sample collection, this is not often the case among inpatients. Additionally, samples are collected throughout the day in both outpatient and inpatient settings.

Calorie restriction (fasting) is helpful for selected tests examples being triglycerides and glucose in the assessment of hypertriglyceridemia and hyperglycemia or hypoglycemia respectively. Fasting for those tests is common and not exclusive. For instance, for triglycerides, recent professional societies guidelines state that fasting is not required routinely for assessment of lipid profile and that when initial nonfasting triglycerides >440 mg/dL (5.0 mmol/L), consideration should be given to repeating lipid profile testing in a fasting state. Additionally, it is recommended that the clinical laboratory should flag abnormal results for medical attention, e.g., triglycerides >200 mg/dL (2.2 mmol/L).

Nonfasting glucose values that are slightly elevated require a repeat on a confirmed fasting sample, for markedly elevated glucose level and those returned abnormal on fasting triggers an additional investigation for diabetes mellitus and insulin resistance syndromes, and for familial hypertriglyceridemia, and for nephrotic syndrome, etc.

Depending on the meal content, triglycerides increase by about 78% postmeal, aspartate transaminase by about 25%, total bilirubin by about 16%, and glucose and phosphate by about 15% compared to premeal levels. Minor changes even after a light breakfast (about 560 kcal) are seen in potassium, urate, and albumin; however, those are often less than 5%. It is important to note that water intake is not restricted during fasting and that if the patient is severely dehydrated, blood collection may be difficult.

Posture

A change from a supine to an upright posture increases the concentrations of many analytes by about 5%–15%. Water moves from the intravascular space to the interstitial space when changing from a supine to an upright posture, this is due to the difference between capillary filtration pressure

Tutorials in Clinical Chemistry. https://doi.org/10.1016/B978-0-12-822949-1.00016-4

and oncotic pressure. This results in about 12% reduction in plasma volume. A posture change from upright to supine results in fluid movement in the opposite direction. Changes in the concentration of intravascular proteins (molecules >4 nm in diameter) is observed. Proteins (albumin) as well as protein-bound constituents (e.g., calcium) increase by 5%–150% when changing from supine to upright posture. Prolonged supine position results in increased urinary calcium excretion.

Changes to posture are of such significance that it is of diagnostic utility in the measurement of renin, aldosterone, adrenaline, and noradrenaline in the investigation of postural hypotension.

Exercise (activity)

Changes in lifestyle, from a sedentary life to excessive exercise, result in changes in laboratory parameters such as elevated muscle enzyme (creatine kinase) in strenuous exercise.

Observed changes in biochemical parameters secondary to exercise depend on the degree of exercise, mild brisk to intermediate, to strenuous. Mild exercise exhibits minor changes, whereas strenuous exercise leads to muscle damage with markedly elevated creatine kinase (CK), lactate dehydrogenase, and aspartate transaminase (AST). Changes are also secondary to sweating in strenuous exercise, particularly in the unconditioned individual (see later). Fluid redistribution from extravascular to interstitial fluid, the hypovolemia leads to increased albumin, total protein, and urea. An increase in uric acid is observed secondary to reduced renal clearance due to increased lactate concentration.

In the unconditioned individual, marked CK release is secondary to the hypoxia and oxidative damage, whereas the increased capacity to metabolize glucose and fatty acids and ketones in the conditioned muscles is due to the high muscle mass and increased mitochondria content. In the conditioned patient, mitochondrial CKMB isoform does not exceed 5% compared to the unconditioned where the relative proportion is often more than 8%.

For this marked biological variability, it is advisable that the patient refrains from any exercise for at least 72 h prior to blood sample collection.

Diurnal rhythm (time of day)

Several biomarkers, e.g., cortisol, ACTH, and prolactin, exhibit significant circadian rhythm. It is likely that initial blood test investigation and collection is early in the morning following an overnight fast, cortisol is high in the morning with a nadir in the evening; thus, results reported must be accompanied by appropriate reference intervals. It is worth noting that in the development of pathology, it is the diurnal and the pulsatile release of hormones that is

often the first abnormality; however, it is difficult to identify without serial measurements, which is not often practical and requires patient hospitalization.

Stress

Patients may experience anxiety and stress (white coat syndrome) when attending a clinical environment or for blood sample collection. The trip itself may pose a certain degree of stress. Certain hormone biomarker levels are influenced by stress a common example being prolactin when an initial slightly elevated result is misinterpreted as laboratory technical error when a repeat sample collection (now in a more familiar surrounding to the patient) accompanied by a reduced element of stress returns the repeat analysis within the normal intervals.

Samples collection

Patient identification

This remains a significant element of correct patient identification prior to sample collection. Patient misidentification remains the top item among patient safety advocates (Joint Commission—Patient Safety Goals).

The use of two patient identifiers is mandatory before samples are collected.

Name, date of birth, and medical record number are good examples, whereas room number and bed number are not.

Sample type collection and handling

Samples received in the laboratory range from blood, urine, cerebrospinal fluid, pleural fluid, and joints fluid, among others. Depending on the test requirements, blood samples may be centrifuged and plasma (in the presence of anticoagulants) and serum are separated. Other samples may require centrifugation to remove particles and where for some centrifugation deposits cellular material required for the investigation and testing.

Sample quality is important as the quality of the results depends on the quality of the sample. Blood sample collections are at risk of hemolysis. The use of a large needle bore and direct stick reduces the risk of sample hemolysis.

Blood (plasma/serum)

Blood samples are the main sample type collected and received by the clinical biochemistry laboratory.

The use of a tourniquet prevents blood return and helps with identifying a suitable vein for venipuncture. However, the tourniquet must not be left for more than 2 min. Venous stasis (prolonged tourniquet application) and forearm exercise may increase ionized calcium due to a decrease in pH caused by localized production of lactic acid. If a tourniquet is applied for more than 1 min while searching for a vein, release tourniquet and reapply after 2–3 min. Allow the tourniquet to remain in place until blood flow is established and removed prior to needle withdraw. Avoid extra muscle activity, such as clenching and unclenching the fist, which may increase potassium results.

Urine

Urine is a valuable sample. It contains excreted metabolites and provides an integrated snapshot of the ongoing metabolism and thus pathology. It also overcomes some of the limitations mentioned above with regard to diurnal rhythm, and pulsatile production of biomarkers (e.g., cortisol).

Although urine considered an easy-to-obtain sample, it is often cumbersome, for instance, in neonates and pediatrics, and the elderly population. It might be inconvenient for some patients.

The number of urine samples being collected for biochemical testing is declining as more tests are available on blood samples. Urine collections are either a random sample which is often early morning, preferably a second void sample, anytime during the day, or late in the evening. Urine samples may be timed for short periods (e.g., 2–4 h) or often for long periods (24-h collections).

Timed collections

Adherence to timed collection protocols is important, such as timed urine samples (24 h collections) and to timed dynamic test protocols such as glucose tolerance test (complete dosage intake and accurate time of blood collection in relation to the dose), blood sample collection at 8 a.m. following intake of dexamethasone dosage during an overnight dexamethasone suppression test, etc.

Special consideration (chain of custody requirements)

Toxicology testing (e.g., in preemployment) as well as forensic testing requires additional steps to achieve a state of "beyond reasonable doubt." Two items are central to the testing process; (a) chain of custody is mandatory. Record is kept for everybody who handles the specimen until the urine is testing is complete or discarded by the laboratory and (b) compliance with all testing procedures and notification of adulteration. Failure to keep comprehensive and accurate record and or interference with the testing procedure is an offense.

Sample integrity is assured via several steps; the sample was collected from the correct patient by observing collection (this is often unsuitable and not possible (e.g., for passing urine)), alternatively, mark the empty container (urine cup) and give it to the patient and check that the container with the markings is returned. Immediately upon sample receipt ensure the container contains the marking, record sample volume, and check urine sample temperature

(acceptable sample is ±4°C from body temperature). This identifies if a prior stored sample is provided of if, the sample has had tap water added to it. Additionally, measure specific gravity and pH to make sure that no additive was added. The latter may change the urine sample pH (low and high pH disrupts antibody-antigen binding and provides a falsely negative result). All of the above-mentioned checkpoints are now included in the urine cup with reagent strips for the drugs of interest to be tested as well as sample integrity checks (temperature, pH, and specific gravity).

The urine container/blood tube is sealed, and the patients often attests that the specimen was theirs. The maple is transported in a locked container (tamperproof), refrigerated, and delivered to the laboratory under a chain of custody arrangement. Upon receipt at the laboratory for testing, sample details are verified for compliance with the chain of custody process and tested for the required drugs. Samples stored in the laboratory are kept under a lock and key specially designated fridges/freezers as required.

Analytical methods

Most of the clinical biochemistry tests are performed using automated analyzers that facilitate rapid analysis of the large volume of testing. The main driver that determines the type of methods applied is the concentration (level) of the analyte in question (Fig. 1). Additionally, determinants include characteristics of the analyte, that is size, activity, physical property (solubility, stability, photometry, and luminesces) as well as the presence of structural variants and interfering substances and reagents.

Assays performance characteristics

In addition to the limit of blank (LoB), limit of detection (LoD), limit of quantitation (LoQ), analytical measurement range (AMR), clinical reportable range (CRR), and specificity (lack of interference from similar or related analytes), assay characteristics include sample type and handling requirements and reporting format (i.e., quantitative vs qualitative).

Limit of blank (LoB)

This defines the lowest signal generated in a sample without any analyte (in reality the buffer or diluent of the assay). It may be confused for a low analyte concentration, but this represents the background signal produced by the test system and is thus inherent to the test in the absence of the analyte of interest. Replicates of blank samples (without the analyte) were measured in the test system several times. The minimum number of measurements required is 60 (when being established and performed during assay development) or 20 measurements when the assay performance

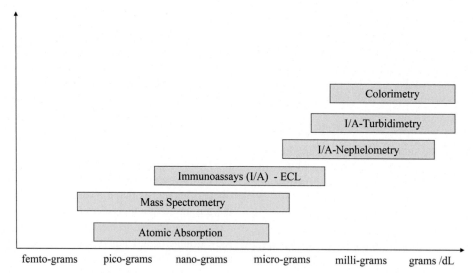

FIG. 1 Analyte concentration-dependent methodologies. *I/A*, immunoassays; *ECL*, electrochemical detection. The method used depends on the concentration of the analyte to be measured as well as on its physical and biochemical characteristics. *(Modified from Fortress Diagnostics Ltd, Northern Ireland, UK.)*

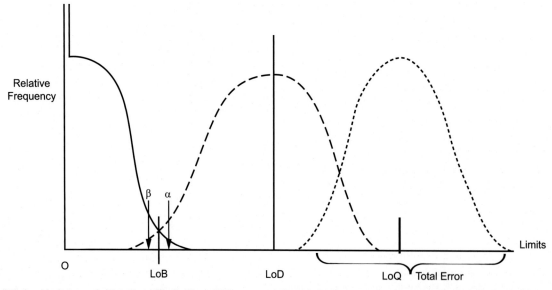

FIG. 2 Relationship between LoB, LoD, and LoQ. The *solid line curve* defines the LoB (analyte-free sample) signal response distribution. The LoB response overlaps with the LoD response *(dashed line)* and thus excludes a small proportion of blank results ("α"). The *dashed line* also represents the scatter (imprecision) of results for a specimen of low concentration. The LoD distribution response overlaps with a small portion of the LoB response ("β") termed type II error. The *dotted line* defines the LoQ and represents the distribution of results for a specimen of low concentration meeting the target for total error (imprecision and bias). It may be that this LoQ total target error is met by a specimen at the LoD concentration in which case LoQ=LoD. Otherwise, LoQ will have to be set after testing a specimen of higher concentration. *(Modified from Tholen DW, Linnet K, Kondratovich M, et al. Protocols for Determination of Limits of Detection and Limits of Quantitation; Approved Guideline. vol. 24(34). ISSN 0273-3099. ISBN 1-56238-551-8.)*

claims are being verified by the end-user clinical laboratory. Assuming a Gaussian distribution of the analytical signal obtained, the formula for determining the LoB is as follows.

$$\text{LoB} = \text{mean}(\text{values obtained}) + 1.645(\text{SD}).$$

For the calculation, the use of the raw analytical signals (provided by the testing system) is preferred (some analyzers may only report analyte value as "zero" at a certain fixed limit below which signals continue to be generated). Assuming a Gaussian distribution of the raw analytical signals, the remaining 5% of values represent an area of response that could be produced by a sample containing a very low concentration of the analyte. This is considered a false positive and is termed a type I (α) error (Fig. 2).

Limit of detection (LoD)

This describes the lowest detectable concentration of the analyte that can be measured by the test system, and at which point it can reliably be distinguished from analytical noise (LoB). The test sample used contains a very low concentration of the analyte, often the lowest calibrator, or a patient's sample with low values of the analytes, or that has been subjected to dilution to low values (using the appropriate diluent to minimize matrix effects). This is a Gaussian distribution, and similar to the overlap seen in LoB, a proportion of very low concentration of the analyte will produce responses less than the LoB upper limit, in statistical terms, this is termed type II (or β) error (Fig. 2). It is calculated using the formula:

$$LoD = LoB + 1.645 (SD \, low \, concentration \, sample).$$

Variations of this approach use the mean plus 3, 4, or even 10 SDs to provide a more conservative LoD.

Limit of quantitation (LoQ)

This takes into consideration the LoB and LoD and describes the lowest concentration that the test system can measure the analyte with a high degree of precision. Typically, an imprecision of <20% is considered acceptable performance. It is at this point that the limit of quantitation (LoQ) is defined. Bias "numerical expression of the degree of trueness" is calculated as the difference ($\pm$) between measured analytes values and actual target values and is concentration dependent.

The LoQ may, however, be equivalent to the LoD or higher. A predetermined acceptable total error (total error = imprecision + bias) must be met for the assay to be acceptable for clinical use (Figs. 2 and 3).

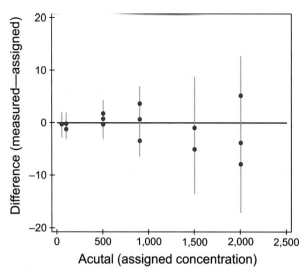

FIG. 3 Example bias (hypothetical) difference between actual (assigned analyte concentration) and measured (estimated). The bias at the lowest concentration is applied to the total error determination. Note that bias is concentration dependent. *(Courtesy: the author's laboratory (Osmolality studies).)*

Analytical measurement range (AMR)

This describes the range (lowest and highest) concentration of the analyte that can reliably be measured by the test system often determined from the assay precision profile and bias plots (Fig. 4).

Clinical reportable range (CRR)

The clinical reportable range (CRR) describes the extended analytical measurement range (AMR) following dilution. It is helpful when reporting an analyte that can be present at

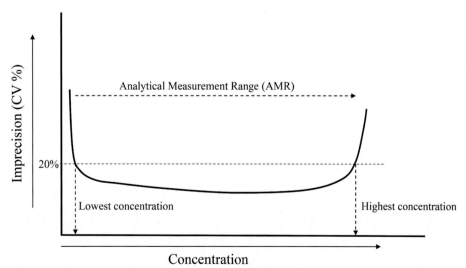

FIG. 4 Precision profile in the determination of the test system analyte measurement range. Note that imprecision is concentration dependent. *(Courtesy: the author's laboratory.)*

usually high concentration (e.g., tumor markers), and absolute values are required for serial samples to monitor response (or lack of) to therapeutic intervention. The common diluent used in clinical laboratory practice is saline (0.9% sodium chloride); however, there is a dilution limit beyond which the sample matrix is so much altered exceeding the test system operating characteristics. Therefore, dilution to an endpoint may not be appropriate for all test systems, and for those a limit of dilution is often imposed (i.e., no dilution beyond 10-fold or so), and analyte values exceeding the AMR at the maximum allowed dilution will be expressed as > (greater than) the highest dilution allowed.

Methods principles

Many method principles are used. They are a function of the analyte being measured. Their chemical, enzymatic, immunological, and chromatographic; properties are observed. The methods are outlined as spectrophotometric, colorimetric, enzymatic system based, antibody based immunoassays (turbidimetric, nephelometric, colorimetric), electropotentiometric (ion selective electrodes), and chromatographic methods (electrophoretic, gel and capillary electrophoresis, and mass spectrometry).

Spectrophotometry/colorimetry

This is the most commonly utilized method. It is often the method used when measuring chemical or enzymatic activity. Colorimetric methods employ fixed wavelength in the visible range (Fig. 6) whereas spectrophotometry employs a range of wavelengths.

Nicotinamide adenine dinucleotides (NAD^+/NADH) are ubiquitous molecules present in all organisms and play important roles as cofactors in fundamental catabolic and anabolic processes. NADH in solution produces a significant absorbance peak at 340 nm compared to its reaction counterpart NAD^+ which has virtually no absorbance at the 340 nm wavelength. This marked distinction is the basis of many numerous assay formations where the reaction is monitored. They act as coenzymes in reversible reactions. Example enzymes are dehydrogenases (e.g., lactate dehydrogenase) and oxidoreductases (e.g., peroxidase, oxidases, hydrolases). Another enzymatic example, the use of enzyme multiplied immunoassay assay (EMIT), where the reagent drug is conjugated to an enzyme often (alkaline phosphates, peroxidase, etc.), This reagent drug-enzyme conjugate competes with drug in patient's sample with reagent antibody, the binding of the enzyme-labeled antigen inhibits enzymatic activity and thus reduces significant color of the enzymatic reaction following addition of substrate, and is inversely proportional to the amount of the drug inpatient sample.

Beer-lambert law states that there is a linear relationship between the concentration of the analyte and the absorbance

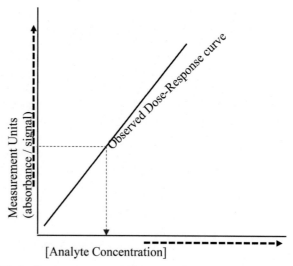

FIG. 5 Dose-response curve. The spectrophotometric response (intensity) positively correlates with analyte concentration or activity.

of the solution (Fig. 5). It is derived as; A (absorbance) $= e$ (extinction coefficient) $\times C$ (concertation) $\times L$ (pathlength). In other words, it describes the attenuation of the incident light by the properties of the sample through which the light is traveling.

An example of a colorimetric method is the reaction of albumin or total protein with a chemical dye (bromocresol green). Albumin in the sample reacts with bromocresol green at acidic pH and forms a colored complex. The reaction is specific to albumin. The intensity of the color is measured using a colorimeter set at 620nm (Fig. 6). The intensity is directly proportional to the albumin concentration in the sample.

Interferences in this methodology format include the presence of metabolites or drug metabolites that also absorb at the same assay-spectrophotometric absorbance range.

Lateral flow chemical tests

Point-of-care strip test (e.g., urinalysis strip test) uses color chemical reactions that are either read by the naked eye by subjective comparison to a color chart or by a colorimeter.

The combination of tests is helpful in the assessment of kidney function, urinary tract infections, carbohydrate metabolism, and liver function.

Substances that cause abnormal urine color, such as drugs containing azo dyes (e.g., Pyridium, Azo Gantrisin, Azo Gantanol), nitrofurantoin (Macrodantin, Furadantin), riboflavin, and visible levels of blood or bilirubin, may affect the ability to accurately read (naked eye or by automated colorimeter) the reagent pads areas on urinalysis reagent strips. The color development on the reagent pad may be masked, or a color reaction may be produced on the pad that could be misinterpreted as a false positive. Levels of ascorbic acid normally found in urine do not interfere.

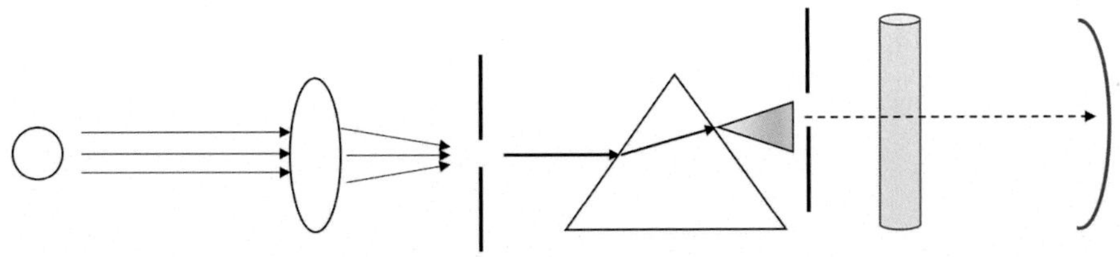

Light Source   Collimator   Entrance Slit   Prizm   Exit Slit Sample   Detector

FIG. 6 Colorimeter components. Light passes through a collimator and entrance slit before beam diffraction at prism. Selected wavelength passes through the sample and absorbance is recorded on a detector. *(Modified from Deverill I, Reeves WG. Light scattering and absorption—developments in immunology. J Immunol Methods. 1980;38(3–4):191–204. https://doi.org/10.1016/0022-1759(80)90267-7. PMID: 7003015 Whicher JT, Price CP, Spencer K. Immunonephelometric and immunoturbidimetric assays for proteins. Crit Rev Clin Lab Sci. 1983;18(3):213–260. https://doi.org/10.3109/10408368209085072. PMID: 6339164.)*

The widespread intake of ascorbic acid (e.g., in vitamin C therapy, as a therapeutical ingredient and stabilizer of numerous medicaments, oxidation inhibitors, and preservatives in food industry) causes a rapid saturation of the organism and renal excretion of the excess. Interfering ascorbic acid concentrations may be reached after the ingestion of fruit juice or plenty of fruit. Therefore, the ascorbic acid test zone minimizes reporting of falsely negative results. The color fields correspond to the following values shown in Table 1.

The reagent strip (dipstick) should be dipped briefly in the urine and excess fluid tapped off. Adherence to the time interval indicated on the container before comparing the resulting color with the color chart. Delayed readings may produce false-positive results.

The "first morning" specimen is the most concentrated and is preferable; however, random collections are acceptable and should be analyzed within 2 h of collection. If testing is delayed, samples may be refrigerated and analyzed within 24 h of collection. Test decision points for detection and grading are shown in Table 1. The test and their respective reactions are discussed.

The albumin test is based on the principle of the "protein error" of indicators, i.e., at a constantly buffered pH, albumin reacts with a tetrabromophenol sulfonephthalein derivative resulting in a color change from yellow-green to green-blue for "positive." The test employs the protein-error-of-indicators principle. A visibly bloody urine may cause falsely elevated results.

Urine dipstick analysis, which largely measures urinary albumin, is the most common method for initial detection of proteinuria. True proteinuria is defined as $\geq$1+ proteinuria when the specific gravity (SG) of the urine sample is $\leq$1.015, or $\geq$2+ proteinuria when the SG of the sample is >1.015. Typically, these findings need to be present in two of three specimens, obtained at least 1 week apart.

Blood detection is based on the pseudoperoxidative activity of hemoglobin and myoglobin, which catalyze the oxidation of an indicator by an organic hydroperoxide, producing a green color. It catalyzes the reaction of diisopropylbenzene dihydroperoxide and 3,3,5,5-tetramethylaminobenzaldehyde in conjunction with a color enhancer. The resulting color ranges from orange through green to dark blue and is related to the degree of blood present (concentration). Differentiation of hemoglobin from erythrocytes can be determined by a color comparison chart on the vial label. Color change due to the presence of red blood cells and hemoglobin can be grouped into hemolyzed and nonhemolyzed reported as Trace, (1+) small, (2+) moderate, and (3+) large. Erroneous results are seen in the presence of Capoten (captopril) which may reduce the test sensitivity. Certain oxidizing contaminants, such as hypochlorite, may produce false-positive results. Microbial peroxidase associated with urinary tract infection may cause a false-positive reaction.

Glucose testing utilizes two enzymes in a sequential manner, in the initial reaction glucose is oxidized by glucose oxidase to gluconic acid and hydrogen peroxide. The latter in the presence of the second enzyme peroxidase reacts with potassium iodide chromogen to colors ranging from green to brown which correlate with the concentration of the glucose. Glucose should not be detectable in normal urine; therefore, the production of any color is positive. The range of values for positive urine glucose is negative, 100, 250, 500, 1000, and $\geq$2000 mg/dL. Ketone bodies reduce the sensitivity of the test; moderately high ketone levels (40 mg/dL) may cause false negatives for specimens containing small amounts of glucose (75–125 mg/dL) but the combination of such ketone levels and low glucose levels is metabolically improbable in screening. An inhibitory effect is produced by gentisic acid. Falsely positive reactions can also be produced by a residue of peroxide-containing cleansing agents.

When testing for ketones, acetoacetic acid, and acetone, react with nitroprusside forming colored product ranging from buff-pink, for a negative result to purple for a positive result. It is important to note that the test does not react with β-hydroxybutyrate formed early in the production of ketones and that a false-negative result misleads clinical management. Specific assays for the measurement of β-hydroxybutyrate are available and should be performed in patients suspected of ketoacidosis. Additionally, the ketone test is subject to the following limitations, false "trace"

TABLE 1 Lateral flow strip (dipstick) tests, and their detection range and limits.

Test	Test reporting ranges		Detection limits
Protein (mg/dL)	NEG, TRACE, 30 (+), 100 (++), 300 (+++), 2000, or more (++++)		15–30 mg/dL albumin
Blood (mg/dL)	Nonhemolyzed	Hemolyzed	0.015–0.062 mg/dL hemoglobin 5–10 erythrocytes/µL
	NEG, TRACE, MOD	TRACE, SM(+), MOD(++), LARGE(+++)	
Leukocytes	NEG, TRACE, SM(+), MOD(++), LARGE(+++)		5–15 white blood cells/hpf
Nitrite	POS, NEG		0.06–0.1 mg/dL nitrite ion
Glucose (mg/dL)	NEG, 100, 250, 500, 1000, 2000, or more neg. (yellow), neg. or normal (greenish), 50, 150, 500, and ≥1000 mg/dL or neg. (yellow), neg. or normal (greenish), 2.8, 8.3, 27.8, and ≥55.5 mmol/L.		75–125 mg/dL glucose
Ketone (mg/dL)	NEG, 5 (TRACE), 15 (SMALL), 40 (MOD), 80 (LG), 160 (LG) 0 (negative), 25 (+), 100 (++), and 300 (+++) mg/dL or 0 (negative), 2.5 (+), 10 (++), and 30 (+++) mmol/L		5–10 mg/dL acetoacetic acid
pH	4.5–9.0 (0.5 pH units increments)		N/A
Specific gravity	1.005, 1.010, 1015, 1.020, 1.025, and 1.030		1.015–1.025; however, it can vary between 1.000 after extreme liquid intake and 1.040 after a longer period of thirst
Bilirubin (mg/dL)	0 (negative), 1 (+), 2 (++), 4 (+++) mg/dL or 0 (negative), 17 (+), 35 (++), 70 (+++) µmol/L.		0.4–0.8 mg/dL bilirubin
Urobilinogen:	normal (0–1), 2, 4, 8, 12 mg/dL or normal (0–17), 34, 70, 140, 200 µmol/L.		0.2 mg/dL (3.5 µmol/L) urobilinogen
Ascorbic acid	0 (negative), 10 (+), and 20 (++) mg/dL (0 (negative), 0.6 (+), and 1.1 (++) mmol/L).		

hpf, high power field; LG, large; MOD, moderate; NEG, negative; SM, slight.
Modified from the author's laboratory using instrument Beckman Coulter iQ Workcell System consists of the ARKRAY AX-4030 and the IRIS iQ200 Elite with iQ200 software.

results may occur with highly pigmented urine specimens or those containing large amounts of levodopa metabolites. Compounds such as 2-mercaptoethane sulfonic acid that contain sulfhydryl groups may cause false-positive results or an atypical color reaction.

Leukocyte detection is based on granulocytic leukocyte esterase content that catalyzes the hydrolysis of the derivatized pyrrole amino acid ester to liberate 3-hydroxy-5-phenyl pyrrole. This pyrrole then reacts with a diazonium salt to produce a purple product. Normal urine should produce no color reaction. Positive reactions produce a purple color that can be reported as small, moderate, or large. Elevated glucose concentrations (≥3 g/dL) may cause decreased test results. The presence of cephalexin (Keflex), cephalothin (Keflin), or high concentrations of oxalic acid may also cause decreased test results. Tetracycline may cause decreased reactivity, and high levels of the drug may cause a false-negative reaction. Positive results occasionally be due to contamination of the specimen by vaginal discharge.

Nitrite detection is based on the conversion of nitrate (derived from the diet) to nitrite by the action of gram-negative bacteria in the urine. At the acid pH of the reagent area, nitrite in the urine reacts with p-arsanilic acid to form a diazonium compound. This diazonium compound in turn couples with 1,2,3,4-tetrahydrobenzo(h)quinoline-3-ol to produce a pink color. The test is reported as negative or positive. Pink spots or pink edges should not be interpreted as positive results. A negative result does not rule out significant bacteriuria. False-negative results may occur with shortened bladder incubation of the urine, the absence of dietary nitrate, or the presence of nonreductive pathological microbes.

pH measurement is based on a double indicator principle that gives a broad range of colors from orange (acidic) through yellow to blue (alkaline) representing the entire urinary pH range. Range values are: 5, 6, 6.5, 7, 7.5, 8, and 8.5. Bacterial growth by certain organisms in a specimen may cause a marked alkaline shift (pH > 8.0), usually because of urea conversion to ammonia.

Specific gravity test methodology is based on the apparent pKa change of certain pretreated polyelectrolytes in relation to ionic concentration. In the presence of an indicator, colors range from deep blue-green in urines of low ionic strength to green and yellow-green in urines of increasing ionic strength. The range of values is: 1.005, 1.010, 1015, 1.020, 1.025, and 1.030.

Some tests are dependent on ions in urine and results may differ from those obtained with other specific gravity methods when certain nonionic urine constituents, such as glucose, are present. Highly buffered alkaline urines may cause low readings, while the presence of moderate quantities of protein (100–750 mg/dL) may cause elevated readings. Falsely negative results can be produced by high doses of ascorbic acid, by antibiotics therapy, and by very low nitrate concentrations in urine as the result of a low nitrate diet or strong dilution (diuresis). Falsely positive results can be caused by the presence of diagnostic or therapeutic dyes in the urine.

Bilirubin detection is based on the coupling of bilirubin with diazotized dichloroaniline in a strongly acid medium forming azobilirubin a colored product. The color ranges through various shades of tan. No color is reported as negative and the presence of any color is reported as small, moderate, or large. Indican (indoxyl sulfate) can produce a yellow-orange to red color response that may interfere with the interpretation of a negative or positive reading. Metabolites of Lodine (etodolac) may cause false-positive or atypical results. Atypical colors (colors unlike the negative or positive color blocks shown on the color chart) may indicate that bilirubin-derived bile pigments are present in the urine sample and may be masking the bilirubin reaction. These colors may indicate bile pigment abnormalities and the urine specimen should be tested further.

Since colors are difficult to interpret and subject to masked and false-positive reactions with reagent strips, it has been recommended to confirm all-positive reactions with another method, such as the ICTOTEST reagent tablets.

Urobilinogen testing is based on the Ehrlich reaction in which p-diethylaminobenzalde in conjunction with a color enhancer reacts with urobilinogen in a strongly acid medium to produce a pink-red color. Values up to 1 mg/dL (1 mg/dL = 1 Eu/dL) are usually considered normal. No color was reported as 0.2 mg/dL and the presence of any color graded as 1.0, 2.0, 4.0, or 8.0 mg/dL.

The test pad may react with interfering substances known to react with Ehrlich's reagent, such as p-aminosalicylic acid and sulfonamides. Atypical color reactions may be obtained in the presence of high concentrations of p-aminobenzoic acid. False-negative results may be obtained if formalin is present. Strip reactivity increases with temperature; the optimum temperature is 22–26°C (72–79°F). The test is inhibited by higher concentrations of formaldehyde. Longer exposure of the urine to light leads to lowered or falsely negative results. Higher, or falsely positive results, can be caused by the presence of diagnostic or therapeutic dyes in the urine. Larger amounts of bilirubin produce a yellow coloration. The test is not a reliable method for the detection of porphobilinogen.

Some kits contain a creatinine test pad to aid with detection of a dilute urine sample and to semiquantitatively index other parameters to creatinine. Creatinine reacts with dinitrobenzoic acid producing a colored product ranging from yellow-brown to blue-black depending on the creatinine concentration. Following the determination of albumin and creatinine levels, the albumin/creatinine ratio can be derived.

Some reagent strips include a test pad for ascorbic acid (vitamin C). It is detected based on the discoloration of Tillman's reagent. The blue-colored 2,6-dichlorophenol indophenol sodium salt is reduced to the colorless leuko form by ascorbic acid. In the presence of ascorbic acid, a color change takes place from blue to red.

Antibody-based assays (immunoassays)

Assays utilizing antibodies as reagents have been in routine use for a long time. In addition to increased assay sensitivity, it affords a higher degree of specificity. The antibodies are either monoclonal (often mouse origin) or polyclonal (often goat, or sheep). The antibodies as reagents are conjugated to either Sepharose beads to improve their sensitivity (as in turbidimetric and nephelometric methods) or to widely used biotin. The latter is used in a second reaction with avidin that is labeled with peroxidase, another common use reagent.

Other established immunoassays detection systems include electrochemiluminescence where a ruthenium II tris(bipyridyl) bound assay reagent (often an antibody) with tripropylamine, following reaction with the analyte, the complex is held at an electrode surface. The assay reagent beads are held at an electrode magnetically following an electrochemiluminescence reaction light emitted at (620 nm) and captured by an adjacent photomultiplier tube. The signal response is proportional to the concentration of the analyte. Another commonly used detection system is chemiluminescence, which describes light emitted during a chemical reaction. Examples are acridinium esters and isoluminol.

Oxidation of isoluminol by hydrogen peroxide in the presence of peroxidase enzyme produces a long-lived light emission at 425 nm. Oxidation of acridinium esters by alkaline hydrogen peroxide in the presence of detergent (triton x100) produces a rapid flash of light at 429 nm.

One step: Homogenous immunoassays

There is no separation step between reagents and sample reactants. This format affords speed (eliminates time for washing and removal of unbound material) at the expense of reduced sensitivity (increased background noise (LoB)). Two steps: heterogeneous immunoassays: this involves the separation of what has and has not bound.

Turbidimetric/nephelometric based

In the turbidimetric and nephelometric methoddes, the test principles are the same; however, the difference in terminology relates to the detection component. In the turbidimetric method, the detector is placed directly in the path of the incident and transmitted light, whereas in the nephelometric methods, the detector is placed at an angle (45–90 degrees) to the incident and transmitted light, this step detects deflected light and affords a high degree of sensitivity compared to the turbidimetric set up (Fig. 7).

In the nephelometric assays, light diffracted by the reaction complex (antibody-antigen) is measured at an angle (Fig. 7). This affords higher sensitivity when compared with turbidimetric assays.

In one assay formulation, e.g., C-reactive protein (CRP), the binding of the sample CRP to the reagent anti-CRP antibody increases the turbidity of the sample and is related to the concentration of the CRP in the sample. When the anti-CRP antibody reagent is conjugated to Sepharose beads and allowed to react with CRP as usual, the degree of turbidity is higher due to the presence of beads (conjugated to the anti-CRP antibody—particle enhanced). Furthermore, if the detector was placed at an angle, the diffracted light affords a higher sensitivity, and lower concentrations of CRP are now detectable.

In another example of a different setup, the antibody binding to drugs either causes a decrease or increase in turbidity that is proportional to the amount of drugs. Examples of assay formations include KIMS (Kinetic Interaction of Molecules in Solution) where in the absence of the drugs, the reagent antibodies bind to a latex-attached reagent antigen. This causes aggregation and an increase in turbidity, whereas in the presence of drug, the binding of the antibody preferentially to the free drug (in patients' sample) and not to the latex-bound reagent drug forms no aggregates and thus no turbidity, degree of which is related to the level of the drug in the patient sample.

Utilizing antibody binding and various detection techniques

The binding properties of antibodies in addition to the characteristics of different detection systems developed and patented by various manufacturers. They have been discussed in detail in Chapter 16 on aspects of laboratory management. They are summarized below.

In the enzyme multiplied immunoassay (EMIT), the antianalyte antibody inhibits the enzymatic activity of an enzyme (usually glucose-6-phosphate dehydrogenase) coupled to the target analyte. The binding of the antibody to the enzyme-labeled analytes causes a steric hindrance or conformational changes inhibiting the enzyme activity and hence no substrate reaction and no color development. In the absence of the analyte of the analyte, the antibody freely binds to the reagent analyte-enzyme complex and color (or reduced color obtained), whereas in the presence of the analyte (from the patient sample) the analyte preferentially binds to the antibody leaving the reagent analyte-enzyme complex free to react with substrate and produce color. Thus, the color intensity is directly related to the analyte concentration. A technique is known as enzyme-multiplied immunoassay test (EMIT) (Fig. 8).

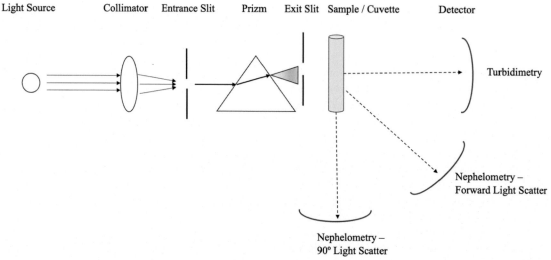

FIG. 7 Turbidimetric and nephelometric assays. The detector is located at an angle to the incident light. Deflected light is measured. This approach offers higher sensitivity compared to turbidimetric methods. *(Modified from Deverill I, Reeves WG. Light scattering and absorption—developments in immunology. J Immunol Methods. 1980;38(3–4):191–204. https://doi.org/10.1016/0022-1759(80)90267-7. PMID: 7003015.)*

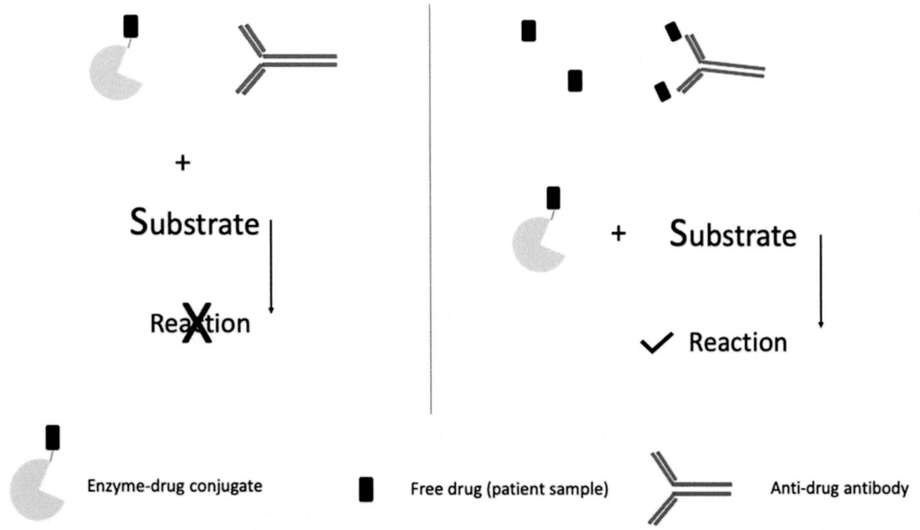

FIG. 8 Principle of the EMIT-based assay. *(Modified from Milone MC. Analytical techniques used in therapeutic drug monitoring. In: Dasgupta A, ed. Therapeutic Drug Monitoring. Academic Press; 2012:49–73. ISBN 9780123854674. https://doi.org/10.1016/B978-0-12-385467-4.00003-8. https://www.sciencedirect.com/science/article/pii/B9780123854674000038. [chapter 3]. From Reisfield GM, Bertholf RL. Drug testing in pain management. In: Dasgupta A, ed. Critical Issues in Alcohol and Drugs of Abuse Testing. 2nd ed. Academic Press; 2019:343–358. ISBN 9780128156070. https://doi.org/10.1016/B978-0-12-815607-0.00025-3. https://www.sciencedirect.com/science/article/pii/B9780128156070000253. [chapter 25].)*

Fluorescence polarization immunoassay (FPIA)

The method is based on the relationship between fluorescence lifetime, and the rotational relation time of a fluorescence-labeled drug. When a fluorescence-labeled drug is excited by plane-polarized light, it rotates freely, and emitted fluorescence photon may not be in the same orientation, thus emitted fluorescence is not polarized in a single plane. However, when bound to an antibody, the drug-antibody complex is significantly larger, and this reduced rotation by about 100-fold. This means that the emitted fluorescence photon is more likely to be in the same polarized plane as that of the incident light. When the reagent antibody binds to the drug in the patient sample, the fluorescence-labeled reagent drug is unbound and thus freely rotating. Thus, the degree of depolarization of the emitted fluorescence is directly proportional to the amount of drug in the patient sample (Fig. 9).

Whereas in the conventional turbidimetric/nephelometric assays, the binding of the antibody to the analyte makes a larger aggregate complex contributing to sample turbidity or light diffraction (in the case of nephelometry) the degree of which is related to the amount concentration of the analytes. In a different manufacturer approach, the reagent analyte is linked to microparticles (e.g., Sepharose beads). In the absence (or presence of low amount) of the analyte, the reagent antibody freely binds to the microparticles conjugated reagent analyte, and the aggregate formed causes a reduction in the light absorbance (more of the incident light is transmitted). In the presence of a patient analyte, this competes for binding to the reagent antibody. The now free reagent analyte (coupled to microparticles) is at a higher

concentration causing a lower degree of light transmission. In other words, the degree of light transmitted is inversely proportional to the amount of analyte in the patient sample, this method principle is termed Kinetic Interaction of Molecules in Solution (KIMS) (Fig. 10).

Two steps immunoassays

Two steps: Heterogeneous immunoassays: this involves the separation of what has and has not bound.

In the initial step, the patient sample (sample analyte) and the reagent analyte (coated with a microparticle-paramagnetic). The two analytes compete for binding to reagent antibody directed against the analyte. Following a short time incubation, the paramagnetic particles are held in place (via an electric magnet), and nonreacting and nonbound sample analyte and reagent components are washed away. Following washing a detection reagent is added (e.g., acridinium-labeled conjugate is added in the second step in addition to the required trigger solutions and the resulting chemiluminescent reaction is measured). A direct relationship exists between the amount of antigen in the sample and the relative light units generated (Fig. 5).

Lateral flow-based immunoassay

Similar to that described above for urine reagent strips (dipstick chemical lateral flow test), lateral flow reaction strips are used in an immuno-based setup. Antibodies directed against specific proteins/hormones, e.g., β-hCG (pregnancy test), hemoglobin (fecal occult blood), infectious

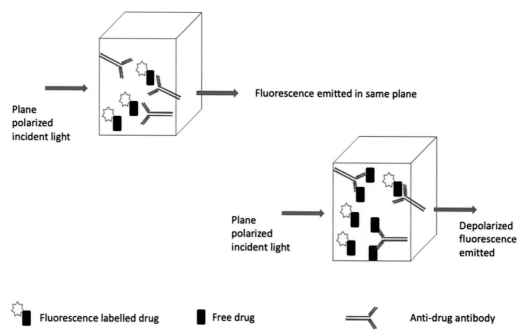

FIG. 9   Principles of the FPIA-based assay. *(Modified from Nishiyama K, Fukuyama M, Maeki M, et al. One-step non-competitive fluorescence polarization immunoassay based on a Fab fragment for C-reactive protein quantification. Sens Actuators B Chem. 2021;326:128982. ISSN 0925-4005. https://doi.org/10.1016/j.snb.2020.128982. From Reisfield GM, Bertholf RL. Drug testing in pain management. In: Dasgupta A, ed. Critical Issues in Alcohol and Drugs of Abuse Testing. 2nd ed. Academic Press; 2019:343–358. ISBN 9780128156070. https://doi.org/10.1016/B978-0-12-815607-0.00025-3. https://www.sciencedirect.com/science/article/pii/B9780128156070000253. [chapter 25].)*

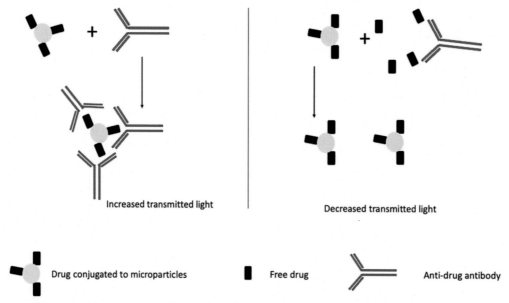

FIG. 10   Assay principle for the KIMS method. *(Modified from Reisfield GM, Bertholf RL. Drug testing in pain management. In: Dasgupta A, ed. Critical Issues in Alcohol and Drugs of Abuse Testing. 2nd ed. Academic Press; 2019:343–358. ISBN 9780128156070. https://doi.org/10.1016/B978-0-12-815607-0.00025-3. https://www.sciencedirect.com/science/article/pii/B9780128156070000253. [chapter 25].)*

agents (structural proteins and/or their respective human immune response—serology testing). hCG will be used as an example.

Antibodies directed against hCG are fixed onto a lateral flow strip. This is the reaction line. Labeled second antibody reagent is located on the sample application pad. Upon ap-

plication of the sample (urine), hCG in the sample reacts with the second labeled antibody as it travels to the reaction site (location of the immobilized first antibody). The hCG and antibody complex reacts with the immobilized antibody forming a sandwich and a colored line appears and indicates a positive reaction (hCG positive) and that in the absence of hCG (negative sample), no antigen-antibody sandwich is formed and no color appears at the test site. A second test site is an integral component of the lateral flow strip and represents a control line. A color-conjugated antibody travels with the sample and antibody directed against the control line, where it deposits and a positive line is observed. This indicates that the test performance was successful (Fig. 11A).

Whereas in some assays, a line at the test line indicates a positive test and the absence of the test line indicates a negative test result (Fig. 11B), it is important to realize that in some lateral flow methods set up the reverse is true, where the absence of test line is a positive finding (Fig. 11B). The lack of QC line indicates an invalid result (Fig. 11A,B).

A number of assays are commercially available mostly as over-the-counter item in pharmacies. Some assays detect intact hCG only and not the free β-hCG subunit nor β core fragments. For those test samples, reduced urine content of intact hCG after 8 weeks gestation may result in poor performance and false-negative results.

The utility of the lateral flow-based tests is often limited and is influenced by molecular heterogeneity of the target hormone/protein and the relative concentration of the urine sample. Laboratory-based quantitative assays used to detect hCG may be detecting hCG degradation products, and

therefore may disagree with the results of some lateral flow-based assays (often a point of debate between laboratory and clinic personnel).

Methodological approaches to detect molecular variants (including free/bound)

Measuring variants such as molecular weight variants (macroprolactin), free thyroid hormones, free testosterone, total (bound and free), and free drugs, e.g., phenytoin, etc.

Molecular (heterogeneity) variants

Circulating proteins (including hormones) may exhibit posttranslational modification in the form of aggregates or binding to autoantibodies. The result is a high molecular weight variant that may exhibit variable reactions (immunological, enzymatic). This results in inaccurate results.

Common laboratory methods in their investigation is use of PEG precipitation.

Examples include macroprolactin, following sample treatment with polyethylene glycol (PEG) precipitation, recovery of <40% postprecipitation with PEG suggests the presence of macroprolactin (high molecular weight prolactin variants) where recovery of >60% suggests the absence

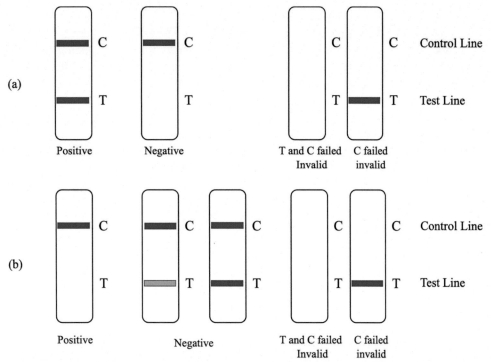

FIG. 11   Example lateral flow test comprising two reaction sites, a test site, and a control site. (A) A control line must always be detected for the test to be valid, regardless of the test line outcomes. A line at the test line indicates a positive test and the absence of the test line indicates a negative test result. It is important to realize that some lateral flow methods set up the reverse is true, where the above test line is a positive finding (B). *(Modified from First Sign® Drug of abuse Cup Test instructions in use by the author's laboratory from Hemosure, Inc., Irwindale, CA 91706. www.hemosure.com. From Jiang N, Ahmed R, Damayantharan M, Ünal B, Butt H, Yetisen AK. Lateral and vertical flow assays for point-of-care diagnostics. Adv Healthc Mater. 2019;8(14):e1900244. https://doi.org/10.1002/adhm.201900244. Epub 2019 May 13. PMID: 31081270.)*

of high molecular weight variants, values between 60% and 40% are often classified as indeterminant gray zone.

Analytes are commonly found in free and protein-bound format in circulation and the free form represents the biologically active form often present in smaller amount (<10%) and thus imposes a requirement of increased sensitivity.

There are two formulations in the measurement of free forms of the analytes. A two-step format includes that a reagent labeled analyte is incubated with a patient sample and competes for binding with the reagent antibody. Measurement is obtained following removal of the unbound analyte (Fig. 12A). In the second format, a chemically modified analyte analog is used in place of the labeled analyte. The addition of labeled analog requires the use of high avidity antibodies and a short second incubation period and that the analog cannot bind to the binding proteins (Fig. 12B,C). An one-step method format with the advantage of shorter testing time is also available (Fig. 12C). Thyroid homone assays are used as an example (Fig. 12).

Equilibrium dialysis

Equilibrium dialysis and ultrafiltration have been considered reference methods for a number of analytes. For instance, it is used to determine the concentration of free drugs such as free phenytoin.

A diluted sample is placed in a chamber and separated by a semipermeable membrane allowing diffusion of free drug across a dialysis membrane. The sample is allowed to equilibrate over a period of time, often overnight, and an aliquot of the dialysate (containing the free drug) is analyzed using LC-MSMS. The latter affords both required

sensitivity and specificity. The technique is cumbersome and time-consuming and thus not amenable to routine clinical practice and thus often performed at reference laboratories. Additionally, there is a lack of standardization. However, the method is valuable when measuring free drugs that exhibit a high degree of protein binding and that changes (both physiological and pathological) cause a change in relative distribution of both bound and free drugs and thus the poor correlation between total drug measurements (often by immunoassays) and clinical symptoms.

Chromatography-based assays

The assays separate parent drug and metabolites using their physiochemical properties and differences and thus be able to reliably quantify their levels. The methods are liquid chromatography coupled to mass spectrometry for detection and quantitation (Fig. 13). The chromatographic assay methodologies require sample preparation prior to analysis, from minimal sample dilution to extensive chemical extractions. The assays are laboratory-based, require relatively expensive instrumentation, time-consuming takes often hours, and are often performed in the batch analysis compared to immunoassay-based assays which often few minutes by point of care to less than an hour by a laboratory-based assays.

Protein electrophoresis

Capillary system

It is designed for the separation of human serum and urine proteins in an alkaline buffer (pH 9.9) by capillary electrophoresis.

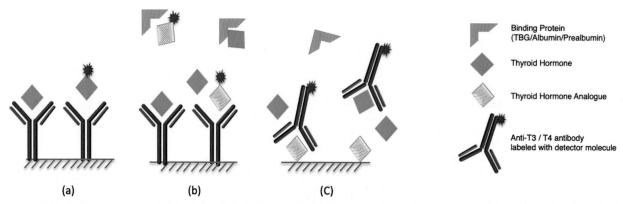

FIG. 12 Thyroid hormone assays configurations. (A) Solid-phase antibody sequesters a small fraction of free hormone. After washing, the labeled hormone (analog) is then added. Measure labeled hormone bound to the solid phase. (B) Free hormone in serum competes with labeled hormone analog for solid-phase antibody binding sites. Measure labeled analog. Hormone analog must bind antibodies but not interact with binding proteins. (C) Free hormone in serum competes with solid-phase analog hormone for binding labeled antibody. Coupling of the analog hormone to solid phase further reduces interactions with binding proteins.

In the labeled antibody format, labeled antibodies compete with sample-free hormone with solid-phase-bound hormone. Coupling of the hormone analog to the solid phase reduces interaction with binding proteins. *(Modified from Koulouri O, Moran C, Halsall D, Chatterjee K, Gurnell M. Pitfalls in the measurement and interpretation of thyroid function tests. Best Pract Res Clin Endocrinol Metab. 2013;27(6):745–762. https://doi.org/10.1016/j.beem.2013.10.003.)*

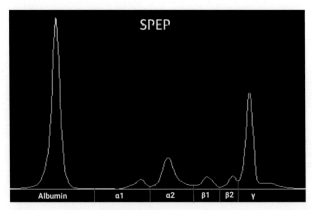

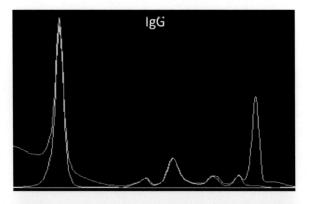

FIG. 13 Capillary protein electrophoresis profile showing an anodal albumin band, alpha 1, 2, beta 1, 2, and gamma globulin regions. This pattern also shows a marked peak in the gamma region. The peak suggests the presence of a monoclonal component. Immunotyping was required and is shown in Fig. 14. *SPEP*, serum protein electrophoresis. *(Courtesy: the author's laboratory.)*

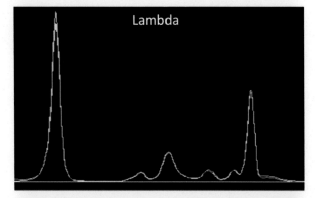

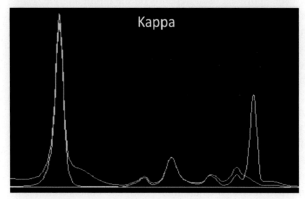

The proteins, separated in silica capillaries, are directly detected at an absorbance of 200 nm. The electropherograms can be interpreted visually to screen for any pattern abnormalities. Direct detection provides accurate relative quantification of individual protein fractions charged molecules are separated by their electrophoretic mobility in an alkaline buffer.

Separation occurs according to the electrolyte pH and electroosmotic flow. A high-voltage protein separation is then performed, and direct detection of the proteins is made at 200 nm at the cathodic end of the capillary.

Proteins are detected in the following order: gamma globulins, beta-2 globulins, beta-1 globulins, alpha-2 globulins, alpha-1 globulins, and albumin (Fig. 13). This pattern also shows a marked peak in the gamma region. The peak suggests the presence of monoclonal component. Immunotyping was required and is shown in Fig. 14. The sample peak (green) was reduced in relation to the original reference pattern (yellow) in the IgG and Kappa reaction profile. This indicates that the monoclonal component is present in the gamma globulin region and is typed as IgG Kappa.

FIG. 14 Capillary immunotyping of the sample in Fig. 12. The sample was incubated with IgG K, and free Kapp and Free Lambda antibodies. The sample peak *(green)* was reduced in relation to the original reference pattern *(yellow)* in the IgG and Kappa reaction profile. This indicates that the monoclonal component is present in the gamma globulin region and is typed as IgG Kappa. *(Courtesy: the author's laboratory.)*

Liquid chromatography-mass spectrometry (LC-MSMS)

Liquid chromatography coupled with mass spectrometric detection (LC-MSMS or tandem MS) has become a widely applied technique in clinical chemistry laboratories (Fig. 15).

It is used for the quantitative analysis of small molecules (i.e., <1000 Da), such as steroids and related hormones (e.g., testosterone and vitamin D metabolites) and drugs and their metabolites.

It is highly sensitive, coupled with sample preparation techniques, and often achieves limits of detection comparable with immunoassays. However, it has the added chromatographic separation with mass-to-charge (m/z) ratio detection which provides a specificity of LC-MSMS that is far superior to that of immunoassays. The LC-MSMS analysis of proteins and peptides can be done either directly using the intact analyte(s) in a so-called "top-down" approach, or in a "bottom-up" approach following digestion with a protease

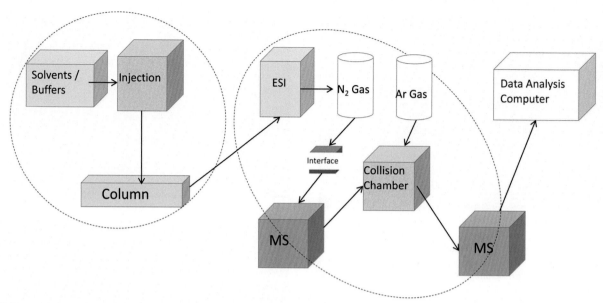

FIG. 15 System components: All *in service* to the column and the detector. *(Modified from the instruments in use by the author; LC-MSMS TQD, Waters Corporation, MA, USA.)*

such as trypsin, and by monitoring specific (tryptic) peptides as surrogate markers.

The approach used depends on the target analyte. Large proteins with m/z values exceeding the operating range of the mass spectrometry instrument require proteolytic digestion. In the bottom-up approach, some tryptic peptides offer better ionization efficiency or better chromatographic peak shape than the intact species.

The LC-MSMS assays although cumbersome to develop and labor-intensive offer enhanced sensitivity and specificity compared to immunoassay-based methods. Methods often involve extensive sample preparation prior to analysis, whereas some methods offer what is termed "dilute and shoot" minimum sample preparation. Peaks of drugs and their metabolites are integrated, and concentrations are determined. The example below is for the measurement of antifungal drugs (voriconazole, posaconazole, itraconazole, and its metabolite hydroxyitraconazole) in the author's clinical laboratory (Fig. 16).

Instrumentation and reagents: Instrument, LC-MSMS (Waters Acquity TQD UPLC-MSMS system), using C-18 column (Waters Acquity UPLC BEH C18 1.7 μm, 2.1 × 100 mm), nitrogen and argon gases. LC-MS grade; acetonitrile, formic acid, and methanol. Standards (itraconazole, hydroxyitraconazole, posaconazole, and voriconazole) and deuterated internal standards (itraconazole—d4, hydroxyitraconazole—d4, posaconazole—d4, and voriconazole—d3).

Methods mobile phase are (0.1% formic acids in water and 0.1% formic acid in acetonitrile).

Sample preparation: Allow samples and reagents to reach room temperature. Prepare 1:50 dilution using the stock internal standard solution and methanol. Prepare the standards and patient samples into working internal standard and add zinc sulfate. Mix and centrifuge before applying the supernatant to the LC-MSMS. The following chromatograms are examples obtained for the standards and internal standards. Internal standards help to identify the compounds and their metabolites as well as allow for compensation and correction for material loss during sample preparation.

The molecular species of the analyte are fragmented and ionized. The most common ionization method is electrospray ionization (ESI), other modalities are atmospheric pressure chemical ionization (APCI), and matrix assisted lazer desorption/ionization (MALDI), etc.

ESI based methods are most common. As the sample elutes out of the LC column, it passes through a narrow highly charged (+ or −ve) capillary electrode. The small internal diameter causes the spray of liquid into a charged mist. This technique is widely used for easily ionized molecules (drugs of abuse, catecholamines, immunosuppressant drugs).

Common interference related to ionization is ion suppression. It describes the suppression of ions produced by the analyte of interest by other materials, for example, the presence of less volatile compounds (salts and ion-pairing agents) affecting the efficiency of droplet formation or droplet evaporation. The signal is suppressed due to less ions reaching the detector which leads to false-negative results or poor quantification.

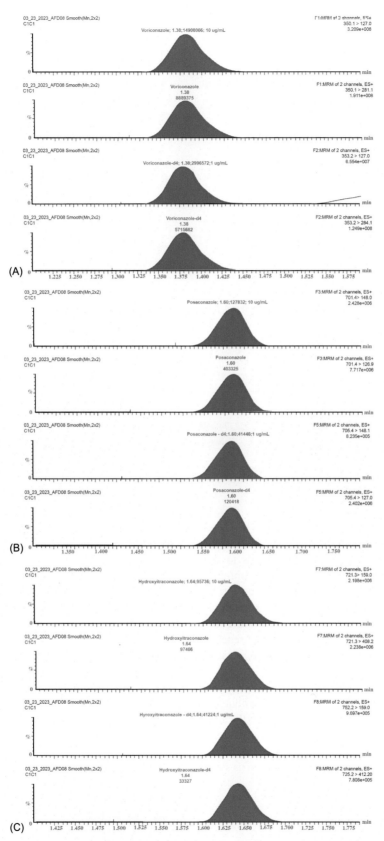

FIG. 16 LC-MSMS example chromatograms for antifungal drugs standards and internal standards. (A) Voriconazole and deuterated voriconazole elution profile. (B) Posaconazole and deuterated posaconazole elution profile. (C) Hydroxyitraconazole and deuterated hydroxyitraconazole elution profile.

(Continued)

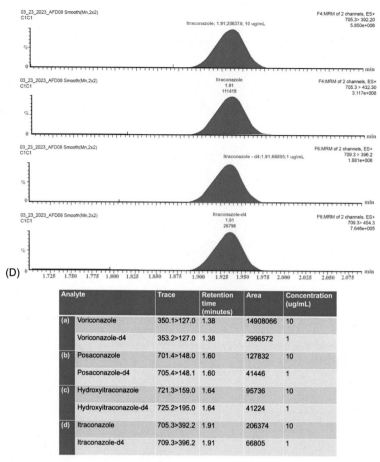

FIG. 16, CONT'D (D) Itraconazole and deuterated itraconazole eluion profile. *(Courtesy: the author's laboratory.)*

Analyte		Trace	Retention time (minutes)	Area	Concentration (ug/mL)
(a)	Voriconazole	350.1>127.0	1.38	14908066	10
	Voriconazole-d4	353.2>127.0	1.38	2996572	1
(b)	Posaconazole	701.4>148.0	1.60	127832	10
	Posaconazole-d4	705.4>148.1	1.60	41446	1
(c)	Hydroxyitraconazole	721.3>159.0	1.64	95736	10
	Hydroxyitraconazole-d4	725.2>195.0	1.64	41224	1
(d)	Itraconazole	705.3>392.2	1.91	206374	10
	Itraconazole-d4	709.3>396.2	1.91	66805	1

The presence of suspected ion suppression can be tested as follows; prepare calibrators in the mobile phase, extract few samples without any analyte, add calibrators to the extracts, and run samples. Compare peaks for calibrators in the mobile phase versus in sample matrix. The difference is due to the presence of ion suppression. An alternative approach is to infuse the analyte directly into the MS and inject extract through HLPC. When the extract reaches the detector, it causes a suppression in the analyte infusion pattern.

Ion suppression can be minimized by changing the ion-pairing agent (trifluoro-acetic acid/heptafluorobutyric acid), changing chromatographic properties so that the analyte does not co-elute with the ion suppressor, changing the ionization technique (ESI is more prone to ion suppression). If recovery remains poor, an alternate analysis such as standard dilution can be used.

Ion-selective electrodes (ISEs)

Ion-selective electrodes measure the potential difference (potentiometry) between a reference electrode and an ion-specific electrode in the presence of that particular ion (e.g., sodium, potassium, chloride, calcium, or magnesium).

The potential difference generated is proportional to the logarithmic concentration of the ion being measured governed by the Nernst equation ($E = E_0 + S \log kc$) where E, electrode potential; E_0, a constant dependent on the electrode system; S, the slope of the electrode (i.e., change in mV produced for a given change in the activity of an ion); k, activity coefficient of an ion ($= 1$ for an ion in an infinitely dilute solution); c, the concentration of the ion.

The ISEs are available in automated clinical chemistry laboratory-based analyzers, point-of-care devices (e.g., Abbott iSTAT), and in blood gases instruments.

The essential component of the electrode system (Fig. 17) is the selectivity of the membrane to the ions to be measured. Selectivity, and thus specificity, is achieved by the use of membranes. The membranes are made up of either porous glass, crystalize, or polymeric material. Although glass membranes are frequently used for pH measurement, polymeric membranes are widely used for the

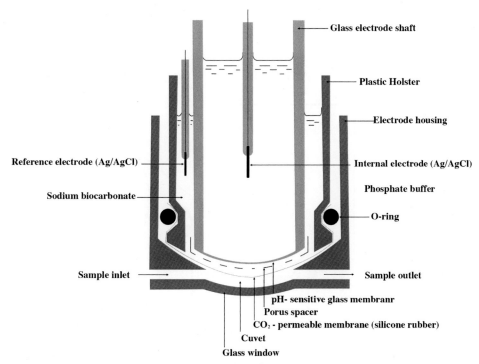

Glass electrode shaft

Plastic Holster

Electrode housing

Reference electrode (Ag/AgCl)

Internal electrode (Ag/AgCl)

Phosphate buffer

Sodium biocarbonate

O-ring

Sample inlet

Sample outlet

pH- sensitive glass membranr
Porus spacer
CO₂ - permeable membrane (silicone rubber)
Cuvet
Glass window

FIG. 17 The basic components of a gaseous electrode highlight the important characteristics and components. Minor differences are present (e.g., CO_2 permeable membrane) to account for analyte-specific measurements. Modification of the pH electrode is used in the pCO_2 electrode. The pH of the internal buffer solution is influenced by diffused sample CO_2 and applying the Henderson-Hasselbalch equation, the change in pH is mathematically linked to pCO_2. *(Modified from Siggard-Andersen O. The Acid-Base Status of the Blood. 4th ed. Williams & Wilkins Company; 1974. ISBN-10: 8716015673, ISBN-13: 978-8716015679.)*

measurement of sodium, potassium, chloride, ionized calcium, and magnesium.

The mechanism of operation is characterized by use of either charged dissociated ion exchanger, charged ion carrier, or ionophore (neutral ion carrier). A polymeric ion-exchange resin is used for the measurement of ionized calcium, a neutral carrier (antibiotic valinomycin) selectively binds potassium, and a number of neutral ionophores have been developed for sodium and magnesium. Dissociated ion exchanges are used for chloride measurement. Selectivity is via extraction of chloride into the liquid phase of the membrane due to its lipophilic property. This suggests that interference by more lipophilic ions may occur suggesting a possible lack of specificity. Therefore, ions of higher lipophilic characteristic than chloride such as bromide and iodine may interfere with chloride measurement but are present in low concertation in blood, thus do not pose significant sources of errors.

However, substances like heparin will diminish the electrode sensitivity to chloride over time when the negatively charged heparin is extracted in place of chloride. Interestingly drugs such as salicylate cause positive interference in chloride electrodes. The development of the polymeric polyvinyl chloride (PVC) membrane with the chemicals needed for the exchange/binding of selective ions

is known as a liquid electrode and is widely used in automated immunoassay. An example of electrode components is shown in Fig. 17.

The pO_2 electrode (Fig. 18) comprises a thin platinum wire fused onto a glass rod. Oxygen reduction at the electrode produces an electric current that is proportional to the level of pO_2. The electrode was developed by Leland Clark in 1954. It uses the Nernst equation to calculate the pO_2 sample content where the electrical potential gradient following oxygen reduction is proportional to O_2 content. An optical-based electrode system is also in use where sample oxygen reduces the intensity and decay time of a phosphorescent dye incorporated within the electrode.

In electrodes for the measurement of lactate levels, the membrane electrode contains lactate oxidase which catalyzes the conversion of sample lactate to pyruvate. Hydrogen peroxide (H_2O_2) generated by the reaction is converted to oxygen by peroxidase. The latter oxidizes at the electrode surface (Fig. 18). The degree of electric current generated (amperometry) is proportional to the sample lactate concentration.

The ion-selective electrodes are all subject to what is termed the exclusion effect. The plasma water which contains dissolved ions and metabolites to be measured is

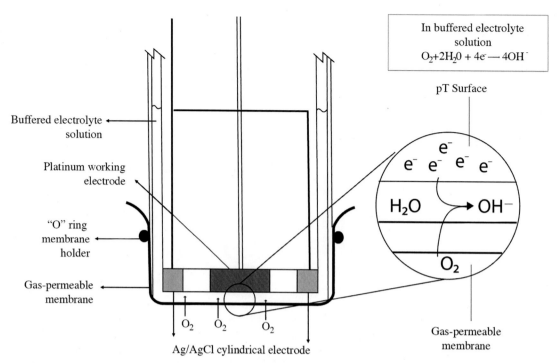

In buffered electrolyte
solution
$O_2 + 2H_2O + 4e^- \longrightarrow 4OH^-$

pT Surface

Buffered electrolyte
solution

Platinum working
electrode

"O" ring
membrane
holder

Gas-permeable
membrane

$O_2 \quad O_2 \quad O_2$

Ag/AgCl cylindrical electrode

Gas-permeable
membrane

FIG. 18 Principles and components of O_2 electrode (Clark pO_2 electrode). Use of membrane containing lactate oxidase catalyzes the conversion of lactate to pyruvate and H_2O_2 which is converted to O_2 by peroxidase and oxidizes at the electrode surface. The current produced is proportional to lactate concentration. *(Modified from D'Orazio P, Meyerhoff ME. Electrochemistry and chemical sensor. In: Tietz Textbook of Clinical Chemistry and Molecular Diagnostics. 4th ed. 2006. P104.)*

influenced by the amount of protein and lipids. The latter excludes water and thus the analytes are in a relatively smaller volume, this effect is exaggerated when an indirect method is applied. That is a small volume of sample is diluted with a larger volume of diluent to mitigate the sample matric effect and the speeds of the electrode measurement exaggerate the size exclusion effects due to proteins and lipids. This is not apparent in the directed method where samples are not diluted prior to analysis (Fig. 19).

Osmolality

Osmometers measure the freezing point of an aqueous solution to determine solute concentration. They utilize high-precision thermistors to sense the sample temperature, control the degree of supercooling and freeze induction, and measure the freezing point of the sample.

Freezing point depression is the widely used method in the assessment of serum and urine osmolality.

Additives such as anticoagulants from collection tubes may contribute to the measured osmolality.

When a solute is dissolved in a pure solvent, the following changes in the solution's properties occur: (a) freezing

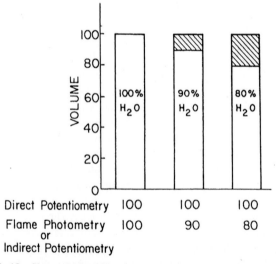

| | Direct Potentiometry | 100 | 100 | 100 |
| Flame Photometry or Indirect Potentiometry | 100 | 90 | 80 |

FIG. 19 Size exclusion effect by proteins and lipids on measurement of analysis by ion selective electrode. The effect is more apparent and exaggerated when an indirect approach is applied to the measurement of the analyte (i.e., sample dilution prior to measurement) often practiced in many automated analyzers to reduce matrix effect and speed the electrode measurement time. *(Modified from Fortgens P, Pillay TS. Pseudohyponatremia revisited: a modern-day pitfall. Arch Pathol Lab Med. 2011;135(4):516–519. https://doi.org/10.5858/2010-0018-RS.1. PMID: 21466372.)*

point is depressed, (b) boiling point is raised, (c) osmotic pressure is increased, and (d) vapor pressure is lowered.

These are the so-called "colligative" or concentrative properties of the solution which, within reasonable limits, change in direct proportion to the solute concentration (the number of particles in the solution). Of the colligative properties, measurement of the freezing point easily permits the precise determination of the concentration of an aqueous solution.

The freezing point of pure H_2O is precisely $+0.010°C$. One mole of a nondissociating solute (a substance that does not dissociate into ionic species), such as glucose dissolved in 1 kg of water, depresses the freezing point of the water by $1.858°C$. This change is known as the freezing point depression constant for water. The freezing point depression also depends on the degree of dissociation of the solute. If the solute is ionic, each ionic species depresses the freezing point by $1.858°C$. For example, if 1 mol of sodium chloride (NaCl) were to completely dissociate into two ionic species (Na^+ and Cl^-) in 1 kg of water, the freezing point would be depressed by $3.716°C$. However, dissociation is never complete. Interference between solute molecules reduces dissociation by a factor called the osmotic coefficient.

In a simple solution (i.e., glucose or sodium chloride in water), the freezing point can be measured, and the unit concentration is easily determined from an equation or a reference table. However, the equation is unique for each solute. In a more complex solution, all ionized and nondissociated species contribute to the freezing point depression. The concentration of each solute cannot be easily determined.

Each of the colligative properties has a similar problem. Though each of the colligative properties changes in direct proportion to the solute concentration, each requires a different mode and unit of measurement. Osmolality is a common unit of concentration measurement that relates all the colligative properties to each other, and other concentration units. Because of its universality, most osmometry applications regularly use osmolality, expressed as "mOsmol/L H_2O," as the common unit of concentration rather than applying further conversion factors.

For blood, a serum sample is the preferred sample type. Plasma samples (blood collected in the presence of an anticoagulant) are not an acceptable sample type. For urine samples, random samples collected in the preservatives-free container are suitable. Specimens should be centrifuged and tested as soon as possible after collection to obtain accurate osmolality results.

When immediate processing of urine specimens is not possible within 2 h of collection, samples may be refrigerated for up to 24 h and can be tested for osmolality without significant bias. This is rare as most osmolality testing is often urgent. All refrigerated samples (serum and/or urine) must be brought to room temperature prior to analysis.

Microscopic analysis

The clinical biochemistry laboratory will often perform microscopic analysis of urine and joint fluids. Urine is examined for cellular and protein casts and joint fluids for the presence of crystals.

Urine crystals

Crystals are formed in supersaturated urine or when solubility is exceeded, and constituents drop out of the solution.

Crystals formation is pH dependent, thus proper sample storage and handling (timely analysis to avoid changes in pH over time (secondary to bacterial growth). If pH is ≥8.5, it suggests a delayed sample and a repeat sample are preferred. Specimens that are >2 h old from collection are not suitable and that specimens from distant sites should be refrigerated and processed within 24 h. Urine crystals are usually not found in freshly voided samples but appear on standing. Particulate matter (normally eliminated by centrifugation/filtration) may cause premature crystallization.

Crystals can be identified by their appearance, but all clinically significant crystals must be confirmed by their solubility characteristics (see Table 2) chart on crystals.

Microscopy joint fluid crystals

Birefringence and intensity (brightness) are diagnostic in joint fluid crystal analysis (small sample volume), no solubility tests are performed tests as in urine sediments.

Consideration when performing joint fluid crystals analysis. Uric acid (monosodium urate) crystals may coexist with calcium pyrophosphate and cholesterol crystals. Calcium pyrophosphate crystals can often be seen in Wright-stained smears. Often, few crystals are seen despite dramatic acute inflammation. Searching for as long as 10–20 min in several slides is occasionally needed to find crystals. The dehydration process of joint fluid can cause cellular disruption and de novo precipitation of uric acid crystals in a fluid having high urate concentration. Uric acid crystals may become nonbirefringent after long-delayed storage. Crystals tend to be embedded in fibrin, so always place a small and thin piece of fibrin on a slide to check for the presence of crystals. If multiple fibrin strands are seen, prepare slides using different strands or from different drops of the sample if the volume is adequate. Some pathologic crystals tend to decrease and may even disappear with storage, whereas several types of artefactual crystals may appear. If crystals are embedded in fibrin, they are considered extracellular (Table 3).

TABLE 2 Urine crystal physical and chemical characteristics.

Crystal	Acid/alkaline	Morphology	Color	NaOH	HCl	Acetic acid	Isopropanol	Heat	Other
Uric acid	Acid	Pleomorphic. Often flat, diamond, or lemon-shaped; may layer or form rosettes; color varies with thickness.	Yellow to brown	S	I	I	I	±	
Amorphous urates	Acid	Granular	Brick dust or yellow-brown	S	I	I		S	
Calcium oxalate	Acid/neutral	Envelopes, dumbbells, or ovoid	Colorless	±	S	I			Nitric acid
Amorphous phosphates	Alkaline/neutral	Granular white sediment	White colorless	I	S	S		I	
Calcium phosphates	Alkaline/neutral	Prisms, wedges, or broken sheets of ice.	Colorless	I	S	S		I	
Triple phosphates	Alkaline	Coffin lids or prisms	Colorless	I	S	S			
Ammonium biurate	Alkaline	Thorny apple	Colorless	S w/gas	±	S w/heat		Slow	
Calcium carbonate	Alkaline	Dumbbells or granules	Colorless	I	S w/gas	S w/gas		I	
Cystine	Acid	Hexagonal plate	Colorless	S	S	I	I		Ammonium hydroxide ± in boiling water
Cholesterol	Acid	Flat plate with notch	Colorless	I	I	I	S (Hot)		Soluble in chloroform and ether.
Leucine	Acid	Spheres with central striation		Yellow or oily brown (S)	I	I	S (Hot)	S (Hot)	Insoluble in ether.
Tyrosine	Acid/neutral		Colorless-yellow	S	S	I	I	S	Insoluble in ether. Soluble in dilute mineral oil.
Bilirubin	Acid	Granules, needles in clusters	Yellow to brown	S	S	S			Soluble in acetone and chloroform. Insoluble in alcohol and ether. Ictotest=pos
Sulfonamides	Acid/neutral	Shocks of wheat, rosettes, and fan-shaped	Green, colorless, or greenish brown	S	I	S			Acetone lignin test=pos
X-ray dyes	Acid/neutral		Colorless	S	S				SG >1.040
Ampicillin	Acid/neutral		Colorless						Refrigeration forms bundles
Sodium urates	Acid						Slightly S	S	
Hippuric acid	Acid/neutral/sl alkaline	Six-sided prisms, needles, or rhombic plates	Yellow or colorless	S	I	I	S	S	Soluble in ether and hot water.

I, insoluble; *S*, soluble.

Modified from Lee AJ, Yoo EH, Bae YC, Jung SB, Jeon CH. Differential identification of urine crystals with morphologic characteristics and solubility test. *J Clin Lab Anal*. 2022;36(11):e24707. https://doi.org/10.1002/jcla.24707. Epub 2022 Sep 26. PMID: 36164743; PMCID: PMC9701861.

TABLE 3 Microscopy of joint fluids. Characteristics of crystals, their morphology and significance.

Crystal	Birefringence	Brightness (intensity)	Morphology	Significance	Size (estimates)
MSU (monosodium urate) or uric acid	Negative Elongation	Strong	Rod, spherule	Pathologic	Submicroscopic—40 μm
CPPD (calcium pyrophosphate deposition) or calcium	Positive Elongation	Weak	Rod, rhomboid	Pathologic	Submicroscopic—40 μm
HA (hydroxyapatite)			Hexagonal individual crystals	Pathologic	Submicroscopic (240 A) to clusters
			Cluster of shiny coins		1.9–15.6 μm
Calcium Hydrogen Phosphate Dehydrate CaHPO$_4$2H$_2$O	Positive	Strong	Rod	Pathologic	
Cholesterol	Negative detection difficult	Weak	Plates (notched corners)	Pathologic	5–40 μm
	Detection difficult		Few rods		
Lipid inclusions	Maltese cross		Round intracellular inclusions (oval fat bodies)	Pathologic	0.5–1 μm
Lipid liquid	Maltese cross		Round intracellular (free fat bodies)	Pathologic	
Calcium oxalate	Positive	Variable	Tetrahedron	Pathologic	
	Detection difficult	Weak	Rods		
Lithium heparin	Positive	Weak	Polymorphic	Artifact	2–5 μm
Talc	Maltese cross	Strong	Ovoid	Artifact	
Corticosteroid	Variable	Usually strong	Polymorphic	Artifact	1–40 μm
Nail polish	Positive	Strong	Rod	Artifact	5–10 μm
Immersion oil	Positive	Strong	Polymorphic	Artifact	1–5 μm

Modified from Faryna A, Goldenberg K. Joint fluid. In: Walker HK, Hall WD, Hurst JW, ed. *Clinical Methods: The History, Physical, and Laboratory Examinations*. 3rd ed. Boston: Butterworths; 1990. Available from: https://www.ncbi.nlm.nih.gov/books/NBK274/. [chapter 166]. Pascual E, Sivera F, Andrés M. Synovial fluid analysis for crystals. *Curr Opin Rheumatol.* 2011;23(2):161–169. https://doi.org/10.1097/BOR.0b013e328343e458.

Interferences

Laboratory test measurements can be affected by endogenous and exogenous material (interferents) present in the sample. Some of these potentially interfering factors can be recognized in the preanalytical phase by the colored appearance of the sample. Interference due to lipemia (turbidity), hemolysis, and icterus (bilirubin) is difficult to predict because of their strong method dependence (Table 4). The limits at which the analysis can be made are described for each method subject to that interference. Serum indices results are very useful for monitoring the degree of potential interference due to lipemia (turbidity), hemolysis, and icterus (bilirubin).

Interference is defined as;

(A) The systematic error of measurement caused by a sample component that by itself does not produce a signal in the measuring system.
(B) The effect of a substance upon any step in the determination of the concentration or catalytic activity of the analyte.
(C) The effect of a substance present in the sample that alters the correct value of the result, usually expressed as concentration or activity for an analyte.

Interference in assays can be seen at different stages of the testing cycle. It is both test and methodology specific. For instance, when measuring glucose using a hexokinase methodology, the presence of a hexose in the sample will also be measured and

TABLE 4 Example limits for hemoglobin (hemolysis), bilirubin (icterus), and turbidity (lipemia) limits beyond which significant interference is observed for the selected assays.

Analyte	Hemolysis (H)	Icterus (I)	Lipemia (L)
Alpha-fetoprotein/PSA	2200	65	1500
Albumin	1000	60	1500
Alkaline phosphatase	200	60	2000
ALT	170	60	150
Ammonia	200	10	50
Amylase	500	60	1500
Cortisol	500	25	1500
Creatinine	800	15	2000
Ferritin	500	65	3300
Folate	100	29	1500
Free T3	1000	66	2000
Free T4	1000	41	2000
FSH	1000	64	1900
GGT	200	50	1500
Haptoglobin	10	60	200
hCG	1000	24	1400

In use by the authors laboratory (complied from manufacturers' kit inserts) and from Ho CKM, Chen C, Setoh JWS, Yap WWT, Hawkins RCW. Optimization of hemolysis, icterus and lipemia interference thresholds for 35 clinical chemistry assays. *Pract Lab Med.* 2021;25:e00232. https://doi.org/10.1016/j.plabm.2021.e00232. PMID: 34095417; PMCID: PMC8145753. Farrell CJ, Carter AC. Serum indices: managing assay interference. *Ann Clin Biochem.* 2016;53(Pt 5):527–538. https://doi.org/10.1177/0004563216643557. Epub 2016 May 3. PMID: 27147624.

erroneously recorded as glucose. The use of glucose-specific glucose oxidase enzyme eliminates the interference.

When analytical interference is suspected, the following may be performed by laboratory personnel:

Review the following: quality control data and calibration, instrument errs, or flags. Including abnormal blanks/reaction rate by the analyzer, delta check (previous results), patient medication/iv lines contamination, manufacturer's package inserts, and literature/publications.

Use a different assay (same/different reaction) and contact manufacturers/suppliers for more recent information or publications.

Selected specific examples

Common interference encountered is selected for discussion; however, this is not meant to indicate that those were the only interferences known, but only those of known significance and are commonly encountered are discussed. The field of inference studies continues to expand as the reader must note that not all possible causes of interference have been identified and this continues to be identified with advancement in methodologies and availability of reported cases in the literature.

The interference is variable, method dependent, and rarely advantageous where it can be an indication of other patronesses. Common interferents are hemoglobin causing spectral interference. It is a marker of RBC rupture and thus an indication of false hyperkalemia. Bilirubin and acetoacetate interfere in the alkaline picrate creatinine method (Jaffe method), among many others (Table 5).

Endogenous interferents

Hemoglobin

Sample hemolysis (in vivo or in vitro) results in the release of intracellular hemoglobin. The high concentration of free hemoglobin interferes in many biochemical assays either via interference with spectral measurement or by quenching the electrochemiluminescence signal in assays with electrochemical detection.

Bilirubin

Similar to hemoglobin, bilirubin interferes in a number of assays. It may interfere with the spectral measurement or participate in oxidative reduction reactions.

Lipids/proteins

The high degree of turbidity caused by circulating lipid particles (micelles) interferes with turbidimetric and nephelometric-based assays. It may also interfere with protein binding and may displace analytes from their binding proteins. The lipids may also potentiate the interference caused by hemoglobin and bilirubin described above.

It is worth noting the lack of correlation between the lipemia index and the triglycerides levels. In vitro diagnostic companies often use intralipid for turbidity interference testing which does not reflect the dynamic nature of lipid micelles.

High levels of lipids and proteins lead to water displacement (pseudo hyponatremia) and also affect the sample matrix viscosity and thus interfere with both reactions, antibody binding, mechanical pipetting, and aspiration of the sample.

Matrix viscosity

Samples with extremely high total protein concentrations (seen in multiple myeloma, lymphoma, Waldenström's macroglobulinemia) exhibit marked matrix viscosity and are often not suitable for analysis (the high sample viscosity impairs automated pipetting (impairs probe pressure transducer function)). The sample may be rescued for analysis if subjected to warming (to 37°C for 30 min) and by using manual pipetting and diluting the samples to reduce the

TABLE 5 Examples of often observed interference by selected interferents, their target analyte, and possible mechanism.

Interferant	Assays	Mode of interference
Hemoglobin	Many assays (direct bilirubin diazo method)	Spectral interference Signal quenching
Bilirubin	Many assays (creatinine Jaffe method)	Spectral Redox reactions
Lipids	Many assays (proteins, electrolytes)	Turbidity (absorbance) Volume displacement
Paraproteins	Many assays	Matrix viscosity Immunoassays interference
Ketones (acetoacetate)	Creatinine (Jaffe method)	Chemical reaction interference
Antidigoxin antibody fragments (DigiBind)	Digoxin	Digitalis intoxication treated with antidigoxin fab (DigiBind)
Total parenteral nutrition	Uric acid, iron, bilirubin, CRP	Turbidity
Acetylcysteine (TPN).	with a urine test for ketones	False positive. Reduces the iron moiety
Sodium fluorescein	T4, T3U FPIA assays	False negative. Background interference
High lactate and LDH	Ethanol	False +ve alcohol results by enzymatic assays
Prednisolone/fludrocortisone	Cortisol	False high. Immuno-cross refractivity. Prednisolone: (>700% cross-reactivity), Fludrocortisone (320% cross-reactivity).
Cyclosporin	50% higher cyclosporin level by immunoassay compared to LC-MSMS	Cross-reactivity of the monoclonal antibody with metabolites AM1, AM9
Codeine	Opiate result (morphine)	Endogenous metabolism to morphine
Ephedrine/pseudoephedrine	False +ve amphetamine assay.	Antibody cross-reactivity
Estrogen	Total T4	Upregulates binding proteins (TBG)
Anticonvulsants	Microsomal enzymes (α-glutamyl transferase, alkaline phosphatase).	Activation of microsomal enzymes.

Modified from Ghazal K, Brabant S, Prie D, Piketty ML. Hormone immunoassay interference: a 2021 update. *Ann Lab Med.* 2022;42(1):3–23. https://doi.org/10.3343/alm.2022.42.1.3. PMID: 34374345; PMCID: PMC8368230.

protein concentration (viscosity) before re-intruding to automated analysis and multiplying results by the dilution factor.

Indices

Automated assessment of serum indices. The assay is based on calculations of absorbance of diluted samples (plasma, serum, urine) recorded at different bi-chromatic wavelength pairs. Indices methods are not designed for the quantitative determination of triglycerides, hemoglobin, or bilirubin. Semiquantitative estimation of levels of lipemia, hemolysis, and icterus is obtained. An aliquot of the specimen is auto-diluted using sodium chloride (0.9%) and absorbance for lipemia at 660 nm (primary wavelength) and 700 nm (secondary wavelength), for hemolysis at 570 nm (primary wavelength) and 600 nm (secondary wavelength), and for icterus at 480 nm (primary wavelength) and 505 nm (secondary wavelength) (Table 4).

Thresholds for hemolysis, icterus, and lipemia are based on scaling factors for conventional units. The following respective factors are applied when reporting analytes in international units (each test has its HIL indices and indices limits are applicable to the test reporting units).

$$H\,limit\,(international\,units) = H\,limit\,(conventional\,units) \times 0.621$$

$$I\,Limit\,(international\,units) = I\,Limit\,(conventional\,units) \times 17.1$$

No recalculation for the L limit is required.

With the use of the scaling factors for conventional units or international units, the displayed values for H and I correspond to an approximate concentration of hemoglobin and bilirubin in mg/dL, or μmol/L respectively.

There is, however, a poor correlation between the L index (corresponds to turbidity) and triglycerides concentration.

Exogenous interferents

Drugs are common causes of interference in laboratory testing, similarly radiocontrast and diagnostic media. The likelihood of interference increases with the number of drugs being administered (Table 6). Biochemistry tests (blood and urine) are the most affected (75%) compared to hematology tests (25%).

Endogenous autoantibodies

Endogenous autoantibodies (interfere with analyte to which the antibody crossreacts). Examples are antibodies against the intrinsic factor. The latter is typically used as the binding protein in serum vitamin B12 assays, antiintrinsic factor antibodies (which are common in pernicious anemia) can lead to elevated vitamin B12 measurement values. Therefore, some vitamin B12 assays are ideally designed to avoid interference from antiintrinsic factor antibodies.

Rheumatoid factors can interfere with some assays and manufacturers often assure a lack of interference from rheumatoid factor up to a concentration of 1500 U/mL.

Heterophile antibodies

Heterophilic antibodies may usually develop as a result of infections, autoimmune disorders, and polyclonal activation (e.g., rubella, measles, adeno-, entero-, and varicella-zoster viruses). The frequency of heterophilic antibodies can be as high as 12%, with nearly equal prevalence of IgG and

IgM. The term "heterophilic" derives from the Greek words "hetero" and "phile," which, respectively, mean "different" and "affinity."

The antibodies produced against poorly defined antigens are generally weak. In contrast, HAMA antibodies usually develop after exposure to animal immunoglobulins and/or proteins. The antibodies have well-defined targets (antibodies constituents of immunoassay) and exhibit high affinities (see below).

Human antimouse antibodies (HAMA)

Human antibodies against animal antibodies cause interference in immunoassays. Circulating HAMA interferes with immunoassay systems employing mouse monoclonal antibodies (which are practically the majority of immunoassays). The antibodies are often IgG and IgM. The incidence of HAMA is variable 10%–40% and depends on the population. It is higher in those with exposure to animals (e.g., those with regular exposure to animals, animal house technicians, veterinarians, and animal handlers) with up to 20% of patients harboring HAMA.

Patients receiving monoclonal antibodies therapeutics or as part of diagnostic (imaging studies) are also at risk of developing HAMA. The frequency may decline as therapeutic and diagnostic monoclonal antibodies are developed as humanized. Chimeric (mouse Fc-region replaced with a human Fc, suffix -ximab) or have been humanized (>95% of mouse sequence replaced with human sequence, suffix -zumab). These modifications certainly lower the risk of patients developing problematic antimouse antibodies.

The mechanism of interference is a "bridging effect" between HAMA and the assay capture and detection antibody (Fig. 19), which is ultimately responsible for abnormal readings and false-positive results.

Antibodies are not species-specific (i.e., polyclonal and monoclonal antibodies) and can be mixed population of antibodies. The degree of interference varies from sample to sample and may vary within a patient over time. Labeled antibody assays are more susceptible than labeled antigen competitive assays (possibly a result of possible modification of the Fc region during antibody labeling/conjugation) (Fig. 20).

In the example of serum hCG interference, measure urinary hCG as HAMA and heterophile antibodies do not appear in the urine. Retest using a different assay (test system).

Perform serial dilutions (has limited value) as a linear dilution may give false confirmation of the reported results in the presence of heterophile antibodies, similarly, lack of linearity in dilution may indicate the presence of heterophile antibodies, but may also be a reflection of the assay that do not necessarily exhibit a linear dilution response.

TABLE 6 The relationship between the number of drugs (therapeutics) being taken and the likelihood of interference.

No. of drugs	Interference detected (% of samples)
1	7.0
2	16.7
3–4	66.7
5	100

It increases with the number of drugs being administered.
Modified from Cascorbi I. Drug interactions—principles, examples and clinical consequences. *Dtsch Arztebl Int.* 2012;109(33–34):546–555; quiz 556. https://doi.org/10.3238/arztebl.2012.0546. Epub 2012 Aug 20. PMID: 23152742; PMCID: PMC3444856.

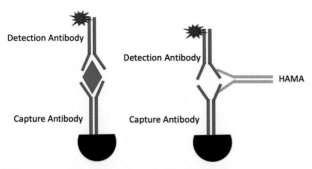

FIG. 20 Possible configurations for HAMA interference. *(Instruction sheet, HBR 1, Purified (Heterophilic Blocking Reagent 1), Cantibodies Laboratory, Inc. CA, USA. From Bolstad N, Warren DJ, Nustad K. Heterophilic antibody interference in immunometric assays. Best Pract Res Clin Endocrinol Metab. 2013;27(5):647–661. https://doi.org/10.1016/j.beem.2013.05.011. Epub 2013 Jun 20. PMID: 24094636.)*

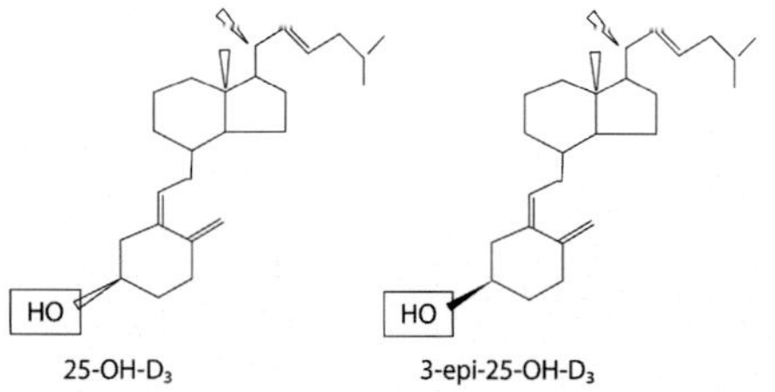

The addition of irrelevant animal immunoglobulin to the sample prior to reassaying is a commonly used strategy to neutralize interfering antibodies. Logically, if a patient sample contains heterophilic antibodies that cross-link the mouse IgG1 assay antibodies, the addition of mouse IgG1 to the sample can neutralize the heterophilic antibodies and prevent interference.

Biotin interference

The high binding avidity between avidin and biotin and ease of conjugating biotin to antibodies and proteins makes the avidin-biotin system a very attractive component in multireagent assay formulation. An example formulation is when an initial incubation of a biotinylated monoclonal hCG-specific antibody and a monoclonal hCG-specific antibody labeled with a ruthenium complex react to form a sandwich complex. In the second incubation step, with the addition of streptavidin-coated microparticles, the complex becomes bound to the solid phase via the interaction of biotin and streptavidin.

Circulating biotin in patients taking high dosage biotin (i.e., >5 mg/day) interferes with the avidin-biotin-based assay formulations and although recent modification of the assay formulation by some manufacturers are in effect, abstinence of >8 h from biotin intake removes the risk of interference.

The avidin-biotin formulation is the basis for many ELISA and research-based reagents and despite the risk of interference, the methodology is likely to remain in use. Precautions must, however, be afforded by stopping biotin intake at least 8 h prior to blood ample collection.

Interference in LC-MSMS

Interference is also seen in LC-MSMS (often chosen as a confirmatory test for interferences suspected in other test

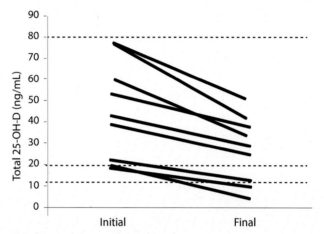

FIG. 21 Chemical structure of 25-OH-vitamion D3 and 3-epimer-25-OHD3. The only structural difference is the orientation of the hydroxyl group. *(Modified from Al-Zohily B, Al-Menhali A, Gariballa S, Haq A, Shah I. Epimers of vitamin D: a review. Int J Mol Sci. 2020;21(2):470. https://doi.org/10.3390/ijms21020470. PMID: 31940808; PMCID: PMC7013384.)*

FIG. 22 Interference of 3-epi-25-OH-D in reportable Vit D results. *(Courtesy: the author's laboratory.)*

methodologies); however, LC-MSMS methods are also subject to interference. For example, in a common vitamin D method by LC-MSMS, an epimer metabolite (3-epi-25-OH Vitamin D_3) (Fig. 21) interferes in 25-OH-vitamin D assays by LC-MSMS. The presence of the epimer leads to falsely elevated vitamin D result, causing falsely elevated Vit D levels with significant differences by as much as twofold (Figs. 21 and 22). It is a metabolite of uncertain biological significance. It is present in all ages (thought to be present in approximately 20% of children under 1 year). It correlates with 25-OH D_3 levels and expresses variable detection by immunoassay and even LC-MSMS.

Formulas and derived calculations

Calculations and formulas are in common use in the clinical biochemistry laboratory and are shown in Table 7. They are used in the derivation of reportable laboratory results and the validation of the testing system and assurance of results validity.

TABLE 7 Common applied formulas in clinical biochemistry laboratories.

Tests	Units	Equation
Anion gap	mmol/L	$Na - (Cl + CO_2)$
Total iron binding capacity (TIBC)	µg/dL	$UIBC + IRON$
% Saturation	%	$IRON/TIBC \times 100$
Calculated LDL-cholesterol	mg/dL	(Total cholesterol − HDL-cholesterol) − (triglycerides /5) (divide by 2.2 if reported in mmol/L)
Calculated osmolality	mOsmol/L	$2(Na) + (GLU/18) + (BUN/2.8)$
Osmolal gap		Measured osmolality—calculated osmolality
Urine amylse, 12 h	U/h	$AMYL (U/L) \times VOLUME (mL)/(1000 \times 12)$
Creatinine, clearance	mL/min	$$\frac{VOL(mL) \times UCRT(mg/dL) \times 1.73}{serum\ creat(mg/dL) \times (hrs \times 60min) surface\ area}$$
Body surface area (BSA)		$\sqrt{(height \times weight)} + 3131$
Urine protein, 24 h	mg/24 h	protein (mg/dL) × volume (mL)/100
Urine calcium excretion, 24 h	mg/24 h	calcium (mg/dL) × volume (mL)/100
Urine amylase, 24 h	U/24 h	AMYL (U/L) × VOLUME (mL)/1000
Urine sodium, 24 h	mmol/24 h	sodium (mmol/24 h) × volume (mL)/1000
Urine potassim, 24 h	mmol/24 h	potassium (mmol/24 h) × volume (mL)/1000
Urine chloride, 24 h	mmol/24 h	chloride (mmol/24 h) × volume (mL)/1000
Urine creatinine, 24 h	g/24 h	creatinine (mg/dL) × volume (mL)/100,000
Urine albumin (microalbumin), 24 h	µg/min	Albumin (macroalbumin) (mg/L) × volume (mL)/(hrs × 60 min)
Urine uric acid, 24 h	mg/24 h	uric acid (mg/dL) × volume (mL)/100
Urine urea nitrogen, 24 h	g/24 h	urea (mg/dL) × volume (mL)/100,000
Urine phosphate, 24 h	g/24 h	phosphorus (mg/dL) × volume (mL)/100,000
Urine albumin (microalbumin)/creatinine ratio	mg Alb/g cr	Albumin (microalbumin) (mg/L)/creat (mg/dL) × 100
Urine protein/creatinine ratio	mg Prot/mg cr	urine protein (mg)/creat (mg)

AGAP, anion gap; *AMY*, amylase; *CA*, calcium; *CREAT*, creatinine; *LDL-CALC*, calculated LDL-cholesterol; *MALB*, microalbumin; *OMSMC GAP*, osmotic gap; *OSMO CALC*, calculated osmolality; *PRO*, protein; *TIBC*, total iron binding capacity; *UUN*, urine urea nitrogen.
In use by the authors laboratory. Modified from Curren, AM, Witt MH. *Curren's Math for Meds: Dosages and Solutions*. 11th ed. Cengage Learning; 2014. ISBN-10: 1111540918. ISBN-13: 978-111154091. Chawla R. *Practical Clinical Biochemistry: Methods and Interpretations*. Jaypee Brothers Medical Pub; 2019. ISBN-10: 9389188768. ISBN-13: 978-9389188769. Mosteller RD. Simplified calculation of body-surface area. *N Engl J Med*. 1987;317(17):1098. https://doi.org/10.1056/NEJM198710223171717. PMID: 3657876.

Summary

– Many if not most of the biomarkers are influenced by physiological and environmental factors such as patient prandial status.
– Several biomarkers, e.g., cortisol exhibits significant circadian rhythm.
– A change from a supine to an upright posture increases the concentrations of many analytes by about 5%–15%.
– Changes in lifestyle. Changes from a sedentary life to excessive exercise result in changes in laboratory parameters. Such as elevated muscle enzyme (creatine kinase) in strenuous exercise.
– The use of two patient identifiers is mandatory before samples are collected.
– Sample quality is important as the quality of the results depends on the quality of the sample.
– The main driver that determines the type of methods applied is the concentration (level) of the analyte in question.
– The clinical reportable range describes the extended analytical measurement range (AMR) following dilution.

- Many method principles are used. They are a function of the analyte being measured. Their chemical, enzymatic, immunological, and chromatographic properties.
- Point-of-care strip test (e.g., urinalysis strip test) use color chemical reactions that are either read by the naked eye by subjective comparison to a color chart or by a colorimeter.
- In the turbidimetric method, the detector is placed directly in the path of the incident and transmitted light, whereas in the nephelometric method, the detector is placed at an angle (45–90 degrees).
- Two steps: heterogeneous immunoassays: this involves the separation of what has and has not bound.
- Laboratory test measurements can be affected by endogenous and exogenous material (interferents) present in the sample.
- Sample hemolysis (in vivo or in vitro) results in the release of intracellular hemoglobin.
- Similar to hemoglobin, bilirubin interferes in a number of assays.
- The high degree of turbidity caused by circulating lipid particles (micelles) interferes with turbidimetric and nephelometric-based assays.
- Samples with extremely high total protein concentrations (seen in multiple myeloma, lymphoma, and Waldenström's macroglobulinemia) exhibit marked matrix viscosity.
- Drugs are common causes of interference in laboratory testing. Similarly radiocontrast and diagnostic media.

- Heterophilic antibodies may usually develop as a result of infections, autoimmune disorders, and polyclonal activation.
- Circulating biotin in patients taking high dosage biotin (i.e., >5 mg/day) interferes with the avidin-biotin-based assay.
- Human antibodies against animal antibodies cause interference in immunoassays.
- The incidence of HAMA is variable 10%–40% and depends on the population.

Further reading

Farrell CJ, Carter AC. Serum indices: managing assay interference. *Ann Clin Biochem.* 2016;53(Pt 5):527–538.

Nguyen KQN, Langevin R, Fankhauser K, Hashim IA. Assessment of risk for interference by circulating biotin in samples received for high sensitivity troponin-T, thyrotropin, and for prostate specific antigen testing by immunoassays. *Clin Lab.* 2020;66(1).

Armbruster DA, Pry T. Limit of blank, limit of detection and limit of quantitation. *Clin Biochem Rev.* 2008;29(suppl 1):S49–S52.

Lippi G, Aloe R, Meschi T, Borghi L, Cervellin G. Interference from heterophilic antibodies in troponin testing. Case report and systematic review of the literature. *Clin Chim Acta.* 2013;426:79–84.

Lima-Oliveira G, Volanski W, Lippi G, Picheth G, Guidi GC. Pre-analytical phase management: a review of the procedures from patient preparation to laboratory analysis. *Scand J Clin Lab Invest.* 2017;77(3):153–163.

Nordestgaard BG, Langsted A, Mora S, et al. Fasting is not routinely required for determination of a lipid profile: clinical and laboratory implications including flagging at desirable concentration cutpoints—a joint consensus statement from the European Atherosclerosis Society and European Federation of Clinical Chemistry and Laboratory Medicine. *Clin Chem.* 2016;62(7):930–946.

Index

Note: Page numbers followed by *f* indicate figures and *t* indicate tables.

Glycated hemoglobin (A1c)
  average glucose values, 173, 173*t*
  interference, 173–176
  nonenzymatic reaction, 172, 172*f*
Glycerol, 157
Glycerol kinase method, 79
Glycogen branching enzyme deficiency, 342
Glycogen storage disorders, 249, 250*t*, 341–342
Glycols, 431*t*
Glycolysis, 104–105
GOLD MARK mnemonic, 431*t*
Gonadotrophins, 22–23
Gonadotropin releasing hormone (GnRH),
  22–23, 28
Gonads, 48–49
  ovarian dysfunction
    characteristics, 46
    delayed puberty, 48
    feedback suppression, 46
    gynecomastia, 48
    hirsutism, 47–48
    hypogonadotropic hypogonadism
     syndrome, 46
    polycystic ovary syndrome (PCOS), 46, 46*t*
    precautious puberty, 48
    primary ovarian failure, 46
    puberty, 48
    secondary ovarian failure, 46
  ovaries
    anti-Mullerian hormone (AMH), 45–46
    structure/function, 45, 45*f*
  testicular dysfunction
    characteristics, 44
    primary and secondary dysfunction, 44
    semen analysis, 44–45
    testicular hypogonadism, 44
  testis, 42
    structure/function, 42–43
    testosterone, 43–44
Graphite furnace atomic absorption
  spectroscopy (GFAAS), 79
Graves' disease, 8–9, 11
Growth hormone (GH), 159
  anterior hyperpituitarism, 26–27
  anterior pituitary, 23
  deficiency, 28–29, 29*t*
Gynecomastia, 48–49

H

Hair testing, 412–413
HAMA. *See* Human antimouse antibodies
  (HAMA)
Haptic dysfunction markers, 394
Haptoglobin, 276–277
hCG. *See* Human chorionic gonadotropin
  (hCG)
Healthcare system network model, 480, 480*f*
Heart failure (HF)
  biomarkers, 206, 209
  causes, 207
  definition, 206
  and diabetes mellitus, 207–209
  in diabetic patients, 169
  early stages, 207, 208*f*

Heavy elements toxicity, 400–401, 400*t*
Hematuria, 98–99
Hemochromatosis, 325–326, 326*t*
Hemoglobin, 424, 424*f*, 432
  by blood gas analyzers, 432–433
  interferes, 508
Hemoglobinopathies, 173–176
Hemolysis, icterus, and lipemia (HIL) serum
  indices, 454–456, 455–456*t*
Hemolytic anemia, 324–325
Hemopexin, 278–279
HemoQuant, 324
Hemosiderin, 322
Henderson-Hasselbalch equation, 426–427
Hepatic dysfunction and biomarkers
  acute liver dysfunction, 119
  cholestatic hepatic dysfunction, 121–122
  chronic liver dysfunction, 119
  hepatocellular dysfunction
    alanine aminotransferase (ALT) enzyme,
     119–120
    alkaline phosphatase (ALP), 120
    aspartate transaminase (AST) enzyme,
     119–120
    gamma glutamyl transferase (γGT), 120
    hepatitis, 120–121
    5′-nucleotidase (5′NT) enzyme, 120
  hepatorenal syndrome, 122
Hepatic encephalopathy, 247
Hepatic fibrosis, 122–125, 124*t*
Hepatitis
  alcoholic hepatitis, 121, 121*t*
  autoimmune hepatitis, 121
  chronic hepatitis, 121
  toxic/ischemic hepatitis, 120
  viral hepatitis, 121, 121*t*
Hepatocellular carcinoma (HCC), 125, 356
Hepatocytes, 376
Hepatoerythropoietic porphyria (HEP), 328
Hepatoma, 125
Hepatorenal syndrome, 122
Hepcidin, 321
Herbal supplements, and interference, 394
Hereditary amyloidosis, 287
Hereditary fructose intolerance, 340
Hereditary hemochromatosis, 125
Hers' disease. *See* Liver glycogen phosphorylase
  deficiency
Heterophile antibodies, 146, 215, 510
Hexokinase-based methods, 170, 170*f*
High-density lipoprotein (HDL), 182*t*, 184–185
High sensitivity C-reactive protein (hsCRP), 210
Hirsutism, 47–49, 224
Hoffman's approach, 465
Homocysteine, 210, 256
Homocysteine metabolism defect, 339, 339*f*
Hormone receptors, 364
Hormones, 109
H. pylori, 298, 310
Human antimouse antibodies (HAMA), 8–9, 9*f*,
  17, 146, 215, 510–511, 511*f*
Human chorionic gonadotropin (hCG),
  213–215, 351–352, 351*f*, 353*f*
  ectopic, 353
  isoforms, 352–353, 352*t*

Human placental lactogen (HPL), 355
Humeral hypercalcemia, 144
Hydrogen breath test, 309
Hydrogen ion metabolism, 426
Hydrogen ion regulation, 419–420
1,25 Hydroxy cholecalciferol (1,25-OH-
  vitamin D), 91
5-Hydroxyindole acetic acid (5-HIAA), 370
21-Hydroxylase deficiency, 38
Hydroxylysine, 135
Hydroxyproline, 135
1,25 Hydroxy vitamin D, 71
25-Hydroxy vitamin D, 109
Hyperaldosteronism, 63
Hyperandrogenism, 47
Hyperbilirubinemia, 111, 113
Hypercalcemia, 17–18, 66–67, 67*t*, 371, 384
  associated biochemical measurements, 141,
   142*t*
  biochemical investigation of, 67–69, 68*f*
  classification, causes of, 141, 142*t*, 143
  definition, 141–142
  diagnosis of, 141
  endocrine causes, 144
  humeral hypercalcemia, of malignancy, 144
  inappropriately high/normal PTH, presence
   of, 144, 145*f*
  investigations of, 142–143, 143*f*
  in malignancy, 142
  management, 143
  prevalence, 141
  primary hyperparathyroidism, 141, 143
  PTH related/non-PTH hypercalcemia, 141
  symptoms, 141
Hyperchloremia, 61
Hypercholesterolemia secondary to lysosomal
  acid lipase deficiency, 195
Hyperchylomicronemia syndrome, 196
Hyperglycemia, 57, 105, 234–235, 249
Hyperglycemic hyperosmolar syndrome (HHS),
  166
Hyper gonadotrophic hypergonadism, 46
Hyperkalemia, 59–60
  biochemical investigation of, 64
  definition, 64
Hypermagnesemia, 74–75, 151, 384
Hypernatremia, 62, 62*t*
Hyperosmolar nonketotic (HONK), 167
Hyperparathyroidism, 18–19, 21, 143–144
Hyperphosphatemia, 71–72, 72*f*, 149–150, 149*f*
Hyperprolactinemia, 28, 221
Hyperproteinemia, 171
Hypersensitivity, 391
Hyperthyroidism, 19
  biochemical follow-up, 11
  Graves' disease, 11
  incidence of, 11
  mild hyperthyroidism, 13
  subclinical hyperthyroidism, 14
  symptoms, 11
  thyroid storm, 12
  toxic multinodular goiter, 11
  treatment of, 11
  TSH adenomas, 12
  T3 thyrotoxicosis, 11

Printed in the United States
by Baker & Taylor Publisher Services